Neurologic Aspects
of Pediatrics

Neurologic Aspects of Pediatrics

Edited by Bruce O. Berg, MD
Professor of Neurology and Pediatrics
Director, Child Neurology
University of California, San Francisco

With 40 Contributing Authors

Butterworth–Heinemann
Boston London Oxford Singapore Sydney Toronto Wellington

Every effort has been made to ensure that the drug dosage schedules within this text are accurate and conform to standards accepted at time of publication. However, as treatment recommendations vary in the light of continuing research and clinical experience, the reader is advised to verify drug dosage schedules herein with information found on product information sheets. This is especially true in cases of new or infrequently used drugs.

 Recognizing the importance of preserving what has been written, it is the policy of Butterworth–Heinemann to have the books it publishes printed on acid-free paper, and we exert our best efforts to that end.

Library of Congress Cataloging-in-Publication Data
Neurologic aspects of pediatrics / edited by Bruce O. Berg;
  with 40 contributing authors.
        p.   cm.
  Includes bibliographical references and index.
  ISBN 0-7506-9054-2 (case bound : alk. paper)
  1. Neurologic manifestations of general diseases.
2. Pediatric neurology. I. Berg, Bruce O.
  [DNLM: 1. Neurologic Manifestations—in infancy &
  childhood. WS 340 N4924]
RJ486.N485   1992
618.92—dc20
DNLM/DLC
for Library of Congress   91-20497
                                         CIP

British Library Cataloguing in Publication Data
Berg, Bruce O.
  Neurologic aspects of pediatrics.
  I. Title
  618.928
  ISBN 0-7506-9054-2

Butterworth–Heinemann
80 Montvale Avenue
Stoneham, MA 02180

10 9 8 7 6 5 4 3 2 1

Printed in the United States of America

Contents

Contributing Authors

Jeffrey C. Allen, MD
Associate Professor of Neurology, New York University Medical Center, New York, NY

Stephen Ashwal, MD
Professor of Pediatrics and Neurology, Attending in Child Neurology, Loma Linda University School of Medicine, Loma Linda, CA

James F. Bale, Jr., MD
Professor of Neurology and Pediatrics, University of Iowa College of Medicine, Iowa City, IA

Dennis W. Bartholomew, MD
Division of Medical Genetics, Department of USAF Medical Center, Keesler AFB (ATC), MI

Elizabeth Martina Bebin, MD
Assistant Professor Departments of Neurology and Pediatrics, University of Virginia, Charlottesville, VA

Roscoe O. Brady, MD
Chief, Developmental and Metabolic Neurology Branch, National Institute of Neurology and Communicative Disorders and Stroke, National Institutes of Health, Bethesda, MD

Saul W. Brusilow, MD
Professor of Pediatrics, Johns Hopkins School of Medicine, Baltimore, MD

Ian J. Butler, MB, BS, FRACP
Professor of Neurology and Pediatrics, University of Texas Medical School at Houston; Consultant in Neurology, Hermann Children's Hospital, Houston, TX

Raymond W. M. Chun, MD
Professor Emeritus, Department of Neurology and Pediatrics University of Wisconsin Medical School, University Hospitals and Clinics, Madison, WI

Philip H. Cogen, MD, PhD
Assistant Professor of Neurological Surgery and Pediatrics, University of California, San Francisco, San Francisco, CA

Bruce H. Cohen, MD
Director, Pediatric Neuro-Oncology, Cleveland Clinic Foundation, Cleveland, OH

Carl J. Crosley, MD
Associate Professor of Neurology and Pediatrics, State University of New York Health Sciences Center at Syracuse; Attending Physician, University Hospital, Syracuse, NY

Francis J. DiMario, Jr., MD
Assistant Professor of Neurology and Pediatrics, University of Pennsylvania School of Medicine, Philadelphia, PA

Paul R. Dyken, MD
Professor of Neurology, Pediatrics, and Pathology, Chairman, Department of Neurology, University of South Alabama; Chief of Neurology and Electroneurodiagnosis, University of South Alabama Hospitals and Clinics, Mobile, AL

Michael S. B. Edwards, MD
Professor of Neurological Surgery and Pediatrics, Director, Division of Pediatric Neurosurgery, University of California, San Francisco, San Francisco, CA

Donna M. Ferriero, MD
Assistant Professor of Neurology and Pediatrics, University of California, San Francisco; Attending Child Neurologist, San Francisco General Hospital, San Francisco, CA

Manuel R. Gomez, MD
Professor of Neurology and Pediatrics, Mayo Clinic, Rochester, MN

Warren D. Grover, MD
Professor of Neurology and Pediatrics, Temple University School of Medicine; Director of Child Neurology, St. Christopher's Hospital for Children, Philadelphia, PA

Christian Guilleminault, MD
Director, Psychiatry and Behavioral Sciences, Stanford University School of Medicine; Assistant Director, Sleep Disorders Clinic and Research Center, Stanford University Medical Center, Stanford, CA

Richard H. Haas, MD
Associate Professor of Pediatrics and Neurosciences, University of California, San Diego, San Diego, CA

William G. Johnson, MD
Associate Professor of Clinical Neurology, Columbia University College of Physicians and Surgeons; Associate Attending Neurologist, Presbyterian Hospital, New York, NY

Thomas K. Koch, MD
Associate Professor of Clinical Neurology and Pediatrics, University of California, San Francisco, San Francisco, CA

William L. Nyhan, MD, PhD
Professor of Pediatrics, University of California, San Diego, La Jolla, CA

Daniel R. Pack, MD
Visiting Assistant Professor of Neurology, Albert Einstein College of Medicine, Bronx, NY

Roger J. Packer, MD
Chairman, Department of Neurology, Children's National Medical Center, Washington, DC

Theodore Page, MD
Assistant Research Biochemist, University of California, San Diego, La Jolla, CA

Martin S. Polinsky, MD
Associate Professor of Pediatrics, Temple University School of Medicine; Attending Nephrologist and Director, Dialysis Unit, St. Christopher's Hospital for Children, Philadelphia, PA

Sanford Schneider, MD
Professor of Neurology and Pediatrics, Head, Division of Child Neurology, Loma Linda University School of Medicine, Loma Linda, CA

W. Donald Shields, MD
Chief, Division of Child Neurology, University of California at Los Angeles School of Medicine, Los Angeles, CA

Roger P. Simon, MD
Professor of Neurology, University of California, San Francisco, Chief, Department of Neurology, San Francisco General Hospital, San Francisco, CA

S. Robert Snodgrass, MD
Professor of Neurology and Pediatrics, University of Southern California School of Medicine, Children's Hospital of Los Angeles, Los Angeles, CA

Russell D. Snyder, MD
Professor of Neurology and Pediatrics, University of New Mexico School of Medicine, Albuquerque, NM

Alfred J. Spiro, MD
Professor of Neurology and Pediatrics, Director, Pediatric Neurology, Albert Einstein College of Medicine, Bronx, NY

Dennis M. Styne, MD
Professor and Chairman Department of Pediatrics, University of California, Davis, Davis, CA

Lawrence Sweetman, PhD
Professor of Pediatrics and Pathology, University of Southern California; Director, Biochemical Genetics Laboratory, Children's Hospital of Los Angeles, Los Angeles, CA

Doris A. Trauner, MD
Professor of Pediatrics and Neurosciences, Chief, Pediatric Neurology, University of California, San Diego, San Diego, CA

Richard S. K. Young, MD
Associate Professor of Neurology and Pediatrics, Yale University School of Medicine, New Haven, CT

Donald P. Younkin, MD
Associate Professor of Neurology, Pediatrics, Biochemistry, and Biophysics, University of Pennsylvania School of Medicine, Philadelphia, PA

Hiroaki Yoshidome, MD
Post-Doctoral Fellow, Columbia University College of Physicians and Surgeons, Presbyterian Hospital, New York, NY

Mary L. Zupanc, MD
Associate Professor of Neurology and Pediatrics, University of Wisconsin Medical School, University Hospitals and Clinics, Madison, WI

Preface

During the last several decades there has been an enormous expansion of our knowledge of medical sciences, and physicians have had to struggle to keep up with available current information. The advent of ultrasonography, computed tomography, and magnetic resonance imaging has enabled us to visualize as never before the structure of soft tissue and bone; moreover, great strides have been made in our understanding of the biochemical basis of many disease processes. Molecular biology, too, has provided newer information regarding multiple genetic diseases.

This burgeoning information has resulted in greater medical specialization, probably no more apparent than in pediatrics. Physicians, not surprisingly, have tended to remain in touch with their own specialty areas, having little contact with others outside those areas of interest and expertise. Pediatricians, perhaps uneasy about neurology because of the complexities of neuroanatomy and physiology, tend to avoid neurologic problems, and neurologists, too, tend to avoid other areas of pediatrics.

It is my hope that this text will provide for all physicians a readily available source of information regarding the neurologic aspects of pediatric diseases. The book is not intended to be a neurology text but rather to embrace the two specialties, neurology and pediatrics, with topics considered at greater depth than in usual textbooks.

I am most grateful to the contributors to this text who patiently endured my editorial tyranny only to realize a delay in publication because of unanticipated quirks of the not so "benign indifference of the Universe." I am particularly grateful to Mr. Christopher Davis and Ms. Kathleen Higgins of Butterworth–Heinemann Publishers who were ever helpful and patient in guiding the manuscript to its completion, as well as to Michael J. Aminoff, colleague and friend, who listened, laughed with me, and offered constructive criticism when necessary. As always, I extend my love and gratitude to my wife, Linda, and our daughters, Kate and Sarah, who not only encouraged and supported this endeavor but put up with the many hours of my absence.

Bruce O. Berg, M.D.

Part I

Neurologic Manifestations of Metabolic Diseases

Chapter 1
Abnormalities of Amino-Acid Metabolism

Lawrence Sweetman and Richard H. Haas

Inborn errors of amino-acid metabolism frequently produce neurologic disease. This might be expected because of the important role of many amino acids in brain function and metabolism. Some amino acids, such as glutamate, aspartate, and glycine, are putative neurotransmitters.

Free amino acids in brain tissue exist in several different pools that differ in their metabolic fate. This property seems unique to the brain and appears to develop in parallel with glial cell proliferation. Neonatal animals do not display brain amino acid compartmentalization. Early studies with radio-labeled glutamate demonstrated that specific activity of glutamine exceeded that in brain glutamate by fourfold to fivefold within a few minutes (1). The glial cell pool of glutamate seems to be responsible for such rapid conversion to glutamine, and the much larger neuronal pool is more closely linked to the citric acid cycle.

Amino acids must cross the blood-brain barrier to enter the brain, and because of their poor lipid solubility, specific active transport mechanisms exist. Families of amino acids share common transport mechanisms, and at least seven different amino-acid transport systems are known. Competition for uptake at the blood-brain barrier has been noted within families of amino acids. Such a mechanism is thought to contribute to the brain amino acid imbalance in phenylketonuria where high phenylalanine plasma levels inhibit the uptake of other aromatic amino acids such as tyrosine. Abnormal ratios of amino acids within the brain will affect protein synthesis as well as neurotransmitter function. Primary transport disorders underlie the accumulation of amino acids in a number of classic amino acidopathies, including Hartnup disease and cystinosis. In hypoglycemia and hypoxic/ischemic injury, release of the excitator in neurotransmitter glutamate is known to stimulate the N-methyl-D-aspartate (NMDA) receptor, producing persistent depolarization of neuronal membranes. This mechanism is thought to be important in neuronal death in these conditions. Potentiation of neurotransmitter effects at

Table 1.1 Aminoacidopathies related to nervous system dysfunction

---

Aromatic amino acids

  Phenylketonuria (PKU)
  Tyrosinemia
  Hawkinsinuria
  Alkaptonuria

Branched-chain amino acids

  Maple syrup urine disease (MSUD)

Sulfur amino acids

  Homocystinuria
  Cystathioninuria
  3-mercaptolactate-cysteine disulfiduria
  Hypermethioninemia

Glycine metabolism

  Nonketotic hyperglycinemia

---

the NMDA receptor may underlie some of the devastating neurotoxicity in nonketotic hyperglycinemia (2).

As in the case of the organic acidemias, primary and secondary effects of inborn errors of amino-acid metabolism can have serious consequences for brain maturation and function. Abnormalities of myelin formation are a common finding in neuropathologic studies in amino acidopathies (Table 1.1).

AROMATIC AMINO ACIDS

Phenylketonuria

Phenylketonuria (PKU) was first identified by Fölling as a result of studying the urine of two mentally retarded siblings. It was not until 1953 that the defect of hepatic phenylalanine hydroxylase was identified as the cause of classic

PKU. A review article summarizes the pioneering work and more recent progress (3). It is now known that classic PKU accounts for only 70% to 95% of the total patients with hyperphenylalaninemia. The overall incidence of hyperphenylalaninemia is 1 in 10,000 births, although there are significant population and ethnic differences. Milder forms of phenylalanine hydroxylase deficiency may not produce phenylketones in the urine, and this group has been termed non-PKU hyperphenylalaninemia. This variation accounts for between 5% and 30% of the overall number of hyperphenylalaninemic patients. Between 1% and 2% of these individuals have a generally more severe disease as a result of abnormalities of tetrahydrobiopterin synthesis. Despite over a half-century of experience with PKU, the pathophysiology underlying the classic and variant phenotypes remains uncertain. The recognition of the consequences for the embryo in untreated maternal PKU serves to remind us that even well-understood metabolic disorders may hold surprises (4).

Biochemistry

Phenylalanine is an essential amino acid and is normally metabolized to the amino acid tyrosine by phenylalanine hydroxylase, which is found only in liver and perhaps kidney (5,6). This enzyme uses oxygen and tetrahydrobiopterin to introduce the hydroxyl group (Figure 1.1). In the process, tetrahydrobiopterin is oxidized to dihydrobiopterin and must be recycled by reduction with nicotinamide-adenine dinucleotide phosphate (NADH) catalyzed by dihydropteridine reductase. The required biopterin is synthesized from guanosine triphosphate (7). In brain, tyrosine hydroxylase can also oxidize phenylalanine to tyrosine (8). A deficiency of phenylalanine hydroxylase results in elevated levels of phenylalanine in plasma of greater than 120 μM/L (2 mg/dL) with normal intake of phenylalanine in the diet. When phenylalanine is highly elevated, it is transaminated to phenylpyruvic acid (the phenylketone of PKU), which can be reduced to phenyllactic acid (See Figure 1.1). Additional metabolites found in urine include 2-hydroxyphenylacetic acid and phenylacetylglutamine (9). Patients with moderate elevations of phenylalanine do not excrete these metabolites. The cause of the neurologic consequences of hyperphenylalaninemia is the elevated phenylalanine itself, which has various secondary effects on brain tissue (10,11). Since phenylalanine is an essential amino acid, the plasma levels can be controlled by special diets low in phenylalanine, which is the basis for treatment.

The most common cause of hyperphenylalaninemia is a deficiency of phenylalanine hydroxylase. The amount of residual activity in liver ranges from 1% to 35%, with the most severe deficiency giving the PKU phenotype and the milder deficiencies giving the non-PKU phenotype (12). In vivo activity of phenylalanine hydroxylase has been determined by the oxidation of stable isotopically labeled phen-

ylalanine with lower activity correlating with the PKU phenotype (13).

Because of the importance of early diagnosis and treatment to prevent mental retardation, screening newborns for elevated phenylalanine has become common. The phenylalanine level in dried blood spots is determined by the Guthrie bacterial inhibition test (14) or by a fluorometric assay (15). Levels above about 0.24 mM/L (4 mg/dL) suggest hyperphenylalaninemia and are followed up with quantitative determinations of phenylalanine in plasma. The human gene for phenylalanine hydroxylase has been cloned (16), and a number of restriction fragment length polymorphism haplotypes have been identified in Caucasians (17). These polymorphism linkages can provide information for prenatal diagnosis of PKU in about 75% of families (18). Haplotype analysis of DNA from families with PKU has permitted the identification of individual phenylalanine hydroxylase alleles and revealed correlations between the haplotypes and clinical phenotypes (17,19). In some Northern European populations as many as 90% of the mutant alleles for phenylalanine hydroxylase are accounted for by only four haplotypes (17) (See Figure 1.1).

A small percentage of patients with hyperphenylalaninemia have defects in biopterin metabolism rather than in phenylalanine hydroxylase (20). These include deficiencies of dihydropteridine reductase (21), guanosine triphosphate (GTP) cyclohydrolase (22), or dihydrobiopterin synthetase (23). These result in a deficiency of tetrahydrobiopterin, which is a required cofactor for phenylalanine hydroxylase. In addition, tetrahydrobiopterin is a required cofactor for the hydroxylation of tyrosine for dopamine synthesis and hydroxylation of tryptophan for serotonin synthesis. Because the synthesis of these neurotransmitters is decreased, these disorders have more profound neurologic problems than PKU, and they do not respond to control of phenylalanine plasma levels by a low phenylalanine diet. Additional modes of therapy include administration of dopamine and 5-hydroxytryptophan (5HT) to compensate for the decreased synthesis, together with carbidopa, an inhibitor of peripheral decarboxylases that slows the metabolism of these compounds and enables more to reach the central nervous system (CNS) (21). Since dihydropteridine reductase also has some activity with dihydrofolate, folinic acid has also been given to patients with a deficiency of this enzyme. In the biopterin synthesis defects, treatment with large amounts of biopterin or analogs that may more effectively reach the CNS have been used (20,21).

Clinical and Neurologic Features

Untreated classic PKU patients have considerable neurologic deficit. Intelligence quotients (IQs) are generally less than 60. The clinical picture is characterized by growth retardation and global developmental delay. Twenty-five percent of patients have an eczematous dermatitis, which may have the typical flexural distribution of atopic dermatitis or a poorly defined nonspecific eczema. Photosensi-

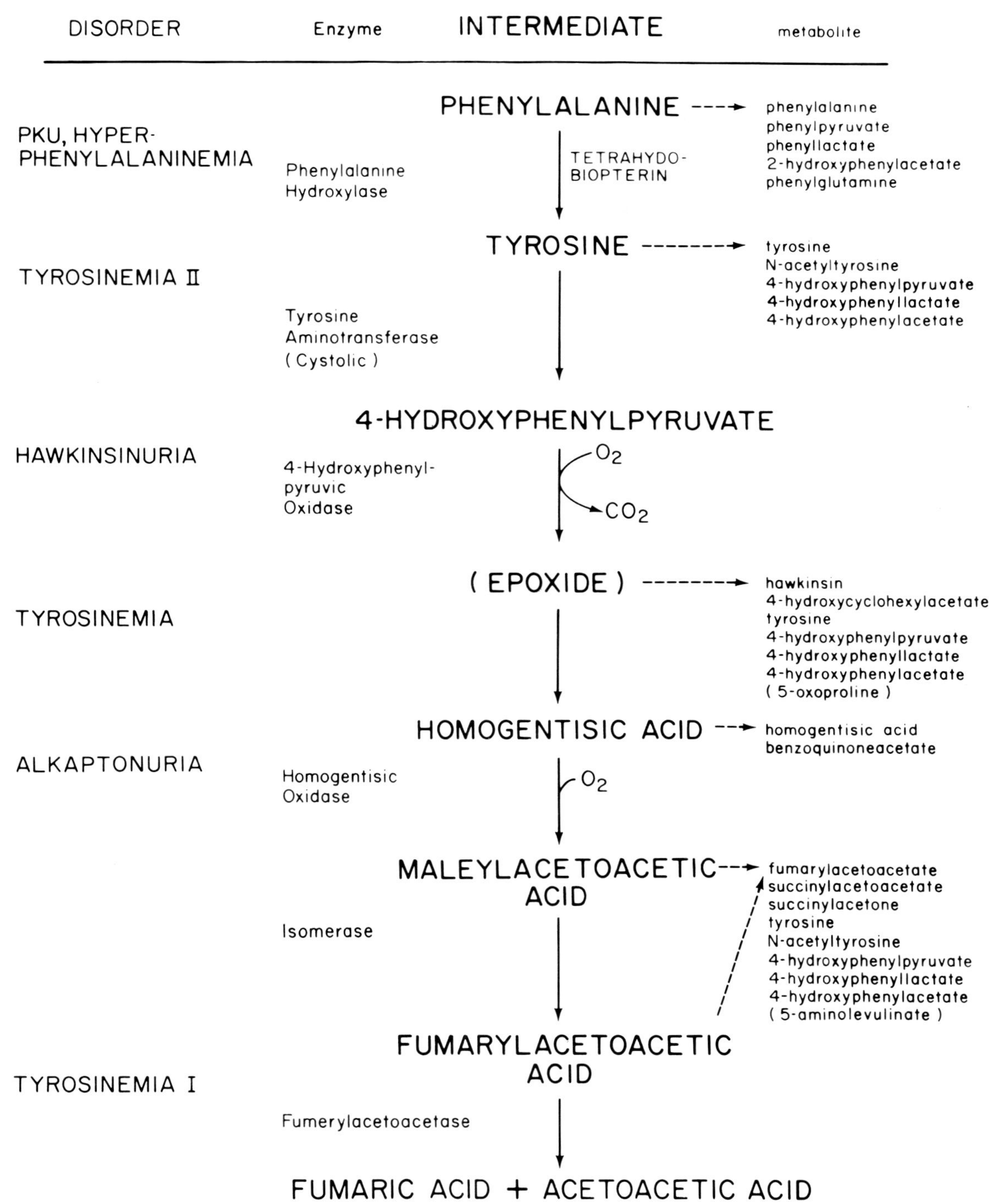

FIGURE 1.1   Metabolism of the aromatic amino acids, phenylalanine, and tyrosine.

tivity, sclerodermoid changes, and hypopigmentation, particularly of the hair, may be seen (24). Three untreated PKU patients died from intercurrent illnesses at 19, 35, and 60 years of age, respectively. Two were microcephalic, and all were hypertonic with brisk deep tendon reflexes. One was severely retarded, unable to stand on his own, and had no speech. Two were hyperkinetic but ambulatory with spastic gaits. The eldest patient developed myoclonic seizures at 59 years of age (25). Parkinsonian-like extrapyramidal symptoms and signs have been reported (26). Although 50% of untreated patients develop hyperreflexia, in one study of 24 phenylketonurics extensor plantor responses were never elicited (27). Hyperkinetic behavior is a well-known feature of PKU. Some patients become psychotic and are usually diagnosed as schizophrenic; however, in one study urine tests for phenylpyruvic acid were negative in 786 psychotic patients on admission to a mental institution (28). PKU with progressive CNS deterioration is well known and is usually due to a defect in biopterin metabolism. Rare patients with classic PKU seem to deteriorate (29).

Untreated PKU usually leads to severe mental retardation; however, patients with normal IQs are described. These patients are usually identified as a result of screening relatives. In one study of asymptomatic affected siblings, 10 of 17 patients were biochemically atypical. Six had lower levels of urinary metabolites and 4 had lower blood levels of phenylalanine than retarded siblings. Although classed as normal, these individuals are generally in the low normal IQ range. Of the 17 affected asymptomatic patients reported, none had IQs greater than 100 and most were in the 80s (30).

It has become increasingly apparent that even well-controlled patients with PKU who were treated early in life have some neurologic deficit. In one study, treated PKU children were found to have more rhythmic motor activity, and were more intense and less persistent than their normal siblings. A significant correlation was noted between decreased persistence and the level of blood phenylalanine (31). Twenty-seven PKU children who had been treated from early infancy were compared with controls with a mean age of 9 1/2 years in both groups. Measurements of coordination and motor skills were identical with controls, but the PKU children showed lower IQs and had lower school achievement with problems noted in concept formation and tactile motor problem-solving abilities. Early serum phenylalanine levels prior to the age of 2 years were not correlated with these deficits, but the serum phenylalanine on the day of testing was positively correlated (32). Problems with information processing, particularly with spatial activities, were noted in a study of 16 early treated PKU children compared with 11 sibling controls. Response time was slower in the PKU patients. Wechsler Intelligence Scale for Children (WISC) full-scale IQ scores were 99.8 (verbal 99.5, performance 100.5) in the PKU children compared with a full-scale IQ of 117.5 (119.6 verbal, 122.8 performance) in controls. When correction was made for the IQ differences between PKU children and their siblings, the observed abnormalities in the PKU group disappeared. The authors concluded that problem-solving strategy, attention span, and accuracy of mental representation may be defective in PKU patients despite efforts to maintain good phenylalanine levels in blood (33).

Untreated maternal PKU has a devastating effect on the fetus. An excellent review points out that in classic cases, 92% of the offspring are mentally retarded, 73% have microcephaly, 40% are growth retarded at birth, and 12% have congenital cardiac anomalies (4). In one study, in addition to the high incidence of major anomalies, minor malformations were found in 18% of 34 children. Twenty-three percent had seizures and 20% strabismus. Low maternal phenylalanine plasma levels in the first trimester are particularly important in preventing congenital anomalies; however, even good control as early as the 5th week may not prevent congenital heart disease and microcephaly in the fetus (34). Phenylalanine itself may not be the only teratogenic agent. Other metabolites may also be important in the production of fetal malformation. However, the IQ of the offspring is significantly correlated with the maternal IQ and the maternal blood phenylalanine level, suggesting that phenylalanine itself plays a major role. Mental retardation in infants of PKU mothers was seen only when the maternal blood level was greater than 1100 µM/L. Microcephaly was observed only when the maternal phenylalanine plasma level was greater than 1200 µM/L (35). A transplacental gradient that raises the fetal blood phenylalanine level above maternal by a factor of 1.25 to 2.5 is thought to be important in teratogenesis (35).

Neurophysiology

Seizures are common in untreated PKU patients. In one Russian study, 19 of 37 patients had seizures that were generally of mixed variety, with paroxysms of staring, head nodding, nystagmoid eye movements, absence, and generalized clonic seizures. Twenty-one of 37 electroencephalograms (EEGs) showed paroxysmal activity with changes more marked in patients with profound intellectual deficit (an IQ of 35 or less). EEGs of all patients were abnormal showing low-voltage dysrhythmia and poor differentiation (36). In a Polish study, 350 sleep EEGs were carried out on PKU children in the 1st year of life; 60% were on treatment. Overall, 70% of records tended to be normal in the treated children in this age group. Abnormalities were less severe in children who were treated and tended to be generalized and nonparoxysmal changes, such as slowing that was occasionally focal with sharp wave activity. Abnormal tracé alternant and loss of sleep features with paroxysmal activity were seen in untreated children (37). In a further study of 335 sleep records of PKU children, 211 of whom were treated and 124 untreated, no significant differences in EEG sleep maturation were noted between PKU and normal children. Sleep spindle activity appeared earlier in the PKU patients and tracé alternant activity persisted slightly longer in PKU. There was no difference in the time of occurrence of hypnogogic hypersynchrony between the groups (38). Studies of 10 children with classic PKU and 5 with variant forms of hyperphenylalaninemia, all under the age of 1 year, showed a high correlation between epileptiform abnormality and phenylalanine blood levels in the first 90 days of life. Thus, electrographic seizure activity seemed to correlate with delay in the institution of dietary therapy (39). Hypsarrhythmia is common in untreated PKU patients, and this tends to evolve into generalized sharp and slow wave paroxysmal activity in older untreated children. In a study of the effect of cessation of dietary therapy, spectral EEG analysis was carried out. No EEG changes were observed when the diet was discontinued at the age of 8 years, but minor changes were seen in early treated patients with more marked changes in later treated patients, whether or not the diet was discontinued. In this study of older children, no correlation was found between the EEG and blood phenylalanine levels on the day of the recording (40).

Pattern visual evoked responses may be more sensitive than the EEG in detecting neurophysiologic derangement. Prolongation of P100 waves and abnormal patterns were seen in 6 of 14 children on a low phenylalanine diet; whereas, EEG abnormalities consisting of slow wave and sharp wave activity was seen only in 3 patients. Six of 9 patients with high mean phenylalanine levels (> 10 mg/dL) and 5 of 8 patients whose diet started after the 2nd month of life had abnormal pattern visual evoked responses (41).

Neuroimaging

Echoencephalography was carried out in 12 patients with untreated PKU and all had cerebral atrophy with mild ventriculomegaly (36). Three women with classic untreated PKU were reported from Japan; all presented with mentally retarded children who were found to have cataracts. One 40-year-old woman had abnormal calcification in the frontal lobes on computed tomographic (CT) scan, but this patient also had a complex chromosome anomaly. No CT calcifications were seen in the other two patients, both women, ages 34 and 24 years, respectively. Cranial calcification similar to that induced by methotrexate toxicity has been reported in patients with abnormal biopterin metabolism (42).

Positron emission tomography (PET) studies were reported in three patients with hyperphenylalaninemia (43). In all cases, decreased glucose utilization was found in the caudate and putamen. Two patients with dihydrobiopterin reductase deficiency were siblings, and both had basal ganglial calcification on CT head scans. The other patient had classic PKU and was under good control without calcification on CT. Such metabolic changes in PKU may underlie extrapyramidal features of this disease (26).

Neuropathology

Early neuropathologic studies of PKU noted nonspecific changes consisting of microcephaly, variable myelin defects, and gliosis. In a study of 8 cases, distinct structural alterations of myelin were found in all, varying from spongy changes to demyelinating lesions. These changes were correlated with the age of the patients. Pediatric patients showed white matter spongiosus with mild gliosis widely spread throughout the brain, including the periventricular and gyral white matter, as well as the cerebellum, brain stem, and optic tracts. Demyelination was seen in 2 of 5 adult cases in a widespread distribution (44). Decreased lipid content of white matter was reported and seemed compatible with earlier reports of retarded myelination (45). Neuropathologic studies of three profoundly retarded adult males with untreated PKU showed pallor of later myelinating areas of the brain compared to controls, but the sequence of myelination appeared normal. There was generalized retarded development of the cytoarchitectonic cortical plate with increased density of cell packing and decreased nerve cell size, with poor distinction between cortical laminations. Areas known to be fully developed at birth, such as the oculomotor nucleus and the nucleus basalis of Mynert, had normal Nissl granulation; but later developing areas, in particular cortical pyramidal cells, had decreased Nissl substance. In addition, a paucity of dendritic arborization and synaptic spines were found in Golgi preparations of pyramidal neurons (25).

Pathophysiology

The cause of the various CNS features of PKU is multifactorial. Phenylalanine hydroxylase is confined to liver; hence, CNS effects are thought to be due to hyperphenylalaninemia, as well as increased levels of various metabolites. Low brain levels of tyrosine provide partial explanation for the decreased neurotransmitter levels found in brain; however, early studies showed that elevated plasma phenylalanine levels inhibit incorporation of tyrosine and branch-chain amino acids into brain protein. In animal models phenylalanine inhibits decarboxylation of dihydroxyphenylalanine and 5HT. In the presence of elevated phenylalanine, serum levels of other essential amino acids are reduced. This effect, together with inhibition of phenylalanine on carrier-mediated transport of large neutral amino acids into brain contributes to the amino-acid imbalance. An imbalance of protein synthesis, increased RNAase activity and polyribosome disaggregation, altered *t*RNA coupling to amino acids, impaired amino-acid incorporation into proteins, and changed structure of neuronal proteins have all been demonstrated in animal models (46).

Studies of rat brain synaptosomes have shown decreased ATPase activity at high concentrations of phenylalanine and its deaminated metabolites phenylpyruvate, phenylacetate, and phenyllactate (47). Phenylalanine inhibits tyrosine transport by rat brain synaptosomal membranes, which presumably contributes to catecholamine depletion (48). Phenylalanine inhibition of tryptophan uptake by rat brain synaptosomal vesicles has also been demonstrated, providing a possible explanation for the depletion of 5HT noted in PKU brain (49). In biopterin deficiencies, the deficiency of tetrahydrobiopterin affects not only phenylalanine hydroxylase but also tyrosine and tryptophan hydroxylase for which it is a cofactor (21). The more dramatic neurologic disease in biopterin deficiencies may reflect a more widespread inhibition of neurotransmitter synthesis than occurs in classic PKU.

The decreased glucose utilization demonstrated in the region of the basal ganglia by PET scanning in one PKU patient raises the question of oxidative metabolic defects in PKU (43). In brain mitochondria, phenylalanine and phenylpyruvate were shown to inhibit state 3 oxidative phosphorylation for first site substrates. In addition, an inhibition of uptake and exchange of beta-hydroxybutyrate and pyruvate across the mitochondrial membrane was found (50).

Anatomic abnormalities in brain maturation and development found in hyperphenylalaninemic rats are changes similar to human findings (25,46). Histologic maturation of the neocortex in phenylketonuric rats was found with decreases in the number and span of dendritic basilar processes of large pyramidal cells, accompanied by an abnormal orientation of these cells in the cerebral cortex (51). Curiously, dendritic spine numbers were increased in the hippocampus in phenylalanine-treated rats (52).

Phenylalanine-treated rats provide a good model for teratogenesis. In humans, mental retardation, microcephaly, congenital heart disease, and low birth weight seem related to the degree of maternal hyperphenylalaninemia (35). In the fetal rat brain exposed to high phenylalanine levels at days 14 to 21 of embryogenesis, a delay in cortical development is seen with catch-up development during the neonatal period (53). Twenty-one-day-old rats treated with phenylalanine had an increased turnover of myelin protein leading to a 15% decrease in the total amount of myelin protein (54). It seems likely that phenylalanine itself is the major culprit in the teratogenesis seen with untreated maternal PKU.

Treatment

Early therapeutic attempts with severe restriction of phenylalanine intake led to growth retardation. This was found to occur if plasma phenylalanine levels were maintained at less than 4 mg/dL. In a study of 132 PKU children, plasma levels of 12 mg/dL resulted in normal growth and apparently normal IQ if treatment was started before 21 days of age (55). Phenylalanine restriction is known to reverse all of the biochemical abnormalities, including elevation of plasma phenylalanine levels and urinary excretion of the various metabolites. The skin and hair darken, behavior improves with less restlessness and irritability, and attention span increases. Motor performance improves, brisk deep tendon reflexes diminish, and there is a decrease in abnormal muscle tone. It was demonstrated early on that relaxation of phenylalanine restriction led to a return of neurologic symptoms in young children. In more recent years there has been a tendency to relax the diet in children around the age of 8 years. However, studies have shown a fall-off in IQ and academic problems in children on unrestricted diets. In one study of 14 patients who were treated early in life but who discontinued therapy between the ages of 5 and 6 years of age, a fall in IQ from a mean of 104 to 90 was observed, with the development of attentional deficit and academic school problems in several children. Two patients with previously normal EEGs developed abnormalities. The most common learning problems were visual-motor integration and cognitive problem-solving difficulties (56). Rat studies demonstrating increased myelin and decreased myelin protein in mature rats treated with phenylalanine provide evidence against the practice of relaxing the diet in PKU children in the early years of life (57). A long-term study of the IQ and EEG in 34 children with early treated PKU showed that the children under strict control had significantly higher IQs than those whose phenylalanine levels were loosely controlled. Abnormal EEGs showing generalized slowing and paroxysmal activity were more frequent in PKU children than in controls; these abnormalities increased with advancing age independent of the IQ, age at start of treatment, and quality of control, supporting other studies showing functional abnormalities in even well-treated PKU patients (58). The most comprehensive data come from the PKU collaborative study in which early treated PKU patients were matched to normal siblings at the age of 8 years. Fifty-five PKU children had a mean Wechsler Intelligence Scale for Children (WISC) full-scale IQ of 100, compared with 107 in their siblings. The IQ was correlated with the maximum diagnostic plasma phenylalanine level and the phenylalanine level at ages 6 and 8 years. When patients were grouped according to their dietary status at the age of 8 years, those on the PKU diet scored at or above their siblings' level on all three scales of the WISC and all three Wide Range Achievement Test (WRAT) subtests. Children off the diet scored 7 to 13 points below their siblings on all measures. The conclusion was that PKU dietary therapy is necessary at least during the school years (59). These data, together with the severe fetal effects of untreated maternal PKU, suggest that lifelong treatment, at least for female patients, may be the best approach. Drug therapy is not usually required in the PKU patient; however, patients with extrapyramidal symptoms may improve with dopaminergic agents. A 14-year-old patient with inadequate diet control presented with tremor of both arms resulting in writing difficulty and in spilling while drinking. The patient improved with Sinemet (Merk, Sharp & Dohme, Westpoint, PA) and worsened when the treatment was stopped (26).

In PKU, tyrosine becomes an essential amino acid. Any dietary therapy must provide adequate amounts of tyrosine and the other neutral amino acids that may have to compete with phenylalanine for brain uptake.

Tyrosinemia

At this time, five different disorders have been described in which tyrosinemia occurs. The most florid neurologic disorders are found in tyrosinemia II (Richnert-Hanhart syndrome). This condition is also called *oculocutaneous tyrosinemia* and is due to a deficiency of cytosolic tyrosine aminotransferase (See Figure 1.1). Mental retardation is common. Tyrosinemia I (hepatorenal tyrosinemia) is due to a deficiency of fumarylacetoacetate hydrolase. The severe form of this predominantly liver disease produces death within the first year of life. Chronic tyrosinemia due to 4-hydroxyphenylpyruvate oxidase deficiency has been described with variable neurologic features ranging from infantile spasms to acute intermittent ataxia. Transient neonatal tyrosinemia is a common problem in preterm infants given high-protein diets. Lethargy and swallowing difficulties, as well as impaired motor activity, have been described, and mild mental retardation may occur in some infants. An infant with the clinical features of type I hereditary tyrosinemia was found to have low maleylacetoacetate isomerase activity in liver and cultured skin fibroblasts. This has been termed *type I b tyrosinemia.*

Blood levels of tyrosine are generally highest in type II tyrosinemia. Patients with high plasma levels of tyrosine and normal IQs are described, implying that elevated levels of tyrosine alone are not the only factor causing CNS injury.

Biochemistry

The liver is the primary organ involved in the catabolism of tyrosine to fumaric acid and acetoacetic acid (See Figure 1.1). The kidney is the only other organ that can catabolize tyrosine. Catabolism is initiated by the transamination of tyrosine to 4-hydroxyphenylpyruvate by soluble tyrosine aminotransferase, which is primarily a liver enzyme (60,61). Hepatic and kidney 4-hydroxyphenylpyruvate oxidase then forms homogentisic acid (62). Further oxidative cleavage of the ring by homogentisic oxidase (63) forms maleylacetoacetic acid, which is isomerized to fumarylacetoacetic acid. This is cleaved by fumarylacetoacetase present in a variety of tissues to yield fumaric acid and acetoacetic acid, which enter general metabolism (64,65). Either maleylacetoacetic acid or fumarylacetoacetic acid can be reduced to succinylacetoacetate, which decarboxylates to give succinylacetone.

The biochemical defect in tyrosinemia type II or oculocutaneous tyrosinemia is a deficiency of the soluble liver tyrosine aminotransferase (60,66). This results in elevated tyrosine, some of which is acetylated to N-acetyltyrosine and excreted (67). Some of the elevated tyrosine is transaminated by mitochondrial aspartate aminotransferase to 4-hydroxyphenylpyruvate in a variety of tissues. In the liver, and to a lesser extent, the kidney, this can be metabolized by the normal catabolic pathway. However, in other tissues that do not contain 4-hydroxyphenylpyruvate oxidase, this compound accumulates and is excreted together with its reduced form, 4-hydroxyphenyllactate and its decarboxylation product, 4-hydroxyphenylacetate (68). This accounts for the somewhat surprising finding that a deficiency of the soluble tyrosine aminotransferase, which would be expected to prevent synthesis of 4-hydroxyphenylpyruvate, actually leads to excretion of elevated amounts of this acid and its metabolites. The elevated plasma tyrosine can be decreased by dietary restriction of phenylalanine and tyrosine, resulting in clinical improvement (69,70).

Transient neonatal tyrosinemia is not an inherited disorder, but is the most common cause of tyrosinemia, especially in premature and low-birth-weight infants (71). Studies of the development of tyrosine aminotransferase and 4-hydroxyphenylpyruvate oxidase activities in fetal

and neonatal human liver showed that the oxidase activity in the fetus is the same as in the adult, but that the transaminase was much lower in the fetus (72). This suggests that the rate-limiting enzyme is tyrosine aminotransferase and that transient neonatal tyrosinemia is due to delayed induction of this enzyme. This leads to excretion of 4-hydroxyphenylpyruvate and 4-hydroxyphenyllactate without succinylacetone by the same mechanism as in oculocutaneous tyrosinemia.

Some patients with tyrosinemia may have a primary deficiency of 4-hydroxyphenylpyruvate oxidase (73,74). Hawkinsinuria, which can cause tyrosinemia, may be due to a block in a step of the complex reaction sequence of this enzyme. A deficiency of homogentisic acid oxidase results in ochronosis and homogentisic aciduria without tyrosinemia.

The majority of patients with hereditary tyrosinemia have tyrosinemia type I or hepatorenal form. This is not due to a primary deficiency of 4-hydroxyphenylpyruvate oxidase, but rather to a deficiency of fumarylacetoacetic acid hydrolase later in the catabolic pathway for tyrosine (See Figure 1.1) (64,65). This leads to the accumulation of fumarylacetoacetic acid and additional metabolites, succinylacetoacetic acid and its decarboxylation product, succinylacetone, which is unique to this form of tyrosinemia (75,76). These metabolites do not inhibit 4-hydroxyphenylpyruvate oxidase (77), but by some unknown mechanism a deficiency of fumarylacetoacetase results in a secondary deficiency of 4-hydroxyphenylpyruvate oxidase (78). As a consequence, there is an accumulation and excretion of 4-hydroxyphenylpyruvate, 4-hydroxyphenyllactic acid, and 4-hydroxyphenylacetate, as well as N-acetyltyrosine. There are additional toxic effects of the accumulated metabolites, leading to liver damage, elevated serum alpha-fetoprotein, elevated plasma methionine, renal tubular disease, and hepatoma. Succinylacetone and fumarylacetoacetate are strong inhibitors of 5-aminolevulinic dehydratase (77), and this decreases porphyrin synthesis, causing increased excretion of 5-aminolevulinic acid. Fumarylacetoacetate, but not succinylacetone, is an inhibitor of methionine adenosyltransferase, which may account for the hypermethioninemia of hepatorenal tyrosinemia (77). Fumarylacetoacetate can react with sulfydryl compounds, and a deficiency of glutathione has been found in hepatorenal tyrosinemia (79). It is not known what compounds may be responsible for the renal tubular damage, but a correlation between proteinuria and succinylacetone excretion has been found (80). The mechanism of hepatic carcinogenesis is unknown.

The excretion of succinylacetone is diagnostic for hepatorenal tyrosinemia (75). An assay for succinylacetone based on the inhibition of 5-aminolevulinate dehydratase has been used for newborn screening (76). The deficiency of fumarylacetoacetase is readily demonstrated in fibroblasts and lymphocytes (81,82). Prenatal diagnosis of hepatorenal tyrosinemia can be done by detecting elevated succinylacetone in amniotic fluid (83,84) or by determining a deficiency of fumarylacetoacetase in cultured amniocytes (82,85) or chorionic villous samples (82).

Clinical and Neurologic Features

Type II, or oculocutaneous tyrosinemia, exhibits florid dermatologic features. The condition was first described in Switzerland in the 1930s by Richnert, an ophthalmologist, and Hanhart, a geneticist. High levels of plasma tyrosine up to 68 mM/dL are seen. Painful keratoses on the palms and digits are noted as well as herpetiform corneal ulcers and variable mental retardation. This condition is inherited as an autosomal recessive trait. An 11-year-old girl, studied in San Diego, first developed bilateral photophobia and conjunctival infection at 6 months of age. The episodes were recurrent, usually occurring in the fall and winter months, and at the age of 7 years, a recurrence of erythematous dry scaly lesions over the toes and soles was noted. The child had a learning disability and Stanford-Binet testing at the age of 7 years revealed an IQ of 66 but with a reading ability above her chronologic age. Plasma tyrosine levels were ten times normal with normal phenylalanine (70). In one other patient, a 10-month-old Japanese female, onset of erythematous blisters developed on the palmar aspects of the fingertips and plantar aspects of the toes. One month later, she had red eyes and photophobia. The lesions spontaneously resolved, but then recurred. Interestingly, an elder brother had adrenogenital syndrome without tyrosinemia. This child was described at the age of 2 years 8 months, at which time somatic, neurologic, and developmental parameters seemed normal (69). A low phenylalanine-tyrosine diet controlled ocular and dermatologic symptoms and signs in both patients.

Follow-up information of 4 Yugoslav patients from the same family with type II tyrosinemia is now available (86). These patients were first described in 1963, and at that time neurologic symptoms were found in only 1. At follow-up examination, 2 were intellectually retarded and one had seizures. No dietary therapy was described in these patients, and it may be that the apparent neurologic progression could have responded to restriction of tyrosine and phenylalanine. CNS features seemed absent in three individuals from a North Carolina kindred, although the youngest child was treated early and a 55-year-old patient did not obtain schooling because of eye lesions (87).

It is clear that in type II tyrosinemia, high tyrosine plasma levels have been observed in a number of patients with normal IQs. In a 1983 review of the literature (70), 14 patients were identified: 5 were mentally retarded, 2 had low normal IQs, and 2 patients appeared neurologically normal. Experience with long follow-up of the Yugoslav kindred suggests that without treatment neurologic symptoms and signs may be progressive (86).

Type I tyrosinemia (hepatorenal tyrosinemia) has two major presentations. The severe infantile form is usually fatal within the first year of life. The juvenile presentation is characterized by chronic hepatic failure and the later development of hepatoma. Liver transplantation has been advocated in these patients (88). In both the infantile and juvenile forms of the disease, a deficiency of fumarylacetoacetate hydrolase can be found. Generalized amino aciduria occurs in this condition, resulting in the deToni-Fanconi syndrome. Hypophosphatemia with rickets results from this renal tubular dysfunction. Hypertrophic obstructive cardiomyopathy has also been described. Neurologic features in type I tyrosinemia result from hepatic failure. A child presenting at 3 months of age with acute hepatic failure, hypoglycemia, and hyperammonemia was thought to have Reye syndrome. Uncontrolled seizures required barbiturate coma (89). Porphyric symptoms with recurrent abdominal pain and polyneuropathy have been described in a number of patients, leading to the suggestion that analysis of whole-blood 5-aminolevulinic acid dehydratase activity may be diagnostically helpful (89). Tyrosinemia type I has a high incidence in the Lac–St. Jean region of Quebec, where 1 child in 685 is born with the disease. In Scandinavia the prevalence is much lower, in the order of 1 in 100,000.

An infant with the clinical features of hereditary tyrosinemia type I was described with normal fumarylacetoacetate hydrolase activity in liver. A complete deficiency of maleylacetoacetate isomerase was found in liver and skin fibroblasts. Normal levels of succinylacetone were found in the urine, helping to differentiate this "type I b" variety from the more common type I hereditary tyrosinemia (90).

Striking neurologic signs and symptoms occur in 4-hydroxyphenylpyruvate oxidase deficiency. A child with intractable seizures beginning at 10 months of age as right partial motor status epilepticus developed jaundice and hepatosplenomegaly at 23 months of age (91). Occasional multifocal myoclonic seizures continued in spite of anticonvulsant therapy. The EEG showed left peritemporal spike and slow wave complexes, and a CT head scan was normal. At 15 months of age the child was mildly developmentally delayed, with hypotonia and intention tremor of the left arm, but at 20 months she presented in coma with recurring seizures. She became vegetative with generalized hypertonia, hyperreflexia, and dyskinesia, and died at 25 months of age. A 17-month-old girl presented with acute intermittent ataxia and drowsiness; she had high plasma levels of tyrosine (62 mmol/dL). Her psychomotor development, EEG, and skull x-ray films were reportedly normal, but plasma tyrosine levels remained high, despite protein restriction (73). The clinical phenotype extends to include a short (less than the third percentile), retarded (IQ 46) adult, with no eye or skin lesions who develops a tremor with L-dopa administration.

Neonatal tyrosinemia is generally asymptomatic, occurring in preterm infants receiving high protein intake. However, mild mental retardation and decreased psycholinguistic ability has been associated with neonatal tyrosinemia (92). Corneal tyrosine crystals have been described (93). This condition is thought to be due to immaturity of the tyrosine aminotransferase or 4-hydroxyphenylpyruvate oxidase enzyme, and it is rapidly corrected by a decreased protein intake and vitamin C supplementation. In a follow-up study of 9 infants with transient neonatal tyrosinemia, 4 continued to have mild metabolic acidosis; some also display hawkinsinuria (94).

Neuropathology

Little neuropathologic information is available. A female infant with type I tyrosinemia died at 6 weeks of age during the acute illness (95). The cerebral gray matter was found to be normal apart from anoxic changes; slight delay in myelination was seen in the cerebral hemispheres, optic chiasm, and spinal nerve roots. The internal capsule, optic tracts, brain stem tegmentum, cerebellar nuclei, and spinal columns showed fibrillary gliosis; marginal spongiform changes were seen in deep subcortical parts of the occipital lobe. A child who died at 25 months of age following a course of intractable seizures had 4-hydroxyphenylpyruvate oxidase deficiency. The cerebral cortex was only 70% of expected size, whereas the cerebellum and brain stem were normal. Microscopic examination showed gliosis in the cerebral cortex and white matter, with Alzheimer type II cells in the pyramidal layer of the precentral gyrus and the occipital cortex. Marked vascularity was observed in the superior colliculi, and hippocampal neurons showed eosinophilia (91).

Pathophysiology

A mink model of tyrosinemia type II is identified as an autosomal recessive trait as in the case of the human disorder. Ocular and skin lesions are associated with blood tyrosine levels 35 to 40 times normal, and hepatic tyrosine aminotransferase activity is very low. These animals have onset of clinical disease as early as 6 weeks of age; an intermediate form may occur at 3 months, and a later form at 6 months. Tyrosinemia can be produced in rats by feeding a low-protein diet with excess tyrosine. Corneal erosions, edema, alopecia, brown urine, and joint swelling are found. Younger rats are more seriously affected. Age-related maturation of the enzymes concerned with tyrosine metabolism seems likely. In humans, blood tyrosine levels between birth and 7 years of age are 2 times those found later in life. This may result from enzyme immaturity, perhaps resulting from a relative 4-hydroxyphenylpyruvate oxidase deficiency. In Canadian Inuit Indians who are breastfed, there is a high incidence of neonatal tyrosinemia (between 6% and 15%), associated with low thyroxine levels that may delay enzyme maturation.

Although data are lacking, it would be expected that blood tyrosine levels will inhibit uptake of other neutral amino acids in a similar manner to the effects of phenylala-

nine in PKU. Phenylalanine itself is elevated in tyrosinemia and may contribute to such an effect. Imbalances in amino-acid composition may affect brain protein synthesis in an analogous way to that demonstrated for PKU. The autopsy data described earlier in 4-hydroxyphenylpyruvate oxidase deficiency demonstrate high blood levels of tyrosine, methionine, and glutamine. Methionine and tyrosine were higher in cerebrospinal fluid (CSF) than plasma, suggesting that brain production of these amino acids may be more important than accumulation from peripheral sources. Patients with deToni-Fanconi syndrome might be expected to have further disorders in plasma and tissue amino acids as a result of the renal tubular leak. Clearly, there are complex factors involved in the CNS features of tyrosinemia as a number of patients with high tyrosine levels have been described with normal intellectual function.

Treatment

Dietary therapy limiting tyrosine and phenylalanine intake is the mainstay of treatment for type II tyrosinemia. Pyridoxine, a cofactor for tyrosine aminotransferase, was found to have no effect in a 7-year-old girl with type II tyrosinemia whose skin and eye lesions responded to restricted tyrosine and phenylalanine (70). A low phenylalanine diet alone does not improve eye lesions. In type I tyrosinemia, treatment initially involved restriction of dietary phenylalanine and tyrosine, which decreased renal tubular damage but did not prevent the liver disease (78). A low phenylalanine-tyrosine diet can normalize the serum tyrosine, but overly zealous restriction can result in an amino-acid deficiency state with growth failure, anorexia, lethargy, and hypotonia. Low plasma cysteine and erythrocyte glutathione levels have led to treatment of some patients with cysteine supplementation and penicillamine, but adequate trials of these therapies have not been carried out. Treatment with blood exchange transfusions has been effective in some patients in lowering tyrosine and its metabolite levels (96). Liver transplantation has been used in a number of tyrosinemia type I patients, particularly in patients who have developed hepatomas (88). Following liver transplantation in 3 patients with hepatorenal tyrosinemia, the urinary phenolic acids derived from tyrosine decreased to normal, and although succinylacetone plus succinylacetoacetate decreased markedly, it was normal in only 1 patient (97). 5-Aminolevulinate excretion also decreased but remained slightly elevated. The kidney is presumably the source of the succinylacetone and succinylacetoacetate excreted following liver transplantation. A patient with chronic tyrosinemia due to 4-hydroxyphenylpyruvate oxidase deficiency did not experience a change in tyrosine blood levels with protein restriction and vitamin C therapy. However, infants with transient neonatal tyrosinemia respond quickly to protein restriction, to 2 g/kg/day and ascorbic acid supplementation at 100 mg four times a day. Corneal tyrosine crystals were shown to respond in a 4-week-old infant within 5 days with phenylalanine and tyrosine restriction and vitamin C supplementation (93).

Hawkinsinuria

Biochemistry

Although rare, hawkinsinuria is a very interesting metabolic disorder because it is inherited as a dominant trait. The affected patients so far described are thus heterozygotes, and other family members have been shown to excrete hawkinsin in the urine. The concept of an enzymatic defect producing a reactive intermediate that has secondary effects responsible for a disease process is an interesting, previously unsuspected mechanism of disease. The first patient excreted large amounts of an unusual sulfur-containing amino acid identified as hawkinsin (2-L-cystein-S-yl-1,4-dihydroxycyclohex-5-en-1-yl)acetic acid (98) as well as small amounts of two isomers of 4-hydroxycyclohexylacetic acid (See Figure 1.1) (99). The second patient with hawkinsinuria was also noted to excrete large amounts of 5-oxoproline, consistent with a disturbance of glutathione metabolism (100). Identified asymptomatic children and adults excrete large amounts of hawkinsin and small amounts of 4-hydroxycyclohexylacetic acid.

Clinical and Neurologic Features

The two patients described in the literature suffered from failure to thrive and irritability in infancy. In both cases, symptoms were noted following discontinuation of breast feeding. In the first male infant, this occurred at 6 weeks of age (101), and in the second case symptoms developed at 2 weeks of age (94). In the first patient, persistent tyrosinuria was noted and treatment with protein restriction coupled with an additional restriction of phenylalanine and tyrosine resolved the acidosis. This child walked at 17 months of age and had a vocabulary of 10 to 12 words at that time. There is no reported evidence of neurologic injury. Following a 5-month history of failure to thrive, irritability with regurgitation, and tachypnea, as well as a swimming pool-like body odor, the second infant had a metabolic acidosis confirmed at 6 months of age. There was no elevation of tyrosine. At that time, weight and length were less than the third percentile, although head growth was relatively preserved on the 50th percentile. There were no abnormal neurologic signs. Initial clear fluids administered intravenously followed by diluted breast milk led to normal feedings without body odor at 13 months of age.

Pathophysiology

The postulated abnormality in hawkinsinuria is a dysfunction of the enzyme 4-hydroxyphenylpyruvate oxidase, the

enzyme that is also deficient in some cases of tyrosinemia. In the case of hawkinsinuria, the enzyme is thought to be unable to break down a reactive epoxide intermediate, which conjugates with glutathione to produce hawkinsin in the urine (See Figure 1.1). Glutathione deficiency probably explains the formation of pyroglutamic acid, which was excreted by both patients; the second patient was mildly anemic with a reticulocytosis, which may indicate hemolysis due to glutathione deficiency. 4-Hydroxycyclohexylacetic acid was also excreted in the urine of the mothers of both reported patients and the other affected family members of the second patient, as well as in the patients themselves after the first year of life. It is postulated that this compound collects after infancy because of the late development of hepatic epoxide hydrolase.

Treatment

Both reported patients responded to a low-protein diet. In the second patient, this was achieved by diluted breast milk. The affected family members in the second case had all been breastfed for the first 8 to 12 months of life and developed no symptoms in infancy. In the second reported case, treatment with ascorbic acid, 500 mg to 1g/day, appeared to be helpful. Ascorbic acid is thought to protect the 4-hydroxyphenylpyruvate oxidase enzyme from degradation.

Alkaptonuria

There are no known neurologic manifestations of alkaptonuria. The occasional patient reported with a seizure disorder and the single report of Parkinson disease likely represent the coincidental occurrence of different disorders. Alkaptonuria plays an important role in the history of metabolic diseases. The concept of autosomal recessive inheritance was first suggested by Garrod in 1902 with reference to alkaptonuria (102,103).

Biochemistry

The biochemical abnormality in alkaptonuria is a large excretion of homogentisic acid due to a deficiency of homogentisic acid oxidase, which normally converts homogentisic acid to maleylacetoacetate (See Figure 1.1) (104). The enzyme that is normally present in liver and kidney is deficient in these organs in alkaptonuria (105). There is no accumulation of 4-hydroxyphenylpyruvate or tyrosine since the formation of homogentisic acid by 4-hydroxyphenylpyruvate oxidase is irreversible. Homogentisic acid in urine is readily oxidized, especially in alkaline solution, to pink, brown, or black products, and urine from alkaptonuric patients can give many erroneous results in clinical chemistry tests (106).

Homogentisic acid is oxidized by a polyphenol oxidase to benzoquinoneacetic acid, which forms colored polymers in connective tissue, causing ochronosis (107), generally in adulthood. Patients develop severe osteoarthritis (108). Auto-oxidation of homogentisic acid produces free radicals and causes degradation of hyaluronic acid (109).

Clinical Features

Children with alkaptonuria are not symptomatic apart from the observation of urine that darkens on standing, and cerumen that similarly darkens when exposed to the atmosphere. Symptoms of this disease usually begin in the fourth decade. The classic triad of symptoms includes ochronotic arthropathy, skin involvement, and cardiac involvement. Renal calculi occur leading to occasional descriptions of chronic renal failure (110). These findings may represent chance association, as was demonstrated in a 50-year-old man who suffered diabetic renal failure (111).

Symptoms of alkaptonuria extend over decades resulting from deposition of polymerized homogentisic acid. The arthropathy may be painful and severe, resembling osteoarthritis on radiographs, with the exception that the shoulder joint is severely affected. Degenerative intervertebral disk disease commonly occurs with calcification, which may result in an ankylosing spondylitis-like clinical picture. Neurologic symptoms and signs of intervertebral disk and spine disease might be expected but have not been reported. Ocular involvement is usual, but this is generally asymptomatic with ochronotic scleral and conjunctival deposits. Cutaneous manifestations can be striking with gray to slate-blue skin, but some patients have no dermal manifestations. Deafness has been reported due to arthritis of the ossicular joints in the inner ear.

CT head scans have been reported as normal in two alkaptonuric children suffering seizures (112,113). Two siblings with alkaptonuria had epileptiform discharges on EEG and one, an 8-year-old boy, suffered occasional generalized tonic-clonic seizures (113). A 2 1/2-year-old child with alkaptonuria had a normal EEG apart from postictal slowing, in spite of having had two generalized seizures. In all cases, the CNS examination was normal. A mentally retarded 5-year-old girl was the product of a consanguineous relationship. She had congenital cataracts and an anterior megalophthalmos, in addition to alkaptonuria (114). This was presumably a chance association of two recessive disorders.

The incidence of alkaptonuria ranges between 1 in 25,000, being highest in the Czechoslovakian population, to a low value of 1 in 10,000,000 in other European groups (115). The prevalence of ochronosis in one Czechoslovakian study was 36 out of 119 patients (116). In spite of cardiac, renal, and vertebral problems, which might be expected to limit life expectancy, there is no evidence that the life span is foreshortened in patients with alkaptonuria (117).

BRANCHED-CHAIN AMINO ACIDS

Maple Syrup Urine Disease

Maple syrup urine disease (MSUD), was described in 1954 by Menkes et al. (118). Four of six siblings died from what is now referred to as the classic or neonatal presentation of the disease. The urine was noted to have a characteristic maple syrup odor. The biochemical defect was later shown to be deficient branched-chain alpha-keto acid dehydrogenase (Figure 1.2). Other presentations of this variable clinical phenotype are described as an intermediate form, an intermittent form, and a thiamine responsive variant. Patients who display improvement with oral thiamine therapy have residual enzyme activity and generally have an intermediate or intermittent presentation. Like other keto acid dehydrogenases, the branched-chain alpha-keto acid dehydrogenase is an enzyme complex composed of three major subunits, E_1, E_2, and E_3. To date a few individual patients have been described in whom their MSUD was found to be due to E_1-beta deficiency, E_2 deficiency, or E_3 deficiency, respectively. The described E_3-deficient patients also had lactic acidemia with deficient activity of other keto acid dehydrogenases.

MSUD is inherited as an autosomal recessive trait with an incidence varying between 1 in 760 in a Pennsylvania Mennonite group to 1 in 290,000 in the New England Newborn Screening Program. Treatment with a low-protein diet and branched-chain amino acid restriction has been effective in limiting CNS involvement and improving the longevity of patients with MSUD.

Biochemistry

MSUD is caused by a deficiency of branched-chain alpha-keto acid dehydrogenase (BCKD) (119). This is a complex of enzymes located on the inner mitochondrial membrane of most tissues (120,121) with the highest activity in the liver and kidneys (122). The substrates for the complex are the three branched-chain keto acids derived from the essential branched-chain amino acids, isoleucine, leucine, and valine. Several transaminase isozymes catalyze the transamination of all three amino acids (123). Since this reaction is readily reversible, the branched-chain keto acids that accumulate in MSUD as a result of a deficiency of BCKD are accompanied by elevated branched-chain amino acids (124). The elevated keto acid derived from isoleucine undergoes spontaneous keto-enol tautomerism to form a second diastereomer that can also be transaminated, forming allo-isoleucine, which is unique to MSUD (125).

The components of BCKD are E_1 or branched-chain keto acid decarboxylase, composed of two subunits, E_1-alpha and E_1-beta, E_2 or acyl transferase, and E_3 or dihydrolipoyl dehydrogenase (See Figure 1.2) (126). The cofactor of E_1 is thiamine pyrophosphate, which is involved in the decarboxylation reaction. E_2 contains covalently bound lipoic

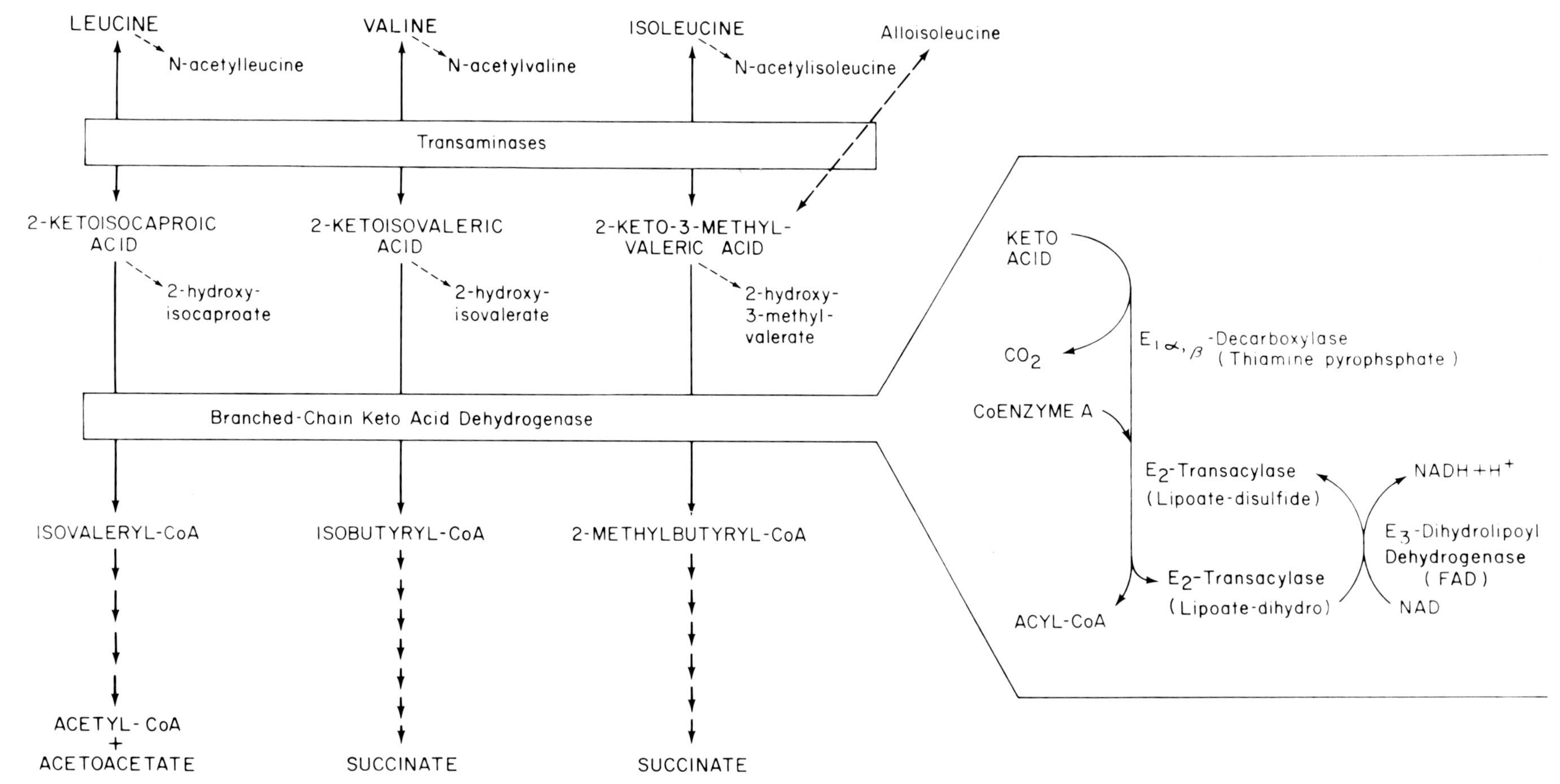

FIGURE 1.2 Metabolism of the branched-chain amino acids, leucine, isoleucine, and valine, in maple syrup urine disease.

acid to which the acylgroup formed by E_1 is transferred. This is then transferred to coenzyme A to form the acyl-coenzyme A product. E_3, which contains flavin adenine dinucleotide, utilizes NAD to reoxidize dihydrolipoate in E_2 to the disulfide. E_3 is also a component of pyruvate dehydrogenase and 2-oxoglutarate dehydrogenase. BCKD activity is regulated by phosphorylation/dephosphorylation. A kinase phosphorylates the E_1 component, causing inactivation (127), while activity is restored by phosphatase (128). The liver BCKD is primarily in the active form, whereas the muscle BCKD is primarily in the phosphorylated inactive form (129). The three branched-chain keto acids and thiamine pyrophosphate inhibit the kinase, resulting in increased activity of BCKD (130).

MSUD can be detected in newborn screening programs by the elevation of leucine in dried blood spots (14). The confirmation of the diagnosis and treatment with a diet restricted in the branched-chain amino acids should be done promptly (131). The diagnosis of MSUD can be made from the elevations of the branched-chain amino acids, including allo-isoleucine, in plasma or the elevation of the branched-chain 2-keto acids in urine or plasma (132). In addition, N-acetyl branched-chain amino acids have been found in urine (133,134). However, in the intermittent forms of MSUD, the branched-chain amino acids and keto acids may not be elevated between episodes. The deficiency of activity of BCKD can be measured in lymphocytes (119), fibroblasts (135), or lymphoblasts (136). A rapid micro assay has been developed (137). There is some correlation between the degree of enzyme deficiency and the clinical severity of the disease (135,136). Heterozygotes can be detected (138) and prenatal diagnosis accomplished by assay of BCKD in cultured amniocytes (139) or in chorionic villous samples (140). The branched-chain amino acids and branched-chain organic acids are not elevated in amniotic fluid with an affected fetus (141).

Specific abnormalities in components of the BCKD are being identified. Some patients lack the E_2 or acyl-transferase protein (142). Further characterization of these mutants should follow the cloning of the complementary DNA (cDNA) for E_2 (143). Other patients have been found to be deficient in the beta subunit of E_1 or decarboxylase (144). The cDNA for the alpha subunit of E_1 has been cloned and used to characterize the deficiency of E_1 in cells from patients (145,146).

Some patients respond to treatment with large doses of thiamine (147,148). The mechanism of the response may involve decreased affinity of the mutant enzyme for thiamine pyrophosphate (149,150) or increased stabilization of the enzyme by thiamine pyrophosphate (151) with the latter more likely since there is a lag of several weeks in clinical response to thiamine treatment.

Clinical and Neurologic Features

The classic disease presents in the neonatal period. Infants are initially normal, but within a few days develop feeding difficulties, vomiting, lethargy, respiratory difficulties, and hypotonia. Some patients are described with alternating periods of irritability and restlessness with high-pitched cry and stupor. Extensor hypertonicity with opisthotonos has been frequently described. Deep tendon reflexes are generally depressed during the acute illness. If untreated, patients become comatose, proceeding to death in most cases. Rare untreated survivors have severe neurologic damage and recurrent episodes of ketoacidosis. Generalized seizures may occur, and hypoglycemia can be prominent. The high incidence of classic MSUD in the Mennonites of Pennsylvania, where a frequency as high as 1 in 176 births has been seen, has allowed the prospective treatment of at-risk newborns. Three of four affected MSUD patients were found to have normal branched-chain amino acids in cord blood, but leucine levels were significantly elevated in the plasma by 4 to 14 hours of age. Thus, classic MSUD can be identified within 48 hours of birth by serum leucine analysis, even in treated patients (152). Patients appear phenotypically normal, although later in the course of MSUD, orthopedic complications such as rapidly progressive scoliosis may be seen (153).

Patients with the intermediate form of MSUD may present from infancy to adulthood. Generally, these patients suffer from failure to thrive and developmental delay. Ataxia may be present, acidosis is usually not marked, and infections may precipitate bouts of keto-acidosis. These patients can be diagnosed by elevated plasma levels of the branched-chain amino acids. Typically, patients are developmentally normal in the first few months of life, but then develop symptoms of lethargy, irritability, and feeding difficulties. Growth delay and developmental delay become apparent. If diagnosed and treated early, patients with intermediate MSUD may subsequently develop normally.

Brain CT head scan changes of increased attenuation in the cerebral white matter and cerebellum are also reversed by treatment (154–156). Patients with the intermediate phenotype generally have residual branched-chain keto acid dehydrogenase deficiency on fibroblast or white cell studies. However, one patient with E_1 deficiency had no branched-chain keto acid dehydrogenase activity, although the presentation was at 10 months of age with ketoacidotic coma following a history of irritability, poor feeding, and delay in growth and development. This patient responded to protein and branched-chain amino acid restriction without subsequent serious ketoacidotic episodes and at the age of 3 1/2 years a Stanford-Binet IQ was 92 (157).

The intermittent presentation of MSUD is milder than the classic disease. Patients may be developmentally and intellectually normal, but suffer episodes of intermittent ataxia and ketoacidosis under stress conditions such as infection or surgery. Episodes of metabolic decompensation may be severe in these patients and even fatal (158).

A report of two different forms of MSUD within a single family suggested the coexistence of the classic form and a variant allele. The two sisters of a girl presenting with the acute neonatal form of the disease were asymptomatic with IQs of 115 and 105, respectively, when measured at 12 and 4 1/2 years of age. These girls spontaneously maintained themselves on a low-protein diet. The mother had 6.7% of control activity on ^{14}C leucine decarboxylation studies.

A number of reported patients have responded to supplemental thiamine at doses between 10 and 300 mg/day, given orally in addition to the maintenance of a low-protein diet and branched-chain amino acid restriction. All cases described thus far have had residual branched-chain keto acid dehydrogenase activity, although 2 of 3 such patients presented with classic disease in infancy with recurrent ketoacidosis (148).

A patient with E_3 (dihydrolipoyl dehydrogenase deficiency) presented with a history of feeding difficulties in the first week of life accompanied by vomiting, constipation, and failure to thrive. Severe developmental delay was apparent at 6 months with hypotonia and very poor head control. At 8 months of age, the patient had respiratory distress with acidosis and a plasma lactic acid level of 10 mM/L. He died following a liver biopsy at 18 months of age during a bout of severe acidosis. This patient had confirmed deficiencies of pyruvate dehydrogenase and 2-oxoglutarate dehydrogenase as well as branched-chain keto acid dehydrogenase deficiency (159).

Neurophysiology

EEGs in patients with MSUD are frequently normal, although during episodes of ketoacidotic coma, generalized slowing suggestive of encephalopathy and paroxysmal discharges may be seen. Of three patients reported with classic MSUD, one had generalized slowing and dysrhythmia, another had numerous spike wave discharges, and a third had a normal EEG despite a clinical presentation of coma at 9 days of age. The EEG was normal in an 18-month-old with developmental delay and decreased attenuation in the white matter of the cerebral and cerebellar cortex on CT brain scan (154). A comb-like rhythm with pseudoperiodic background recorded over the central regions has been suggested as a specific EEG finding of MSUD; however, no other authors have reported this finding (160).

Neuroimaging

CT brain scan findings of patients with untreated MSUD have been reported by a number of authors. A common finding is a generalized decrease in attenuation of white matter in both cerebral hemispheres and cerebellum (154–156,161). In all cases described, this appearance has resolved following treatment with branched-chain amino acid restriction. In one case, repeat CT brain scan 40 days after the institution of therapy showed complete resolution of the white matter lucency and enlargement of ventricular

size (161). It is generally believed that the CT head scan appearance of the untreated MSUD is the result of cerebral edema. We have carried out magnetic resonance imaging (MRI) brain scans in two patients, the first of which presented in the neonatal period with classic disease. In this child, an MRI carried out at 1 month of age showed a striking decrease in intensity of all white matter with normal ventricular size. A follow-up scan after treatment for 1 year, showed a marked improvement in signal intensity on T1-weighted images so that the findings were considered normal. However, on T2-weighted images scattered areas of high T2 signal within white matter were noted. The second patient was studied at 6 years of age. This child had a seizure disorder and mild learning impairment. His MSUD is well controlled on treatment. The MRI was normal apart from slight ventriculomegaly and several equivocal minute foci of hyperintensity within the deep cerebral white matter.

Pathology

A number of neuropathology reports are available. Two cases in the original description of MSUD came to autopsy (118), and in both cases there was cerebral edema with suggestion of myelination delay in the brain stem in one case and in the spinal cord in the other. These patients died at 11 and 14 days, respectively. Autopsies from older patients who survived neonatal disease generally reported widespread status spongiosis of the white matter. These changes have been described in patients dying from nine months to 4 1/2 years of age; however, in one case, an infant who died at 12 days, spongiform changes were observed in the white matter, as well as generalized edema (162). Two other cases were reported with spongiform white matter changes apparent at 4 days and 5 weeks, respectively (95). An excellent review of the early pathologic reports is available (95). It was originally thought that myelination delay was present; however, in one reported case subcortical white matter contained more myelin than the central white matter and internal capsule, which argues against myelination delay.

Muscle biopsies were found to be abnormal in three patients with classic neonatal disease. The biopsies were carried out at 1 day of age, 30 days, and 63 days. In the last patient, there were myopathic changes at electromyography (EMG), but in the first case the EMG and nerve conduction velocities were normal. Determinations of serum creatine kinase (CK) were mildly elevated in 2 of the 3 cases. In all cases, variation of fiber size was noted with type 2 fiber predominance in the eldest case. Some fibers were angulated. The most interesting finding, however, was diffuse multifocal myofibrillar destruction, which could be found both centrally and in the subsarcolemmal area. Electron microscopy showed Z-band disruption resembling rod bodies (163).

Pathophysiology

An animal model of MSUD, inherited as a recessive trait, has been described in Hereford calves (164–166). The calves are normal at birth and able to stand and feed well, but within 3 days they become recumbent. By 5 days they are opisthotonic or dead. Various tissues studied show increased branched-chain amino acids in all cases. Ketonuria with urine that smelled like burnt sugar was described. The brain shows widespread vacuolation (status spongiosis) of white matter and associated gray matter. Electron microscopy reveals intramyelinic vacuole formation, confirming myelin edema (167). In spite of the availability of this model, however, it is unclear how the metabolites that accumulate in MSUD cause CNS symptoms and signs of disease.

Degradation of rat brain proteins by MSUD metabolites has been shown after injection directly into the brain. Alpha-ketoisocaproate seems to be the major myelinotoxic agent. Significant loss of myelin proteins was found in this study of developing rats (168). Ketoacids have also been shown to be toxic in vitro in myelinating cerebellar explants (168).

Leucine has been found to be an allosteric regulator of the blood-brain barrier uptake system that transports brain peptides TyrMIF-1 and the encephalins out of the CNS. It is postulated that inhibition of peptide transport would lead to elevation of the encephalins and TyrMIF-1 in the brain of MSUD patients, and that some of the toxic effects of leucine could be due to increased quantities of brain peptides (169).

Alpha-keto acids cause selective in vitro decrease of alpha-adrenergic and beta-adrenergic receptor binding in rat brain synaptosomes. No effect was seen on cholinergic, gamma-aminobutyric acid (GABA), or dopamine receptors. The branched-chain amino acids themselves did not produce this effect (170).

A number of effects from alpha-keto acids have been demonstrated in the oxidative metabolism of carbohydrates. Pyruvate oxidation in isolated brain mitochondria is inhibited (171). Pyruvate transport into mitochondria is compromised. Alpha-ketoglutarate dehydrogenase and pyruvate dehydrogenase complex activity is inhibited in some preparations. An inhibition of both glucose and pyruvate utilization in brain slices, along with an inhibition of acetylcholine synthesis has been reported (172).

Therapy

Prenatal diagnosis and the possibility of diagnosis in the neonatal period with plasma amino-acid analysis allows some patients to be treated in the newborn period. The successful management of one patient with a modified milk formula providing low branched-chain amino acid intake supplemented with a branched-chain free amino acid mixture is reported (173). The outcome of optimal treatment prior to damaging ketoacidosis episodes can be a normal brain and development (174). Patients presenting with the neonatal form of the disease with lethargy or coma should be aggressively treated with intravenous administration of dextrose and electrolyte solutions, exchange transfusion, or peritoneal dialysis. Once the acute episode is controlled, protein and branched-chain amino acid intake is limited to provide the minimum quantity of branched-chain amino acids necessary for growth. The patients must be carefully followed with repeated plasma amino-acid determinations. For most infants, approximately 50 mg/kg/day of leucine, isoleucine, and valine is adequate. Branched-chain amino acid free formulas such as Mead-Johnson (Evansville, IN) MSUD diet powder are commercially available. Thiamine-sensitive patients require life-long supplementation. A review of MSUD treatment is available (175).

SULFUR AMINO ACIDS

A number of different metabolic defects result in homocysteine accumulation in the blood and increased urine excretion of homocysteine. Most described patients suffer from cystathionine beta-synthase deficiency (Figure 1.3). Homocystinuria was first described in 1962 (176) and cystathionine beta-synthase was identified as the enzyme defect in these early cases soon afterward (177). Defects of cobalamin and folate metabolism can also cause homocystinuria; disorders cblC, cblD, cblE, and cblG are discussed in the section on methylmalonic acidemia. In addition, nutritional and absorptive deficiencies of vitamin B_{12} and folate may produce homocystinuria as can drugs acting as inhibitors of pyridoxine (vitamin B_6) metabolism. Finally, artifactual elevations of homocysteine may be seen as the result of bacterial activity on urine cystathionine.

Cystathionine Beta-Synthase Deficiency

This disorder of methionine metabolism is inherited as an autosomal recessive trait and occurs with a frequency between 1 in 50,000 in New England and Ireland to 1 in 1,000,000 in Japan. Four major organ systems are affected in this disorder: the eye, the brain, the cardiovascular system, and the skeletal system. Affected infants may be identified through neonatal screening programs; if undetected, most patients will have psychomotor developmental delay and lens dislocation in the first decade. This disorder produces progressive neurologic impairment that is thought to be due to homocysteine accumulation as well as the later effects of cerebrovascular disease. The genetic defect underlying cystathionine beta-synthase deficiency is heterogeneous but tends to be constant within sibships. Most patients who are responsive to pyridoxine have residual enzyme activity. This was found in 31 of 39 fibroblast cell lines studied from these patients. Affected individuals with

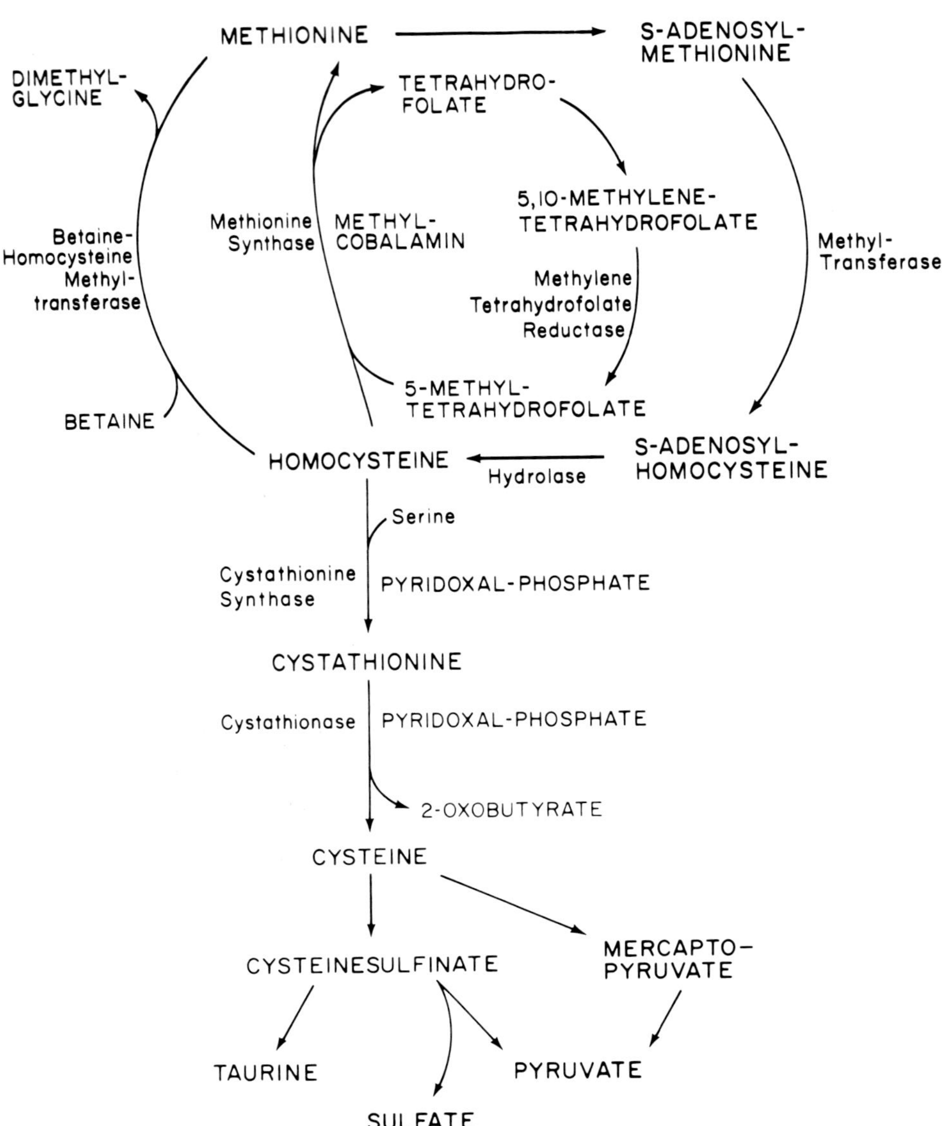

FIGURE 1.3 Metabolism of the sulfur amino acids, methionine, homocysteine, cysteine, and cystathionine.

homocystinuria have been shown to have 0% to 10% of cystathionine beta-synthase activity in fibroblasts, with decreased activity also found in liver and brain.

Biochemistry of Homocysteine and Methionine

Homocysteine occupies a key site in the metabolic interrelationships of the sulfur amino acids methionine and cysteine (See Figure 1.3). Homocysteine and cysteine contain a free sulfydryl group that is readily oxidized to form the disulfides, homocystine, and cystine as well as the mixed disulfide, homocysteine-cysteine disulfide. Generally, the compounds that are measured in plasma and urine are the disulfides, but in addition homocysteine can form disulfides with cysteine residues of plasma proteins, giving significant amounts of protein-bound homocysteine (178).

The biochemistry of the sulfur amino acids has been reviewed in detail (179) and will be only briefly summarized. In humans, methionine is an essential amino acid, whereas cysteine is not, provided that adequate amounts of methionine are available. Methionine adenosyltransferase converts methionine to S-adenosylmethionine, which is a methyl donor for many biochemical reactions as well as a substrate for polyamine synthesis. When the methyl group is transferred, the product is S-adenosylhomocysteine, which is hydrolyzed to homocysteine. Homocysteine can be converted back to methionine by methionine synthase with the methyl group provided by 5-methyltetrahydrofolate in a methyl cobalamin requiring reaction. The major source of the 5-methyltetrahydrofolate is the metabolism of serine to glycine with the formation of 5,10-methylenetetrahydrofolate, which is then converted to 5-methyltetrahydrofolate by methylenetetrahydrofolate reductase (See Figure 1.3).

An alternative fate for homocysteine is the transsulfuration pathway in which cystathionine synthase condenses serine and homocysteine. The product cystathionine is then cleaved by cystathionase to form cysteine and 2-oxobutyrate. Both of these enzymes require pyridoxal phosphate as a cofactor. Cysteine can be metabolized to cysteine sulfinate, which can be further metabolized to either taurine or sulfate. Cysteine can also be metabolized to 3-mercaptopyruvate and then to sulfate.

A number of inherited disorders can result in homocystinuria and elevated homocystine in plasma. Deficiencies in the methylation of homocysteine to methionine result in normal or low levels of methionine in plasma and elevated homocysteine in plasma and urine. This can be due to defects in cobalamin metabolism that cause combined homocystinuria and methylmalonic aciduria, or defects in methylcobalamin metabolism that cause homocystinuria without methylmalonic aciduria (180). A deficiency of methylenetetrahydrofolate reductase also decreases methylation of homocysteine resulting in homocystinuria with normal or low methionine in plasma (181,182).

The most common cause of homocystinuria is a deficiency of cystathionine synthase (177,183). Plasma methionine is usually elevated as a result of increased methylation of the accumulated homocysteine, and plasma cysteine is low as a result of the lack of the transsulfuration pathway for its synthesis. Considerable amounts of the homocysteine in plasma is bound to protein, and in treated patients there may be very little free homocysteine (178). Methionine is generally normal in the urine, but homocystine is elevated in urine.

A simple screening test with cyanide and nitroprusside readily detects elevated homocystine in urine, but also reacts with cystine. A more specific screening test for homocystine in urine uses silver nitroprusside (184). Newborn screening for homocystinuria can be done by detecting elevated methionine in dried blood spots (14), but positive tests must be studied further to distinguish homocystinuria from other disorders with elevated methionine. A deficiency of cystathionine synthase can be assayed in a variety of tissues from patients, including cultured fibroblasts (185), lymphoblasts, and amniocytes (186). Some 85% to 90% of carriers for homocystinuria can be detected by measuring peak plasma homocystine levels after an oral load of methionine or by assay of cystathionine synthase in cultured fibroblasts (187). Prenatal diagnosis for homocystinuria can be accomplished by detecting a deficiency of cystathionine synthase activity in cultured amniocytes (188).

The biochemical basis for dietary management of homocystinuria is directed at reducing the methionine and homocystine plasma levels by restricting methionine and raising the cystine levels by increasing cystine (189). It is believed that homocysteine rather than methionine is responsible for the complications of homocystinuria, and betaine has been used to increase the methylation of homocysteine to methionine and, thus, lower plasma homocystine levels (190,191). The increased methylation of homocysteine to methionine with betaine makes use of an alternative pathway involving betaine-homocysteine methyltransferase.

Pyridoxal phosphate is a cofactor for cystathionine synthase, and pharmacologic doses of pyridoxine have been found to be effective in lowering homocysteine levels in more than a third of the patients with homocystinuria (183). Biochemical heterogeneity is found in studies of the activity and thermostability of cystathionine synthase and its affinity for pyridoxal phosphate in cultured fibroblasts (192,193). The majority of patients nonresponsive to pyridoxine have no detectable cystathionine synthase activity in fibroblasts, while the majority of the responders do have residual activity that showed a greater percentage stimulation with pyridoxal phosphate than normals, although there was not complete concordance (194).

Clinical and Neurologic Features

An extensive review of 600 patients from around the world has provided valuable information about the natural history of homocystinuria (183). The ocular involvement in homocystinuria has been well characterized (183,195). Only 3% of patients with untreated disease have both lenses in place by 38 years of age; 35% have lens subluxation by age 5 years, and 90% by 25 years of age. Other complications include myopia, pupil block glaucoma, and rarely optic atrophy. Lens subluxation may progress in spite of adequate pyridoxine treatment in responsive patients (196). Electron microscopy of the lens shows partially broken zonules, abnormal zonular attachment, and a spongy appearance to the capsule (195).

CNS involvement is often manifested as mental retardation. In the survey of 600 patients (183), IQs ranged from 10 to 138, with a median IQ of 64. Patients who were responsive to pyridoxine had a median IQ of 78 compared to nonresponsive patients. There tended to be clustering of IQ values within sibships. Seizures occurred in up to 21% of patients if not treated from early infancy. Abnormal EEGs with electrographic seizures were frequently seen, even in the absence of clinical seizure disorders. Psychiatric disorders are common in homocystinuric patients. In a report on 63 classic homocystinuric patients, 51% had significant psychiatric disorders (197). The mean age of these patients at diagnosis was 19 years. Ten percent had episodic depression, 12% had chronic behavioral problems, 5% had obsessive-compulsive problems, and 19% had personality disorder. Early case reports suggested a high incidence of relatives were diagnosed as schizophrenic and noted schizophrenia as a fairly common manifestation of homocystinuria. In fact, these were probably incorrect diagnoses; a literature review revealed only three well-documented cases of schizophrenia in homocystinuria (197). One of these patients suffered from 5,10-methylenetetrahydrofolate reductase deficiency. In homocystinuric patients, aggressive behavior and conduct disorders are particularly common among the mentally retarded group and those who are unresponsive to pyridoxine (197). Cerebrovascular disease is a serious complication of homocystinuria, and one third of 147 patients suffered thromboembolic events. Ten percent of this group of patients suffered myocardial infarcts, 11% peripheral arterial occlusions, and 51% peripheral venous occlusions, including 32 who had pulmonary emboli (183). Homocystinuria is one of the more common causes of stroke in childhood.

There are reports of widespread thromboembolism following surgical procedures (198). In spite of the substantial risk of thromboembolism, surgery is relatively safe if patients are adequately hydrated and maintained on pyridoxine if responsive, and if consideration is given to the use of platelet anticoagulants. Only 14 postoperative thromboembolic events were recorded in 241 major surgical procedures in affected patients (183). Cerebral venous thrombosis is a reported thromboembolic complication (199). Angiographic findings were reported in two female siblings with homocystinuria at 21 and 28 years, respectively (200). In the younger patient, there was severe arterial narrowing with numerous small aneurysms in the interlobar arteries of both kidneys, the common hepatic artery, and left gastric arteries, with distal occlusions and narrowing of the superior mesenteric artery. Her older mentally retarded sibling had irregularity of the aortic arch at the origin of the right internal carotid artery with a severe distal stenosis as well as irregularity and aneurysmal dilatation of the splenic artery.

The high incidence of arteriosclerosis in homocystinuric patients has led to considering the possibility that the heterozygous state may also be associated with an increased risk of arteriosclerosis. In 19 patients with arteriosclerotic cerebrovascular disease, presenting between the ages of 34 and 63 years, 18 had transient ischemic attacks and one had progressive stroke. Significantly elevated plasma homocysteine was found following an overnight fast and methionine load (201). In another larger survey, 7 of 25 patients with occlusive peripheral arterial disease and 7 of 25 patients with progressive cerebrovascular disease were found to be heterozygous for cystathionine synthetase. These patients had no abnormalities with methionine loading. A further 25 patients with myocardial infarction had no association with the heterozygous state (202). Heterozygosity for cystathionine beta-synthase may be as high as 1 in 70 of the population.

Skeletal changes are common in homocystinuria. Fifty percent of patients have osteoporosis by the end of the second decade. This is generally evident in long bones; however, osteoporosis may lead to collapse of vertebral bodies and scoliosis is common (183).

Abnormal neurologic findings in homocystinuria, when present, are usually due to cerebrovascular disease. However, a number of patients have been described with dystonia. Three patients with cystathionine beta-synthase deficiency developed dystonia at 18 years, 9 years, and 10 years of age, respectively. The first patient was mentally retarded with a marfanoid habitus, developing osteoporosis, and bilateral lens dislocation. This patient was resistant to pyridoxine. He developed spasmodic torticollis progressing to truncal and upper limb dystonia, responding only partially to bromocriptine. Rapid progression was ultimately fatal. Two other children developed dystonia of the trunk, limb, and neck that was slowly progressive despite treatment. In no case did neuroimaging or autopsy studies reveal definable evidence of basal ganglial pathology or cerebrovascular disease. The literature contains other patients with homocystinuria who developed rapidly progressive dystonia in the late teens (203). This infrequent finding is postulated to be due to neurotransmitter imbalance.

Methylenetetrahydrofolate Reductase Deficiency

Homocystinuria due to 5,10-methylenetetrahydrofolate reductase deficiency is inherited as an autosomal recessive trait. CNS manifestations tend to be more striking than in cystathionine beta-synthase deficiency. A boy died at 7 1/2 years of age with severe mental retardation, spasticity, and intractable seizures following a rapid deterioration in the previous 6 months (204). Low cerebrospinal fluid (CSF) folate levels are usually found with normal methionine in plasma and CSF. Some patients are responsive to folate. One 15-year-old mentally retarded girl presented with a schizophrenia-like picture characterized by progressive withdrawal, hallucinations, anorexia, and tremors. Her early growth and development had been normal. Treatment with 300 mg of pyridoxine a day had no effect on homocystine urinary excretion but produced peripheral neuropathy. The psychosis and homocystinuria improved with folate treatment (205).

A patient with the cobalamin G defect presented at the age of 21 years with neurologic findings of subacute combined degeneration. This woman had a wide-based gait with positive Romberg sign, brisk deep tendon reflexes, decreased perception of vibration and pin prick, and horizontal rotatory nystagmus. She had homocystinuria but no elevation of methylmalonate (206).

Neurophysiology

As noted, seizures occur in up to 21% of patients with homocystinuria. Although these are generally tonic-clonic in type, unusual seizure types have been reported. Three children with folate-responsive periodic behavior abnormalities have been reported (207,208). A 4-year-old patient with rage attacks had no other clinical evidence of seizures. His EEG showed polyspike and irregular generalized spike wave activity. A 3-year-old girl with tonic seizures and episodic repetitive behavioral changes suggesting complex partial seizures had generalized bursts of polyspike activity during sleep (207).

Neuroimaging

Computed tomographic (CT) brain scans are described in a number of case reports. Neuroimaging is generally normal unless cerebrovascular abnormalities are present. In the case of a 10-year-old girl presenting with left hemiparesis and bilateral papilledema, a CT brain scan showed a right temporo-occipital low-density lesion suggesting an infarct, and with contrast enhancement an empty delta sign was seen in the sagittal sinus. The diagnosis of cerebral venous and dural sinus thrombosis was confirmed by digital subtraction angiography (199). CT brain scans in patients presenting with dystonia have revealed no abnormality (209).

Pathology

A number of pathologic studies of the nervous system have been reported in homocystinuria (210–212). Occlusion of small vessels with both fresh and old thrombi and cortical infarcts secondary to vascular occlusion are frequently seen. In addition, however, neuronal loss in the cortex and hippocampus has been reported (210), and in one case extensive spongy degeneration of the white matter throughout the brain was observed (212). These changes have not been found in other neuropathology reports. The brain was normal in a homocystinuric patient dying 3 years after the onset of dystonia at 18 years of age (209).

Pathophysiology

The pathologic findings of neuronal and white matter changes disproportionate to vascular occlusion (210) provided an early suggestion that brain pathology in homocystinuria occurs independently of cerebrovascular disease. Homocysteine accumulates and homocysteic acid (the oxidation product of homocysteine) is a well-established excitotoxic agent. This compound appears to stimulate the NMDA receptor, providing a possible mechanism for neuronal destruction. It has been postulated that dystonia may result from abnormal glutamate receptor stimulation in the basal ganglia (209). As methionine levels are low in cystathionine beta-synthase deficiency, taurine production is likely to be inhibited. Taurine is a putative neurotransmitter acting as an inhibitor, and it may play a role in the release of dopamine and other neurotransmitters. Folate deficiency can affect catecholamine production as tyrosine hydroxylase uses tetrahydrofolate as a cofactor. This enzyme is the rate limiting step in catecholamine synthesis. One patient with 5,10-methylenetetrahydrofolate reduc-

tase deficiency has been reported with parkinsonian symptoms (213). The high infinity uptake of taurine by rat brain synaptosomes was inhibited by L-homocysteine as was the taurine uptake in mouse astrocyte cultures but not in cultured neurons. In this study, GABA uptake in astrocytes was inhibited also (214). Cystathionine is a putative neurotransmitter present in high concentrations in normal brain (215); its deficiency can be expected in homocystinuria.

The etiology of arteriosclerosis is probably multifactorial. Vascular intimal changes are seen even in young children. Soluble factors in the blood are thought to contribute to arteriosclerotic tendencies, but abnormal platelet function due to methionine elevation may play the major role (216). It should be emphasized that the etiology of mental retardation in homocystinuria is not simply due to cerebrovascular disease. Most mentally retarded homocystinuric patients have no evidence of stroke.

Diagnosis and Treatment

Neonatal screening for homocystinuria is based upon the accumulation of methionine in blood. Levels may be falsely low in the first few days of life. The urinary cyanide nitroprusside reaction is positive in homocystinuric patients if the urine is fresh. False-positive results may occur; patients taking multivitamin supplements containing pyridoxine may produce false-negative results. Treatment varies depending on the age of the patient. Patients with pyridoxine sensitivity should be treated with pyridoxine supplementation, and treatment with 500 to 1000 mg/day for several weeks is needed before an individual can be considered pyridoxine resistant. Caution is required as very large doses of pyridoxine (greater than 2 g/day) produce a sensory neuropathy. Children not sensitive to pyridoxine, particularly neonates, can be treated with methionine restriction. This treatment has been shown to be effective in preventing seizures and mental retardation. Methionine restriction to maintain blood levels within or near the normal range and the absence of homocysteine in the urine represents optimal management. Unfortunately, methionine-restricted diets are unpalatable and usually not tolerated by older children and adults.

Cystathioninuria

Biochemistry and Clinical Features

After cystathionine is synthesized from homocysteine and serine in the transsulfuration pathway, it is cleaved by cystathionase to cysteine and 2-ketobutyric acid (See Figure 1.3). A deficiency of cystathionase results in cystathioninuria (217,218). A number of the initial patients were mentally retarded, but subsequently normal individuals were diagnosed with cystathioninuria, and it is now considered a benign condition (219,220). Interestingly, cystathioninuria was the first disorder to be shown to be responsive to pyridoxine treatment, with a decrease in cystathionine excretion (218).

3-Mercaptolactic-Cysteine Disulfiduria

Biochemistry and Clinical Features

A minor pathway for cysteine metabolism is the transamination to 3-mercaptopyruvate, which can be metabolized by mercaptopyruvate sulfur transferase to various sulfur products. A deficiency of this enzyme results in accumulation of mercaptopyruvate, which is reduced to mercaptolactate by lactate dehydrogenase and then forms a mixed disulfide with cysteine. 3-Mercaptolactate cysteine disulfiduria is a very rare disorder, and 5 cases have been reviewed (221). Two patients were mentally retarded and three were normal, suggesting that mental retardation is not related to the enzyme deficiency. One pedigree has been studied in detail (222).

Hypermethioninemia

Biochemistry and Clinical Features

A deficiency of hepatic methionine adenosyltransferase results in the accumulation of methionine and hypermethioninemia without homocystinuria (See Figure 1.3) (223,224). The enzyme is normal in erythrocytes, lymphocytes, and fibroblasts. There are no neurologic consequences of this enzyme deficiency.

GLYCINE METABOLISM

Nonketotic Hyperglycinemia

Plasma and urine glycine are elevated in a number of organic acidemias. It was realized early on, however, that most of the disorders in which glycine accumulation occurred as a secondary phenomenon were associated with ketosis. Thus, hyperglycinemic conditions were segregated into ketotic and nonketotic hyperglycinemia (NKH) (225). The mechanism underlying the secondary hyperglycinemia seen in disorders such as propionic acidemia and methylmalonic acidemia remains unclear but may relate to glycine mitochondrial transport. In NKH the defect lies in the glycine cleavage system (Figure 1.4) (226). Defects in three of the four specific proteins in this enzyme system have been identified in patients with NKH; patients with classic disease have generally had deficiency of the P protein. Although the usual presentation of this disorder is a devastating neonatal seizure disorder following which little or no neurologic development occurs, milder presentations,

including an adult phenotype, have been described. A description of transient NKH in neonates expands the clinical phenotype further (227,228).

Biochemistry

Glycine is metabolized by a complex enzyme system, the glycine cleavage system, to ammonia, carbon dioxide, and hydroxymethyl tetrahydrofolate (229,230). The reaction localized in the mitochondria is reversible and can either synthesize or degrade glycine (231). The glycine cleavage system is composed of four proteins labeled P, H, T, and L (See Figure 1.4). The P protein contains pyridoxal phosphate and has glycine decarboxylase activity. The H protein is a lipoic acid containing protein that accepts the aminomethyl group from glycine decarboxylation. The T protein is a tetrahydrofolate requiring flavoprotein that forms hydroxymethyl-tetrahydrofolate and ammonia, leaving the lipoic acid of the H protein as the disulfide. The L protein is dihydrolipoyl dehydrogenase, which utilizes NAD to oxidize the lipoic acid of the H protein to the disulfide. The hydroxymethyl-tetrahydrofolate can enter the 1-carbon pool or be used to synthesize serine. The enzyme hydroxymethyltransferase catalyzes the reversible formation of serine from hydroxymethyl-tetrahydrofolate and glycine and is localized in the mitochondria together with the glycine cleavage system (231). Serine can be converted to pyruvate by serine dehydratase and metabolized through the tricarboxylic acid cycle (See Figure 1.4).

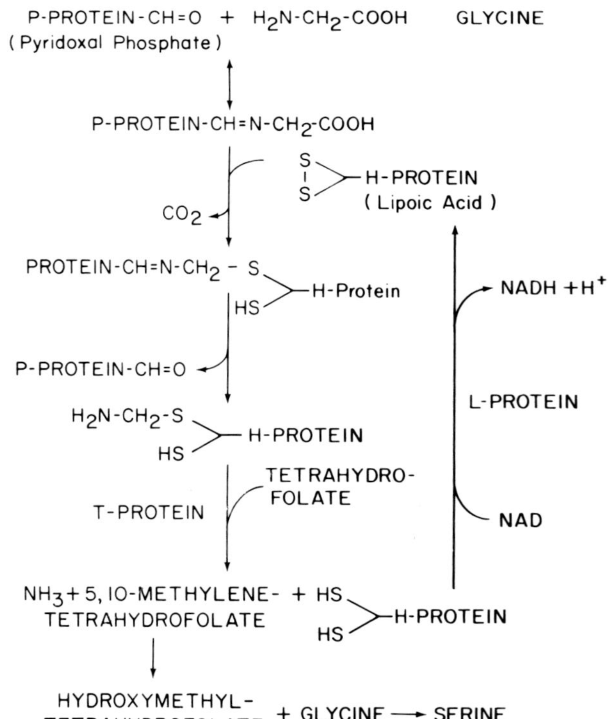

FIGURE 1.4 Reactions and components of the glycine cleavage system, which is deficient in nonketotic hyperglycemia.

The basic biochemical defect in nonketotic hyperglycinemia was shown to be deficiency of the glycine cleavage system in liver (232,233) and in brain (234,235). A summary of the abnormalities of the glycine cleavage system in 14 patients showed that most had an abnormal P protein while others had an abnormal T protein (236). Immunotitration has shown an absence of P protein in one patient (237).

A deficiency of the glycine cleavage system generally results in elevated glycine in urine, plasma, and CSF (234,236,238). However, the excretion of glycine is not always increased, and glycine in plasma may not always be elevated (239). In addition, glycine in these fluids may be elevated in ketotic hyperglycinemia due to propionic or methylmalonic acidemia. The most reliable biochemical parameter for the differential diagnosis of nonketotic hyperglycinemia is the ratio of CSF glycine to plasma glycine (234,236,238). The normal ratio is less than 0.04, while the typical ratio for nonketotic hyperglycinemia is greater than 0.20 (units for glycine in μM/L). In two reports, transient nonketotic hyperglycinemia with elevated CSF/plasma glycine ratios were found in neonates that normalized with time (227,228). It is unlikely that these four patients have defects in the glycine cleavage system, although they may have had immaturity of this system. In the diagnosis of nonketotic hyperglycinemia in neonates, serial determinations of the CSF/plasma glycine ratio would be prudent. Persistent elevation would indicate a defect in the glycine cleavage system.

The glycine cleavage system is not expressed in cultured normal fibroblasts, and demonstration of a deficiency for definitive diagnosis is usually done with liver or brain specimens (236). The activity has been found in normal chorionic villi, and a deficiency was demonstrated in chorionic villi from a pregnancy at risk for nonketotic hyperglycinemia that was terminated at 12 weeks (240). Thus, it may be possible to obtain prenatal diagnosis from chorionic villous samples. Although it had been reported that an elevated ratio of glycine to serine in amniotic fluid was found with a fetus affected with nonketotic hyperglycinemia (241), this has been questioned (242) and is not considered reliable for prenatal diagnosis.

One approach to the treatment of nonketotic hyperglycinemia is to lower the glycine levels by administering benzoate. The biochemical rationale for this is that benzoate is conjugated with glycine by glycine N-acylase to form hippuric acid, which is excreted (243,244).

Clinical and Neurologic Features

More than 80% of NKH patients present in the neonatal period (236,245), usually within the first 48 hours, with intractable myoclonic and other generalized seizures. Hiccups are common. Following the onset of symptoms, a rapid progression to coma occurs, often with apnea, and death ensues unless artificial ventilation is provided. Most patients die in the neonatal period, even if intensive care is available. In survivors, apnea resolves, but there is virtual total psychomotor developmental arrest. Intractable seizures continue, and death within the first year of life is common. Following neonatal hypotonia, survivors generally develop a spastic quadriparesis, frequently with opisthotonos. The clinical and biochemical features of 120 patients have been reviewed (236). Quantitative urinary organic acid analysis is essential in patients presenting with the neonatal presentation in order to exclude the organic acidemias. The CSF/plasma glycine ratio provides important diagnostic information. This ratio is elevated above 0.04 in NKH patients.

Milder clinical presentations offer a greater diagnostic challenge. A patient under our care developed tonic-clonic seizures at 3 days of age that were controlled by phenobarbitol and phenytoin. Anticonvulsants were stopped at 4 1/2 months of age and normal seizure free development continued until 9 months. Following a third diphtheria-pertussis-tetanus (DPT) immunization, intractable seizures developed that were both tonic-clonic and myoclonic in type with associated choreoathetosis. Loss of motor and language milestones occurred (246). The clinical presentation may be consistent with a neurodegenerative disease following a period of normal development for the first 6 months. The clinical features with rapid development of decerebrate rigidity and early death have suggested a neurolipidosis (247). Most affected siblings with this autosomal recessive disease present similar phenotypes, although in one family a child with the severe neonatal signs and symptoms had a sibling with only mild developmental delay at 1 year of age (233).

An adult variant presentation with psychomotor retardation and rare seizures has been described in a 22-year-old man (248). This patient had hypotonic arms with spasticity of the legs (248). Global developmental delay with seizures beginning at 11 months of age were the early clinical features in a 34-year-old demented woman with generalized hyperreflexia, athetosis, and poor articulated speech (249). A different adult presentation with signs and symptoms of a spinocerebellar degeneration and optic atrophy has been described, and has also been reported in a 15-year-old boy (250). These patients have normal development without seizures; CSF glycine levels are normal or only slightly elevated (250). Two neonates presenting with transient NKH were reported (227); both patients were hypotonic and had intractable seizures with high CSF levels of glycine. In the first patient, who also had a dilated cardiomyopathy, CSF glycine levels were normal within 7 days. In the second infant the CSF glycine was still 20 times normal at 45 days of age. Two other neonates with transient hyperglycinemia have been described (228).

Neurophysiology

EEG changes are marked in the classic form of this disease, and findings have been reported in three patients with the neonatal presentation (246). An EEG recorded on the second day in one comatose neonate with NKH showed prolonged multifocal seizures with a burst suppression pattern. At the age of 5 1/2 months this same patient continued to show bilateral seizure activity with burst-suppression pattern. Widespread focal epileptiform discharges with long runs of electrographic seizure activity are typical, although some patients show a pseudoperiodic record (251,252). One 3-month-old showed bursts of period synchronous high-voltage single or multiple spike and sharp wave activity superimposed on a fairly normal background. Bursts occurred at 2- to 6-second intervals without clinical seizure activity; however, clinical seizures were correlated with periods of high amplitude, fast 4- to 5-second spike wave activity in the right temporal and parietal area lasting up to 30 seconds in duration. This activity was associated with clinical focal clonic seizure activity. This patient showed some improvement in background activity at 4 months but electrographic and clinical seizures continued. Vertex spikes elicited with tactile stimuli were observed in a 38-week gestation neonate with NKH who displayed stimulus-provoked myoclonus starting at 2 hours of age. This electrographic midline seizure activity was associated with a burst-suppression background pattern. Brain stem auditory evoked responses recorded on the second day of life showed prolonged latencies in waves III and V.

Older patients with clinical seizures also have abnormal EEGs, and hypsarrhythmia has been described in some patients. A 3 1/2-year-old patient who initially presented in the neonatal period continued to have 20 tonic-clonic seizures a day. The EEG showed numerous paroxysmal multifocal spike discharges with bursts of delta and alpha activity. We have seen an 11-month-old girl who briefly experienced neonatal seizures, but then developed normally until the onset of intractable seizures at 9 months of age. Her EEG showed multifocal epileptiform discharges with long runs of electrographic seizure activity. Clinical seizures were unusual and manifested by myoclonus and athetoid arm movements. The two patients described with transient nonketotic hyperglycinemia had EEGs in the first few days of life that were "grossly distorted with multifocal seizure spikes" (227).

Electroretinograms (ERG) were reported in two siblings with neonatal NKH. One of these children showed reduced flash ERG amplitudes (253).

Neuroimaging

Brain CT findings have been described in a number of case reports. Older patients with classic disease show decreased white matter attenuation and cortical atrophy. Mildly affected patients, however, may have normal CT brain scans in spite of global psychomotor delay (249). A review of CT and pathologic reports included: 5 of 15 patients with ventricular enlargement; hypoplasia of the cerebellum found in 2 of 16; gyral malformations noted in 6 of 14; and

hypoplasia or complete absence of corpus callosum was found in 6 of 15 cases. Seven of 12 patients had small brains. Retarded myelination was noted in 6 of 11 cases, and all 13 patients in whom data were available showed spongy myelinopathy (254).

We have published a series of MRI brain scans in NKH patients (255). Six patients in this series suffered the severe neonatal form and one presented at 9 months of age with intractable seizures. Myelination patterns in NKH patients assessed by MRI were normal in the subjects less than 4 months of age, but decreased or absent supratentorial white matter myelination was found in patients older than 10 months. Varying degrees of myelination were found in the internal capsule, corona radiata, centrum semiovale, corpus callosum, and subcortical white matter tracts. Compared to age-matched controls, the corpus callosum was abnormally thin in 6 of 7 subjects. No patients had partial or complete agenesis of the corpus callosum in this series. It is likely that many of the reported patients with agenesis of the corpus callosum who were assessed only by CT did, in fact, have hypoplastic but not completely absent corpus callosi (Figure 1.5).

Pathology

Autopsy studies in NKH are similar to findings observed in severe cases of propionic acidemia, methylmalonic acidemia, and MSUD. Spongy myelinopathy is commonly

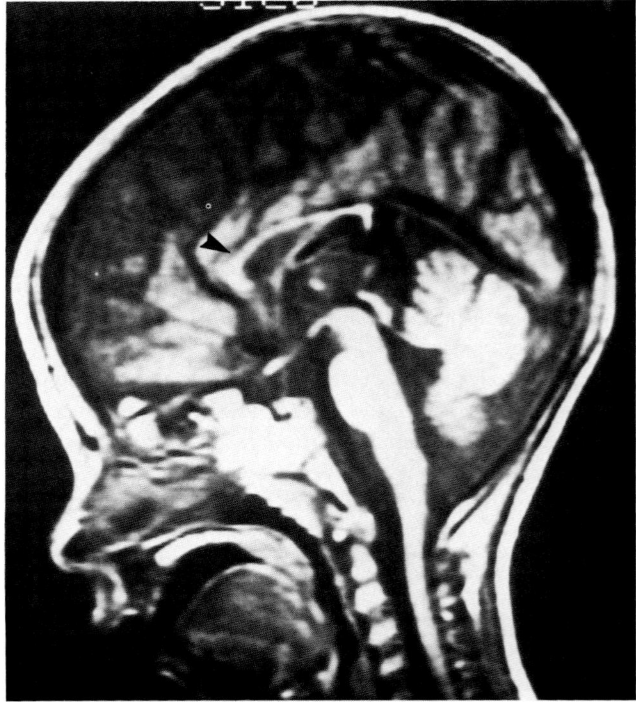

FIGURE 1.5   T1-weighted MRI sagittal brain scan of a 2-year-old patient with nonketotic hyperglycinemia. The arrow indicates a thin hypoplastic corpus callosum. Cortical atrophy is also present.

(256). In one of these patients, however, there was almost total loss of Purkinje and granule cells in the cerebellum; these changes have not been described in other reported cases. A patient presenting with a neurodegenerative course following normal development was found to have extensive spongiform change with white matter vacuolation (247). Electron microscopic studies of brain were reported in four neonatal deaths (257), showing normal amounts of white matter in the spinal cord, brain stem, and cerebrum compared to controls; however, spongiform changes were found in the areas containing myelin. Vacuoles were observed within myelin sheaths. Autopsy studies of brain were normal in three Finnish infants who died within the first 10 days of life (251). Throughout the neuropathology literature it is clear that white matter changes are predominant in hyperglycinemia and that these changes are more evident in older patients.

Pathophysiology

The mechanism underlying the neuropathologic changes in NKH is uncertain. It is likely that elevated brain glycine plays a major role in the pathophysiology. Glycine is a putative neurotransmitter in the CNS, largely playing an inhibitory role. It is postulated that excessive postsynaptic inhibition may be caused by swamping of synaptic clefts with glycine. Glycine is neurotoxic, more so in neonatal animals than older animals.

In one patient with a neonatal presentation of the disease who died with myoclonic seizures and elevated CSF and brain glycine, the low affinity glycine transport system was found to be absent in the brain, with altered transport in the spinal cord involving both high and low affinity glycine transport systems (258).

A plausible mechanism for the neurotoxicity of glycine, the seizures, and brain damage in NKH involves the NMDA receptor. Glycine has been found to potentiate the NMDA response in mouse brain neurons (2). Thus, glutamate and the NMDA receptor may be involved in neuronal injury in NKH as is the case in hypoxic ischemic injury and hypoglycemia (259).

Treatment

The major management problem in NKH is intractable seizure activity. Administration of anticonvulsants is rarely effective. Sodium benzoate has been used for 10 years, initially because of its effects in decreasing CSF and plasma glycine (260–262). More recently, however, sodium benzoate has been shown to have an anticonvulsant activity in its own right in NKH patients. Three patients were reported to have dramatically decreased seizure activity in response to oral administration of sodium benzoate in the maximum tolerated dosages (up to 900 mg/kg/day) (246). Sodium benzoate encourages excretion of glycine as hippurate in the urine. Diazepam has been advocated as helpful in the control of seizures. This was effective in two patients with intractable seizures when combined with choline and sodium benzoate (263). A few patients have seemed to respond to strychnine, which blocks glycine inhibition in the spinal cord (252,264). Other authors have reported failure of strychnine treatment in the neonatal period (265), and it is generally believed that more severely affected patients do not respond to this agent. Valine sensitivity was noted in one NKH patient but dietary restriction had no effect on the development of severe mental retardation (266). No treatment utilized to date has affected the severe mental retardation that accompanies classic NKH.

REFERENCES

1. Berl S, Lajtha A, Waelsh H. Amino acid and protein metabolism-VI. Cerebral compartments of glutamic acid metabolism. J Neurochem 1961;7:186–197.
2. Johnson JW, Ascher P. Glycine potentiates the NMDA response in cultured mouse brain neurons. Nature 1987;325:529–531.
3. Guttler F. Phenylketonuria: Fifty years since Fölling's discovery and still expanding our clinical and biochemical knowledge. Acta Paediatr Scand 1984;73:705–716.
4. Hanley WB, Clarke JT, Schoonheyt W. Maternal phenylketonuria (PKU)—A review. Clin Biochem 1987; 20:149–156.
5. Kaufman S. The phenylalanine hydroxylating system from mammalian liver. Adv Enzymol 1971;35:245–319.
6. Kaufman S. Enzymology of the phenylalanine-hydroxylating system. Enzyme 1987;38:286–295.
7. Curtius HC, Heintel D, Ghisla S, et al. Biosynthesis of tetrahydrobiopterin in man. J Inherited Metab Dis 1985;8 Suppl 1:28–33.
8. Katz I, Lloyd T, Kaufman S. Studies on phenylalanine and tyrosine hydroxylation by rat brain tyrosine hydroxylase. Biochim Biophys Acta 1976;445:567–578.
9. Chalmers RA, Watts RWE. Quantitative studies on the urinary excretion of unconjugated aromatic acids in phenylketonuria. Clin Chim Acta 1974;55:281–294.
10. Krause W, Halminski M, McDonald L, et al. Biochemical and neuropsychological effects of elevated plasma phenylalanine in patients with treated phenylketonuria. A model for the study of phenylalanine and brain function in man. J Clin Invest 1985;75:40–48.
11. Waisbren SE, Mahon BE, Schnell RR, et al. Predictors of intelligence quotient and intelligence quotient change in persons treated for phenylketonuria early in life. Pediatrics 1987;79:351–355.
12. Bartholome K, Lutz P, Bickel H. Determination of phenylalanine hydroxylase activity in patients with phenylketonuria and hyperphenylalaninemia. Pediatr Res 1975;9:899–903.
13. Trefz FK, Bartholome K, Bickel H, et al. In vivo residual activity of the phenylalanine hydroxylating system in phenylketonuria and variants. J Inherited Metab Dis 1981;4:101–102.
14. Levy HL. Neonatal screening for inborn errors of amino acid metabolism. Clin Endocrinol Metab 1974;3:153–166.

15. Spierto FW, Hearn TL, Gardner FH, et al. Phenylalanine analyses of blood-spot control materials: preparation of samples and evaluation of interlaboratory performance. Clin Chem 1985;31:235–238.

16. DiLella AG, Kwok SC, Ledley FD, et al. Molecular structure and polymorphic map of the human phenylalanine hydroxylase gene. Biochemistry 1986;25:743–749.

17. Guttler F, DiLella AG, Ledley FD, et al. Molecular biology of phenylketonuria. Eur J Pediatr 1987;146:A5–11.

18. Woo SL, Lidsky AS, Guttler F, et al. Prenatal diagnosis of classical phenylketonuria by gene mapping. JAMA 1984;251:1998–2002.

19. Guttler F, Ledley FD, Lidsky AS, et al. Correlation between polymorphic DNA haplotypes at phenylalanine hydroxylase locus and clinical phenotypes of phenylketonuria. J Pediatr 1987;110:68–71.

20. Smith I, Hyland K, Kendall B, et al. Clinical role of pteridine therapy in tetrahydrobiopterin deficiency. J Inherited Metab Dis 1985;8 Suppl.1:39–45.

21. Kaufman S. Hyperphenylalaninaemia caused by defects in biopterin metabolism. J Inherited Metab Dis 1985;8 Suppl 1:20–27.

22. Niederwieser A, Blau N, Wang M, et al. GTP cyclohydrolase I deficiency, a new enzyme defect causing hyperphenylalaninemia with neopterin, biopterin, dopamine, and serotonin deficiencies and muscle hypotonia. Eur J Pediatr 1984;141:208–214.

23. Niederwieser A, Leimbacher W, Curtius HC, et al. Atypical phenylketonuria with "dihydrobiopterin synthetase" deficiency: Absence of phosphate-eliminating enzyme activity demonstrated in liver. Eur J Pediatr 1985;144:13–16.

24. Lee EB. Metabolic diseases and the skin. Pediatr Clin North Am 1983;30:597–608.

25. Bauman ML, Kemper TL. Morphologic and histoanatomic observations of the brain in untreated human phenylketonuria. Acta Neuropathol (Berl) 1982;58:55–63.

26. MacLeod MD, Munro JF, Ledingham JG, et al. Management of the extrapyramidal manifestations of phenylketonuria with L-dopa. Arch Dis Child 1983;58:457–458.

27. Atwell RA, Berlin SJ. Lower extremity manifestations of phenylketonuria. J Foot Surg 1983;22:3–8.

28. Reveley AM, Reveley MA. Screening for adult phenylketonuria in psychiatric inpatients. Biol Psychiatry 1982;17:1343–1345.

29. Westwood A, Barr DG. Phenylketonuria with a progressive neurological disorder not responsive to tetrahydrobiopterin. Acta Paediatr Scand 1982;71:859–861.

30. Primrose DA. Phenylketonuria with normal intelligence. J Ment Defic Res 1983;27:239–246.

31. Koch R, Blaskovics M. Four cases of hyperphenylalaninaemia: studies during pregnancy and of the offspring produced. J Inherited Metab Dis 1982;5:11–15.

32. Brunner RL, Jordan MK, Berry HK. Early-treated phenylketonuria: Neuropsychologic consequences. J Pediatr 1983;102:831–835.

33. Brunner RL, Berch DB, Berry H. Phenylketonuria and complex spatial visualization: An analysis of information processing. Dev Med Child Neurol 1987;29:460–468.

34. Nevin NC, Carson NA. Severe mental retardation due to maternal phenylketonuria. Ulster Med J 1982;51:133–135.

35. Levy HL, Waisbren SE. Effects of untreated maternal phenylketonuria and hyperphenylalaninemia on the fetus. N Engl J Med 1983;309:1269–1274.

36. Barashnev YI, Korneichuk VV, Klembovsky AI, et al. Role of the liver in the pathogenesis of cerebral disorders in phenylketonuria. J Inherited Metab Dis 1982;5:204–210.

37. Koslacz Folga A, Jackowska K, Pakszys M. Characteristics of sleep EEG abnormalities in children with phenylketonuria during the first year of life. Probl Med Wieku Rozwoj 1979;8:36–46.

38. Koslacz Folga A, Pakszys M, Cabalska B, et al. Evaluation of the maturity of the bioelectrical activity of the brain of infants with phenylketonuria during sleep. Probl Med Wieku Rozwoj 1982;11:27–37.

39. De Giorgis GF, Antonozzi I, Del Castello PG, et al. EEG as a possible prognostic tool in phenylketonuria. Electroencephalogr Clin Neurophysiol 1983;55:60–68.

40. Behbehani AW. Termination of strict diet therapy in phenylketonuria. A study on EEG sleep patterns and computer spectral analysis. Neuropediatrics 1985;16:92–97.

41. Landi A, Ducati A, Villani R, et al. Pattern-reversal visual evoked potentials in phenylketonuric children. Childs Nerv Syst 1987;3:278–281.

42. Smith I, Leeming RJ, Cavanagh NP, et al. Neurological aspects of biopterin metabolism. Arch Dis Child 1986;61:130–137.

43. Yanai K, Iinuma K, Matsuzawa T, et al. Cerebral glucose utilization in pediatric neurological disorders determined by positron emission tomography. Eur J Nucl Med 1987;13:292–296.

44. Malamud N. Neuropathology of phenylketonuria. J Neuropathol Exp Neurol 1966;25:254–268.

45. Alejandre MJ, Marco C, Ramirez H, et al. Lipid composition of brain myelin from normal and hyperphenylalaninemic chick embryos. Comp Biochem Physiol [B] 1984;77:329–332.

46. Huether G, Neuhoff V, Kaus R. Brain development in experimental hyperphenylalaninaemia: Disturbed proliferation and reduced cell numbers in the cerebellum. Neuropediatrics 1983;14:12–19.

47. Dwivedy AK, Shah SN. Effects of phenylalanine and its deaminated metabolites on Na^+,K^+-ATPase activity in synaptosomes from rat brain. Neurochem Res 1982;7:717–725.

48. Aragon MC, Gimenez C, Valdivieso F. Inhibition by L-phenylalanine of tyrosine transport by synaptosomal plasma membrane vesicles: implications in the pathogenesis of phenylketonuria. J Neurochem 1982;39:1185–1187.

49. Herrero E, Aragon MC, Gimenez C, et al. Inhibition by L-phenylalanine of tryptophan transport by synaptosomal plasma membrane vesicles: Implications in the pathogenesis of phenylketonuria. J Inherited Metab Dis 1983;6:32–35.

50. Clark JB, Land JM. Phenylketonuria and maple syrup urine disease and their association with brain mitochondrial substrate utilization. In: Hommes FA, Van der Berg CJ, eds. Normal and Pathological Development of Energy Metabolism. New York: Academic Press, 1975:177–191.

51. Cordero ME, Trejo M, Colombo M, et al. Histological maturation of the neocortex in phenylketonuric rats. Early Hum Dev 1983;8:157–173.

52. Lacey DJ. Hippocampal dendritic abnormalities in a rat model of phenylketonuria. Ann Neurol 1984;16:577–580.

53. Spero DA, Yu MC. Effects of maternal hyperphenylalaninemia on fetal brain development: a morphological study. Exp Neurol 1983;79:655–665.

54. Taylor EH, Hommes FA. Effect of experimental hyper-

phenylalaninemia on myelin metabolism at later stages of brain development. Int J Neurosci 1983;20:217–227.

55. The dietary treatment of phenylketonuria. Nutr Rev 1983;41:11–14.

56. Seashore MR, Friedman E, Novelly RA, et al. Loss of intellectual function in children with phenylketonuria after relaxation of dietary phenylalanine restriction. Pediatrics 1985;75:226–232.

57. Hommes FA, Eller AG, Taylor EH. Turnover of the fast components of myelin and myelin proteins in experimental hyperphenylalaninemia. Relevance to termination of dietary treatment in human phenylketonuria. J Inherited Metab Dis 1982;5:21–27.

58. Pietz J, Benninger C, Schmidt H, et al. Long-term development of intelligence (IQ) and EEG in 34 children with phenylketonuria treated early. Eur J Pediatr 1988;147:361–367.

59. Koch R, Azen C, Friedman EG, et al. Paired comparisons between early treated PKU children and their matched sibling controls on intelligence and school achievement test results at eight years of age. J Inherited Metab Dis 1984;7:86–90.

60. Fellman JH, Vanbellinghen PJ, Jones RT, et al. Soluble and mitochondrial forms of tyrosine aminotransferase. Relationship to human tyrosinemia. Biochemistry 1969;8:615–622.

61. Anderson SM, Pipsa JP. Purification and properties of human liver tyrosine aminotransferase. Clin Chim Acta 1982;125:117–123.

62. Fellman JH, Fujita TS, Roth ES. Assay, properties and tissue distribution of p-hydroxyphenylpyruvate hydroxylase. Biochim Biophys Acta 1972;284:90–100.

63. LaDu BN, Zannoni VG, Laster L, et al. The nature of the defect in tyrosine metabolism in alcaptonuria. J Biol Chem 1958;230:251–260.

64. Fallstrom SP, Lindblad B, Lindstedt S, et al. Hereditary tyrosinemia-fumarylacetoacetase deficiency. Pediatr Res 1979;13:78.

65. Berger R, Smit GPA, Stoker-de Vries SA, et al. Deficiency of fumarylacetoacetase in a patient with hereditary tyrosinemia. Clin Chim Acta 1981;114:37–44.

66. Kennaway NG, Buist NRM. Metabolic studies in a patient with hepatic cytosol tyrosine aminotransferase deficiency. Pediatr Res 1971;5:287–297.

67. Jellum E, Horn L, Thoresen O, et al. Urinary excretion of N-acetyl amino acids in patients with some inborn errors of amino acid metabolism. Scand J Clin Lab Invest Suppl 1986;184:21–26.

68. Kennaway NG, Buist NRM, Fellman JH. The origin of urinary p-hydroxyphenylpyruvate in a patient with hepatic cytosol tyrosine aminotransferase deficiency. Clin Chim Acta 1972;41:157–161.

69. Machino H, Miki Y, Kawatsu T, et al. Successful dietary control of tyrosinemia II. J Am Acad Dermatol 1983;9:533–539.

70. Ney D, Bay C, Schneider JA, et al. Dietary management of oculocutaneous tyrosinemia in an 11-year-old child. Am J Dis Child 1983;137:995–1000.

71. Halvorsen S. Screening for disorders of tyrosine metabolism. In: Bickel H, Guthrie R, Hammersen G, eds. Neonatal Screening for Inborn Errors of Metabolism. New York: Springer-Verlag, 1980;45–57.

72. Ohisalo JJ, Laskowska-Klita T, Andersson SM. Development of tyrosine aminotransferase and p-hydroxyphenylpyruvate dioxygenase activities in fetal and neonatal liver. J Clin Invest 1982;70:198–200.

73. Giardini O, Cantani A, Kennaway NG, et al. Chronic tyrosinemia associated with 4-hydroxyphenylpyruvate dioxygenase deficiency with acute intermittent ataxia and without visceral and bone involvement. Pediatr Res 1983;17:25–29.

74. Endo F, Kitano A, Uehara I, et al. Four-hydroxyphenylpyruvic acid oxidase deficiency with normal fumarylacetoacetase: A new variant form of hereditary hypertyrosinemia. Pediatr Res 1983;17:92–96.

75. Lindblad B, Lindstedt S, Steen G. On the enzymatic defects in hereditary tyrosinemia. Proc Natl Acad Sci USA 1977;74:4641–4645.

76. Grenier A, Lescault A, Laberge C, et al. Detection of succinylacetone and the use of its measurement in mass screening for hereditary tyrosinemia. Clin Chim Acta 1982;123:93–99.

77. Berger R, Van Faassen H, Smith GP. Biochemical studies on the enzymatic deficiencies in hereditary tyrosinemia. Clin Chim Acta 1983;134:129–141.

78. Kvittingen EA. Hereditary tyrosinemia type I—an overview. Scand J Clin Lab Invest Suppl 1986;184:27–34.

79. Stoner E, Starkman H, Wellner D, et al. Biochemical studies of a patient with hereditary hepatorenal tyrosinemia: Evidence of glutathione deficiency. Pediatr Res 1984;18:1332–1336.

80. Fallstrom SP, Lindblad B, Steen G. On the renal tubular damage in hereditary tyrosinemia and on the formation of succinylacetoacetate and succinylacetone. Acta Paediatr Scand 1981;70:315–320.

81. Kvittingen EA, Halvorsen S, Jellum E. Deficient fumarylacetoacetate fumarylhydrolase activity in lymphocytes and fibroblasts from patients with hereditary tyrosinemia. Pediatr Res 1983;17:541–544.

82. Kvittingen EA, Brodtkorb E. The pre- and post-natal diagnosis of tyrosinemia type I and the detection of the carrier state by assay of fumarylacetoacetase. Scand J Clin Lab Invest Suppl 1986;184:35–40.

83. Gagne R, Lescault A, Grenier A, et al. Prenatal diagnosis of hereditary tyrosinemia: Measurement of succinylacetone in amniotic fluid. Prenat Diagn 1982;2:185–188.

84. Jakobs C, Dorland L, Wikkerink B, et al. Stable isotope dilution analysis of succinylacetone using electron capture negative ion mass fragmentography: an accurate approach to the pre- and neonatal diagnosis of hereditary tyrosinemia type I. Clin Chim Acta 1988;171:223–231.

85. Kvittingen EA, Steinmann B, Gitzelmann R, et al. Prenatal diagnosis of hereditary tyrosinemia by determination of fumarylacetoacetase in cultured amniotic fluid cells. Pediatr Res 1985;19:334–337.

86. Salamon T, Hrnjica M, Schnyder UW, et al. 4 cases of Richner-Hanhart syndrome (tyrosinemia type II) with neurological symptomatology in a Yugoslav family. Hautarzt 1988;39:149–154.

87. Goldsmith LA. Tyrosinemia II. A large North Carolina kindred. Arch Intern Med 1985;145:1697–1700.

88. Starzl TE, Zitelli BJ, Shaw BW Jr, et al. Changing concepts: liver replacement for hereditary tyrosinemia and hepatoma. J Pediatr 1985;106:604–606.

89. Goulden KJ, Moss MA, Cole DE, et al. Pitfalls in the initial diagnosis of tyrosinemia: Three case reports and a review of the literature. Clin Biochem 1987;20:207–212.

90. Berger R, Michals K, Galbraeth J, et al. Tyrosinemia type Ib caused by maleylacetoacetate isomerase deficiency: A new enzyme defect. Pediatr Res 1988;23:328A.

91. Seshia SS, Perry TL, Dakshinamurti K, et al. Tyrosinemia and intractable seizures. Epilepsia 1984;25:457–463.

92. Mamunes P, Prince PE, Thornton NH, et al. Intellectual deficits after transient tyrosinemia in the term neonate. Pediatrics 1976;57:675.

93. Driscoll DJ, Jabs EW, Alcorn D, et al. Corneal tyrosine crystals in transient neonatal tyrosinemia. J Pediatr 1988;113:91.

94. Wilcken B, Hammond JW, Howard N, et al. Hawkinsinuria: A dominantly inherited defect of tyrosine metabolism with severe effects in infancy. N Engl J Med 1981;305:865–868.

95. Martin JJ, Schlote W. Central nervous system lesions in disorders of amino-acid metabolism: A neuropathological study. J Neurol Sci 1972;15:49–76.

96. Lindblad B, Friden J, Greter J, et al. Treatment of hereditary tyrosinaemia (fumarylacetoacetase deficiency) by enzyme substitution. J Inherited Metab Dis 1986;9 Suppl 2:257–261.

97. Tuchman M, Freese DK, Sharp HL, et al. Contribution of extrahepatic tissues to biochemical abnormalities in hereditary tyrosinemia type I: study of three patients after liver transplantation. J Pediatr 1987;110:399–403.

98. Niederwieser A, Matasovic A, Tippett P, et al. A new sulfur amino acid, named hawkinsin, identified in a baby with transient tyrosinemia and her mother. Clin Chim Acta 1977;76:345–356.

99. Niederwieser A, Wadman SK, Danks DM. Excretion of cis- and trans-4-hydroxycyclohexylacetic acid in addition to hawkinsin in a family with a postulated defect of 4-hydroxyphenylpyruvate dioxygenase. Clin Chim Acta 1978;90:195–200.

100. Hocart CH, Halpern B, Hick LA, et al. Hawkinsinuria—identification of quinolacetic acid and pyroglutamic acid during an acidotic phase. J Chromatogr 1983;275:237–243.

101. Danks DM, Tippett P, Rogers J. A new form of prolonged transient tyrosinemia presenting with severe metabolic acidosis. Acta Paediatr Scand 1975;64:209–214.

102. Garrod AE. The incidence of alkaptonuria: A study in chemical individuality. Lancet 1902;2:1616–1620.

103. Garrod AE. The Lancet. The incidence of alkaptonuria: A study in chemical individuality. Nutr Rev 1975;33:81–83.

104. Christensen K, Manthorpe R. Alkaptonuria and ochronosis. A survey and 5 cases. Hum Hered 1983;33:140–144.

105. Zannoni VG, Seegmiller JE, LaDu BN. Nature of the defect in alcaptonuria. Nature 1962;193:952–953.

106. Koska L. Artifacts produced by homogentisic acid in the examination of urine from alkaptonurics. Ann Clin Biochem 1986;23:354.

107. Zannoni VG, Lomtevas N, Goldfinger S. Oxidation of homogentisic acid to ochronotic pigment in connective tissue. Biochim Biophys Acta 1969;177:94–105.

108. Schumacher HR, Holdsworth DE. Ochronotic arthropathy. I. Clinicopathologic studies. Semin Arthritis Rheum 1977;6:207–246.

109. Martin JP Jr, Batkoff B. Homogentisic acid autoxidation and oxygen radical generation: Implications for the etiology of alkaptonuric arthritis. Free Radic Biol Med 1987;3:241–250.

110. Nora JR, Nora GE, Fitzgerald M. Alkaptonuria: Report of six cases. Ill Med J 1967;132:681–685.

111. Abreo K, Abreo F, Zimmerman SW, et al. A fifty-year-old man with skin pigmentation, arthritis, chronic renal failure and methemoglobinemia. Am J Med Genet 1983;14:97–114.

112. Van den Doel EM, Van Nieuwenhuizen O, Willemse J. Alcaptonuria with seizures [letter]. J Neurol Neurosurg Psychiatry 1985;48:1072.

113. Bhaskar PA, Neelakandan B. Alcaptonuria with seizures [letter]. J Neurol Neurosurg Psychiatry 1983;46:98.

114. Rao VA. Anterior megalophthalmos associated with lamellar cataract on alkaptonuria. Indian J Ophthalmol 1982;30:109–110.

115. Gaines JJ Jr. The pathology of alkaptonuric ochronosis. Hum Pathol 1989;20:40–46.

116. Cerenansky J, Sitaj S, Urbanek T. Alkaptonuria and ochronosis. J Bone Joint Surg [Am] 1959;41A:1169–1182.

117. Srsen S, Vondracek J, Srsnova K, et al. Analysis of the life span of alkaptonuric patients. Cas Lek Cesk 1985;124:1288–1291.

118. Menkes JH, Hurst PL, Craig JM. New syndrome: Progressive infantile cerebral dysfunction associated with unusual urinary substance. Pediatrics 1954;14:462–466.

119. Dancis J, Hutzler J, Levitz M. The diagnosis of maple syrup urine disease (branched-chain ketoaciduria) by the in vitro study of the peripheral leukocyte. Pediatrics 1963;32:234–238.

120. Pettit FH, Yeaman SJ, Reed LJ. Purification and characterization of branched chain alpha-keto acid dehydrogenase complex of bovine kidney. Proc Natl Acad Sci USA 1978;75, No. 10:4881–4885.

121. Danner DJ, Lemmon SK, Besharse JC, et al. Purification and characterization of branched chain alpha-ketoacid dehydrogenase from bovine liver mitochondria. J Biol Chem 1979;254, No. 12:5522–5526.

122. Khatra BS, Chawla RK, Sewell CW, et al. Distribution of branched-chain alpha-keto acid dehydrogenases in primate tissues. J Clin Invest 1977;59:558–564.

123. Goto M, Shinno H, Ichihara A. Isozyme patterns of branched chain amino acid transaminase in human tissues and tumors. Jpn J Cancer Res (GANN) 1977;68:663–667.

124. Langanbeck U, Wendel U, Mench-Hoinowski A, et al. Correlations between branched-chain amino acids and branched-chain alpha-keto acids in blood in maple syrup urine disease. Clin Chim Acta 1978;88:283–291.

125. Matthews DE, Ben-Galim E, Haymond MW, et al. Alloisoleucine formation in maple syrup urine disease: Isotopic evidence for the mechanism. Pediatr Res 1980;14:854–857.

126. Heffelfinger SC, Sewell ET, Danner DJ. Identification of specific subunits of highly purified bovine liver branched-chain ketoacid dehydrogenase. Biochemistry 1983;22:5519–5522.

127. Paxton R, Kuntz M, Harris RA. Phosphorylation sites and inactivation of branched chain alpha-ketoacid dehydrogenase isolated from rat heart, bovine kidney, and rabbit liver, kidney, heart, brain and skeletal muscle. Arch Biochem Biophys 1986;244:187–201.

128. Damuni Z, Merryfield ML, Humphreys JS, et al. Purification and properties of branched chain alpha-ketoacid dehydrogenase phosphatase from bovine kidney. Proc Natl Acad Sci USA 1984;81:4335–4338.

129. Block KP, Aftring RP, Buse MG, et al. Estimation of branched-chain alpha-keto acid dehydrogenase activation in mammalian tissue. In: Harris RA, Sokatch JR, eds. Methods in enzymology, Vol. 166. San Diego: Academic Press, 1988:201–213.

130. Paxton R, Harris RA. Regulation of branched chain alpha-ketoacid dehydrogenase kinase. Arch Biochem Biophys 1984;231:48–57.

131. Fernhoff PM, Fitzmaurice N, Milner J, et al. Coordinated system for comprehensive newborn metabolic screening. South Med J 1982;75:529–532.

132. Snyderman SE, Goldstein F, Sansaricq C, et al. The relationship between the branched chain amino acids and their alpha-ketoacids in maple syrup urine disease. Pediatr Res 1984;18:851–853.

133. Lehnert W, Werle E. Elevated excretion of N-acetylated branched-chain amino acids in maple syrup urine disease. Clin Chim Acta 1988;172:123–126.

134. Hagenfeldt L, Naglo AS. New conjugated urinary metabolites in intermediate type maple syrup urine disease. Clin Chim Acta 1987;169:77–83.

135. Dancis J, Hutzler J, Cox RP. Maple syrup urine disease: branched-chain keto acid decarboxylation in fibroblasts as measured with amino acids and keto acids. Am J Hum Genet 1977;29:272–279.

136. Indo Y, Akaboshi I, Nobukuni Y, et al. Maple syrup urine disease: A possible biochemical basis for the clinical heterogeneity. Hum Genet 1988;80:6–10.

137. Wendel U, Wohler W, Goedde HW, et al. Rapid diagnosis of maple syrup urine disease (branched chain ketoaciduria) by micro-enzyme assay in leukocytes and fibroblasts. Clin Chim Acta 1973;45:433–440.

138. Chuang DT, Ku LS, Kerr DS, et al. Detection of heterozygotes in maple syrup urine disease: Measurements of branched-chain alpha-keto acid dehydrogenase and its components in cell cultures. Am J Hum Genet 1982;34:416–424.

139. Cox R, Hutzler J, Dancis J. Antenatal diagnosis of maple syrup urine disease. Lancet 1978;2:212.

140. Kleijer WJ, Horsman D, Mancini GM, et al. First-trimester diagnosis of maple syrup urine disease on intact chorionic villi [letter]. N Engl J Med 1985;313:1608.

141. Wendel U, Claussen U, Langenbeck U. Pattern of branched-chain alpha-keto acids in amniotic fluid. Clin Chim Acta 1980;120:267–269.

142. Danner DJ, Armstrong N, Heffelfinger SC, et al. Absence of branched chain acyl-transferase as a cause of maple syrup urine disease. J Clin Invest 1985;75:858–860.

143. Hummel KB, Litwer S, Bradford AP, et al. Nucleotide sequence of a cDNA for branched chain acyltransferase with analysis of the deduced protein structure. J Biol Chem 1988;263:6165–6168.

144. Indo Y, Kitano A, Endo F, et al. Altered kinetic properties of the branched-chain alpha-keto acid dehydrogenase complex due to mutation of the beta-subunit of the branched-chain alpha-keto acid decarboxylase (E1) component in lymphoblastoid cells derived from patients with maple syrup urine disease. J Clin Invest 1987;80:63–70.

145. Hu CW, Lau KS, Griffin TA, et al. Isolation and sequencing of a cDNA encoding the decarboxylase (E1) alpha precursor of bovine branched-chain alpha-keto acid dehydrogenase complex. Expression of E1 alpha mRNA and subunit in maple syrup urine disease and 3T3-L1 cells. J Biol Chem 1988;263:9007–9014.

146. Fisher CW, Chuang JL, Griffin TA, et al. Molecular phenotypes in cultured maple syrup urine disease cells: Complete E1alpha cDNA sequence and mRNA and subunit contents of the human branched chain alpha-keto acid dehydrogenase complex. J Biol Chem 1989;264:3448–3453.

147. Duran M, Wadman SK. Thiamine-responsive inborn errors of metabolism. J Inherited Metab Dis 1985;8:70–75.

148. Fernhoff PM, Lubitz D, Danner DJ, et al. Thiamine response in maple syrup urine disease. Pediatr Res 1985;19:1011–1016.

149. Chuang DT, Ku LS, Cox RP. Biochemical basis of thiamin-responsive maple syrup urine disease. Trans Assoc Am Physicians 1982;95:196–204.

150. Chuang DT, Ku LS, Cox RP. Thiamin-responsive maple syrup urine disease: Decreased affinity of the mutant branched-chain alpha-keto acid dehydrogenase for alpha-ketoisovalerate and thiamin pyrophosphate. Proc Natl Acad Sci USA 1982;79:3300–3304.

151. Danner DJ, Wheeler FB, Lemmon SK, et al. In vivo and in vitro response of human branched chain alpha-ketoacid dehydrogenase to thiamine and thiamine pyrophosphate. Pediatr Res 1978;12:235–238.

152. DiGeorge AM, Rezvani I, Garibaldi LR, et al. Prospective study of maple syrup urine disease for the first four days of life. N Engl J Med 1982;307:1492–1495.

153. Herndon WA. Scoliosis and maple syrup urine disease. J Pediatr Orthop 1984;4:126–128.

154. Verdu A, Lopez Herce J, Pascual Castroviejo I, et al. Maple syrup urine disease variant form: Presentation with psychomotor retardation and CT scan abnormalities. Acta Paediatr Scand 1985;74:815–818.

155. Suzuki S, Naito H, Abe T, et al. Cranial computed tomography in a patient with a variant form of maple syrup urine disease. Neuropediatrics 1983;14:102–103.

156. Mantovani JF, Naidich TP, Prensky AL, et al. MSUD presentation with pseudotumor cerebri and CT abnormalities. J Pediatr 1980;96:279–281.

157. Gonzalez Rios MC, Chuang DT, Cox RP, et al. A distinct variant of intermediate maple syrup urine disease. Clin Genet 1985;27:153–159.

158. Goedde HW, Langelbeck V. Clinical and biochemical genetic aspects of intermittant branched-chain ketoaciduria. Acta Paediatr Scand 1970;59:83–87.

159. Munnich A, Saudubray JM, Taylor J, et al. Congenital lactic acidosis, alpha-ketoglutaric aciduria and variant form of maple syrup urine disease due to a single enzyme defect: dihydrolipoyl dehydrogenase deficiency. Acta Paediatr Scand 1982;71:167–171.

160. Estivill E, Sanmarti FX, Vidal R, et al. Comb-like rhythm: An EEG pattern peculiar to leucinosis. An Esp Pediatr 1985;22:123–127.

161. Romero FJ, Ibarra B, Rovira M, et al. Cerebral computed tomography in maple syrup urine disease. J Comput Assist Tomogr 1984;8:410–411.

162. Menkes JH, Philippart M, Fiol RE. Cerebral lipids in maple syrup urine disease. J Pediatr 1965;66:584–594.

163. Ferriere G, de Castro M, Rodriguez J. Abnormalities of muscle fibers in maple syrup urine disease. Acta Neuropathol (Berl) 1984;63:249–254.

164. Healy PJ, Harper PA, Dennis JA. Diagnosis of neuraxial oedema in calves. Aust Vet J 1986;63:95–96.

165. Duffell SJ, Harper PA, Healy PJ, et al. Congenital hypomyelinogenesis of Hereford calves. Vet Rec 1988;123:423–424.

166. Harper PA, Healy PJ, Dennis JA. Maple syrup urine disease as a cause of spongiform encephalopathy in calves. Vet Rec 1986;119:62–65.

167. Harper PA, Healy PJ, Dennis JA. Ultrastructural findings in maple syrup urine disease in Poll Hereford calves. Acta Neuropathol (Berl) 1986;71:316–320.

168. Tribble D, Shapira R. Myelin proteins: Degradation in rat brain initiated by metabolites causative of maple syrup urine disease. Biochem Biophys Res Commun 1983;114:440–446.

169. Banks WA, Kastin AJ. Interactions between the blood-brain barrier and endogenous peptides: Emerging clinical implications. Am J Med Sci 1988;295:459–465.

170. Dwivedi C, James EC, Parmar SS. Effects of abnormal metabolites of maple syrup urine disease on neurotransmitter receptor binding. Biochem Med Metab Biol 1986;35:275–278.

171. Lysiak W, Stepinski J, Angielski S. Acta Biochim Pol 1970;17:131–141.

172. Gibson GE, Blass JP. Inhibition of acetylcholine synthesis and of carbohydrate utilization by maple-syrup-urine disease metabolites. J Neurochem 1976;26:1073–1078.

173. Naughten ER, Saul IP, Roche G, et al. Early diagnosis and dietetic management in newborn with maple syrup urine disease. Birth to six weeks. J Inherited Metab Dis 1985;8:131–132.

174. Clow CL, Reade TM, Scriver CR. Outcome of early and long-term management of classical maple syrup urine disease. Pediatrics 1981;68:856–862.

175. Snyderman SE. The dietary therapy of inherited metabolic disease. Prog Food Nutr Sci 1975;1:507–530.

176. Field CMB, Carson NAJ, Cusworth DC, et al. Homocystinuria: A new disorder of metabolism [abstract]. Tenth Int Cong Paediatr 1962;274.

177. Mudd SH, Finkelstein JD, Irreverre F, et al. Homocystinuria: An enzymatic defect. Science 1964;143:1443–1445.

178. Wiley VC, Dudman NP, Wilcken DE. Interrelations between plasma free and protein-bound homocysteine and cysteine in homocystinuria. Metabolism 1988;37:191–195.

179. Cooper AJL. Biochemistry of sulfur-containing amino acids. Ann Rev Biochem 1983;52:187–222.

180. Mahoney MJ, Bick D. Recent advances in the inherited methylmalonic acidemias. Acta Paediatr Scand 1987;76:689–696.

181. Shih VE, Salam MZ, Mudd SH, et al. A new form of homocystinuria due to N5-10-methylenetetrahydrofolate reductase deficiency. Pediatr Res 1977;6:395.

182. Freeman JM, Finkelstein JD, Mudd SH, et al. Homocystinuria presenting as reversible "schizophrenia." A new defect in methionine metabolism with reduced methylenetetrahydrofolate-reductase activity. Pediatr Res 1972;6:423.

183. Mudd SH, Skovby F, Levy HL, et al. The natural history of homocystinuria due to cystathionine beta-synthase deficiency. Am J Hum Genet 1985;37:1–31.

184. Spaeth GL, Barber GW. Prevalence of homocystinuria among the mentally retarded: Evaluation of a specific screening test. Pediatrics 1967;40:586–589.

185. Uhlendorf BW, Conerly EB, Mudd SH. Homocystinuria: Studies in tissue culture. Pediatr Res 1973;7:645–658.

186. Fleisher LD, Beratis NG, Tallan HH, et al. Homocystinuria due to cystathionine synthase (CS) deficiency: Investigation in cultured long-term lymphocytes, fetal skin fibroblasts and amniotic fluid cells. Pediatr Res 1974;8:388.

187. Boers GH, Fowler B, Smals AG, et al. Improved identification of heterozygotes for homocystinuria due to cystathionine synthase deficiency by the combination of methionine loading and enzyme determination in cultured fibroblasts. Hum Genet 1985;69:164–169.

188. Fowler B, Brresen AL, Boman N. Prenatal diagnosis of homocystinuria [letter]. Lancet 1982;2:875.

189. Poole JR, Mudd SH, Conerly EB, et al. Homocystinuria due to cystathionine synthase deficiency: Studies of nitrogen balance and sulfur excretion. J Clin Invest 1975;55:1033–1048.

190. Wilcken DE, Wilcken B, Dudman NP, et al. Homocystinuria—The effects of betaine in the treatment of patients not responsive to pyridoxine. N Engl J Med 1983;309:448–453.

191. Wilcken DE, Dudman NP, Tyrrell PA. Homocystinuria due to cystathionine beta-synthase deficiency—The effects of betaine treatment in pyridoxine-responsive patients. Metabolism 1985;34:1115–1121.

192. Fleisher LD, Longhi RC, Tallan HH, et al. Cystathionine beta-synthase deficiency: Differences in thermostability between normal and abnormal enzyme from cultured human cells. Pediatr Res 1978;12:293–296.

193. Fowler B, Kraus J, Packman S, et al. Homocystinuria: Evidence for three distinct classes of cystathionine beta-synthase mutants in cultured fibroblasts. J Clin Invest 1978;61:645–653.

194. Fowler B. Recent advances in the mechanism of pyridoxine-responsive disorders. J Inherited Metab Dis 1985;8 Suppl 1:76–83.

195. Michalski A, Leonard JV, Taylor DS. The eye and inherited metabolic disease: A review. J R Soc Med 1988;81:286–290.

196. Blika S, Saunte E, Lunde H, et al. Homocystinuria treated with pyridoxine. Acta Ophthalmol (Copenh) 1982;60:894–906.

197. Abbott MH, Folstein SE, Abbey H, et al. Psychiatric manifestations of homocystinuria due to cystathionine beta-synthase deficiency: Prevalence, natural history, and relationship to neurologic impairment and vitamin B$_6$-responsiveness. Am J Med Genet 1987;26:959–969.

198. Jackson GM, Grisolia JS, Wolf PL, et al. Postoperative thromboemboli in cystathionine beta-synthase deficiency. Am Heart J 1984;108:627–628.

199. Schwab FJ, Peyster RG, Brill CB. CT of cerebral venous sinus thrombosis in a child with homocystinuria. Pediatr Radiol 1987;17:244–245.

200. Wicherink Bol HF, Boers GH, Drayer JI, et al. Angiographic findings in homocystinuria. Cardiovasc Intervent Radiol 1983;6:125–128.

201. Brattstrom LE, Hardebo JE, Hultberg BL. Moderate homocysteinemia—A possible risk factor for arteriosclerotic cerebrovascular disease. Stroke 1984;15:1012–1016.

202. Boers GH, Smals AG, Trijbels FJ, et al. Heterozygosity for homocystinuria in premature peripheral and cerebral occlusive arterial disease. N Engl J Med 1985;313:709–715.

203. Davous P, Rondot P. Homocystinuria and dystonia [letter]. J Neurol Neurosurg Psychiatry 1983;46:283.

204. Haan EA, Rogers JG, Lewis GP, et al. 5,10-Methylenetetrahydrofolate reductase deficiency. Clinical and biochemical features of a further case. J Inherited Metab Dis 1985;8:53–57.

205. Editorial. Folate-responsive homocystinuria and "schizophrenia." Nutr Rev 1982;40:242–245.

206. Carmel R, Watkins D, Goodman SI, et al. Hereditary defect of cobalamin metabolism (cblG mutation) presenting as a neurologic disorder in adulthood. N Engl J Med 1988;318:1738–1741.

207. Murphy JV, Thome LM, Michals K, et al. Folic acid responsive rages, seizures and homocystinuria. J Inherited Metab Dis 1985;8:109–110.

208. Freeman JM, Finkelstein MD, Mudd SH. Folate-responsive homocystinuria and "schizophrenia." A defect in methylation due to deficient 5,10-Methylenetetrahydrofolate reductase activity. N Engl J Med 1975;292:491–496.

209. Kempster PA, Brenton DP, Gale AN, et al. Dystonia in homocystinuria. J Neurol Neurosurg Psychiatry 1988;51:859–862.

210. Carson NAJ, Dent CE, Field CMB, et al. Homocystinuria: Clinical and pathological review of 10 cases. J Pediatr 1965;66:565–583.

211. Dunn HG, Perry TL, Dorman CL. Homocystinuria. Neurology 1966;16:407–420.

212. Chou SM, Waisman HA. Spongy degeneration of the nervous system: Case of homocystinuria. Arch Pathol 1965;79:357–363.

213. Clayton PT, Smith I, Harding B, et al. Subacute combined degeneration of the cord, dementia and Parkinsonism due to an inborn error of folate metabolism. J Neurol Neurosurg Psychiatry 1986;49:920–927.

214. Allen IC, Schousboe A, Griffiths R. Effect of L-homocysteine and derivatives on the high-affinity uptake of taurine and GABA into synaptosomes and cultured neurons and astrocytes. Neurochem Res 1986;11:1487–1496.

215. Tudball N, Beaumont A. Studies on the neurochemical properties of cystathionine. Biochim Biophys Acta 1979;588:285–293.

216. Bose R, Dutta A. Hemiplegia in homocystinuria [letter]. J Assoc Physicians India 1986;34:674.

217. Frimpter GW. Cystathioninuria: Nature of the defect. Science 1965;149:1095–1096.

218. Frimpter GW, Haymovitz A, Horwith M. Cystathioninuria. N Engl J Med 1963;268:333–339.

219. Scott CR, Dassell SW, Clark SH, et al. Cystathioninemia: A benign genetic condition. J Pediatr 1970;76:571–577.

220. Perry TL, Hardwick DF, Hansen S, et al. Cystathioninuria in two healthy siblings. N Engl J Med 1968;278:590–592.

221. Crawhall JC. A review of the clinical presentation and laboratory findings in two uncommon hereditary disorders of sulfur amino acid metabolism, beta-mercaptolactate cysteine disulfiduria and sulfite oxidase deficiency. Clin Biochem 1985;18:139–142.

222. Hannestad U, Martensson J, Sjodahl R, et al. 3-Mercaptolactate cysteine disulfiduria: Biochemical studies on affected and unaffected members of a family. Biochem Med 1981;26:106–114.

223. Gaull GE, Tallan HH, Lonsdale D, et al. Hypermethioninemia associated with methionine adenosyltransferase deficiency: Clinical, morphologic, and biochemical observations on four patients. J Pediatr 1981;98:734–741.

224. Gaull GE, Tallan HH. Methionine adenosyltransferase deficiency: New enzymatic defect associated with hypermethioninemia. Science 1974;186:59–60.

225. Nyhan WL, Ando T, Gerritsen T. Hyperglycinemia. In: Nyhan WL, ed. Amino Acid Metabolism and Genetic Variation. New York: McGraw-Hill, 1967:255–265.

226. Hiraga K, Kochi H, Hayasaka K, et al. Defective glycine cleavage system in nonketotic hyperglycinemia occurrence of a less active glycine decarboxylase and an abnormal aminomethyl carrier protein. J Clin Invest 1981;68:525–534.

227. Luder AS, Davidson A, Goodman SI, et al. Transient nonketotic hyperglycinemia in neonates. J Pediatr 1989;114:1013–1015.

228. Schiffmann R, Kaye EM, Willis JK III, et al. Transient neonatal hyperglycinemia. Ann Neurol 1989;25:201–203.

229. Motokawa Y, Kikuchi G. Isolation and partial characterisation of the components of the reversible glycine cleavage system of rat liver mitochondria. J Biochem 1972;72:1281–1284.

230. Motokawa Y, Kikuchi G. Glycine metabolism by rat liver mitochondria: Isolation and some properties of the protein-bound intermediate of the reversible glycine cleavage reaction. Arch Biochem Biophys 1974;164:634–640.

231. Motokawa Y, Kikuchi G. Glycine metabolism in rat liver mitochochondria V. Intramitochondrial localization of the reversible glycine cleavage system and serine hydroxymethyltransferase. Arch Biochem Biophys 1971;146:461–466.

232. Tada K, Narisawa K, Yoshida T, et al. Hyperglycinemia: A defect in glycine cleavage reaction. Tohoku J Exp Med 1969;98:289–296.

233. De Groot CJ, Troelstra JA, Hommes FA. Nonketotic hyperglycinemia: An in vitro study of the glycine-serine conversion in liver of three patients and the effect of dietary methionine. Pediatr Res 1970;4:238–243.

234. Perry TL, Urquhart N, MacLean J, et al. Nonketotic hyperglycinemia. Glycine accumulation due to absence of glycerine cleavage in brain. N Engl J Med 1975;292:1269–1273.

235. Perry TL, Urquhart N, Hansen S. Studies of the glycine cleavage enzyme system in brain from infants with glycine encephalopathy. Pediatr Res 1977;11:1192–1197.

236. Tada K. Nonketotic hyperglycinemia: Clinical and metabolic aspects. Enzyme 1987;38:27–35.

237. Hayasaka K, Tada K, Kikuchi G, et al. Nonketotic hyperglycinemia: Two patients with primary defects of P-protein and T-protein, respectively, in the glycine cleavage system. Pediatr Res 1983;17:967–970.

238. von Wendt L, Simila S, Hirvasniemi A, et al. Altered levels of various amino acids in blood plasma and cerebrospinal fluid of patients with nonketotic hyperglycinemia. Neuropadiatrie 1978;9:360–368.

239. Applegarth DA, Poon S. Interpretation of elevated blood glycine levels in children. Clin Chim Acta 1975;63:49–54.

240. Hayasaka K, Tada K, Fueki N, et al. Feasibility of prenatal diagnosis of nonketotic hyperglycinemia: Existence of the glycine cleavage system in placenta. J Pediatr 1987;110:124–126.

241. Garcia Castro JM, Isales Forsythe CM, Levy HL, et al. Prenatal diagnosis of nonketotic hyperglycinemia. N Engl J Med 1982;306:79–81.

242. Mesavage C, Nance CS, Flannery DB, et al. Glycine/serine ratios in amniotic fluid: An unreliable indicator for the prenatal diagnosis of nonketotic hyperglycinemia. Clin Genet 1983;23:354–358.

243. Kolvraa S, Gregersen N. Acyl-CoA: glycine N-acyltransferase: Organelle localization and affinity toward straight- and branched-chain acyl-CoA esters in rat liver. Biochem Med Metab Biol 1986;36:98–105.

244. MacDermot KD, Nelson W, Soutter V, et al. Glycine and benzoate conjugation and glycine acyltransferase activity in the developing and adult rat: possible relationships to nonketotic hyperglycinemia. Dev Pharmacol Ther 1981;3:150–159.

245. Langan TJ, Pueschel SM. Nonketotic hyperglycinemia: clinical, biochemical, and therapeutic considerations. Curr Probl Pediatr 1983;13:1–30.

246. Wolff JA, Kulovich S, Yu AL, et al. The effectiveness of benzoate in the management of seizures in nonketotic hyperglycinemia. Am J Dis Child 1986;140:596–602.

247. Trauner DA, Page T, Greco C, et al. Progressive neurodegenerative disorder in a patient with nonketotic hyperglycinemia. J Pediatr 1981;98:272–275.
248. Singer HS, Valle D, Hayasaka K, et al. Nonketotic hyperglycinemia: studies in an atypical variant. Neurology 1989;39:286–288.
249. Flannery DB, Pellock J, Bousounis D, et al. Nonketotic hyperglycinemia in two retarded adults: A mild form of infantile nonketotic hyperglycinemia. Neurology 1983;33:1064–1066.
250. Steiman GS, Yudkoff M, Berman PH, et al. Late-onset nonketotic hyperglycinemia and spinocerebellar degeneration. J Pediatr 1979;94:907–911.
251. von Wendt L, Simila S, Saukkonen AL, et al. Prenatal brain damage in nonketotic hyperglycinemia. Am J Dis Child 1981;135:1072.
252. Arneson D, Chien LT, Chance P, et al. Strychnine therapy in nonketotic hyperglycinemia. Pediatrics 1979;63:369–373.
253. Hayasaka S, Setogawa T, Hara S, et al. Nystagmus and subnormal electroretinographic response in nonketotic hyperglycinemia. Graefes Arch Clin Exp Ophthalmol 1987;225:277–278.
254. Dobyns WB. Agenesis of the corpus callosum and gyral malformations are frequent manifestations of nonketotic hyperglycinemia. Neurology 1989;39:817–820.
255. Press GA, Barshop BA, Haas RH, et al. Abnormalities of the brain in nonketotic hyperglycinemia: MR manifestations. AJNR 1989;10:315–321.
256. Shuman RM, Leech RW, Scott CR. The neuropathology of the nonketotic and ketotic hyperglycinemias: Three cases. Neurology 1978;28:139–146.
257. Agamanolis DP, Potter JL, Herrick MK, et al. The neuropathology of glycine encephalopathy: A report of five cases with immunohistochemical and ultrastructural observations. Neurology 1982;32:975–985.
258. Mayor F Jr, Martin A, Rodriguez Pombo P, et al. Atypical nonketotic hyperglycinemia with a defective glycine transport system in nervous tissue. Neurochem Pathol 1984;2:233–249.
259. Rothman SM, Olney JW. Glutamate and the pathophysiology of hypoxic-ischemic brain damage. Ann Neurol 1986;19(2):105–111.
260. Baumgartner R, Ando T, Nyhan WL. Nonketotic hyperglycinemia. J Pediatr 1969;75:1022–1030.
261. Krieger I, Winbaum ES, Eisenbrey AB. Cerebrospinal fluid glycine in nonketotic hyperglycinemic: Effect of treatment with sodium benzoate and a ventricular shunt. Metabolism 1977;26:517–524.
262. Wadman SK, Duran M, Ketting D, et al. D-Glyceric acidemia in a patient with chronic metabolic acidosis. Clin Chim Acta 1976;71:477–484.
263. Matalon R, Naidu S, Hughes JR, et al. Nonketotic hyperglycinemia: Treatment with diazepam—A competitor for glycine receptors. Pediatrics 1983;71:581–584.
264. Gitzelmann R, Steinmann B, Otten A, et al. Nonketotic hyperglycinemia treated with strychnine, a glycine receptor antagonist. Helv Paediatr Acta 1978;32:517–525.
265. von Wendt L, Simila S, Saukkonen AL, et al. Failure of strychnine treatment during the neonatal period in three Finnish children with nonketotic hyperglycinemia. Pediatrics 1980;65:1166–1169.
266. Krieger I, Hart ZH. Valine-sensitive nonketotic hyperglycinemia. Case report. J Pediatr 1974;85:43–48.

Chapter 2
Abnormalities of Urea Cycle and Ammonium

Dennis W. Bartholomew[*] and Saul W. Brusilow

UREA CYCLE DEFICIENCIES

Urea is a highly soluble organic compound whose formation represents the final step in waste nitrogen disposal for humans and other ureotelic mammals. The presence of urea in human urine was first demonstrated by Hilaire Marie Rouelle in 1773 and was shown to be a normal excretion product 70 years later. In 1932 Krebs and Henseleit postulated a pathway for ureagenesis based on their observations of increased urea production in animals exposed to high doses of arginine and ornithine. Our present understanding of the urea cycle was further refined by Ratner and Cohen.

Urea is generated almost entirely in the hepatocytes under the control of six enzymes. It is subsequently excreted by the kidneys; less than 5% is lost in the feces. About 80% of the nitrogen excreted in humans is processed in this manner (1). In addition to its role in waste nitrogen disposal, the urea cycle serves both to synthesize and to degrade arginine, as well as generate ornithine, a necessary precursor for proline and polyamine biosynthesis (2).

Nitrogen destined for excretion as urea is generated from ammonium and aspartate (Figure 2.1). One source of mitochondrial ammonium for processing into carbamyl phosphate is derived from the intestinal deamination of glutamine (3). The direct deamination of other amino acids including histidine, threonine, and lysine may also contribute to this pool. Extrahepatic sources of glutamine include the intestines and muscle. Renal glutaminase activity may also provide free ammonium for ureagenesis (4). The regeneration of ornithine by the action of cytosolic arginase and its subsequent active transport back into the mitochondria permits the cyclic nature of urea production to continue. Each turn of the cycle results in the synthesis of one molecule of urea at a cost of three molecules of adenosine triphosphate (ATP).

[*]The views expressed are solely those of the authors and do not necessarily reflect those of the Department of Defense.

Enzyme Biology and Molecular Genetics

Carbamyl Phosphate Synthetase

The formation of carbamyl phosphate from bicarbonate and ammonium is the first committed step in the urea cycle. It is an ATP-dependent reaction catalyzed by the enzyme carbamyl phosphate synthetase I (CPS I) in the mitochondrial matrix. The enzyme exists in both monomeric and dimeric forms, but in vitro it is active primarily as a monomer in the presence of its allosteric activator, N-acetylglutamate (NAG). The absence of NAG renders CPS I inactive. NAG is synthesized in the hepatocyte mitochondria by the action of NAG synthetase, and probably acts by inducing a conformational change in CPS I. A deficiency of NAG synthetase has been reported in two cases presenting with neonatal hyperammonemia (5).

CPS I is the most abundant protein in the hepatocyte mitochondria, comprising about 20% of the protein in that organelle. On the other hand, CPS II is a cystosolic enzyme that constitutes a heteromeric complex of the enzymes CPS, aspartate transcarbamylase, and dihydroorotase in a single functional unit that catalyzes the initial three steps in pyrimidine synthesis. In this case, the substrate nitrogen is derived from glutamine rather than free ammonium. CPS II has no requirement for NAG or other activators and is encoded by a separate genetic locus. It does not play a direct role in the routine production of urea in humans (6).

Despite the abundance of CPS I in the liver, analysis of mRNA from human liver libraries suggests that the rate of CPS I synthesis is low, though it is inducible, particularly by starvation. Somatic cell hybrid studies using Chinese hamster ovary cells have revealed only a single locus on the short arm of chromosome 2 (7).

Like other mitochondrial proteins encoded by nuclear genes, CPS I is synthesized as a precursor with a 38-residue leader sequence, which functions in the recognition of this enzyme by a putative mitochondrial membrane receptor.

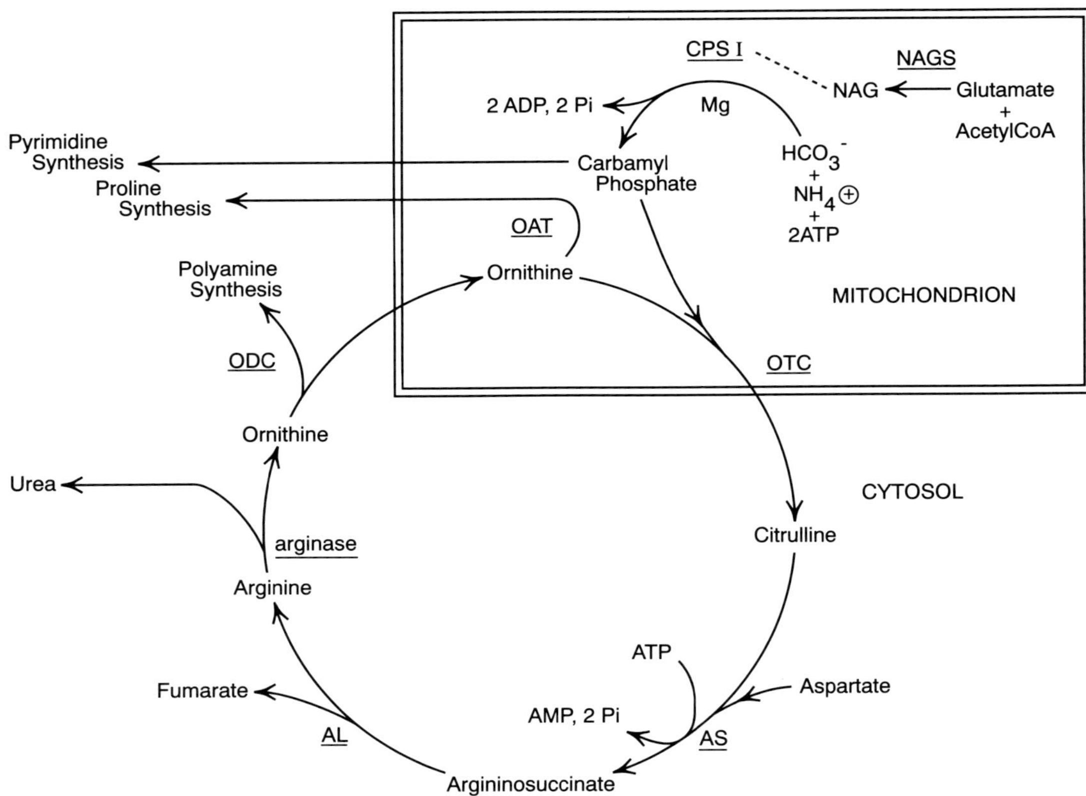

FIGURE 2.1 The urea cycle serves to dispose of waste nitrogen, as well as contribute precursors for the endogenous biosynthesis of proline, pyrimidines, and polyamines. Only carbamyl phosphate synthetase I (CPS I) has a requirement for an allosteric activator, N-acetylglutamate (NAG). The enzymes necessary for ureagenesis are abbreviated and underlined: NAGS, N-acetylglutamate syn-thetase; OTC, ornithine transcarbamylase; AS, argininosuccinic acid synthetase; AL, argininosuccinic acid lyase. Two enzymes that utilize ornithine for biosynthesis of other compounds are ornithine decarboxylase (ODC) and ornithine aminotransferase (OAT).

This highly, positively charged sequence is cleaved and degraded following translocation of the enzyme into the mitochondrial matrix.

The gene itself has not been completely characterized in humans but appears to be highly homologous to CPS I in rats. Several more recently identified Bgl I gene-linked restriction fragment-length polymorphisms (RFLPs) have proved useful in the prenatal diagnosis of this disorder (8). To date no deletions, insertions, or base substitutions have been identified at the molecular level in patients with proved CPS I deficiency (CPSD).

Ornithine Transcarbamylase

The formation of citrulline from the precursors ornithine and carbamyl phosphate occurs in the mitochondria under the control of the enzyme ornithine transcarbamylase (OTC). Inorganic phosphate is released and the citrulline molecule diffuses into the cytoplasm where the remaining steps of ureagenesis occur. OTC exists functionally as a trimer; each identical subunit has a molecular weight of about 36,000 daltons (9). It is expressed only in the liver and intestinal mucosa and does not require a cofactor for activity. In contrast to CPS, OTC is present in relatively small quantity, comprising less than 1% of protein content of liver mitochondria.

OTC is assembled on free ribosomes as a precursor about 4000 daltons larger than the mature subunit. A highly basic leader sequence of 32 amino acids directs entry of the enzyme into the mitochondria, during which the leader is cleaved and degraded in the matrix (10). Elegant studies have shown that the region between residues 8 and 22 of the leader sequence are sufficient in themselves to direct mitochondrial localization and processing of the protein, and that the highly conserved arginine residues play a crucial role in this function (11).

Somatic cell hybridization studies have confirmed the localization of the OTC gene to the X chromosome, as predicted by classic genetic studies of OTC-deficient (OTCD) patients (12). Chromosome deletion analysis has regionalized the locus to Xp21.1. Human OTC cDNA clones have been isolated and indicate that the gene contains 10 exons and is at least 73 kilobases in length. Gene deletions and point mutations have been identified in several OTCD patients, though most cases have not been characterized at the molecular level (13). Polymorphic DNA markers within the OTC locus have been successfully used prenatally to identify affected fetuses in informative pedigrees.

OTC deficiency is the only known urea cycle defect to have an analogous disease in an animal model. The inbred mouse strains, the sparse-fur (spf) and sparse-fur ash (spf-ash), carry a mutant OTC gene on the X chromosome that exhibits less than 20% of normal enzyme activity and have proved useful in the molecular analysis of these defects in humans.

Argininosuccinic Acid Synthetase

The condensation of citrulline with aspartate to form argininosuccinate is catalyzed by the enzyme argininosuccinic acid synthetase (AS). This ATP-dependent cytosolic reaction requires magnesium for full activity, and appears to be the rate-limiting step in vitro for ureagenesis; it is likely that substrate levels determine reaction velocities in vivo. The active form of the enzyme is a homotetramer of 46,000 dalton subunits and is present in most body tissues, though expression is greatest in the hepatocyte (14). AS is a highly basic protein with 21 arginine and 33 lysine residues. Critical arginine and cysteine residues appear to have functional role at the catalytic site. AS is inhibited under physiologic conditions by high levels of arginine (15).

The human AS gene has been localized to the long arm of chromosome 9 in the region 9q-34-qter by somatic cell hybridization. AS has been cloned and sequenced; it is 63 kilobases in length and contains 14 exons, encoding an mRNA of approximately 1600 base pairs. The initial two exons are untranslated. An interesting mRNA splicing variant site excises the second exon from most but not all AS mRNAs. This has no apparent effect on the function of the enzyme product (16).

An unusually large number of processed pseudogenes for AS have been identified in the human genome. Processed pseudogenes lack introns as well as specific upstream promoters and enhancers. These nonfunctional sequences were probably the result of multiple, random insertions of duplicated AS cDNA. Since they are also found in primates, it is likely that they arose at least 10 million years ago, prior to the evolutionary separation of early man from the great apes. Those pseudogenes studied to date appear to have deletions, insertions, multiple termination codons or some combination in all three reading frames, consistent with their nonfunctional status and ancient origin. They have been found on 9 autosomes, as well as the X and Y (17).

Cloned human AS cDNA has been transferred to Chinese hamster, rat, and immortalized citrullinemic (AS-deficient) cell lines using a variety of gene insertion techniques with successful integration as demonstrated by AS gene transcription and low-level translation (18).

An intriguing variant of AS deficiency has been seen in adult Japanese patients who appear to have a tissue-specific regulatory defect in AS expression; that is, the enzyme is grossly deficient in hepatocytes but present and functional in normal amounts in kidney and fibroblasts. This abnormality may be the result of mutations in the upstream untranslated region 5' to the first exon where regulatory sequences for tissue-specific expression are frequently found (19). Most cases of classic neonatal ASD, however, are characterized by lack of detectable AS protein in all tissues studied.

Argininosuccinase

Argininosuccinate is cleaved to fumarate and arginine in the cytosol under the control of argininosuccinase (AL). This enzyme is also a homotetramer and has been found in all tissues, though concentrations are highest in the liver. No required cofactors have been identified. Dissociation of the 5000 dalton subunits is known to dramatically decrease enzyme activity.

A study on the genetic heterogeneity of argininosuccinase deficiency (ALD) in 28 unrelated patients revealed extensive interallelic complementation. Although this phenomenon is not well documented in humans, it is known to be common in bacteria at loci coding for homomultimeric proteins (20). Complementation is thought to result from subunit interaction and conformational changes exposing catalytic sites (21), and suggests that multiple mutations have occurred at the AL locus. Since most affected patients are likely to be compound heterozygotes for ALD, it may be that some will have a functional advantage over true homozygotes in that structural protein differences may improve subunit interaction.

The genetic locus for AL was mapped to chromosome 7 by Naylor et al. (22) using bioautography techniques in 1978. Mouse-human somatic cell hybridization studies using cell lines with a derived chromosome 7 further localized the gene to 7pter-q22. The AL gene was cloned and sequenced in 1986, revealing an open reading frame of 1503 nucleotides. A 4 kilobase fragment of the gene was also found on chromosome 22, but is not transcriptionally active (23).

Over 90% of patients with ALD have immunologically detectable enzyme present. This is consistent with the hypothesis that decreased enzyme activity is most commonly the result of a structural gene abnormality, which affects subunit interaction or the catalytic site (24). A patient with a tissue-specific deficiency of AL, however, was described by Glick et al. (25) in 1976. Assay for AL activity in an infant who died at 6 days of age from hyperammonemia was undetectable in the liver but normal in kidney and brain. A mutation in the regulatory sequence for the AL locus could explain these findings in a manner analogous to previously described Japanese patients with tissue-specific ASD. To date at least two different abnormalities have been described in AL-deficient patients at the molecular level.

Arginase

Arginine is cleaved to form urea and ornithine in the final step of the urea cycle under the control of the cytosolic enzyme arginase I. The enzyme is abundant in the liver but also present in red blood cells (RBCs), kidney, brain, and the gastrointestinal tract. A second enzyme with similar activity, arginase II, differs immunologically from arginase I and is probably encoded by a separate genetic locus (26). Arginase II is a mitochondrial protein found in highest concentration in kidney and brain, constituting about half of the total arginine hydrolysis activity in those tissues, and may play a role in ornithine production for polyamine synthesis. On the other hand, arginase I contributes 98% of the total arginase activity in liver and RBCs; it is this enzyme that is deficient in hyperargininemia.

Arginase I is probably composed of four identical subunits with a total molecular weight of about 115,000 daltons. The gene has been localized to chromosome 6 (6q23) using somatic cell hybridization techniques and exists in a single copy of about 11.5 kilobases with 8 exons (27). No information is yet available on its evolutionary relationship to the gene for arginase II. Abnormalities at the molecular level in arginase-deficient patients have rarely been described. Taq 1 cleavage site mutations have been described in 2 patients, but no major gene deletions or rearrangements have been found to date.

Pathophysiology

Interruption of the urea cycle inevitably results in the accumulation of ammonium, a potent neurotoxin. Other potential mammalian pathways of nitrogen excretion, such as uric acid production, lack the capacity to prevent nitrogen accumulation as ammonium. Studies in primates subjected to infusions of ammonium acetate revealed a progression of signs and symptoms that closely paralleled findings in human hyperammonemic subjects (28). At low levels, animals exhibited lethargy, lack of interest in surroundings or food, emesis, and tachypnea. Higher levels led to coma, seizures, areflexia, and apnea with evidence of increased intracranial pressure. Electroencephalographic findings included prolonged slowing, burst-suppression, and isoelectricity patterns with increasing plasma ammonium levels. Evidence of cerebellar-tonsillar herniation and astrocytic swelling was observed at autopsy, but no neuronal changes were noted. Studies in cats receiving infusions of ammonium acetate suggested that elevations in intracranial pressure resulted in part from two physiomechanical factors: a 30% increase in cerebral blood flow at ammonium levels of 500 μM/L or more, and an increase in the rate of cerebrospinal fluid (CSF) formation that roughly correlated with the plasma ammonium concentration (29).

In humans, extensive neuropathologic data on patients who expired in hyperammonemic coma as a result of a urea cycle disorder are limited. Increased intracranial pressure was suggested to be a consequence of the intracellular-osmotic effect of increased concentration of glutamine in the astrocyte (30). An increase in glutamine is the normal physiologic response to elevated plasma ammonium through the direct amination of glutamate under the control of the enzyme glutamine synthetase; that is, glutamate appears to act as a sink for free ammonium, a form of detoxification. CSF measurement of glutamine in patients dying of hyperammonemic coma may exceed 6 μM/L (31). As will be discussed, elevation of plasma glutamine is frequently the initial laboratory indication of impending hyperammonemia. Studies have consistently documented that ammonium is quickly embodied into brain glutamine in the astrocyte (32).

Some authors have implicated other neurochemicals in the pathogenesis of hyperammonemia-induced neurologic dysfunction. Studies in rats and mice have suggested alterations in tryptophan transport in the central nervous system (CNS) as a consequence of elevations in plasma ammonium and increased levels of 5-hydroxyindole acetic acid (5-HIAA) in cerebral tissue, suggesting serotonin synthesis is enhanced (33). Conversely, 5-HIAA levels are depressed in arginase deficiency, perhaps as a result of competition between arginine and neutral amino acids for receptors (34). While arginine is known to normally utilize a separate carrier for uptake, profound argininemia may result in competitive binding to other carriers, analagous to the circumstances in hyperphenylalaninemia. Abnormalities in gamma-aminobutyric acid (GABA) and other neurotransmitters have also been postulated. The significance of these findings remains unclear.

Autopsy findings are not specific for any of the urea cycle defects; pathologic findings appear to be related to the duration of symptomatic hyperammonemia (35). Infants who expire soon after birth from hyperammonemia exhibit gross signs of brain swelling, and most show a proliferation of Alzheimer type II astrocytes. A prolonged clinical course is correlated with evidence of cortical atrophy, neuronal loss, and extensive gliosis. Case reports have described particular abnormalities in the thalamus, putamen, red nuclei, and cerebellum but these are inconsistent findings (36–38). An apparent defect in myelination has been noted in two cases of AL deficiency (39).

Clinical Presentation

The timing of onset and clinical severity of disorders of ureagenesis are in large part dependent upon the nature of the molecular defect and the degree to which the patient sustains some minimal capacity for waste nitrogen elimination. The spectrum of variability extends from newborns with severe deficiencies of OTC or CPS who present with fulminant irreversible hyperammonemia in the first few days of life to adult females who are heterozygotic for OTCD and virtually asymptomatic. There exists a wide range of clinical involvement in between, and the distinction between early and late onset disease is somewhat arbitrary.

Case Report

Infant male JW weighed 3550 g at birth after a routine gestation and vaginal delivery. His mother was a gravida 2 para 2 female. Apgar scores were 8 at 1 minute and 9 at 5 minutes, and he was moved to the newborn nursery for routine postnatal care. At 36 hours of age, the mother complained that JW was refusing to breastfeed and was difficult to arouse. No abnormalities were noted on physical examination of the infant. Blood glucose level was 62 mg/dL. A sepsis work-up, including complete blood count, blood culture, suprapubic bladder tap for urine culture, spinal tap, and chest radiograph was performed, but the findings were not suggestive of perinatal infection. Intravenous (IV) broad-spectrum antibiotics were administered and breast milk was continued using gavage. He was 48 hours old when the nursing staff reported JW was vomiting his feedings and appeared in respiratory distress. Repeat physical examination revealed a poorly arousable neonate with a respiratory rate of 60/minute, but no other abnormalities. A second chest radiograph was unchanged from the previous normal study. A room-air arterial blood gas sample showed a pH of 7.57, pCO$_2$ of 21 mm Hg, pO$_2$ of 95 mm Hg and a bicarbonate level of 38 meq/L. A plasma ammonium was 252 μM/L (normal < 30 μM/L).

A careful review of the family history with the mother revealed that her first child was a female whose infancy was marked by persistent feeding intolerance, poor growth, and developmental delay. She died suddenly at 21 months of age of Reye syndrome after becoming comatose during the course of a viral illness. The mother admitted to an aversion for foods of high-protein content and was a practicing vegetarian.

JW started on an IV infusion of 10% dextrose and was given a bolus of 10% arginine HCl 2 mL/kg, and then transferred to a tertiary care center for immediate hemodialysis. On arrival he was flaccid, unresponsive to painful stimulation, and tachypneic. Plasma ammonium was 566 μM/L, plasma glutamine was 1680 μM/L (normal 250 to 650 μM/L), and plasma citrulline was undetectable. A random urine sample contained 290 μg orotate/mg creatinine (normal < 10). A provisional diagnosis of OTCD was made. Despite repeated cycles of hemodialysis, plasma ammonium levels remained above 500 μM/L for the next 24 hours. The parents elected to terminate heroic measures and the infant expired the following day. OTC enzyme assay in hepatic tissue obtained at the time of death revealed essentially no activity.

Neonatal

Deficiencies of OTC, CPS, AS, or AL are indistinguishable in neonates on clinical grounds alone. Signs and symptoms of hyperammonemia represent a common pathologic response to interruption of the waste nitrogen excretion pathway. The exception is arginase deficiency, which is rarely symptomatic in the neonatal period.

Urea cycle defects typically present on the second or third day of life with nonspecific signs of neonatal distress in a term infant not known to be at special risk for any major medical complications, such as sepsis, congenital heart disease, or intraventricular hemorrhage. The infant may refuse feedings, be poorly arousable, and have decreased tone; vomiting is common. Even if protein feedings are withdrawn, hyperammonemia is likely to progress as a result of endogenous protein breakdown and poor caloric intake. Hyperventilation will produce marked respiratory alkalosis. Seizures may ensue, and some infants will develop an asterixis-like tremor. The anterior fontanel may be bulging. Ultimately, deep coma develops and the infant becomes areflexic and unresponsive to any stimuli. Breathing patterns are disordered; apnea and cardiovascular collapse soon follow.

The accumulation of ammonium ions has a direct stimulatory effect on the respiratory center in the brain stem resulting in an initial marked respiratory alkalosis. This diagnostic clue suggests a primary disorder of ureagenesis as the etiology for unexplained hyperammonemia, rather than a secondary effect of other disorders that may present with acidosis and hyperammonemia, such as propionic acidemia, methylmalonic acidemia, medium-chain acyl-CoA dehydrogenase deficiency, and glutaric aciduria type II. Hyperammonemia in neonatal urea cycle disorders is inexorably progressive and will terminate in a fatal outcome if early aggressive intervention is not initiated.

Neonatal hyperammonemia has many causes, but early management is not predicated on knowledge of a specific etiology. In addition to a thorough physical examination, initial evaluation should include arterial blood gases, complete blood count, serum electrolytes, blood urea nitrogen (BUN), plasma amino acids, and urine for identification of organic acids and orotate, though the results of the latter tests are seldom immediately available.

Laboratory findings reveal a respiratory alkalosis, often to a profound degree. Aggressive diagnostic steps to identify other causes of neonatal coma are unrewarding. Liver function studies are usually normal, though the transaminases may be mildly elevated. BUN is frequently low. The plasma ammonium level may remain in the high normal range for the first 24 hours of life before increasing rapidly to levels that may exceed 1000 μM/L. Plasma amino acids will show an early increase in glutamine, perhaps before symptoms of ammonium intoxication appear. Plasma glutamine levels may increase to over 2000 μM/L (normal 250 to 650 μM/L) in the terminal stages of urea cycle disorders, and plasma arginine levels are often low. Plasma citrulline may be absent or grossly elevated, depending on the enzyme defect (see case report).

Orotic aciduria in hyperammonemic males should be sought. Computed tomographic (CT) brain scans reveal only nonspecific generalized edema in the early stages of the disease: survivors may exhibit cortical atrophy, loss of gray matter, and mildly dilated ventricles, though these findings may vary from patient to patient (40).

Case Report

A 4-year-old female was electively admitted to the hospital for evaluation of developmental delay, seizures, and recurrent episodes of lethargy and hyperemesis with minor viral infections. She was born at term and had an unremarkable early course until her mother attempted to wean her from the breast to bottle feedings at 8 months of age. Despite the use of a variety of different proprietary infant formulas, the infant would take only small amounts at a time and frequently refused feedings. She was evaluated for failure to thrive after she began to fall off her growth curve but no definite cause was found. She continued to be a picky eater in childhood, refusing meats and milk. Developmental milestones were delayed but gradually acquired. Viral infections frequently resulted in profound illness with repeated emesis and occasionally marked lethargy, from which she recovered slowly. Generalized motor seizures were noted in the second year of life and were controlled with carbamazepine.

Physical examination on admission revealed a thin female whose height and head circumference were at the 25th percentile for age, while her weight was at the 5th percentile. The liver edge was palpable 4 cm below the right costal margin; the examination was otherwise unremarkable. Laboratory evaluation was notable for normal serum concentrations of glucose, electrolytes, arterial blood gases, and a normal complete blood count. Serum liver transaminases were mildly elevated though the serum urea nitrogen level was low. A random plasma ammonium level was 68 μM/L (normal < 30 μM/L). Urine organic acid analysis was unremarkable. Fasting plasma amino acids showed a marked elevation in glutamine, moderate elevation of citrulline, and a depressed level of arginine. Additionally, the chromatogram was remarkable for peaks consistent with significant plasma levels of argininosuccinate and its anhydrides. A preliminary diagnosis of ALD was made, and the child started on a low-protein diet with supplemental arginine. The plasma ammonium level decreased into the normal range and episodes of lethargy did not recur, though the seizure disorder remained unchanged.

Late Onset

Patients with milder mutations may remain asymptomatic during infancy. As their anabolic needs decrease, they may begin to show an aversion to dietary protein. Episodic coma in response to physiologic stresses such as intercurrent infections or excessive protein intake may be misdiagnosed as Reye syndrome. Developmental delay, seizures, and dementia have also been reported (41).

Variants of CPSD have been described in which the affected individual did not manifest symptoms of protein intolerance until later in childhood, suggesting some degree of residual enzyme activity. In families without demonstrated consanguinity, it is likely that most affected members are genetic compounds; that is, they have different mutations at the CPS locus for each allele. Under these circumstances, the possibility of some residual enzyme activity remains.

Rare cases of OTCD in males have escaped detection until later in life. These appear to represent Km mutants or other functional abnormalities in an otherwise intact enzyme and suggest the retention of residual enzyme activity. Similar clinical findings have been noted in both argininosuccinic acid synthetase deficiency (ASD) and ALD. Older children with ALD may exhibit a peculiar, dry, kinky-fragile abnormality of the hair shaft. This may be related to diet and is less common in patients under adequate treatment.

Differential Diagnosis

The development of hyperammonemic coma is a grave prognostic sign. Salvage of intact patients with urea cycle disorders is dependent on the early recognition of symptoms, prompt assessment of the plasma ammonium, and aggressive therapy. The inclusion of acute metabolic disease in the differential diagnosis of a neonate who is not doing well may allow survival in an affected infant who would otherwise have been lost. In addition, a family history of consanguinity or unexplained sibling infant deaths should suggest an inborn error of metabolism to the clinician.

Upon physical examination, there are little data to specifically indicate urea cycle disorders. Hyperammonemic infants will invariably hyperventilate until hemodynamic instability ensues secondary to brain stem compression. AS-deficient infants may have hepatomegaly, which persists throughout childhood but it appears not to be clinically significant. The algorithm for the differential diagnosis of neonatal hyperammonemic coma is summarized in Figure 2.2. Secondary hyperammonemia in infants with sepsis, acute liver failure, and organic acidemias may be differentiated from urea cycle defects by clinical presentation, presence of metabolic acidosis, bone marrow depression, and a plasma amino acid profile that is nonspecific or suggestive of another metabolic abnormality. The entity of transient hyperammonemia of the newborn is limited to premature infants with early respiratory distress and is discussed later.

The absence of citrulline in plasma in the clinical setting of hyperammonemia is highly suggestive of a deficiency of CPS or OTC, both of which interfere with citrulline synthesis. This finding appears to be consistent, even in at-risk neonates being treated under prospective protocols. The urine orotic acid (normal < 10 μg/mg creatinine) is elevated in OTCD as a consequence of the accumulation of unprocessed carbamyl phosphate being shunted into the pyrimidine synthetic pathway in the cytosol. In contrast to OTCD, urine orotic acid is normal in CPSD. Diagnosis may

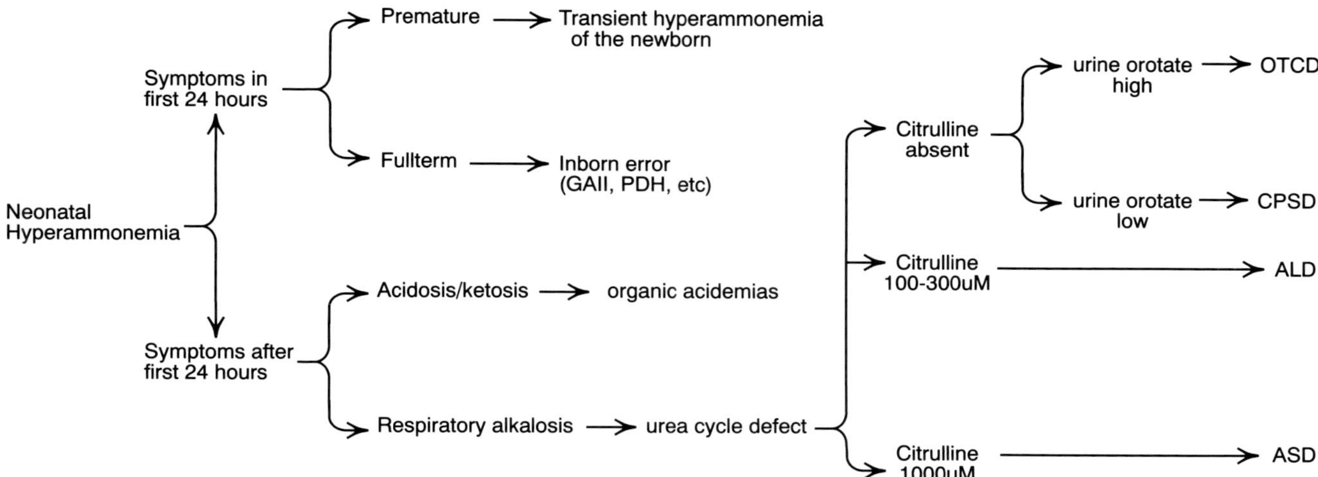

FIGURE 2.2 The differential diagnosis of neonatal hyperammonemia is influenced by its temporal onset, associated acid-base status, plasma citrulline, and urinary orotate concentrations. Additional discriminating factors may include a positive family history of metabolic disease, abnormal odors, and unexplained anion gap. Early (<24 hours) hyperammonemia may result from deficiencies in the pyruvate dehydrogenase (PDH) complex or glutaric aciduria type II in the term infant. Respiratory distress in a setting of prematurity and early hyperammonemia suggests transient hyperammonemia of the newborn. Abbreviations: OTCD, ornithine transcarbamylase deficiency; CPSD, carbamyl phosphate synthetase deficiency; ASD, argininosuccinic acid synthetase deficiency; ALD, argininosuccinic acid lyase deficiency. (Adapted from Brusilow SW, Valle DL. Symptomatic inborn errors of metabolism in the neonate. In: Current Therapy in Neonatal-Perinatal Medicine 1985–1986. Toronto: BC Decker, 1985:207 and reprinted with permission).

be confirmed by assaying CPS and OTC activity in a percutaneous liver biopsy sample after the patient is stabilized on therapy. Open liver biopsy is recommended. Unfortunately, neither enzyme is expressed in white blood cells, amniocytes, or fibroblasts.

Plasma citrulline levels in ASD may exceed 1000 μM/L (normal 8 to 35 μM/L); hence, the common name citrullinemia. Arginine levels may be slightly decreased and argininosuccinate is absent. Glutamine is nonspecifically elevated. Orotic aciduria may occur, but in the presence of a high plasma citrulline level, which offers no problems in differential diagnosis. An enzymatic diagnosis may be confirmed by assay of liver or fibroblasts, though this is invariably unnecessary in view of the high plasma citrulline.

The diagnosis of ALD is suggested by a characteristic plasma amino acid pattern, which shows large peaks on the chromatogram corresponding to argininosuccinate and its anhydrides. Care must be taken in interpreting the amino acid results, since these compounds may co-chromatograph with other amino acids, particularly isoleucine and methionine, and give misleading results. Plasma citrulline is also elevated to 100 to 300 μM/L. Again, plasma glutamine levels are increased, whereas, the plasma arginine level may be low.

Treatment

Early management of acute neonatal hyperammonemic coma is independent of the enzyme deficiency and must be initiated expeditiously while diagnostic studies are underway (Table 2.1). All protein intake should be stopped and the infant made NPO. An IV solution of 10% dextrose should be administered at a maintenance rate to supply protein-sparing calories (42,43). There is little question that hemodialysis is 7 to 10 times more efficient than peritoneal dialysis in removing ammonium and glutamine, and is the single most effective means of lowering the plasma ammonium level acutely (44,45). Cannulation of the femoral or umbilical vessels may allow adequate vascular access. Multiple cycles of dialysis are often necessary. If hemodialysis is not immediately available, peritoneal dialysis may be used while preparing the infant for transport to a tertiary care facility. Exchange transfusion and charcoal hemoperfusion have not been shown to be effective.

Patients with deficiencies of CPS, OTC, AS, and AL have an absolute requirement for L-arginine (46). Interruption of the urea cycle at any of these steps blocks endogenous synthesis of this amino acid. Arginine supplementation will not only slow the increased protein catabolism caused by the deficiency of an essential amino acid, but will continue to supply ornithine precursors to exploit whatever residual urea synthetic capacity remains. The initial therapy of any infant suspected of having a urea cycle disorder should include an IV infusion of 10% arginine HCl 500 mg/kg administered over 90 minutes, followed by a sustaining infusion of the same dose for 24 hours (2 mL/kg/day of 10% arginine HCl). When the infant has been stabilized, oral citrulline 170 mg/kg/day may be substituted for arginine; it has the advantage of contributing one less nitrogen. IV citrulline is not yet routinely available.

It has been known for more than 50 years that in humans, the administration of benzoic or phenylacetic acid

Table 2.1 Management protocols for hyperammonemia secondary to urea cycle disorders

| Disease | Condition | Hemodialysis | Dietary Nitrogen* | | Other | Sodium Benzoate* | Sodium Phenylacetate* | 10% Arginine HCl |
			Essential Amino Acids	Natural Protein				
OTCD CPSD	Acute	Yes	—	—	NPO D1OW IV	Priming Infusion	Priming Infusion[1]	Priming Infusion[2]
OTCD CPSD	Maintenance	No	0.7	0.7	—	0.25	0.25	None (use 0.17 g/kg/d citrulline)
ASD	Acute	Yes	—	—	NPO D10W IV	Priming Infusion[1]	Priming Infusion[1]	Priming Infusion[3]
ASD	Maintenance	No	—	1.0–1.5	——	0.25	0.25	0.5–0.7 g/kg/d
ALD	Acute	Rarely	—	—	NPO D10W IV	—	—	Priming Infusion[3]
ALD	Maintenance	No	—	1.5–2.0	—	—	—	0.5–0.7 g/kg/d

* grams/kilogram/day
[1] 0.25 g/kg IV, mixed in 35 mL/kg D10W and infused over 90 minutes, followed by infusion of 0.5 g/kg over 12 hours. Infusion slowed to 0.25 g/kg/24 hours as plasma ammonium level falls.
[2] 0.21 g/kg (2 mL/kg of 10% solution) over 90 minutes, then 0.21 g/kg/day
[3] 0.63 g/kg (6 mL/kg of 10% solution) over 90 minutes, then 0.63 g/kg/day

or their salts leads to a change in the partition of urinary nitrogen; urea nitrogen decreases with no change in total nitrogen (47). This difference is accounted for by the accumulation of the respective amino acylation products of benzoate and phenylacetate. Such early experiments suggested that these compounds may be useful in states of decreased ureagenesis, and have since proved to be the case in clinical practice. The biochemical mechanisms are summarized in Figure 2.3. Salts of benzoic acid may be activated in vivo by esterification to coenzyme A (CoA) via the enzyme medium-chain fatty-acyl-CoA ligase. Benzoyl-CoA subsequently reacts with the nonessential amino acid glycine to form hippurate under the control of a specific acyltransferase.

Hippurate is rapidly excreted in the urine carrying with it the nitrogen from glycine. In a similar manner, salts of phenylacetic acid are activated and bind with the nonessential amino acid glutamine to form phenylacetylglutamine, which is also cleared rapidly in the urine. Since glutamine contains two nitrogen atoms, it is clear that on a molar basis, phenylacetate will result in twice the nitrogen excretion of benzoate. Glycine and glutamine are rapidly resynthesized resulting in diversion of nitrogen from the defective urea cycle to these alternative pathways. Both drugs are available in oral and intravenous forms, and do not appear to be toxic when used in recommended dosages. Two cases of accidental overdosage have been seen: one child who received 10 times the recommended IV dose of both drugs expired. The efficacy of these drugs is also limited by the capacity of the body to activate them, although the dose above which accumulation occurs has not been

established. The sodium salts of both drugs are used for IV administration. A third investigational agent, phenylbutyrate, is currently under study. Phenylbutyrate is converted to phenylacetate via beta oxidation in vivo and has the advantage of lacking much of the distasteful clinging odor associated with phenylacetate.

Waste nitrogen excretion through the use of sodium benzoate and sodium phenylacetate as a means of bypassing the urea cycle has been shown to be a safe and effective means of controlling mild-to-moderate acute elevations of plasma ammonium (48). These agents are usually not effective for plasma ammonium levels in excess of 500 μM/L, and their administration should not delay the initiation of hemodialysis in acutely ill infants. Sodium benzoate (NaB) and sodium phenylacetate (NaP) are both given in a dose of 250 mg/kg each over 90 minutes in 35 mL/kg of 10% dextrose solution; they may be mixed in the same bottle. Rapid infusion of these drugs may precipitate nausea and emesis. A sustaining infusion of 250 mg/kg of each should be maintained for the following 12 hours or until the plasma ammonium level falls to near normal. Failure to reverse advancing hyperammonemia with IV therapy should prompt immediate hemodialysis.

At present, the long-term therapy of OTCD and CPSD consists of marked dietary protein restriction and the use of other pathways of waste nitrogen excretion. Citrulline administration enhances residual urea cycle activity at a cost of 1 nitrogen added to the free amino acid pool per molecule of citrulline. Sufficient nitrogen is supplied from a combination of natural protein and essential amino acids to meet anabolic needs. A diet consisting of 0.7 g/kg/day of

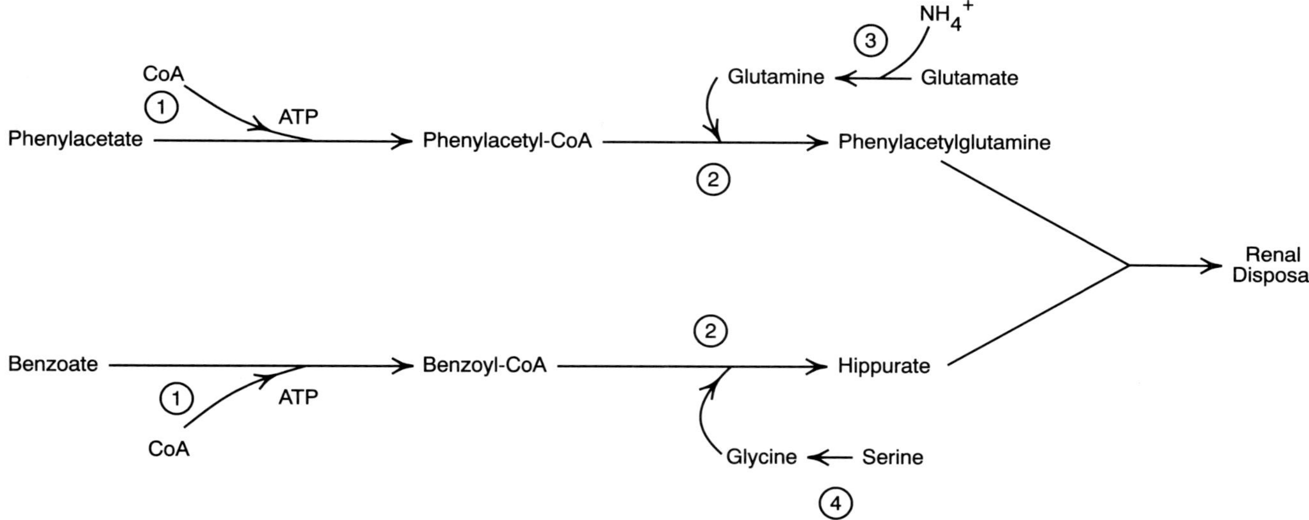

FIGURE 2.3 Benzoate and phenylacetate are esterified with coenzyme A (CoA) in an ATP-dependent reaction catalyzed by medium chain fatty acyl-CoA ligase (1). Each reacts with its target amino acid, glycine and glutamine, respectively, via a specific acyl-transferase (2), and the products are rapidly excreted in the urine. Glutamine is regenerated by the direct amidation of glutamate via glutamine synthetase (3), while glycine is endogenously synthesized by a number of different pathways, the most active of which is the transamination of hydroxypyruvate to serine and its subsequent conversion to glycine (4).

natural protein, 0.7 g/kg/day of essential amino acid mixture, and a nonprotein calorie source, such as Product 80056 (Mead Johnson, Evansville, IN), in quantity sufficient to provide at least 120 kcal/kg/day is recommended. Frequent monitoring of anthropometric, nutritional, and biochemical parameters is required to titrate nitrogen intake to meet the growing infant's changing metabolic needs. Tolerance of protein frequently decreases as the rate of body growth slows after the first year of life.

The utility of citrullinuria as a means of disposing of waste nitrogen in ASD is limited by its poor renal clearance. Notwithstanding this and the presence of only a single nitrogen atom (from carbamyl phosphate) per molecule of citrulline, its urinary excretion remains an important pathway for waste nitrogen disposal in these children. Thus, long-term therapy with high doses of L-arginine (up to 700 mg/kg/day) permits continual synthesis and excretion of citrulline, though this pathway is insufficient to provide the waste nitrogen disposal capacity required, even with the dietary restriction of natural protein to 1.5 g/kg/day. The use of NaB and NaP in the standard dosage of 250 mg/kg/day each permits affected children to be maintained on a more palatable diet by providing other means of disposing of the nitrogen generated by the metabolism of additional dietary protein.

ALD is characterized by markedly increased plasma and urine levels of argininosuccinate. Of the four nitrogen atoms in argininosuccinate, two are normally destined for disposal of urea. Unlike citrulline, the renal clearance of argininosuccinate is comparable to the glomerular filtration rate; hence, the molecule has considerable potential as an adequate replacement for urea in excreting excess nitrogen for patients with ALD. This capacity is clearly dependent on the constant repriming of the cycle with supplemental arginine. Failure to replenish arginine would rapidly deplete the cycle of ornithine precursors and inhibit synthesis of argininosuccinate. A moderate dietary protein intake of 1.25 to 1.75 g/kg/day in combination with high dose L-arginine (500 to 700 mg/kg/day) will provide adequate waste nitrogen disposal capacity in the young child under normal conditions. Benzoate and phenylacetate are not required to prevent recurrences of hyperammonemia. High circulating plasma levels of argininosuccinate are an unavoidable consequence of this therapy; it is uncertain whether this finding has a deleterious effect on outcome.

The use of alpha-keto analogs of amino acids to promote endogenous biosynthesis of amino acids and decrease natural protein anabolic requirements has not been shown to improve outcome in the urea cycle disorders (49).

Future therapeutic measures may alter the grim prognosis of these disorders. Liver transplantation has been successfully performed in one affected male at 19 months of age with an encouraging follow-up 2 years postsurgery (66). The cloning of the human OTC gene and demonstration of appropriate mitochondrial localization and expression in intact yeast cells following transfection with a plasmid containing the gene and a galactose operon promoter are promising suggestions that this disorder may be amenable to gene therapy in the future (50). Mitochondrial expression of OTC in HeLa cells, which are ordinarily devoid of OTC activity, was achieved following insertion of a human OTC gene linked to an SV40 promoter. Sadly, these theoretically curative approaches will be of little benefit to a child who has already been profoundly damaged from hyperammonemic coma.

Outcome

Severe neonatal hyperammonemia secondary to CPSD has a poor prognosis. Less than 50% of affected infants will survive the initial insult. Virtually all survivors have some degree of neurologic handicap (51). The rapid resolution of hyperammonemic coma is the single factor most associated with a good long-term outcome. The prevention of neonatal coma with prospective therapy for infants known to be at risk because of a previously affected sibling with CPSD has been shown to be highly effective in eliminating the neonatal mortality associated with this disease. Preliminary studies also suggest significantly improved long-term neurodevelopmental outcome, even if the child continues to have recurrent episodes of hyperammonemia (52).

Neonatal OTCD appears to have the highest mortality of any of the urea cycle disorders. Many children succumb to repeated episodes of hyperammonemic coma before 36 months of age, and most survivors are severely neurologically impaired. Prospective intervention at birth for at-risk neonates or those who were diagnosed prenatally usually allows survival and may improve long-term outcome, though data on this point are limited (52,69).

The prognosis for survival in children with ASD exceeds that of patients with disorders of the more proximal steps of the urea cycle. This probably occurs as a result of their ability to exploit the urinary loss of citrulline and tolerate additional dietary protein or stressful states such as infections, surgery, or starvation that lead to endogenous protein catabolism. Neurodevelopmental outcome was studied by Msall et al. in 8 AS-deficient patients who survived neonatal hyperammonemic coma (51). The intelligence quotient (IQ) at 12 months of age was 44 ± 10. Seven children had one or more neurologic disabilities. The severity of neurologic damage correlated closely with the duration of neonatal coma. Children at risk for ASD treated from birth under prospective protocols do not develop hyperammonemic coma. Preliminary data suggest that long-term survival and neurodevelopmental outcome is also improved when managed with dietary protein restriction, benzoate, phenylacetate, and supplemental arginine from birth. There is no evidence that high plasma citrulline levels are deleterious.

In contrast to the other urea cycle disorders, neonates with hyperammonemia secondary to ALD are the most likely to recover quickly from coma and with the exception of arginase deficiency, have the fewest recurrences. Intercurrent illness, or lack of compliance with dietary restrictions or arginine supplementation, may lead to a gradual onset of lethargy, nausea, headache, and other nonspecific signs of increased plasma ammonium levels; but they are unlikely to result in coma unless continued over an extended period of time. Even with this advantage, the long-term neurodevelopmental outcome for AL-deficient patients has been disappointing. The IQ at 12 months for 8 survivors of neonatal coma was 50 ± 7 (51). One affected male treated from birth and who has had no subsequent documented episodes of hyperammonemic coma is mildly retarded and has other neurologic problems including seizures. We have seen no evidence of progressive deterioration in patients under the treatment protocol, some of whom have been followed for over 7 years. It is unclear whether this neurologic damage is the result of an in utero process, chronic low-grade hyperammonemia, high circulating levels of arginine and argininosuccinate, or other factors unrelated to the mutant AL genes.

Prenatal Diagnosis

The prenatal diagnosis of CPSD has been complicated by the lack of expression of this enzyme in amniocytes and the absence of diagnostic metabolites in the amniotic fluid of an affected fetus. The cloning of the human CPS gene and the discovery of the Bgl I restriction fragment-length polymorphisms in probes tightly linked to the CPS locus has allowed prenatal diagnosis using these DNA markers in about 50% of at-risk families (8). These studies may be performed on fetal cells obtained by amniocentesis or chorionic villus sampling (CVS). The latter procedure has a slightly higher risk of complications but may be performed as early as the 8th week of pregnancy. Direct in utero diagnosis of both OTCD and CPSD is possible only with fetal liver biopsy, since the protein is not expressed in amniocytes or fetal blood.

Indirect prenatal diagnosis for OTCD is possible in many at-risk families using DNA polymorphic markers tightly linked to the OTC locus. There are three intragenic polymorphisms as well as several flanking markers now available (53–55). A complicating factor is the identification of female carriers. Since about 30% of cases may represent new mutations in a family, DNA diagnosis through linkage analysis is only feasible if the mother is proved to be a carrier. An example of this study is illustrated in Figure 2.4.

AS synthetase is expressed in amniocytes; prenatal diagnosis using enzyme activity assays and determination of amniotic fluid citrulline levels is available. Because of the large number of nonfunctional pseudogenes for AS, only markers that flank the gene or are present in one of its introns would be useful for DNA diagnosis by linkage analysis. At present there is no advantage to indirect linkage studies over direct enzyme assay, except perhaps in families where defects in tissue-specific expression of AS are well documented. Prenatal diagnosis of ALD has been accomplished using amniocyte enzyme activity assays and measurement of argininosuccinate in amniotic fluid.

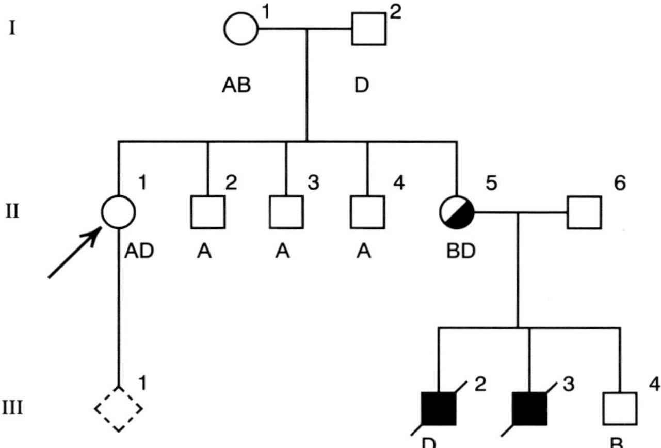

FIGURE 2.4   The consultand (II-1) in this pedigree was 19 weeks pregnant when she requested carrier testing for X-linked OTC deficiency. A sister (II-5) was an obligate carrier and had a positive allopurinol challenge test, but this test could not be performed on the consultand because its reliability in pregnancy is uncertain. A family linkage study was performed and found to be informative for an Msp1 polymorphism in the obligate carrier (II-5), which allowed haplotypes to be assigned using Msp1 and BAMH1 as markers. The mutant OTC allele is linked with haplotype D, which the carrier mother inherited from her father. Since the father (I-2) was not clinically affected, the disease apparently arose as a new mutation in the X chromosome he passed to his carrier daughter. Therefore, the consultand is probably not a carrier for OTCD, even though she also carries the D haplotype. This assumes that individual I-2 is not a germ line mosaic carrier for the OTC mutation. The pregnancy was carried to term and a healthy male infant was delivered. Haplotype analysis on the newborn was not performed.

ARGINASE DEFICIENCY

Arginase deficiency was first described by Terheggen et al. (27), in 1969. It is the rarest of the urea cycle disorders, but has been found in German, Saudi, Mexican-American, Ashkenazim, French Canadian, and other population groups. Despite an almost total inhibition of arginase I activity, affected patients retain substantial capacity for urea synthesis and rarely develop hyperammonemic coma.

Parents of offspring affected with this rare autosomal-recessive disorder are frequently consanguineous. Since hyperammonemia is uncommon, the condition is rarely suspected at birth. Nonspecific symptoms suggesting low-level ammonia intoxication may appear episodically throughout infancy and childhood (56). These include lethargy, irritability, and emesis. Some children will be seen in retrospect to have an aversion to dietary protein. Developmental milestones are delayed, and seizures may occur. Eventually, acquired psychomotor skills are lost and neurologic symptoms become manifest.

The physical examination reveals spasticity, predominantly of the lower extremities. Ataxia and microcephaly have been seen, and most patients are mentally retarded. Electroencephalographic abnormalities may occur but are not specific.

The primary laboratory abnormality is a striking elevation of plasma arginine. Plasma concentration of glutamine may be mildly elevated and ornithine decreased; plasma levels of citrulline are normal. There is a marked increase in urinary excretion of arginine and, to a lesser extent, lysine, ornithine, and cystine. Orotic aciduria probably occurs as a result of intramitochondrial depletion of ornithine and the subsequent shunting of carbamyl phosphate into the pyrimidine synthetic pathway (57). An abnormal urinary excretion of several guanidino compounds secondary to the inhibition of the ornithine-dependent creatine synthetic pathway has been described (58,59). Plasma ammonium is at the upper limits of normal, though it may be pathologically elevated in response to protein loads or intercurrent illness. The diagnosis is confirmed by the determination of arginase activity in RBCs or hepatocytes. Activity in fibroblast samples remains within the normal range owing to the presence of significant amounts of arginase II in that tissue.

The initial therapy for arginase deficiency is the reduction of the dietary intake of protein. Even extreme restrictions in dietary nitrogen, however, are insufficient to ameliorate the clinical deficit, though laboratory parameters are improved. Transfusion of packed RBCs containing normal amounts of arginase has been attempted, but a transient reduction in plasma arginine was the only documented benefit (67). Lysine supplementation has been proposed as a means of competitively inhibiting the tubular reabsorption of arginine, but studies in two affected children resulted in paradoxical increase in plasma arginine, probably as a result of the direct inhibitory effect of lysine on arginase activity (68).

The recommended management of arginase deficiency includes a marked restriction in dietary natural protein intake and the addition of an essential amino-acid supplement, to a total protein equivalent of about 1.0 g/kg/day. In addition, benzoate and phenylacetate administered in the usual dosages may be useful to enhance waste nitrogen excretion. Strict adherence to this regimen may result in improvement in both the intellectual and the neurologic status in some patients.

An intriguing approach to the treatment of arginase deficiency is the manipulation of regulatory elements controlling expression of arginase II. While this course of therapy remains completely speculative, the liver-specific induction of arginase II offers a potential means of bypassing the hepatic deficiency of arginase I in these patients. Unfortunately, no information on these regulatory sequences has been reported.

Prenatal diagnosis of arginase deficiency is possible through the analysis of fetal RBCs for arginase activity. The technique of percutaneous umbilical blood sampling (PUBS) is an established in utero diagnostic procedure at several major centers. Polymorphic DNA markers at the arginase locus to establish linkage have been described and may allow earlier prenatal diagnosis through amniocentesis or CVS.

TRANSIENT HYPERAMMONEMIA OF THE NEWBORN

A transient nonheritable form of hyperammonemia in preterm infants has been recognized for many years. This poorly understood phenomenon occurs in the clinical setting of respiratory distress, usually secondary to hyaline membrane disease, in the first 24 hours of life in a premature infant. Plasma ammonium may be elevated to over 1000 μM/L, and the clinical signs of early hyperammonemia are otherwise indistinguishable from those of urea cycle defects, except by the time of onset and the accompanying respiratory difficulties (60). The family history is noncontributory, and laboratory parameters are not suggestive of a particular disorder of ureagenesis. Aggressive therapy to acutely lower the plasma ammonium and treat the underlying pulmonary disorder is indicated. Neurologic outcome for survivors is dependent on the rapidity of the resolution of coma. Hyperammonemia does not recur. The etiology of this condition is uncertain. Inhibition of one or more of the urea cycle enzymes by an unknown mechanism is likely, though their in vitro activity has been demonstrated to be normal.

Asymptomatic hyperammonemia of the newborn may occur in up to half of prematurely born neonates, and is characterized by a plasma ammonium of twice the level found in term infant controls. It may persist for more than 4 weeks but is not associated with any clinical signs of hyperammonemia. Follow-up evaluation at 30 months of age of 25 preterm infants with plasma ammonium levels ranging from 40 to 72 μM/L during the first weeks of life revealed no significant IQ differences from age-matched preterm controls with normal ammonium levels, suggesting that treatment of asymptomatic low-level hyperammonemia in this age group is not indicated (61).

NEWBORN SCREENING

Large-scale newborn screening programs for the detection of phenylketonuria (PKU) are now mandated in all 50 states in the United States. Other diseases that are commonly screened for include congenital hypothyroidism, galactosemia, hemoglobinopathies, homocystinuria, maple syrup urine disease (MSUD), tyrosinemia, and biotinidase deficiency. Several clinical trials of newborn screening for urea cycle disorders have been performed in the United States, Austria, Japan, New Zealand, Canada, and Australia. Current methods utilize an enzyme-multiple bacterial auxotroph assay on dried filter paper specimens that identifies patients likely to have ASD, ALD, arginase deficiency, and hyperornithinemia (ornithine aminotransferase deficiency) by measurements of the bacterial growth zone around the blood specimen (62). Such screening tests are likely to be of value only to those patients with mild forms of disease, since the more severely affected neonate will have become symptomatic early in the postnatal course.

Detection of Female OTCD Heterozygotes

A particular problem in counselling families with an affected OTCD male is the identification of at-risk carrier females. The protein tolerance test (ingestion of a standard quantity of protein followed by a urine collection for measurement of orotic acid output) for females has been largely supplanted by the allopurinol challenge test. This technique takes advantage of the fact that an allopurinol metabolite interacts with the pyrimidine biosynthetic pathway by inhibiting the enzyme orotidine monophosphate decarboxylase. Approximately 90% of adult OTCD carrier females will show an increased excretion of orotodine in the urine following a standard dose of 300 mg of allopurinol, demonstrating increased flux through pyrimidine pathway due to excessive substrate, carbamyl phosphate. The advantage of this test is that it is simple, reproducible, and will not induce nausea and symptoms of hyperammonemia in affected women. The test may also be useful for testing at-risk males who were treated prospectively and did not develop orotic aciduria (63).

Female infants who inherit the abnormal OTC allele from carrier mothers are frequently asymptomatic during the newborn period, but may present later in childhood with episodic hyperammonemia, recurrent Reye syndrome, protein intolerance, and a variety of soft neurologic signs including learning disorders (64). The wide variation in symptoms in carrier females is typical of many X-linked recessive diseases, where the degree of lyonization as well as the underlying molecular defect will influence the phenotype. About one third of female cases represent new mutations, in accordance with Haldane's hypothesis for X-linked recessive disorders with a reproductive fitness of zero.

The need for treatment in heterozygotic females must be assessed on an individual basis. There are data to indicate that even asymptomatic carrier females may have some degree of intellectual impairment. The benefits of therapy with protein restriction, benzoate, phenylacetate, and citrulline are well established in this group (65).

CONCLUSION

Urea cycle disorders are a significant and life-threatening cause of hyperammonemia in infants and children. Early recognition of signs and symptoms, prompt diagnostic evaluation, and aggressive management are mandatory if the infant is to survive. Regardless of etiology, survivors of prolonged neonatal hyperammonemic coma incur severe irreversible neurologic damage. Long term treatment of all the urea cycle disorders is available, but places an enormous burden on the physician. Recurrences of episodic hyperammonemia are frequent in OTCD and CPSD and may terminate in a fatal outcome despite optimal therapy.

Prenatal diagnosis is available for most families known to be at risk for urea cycle disorders, either through direct enzyme analysis or linkage with polymorphic DNA markers. Further analysis of the molecular biology of these genes and their regulatory elements may provide novel insights into the process of gene production expression. Moreover, such developments may suggest as yet unavailable methods of intervention using somatic gene therapy.

REFERENCES

1. Rodwell VW. Catabolism of amino acid nitrogen. In: Martin DW, Mates PA, Rodwell VW, et al., eds. Harper's Review of Biochemistry. Los Altos: Lange, 1985:283–292.
2. Brusilow SW, Horwich AL. Urea cycle enzymes. In: Scriver C, Beaudet A, Sly W, eds. The Metaboblic Basis of Inherited Disease. New York: McGraw-Hill, 1989;629–663.
3. Haussinger D. Regulation of hepatic ammonia metabolism: The intercellular glutamine cycle. Adv Enzyme Regul 1986; 25:159–180.
4. Windmueller HG, Spaeth AE. Source and fate of circulating citrulline. Am J Physiol 1981;241:E473–E480.
5. Bachmann C, Colombo JP, Jaggi K. N-acetylglutamate synthetase (NAGS) deficiency: Diagnosis, clinical observations and treatment. Adv Exp Med Biol 1981;153:39–45.
6. Cheung CW, Raijman L. Arginine, mitochondrial arginase and the control of carbamyl phosphate synthesis. Arch Biochem 1981;209:643–649.
7. Adcock MW, O'Brien WE. Molecular cloning of cDNA for rat and human carbamyl phosphate synthetase I. J Biol Chem 1984;259:13471–13476.
8. Fearon ER, Mallonee RL, Phillips JA, et al. Genetic analysis of carbamyl phosphate synthetase I deficiency. Hum Genet 1986;70:207–210.
9. Horwich AL, Fenton WA, Williams KR, et al. Structure and expression of a complementary DNA for the nuclear coded precursor of human mitochondrial ornithine transcarbamylase. Science 1984;224:1068–1074.
10. Horwich AL, Kalousek F, Fenton WA, et al. Targeting of pre-ornithine transcarbamylase to mitochondria: Definition of critical regions and residues in the leader peptide. Cell 1986;44:451–459.
11. Horwich AL, Fenton WA, Firgaira FA, et al. Expression of amplified DNA sequences for ornithine transcarbamylase in HeLa cells: Arginine residues may be required for mitochondrial import of enzyme precursor. J Cell Biol 1985; 100:1515–1521.
12. Lindgren V, DeMartinville B, Horwich AL, et al. Human ornithine transcarbamylase locus mapped to band Xp21.1, near the Duchenne muscular dystrophy locus. Science 1984; 226:698–700.
13. Rozen R, Fox J, Fenton WA, et al. Gene deletion and restriction fragment length polymorphisms at the human ornithine transcarbamylase locus. Nature 1985;313:815–817.
14. Sase M, Kobayashi K, Inamura Y, et al. Level of translatable messenger RNA coding for arginosuccinate synthetase in the liver of patients with quantitative-type citrullinemia. Hum Genet 1985;69:130–134.
15. Jackson MJ, Beaudet AL, O'Brien WE. Mammalian urea cycle enzymes. In: Campbell A, Herskowitz I, Sandler L, eds. Annual Review of Genetics. Palo Alto: Annual Reviews, 1986;20:431–464.
16. Beaudet AL, O'Brien WE, Bock HO, et al. The human argininosuccinate synthetase locus and citrullinemia. In: Harris H, Hirschorn K, eds. Advances in Human Genetics. New York: Plenum Publishing, 1986;161–196.
17. Su TS, Nussbaum RL, Airhart S, et al. Human chromosomal assignments for 14 argininosuccinate synthetase pseudogenes: cloned DNAs as reagents for cytogenetic analysis. Am J Hum Genet 1984;36:954–964.
18. Wood PA, Partridge CA, O'Brien WE, et al. Expression of human argininosuccinate synthetase after retroviral-mediated gene transfer. Somat Cell Mol Genet 1986;12:493–500.
19. Matsudo Y, Tsuji A, Katunuma N. Qualitative abnormality of liver argininosuccinate synthetase in a patient with citrullinemia. Adv Exp Med Biol 1982;153:77–82.
20. McInnes RR, Shih V, Chilton S. Interallelic complementation in an inborn error of metabolism: genetic heterogeneity in argininosuccinate lyase deficiency. Proc Natl Acad Sci USA 1984;81:4480–4484.
21. Crick FHC, Orgel LE. The theory of interallelic complementation. J Mol Biol 1964;8:161–165.
22. Naylor SL, Klebe RJ, Shows TB. Argininosuccinic aciduria: Assignment of the argininosuccinate lyase gene to the pter-q22 region of human chromosome 7 by bioautography. Proc Natl Acad Sci USA 1978;75:6159–6162.
23. O'Brien WE, McInnes RR, Kalumuck K, et al. Cloning and sequence analysis of cDNA for human argininosuccinate lyase. Proc Natl Acad Sci USA 1986;83:7211–7215.
24. Kobayashi K, Itakura Y, Saheki T, et al. Absence of argininosuccinate lyase protein in the liver of two patients with argininosuccinic aciduria. Clin Chim Acta 1986;159:59–67.
25. Glick NR, Snodgrass PJ, Schafer IA. Neonatal argininosuccinate lyase activity. Am J Hum Genet 1976;28:22–30.
26. Spector EB, Kern RM, Haggerty DF, et al. Differential expression of multiple forms of arginase in cultured cells. Mol Cell Biochem 1985;66:45–53.
27. Terheggen HG, Lowenthal A, Colombo JP. Clinical and biochemical findings in argininemia. Adv Exp Med Biol 1982;153:111–119.
28. Voorhies TM, Ehrlich ME, Duffy TE, et al. Acute hyperammonemia in the young primate: Physiologic and neuropathologic correlates. Pediatr Res 1983;17:970–975.
29. Chodobski A, Szmydynger-Chodobska J, Orbanska A, et al. Intracranial pressure, cerebral blood flow and cerebrospinal fluid formation during hyperammonemia in the cat. J Neurosurg 1986;65:86–91.
30. Brusilow SW, Traystman R. Hepatic encephalopathy. N Engl J Med 1986;314:784.

31. Hourani BT, Hamlin EM, Reynolds TB. Cerebrospinal fluid glutamine as a measure of hepatic encephalopathy. Arch Intern Med 1971;127:1033–1036.

32. Gjedde A, Lockwood AH, Duffy TE, et al. Cerebral blood flow and metabolism in chronically hyperammonemic rats: effect of an acute ammonia challenge. Ann Neurol 1978; 3:325–330.

33. Bachman C, Colombo JP. Increased tryptophan uptake into the brain in hyperammonemia. Life Sci 1983;33:2417–2424.

34. Hyland K, Smith I, Clayton PT. Impaired neurotransmitter amine metabolism in arginase deficiency. J Neurol Neurosurg Psychiatry 1985;48:1188–1189.

35. Martin JJ, Schlote W. Central nervous system lesions in disorders of amino acid metabolism. J Neurol Sci 1972; 15:49–76.

36. Harding BN, Leonard JV, Erdohazi M. Ornithine carbamoyl transferase deficiency: A neuropathological study. Eur J Pediatr 1984;141:215–226.

37. Ebels EJ. Neuropathological observations in a patient with carbamylphosphate-synthetase deficiency and in two sibs. Arch Dis Child 1972;47:47–51.

38. Lewis PD, Miller AL. Argininosuccinic aciduria: A case report with neuropathological findings. Brain 1970;93:413–422.

39. Solitaire GB, Shih VE, Nelligan DJ, et al. Argininosuccinic aciduria: clinical, biochemical, anatomical, and neuropathological observations. J Ment Defic Res 1969;13:153–170.

40. Kendall BE, Kingsley DPE, Leonard JV, et al. Neurological features and computed tomography of the brain in children with ornithine carbamoyl transferase deficiency. J Neurol Neurosurg Psychiatry 1983:46:28–34.

41. Dimagno EP, Lowe JE, Snodgrass PJ, et al. Ornithine trans-carbamylase deficiency—a cause of bizarre behavior in a man. N Engl J Med 1986;315:744–747.

42. Brusilow SW, Valle DL. Symptomatic inborn errors of metabolism in the neonate. In: Nelson N, ed. Current Therapy in Neonatal-Perinatal Medicine. Toronto: BC Decker, 1985–1986;207.

43. Brusilow SW, Danney M, Waber LJ, et al. Treatment of episodic hyperammonemia in children. N Engl J Med 1984; 310:1630–1634.

44. Donn SM, Swartz RD, Thoene JG. Comparison of exchange transfusion, peritoneal dialysis and hemodialysis for the treatment of hyperammonemia in an anuric infant. J Pediatr 1979;95:67–70.

45. Brusilow SW. Personal Communication.

46. Brusilow SW. Arginine, an indispensable amino acid for patients with inborn errors of urea synthesis. J Clin Invest 1984;74:2144–2148.

47. Lewis HB. Studies in the synthesis of hippuric acid after benzoate ingestion in man. J Biol Chem 1914;18:225–231.

48. Batshaw ML, Brusilow SW. Treatment of hyperammonemic coma caused by inborn errors of urea synthesis. J Pediatr 1980;97:893–900.

49. Brusilow SW, Batshaw ML, Walser M. Use of keto-acids in inborn errors of urea synthesis. In: Winick M, ed. Nutritional Management of Genetic Disorders. New York: John Wiley and Sons, 1979;65–75.

50. Cheng MY, Pollock RA, Hendrick JP, et al. The cytoplasmi-cally-synthesized subunit precursor of human mitochondrial ornithine transcarbamylase can be imported and proteolyti-cally processed to an enzymatically active form by mitochondria of S.cerevisiae. Proc Natl Acad Sci USA 1987; 84:4063–4067.

51. Msall M, Batshaw ML, Suss R, et al. Neurologic outcome in children with inborn errors of urea synthesis. N Engl J Med 1984;310:1500–1505.

52. Bartholomew DW, Reichel R, Brusilow SW. Prospective diagnosis and treatment of urea cycle disorders. Pediatr Res 1987;21:288A.

53. Fox J, Hack AM, Fenton WA, et al. Prenatal diagnosis of ornithine transcarbamylase deficiency with use of DNA polymorphisms. N Engl J Med 1986;315:1205–1208.

54. Old JM, Purvis-Smith S, Wicken B, et al. Prenatal exclusion of ornithine transcarbamylase deficiency by direct gene analysis. Lancet 1985;1:73–75.

55. Rozen R, Fox JE, Hack AM, et al. DNA analysis for ornithine transcarbamylase deficiency. J Inherited Metab Dis 1986;9 (Suppl 1):49–57.

56. Snyderman SE, Sansaricq C, Chen WJ, et al. Argininemia. J Pediatr 1977;90:563–568.

57. Qureshi IA, Letarte J, Ouellet R, et al. Ammonia metabolism in a family affected by hyperargininemia. Diabetes Metab Rev 1981;7:5–11.

58. Marescau B, Qureshi IA, De Deyan P, et al. Guanidino compounds in plasma, urine and cerebrospinal fluid of hyper-argininemic patients during therapy. Clin Chim Acta 1985; 146:21–27.

59. Weichert P, Mortelmans J, Lavinha F, et al. Excretion of guanidino derivatives in urine of hyperargininemic patients. J Genet Hum 1976;24:61–72.

60. Hudak ML, Jones MD, Brusilow SW. Differentiation of transient hyperammonemia of the newborn and urea cycle enzyme defects by clinical presentation. J Pediatr 1985;107:712–719.

61. Batshaw ML, Wachtel RC, Cohen L, et al. Neurologic outcome in premature infants with transient asymptomatic hyperammonemia. J Pediatr 1986;108:271–275.

62. Naylor EW. Newborn screening for urea cycle disorders Adv Med Biol 1982;153:9.

63. Brusilow SW, Valle D. Allopurinol (AP) induced orotidinuria (ODNU): A test of heterozygosity for ornithine transcarbamylase deficiency. Pediatr Res 1987;21:289A.

64. Rowe PC, Newman SL, Brusilow SW. Natural history of symptomatic partial ornithine transcarbamylase deficiency. N Engl J Med 1986;314:541–547.

65. Brusilow SW. Disorders of the urea cycle. Hosp Pract 1985;Oct 15:65–72.

66. Korson MS, Lillehei CW, Vacanti JP, Levy HL. Liver transplantation for ornithine transcarbamylase deficiency (OTCD) (Abstract). Am J Hum Genet 1989;45 (Suppl):A8.

67. Michels V, Beaudet AL. Arginase deficiency in multiple tissues in argininemia. Clin Genet 1978;13:61–63.

68. Snyderman SE, Sansaricq C, Norton PM, Goldstein F. Argininemia treated from birth. J Pediatr 1979;95:61.

69. Maestri NE, Hauser ER, Hamosh A, Bartholomew D, Brusilow S. Prospective treatment of urea cycle disorders. J Pediatr, in press.

Chapter 3
Disorders of Organic Acids

Richard H. Haas and William L. Nyhan

Inborn errors of metabolism in which organic acids accumulate are found in many different areas of cellular metabolism. An organic acid in this context is a compound characterized by the presence of one or more carboxylic acid groups or acidic phenolic groups but with the absence of basic amino groups (1). In many cases, organic acid disorders are the result of defects of mitochondrial metabolism, and they produce either primary or secondary effects on oxidative metabolism. Brain cells (neurons, glia, and the capillary endothelial cells that contribute to the blood-brain barrier) are highly energy-dependent for normal function. The major substrates for brain metabolism are glucose and ketone bodies. These undergo intramitochondrial oxidative metabolism leading ultimately to the production of carbon dioxide, water, and adenosine triphosphate (ATP); 38 molecules of ATP are produced for each molecule of glucose fully oxidized. Brain dependence on the integrity of oxidative metabolism arises because of the combination of energy need, the inefficiency of glycolysis as an ATP-generating system (2 ATP molecules produced for each glucose molecule metabolized to lactate), and low substrate stores in the brain. There is very little reserve of glycogen or glucose in the brain, so that by 1 minute of complete ischemia in mice, glycogen and glucose fall to zero and the high-energy compounds creatine phosphate and ATP drop to 1% and 5% of controls, respectively (2).

The inborn errors that produce organic-acid accumulation may affect neuronal metabolism directly when the defect is located in a major metabolic pathway. Such defects often produce severe encephalopathies. The cytochrome chain is the final common pathway for glial and neuronal oxidative metabolism. Electron transport chain defects are increasingly being identified in the group of mitochondrial encephalomyopathies (3). In many disorders, organic-acid accumulation results in secondary mitochondrial dysfunction. Many organic acids and especially fatty acids are mitochondrial toxins producing both uncoupling and inhibition of oxidative phosphorylation. Such toxic effects may underlie the Reye-like encephalopathies seen in some organic acidemias and may play a part in the encephalopathy of Reye syndrome itself (4). Carnitine may be protective to the brain in such circumstances. This amino acid plays an important role as a transport molecule, allowing long-chain fatty acids to cross the mitochondrial matrix membrane, although the extent and importance of this function in the brain is unclear (5). Carnitine also functions as a buffering molecule, removing potentially toxic organic acids and sequestering them as carnitine esters. Carnitine ester excretion is high in organic-acid disorders, and supplemental carnitine is therapeutically helpful (6).

Although organic acids are generally weak acids, accumulation may exceed tissue-buffering capacity. Most enzymatic reactions are pH-sensitive, and a reduction of intracellular or intramitochondrial pH will render many metabolic steps inefficient. Such mechanisms are proposed to underlie the neurotoxicity accompanying lactic-acid accumulation (7).

Neurotransmitter synthesis and reuptake is an important function of neurons and glia. It has become apparent that accumulation of neurotransmitters can be toxic. The toxic effects of the putative excitatory neurotransmitter glutamate are the most clearly defined. Pools of glutamate can be found in brain associated with the neuronal and the glial elements. These large stores of glutamate are a potential substrate and source of carbon skeleton for oxidative metabolism. Through its action on the N-methyl-D-aspartate (NMDA) receptor, glutamate has been shown to play a major role in the neuronal damage resulting from hypoxic/ischemic injury, status epilepticus, and hypoglycemia. Defects in neurotransmitter synthesis, release, and reuptake may underlie some of the functional and anatomic changes that occur when organic-acid accumulation disrupts efficient brain energy production.

CLASSIC ORGANIC ACIDEMIAS

Propionic Acidemia

Propionic acidemia is the prototype organic acidemia, and as such it will be described at length. The earliest description of a patient with propionic acidemia in 1961 (8) preceded the later distinction between the ketotic and nonketotic hyperglycinemias (9) and the later identification of propionyl CoA carboxylase deficiency as the biochemical defect. There are many similarities in the central nervous system (CNS) findings in nonketotic hyperglycinemia and the organic acidemias that comprise the ketotic hyperglycinemic group—propionic acidemia, methylmalonic acidemia, isovaleric acidemia, and 3-oxothiolase deficiency. Because the features of the neonatal presentation in these disorders are nonspecific and frequently fatal, it is clear that many patients die undiagnosed. An earlier sibling death is often found in the family history.

The usual presentation of propionic acidemia in infancy with a picture similar to overwhelming sepsis provides ample opportunity for CNS injury as a result of hypoxia, ischemia, and hypoglycemia (a particularly common feature of methylmalonic acidemia). Patients are hypotonic, lethargic, frequently have seizures, and, if treatment is unsuccessful, progress to coma and death. Repeated relapses characterize these metabolic disorders, and an opportunity for CNS injury accompanies each episode. Overzealous treatment with severe and prolonged protein restriction may irreversibly limit brain growth and development as a consequence of protein malnutrition. Supplementation with leucine has been reported to improve hypotonia, somatic growth, and developmental quotient (DQ); one reported patient showed a DQ improvement from 65 at 18 months of age to 78 at 25 months of age (10).

A review of the clinical features of 65 patients with propionic acidemia revealed neurologic symptoms and signs in the majority of patients (11) (Table 3.1). The out-

Table 3.1 Neurologic abnormalities in 65 patients with propionic acidemia

	Patients initially presenting (%)	Patients ever exhibiting (%)
Lethargy	51	63
Feeding difficulties (vomiting, refusing food)	49	65
Hypotonia	48	54
Seizures	23	43
Myoclonus	12	20
Coma	15	28
Hypothermia	6	6

Modified from Wolf et al. 1981 (11)

look for the CNS is not always dismal, however. Three adolescent girls in this series were reported with above-average intelligence, and one of these was completely asymptomatic, having been detected by routine screening following identification of an affected sibling (12). The first reported patient, who died of pneumonia at the age of 7 years, was microcephalic and severely retarded. The importance of early diagnosis and careful therapy in order to optimize CNS development was highlighted by a report of the disease course in his sister (13). This girl avoided the early episodes of severe metabolic decompensation with hyperammonemia exhibited by her brother and at the age of 7 years 8 months, she was found to be neurologically normal, with a full-scale Wechsler Intelligence Scale for Children (WISC) IQ of 125 and normal results on the Goodenough Tests. The reported asymptomatic teenage patient (12) compared with the usually severe neonatal presentation highlights the clinical spectrum of propionic acidemia.

The existence of asymptomatic patients together with the favorable CNS outcome in patients who are optimally managed indicates that a defect in propionyl CoA carboxylase itself does not damage the brain. Accumulated evidence suggests that CNS symptomatology in propionic acidemia is the result of metabolic decompensation and the accumulation of neurotoxic agents together with hypoxic/ischemic injury. Ammonia, glycine, and propionyl CoA are the most likely neurotoxic agents, but abnormal metabolites such as tiglylglycine and methyl citrate may also play a part in CNS dysfunction.

Clinical and Neurologic Features

The clinical spectrum of propionic acidemia extends from normality to severe CNS damage with microcephaly, hypotonia that may progress to spastic quadriparesis, mental retardation, and seizures. The severity of CNS damage seems related to the occurrence of episodes of metabolic decompensation with acidosis and coma. Infants presenting with the classic presentation of ketoacidotic coma with hyperglycinemia and hyperammonemia usually suffer significant CNS injury.

Electroencephalogram.   The electroencephalogram (EEG) during acute episodes will show nonspecific slowing. Electrographic seizures may be seen with or without clinical correlates. In hyperammonemic patients, triphasic waves may be seen.

Neuroimaging.   Neuroimaging studies may be normal, but diffuse edema in white matter has been reported during an acute episode (14). Generalized cortical atrophy may be apparent on magnetic resonance imaging (MRI) or computed tomography (CT) studies of patients surviving episodes of neonatal coma (Figure 3.1). In general, neuroimaging studies correlate well with the neurologic status of the patient. Patients without neurologic findings will often have normal neuroimaging studies.

Neuropathology.   Spongiform degeneration of the CNS was noted in a child with propionyl CoA carboxylase deficiency who died following recurrent episodes of hyperglycinemia and acidosis without ketosis (15).

The similarity of the neuropathologic findings in two children with nonketotic hyperglycinemia and one case of propionic acidemia was noted by Schumann et al. (16). Dysmyelination was found in all cases. This propionic acidemic patient died at 26 days of age following the onset of

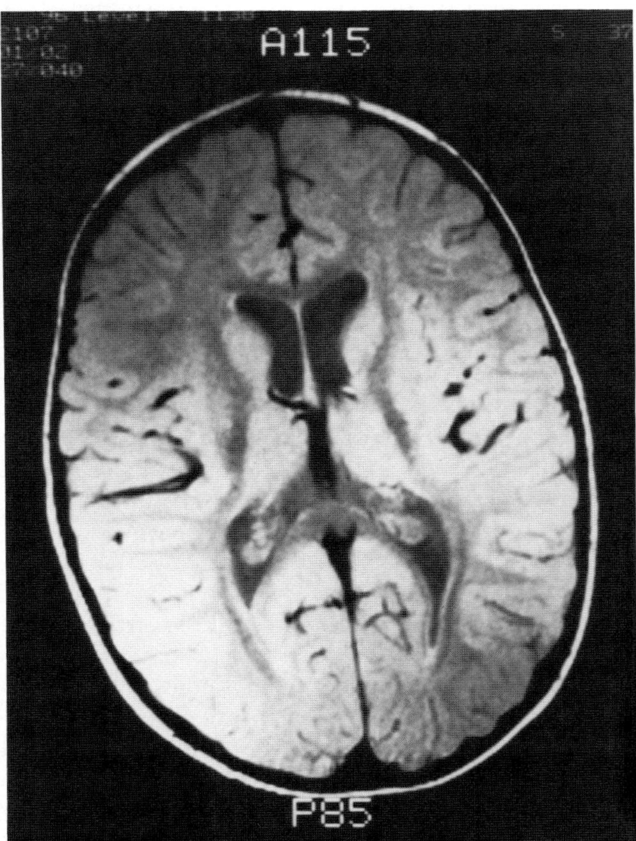

FIGURE 3.1   T1-weighted MRI brain scan of a 5-year-old child with propionic acidemia. There is moderate ventriculomegaly due to cortical atrophy.

profound acidosis on the fifth day of life. She remained acidotic and developed intractable tonic-clonic seizures at day 20. Brain weight was normal without gross abnormality. Microscopic infarctions were found in the cingulate gyrus and the globose nucleus of the cerebellum. Pale staining and diffuse vacuolation of myelin was noted in the internal capsule, globus pallidus, and ascending and descending tracts of brain stem tegmentum, as well as posterior columns of spinal cord. Autopsy findings were reported on a 5 1/2-month-old male infant who died following recurrent episodes of coma, acidosis, and hyperammonemia with onset at 10 days of age (17). A microvacuolar spongy degeneration of subcortical and deep cortical layers was found. The vacuoles were seen interstitially and in association with myelin sheaths. In this case, the internal capsules and brain stem white matter tracts, as well as spinal cord, were spared. The cerebellum, however, showed striking atrophy and almost total absence of the external granular layer with decreased neuronal density in the internal granular layer, molecular, and Purkinje cell layers. A small area of neuronal loss and gliosis was noted in the putamen. Alzheimer type II astrocytes were seen in the areas of cortex affected by spongiform changes.

Neuropathologic findings differed in two fatal cases of propionic acidemia (14). The first infant, who was microcephalic, died at 12 days of age following the onset at 4 days of hypothermia, shock, and a brief cardiorespiratory arrest. Severe metabolic acidosis and a blood ammonia of 1600 μM was noted. Thrombocytopenia persisted despite platelet transfusions. As in the patient described earlier, neuropathologic changes included spongy rarefaction at the gray-white matter interface, but these changes were restricted to the temporal lobe. Basal ganglia and internal capsules as well as the thalamus demonstrated multiple discrete foci of status spongiosis with Alzheimer type II astroglia present in the basal ganglia. Midbrain, pontine, and medullary white matter tracts displayed status spongiosis; the hila of the olives and the intracranial courses of several cranial nerves showed spongiform myelin changes, but still unmyelinated fiber tracts were unaffected. Severe loss of the external granular layer of cerebellum along with patchy loss of Purkinje cells and spongy rarefaction of deep subcortical cerebellar myelinated fibers were seen. There was a localized subarachnoid hemorrhage over the right cerebellar hemisphere. The second patient died at 23 months with a developmental age of approximately 7 months. There were recurrent hospital admissions for metabolic acidosis, the first occurring at 18 hours of age. A serum ammonia of 457 μM was documented. In this patient, no spongiform changes were seen in the myelin, although occasional regions of focal perivascular spongiform rarefaction were seen in the caudate nucleus. Cerebellar Purkinje cells were depleted, and early anoxic changes were seen in cortical and cerebellar neurons.

Neuropathologic findings in propionic acidemic patients may be summarized as ranging from normal to spongiform white matter changes most marked in the basal ganglia and at the gray-white matter junctions. In several cases, severe depletion of the external granular layer of the cerebellum has been noted. Spongiform changes are most striking in patients dying within the first year of life, and it is possible that these microcysts are age-related, disappearing later. Some support for this hypothesis comes from the fact that spongiform changes are most marked in patients dying early in the course of phenylketonuria as well as nonketotic hyperglycinemia. The "quaking" mutant mouse displays myelin vacuolation at 3 weeks of age, but by 7 weeks few vacuoles are seen (18).

Pathophysiology

Brain damage in propionic acidemia seems related to the frequency and severity of episodes of metabolic decompensation. Hyperammonemia is a common, but not invariable, accompaniment of coma in propionic acidemia. The mechanism is uncertain, but it is likely that deficiency of N-acetylglutamate, which is a promoter of the carbamylphosphate synthetase (CPS) reaction, plays an important role. Propionyl CoA, itself, inhibits the CPS enzyme. In addition to inhibition of the formation of N-acetylglutamate, there may be a direct inhibitory effect on CPS itself. Decreased CPS activity has been noted in both propionic and methylmalonic acidemia (19). Close correlations between serum organic acid levels and blood ammonia have been reported for patients with propionic acidemia (20,21), isovaleric acidemia (20,22), and methylmalonic acidemia (22), supporting the concept that ammonia toxicity may be a common mechanism of injury in the organic acidemias. In a wide variety of conditions associated with hyperammonemia, specific pathologic changes in the brain have been found. Alzheimer type II cells are commonly seen in hepatic encephalopathy as well as hyperammonemia due to the organic acidemias. These astrocytes have swollen irregular nuclei with prominent nucleoli. Similar astrocytic changes are seen in primates exposed to hyperammonemia (23). Oligodendroglia also show histologic changes in the presence of hyperammonemia characterized by fibrillary aggregations (23). Although Alzheimer type II changes are seen in diseases without documented hyperammonemia, they are regularly found in hyperammonemic states. EEG changes in hepatic encephalopathy vary from abnormalities of the alpha rhythm to a generalized slowing, and there is a correlation between severity of coma and EEG changes as well as blood ammonia levels (24). Causes and effects of hyperammonemia were comprehensively reviewed by Hsia (25). Biochemical mechanisms underlying ammonia toxicity in the brain are unclear, but inhibition of oxidative phosphorylation with mitochondrial swelling (26), glutamate and glutamine accumulation with depletion of 2-oxoglutarate (27), and inhibition of mitochondrial respiration when citrate and isocitrate are used as substrates (28) may all be important factors in the neurotoxicity of ammonia.

Propionate accumulation, itself, is toxic. Propionyl CoA is the likely agent responsible for the uncoupling of oxidative phosphorylation and inhibition of state 3, observed when propionate is incubated with isolated mitochondria. Propionyl CoA inhibits the enzyme succinyl CoA ligase (4,29). Reduction of cytochrome oxidase activity has also been observed in both propionic acidemia and methylmalonic acidemia (30). Hyperglycinemia accompanies most episodes of metabolic decompensation in propionic acidemia, and glycine itself may be neurotoxic. Glycine has been shown to potentiate the NMDA response in cultured mouse brain neurons (31). A potentiation of NMDA receptor-mediated depolarization may be an important mechanism of glycine toxicity. The abnormal metabolites, 2-methylcitrate and tiglylglycine accumulate in patients with propionic and methylmalonic acidemia. 2-Methylcitrate inhibits a number of enzymes in the citric acid cycle including citrate synthetase, aconitase, and isocitrate dehydrogenase. In addition, phosphofructokinase is inhibited (32).

The pathophysiology of brain damage in propionic acidemia is complex and probably involves a number of mechanisms. It is likely that damage occurs only during episodes of severe metabolic decompensation, which are usually associated with coma and hyperammonemia. Compromise in oxidative metabolism at several points including glycolysis, the citric acid cycle, and the cytochrome chain, may be important mechanisms of neurotoxicity. In addition, hyperammonemia and hyperglycinemia are likely to contribute as neurotoxins. All of these biochemical changes are likely to be more severe in the presence of hypoxic/ischemic injury in which mitochondrial function is already compromised.

Biochemical Characteristics

The patient with propionic acidemia displays a rich variety of metabolic consequences of the deficiency of the fundamental enzyme. Among the most important for the diagnosis of the disorder is the formation of methylcitrate (33). This unique metabolite is present in appreciable quantity and is very stable. Its detection is the most reliable method for the diagnosis.

The disorder is often first suspected following the detection of large quantities of glycine in blood or urine (8). The urine of any hyperglycinemic child should be studied for methylcitrate, because propionic acidemia is treatable and nonketotic hyperglycinemia is essentially not treatable. The pathophysiology of the accumulation of glycine is inhibition of the synthesis of a protein subunit of the glycine cleavage enzyme by propionyl CoA (34,35). Patients with propionic acidemia develop lactic acidosis at times of acute illness (11). Patients with lactic acidosis should also be studied for a diagnosis of propionic acidemia. The accumulation of 2-methylacetoacetate and 2-methyl-3-hydroxybutyrate (36) may mistakenly suggest a diagnosis of oxothiolase deficiency. More serious, the detection of 3-hydroxyisovalerate (36) and especially its disappearance with fluid therapy might mistakenly suggest a diagnosis of multiple carboxylase deficiency, because patients with that disorder, unlike patients with propionic acidemia, tolerate large amounts of protein when treated with biotin. These problems should readily be resolved by quantification of organic acids (1).

Among the most important consequences of propionic acidemia from the point of view of the generation of clinical illness is the propensity for ketogenesis (8). At times of acute crisis, in response to the administration of the usual amounts of dietary protein or to infection, these patients generate large amounts of acetoacetate and 3-hydroxybutyrate, much like a ketoacidotic diabetic. Massive ketosis leads to acidosis, dehydration, coma, and death. Mechanisms for the ketosis include inhibition of oxidative enzymes (29, 30) and the depletion of oxaloacetate by condensation with propionyl CoA to form methylcitrate (33). Inhibition of the citric acid cycle and the entry of acetyl CoA would lead to condensation with itself to form acetoacetate. The hyperammonemia may also be an important factor in the causation of clinical abnormalities, especially in the nervous system. Levels may be as high as those of patients with disorders of the urea cycle, and this may lead to problems in diagnosis (37). Fortunately, there is an ontogeny to the hyperammonemia, and though it is often a serious problem in the initial neonatal episode, it is rarely encountered even in severe acidosis in later infancy and childhood (38). Patients with propionic acidemia and methylmalonic acidemia also accumulate odd-chain fatty acids, which are laid down in lipids.

The molecular defect in propionic acidemia is in the enzyme propionyl CoA carboxylase (E.C.6.4.1.3.) (Figure 3.2), which catalyzes the conversion of propionyl CoA to methylmalonyl CoA and ultimately to intermediates of the citric acid cycle. All of the metabolic abnormalities observed in patients with propionic acidemia stem from this fundamental defect. In most patients, there is some, but very little, demonstrable activity: certainly less than 5% and often less than 1% of the control level. The defect is demonstrable in freshly isolated leukocytes, cultured fibroblasts, liver, and other tissues (15, 39–43). The defect can readily be demonstrated in vitro by measuring the conversion of ^{14}C-propionate to ^{14}CO$_2$ (41). A similar defect in conversion to expiratory CO$_2$ has been demonstrated in vivo (44).

The enzyme is mitochondrial. It requires biotin covalently bound to the enzyme, ATP, and magnesium. It is a tetrameric protein containing four identical proteins, each with two nonidentical subunits in an alpha-4 and beta-4 structure. Biotin binds to the larger alpha subunit. Although biotin may increase levels of activity of the enzyme in cells of some patients (45), none have been observed to benefit clinically from treatment with biotin.

In studies of cultured fibroblasts, two complementation groups have been documented, pccA and pccC, indicating at least two loci for mutation in the alpha and beta subunits, respectively (46). The enzyme in group A is heat labile and has a low affinity for potassium. Immunotitration studies using antisera against human or porcine propionyl CoA carboxylase indicated that neither pccA nor pccC fibroblast extracts contain any detectable cross-reacting material (CRM) (47). From these studies it was concluded that residual activity measured in cells of patients may represent another carboxylase capable of utilizing propionyl CoA as substrate. cDNA clones have been isolated, which code for alpha and beta subunits of human propionyl CoA carboxylase (48). The gene for the alpha chain has been localized to chromosome 13 and that for the beta to chromosome 3. Each displayed restriction fragment length polymorphism (RFLP). The gene for the beta chain has been further localized to 3ql3.3–22 (49).

Genetics

The inheritance of propionic acidemia is an autosomal-recessive trait. Reduced levels of activity of propionyl CoA

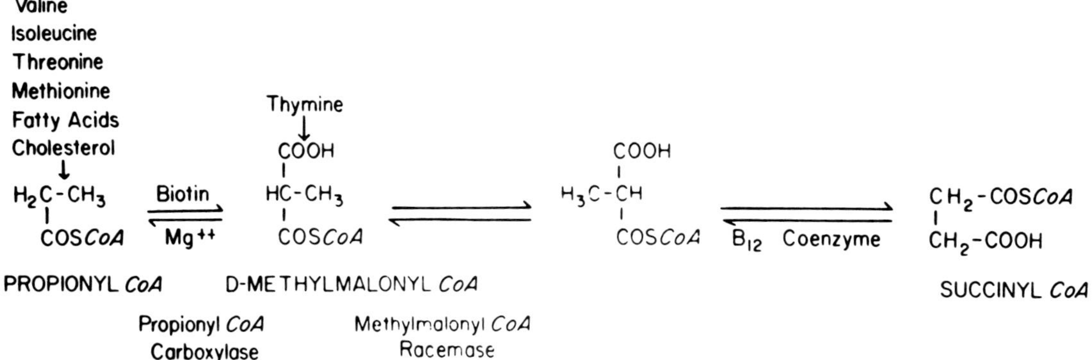

FIGURE 3.2 Metabolism of propionic acid. Propionyl CoA carboxylase is the site of the defect in propionic acidemia. (Reprinted with permission from Nyhan WL. Abnormalities in amino acid metabolism in clinical medicine. Norwalk, CT: Appleton Century Crofts, 1984)

carboxylase may be found in leukocytes or fibroblasts of carriers, but this is not reliable because some heterozygotes have normal levels (43, 50).

Prenatal diagnosis is available by assay of the enzyme in cultured amniocytes or chorionic villus cells (51, 52) or by the incorporation of ^{14}C-propionate into precipitable protein (53, 54). The most reliable and quickest method is the determination of methylcitrate in amniotic fluid (55–57). This method avoids the documented pitfall of enzymatic diagnosis, the overgrowth of maternal, not fetal, cells during the long periods in culture required for most enzyme assays (58).

Treatment

Treatment in patients with propionic acidemia must be considered under the headings of management of the acute episode of life-threatening illness and chronic management designed to prevent or minimize acute episodes and optimize developmental progress.

The acute episode requires intensive care, often including assisted ventilation at least in the initial hyperammonemic episode. The hyperammonemia and propionic acidemia may respond to multiple exchange transfusions or peritoneal dialysis (59,60) or the intravenous infusion of sodium benzoate or phenylacetate. The most effective method is hemodialysis (61). Large amounts of fluid-containing electrolytes and glucose are required to meet deficits and continuing losses. Isotonic sodium bicarbonate containing glucose and potassium acetate is conveniently administered in initial doses as high as 200 mL/kg/day. Once hyperammonemia is absent, 0.25 to 0.5 g/kg of protein or amino acids may spare further catabolism of body proteins.

Chronic management depends on the dietary reduction of the intake of protein containing isoleucine, valine, threonine, and methionine. We restrict intake to the minimal amounts required for growth (62). The amounts are usually below 1 g/kg of protein per day, but each patient must be treated individually (63). There appeared to be little difference whether the day's protein was provided as a single meal or distributed evenly (64); nitrogen balances were the same, but fasting concentrations of cystine, methionine, isoleucine, leucine, and threonine, as well as most of the nonessential amino acids, were higher when protein intake was evenly distributed. The remaining calories are provided as carbohydrate and fat. Mead Johnson Product No. 80056 (Mead Johnson, Evansville, IN) is convenient for the generation of diets for infants and also provides vitamins and minerals. Parents are taught to monitor the urine for ketones. Patients are monitored at the University of California, San Diego, Medical Center for growth and development, nitrogen balance, electrolyte status, and the concentrations of amino acids in blood and organic-

acid metabolites in urine. A particularly low level of an individual essential amino acid, especially if growth falls off, provides an argument for specific supplementation. Supplementation with leucine in an 18-month-old girl who was failing to thrive was followed by catch-up growth, improvement in muscular hypotonia, and restoration of the plasma concentration of leucine (10). We have also obtained data indicating that leucine may be limiting in infants receiving such restricted diets (62). We and others have reassured ourselves that leucine is not toxic in propionic acidemia, despite early indications to the contrary (8).

The addition of carnitine to the therapeutic regimen has made a major difference in the management of propionic acidemia. Patients with propionic acidemia all develop secondary deficiency of carnitine (65, 66), and treatment readily returns levels of free carnitine to normal. These patients are not hypoketotic as one might expect in the absence of carnitine, however. Instead, they have abnormally active ketogenesis, which is the major factor in morbidity and mortality. Treatment with carnitine modulates down in a dose-response fashion this propensity for ketogenesis (6). This effect appears to be the result of the formation and excretion of propionylcarnitine ester (67–69). Although there is a renal threshold for free carnitine, there does not appear to be one for carnitine esters. The major effect of carnitine is a detoxifying one. Doses range from 50 to 300 mg/kg.

Methylmalonic Acidemia

The clinical features of methylmalonic acidemia vary widely, from asymptomatic neurologically normal individuals to children with severe illness in infancy characterized by recurrent episodes of ketoacidotic coma. The severely affected patients generally have neurologic disease characterized by hypotonia, seizures, and developmental delay with subsequent mental retardation and spasticity with or without features of basal ganglia damage. All patients with methylmalonic acidemia have deficient methylmalonyl CoA mutase activity, and in approximately 50% this is due to either absence (Mut°) or functional abnormality (Mut⁻) of the apoenzyme itself. The other patients have deficiencies of adenosylcobalamin synthesis with secondary effects on methylmalonyl CoA mutase. The bulk of these patients fall into the groups CblA and CblB, determined by complementation studies. A minority of patients, however, with concomitant homocystinuria have been described (CblC and CblD). One family with an apparent defect of methionine synthetase (CblE) (71) and one patient with an intracellular cobalamin transport defect (CblF) (72) have been described.

An excellent review of the clinical features of the major categories of methylmalonic acidemia has been published (70) (Table 3.2).

Table 3.2 Clinical and laboratory features of methylmalonic acidemia in 45 patients.

Presenting Clinical Features	Patients (%) (n = 45)	Presenting Laboratory Features	Patients (%) (n = 45)
Lethargy	84	Normal serum cobalamin	100
Failure to thrive	73	Metabolic acidosis	92
Recurrent vomiting	73	Ketosis	81
Dehydration	71	Hyperammonemia	71
Respiratory distress	67	Elevated glycine	68
Developmental delay	63	Leukopenia	60
Hepatomegaly	41	Anemia	55
Coma	40	Thrombocytopenia	50

Matsui et al. 1983 (70)

Clinical and Neurologic Features

The severe neonatal presentation that is associated with a marked risk of neurologic impairment is seen in most patients with the Mut° class. However, patients with Mut⁻ and CblA and CblB complementation categories also frequently present in the neonatal period. The typical neonatal presentation is indistinguishable from that described in propionic acidemia. Severe ketoacidosis with a clinical picture suggesting sepsis is accompanied in most patients by marked hyperammonemia. Hypoglycemia may also be found. Neutropenia is generally seen, and thrombocytopenia may occur. Patients may present with mucocutaneous candidiasis because of the particular susceptibility of the Candida T-cell response to methylmalonate and other metabolites (73). Failure to thrive, severe anorexia, and osteoporosis are commonly found. Hyperuricemia and hyperglycinemia are usually present during episodes of metabolic decompensation or periods of poor metabolic control. The common neurologic findings are listed in Table 3.2 and include profound hypotonia, developmental retardation, lethargy, and coma during periods of ketoacidosis and hyporeflexia, which may develop into hyperreflexia with spasticity. Clinical features of basal ganglia involvement have been described in several patients. The findings are predominantly those of dystonia with choreiform movements in some (74).

Neurologic outcome depends not only on the presence or absence of a severe neonatal presentation, but also on the response to B₁₂ therapy and protein restriction. Initial presentation in late infancy is common in methylmalonic acidemia. This presentation is seen in 40% of the patients with the Mut⁻ variant, and later presentations are seen in approximately 50% of patients with CblA and CblB. Although the presentation is later, neurologic injury is common during episodes of ketoacidosis. Four patients with acute extrapyramidal syndromes have recently been described. Only one had a neonatal presentation; the other three developed ketoacidosis at 14, 15, and 20 months,

respectively. All patients showed globus pallidus lesions (74). It has been well documented that hyperammonemia is not usually seen in methylmalonic acidemia when patients present with ketoacidosis outside of the neonatal period (38).

Patients with CblD have lower levels of methylmalonic acid and do not develop ketoacidosis. They may present in the neonatal period with failure to thrive, anorexia, and developmental delay. Hypotonia, microcephaly, seizures, and retinopathy have been described (70, 75, 76). Patients with CblC, in particular, have had a poor outcome despite cobalamin treatment. Macrocytic anemia is usually seen. A number of cases of later-onset CblC have been described. These children presented between the ages of 4 and 14 years with lethargy and a dementing picture over a few months. The clinical presentation of a patient with CblD was also predominantly neurologic: mental retardation, psychosis, nystagmus, and hyperactive reflexes were seen in one boy who presented at 14 years of age. This patient had recurrent thromboemboli despite cobalamin treatment. A younger brother was less severely affected, but had learning disability (77).

The CblE defect was described in a single family. The proband presented with anorexia, bloody diarrhea, and vomiting at 9 weeks of age along with hypotonia, developmental delay, and megaloblastic anemia. The homocystinuria resolved and plasma amino acid levels returned to normal with cobalamin therapy, but the child remained developmentally delayed. A sibling was started on cobalamin prenatally and had no biochemical or clinical defects.

The patient described with the ClbF defect presented at 12 days of age with hypotonia, seizures, feeding difficulties, and stomatitis with glossitis. At follow-up, global developmental delay and seizures persisted.

A defect termed CblG has been identified in a family with homocystinuria and megaloblastic anemia without methylmalonic aciduria. This defect in methionine synthetase activity has produced developmental delay in all untreated patients and neurologic disease in an adult family member (78).

Electroencephalography. EEG findings are nonspecific. As in the case of propionic acidemia, generalized slowing may be seen during episodes of ketoacidotic coma. A periodic burst-suppression pattern was found in one neonate who died at 6 days of age in hyperammonemic ketoacidotic coma (79). In patients who recover, the EEG may become normal (80, 81), but the background may remain slow and disorganized. Multifocal sharp waves and epileptiform discharges may be seen.

Neuroimaging. The initial description of CT brain scan findings in two patients with methylmalonic acidemia noted diffuse decreased attenuation of white matter in one patient who presented in infancy. This progressed to a generalized atrophy at 1 year of age. The second patient presented later with spastic quadriparesis and developmental delay. CT brain scan at 1 year of age showed focal white matter lucencies in the posterior limbs of the internal capsules (82). A 19-month-old girl with CblA methylmalonic acidemia presented with ketoacidotic coma. CT scan showed symmetrical decreased attenuation in the globus pallidi (80). These changes were attributed to basal ganglia necrosis of undetermined cause, with hypoxia or cyanide accumulation due to cyanocobalamin treatment raised as possibilities (80). A patient of 20 months of age with acidosis and lethargy was reported, however, with symmetrical globus pallidus necrosis on CT during the acute presentation of methylmalonic acidemia. This patient was documented as not being hypoxic, and the lesions were noted prior to B$_{12}$ therapy. The lesions were confirmed by follow-up CT and MRI brain scans (83). Four cases of methylmalonic acidemia, two of which had documented CblA defects, were reported with bilateral destruction of the globus pallidus and variable involvement of internal capsules as demonstrated on CT. These patients all presented with acute extrapyramidal syndromes following episodes of ketoacidosis. None of the patients received cyanocobalamin before or during the acute episodes (74). The authors noted that symmetrical lesions within the globus pallidi sparing other basal ganglial structures seem unique to methylmalonic acidemia and propionic acidemia. We have noted symmetrical high T2 signal in the globus pallidi in 2 of 3 patients with methylmalonic acidemia studied by MRI scans. In addition, more diffuse white-matter changes were suggested by the finding of high T2 signal diffusely within cortical white matter in one patient and focally within periventricular white matter in another.

Neuropathology. Autopsy data are available in several patients with severe forms of methylmalonic acidemia. In one case with a neonatal presentation, autopsy at 4 years of age showed diffuse cerebral and cerebellar atrophy, which was most marked in the white matter (82). Multifocal cerebellar hemorrhage has been reported in an infant who died of methylmalonic acidemia at 17 days of age following severe ketoacidosis with hyperammonemia (79). Diffuse gliosis of the white matter and scattered Alzheimer type II astrocytes were found in the cerebral cortex and cerebellum. The pathologic substrate of the high T2 signal observed on MRI in the globus pallidus and the decreased attenuation seen on CT in methylmalonic acidemia patients has not yet been clearly elucidated. Basal ganglial changes were noted at autopsy, however, in two infants who died of methylmalonic acidemia (84). One died at 1 month of age with putaminal necrosis and gliosis noted in the globus pallidus but with minimal neuronal loss. The other child died at 9 months with spongiform change and astrocytic hypertrophy of the globus pallidus, also with minimal neuronal loss.

Pathophysiology

The brain damage usually sustained following the neonatal presentation of methylmalonic acidemia with hyperammonemic ketoacidosis is probably the result of a combination of hyperammonemic damage, severe acidosis, and hypoxic/ischemic injury. Accumulation of toxic metabolic intermediates like propionyl CoA may also play a role in injury to the nervous system sustained during metabolic decompensation. It is interesting that in methylmalonic acidemia, hyperammonemia has not been reported outside of the neonatal period. So this mechanism is not responsible for injury sustained during later episodes of ketoacidosis. As in the case of propionic acidemia, reduced cytochrome oxidase activity has been reported in the liver in methylmalonic acidemic patients (30). Thus, secondary mitochondrial changes may precipitate a damaging failure of oxidative metabolism. The apparently unique globus pallidus lesions observed in methylmalonic acidemia suggest a differential sensitivity to or local accumulation of toxic metabolites.

Methylmalonic acid, itself, may be neurotoxic. A 16% reduction in ganglioside N-acetylneuraminic acid was noted in the cerebellum of young rats following chronic administration of methylmalonic acid. This ganglioside is thought to be important in synaptogenesis (85). Hyperglycinemia frequently accompanies episodes of ketoacidosis in methylmalonic acidemia, and, as in the case of propionic acidemia, glycine facilitation of excitation at the NMDA receptor may play a part in neuronal injury (31). Hypoglycemia (86) can occur in ketoacidotic episodes, particularly in the neonatal period, and the mechanism of injury may, in this case also, involve the NMDA receptor.

Biochemical Characteristics

The fundamental abnormality in methylmalonic acidemia is defective activity in the enzyme methylmalonyl CoA mutase, which catalyzes the conversion of methylmalonate to succinyl CoA (See Figure 3.2). This may result from defects in the apoenzyme itself in the so-called Mut complementary groups, which have been subdivided into the Mut° group, in which the mutation has resulted in no detectable activity in vitro, and the MUT$^-$ group, in which there is some residual activity (87–89). The relationship of the other complementation groups to the transformations of cobalamin and particularly its synthesis into 5'-deoxyadenosylcobalamin, which is an obligatory cofactor of the mutase enzyme, is shown in Figure 3.3.

Patients with defective adenosylcobalamin synthesis respond clinically to treatment with vitamin B$_{12}$. Patients in the CblC and D groups who have homocystinuria as well as methylmalonic acidemia because they cannot make either methylcobalamin or deoxyadenosylcobalamin, do not. Among patients in the Mut° group, immunotitration stud-

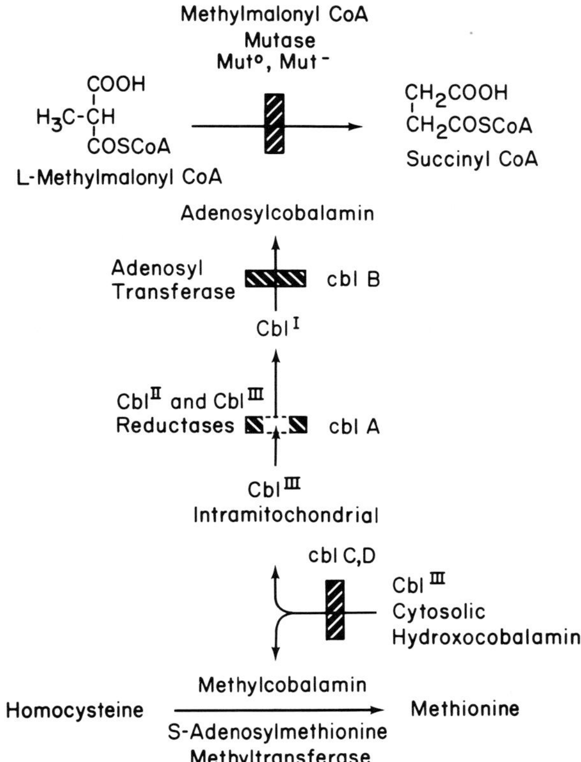

FIGURE 3.3 Metabolic transformations of cobalamin and its role in the methylmalonyl CoA mutase reaction and that of methionine synthetase. The sites of the various complementation groups are shown. (Reprinted with permission from Nyhan WL, Sakati NA, eds. Diagnostic recognition of genetic diseases. Philadelphia: Lea & Febiger, 1987)

ies have revealed some to have some CRM, albeit reduced, while others had none (89). Immunochemical studies have detected an enzyme mutation that interferes with the transport of the enzyme into the mitochondria. The gene for the mutase enzyme has been cloned (90), and its locus has been mapped to chromosome 6 (91).

In fibroblasts of patients in CblA and B, the content of deoxyadenosylcobalamin is reduced, as is their ability to convert ^{57}Co-hydroxycobalamin to ^{57}Co-deoxyadenosyl-cobalamin (92,93). The two groups are most readily distinguished by complementation analysis (94,95). The A variants appear to have a defect in Cbl(III) reductase, because when reducing conditions are established that bypass this step, cells can synthesize deoxyadenosylcobal-amin from the cobalt-labeled precursor, whereas the B variants are defective in the adenosyltransferase reaction (96). Patients with CblA regularly respond clinically to B₁₂, whereas some CblB patients do, and others, probably those with a complete defect in the transferase enzyme, do not.

The metabolic consequences of defective activity of the mutase enzyme are similar to those seen in propionic acidemia. Methylmalonyl CoA and propionyl CoA accumulate and are converted to methylmalonate and propi-onate and to methylcitrate. The same four essential amino acids are catabolized imperfectly and must be limited in intake, or they will be converted to toxic organic acids. The excretion of methylmalonate in this disease is a very precise mirror of metabolic status, more so than the intermediates observed in propionic acidemia or any other metabolic disease. As the dietary intake of the precursor amino acids is raised above the amounts recommended for growth and anabolism, the relationship between precursor excess and methylmalonate in the urine is mole for mole (62).

Further metabolic consequences of the accumulation of these organic acids in intermediates are, as in propionic acidemia ketogenesis, hyperglycinemia, lactic acidemia, and hyperuricemia. Urate nephropathy and renal failure may occur (97) as may renal tubular acidosis (98).

Genetics

Methylmalonic acidemia, in each of its variant forms, is transmitted as an autosomal-recessive trait. Heterozygote detection is not reliable. Routine neonatal screening in the state of Massachusetts yielded an incidence of 1 in 48,000 (99). It was in the course of this screening program that the phenotype of asymptomatic patients with methylmalonic acidemia was discovered (100). These eight individuals excreted very small amounts of methylmalonic acid; they appeared to be examples of the Mut⁻ group in which the residual activity of the enzyme in vivo is very high. In the initial report seven patients were found to be B₁₂-responsive.

Prenatal diagnosis has been accomplished by assay of mutase activity in cultured amniocytes (101). Methyl-malonic acid may also be detected in maternal urine, but this is reliable only too late in gestation to be useful for prenatal diagnosis (102). The best and most rapid methods utilize the direct quantitation of methylcitrate, methyl-malonate, or both, in amniotic fluid (56,57,103,104). Effective prenatal treatment with B₁₂ of a B₁₂-responsive fetus has been reported following prenatal diagnosis (105); the patient was a healthy teenager at most recent follow-up.

Treatment

Patients with B₁₂-responsive methylmalonic acidemia should be treated with B₁₂. The usual dosage is 1 mg of cyanocobalamin daily. It can be given by mouth. Dosage should be adjusted to keep the level of excretion of methyl-malonate minimal. This is the single most important ele-ment in prognosis. In general, patients who respond to B₁₂ do well, and a substantial number are neurologically and mentally normal; whereas most of the mutase apoenzyme deficient patients die, and the survivors are mostly impaired (70,106).

Dietary restriction of protein containing isoleucine, valine, threonine, and methionine is necessary for all but the asymptomatic phenotypes; it needs to be much less rigid in B_{12}-responsive patients. It must be very rigid in Mut° patients. Most of these patients are so anorexic, that tube feeding is required. The amino-acid precursor intake is ideally carefully limited, so that growth and nitrogen retention take place, but methylmalonate excretion is at a minimal plateau level (107). Alanine supplementation may be helpful in patients receiving these very restricted diets (108). Oral neomycin may be helpful, particularly for short periods, in removing sources of methylmalonate arising from propionic acid made by intestinal bacteria (109). As in patients with propionic acidemia (6), the addition of carnitine to the therapeutic regimen has made a major difference in management. All of these patients should be treated with carnitine. Doses of 50 to 300 mg/kg are useful, limited only by the possibility of diarrhea at higher doses.

Isovaleric Acidemia

More than 60 patients with this disorder are now described (110). The most common manifestation is as an acute, severe neonatal illness simulating neonatal sepsis. The clinical picture is difficult to distinguish from the neonatal manifestation of other organic acidemias; however, the presence of an offensive odor due to isovaleric acid may suggest the diagnosis. The characteristic odor may not be apparent in patients who have undergone treatment, particularly if this includes hemodialysis. The disease has been estimated fatal in the neonatal period in 60%; survivors tend to have recurrent episodes of vomiting and keto-acidosis. The distinction between the acute neonatal phenotype and the chronic phenotype of a later presentation of metabolic decompensation appears artificial (111). Glycine-conjugating ability may dictate severity of the disease in a particular patient, as levels of isovaleryl CoA dehydrogenase activity are nonpredictive (112).

Clinical and Neurologic Features

In general, patients with isovaleric acidemia are not dysmorphic. One report of dwarfism, cataract, and congenital anomalies reminiscent of rhizomelic chondrodystrophia calcificans congenita appeared to reflect factors distinct from metabolic disease (113). During acute metabolic crises that occur in isovaleric acidemia, CNS injury may occur. Children who survive such episodes without injury and are then consistently treated frequently have a normal intellect without language or motor difficulties. Early and consistent treatment appears to be an important factor in avoiding CNS damage (110,114). In some instances, patients remain intellectually normal without CNS damage despite recurrent episodes of metabolic acidosis. In general, these patients are not hyperammonemic or deeply comatose during such episodes and may have a mild form of the disease (115).

Encephalopathy may often accompany episodes of acute metabolic decompensation in isovaleric acidemia. Poor feeding and vomiting signal an attack. The vomiting may be so severe that pyloric stenosis is diagnosed. Patients become lethargic and may progress to coma. Seizures may occur that can be focal (116) or generalized. An erroneous diagnosis of Reye syndrome may be made (110). In one infant, hyperglycemia and ketosis led to a diagnosis of diabetes mellitus (117). Intraventricular hemorrhage and cerebellar hemorrhage have both been described (110,116), although intracranial hemorrhage is rare. Hyperammonemia is common during acute episodes, but levels are usually less than 400 μM (118). Higher, potentially damaging levels of hyperammonemia have been reported (20,116,119, 120). On recovery from episodes of acute encephalopathy, patients may have transient or permanent evidence of motor injury including ataxia, intention tremor, brisk deep tendon reflexes, and extrapyramidal involuntary movements. Microcephaly may be a long-term consequence (121,122).

With early diagnosis and prompt treatment, many patients are neurologically normal. In the French experience, 2 of 8 patients were retarded, and the other 6 were normal (114). In the Philadelphia series of 9 patients, 4 had normal IQs or DQs, and 5 were moderately to mildly retarded with measured IQs of 49 to 70 (100).

Electroencephalography. In general, the EEG in patients with isovaleric acidemia is normal between episodes. If the brain has been damaged, signs of slowing and disorganization may be seen (121). Even in the presence of CNS injury, the EEG may be normal—this was reported in a 17-month-old child with spastic diplegia (111). We have obtained EEGs in two siblings with later onset of mild disease: one, a 5-year-old, had mild truncal ataxia with an EEG, which was slow for her age, but otherwise normal. Her 18-month-old sister was neurologically normal and had a normal EEG. No reports of CT or MR brain scans are available in isovaleric acidemia.

Neuropathology. Neuropathologic studies were carried out in a neonate who died at 11 days of age in an episode of severe acidosis (116). Blood ammonia level was 1200 μM. There was diffuse cerebral edema, massive cerebellar hemorrhage, and upward transtentorial herniation. The cerebellar hemorrhages originated in the perivascular regions, becoming confluent and rupturing into the subarachnoid space. Spongiform changes were seen in the white matter with reactive gliosis involving cortex, brain stem, and cerebellum. Glial cells of both gray and white matter showed focal clustering and degeneration. No Alzheimer type II astrocytes were seen. The white-matter changes in this patient seemed compatible with edema and were less severe in this and other reported cases (123–125) than in other organic acidemias (17) or in nonketotic hyperglycinemia (16).

Pathophysiology

Isovaleric acid has been found incorporated in the phospholipids of porpoise brain (126), but such short-chain fatty acids have not been reported as normal brain constituents in other mammals. In the human, isovaleric acid is thought to serve only as a metabolic intermediate in the metabolism of leucine. Isovaleric acid and, in particular, isovaleryl CoA, like other short-chain fatty acids, are toxic to mitochondria. Effects include uncoupling of oxidative phosphorylation (127,128) as well as inhibition of state 3 substrate oxidation (128). In one patient, a high basal metabolic rate was recorded, suggesting that uncoupling of oxidative phosphorylation may be clinically significant (121). As in the case of the other organic acidemias, no single cause explains the brain damage that may occur in episodes of metabolic decompensation. In some patients, high levels of ammonia may be damaging. The mechanism of hyperammonemia, as in the case of propionic acid, appears to involve an inhibition of N-acetylglutamate synthetase (129). In most cases, however, hyperammonemia is less than 400 μM (118), and Alzheimer type II glial cells have not been seen. Secondary effects of accumulation of isovaleric acid include a depletion of free coenzyme A and free carnitine. Accumulation of other branched-chain amino acids may inhibit succinyl CoA oxoacid transferase, resulting in an impairment of ketone utilization. 2-oxoisocaproic acid inhibits pyruvate and 3-hydroxybutyrate uptake into rat brain mitochondria (130).

Biochemical Characteristics

Concentrations of isovaleric acid in the serum are elevated. During acute crises, levels may reach 5 μM; normal individuals have less than 0.005 μM. This is the compound that accounts for the acrid odor characteristic of this disease. Conjugation of isovaleryl CoA with glycine is more efficient than any other organic acid, and therefore analysis of the urine for isovalerylglycine is the most effective method for making a definitive diagnosis (131,132). The compound is nonvolatile, unlike isovaleric acid itself, stable, and excreted in large amounts, even under conditions of remission. The excretion of isovalerylglycine may be as great as 3 g, while in normal persons it is less than 2 mg.

The other organic acid excreted in large quantities is 3-hydroxyisovaleric acid (133). Less common organic acids making up the metabolic pattern include 4-hydroxyisovaleric acid, and methylsuccinic and mesaconic acids (134,135). Lactic acid, acetoacetic acid, and 3-hydroxybutyric acid are found in the urine in acute episodes. Isovalerylglucuronide (136) and isovalerylcarnitine are additional detoxification products.

The molecular defect in isovaleric acidemia is in the enzyme isovaleryl CoA dehydrogenase (137,138), which catalyzes the conversion of isovaleryl CoA to 3-methylcrotonyl CoA. Levels of activity in fibroblasts approxi-

mated 13% of control. The gene for this enzyme has been cloned and has been localized to chromosome 15q 12–15 (139).

Genetics

Isovaleric acidemia is inherited as an autosomal-recessive trait. Heterozygote detection and prenatal diagnosis have been carried out by the study of the oxidation of leucine-2-^{14}C to ^{14}CO$_2$ in cultured cells (138). Prenatal diagnosis may be accomplished directly by the gas chromatography mass spectrometry (GCMS) assay of 3-hydroxyisovaleric acid in amniotic fluid (136).

Treatment

The cornerstone of treatment is the reduction of the dietary intake of protein to the amounts required for growth (140). Supplemental alanine may permit better growth on very low intakes of protein (141). Supplemental glycine may aid in detoxifying accumulated isovaleryl CoA by promoting the formation of isovaleryl glycine. Amounts employed in infants have been 800 mg/day; in addition, 250 mg/kg/day has been used in the management of the acute episode (121,142,143). Carnitine is another useful adjunct. Doses employed have been 60 to 200 mg/kg.

Multiple Carboxylase Deficiency

There are two forms of multiple carboxylase deficiency. The neonatal form is due to holocarboxylase synthetase deficiency. Patients present in the first few days of life with severe metabolic acidosis, with lactic acidemia, hyperammonemia, lethargy, hypotonia, and coma. If the patient survives, alopecia and a red, scaly rash affects the whole body. Brain damage may occur during episodes of acute encephalopathy. All patients so far identified have been biotin-responsive.

Biotinidase deficiency generally presents in later infancy with episodic metabolic acidosis and a less severe, predominantly perioral dermatitis together with partial alopecia. Neurologic features are generally pronounced in biotinidase deficiency and may precede any other findings. They include generalized tonic-clonic seizures, as well as myoclonic epilepsy, developmental delay, and ataxia. Biotinidase deficiency may present with a picture of Leigh encephalopathy (144,145). Patients with biotinidase deficiency respond to biotin.

Clinical expression is not a reliable way to distinguish biotinidase-deficient patients. Biotinidase deficiency is occasionally manifested in early infancy (146). Holocarboxylase deficiency may be manifested as the more indolent form (147). A definitive diagnosis requires enzyme assay. In addition to clinical similarities between these two defects, activity in leukocytes of the carboxylases—pyruvate carboxylase, propionyl CoA carboxylase, and 3-methyl-crotonyl CoA carboxylase—are similarly reduced. World-wide experience suggests that the incidence of biotinidase deficiency varies in different populations from 1 : 20,000 to 1 : 140,000, although only approximately 40 biotinidase-deficient patients have been identified. Biotinidase deficiency appears to be 3 to 4 times more common than is holocarboxylase synthetase deficiency.

Holocarboxylase Synthetase Deficiency

Clinical and Neurologic Features

Most patients with holocarboxylase synthetase deficiency have presented with severe neonatal ketoacidosis. The clinical presentation is a life-threatening illness very similar to propionic acidemia or methylmalonic acidemia. Moderate hyperammonemia is common. Undiagnosed patients progress to coma and may die in the initial episode. If recovery occurs and the condition is not recognized and treated with biotin, recurrent episodes of severe ketoacidosis develop along with whole-body alopecia and an impressive erythematous, scaly dermatitis. Patients generally have characteristic organic aciduria with elevation of lactic acid, 3-methylcrotonyl glycine, 3-hydroxyisovalerate, and methylcitrate, as well as hydroxypropionate. Treatment with biotin may be dramatically effective, and normal neurologic development may follow.

Two infants (147,148) illustrated the typical neonatal presentation. The first had ketonuria and lethargy essentially at birth, and at 7 weeks of age had ketoacidosis and persistent lethargy with an erythematous dermatitis most pronounced in the perioral and perianal areas. The hair was thin. Blood concentration of ammonia was elevated at 228 μM. There was elevation of blood alanine as well as marked lactic acidemia. At 3 1/2 months, the infant developed *Haemophilus influenzae* meningitis and gastrointestinal candidiasis. There was developmental delay. Following treatment with biotin at 4 months of age, all biochemical abnormalities and skin lesions resolved, and at the age of 2 years, somatic and psychomotor development appeared normal. The other child presented on the 2nd day of life with ketonuria and metabolic acidosis and had a 10-times-normal level of lactate. There was hyperammonemia at 234 μM and hypoglycemia. Hypertonicity and irritability progressed to coma. Following the identification of characteristic organic aciduria, treatment with biotin resulted in a rapid recovery. Bailey scale testing at 1 1/2 years of age revealed a discrepancy between mental development index at 123 and psychomotor developmental index at 88. There were defects in shape discrimination and gross motor skills. The phenotypic heterogeneity in holocarboxylase synthetase deficiency is illustrated by an account of a child who presented at 15 months of age with a history of motor developmental delay, severe ketoacidosis with lactic acidemia (147). Recurrent episodes occurred at 22 and 24 months of age. The child was reported to walk late at 17 months with an ataxic gait, and at 20 months of age he developed minor motor seizures that were difficult to control. A sibling had died from ketoacidosis. This presentation of holocarboxylase synthetase deficiency is similar to the typical presentation of biotinidase deficiency.

In addition to irritability, lethargy, hyperreflexia, and the development of coma, patients have been reported with athetoid movements, opisthotonos, and infantile spasms.

Neurophysiology and Neuroimaging. EEGs in infants with holocarboxylase synthetase deficiency are generally described during episodes of ketoacidosis. Descriptions range from diffusely abnormal with focal features to burst-suppression patterns. The EEG generally becomes normal with treatment. CT brain scans may be normal, although decreased white-matter attenuation reminiscent of leukodystrophy has been reported.

Neuropathology and Pathophysiology. Pathologic data are not available in patients with proved holocarboxylase synthetase deficiency. Neuronal injury will occur if severe ketoacidosis with hyperammonemia persists or if hypoglycemia is prolonged. Patients developing coma with apnea may suffer hypoxic/ischemic insults.

Biochemical Characteristics

The disease is usually first suspected on the basis of the clinical picture and the presence of metabolic acidosis with or without hyperammonemia. The diagnosis is usually made by organic acid analysis. The classic pattern is the excretion of 3-hydroxyisovalerate, 3-methylcrotonylglycine, 3-hydroxypropionate, and methylcitrate. In most instances 3-hydroxyisovalerate is excreted in much larger quantities than are the other organic acids (149). Lactate is also found in large quantities (150), and lactic acid concentrations in blood and cerebrospinal fluid (CSF) are elevated. Tiglylglycine may also be detected in the urine.

Deficiency of the three carboxylases, propionyl CoA carboxylase, 3-methylcrotonyl CoA carboxylase, and pyruvate carboxylase is readily demonstrated in leukocytes or in fibroblasts cultured in Eagle's minimal essential medium. On the other hand, growth of fibroblasts in medium containing 100 nM biotin have normal carboxylase activity (151,152).

The fundamental defect is in the enzyme holocarboxylase synthetase, which activates biotin and catalyzes its attachment to an epsilon-amino group of a lysine residue of each apocarboxylase protein. Without the attached biotin, the apocarboxylase is devoid of enzyme activity; with the biotin it is fully active. In each of the cell lines studied to date, the defective enzyme has had some activity and an altered Michaelis constant (Km) for biotin (153,154). The affinity for biotin has ranged from 3 to 70 times less than the normal enzyme kinetics.

Genetics

Current estimates of prevalence are 1 in 60,000 births. Genetic transmission is that of an autosomal-recessive trait. Heterozygote detection has not been possible. Prenatal diagnosis may be accomplished most readily by the gas chromatography mass spectrometry (GCMS) detection of 3-hydroxyisovalerate in amniotic fluid (155). It may also be detected by GCMS analysis for methylcitrate or the assay of carboxylase activity in cultured amniocytes (156).

Biotinidase Deficiency

Clinical and Neurologic Features

The clinical features most often found in this disorder are listed in Table 3.3. It can be seen that considerable clinical heterogeneity exists, and most patients do not display the full clinical picture until late in the course of the disease. The usual time of onset of symptoms is in the second 6 months of life. Ataxia, generalized seizures, and developmental delay may individually, or in combination, precede other features of biotinidase deficiency (146,157). Organic aciduria and metabolic acidosis may not be present early in the disease. A feature present at some time or another in most patients is hypotonia, which may be profound. Approximately 50% of patients suffer from hearing loss or visual impairment (or both). In one review, optic atrophy was found in 4 of 28 reported cases (158). It appears that sensorineural hearing loss and visual impairment are fea-

Table 3.3 Clinical manifestations of biotinidase deficiency

Skin Rash	11/16
Alopecia	12/16
Seizures	11/16
Ataxia	9/16
Hypotonia	8/16
Developmental delay	7/17
Conjunctivitis	4/16
Optic atrophy	2/16
Hearing loss	2/16
Fungal infections	5/16
Metabolic acidosis	13/16
Lactic acidosis	11/14
Organic aciduria	11/15
Hyperammonemia	3/8
Improvement with biotin	14/14
Proved biotinidase deficiency	6/17

Age range (onset of symptoms 3 weeks–24 months)
Adapted from Wolf et al. 1983 (146)

tures that do not respond to biotin treatment, presumably representing irreversible cranial nerve injury. Auditory and visual handicaps seem to be more common if treatment is delayed beyond the first year of life (159). During episodes of metabolic decompensation that are often induced by intercurrent infection, severe life-threatening acidosis may occur. This can be accompanied by coma, hypothermia, severe hypotonia, and areflexia. These episodes are abolished by biotin therapy, and developmental delay may recover. Alopecia and the perioral cutaneous eruption also improve. Cutaneous candidiasis may be seen, and this may be related to T- and B-cell deficiencies that have been reported (160).

Seizures in patients with biotinidase deficiency may be severe and intractable. Infantile spasms may occur, but most patients exhibit generalized tonic-clonic seizures, which may be refractory to anticonvulsant treatment.

Clinical presentation resembling Leigh syndrome has been described (144,145). A 6 1/2-month-old female presented initially with stridorous breathing, which became labored and accompanied by apnea. Lactic and pyruvic acidosis was noted along with psychomotor regression. The child displayed axial hypotonia, very poor head control, and a rapid deterioration over 2 hours with ketosis. There was no skin rash. Following a rapid response to intramuscular biotin and thiamine, the child made a complete recovery and was developmentally normal at 15 months of age (144). A 29-month-old infant presented with truncal and gait ataxia, but only mild dysmetria. There was delayed language development, but otherwise normal developmental milestones. Deep tendon reflexes were brisk. Three months later, a perioral erythematous rash developed that involved the cheek and chest at the time of an upper respiratory tract infection. On the second occasion, characteristic organic aciduria was found, and biotinidase deficiency was confirmed. Although the usual patient presents with a triad of skin lesions, ataxia, and seizures, the two cases described demonstrate the variability in clinical presentation. Biotinidase deficiency should be considered in any infant presenting with any combination of the features listed in Table 3.3.

The progression of biotinidase deficiency when untreated is exemplified by the following reported patient (158). A caucasian boy suffered from developmental delay, conjunctivitis, palpebral eczema, as well as generalized seizures commencing at six months of age. No lactic acidosis was found. At 5 years of age, he had an acidotic episode with mild lactic and pyruvic acidemia. By 6 years of age, seizures, alopecia, keratoconjunctivitis, ataxia, and more severe lactic acidemia were present in addition to hearing loss. At age 7, the boy developed severe acidemia with coma, and at that time he had marked alopecia, mucocutaneous lesions, and optic atrophy. Examination of the urine showed a typical organic aciduria, and biotinidase deficiency was confirmed. Biotin treatment resolved all neurologic symptoms apart from deafness and visual impairment.

Neurophysiology. The EEG is frequently normal in patients with biotinidase deficiency. During episodes of acute acidosis, diffuse slowing may provide evidence of a metabolic encephalopathy. The EEG was normal in a 26-month-old with biotinidase deficiency despite ataxia and language developmental delay (161). A 23-month-old toddler with marked developmental delay, hypotonia, tonic-clonic seizures, normal plasma but an elevated CSF lactate, had an EEG with evidence of diffuse slowing and minimal diffuse convulsive activity. The EEG rapidly became normal with biotin treatment (162). A 19-month-old female infant with alopecia, eczema, hypotonia, brisk deep tendon reflexes, and optic atrophy as well as lactic and pyruvic acidemia had excessive slow waves on her EEG. This child also had poorly formed visual evoked responses in keeping with her marked optic atrophy (163). A 23-month-old infant with hypotonia, sparse hair, labored respirations, and a history of generalized convulsions had widespread mild abnormalities on the EEG, but no paroxysmal activity. An electroretinogram was normal in this child, but visual evoked responses showed reduced amplitude of the early components. This patient also had severe partial hearing loss (163). An infant who presented at 6 months of age with the clinical picture of Leigh syndrome, displayed brief periods of diffuse slow wave activity during episodes of lethargy and acidosis (144).

Neuroimaging. A single report of calcification of the basal ganglia in the absence of neurologic signs and symptoms of basal ganglial disease was reported (161) in a 26-month-old female infant with biotinidase deficiency. Calcification on CT scan was punctate and diffuse. The MRI brain scan was interpreted as showing mild heterogeneity in the cerebral white matter on T2-weighted images, but this was believed to be within the range of normal. A review of CT brain scans reported in the literature in 6 other patients ranging in age from 4 weeks to 36 months reported that 2 were normal, 1 showed cerebral edema, 1 patient had a right parietal cyst, and 2 demonstrated diffuse cortical atrophy with decreased attenuation of the white matter. One patient with a normal CT also had a normal MRI brain scan (161). In no patient has cerebellar pathology been defined by neuroimaging despite the pathologic data suggesting that the cerebellum may demonstrate vermian atrophy and pyramidal cell loss in biotinidase deficiency. In addition, the prominent finding of ataxia has no obvious correlate on neuroimaging studies. It should be noted, however, that to date MRI scan data are incomplete. One patient presenting at 6 months with signs and symptoms similar to Leigh syndrome had diffuse cortical atrophy, but no changes in the basal ganglia (144); however, another child with this presentation had a normal CT brain scan at 12 months, but by 21 months the CT showed symmetrical hypodense areas adjacent to the third ventricle, in the hypo-

thalamus, the rostral pons, and the lamina quadrigemina (145).

Neuropathology. Little information is available about pathologic changes in biotinidase deficiency. An autopsy carried out on a 3 1/2-year-old child with probable biotinidase deficiency showed superior cerebellar vermian atrophy with virtually complete loss of the Purkinje cell layer and moderate gliosis in the white matter of the cerebellum and dentate nuclei. In addition, there was a subacute necrotizing myelopathy. The thalamus had perivascular cuffing of lymphocytes and proliferation of microglia (164). An infant who died at 3 months of age was found to have focal areas of vacuolization and gliosis in the white matter of the cerebral cortex and cerebellum, as well as dysmyelination. Mild gliosis was found in the hippocampal pyramidal cell layer, and evidence of viral encephalopathy was found in the putamen and caudate nucleus (165). A patient who died with the clinical picture of Leigh syndrome had brain pathology of subacute necrotizing encephalopathy with the addition of extensive white-matter spongiform changes and mammillary body involvement (145).

Pathophysiology

Neurologic symptoms are a prominent feature of biotinidase deficiency, and a number of reports have documented elevated concentrations of lactate and pyruvate in the CSF in patients demonstrating neurologic signs and symptoms. This may be found often despite normal blood levels of lactate and pyruvate and the absence of systemic acidosis (162,166–169). Studies of the pattern of organic acids in CSF demonstrate that lactate is elevated preferentially with trace levels of other organic acids found (167). In a later report on another patient, propionate was elevated in parallel with lactate, but other organic acids were not detected (162). This implies that pyruvate carboxylase is the enzyme predominantly affected in the brain in biotinidase deficiency. CSF amino acids were consistent with citric acid cycle depletion, demonstrating low levels of aspartate, glutamate, and glutamine in one patient (167).

Both human and rat brains have much lower biotinidase activity than serum or other tissues. It seems likely that the brain is very inefficient at recycling biotin and thus dependent on biotin transferred across the blood-brain barrier. CSF levels of biotin are 20% of plasma. Biotinidase levels in CSF are 0.01 that in serum. The susceptibility of the human brain to biotinidase deficiency suggests that much of the neurologic symptomatology may be related to accumulation of lactate. Blood flow in the cerebellum is normally 50% of that in other parts of the brain, and for this reason the cerebellum may be more susceptible to local accumulation of toxic metabolites in biotinidase deficiency (170).

Biocytin, the lysine-conjugated form of biotin resulting from carboxylase degradation, accumulates in biotinidase deficiency. This will occur whether or not biotin treatment is available. Biocytin was found in the urine of six patients with biotinidase deficiency; whereas, this material is normally undetectable (171). The idea that biocytin accumulation itself might be responsible for neurologic symptoms has been suggested. Biocytin might compete with biotin itself for sites on carboxylase proteins (172). Because optic atrophy and auditory nerve damage do not improve with biotin treatment of biotinidase deficiency, there is a possibility that biocytin accumulation is responsible for these lesions. As noted, however, biocytin continues to accumulate in biotinidase deficiency. It is not yet clear whether hearing and visual acuity continue to deteriorate in patients treated with adequate quantities of biotin. They certainly have been seen mostly in untreated patients. The possible toxic effect of biocytin remains speculative.

Biochemical Characteristics

The definitive diagnosis of biotinidase deficiency requires the assay of biotinidase activity. This is most readily available as an assay of plasma activity; however, fibroblast biotinidase activity can also be measured. Patients with biotinidase deficiency display normal activity of fibroblast carboxylases whether or not there is biotin in the medium. This has been used to discriminate the disorder from holocarboxylase synthetase deficiency in which low carboxylase activities are found in fibroblasts grown in biotin-deficient media. Carboxylase measurements in freshly isolated lymphocytes are low in biotinidase deficiency, and they become normal when treatment with biotin is initiated.

Biotinidase may be assayed in serum, liver, or cultured fibroblasts (157,173,174). The usual method assesses the cleavage of the artificial substrate N-biotinyl-3-aminobenzoate (173). A radiochemical assay for the cleavage of the natural substrate is available (175). A screening program has been developed suitable for spots of dried blood on filter paper (176).

The pattern of urinary excretion of organic acids is similar in both biotinidase deficiency and holocarboxylase synthetase deficiency. Lactic aciduria occurs along with the excretion of 3-hydroxyisovaleric acid, 3-hydroxypropionic acid, 3-methylcrotonyl glycine, and methylcitric acid. Blood concentrations of lactate, pyruvate, and alanine are elevated, although they may be normal, particularly in the early stages of the disease. CSF lactate and pyruvate may be elevated even when the plasma is normal (145,162, 167,177).

Genetics

Current estimates of prevalence are 1 in 60,000 births. Genetic transmission is autosomal recessive. Parents have approximately 50% of normal activity of biotinidase (173). Prenatal diagnosis should be possible.

Treatment

Patients with biotinidase deficiency require lifelong supplementation with biotin. The usual dose is 10 to 20 mg/day. Biotin supplementation improves all symptoms apart from auditory nerve and optic nerve injury, which seems irreversible. Organic aciduria disappears. There is, however, evidence that physiologic supplementation may not be adequate in some patients with biotinidase deficiency (166).

Other Causes of Multiple Carboxylase Deficiency

Biotin deficiency can result from parenteral nutrition with biotin preparations or faddish ingestion of raw egg. The resulting pattern of ketoacidosis and organic acid excretion is similar to that of multiple carboxylase deficiency. An erythematous skin rash and alopecia develop. The avidin in raw egg complexes with biotin, preventing its absorption. Patients have been described in whom there was no evidence of nutritional compromise and yet they did not fit the categories of holocarboxylase synthetase deficiency or biotinidase deficiency. A 30-year-old woman presented with a gradual onset of ataxia, deafness, myoclonus, seizures, and a right hemiparesis; her EEG showed mild, diffuse slowing and the MRI head scan was normal (168). This patient also developed sensorineural deafness and hypotonia. Arterial pH and lactate levels were normal. CSF levels were not checked; however, the urine showed the typical excretion pattern of multiple carboxylase deficiency. Fibroblast carboxylase activities were normal, but so was biotinidase activity. This patient responded to biotin treatment, and deteriorated whenever treatment was interrupted. The underlying metabolic defect in such patients remains obscure.

3-Oxothiolase Deficiency

3-Oxothiolase, also called beta-ketothiolase, is now known to represent a generic term for a group of different enzymes. Most patients who have been described with 3-oxothiolase deficiency are in fact suffering from deficiency of a potassium-dependent mitochondrial thiolase, 2-methylacetoacetyl CoA thiolase. Other thiolase deficiencies known to cause human disease include mitochondrial acetoacetyl CoA thiolase and cytosolic acetoacetyl CoA thiolase. The nervous system is variably affected in this group of disorders.

Clinical and Neurologic Features

The presentation varies from a neonatal severe ketoacidosis with hyperglycinemia and hyperammonemia, through episodic ketoacidosis manifesting in infancy or childhood, to asymptomatic individuals. There may be severe psychomotor retardation, although in most described patients, normal psychomotor development occurs when a low-protein diet has been instituted. The severe neonatal presentation is clinically indistinguishable from other organic acidemias like propionic and methylmalonic acidemia. Two patients were described demonstrating the clinical heterogeneity of 3-oxothiolase deficiency (178). A 10-month-old was seen on the fourth admission for acidosis and dehydration and had three further hospital admissions for severe metabolic acidosis between 9 and 19 months of age. Three siblings of this Laotian child died of unknown causes before the age of 6 months. During episodes of acidosis, lethargy alternating with agitation was noted. Following diagnosis with an isoleucine challenge test, treatment with a low-protein diet of 1.7 g/kg/day at 19 months resulted in normal growth and development. A 7-year-old girl was seen with 14 previous admissions for vomiting and tachypnea due to severe metabolic acidosis. The first episode occurred at 16 months following the termination of breastfeeding. Seizures with fever occurred at 4 months of age, although an EEG was normal. Developmental milestones were delayed. Good head control was not achieved until the age of 7 months. This child did not sit until the age of 13 months nor walk until 2 1/2 years. At age 7 she was developmentally retarded and had an unstable gait tending to "throw out" her right leg. She was described as constantly in motion with some myoclonus, and she had a left extensor plantar response. Somatic growth parameters were normal (178). A child presenting at 1 year of age with diarrhea and persistent vomiting as well as hepatomegaly was found to have severe ketoacidosis and a spuriously elevated salicylate level due to high acetoacetate in the blood and urine. A sibling died 9 years earlier at 30 months of age during a similar episode. Despite the severity of disease, the proband's development was normal in the first year (179). An 8 1/2-year-old girl died of a congestive cardiomyopathy. She had pernicious vomiting in the neonatal period leading to a pyloromyotomy at 4 weeks of age. At 12 weeks, this child was hypotonic with marasmas and tachypneic along with thrombocytopenia, hyperglycinemia, and hyperammonemia. In addition, ketonuria was documented. Growth was normal when she was given 1.5 g/kg protein diet. This child demonstrated moderate developmental delay, however, with truncal ataxia and incoordination of fine motor movements (180). No other patients have been described with cardiomyopathy. A 10-month-old girl presented with vomiting, lethargy, and seizures associated with a fever. At age 2 she developed lethargy and a marked acidosis with hyperammonemia and hyperglycinemia. Treatment with a 1.5 g/kg/day low-protein diet resulted in normal psychomotor development at 10 years of age. The patient was at that time following her own self-selected, protein-restricted diet (181).

A history of sibling death is common in patients with oxothiolase deficiency, and this highlights the potential severity of this defect in isoleucine metabolism. Diagnosis of this entity can be difficult because the characteristic urine metabolites may be present in small quantities or undetectable between bouts of ketoacidosis (178).

Detailed electrophysiologic, neuroimaging, and pathologic data are not available in this condition. The pathophysiology of CNS damage is unclear, but most likely episodes of severe acidosis and hyperammonemia are the major causes of CNS damage and subsequent psychomotor delay. Many patients are intellectually and neurologically normal following the introduction of a low-protein diet and the cessation of episodes of metabolic decompensation, implying that the enzyme defect itself does not compromise CNS function.

Biochemical Characteristics

The fundamental defect is in the mitochondrial thiolase 2-methylacetoacetyl CoA thiolase, which catalyzes the conversion of this CoA containing product of isoleucine to acetyl CoA and propionyl CoA. The enhancement of activity by potassium is a distinguishing property of this thiolase. The defect is measurable in cultured fibroblasts. Heterogeneity has been observed in that some patients have had virtually no activity whereas others have had as much as 10% of normal activity (178).

Genetics

Genetic transmission is that of an autosomal-recessive trait. Heterozygotes can be detected by enzymatic analysis of cultured fibroblasts (182). Prenatal diagnosis should be possible by assay of the enzyme in cultured amniocytes or GCMS assay for 2-methyl-3-hydroxybutyric acid (183).

Treatment

A diet low in protein appears to be effective. As a consequence of the metabolic block, 2-methylacetate accumulates, but little of this compound is found in the urine. Instead, 2-methyl-3-hydroxybutyric acid and tiglylglycine are the characteristic metabolites (184,185). Unfortunately, these compounds may be masked in the presence of ketosis and may disappear from the urine during periods of wellness (178). An isoleucine challenge test with 100 mg/kg of oral isoleucine followed by an 8-hour urine collection will help in the diagnosis of such patients.

Glutaric Aciduria Type I

This disorder, first described in 1975 (186), displays some clinical heterogeneity, but the phenotype of clinically affected individuals is typically that of a degenerative neurologic disease with an evolving choreoathetoid movement disorder and intellectual impairment in most cases. This autosomal-recessive disorder is due to a specific defect in glutaryl CoA dehydrogenase in the final common pathway of the metabolism of lysine, tryptophan, and hydroxylysine. Glutaric aciduria type II (GA II) is the result of a different metabolic defect that in a number of cases has been found to be due to electron transport factor (ETF) deficiency, or ETF dehydrogenase deficiency, which results in an effective deficiency of a number of acyl CoA dehydrogenases affecting the metabolism of fatty acids, valine, leucine, and isoleucine. In GA II choreoathetosis resulting from basal ganglia damage may also be observed. The phenotype is variable, however. Although glutaric acid is excreted in both types of glutaric acidurias, levels are lower in GA II, and dicarboxylic acids are prominent. GA II is described under the heading Defects of electron transport complexes.

Clinical and Neurologic Features

The first two patients described with Glutaric Aciduria Type I (GA I) were male and female siblings who developed irritability and motor developmental delay at 3 months and 7 months of age, respectively. The more severely affected, the girl, had generalized spasticity without head control, and she could not roll over at 1 year of age. Her brother had similar symptoms at 2 years. By 7 years of age he had developed dystonia with athetosis, facial grimacing, and opisthotonos. These patients appeared mentally retarded; however, subsequent clinical descriptions suggest that mental retardation may be an inconstant feature difficult to assess in many patients with severe motor disability, as well as choreoathetosis and dysarthria. One patient was described in whom progressive athetoid cerebral palsy was associated with an apparently normal intellect (187). The parents were first cousins. This child had developmental delay, he walked at the age of 2 years and had mild ataxia; his brother seemed to have normal development, and walked at 14 months of age. Soon thereafter, the brother developed seizures and an encephalitis-like condition along with petechial rash and coma. By 18 months of age, this child had developed choreiform movements of the arms and neck muscles and could neither sit nor stand. He deteriorated neurologically and developed dystonic extensor and flexor spasms particularly on the left. At the age of 4 years he could say only a few words, but was thought to be intellectually normal. His brother developed increasing choreiform movements, but appeared intellectually normal and does well in school. Both children, in addition to glutaric acid, had elevated levels of beta-hydroxyglutaric acid as well as glutaconic acid, mild hyperglycinemia, and the presence of alpha-aminoadipic acid in the urine. These latter two compounds were not detected in the first cases described (186). A number of cases have been described with bilateral subdural hygromas. There is often marked fluid accumulation in the temporal regions resembling schizencephaly (188–190). This has been accompanied by macrocephaly at birth and raises the question of prenatal neuronal injury in this disorder. In addition to the clinical picture of choreoathetosis, patients are often described as hyperkinetic. One 3 1/2-year-old female was reported who had temporary adrenocortical insufficiency presenting with hypoglycemia (188). The dramatic picture of progressive choreoathetosis with dystonia has prompted the question as to whether the entity known variously as infantile striatal necrosis, familial holotopistic striatal necrosis, or familial striatal degeneration is in fact GA I (191). An encephalitic-like picture with rapid onset of coma has been described in two patients, and one child died with a clinical course similar to Reye syndrome (192). GA I may resemble Leigh encephalopathy (193). It is easy to see how the diagnosis of GA I could be missed in a child diagnosed with athetoid cerebral palsy. The diagnosis will be extremely difficult in the occasional GA I patient with normal urinary organic acids (194).

Electrophysiology. EEG findings reported in patients with GA I are often normal, although patients with acute encephalopathy have generalized slowing. Following recovery from this acute episode, the EEG may normalize, as was the case in a 24-month-old who, on recovery from his second viral-like illness associated with severe lethargy and vomiting, was found to have hypotonia, dystonia, and choreoathetosis. The follow-up EEG was normal, although an EEG during his initial episode of coma at 11 months of age was slow. This patient was also found to have a normal electromyogram, nerve conduction velocities, and brain stem auditory evoked responses (195). The EEG may show epileptiform discharges even in the absence of clinical seizures although this is infrequently reported (196). Despite bilateral frontotemporal fluid collections and the later development of cortical atrophy with gliosis of the basal ganglia, the EEG was normal in one 8-month-old child with GA I (189).

Neuroimaging. The CT brain scan is usually abnormal in patients with GA I. Cortical atrophy with gyral widening and mild ventriculomegaly may be apparent very early in the course of the disease. A number of patients have been described with marked fluid collections in the region of the sylvian fissures and over the frontal cortex, leading to a diagnosis of subdural hygroma (188,189). It has been reported from studies of serial CT brain scans that within days of appearance of symptoms, atrophy of frontal and the anterior aspect of the temporal lobes can be noted. With these early changes, basal ganglia appear normal on CT scan. Atrophic changes of this sort have also been noted in an asymptomatic child with typical urinary changes and proved enzyme defect (190). Decreased attenuation in putamen and caudate nuclei may be seen, and later on caudate atrophy can be defined by CT. Signal changes on MRI scan may be seen in the caudate nucleus prior to atrophy (195).

Pathology. In most cases, the liver shows microvesicular fatty infiltration. In addition, the myocardium and proximal renal tubules may show similar changes (192,197). In two severely affected 1-year-old patients, basal ganglia changes were minimal, but in a 3-year-old and 10-year-old patient, gliosis in the caudate and putamen was marked with extensive neuronal loss (192,198). Spongy degeneration of cortical white matter has also been reported.

Glutaric acid accumulation has been found in the brain, liver, kidneys, skeletal, and cardiac muscle (192,198). In one patient, gamma-aminobutyric acid (GABA) levels were measured and found to be very low in the caudate and putamen. There was extensive neuronal necrosis and low levels of glutamate decarboxylase (GAD) in these areas (198).

Pathophysiology

The mechanism of brain damage in patients with GA I is not known; however, a number of hypotheses relate to the toxicity of metabolites that accumulate in glutaric aciduria. Absent or very low glutaryl CoA dehydrogenase activity is found in all tissues studied including the brain in GA I. 3-Hydroxyglutarate and glutaconic acid accumulate along with glutaric acid. Accumulation of these organic acids may result in nonspecific mitochondrial injury. This mechanism is thought to underlie the microvesicular fat accumulation in liver and other tissues. The basal ganglia are known to be particularly sensitive to mitochondrial dysfunction. Preferential damage in this area occurs in other disorders, such as Leigh syndrome and carbon monoxide intoxication, in which oxidative metabolism is compromised.

The therapeutic effects of a GABA agonist 4-amino-3-(4-chlorophenol)butyric acid (baclofen) and the decreased GAD and GABA concentrations measured in the striatum in one patient (198) may provide an explanation of selective caudate and putamen toxicity. The pathologic picture is similar to Huntington chorea. All three of the organic acids shown to accumulate in tissue in GA I are competitive inhibitors of GAD. This may have a significant effect on GABA synthesis. Other plausible hypotheses postulate an effect of glutaric acid on glutamate receptors including the NMDA receptor. Quinolinic acid, an intermediate in tryptophan metabolism, may accumulate in GA I. This compound is an effective neurotoxin.

Biochemical Characteristics

The basic defect is in the enzyme glutaryl CoA dehydrogenase (199). The defect is demonstrable in leukocytes and cultured fibroblasts as well as in liver (199–201). Heterogeneity has been demonstrated in that some patients have no evident activity whereas others have had some; the latter appear to be less severely affected (200).

The diagnosis is usually made on the basis of finding large amounts of glutaric acid in the urine on analysis of organic acids (186). These patients also excrete 3-hydroxyglutaric and glutaronic acids in the urine (196). In some, concentrations of glycine and 2-aminoadipate were elevated (196).

Genetics

Genetic inheritance is an autosomal-recessive trait. Prenatal diagnosis is possible by direct GCMS assay of glutaric acid in the amniotic fluid (202,203).

Treatment

Most patients are managed with a low-protein diet with particular restriction of lysine. There is good evidence that glutaric acid and excretion of other metabolites fall rapidly with this therapy. A number of patients have been reported to improve clinically somewhat on this treatment, but riboflavin has been reported to have a more pronounced effect. In unblinded studies three children with typical disease were treated with a diet low in lysine and tryptophan. This resulted in an improvement in motor ability and a decrease in hyperkinesia, with improvement in urinary metabolites. Symptoms improved considerably, however, with the addition of riboflavin. Dosages of riboflavin between 100 and 300 mg/day are utilized. Some patients have not responded to riboflavin treatment (193,197). Biotin, thiamine, and pyridoxine supplementation were reported to have no effect in three patients (200). Low carnitine levels can be improved with L-carnitine supplementation, and by analogy, with the treatment of other organic acidemias, L-carnitine may prove clinically helpful. In one patient with a picture of progressive dystonic static encephalopathy associated with basal ganglia degeneration, riboflavin and L-carnitine therapy produced modest clinical improvement and biochemical improvement. GABA levels in the CSF increased on this therapy (195). Several authors have reported beneficial effects with the GABA agonist baclofen (188,189,200). Irritability, temper tantrums, sleeplessness, dystonia, and choreoathetosis have all apparently responded to baclofen treatment in a few patients.

LACTIC ACIDEMIA

The lactic acidemias, as a group, comprise the most common of the organic acidemias in childhood. Lactic acid is the end product of glycolysis when further oxidative metabolism is impaired. Some tissues lacking mitochondria (red cells) or with few mitochondria (white blood cells, fast twitch muscle fibers, renal medulla) produce lactic acid. Lactic acid is the physiologic product of glucose metabolism and accumulates when production exceeds utilization.

Brain itself produces some lactate, and in some neonatal animals the CNS is able to use lactate efficiently as a substrate (5). The brain is highly dependent on oxidative metabolism for normal function. The accumulation of lactic acid implies a defect in mitochondrial oxidative metabolism that compromises brain function, particularly in areas such as the basal ganglia, which have very high metabolic rates. In many patients with lactic acidemia, the CNS bears the brunt of the disease process. Increasingly, patients are recognized in whom CSF lactate and pyruvate are elevated despite only minimal changes in the concentration in blood. This observation highlights the sensitivity of the brain to oxidative defects and the relative inability of the brain (outside of the neonatal period) to metabolize lactate. Lactic acid accumulation is toxic to nervous tissue, and areas with poor blood flow may be particularly sensitive to the effects of lactic acid accumulation, providing one explanation for the differential pathology seen in the lactic acidemias (5).

Lactic acidosis may be physiologic or pathologic. In the pathologic group suffering from inborn errors of metabolism, despite extensive investigation, more than 60% of the patients remain undiagnosed. This large group of idiopathic lactic acidemias remains a challenging problem for diagnosticians and biochemists. It is likely that many patients are suffering from as yet undefinable defects in electron transport. The problem is compounded by the fact that patients with defects in oxidative metabolism may have only mild or intermittent elevations in pyruvate and lactate. The lactate/pyruvate ratio in the blood or CSF may be helpful in identifying abnormalities in the mitochondrial and cytoplasmic NADH/NAD ratio or the redox state. NADH accumulation and thus a high lactate/pyruvate ratio is often seen in defects of the electron transport chain.

The comprehensive evaluation of a patient with lactic acidemia requires the exclusion of secondary and often treatable causes of lactic acidemia. Comprehensive quantitative organic acid analysis in the urine is the major tool for the exclusion of secondary causes of lactic acidemia. Beyond this testing, the evaluation of a lactic acidemic patient requires inpatient study, with an evaluation of the response to fasting and to various carbohydrate challenges. Skin biopsy for fibroblast culture and muscle biopsy are usually necessary. Figure 3.4 details the flow chart approach utilized at the University of California, San Diego for the investigation of patients with lactic acidemia.

A number of clinical syndromes associated with lactate and pyruvate accumulation have been defined. Several biochemical defects have been described in various patients presenting with each of these clinical manifestations. The most common presentations are: (1) severe neonatal or infantile lactic acidemia; (2) Leigh subacute necrotizing

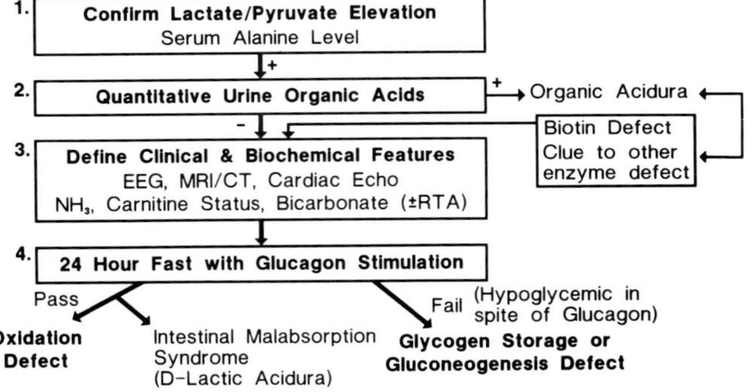
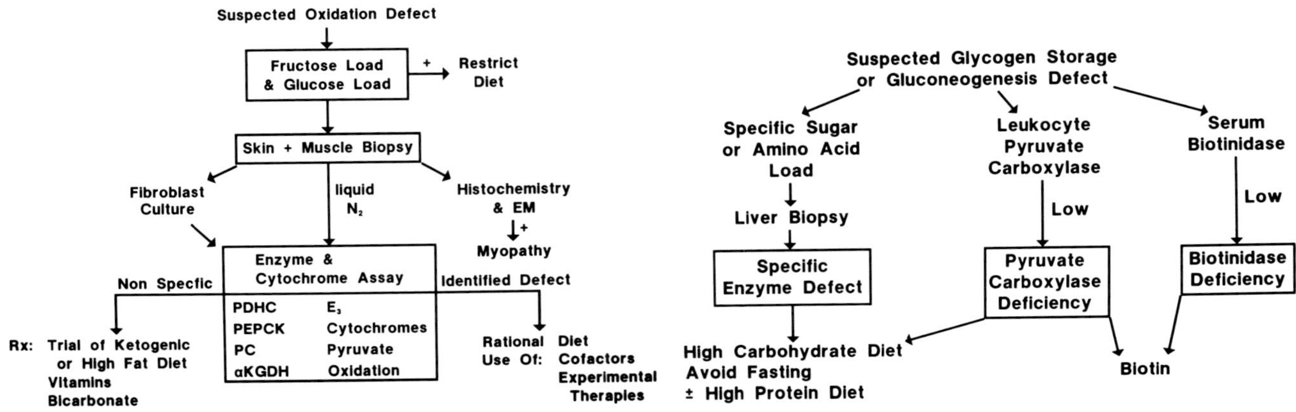

FIGURE 3.4 Flow chart used at the University of California, San Diego for the comprehensive evaluation of primary and secondary causes of lactic acidemia.

encephalomyelopathy; (3) psychomotor delay with static or progressive (i.e., poliodystrophy) CNS disease; (4) intermittent ataxia often with a slow spinocerebellar-type degenerative picture; (5) mitochondrial encephalomyopathies, including mitochondrial encephalomyopathy with lactic acidosis and stroke-like episodes (MELAS), myoclonic epilepsy with ragged red fibers (MERRF), and Kearns-Sayre syndrome; and (6) mitochondrial myopathy.

Because of the biochemical and clinical heterogeneity of the lactic acidemias, along with the striking overlap of different biochemical etiologies with similar clinical pictures, the investigation of lactic acidemia requires a comprehensive approach such as that detailed in Figure 3.4.

Primary Oxidative Defects: Pyruvate Dehydrogenase Deficiency

The pyruvate dehydrogenase (PDH) enzyme is a complex of three major subunits termed E_1, E_2, and E_3. This configuration is common to all three keto acid dehydrogenases, pyruvate dehydrogenase, oxoglutarate dehydrogenase, and branched-chain ketoacid dehydrogenase. The E_3 enzyme is common to all three enzyme complexes, whereas E_2 and E_1 differ. In the case of PDH and the branched-chain keto acid dehydrogenase, E_1 is known to consist of two alpha and two beta subunits. The complexity of the PDH complex goes further in that there are two other important enzymes, a phosphatase, which activates the E_1 enzyme by dephosphorylation, and kinase, which inactivates E_1 by phosphorylation. Similar phosphorylation and dephosphorylation occur with the branched-chain keto acid dehydrogenase. In all cases of human PDH deficiency that have been described, the brain is involved. Patients with E_1 deficiency, E_1 phosphatase deficiency, and E_3 deficiency have all been described. Most of the defined patients have had apparent E_1 deficiency. Indeed, the first patient described with PDH deficiency who presented with intermittent ataxia associated with lactic and pyruvic acidosis was thought to have E_1 deficiency (204). The original PDH assays used by various investigators were suboptimal, but more recent methods for studying fibroblast and tissue PDH activity are much more reliable (205–207). A significant problem still exists, however, in the assay of E_1 activity with ferricyanide, as this assay measures only 0.5% to 1% of the total enzyme activity. Thus E_1 assays should be viewed as indicating the possible site of PDH defect only. The extensive literature reporting E_1 deficiency should be considered with this in mind (Figure 3.5).

In a review of the literature and 30 personal cases, Robinson et al. (207) reported on the clinical phenotype of 54 patients with apparent E_1 deficiency. In general, patients with more severe PDH deficiency have more severe disease. Twenty-five patients with total PDH activity averaging less than 22% of control have died. Thirteen of these had severe lactic acidosis in the neonatal period or the first few months of life and died before 6 months of age. Four of these patients had agenesis of the corpus callosum. The other 12 patients died between the ages of 10 months and 3 years, and this group generally had the clinical and pathologic features of Leigh syndrome.

Living patients with apparent E_1 deficiency and psychomotor retardation accounted for 23 of the total 54 patients (207). Clinical and neuroradiologic features varied from an apparent static or slowly progressive encephalopathy to Leigh syndrome. This group had an average PDH activity of 31.6% of control. Six patients were reported with ataxia and intermittent lactic and pyruvic acidosis. All of these patients were male, and one was the original patient, B.R., described in 1970 (204), who, at the age of 28 years, is a computer programmer with intermittent ataxic symptoms and neurologic findings compatible with a very slowly progressive spinocerebellar degeneration.

Patients with pyruvate dehydrogenase phosphatase deficiency have rarely been reported (211,212). The clinical presentation is varied from severe lactic acidosis in infancy to Leigh syndrome, which was the presentation in three of four patients. Lipoamide dehydrogenase deficiency, or E_3 deficiency, has been reported in six patients (213,214). All had evidence of multiple oxoacid dehydrogenase deficiency with deficiency of PDH, 2-oxoglutarate dehydrogenase and 2-oxo branched-chain dehydrogenase deficiency. Urine organic acids may show a picture of branched-chain amino acid accumulation similar to very mild maple syrup urine disease, and patients generally have moderately severe lactic acidemia. Autopsy data have shown focal involvement of the brain stem and basal ganglia with neuronal and myelin loss (213,214). At least one patient with E_3 deficiency has responded to treatment with oral lipoic acid (215).

Leigh Syndrome

Subacute necrotizing encephalomyelopathy (Leigh syndrome) was first described in 1951 (208), and an excellent review of the clinical features has been published (209). The disorder is usually manifested during the end of the 1st year of life, with failure to thrive and developmental delay. Lactic and pyruvic acidemia are usually present, although elevations may be marginal. Patients may either deteriorate rapidly or follow a course of episodic deterioration, usually associated with infection and metabolic acidosis. Dystonia is common, and later in the course of the disease quadriparetic spasticity is usual. A mixed seizure disorder is common. Patients may display tonic-clonic, myoclonic, and absence seizures as well as akinetic attacks. As the disease progresses, brain stem signs and symptoms become prominent with the development of abnormalities of eye movements and central respiratory failure. Patients often die from apnea. The CT brain scan often shows decreased attenuation of the basal ganglia (210), which is later followed by generalized cortical atrophy and may be accompanied by blotchy areas of low density within the cortex. A typical MRI brain scan is shown in Figure 3.6, the pathologic specimen of brain sectioned at a similar level is also depicted. Pathologically, findings are very similar to Wernicke encephalopathy with capillary proliferation, gliosis, and neuronal loss in affected brain areas. Patients generally succumb within 2 to 3 years of diagnosis, although long-term survivors are common and a few adult patients have been described. The clinical heterogeneity of Leigh syndrome is matched by biochemical heterogeneity. As many as 25% of patients, however, may suffer from PDH deficiency. In addition, patients with cytochrome c oxidase deficiency appear to form another large group. Pyruvate carboxylase deficiency and electron transport chain defects other than cytochrome c oxidase have also been described.

Primary Oxidative Defects: Pyruvate Carboxylase Deficiency

Pyruvate carboxylase (PC) is an important intramitochondrial enzyme generally considered to be the flux-generating

step in gluconeogenesis, as well as a source of 4-carbon skeletons for the citric acid cycle. Pyruvate carboxylase is composed of four identical subunits, each of which covalently binds a biotin molecule that is an essential cofactor. Thus, in multiple carboxylase deficiency due to holocarboxylase synthetase deficiency and in biotinidase deficiency, there is deficient activity of pyruvate carboxylase, and this is particularly important for the brain. Acetyl CoA is an allostearic activator, and a high ATP/ADP ratio also encourages PC activity. Although the highest PC activity is in the liver and kidney, evidence of selectively elevated lactate and pyruvate in the CSF in multiple carboxylase deficiency suggests an important role for PC in the CNS. Its synthetic role is particularly important for the developing brain.

Clinical and Neurologic Features

The first description of PC deficiency in 1968 suggested this abnormality might be the cause of the Leigh syndrome phenotype (216). Three subsequent reports also found PC deficiency in individual patients with Leigh syndrome

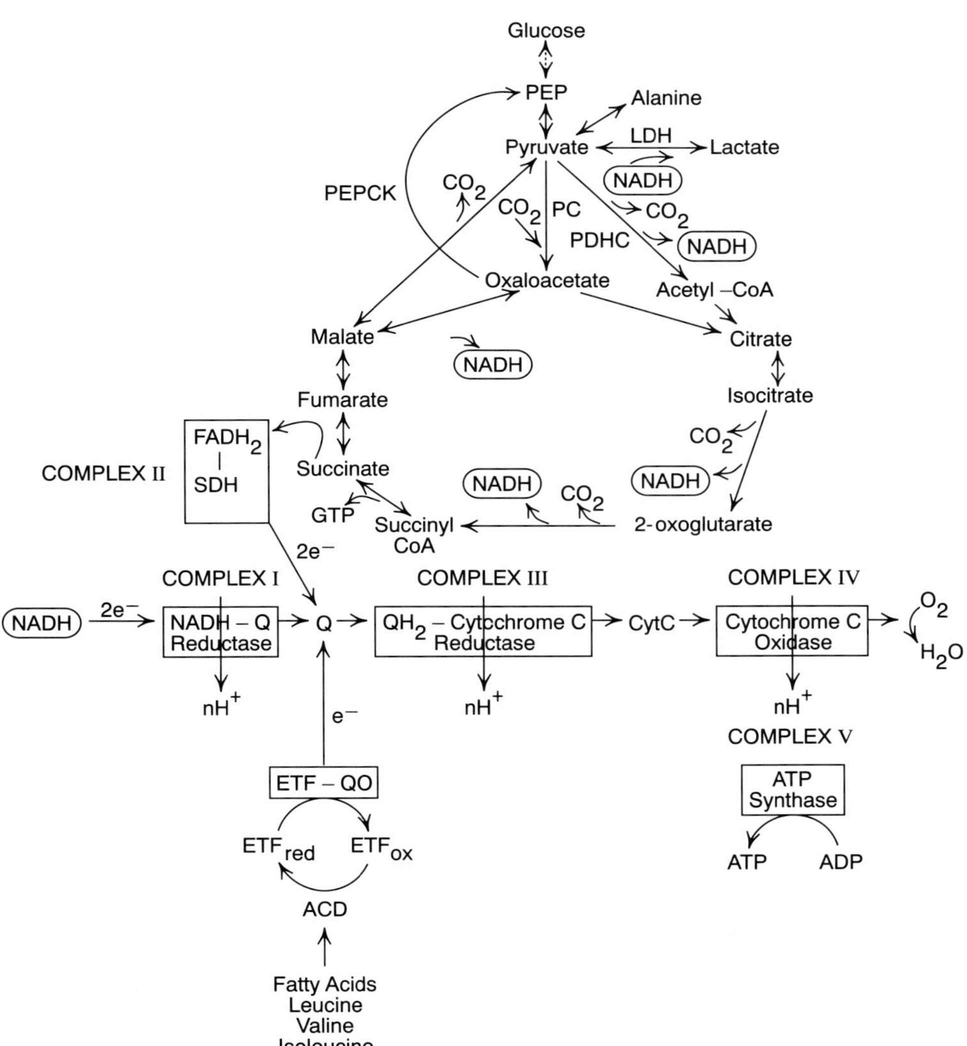

FIGURE 3.5 Overview of oxidative metabolism: PEPCK, phosphoenolpyruvate carboxykinase; LDH, lactic dehydrogenase; PDHC, pyruvate dehydrogenase complex; PC, pyruvate carboxylase; SDH, succinic dehydrogenase: Q, Coenzyme Q10; ETFQO, Electron Transfer Factor coenzyme Q oxidoreductase; ACD, mitochondrial acyl CoA dehydrogenases.

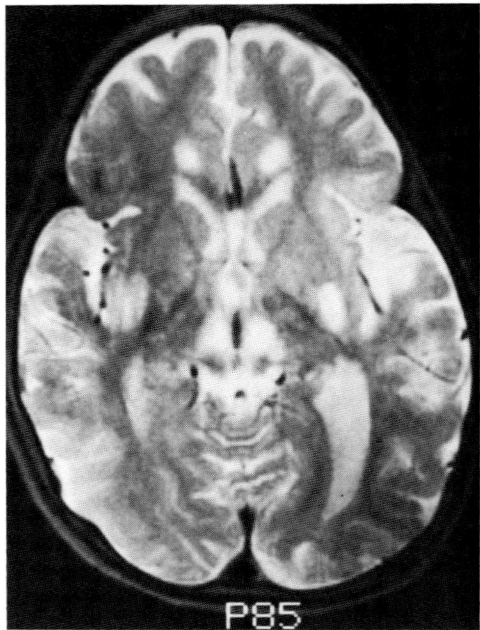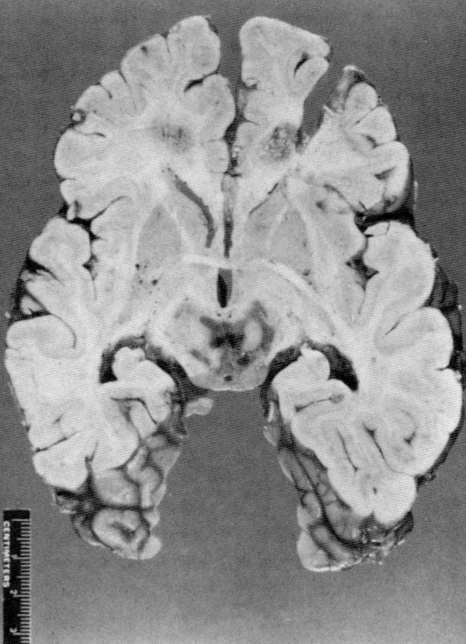

FIGURE 3.6 T2-weighted MRI brain scan of a 2-year-old child with Leigh syndrome (left) with an autopsy specimen of the patient at a similar level (right). Necrotic lesions in deep frontal areas, putamina, thalami, and upper brainstem (sparing the red nuclei) correspond with areas of high T2 MRI signal. There is generalized brain atrophy.

(217–219). In one of these, the E_1 component of pyruvate dehydrogenase was deficient along with an apparent reduction in liver and brain PC activity to 30% of control. These earlier reports are now considered misleading because of the instability of PC in autopsy material. In two cases, antemortem liver biopsy revealed normal PC activity, but reduced levels were found in autopsy material in the same patients (220,221). In studies of liver biopsies in 6 patients with Leigh syndrome and fibroblast assays on 5, PC activity was found to be normal, apart from 1 case in which citrate synthetase was reduced along with PC, suggesting autolytic change (222). The development of a reproducible fibroblast assay for PC (223) has provided a better understanding of the clinical phenotype.

There are two well-documented phenotypes associated with PC deficiency. The severe neonatal manifestation has been reported from Europe. Patients present with severe lactic acidemia, citrullinemia, hyperlysinemia, and hyperammonemia (224–226). In addition, 2-oxoglutaric acid is elevated in urine, and alanine levels are high. All affected patients have died in the first 3 months of life. Patients with the neonatal presentation have elevated lactate/pyruvate ratios and elevated acetoacetate/beta-hydroxybutyrate ratios. These findings suggest a disparity between the mitochondrial and cytosolic redox states.

The juvenile presentation has largely been reported from North America, and most patients have been American Indians. The onset is in the first 6 months of life with episodes of metabolic acidosis caused by lactic acidemia. These are generally precipitated by infection. Patients have severe psychomotor retardation. One patient presented at 3 months of age with fever and tonic-clonic seizures that responded to phenobarbital (227). Between 5 and 9 months

of age, failure to thrive, developmental delay, and a persistent mild metabolic acidosis were noted. At 9 months of age, a bout of severe acidosis with lactic acidemia occurred; this child had proximal renal tubular acidosis. At 46 months, he was microcephalic and severely mentally retarded; he could not sit or feed himself, and he had no expressive language. There were brief sudden episodes of severe metabolic acidosis associated with tachypnea and blotchy cyanosis of the extremities. Glucose response to an alanine load was flat. Hypoglycemia occurred on fasting, associated with lactic acidosis. At autopsy, undetectable PC activity was found in the brain. Levels were 6% of normal in the liver and very low in the kidney. Subsequent studies of lymphocytes and fibroblasts in this patient confirmed PC deficiency (223). The juvenile presentation of PC deficiency has been reported by a number of authors (228–231). In one case, a child considered to have Alpers progressive infantile poliodystrophy was found to have low hepatic PC activity (232). The diagnosis was based only on autopsy material, and thus may be unreliable.

Little neurophysiologic and neuroimaging information is available in PC deficiency. A well-characterized child who died at 46 months of age demonstrated on EEG prominent theta waves and abnormal slow wave activity with abnormal photic stimulation. Nerve conduction velocities and EMG were normal (227). The autopsy findings of deficient myelination, cortical atrophy, and cystic degeneration in the cerebral cortex should be apparent on neuroimaging studies.

There is little information about therapy for PC deficiency. Treatment with biotin supplementation is logical. Because oxaloacetate and aspartate levels are thought to be low, treatment with aspartate has been used with some limited success in one patient (227).

Pathology.   Earlier reports link the pathologic findings of Leigh syndrome to PC deficiency, but as discussed earlier, this association cannot be considered confirmed. In a well-documented case of juvenile PC deficiency, autopsy was available following death at 46 months of age. Cortical atrophy was present with enlargement of the lateral ventricles. Decreased white matter, particularly apparent in the corpus callosum was observed, and symmetric, poorly formed myelin in the cerebellum and corona radiata was apparent. Severe depletion of neurons was observed in the cerebral cortex. Ectopic neurons were found in the white matter and ectopic glia in the subarachnoid space, suggesting effects of PC deficiency in the developing embryo. The liver showed some lipid accumulation, and on electron microscopy (EM) studies of a liver biopsy, hyperplasia of smooth endoplasmic reticulum with faintly osmophilic vacuoles containing granular material thought to be smooth endoplasmic reticulum was seen. There were increased glycogen and paracrystalline inclusions in mitochondria. Muscle obtained at biopsy showed increased lipid and rounding of type I and type II fibers. At autopsy, the kidneys showed diffuse tubular vacuolation, particularly prominent in the distal tubules (227).

Autopsies carried out in two patients with the neonatal presentation revealed poor myelination with cortical atrophy, astrocytic proliferation and gliosis, along with neuronal loss in the cerebral cortex (224,226). In the neonatal form, hepatomegaly is due to hepatocellular lipid accumulation. The child reported with Alpers disease had massive neuronal loss in the cerebral cortex with spongiform change and relative sparing of the white matter (232).

Pathophysiology

PC deficiency profoundly affects the brain. The mechanism is probably twofold. In the developing brain, the role of PC in providing citric acid cycle intermediates is important. Lactic and pyruvic acid accumulation occurs in PC deficiency. Local accumulation of lactic acid is toxic to the brain (7).

There is evidence that PC is predominantly associated with astrocytes (233). The concept that a small astrocytic synthetic compartment is important in the production of citric acid cycle intermediates that are secondarily taken up by neurons helps provide an explanation for amino acid changes reported in PC deficiency and the elevation of 2-oxoglutarate found in the urine of both neonatal and juvenile patients. Amino acid levels were measured in autopsy brain material from a juvenile PC patient who died at 3 years of age (234). Glutamine was greatly diminished in all brain regions. Glutamic acid and proline levels were elevated, and GABA was normal. CSF glutamine levels and plasma glutamine levels were decreased in four living patients who were studied (234). PC deficiency can be expected to produce low levels of oxaloacetate and aspartic acid, which will limit citric acid cycle activity producing profound effects on brain energy metabolism.

Biochemical Characteristics

The major consequences of the metabolic defect is the accumulation of lactic acid. Changes in oxaloacetate, oxoglutarate, and amino acids were considered in the preceding section. PC is a protein in which there are four identical subunits each containing a molecule of biotin attached to an epsilon-amino group of a lysine moiety. In the neonatal and juvenile patients described, levels of enzyme activity have been very low, generally less than 5%. An explanation for the phenotypic variation in PC deficiency comes from immunologic studies of the 125-KD band on electrophoresis, which corresponds to the subunits of pyruvate carboxylase (235,236). One group of patients presenting with the neonatal form of the disease have little or no immunoreactive protein; whereas, in the juvenile presentation the pyruvate carboxylase protein can be identified. Cultured fibroblasts of patients with the neonatal form also have absent PCmRNA (Sq1) (236,237). Partial cDNA clones for normal PC have been obtained (231,237,238).

Genetics

PC deficiency is apparently inherited as an autosomal-recessive trait. Heterozygote detection has not been established. Prenatal diagnosis of an affected fetus has been reported twice (239,240).

Treatment

There is little information about therapy and PC deficiency; however, treatment with biotin supplementation is logical. Oxaloacetate and aspartate levels are thought to be low, and treatment with aspartate has been used with some limited success in one patient (227).

Phosphoenolpyruvate Carboxykinase Deficiency

Phosphoenolpyruvate carboxykinase (PEPCK) is a gluconeogenetic enzyme located in both the cytosolic and mitochondrial compartments. In human fibroblasts, most PEPCK is mitochondrial, and thus patients with documented fibroblast PEPCK deficiencies have a predominant deficiency of the mitochondrial enzyme form. The clinical features of PEPCK deficiency are hepatomegaly and hypoglycemia with associated lactic acidosis and failure to thrive. Two patients described have suffered from hypertriglyceridemia and hypercholesterolemia (241,242). The first description of PEPCK-deficient patients was of two infants who died of uncontrollable hypoglycemia. PEPCK measurements on biopsied liver homogenates were the basis of the diagnosis. There were phenotypic differences in the two patients so far described with well-defined mitochondrial deficiency. In one, the clinical picture was that of a myopathy, with hypotonia and lactic acidemia; the patient survived to 10 years of age (242). The child more recently described died at 6 months of age following a more severe course with liver disease and peripheral edema as well as unexplained episodes of fever (243).

Citric Acid Cycle Defects

Two defined citric acid cycle enzymatic defects have been described. These are fumarase and 2-oxoglutarate dehydrogenase (KDH) deficiency. In addition, a number of patients have been described with ^{14}C-pyruvate oxidation defects, suggesting an abnormality in the citric acid cycle. Patients with both defined and undefined citric acid cycle defects have lactic acidemia and neurologic defects.

Fumarase Deficiency.   Fumarase is the citric acid cycle enzyme responsible for conversion of fumarate to malate. Cytosolic and mitochondrial enzymes exist; however, these two isoenzymes are very similar, and both may be products of the same autosomal gene located on the long arm of chromosome 1 (244). Fumarase deficiency was reported in an infant who died at 8 months of age with failure to thrive, hypotonia, and severe developmental delay (245). Cyanosis and hypothermia occurred on the 1st day of life. At 3 weeks of age, persistent vomiting produced dehydration and lactic acidosis (blood lactate 3.7 mM). By 3 months of age, microcephaly, lethargy alternating with extreme irritability, hypotonia, and hypoactive deep tendon reflexes with poor head control and grasp were present. At 6 months of age, following sepsis, opisthotonic posturing developed. The patient died at home at 8 months of age. Muscle and liver biopsies were obtained at the time of gastrostomy and fundoplication. Slight hepatocellular cytoplasmic vacuolation was seen. The muscle showed type I fiber predominance, and subsarcolemmal mitochondrial accumulation on electron microscopy. Electrophysiologic studies included EEG, which showed abnormal background rhythms with bitemporal spike wave discharges at 3 months of age. Visual evoked responses could not be demonstrated at 5 months. CT brain scans carried out at 3 weeks and at 3 months of age, demonstrated progressive diffuse cerebral atrophy.

Urinary organic acid analysis at 3 months of age showed elevation of fumarate, succinate, and citrate in the urine along with a mild dicarboxylic aciduria. Studies of oxidative metabolism in liver and muscle suggested impaired glutamate and succinate utilization by muscle mitochondria. Substrates were metabolized normally in the liver.

Extensive studies of mitochondrial enzymes were normal apart from fumarase, which was virtually absent in liver and muscle mitochondria and less than 5% in muscle and liver homogenates. These data suggested that the patient had deficiency of both cytosolic and mitochondrial fumarase.

A second patient with fumarase deficiency was the product of a first-cousin marriage. At 1 year of age, this male infant was microcephalic, hypotonic, and severely developmentally delayed. Like the first patient described, there were large amounts of succinate and fumarate in the urine, but this patient also had 2-oxoglutarate excretion (246). Two mentally retarded adults were described with fumaric acid accumulation in the urine; however, blood levels were normal in these patients, and a renal clearance abnormality was postulated. Fumarase activity was not measured.

2-Oxoglutarate Dehydrogenase Deficiency

Oxoglutarate dehydrogenase is a 3-component enzyme complex responsible for the conversion of oxoglutarate to succinyl CoA. Oxoglutarate dehydrogenase may be the flux-controlling step in the citric acid cycle in the brain. As in the case of the pyruvate dehydrogenase complex and branched-chain dehydrogenase, oxoglutarate dehydrogenase has E_1, E_2, and E_3 subunits. At present, there is no evidence, however, of regulation of the E_1 component of oxoglutarate dehydrogenase by phosphatase and kinase, the regulatory enzymes. The E_3 component (lipoamide dehydrogenase) is common to the three dehydrogenase enzymes, and thus E_3 deficiency affects all three enzymes (213,215,247). E_3 deficiency may be manifested as a variant form of maple syrup urine disease (214).

Oxoglutaric aciduria occurs commonly with urinary accumulation of other citric acid cycle intermediates in patients with mitochondrial encephalomyopathies and in particular those presenting with the clinical phenotype of Leigh syndrome. In addition, oxoglutarate is found in the urine when urinary tract infection allows bacterial production of the compound. In two siblings, an apparent isolated deficiency of oxoglutarate dehydrogenase was reported (248). The parents were first cousins. The manifestation was that of a degenerative neurologic disease with delayed early development. These affected children, a boy and girl, both developed the ability to walk unsteadily. By the age of 5 years, the boy was spastic and unable to walk; however, both children appeared to have normal intellect without loss of mentation. Urinary levels of oxoglutarate were markedly elevated in these patients, with mild lactic acidemia in one. Fibroblast oxoglutarate dehydrogenase complex activity was 30% of normal with apparently normal E_1 and E_3 activity.

Undefined Citric Acid Cycle Defects

The first patient described with an unlocalized citric acid cycle defect was reported in 1972 (249). This 3-year-old girl was the product of a consanguineous marriage, and a sibling had died in infancy. The patient was severely retarded, microcephalic, and hypotonic with hyperactive reflexes. She had optic atrophy, strabismus with nystagmoid movements, and ataxia. The palate was high-arched, and there were bilateral epicanthic folds. Despite the retardation and severe neurologic deficits, this girl had a vocabulary of 20 words. EEG was slow for her chronologic age. Urinalysis showed ketonuria and increased alanine, but organic acids were not measured. There was lactic and pyruvic acidemia. Studies in intact fibroblasts showed diminished oxidation of pyruvate, palmitate, and citrate, compared with controls, but isocitrate and glutamate were oxidized at a normal rate. Pyruvate dehydrogenase activity seemed low, although E_1 measurements were normal.

A 3 1/2-year-old child died with the clinical and pathologic findings of Alpers poliodystrophy (250). At 2 1/2 years of age, global development delay was noted. An EEG was normal. At 3 1/2 years a generalized seizure occurred; the child had hypotonia, weakness, areflexia, and almost continuous myoclonic seizure activity. Intermittent respiratory disturbance, and coma ensued, resulting in death from respiratory arrest. EEG showed severe background slowing with generalized and multifocal spike and sharp wave activity. Somatosensory evoked potentials in the median nerve showed normal peak latencies for the first complex, but marked delay in the secondary complex. Brain stem auditory evoked potentials were absent. Visual evoked responses were normal. Nerve conduction velocities and electromyogram were normal. The urine in this child showed an increase in 2-oxoglutarate, succinate, and lactate. There was lactate and pyruvic acidemia, and CSF lactate was elevated during coma with a high lactate/pyruvate ratio at that time. Studies of leukocytes, fibroblasts, and liver homogenate showed very low $^{14}CO_2$ production when $5\text{-}^{14}C$ 2-oxoglutarate was provided as substrate. Studies of other mitochondrial oxidative enzymes and cytochromes were normal. Pathologic findings were typical of Alpers poliodystrophy. There were multiple foci of spongy degeneration within the gray matter with relative sparing of the white matter. Extensive degeneration of the Purkinje cells in the cerebellum was noted. Neuronal loss and gliosis were found in the globus pallidus and some brain stem nuclei. EM studies showed mitochondrial swelling in neurons and astrocytes, but no specific abnormalities.

Four patients with lactic acidemia, but without organic aciduria, were reported in whom decreased oxidation of $3\text{-}^{14}C$ pyruvate to $^{14}CO_2$ was noted (251,252). Studies of pyruvate dehydrogenase and pyruvate carboxylase were normal. Three of these patients were developmentally delayed, two had seizures, and all were ataxic. Two pre-

sented in the 2nd year of life and the other two at 10 and 11 years, respectively.

Electron Transport Chain Defects

Mitochondrial Encephalomyopathy

This term was coined by Shapira (253) in 1977 to encompass a group of disorders in which multisystem disease produced mitochondrial dysfunction in the brain, skeletal muscle, and other organs. The original conditions grouped as mitochondrial encephalomyopathies included: Kearns-Sayre syndrome, Menkes syndrome, Alpers disease, Leigh syndrome, Zellweger disease, Canavan disease, and a small group of disorders characterized by encephalopathy, ragged red fibers (muscle), and apparent defects in the electron transport chain. Two disorders in the original classification were predominantly white-matter diseases: Zellweger disease, which results from an absence of peroxisomes (254), and Canavan disease, which is due to deficiency of the enzyme aspartoacylase (255). The eponymous names applied to these disorders reflected the clinical basis for identification and characterization. Over the past 12 years, considerable progress has been made in biochemical characterization of this group of disorders, although this has not simplified the field because different biochemical defects may underlie similar clinical presentations, and phenotypic variability is itself a hallmark of mitochondrial disease.

Many descriptions of ragged red fiber disease with encephalopathy have been published, and three main clinical phenotypes have emerged: mitochondrial encephalomyopathy with lactic acidosis and stroke-like episodes (MELAS), myoclonic epilepsy with ragged red fibers (MERRF), and Kearns-Sayre syndrome. Defects in the function of the electron transport chain appear to underlie the symptoms in all three of these disorders. An excellent review of the early characterization of these disorders is available (256), and the main features are listed in Table 3.4.

Mitochondrial Encephalomyopathy with Lactic Acidosis, and Stroke-like Episodes

The acronym MELAS was first suggested by Pavlakis et al. (257), who described two patients with normal early development, short stature, episodic vomiting and seizures, recurrent hemipareses, and hemianopia. These two children had partial defects of cytochrome c oxidase in muscle. It now seems, however, that most cases are related to complex I deficiencies (258,259).

Table 3.4 Spectrum of mitochondrial cytopathies with ragged red fibers and encephalopathy

	MELAS	*MERRF*	*Kearns-Sayre*	*Mixed*
Usual age onset	Teens	Teens	Teens	Early child-hood to adult
Probable inheritance	Maternal	Maternal	Sporadic	Various
Most common biochemical defect	Complex I	Complex IV t-RNA lysine defect	Mito DNA deletion	Various
Major discriminating features				
Episodic vomiting	+	−	−	+ / −
Stroke-like episodes	+	−	−	+ / −
Myoclonus	−	+	−	+ / −
Ophthalmoplegia	−	−	+	+ / −
Pigmentary retinopathy	−	−	+	+ / −
CSF protein > 100 mg/dL	−	−	+	+ / −
Heart block	−	−	+	+ / −
Other features				
Short stature	+	+	+	+ / −
Lactic acidemia	+	+	+ / −	+ / −
Cardiomyopathy	−	−	+	+ / −
Hepatomegaly	+ / −	+ / −	−	+ / −
Ataxia	+ / −	+	+	+
Sensorineural deafness	+ / −	+ / −	+	+ / −
Tonic-clonic seizures	+	+	+	+ / −

Clinical and Neurologic Features

In 1975, a brother and sister were described with what came to be known as the MELAS syndrome. Following a period of normal development the girl suffered episodes of vomiting and generalized weakness from the age of 6 years. These were followed by headaches, clonic seizures, and dementia together with episodes of hemiparesis at the age of 15 years. The proband died at the age of 16 years, and autopsy confirmed focal zones of softening in the cerebral cortex with ferrocalcific deposits in the globus pallidus and putamen. The brother suffered a more rapidly progressing similar disease with vomiting from the age of 4 years, weakness at the age of 8 years, seizures by the age of 9 years, and dementia and blindness just prior to death at the age of 10 years. A defect in mitochondrial oxidative metabolism was suspected. A similar case was described with autopsy confirmation of brain infarction (260).

A personal case typifies the more usual course of this condition. This boy was described at the age of 11 years (261) when he had presented with a 7-month history of pounding temporal headaches and visual obscurations. Apart from short stature, he was previously normal and a good student. At the initial evaluation, bilateral sensorineural hearing loss, horizontal nystagmus, palatal dysarthria, and a left-sided afferent pupillary defect were noted. The CT brain scan was normal. Right occipital slowing was present on the EEG; CSF lactate and pyruvate were elevated. Apparent resolution of symptoms with steroid treatment was followed by the development of generalized seizures, dementia, profound sensorineural deafness, and cortical blindness. A cardiomyopathy required treatment with digoxin and hydralazine. He died unexpectedly at the age of 18 years. His CT brain scan 2 years prior to death showed generalized cortical atrophy with extensive basal ganglia calcification and multifocal areas of cortical hypodensity (Figure 3.7).

The mode of inheritance was uncertain in three familial patients who developed symptoms of MELAS in adulthood. The male proband developed rapidly progressive disease following the onset of symptoms at 24 years of age. Multiple cortical infarctions, elevated CSF and serum lactate, seizures, and sensorineural deafness were clinical features. The mother and a sister suffered milder disease with deafness, short stature, and basal ganglia calcification similar to that of the proband. The mother and son both had ragged red fibers on muscle biopsy (262).

Profound muscle cytochrome oxidase (complex IV) deficiency was reported in an infant presenting with features of MELAS (263). Development was normal until 5 months of age. Recurrent seizures and progressive psychomotor deterioration then followed. Microcephaly and intracranial calcifications were noted at 6 months. At 23 months, this child had a transient right hemiparesis followed subsequently by a left hemiparesis. CSF lactate was elevated. Muscle biopsy showed focal subsarcolemmal accumulations of large mitochondria with increased glycogen and lipid. Normal muscle complex I and II-III activity contrasted with very low complex IV activity.

In a review of CT and MRI brain scan findings in patients with MELAS, predominantly posterior hypodense lesions were seen by CT in 8 of 10 patients in the parietal

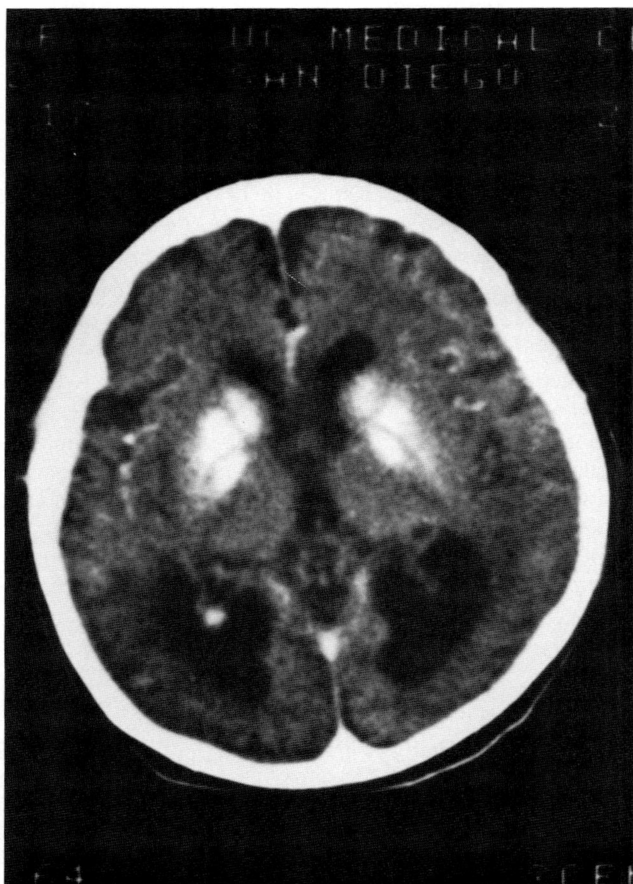

FIGURE 3.7 CT brain scan of a 18-year-old boy with MELAS syndrome. Extensive bilateral basal ganglia calcification and generalized atrophy are striking. Scattered areas of focal low density represent infarctions in a nonvascular distribution. These are most marked in the occipital areas; the patient suffered cortical blindness.

area, with occipital hypodensities in 7 of 10. These lesions were often bilateral, but usually asymmetrical (264). Sequential CT scans showed resolution and sequential appearance of multiple lesions. In two patients, MRI scanning showed high T2 signal indicating focal cerebellar lesions that had not been suspected on CT scan. These lesions were not seen on T1-weighted images. Basal ganglia calcification was reported in most cases. This is generally seen on CT scan and can be missed on MRI. In some cases, basal ganglia calcification was identified only at autopsy (257).

Neuropathology

In discussion of an atypical case, the neuropathology of MELAS was reviewed (265). Inconsistent CNS pathology was found ranging from a severe poliodystrophy with diffuse cortical neuronal loss and spongy degeneration (266) to patients with more focal changes involving the cerebral cortex with neuronal loss, gliosis, and vascular prolifera-

tion (267), areas corresponding to the CT observation of low density focal lesions are indistinguishable from cortical infarcts. There is a loss of neurons with proliferation of macrophages, astrocytes, and capillaries, but lesions do not correspond to any vascular distribution, and no occluded vessels or atheromatous lesions were observed. Autopsy findings in an 18-year-old with the onset of CNS disease at 10 years of age showed extensive cortical atrophy with multifocal and continuous areas of infarction in the cerebral cortex (260). Infarctions were predominantly in the gray and subcortical white matter, sparing deep white matter. Massive calcification in the caudate, globus pallidus, internal capsule, lateral thalamic nuclei, and dentate nucleus was found together with fine mineral deposits elsewhere in the brain.

Myoclonic Epilepsy with Ragged Red Fibers

The MERRF syndrome (269,270) has many characteristics that are similar to MELAS (See Table 3.4). Myoclonic seizures are, however, a striking feature of MERRF, and episodic vomiting with stroke-like episodes are uncommon. Stroke-like episodes have, however, been described. Cerebellar ataxia is striking. Proprioceptive sensory loss is commonly found. Patients frequently have short stature, dementia, optic atrophy, and sensorineural hearing loss.

An early account (269) reported two sisters with myoclonic epilepsy, motor ataxia, diffuse muscle weakness associated with easy fatigability on minimal exertion, sensorineural hearing loss, and average intelligence. An older brother and the mother had limb girdle weakness, but no clinical seizure activity. The EEG, however, showed subclinical paroxysmal spike wave discharges in both the mother and son. The mother and both daughters had high blood and CSF lactate and pyruvate levels. Ragged red fibers were documented on muscle biopsy (269). The clinical heterogeneity of MERRF was demonstrated by studies of a large family in whom the pattern of inheritance was maternal (270). Twenty-nine family members from four generations were studied; 9 of 11 biopsied had mitochondrial myopathy. The patients in this family were classified into four clinical grades depending on severity of CNS disease. The most severely affected individual had pes cavus at birth and deafness in childhood; random muscle jerking developed between 15 and 18 years of age. At 18 years of age, this young woman was ataxic, spastic, and demented. Two moderately affected individuals were intellectually normal, but suffered progressive ataxia, and myoclonus. One had migraine headaches, and another had sensorineural deafness. Four mildly affected patients had sensorineural hearing loss and abnormal EEGs with slowing and spike wave paroxysms, but there was no clinical seizure activity, ataxia, or dementia. Two other individuals with ragged red fiber disease were clinically asymptomatic. The 2 asymptomatic individuals in this kindred had normal EEGs, but the other 7 displayed EEG abnormalities ranging from intermittent rhythmic background slowing to slowing with frequent generalized atypical spike wave discharges. Visual evoked responses were prolonged in the severely affected patient; latencies were normal in the other 8 patients although high amplitudes were found in 6. Brain stem auditory evoked responses were normal in 3 of 4 patients and unobtainable in the deaf, severely affected teenager. Two of 5 patients showed prolonged somatosensory evoked response latencies; EMGs and nerve conduction velocities were normal in all 4 patients tested. Muscle biopsies showed mitochondrial abnormalities in all nine patients studied; in 7 of 9, ragged red fibers were seen. The maternal inheritance pattern in this family strongly supported mitochondrial inheritance involving mitochondrial DNA. Despite this mitochondrial pattern of inheritance, which suggested a likely defect in one of the 13 electron transport chain polypeptides encoded by mitochondrial DNA, in only one patient with MERRF has a partial defect of complex IV been identified. There was considerable variation in complex IV activity from tissue to tissue and from different samples of the same tissue (271). In two siblings, an early atypical presentation of MERRF was associated with low muscle succinate-cytochrome c reductase activity (272). A mitochondrial lysine tRNA mutation has been found in several unrelated MERRF families. Electron transport activities seem lowest in complexes with large numbers of lysine residues.

Kearns-Sayre Syndrome

Kearns-Sayre syndrome was described in 1958 (273). In its classic form, Kearns-Sayre syndrome can be distinguished from ophthalmoplegia-plus (274). This multisystem disorder usually produces symptoms in late childhood with the onset of progressive external ophthalmoparesis, cardiac conduction block, atypical pigmentary degeneration of the retina, and dementia. Basal ganglia calcification and white-matter hypodensities (275) provide some similarities to MELAS; however, CT abnormalities are inconsistent, and hypodensities tend to spare the gray matter. According to Rowland (256) a CSF protein level of over 100 mg/dL is necessary for the diagnosis. Ragged red fiber myopathy is found on biopsy. Similar clinical disorders lack one or other of the cardinal features of Kearns-Sayre disease (mitochondrial myopathy, ophthalmoplegia, atypical pigmentary retinal degeneration, and onset of the disease before the age of 20 years), and are termed ophthalmoplegia-plus. Kearns-Sayre syndrome has been described as a sporadic disorder; whereas, familial cases of ophthalmoplegia-plus have been described.

Reduced coenzyme Q_{10} was found in skeletal muscle and serum in a patient with Kearns-Sayre syndrome together with reduction of all electron transport chain complexes measured in skeletal muscle. Studies of muscle in four patients with Kearns-Sayre syndrome showed normal coupling, but inhibition of complex III respiratory rates with NADH-linked substrates and succinate (276). Cytochrome oxidase activity was also reduced, and in three patients a severe deficiency of cytochrome a and a_3 were found together with an excess of the c cytochromes. The discovery of mitochondrial DNA deletions in 11 of 14 patients studied with typical Kearns-Sayre syndrome as well as 17 of 36 patients with progressive external ophthalmoplegia (277), provides an explanation for the extensive electron transport chain abnormalities reported in Kearns-Sayre patients. It appears that mitochondrial DNA containing a deletion is not functional, and these patients effectively have reduced quantities of active mitochondrial DNA. In one such patient, a severe deficiency of electron transport complex I activity was found together with a partial deficiency of complex IV and V activities. A 4.9-kilobase deletion was found in 50% of the mitochondrial DNA molecules in muscle, but no deletion was found in lymphocytes or platelets. This particular deletion removed 4 genes for subunits of complex I, 1 gene for complex IV, and 2 genes for complex V together with 5 genes for tRNAs (278).

Other Mitochondrial Cytopathies

Many patients with CNS and systemic disease caused by mitochondrial oxidative dysfunction do not fit into the categories of mitochondrial encephalomyopathies described earlier. Some patients appear to have a mixed disorder, with presentation ranging from early childhood to adulthood even within the same kindred. In one family, a 6-year-old girl had intractable tonic-clonic convulsions, progressive dementia, retinal pigmentary degeneration, sensorineural hearing loss and nystagmus with CT findings of calcifications of the caudate nuclei and globus pallidus (279). Other abnormalities included nephrogenic diabetes insipidus and the lack of a growth hormone response to stimulation. This patient's brother aged 8 years was mildly mentally retarded and had muscle wasting and weakness in the distal legs, pigmentary degeneration of the retina, but the CT brain scan was normal. The mother had blepharoptosis from childhood, and at the age of 30 years had arm tremor and deafness. Other affected family members included a 48-year-old with pigmentary degeneration of the retina and a CT scan demonstrating cortical atrophy; a 42-year-old with transient schizophrenic symptoms, seizures, bradykinesia, and weakness, and multiple low density areas of infarction on CT brain scan; and a 53-year-old with seizures, severe mental retardation, diffuse cortical atrophy on CT with focal low densities, and bilateral calcification of caudate and globus pallidus. All five patients biopsied showed ragged red fiber disease.

A 6-year-old girl with marked lactic acidosis had hypotonia, deafness, mental retardation, short stature, cataracts, hypothyroidism, and a deToni-Fanconi-Debré syndrome with carnitine deficiency and ragged red fibers (280). Congenital cataract involving the nucleus, cortex, and capsule of the lens was reported in 7 of 22 children from three unrelated families. These patients had easy fatigability, progressive cardiomyopathy with septal hypertrophy, and lactic acidemia on exercise. A mitochondrial myopathy with storage of lipid, glycogen, and paracrystalline mitochondrial inclusions was found in skeletal and heart muscle (281). A family with apparent maternal inheritance of a mitochondrial cytopathy was characterized by myopathy, neuropathy, ataxia, pathologic EEGs, hyperacusis, and retinitis pigmentosa with disease in nine siblings aged 42 to 64 years. CSF lactate and pyruvate levels were elevated with normal blood measurements (282). In most cases, the biochemical defect underlying these types of mitochondrial cytopathy remains obscure.

A common clinical presentation of mitochondrial cytopathy due to deficiency of electron transport chain constituents is the syndrome of severe lactic acidemia in infancy with degenerative CNS disease. In some cases, the neurologic findings are those of Leigh syndrome. In others, more generalized cortical destruction described as poliodystrophy is found. Most patients presenting with mitochondrial cytopathy of this sort do not have an identified defect. Cytochrome c oxidase deficiency is one well-characterized cause of this clinical picture, however.

Biochemical Characteristics

The electron transport chain is the final common pathway of oxidative metabolism in the mitochondrion (See Figure 3.5). Electrons transported down the respiratory chain release energy that is utilized to pump protons across the intramitochondrial membrane. The chemiosmotic gradient thus established is utilized by the mitochondrion in a number of ways including ATP synthesis. The major entry points for electrons into the electron transport chain are at complex I and complex II. Complex I (NADH coenzyme Q oxidoreductase) receives NADH generated through the activities of a number of oxidative enzymes including components of the citric acid cycle and pyruvate dehydrogenase. These electrons are passed to coenzyme Q. Coenzyme Q also receives electrons from complex II where a flavine adenine dinucleotide is the electron donor and from reduced electron transfer factor (ETF red). Coenzyme Q passes electrons to complex III, which passes them on to cytochrome c. Cytochrome c in turn is oxidized by complex IV, or cytochrome c oxidase. Complex V, the (ATP synthase) is responsible for the production of ATP from ADP. Thirteen of the polypeptides in the electron transport system are encoded by mitochondrial DNA; the remainder (more than 90%) are encoded by nuclear DNA. Assembly of electron transport complexes within the mitochondrion is poorly understood. An abnormality of the assembly of complex III was suggested in one patient with mitochondrial myopathy and lactic acidosis (283). Such assembly

problems may underlie electron transport chain abnormalities in Kearns-Sayre disease. Assembly is presumably under nuclear control.

Mammalian electron transport complexes contain many more subunits than do those of lower animals and yeast. The roles of these additional encoded subunits remain obscure; however, it is likely that a major function involves regulation of electron transport complex activity. Such regulation can provide a mechanism for tissue variability in the activity of various electron transport complexes. In the case of human diseases, heteroplasmy, or the mixture of normal and abnormal mitochondria within individual cells together with a threshold phenomenon, may account for phenotypic and tissue heterogeneity (284).

Mitochondria are inherited from the mother. These organelles replicate rapidly so the multiplication rate of mitochondrial DNA is 10 times that of nuclear DNA. Each cell contains several hundred or thousand mitochondria. Electron transport chain abnormalities encoded by abnormal mitochondrial DNA will be inherited in a nonmendelian fashion. There may be a greater than 50% chance of disease occurrence in offspring, although heteroplasmy and tissue heterogeneity may mitigate the effects of an abnormal mitochondrial complement.

Pathogenesis

Mitochondrial diseases may be inherited or sporadic. Kearns-Sayre syndrome represents a sporadic disease in which the mitochondrial DNA deletion probably occurs at the germ-cell level, affecting some tissues and not others. Electron transport complex assembly is probably dependent on normal mitochondrial DNA as well as nuclear DNA. Transport of nuclear-encoded proteins necessary for mitochondrial replication and assembly is another potential abnormality, which could account for some patients with mitochondrial cytopathy. Point mutations in mitochondrial DNA are known to be responsible for some human mitochondrial diseases. Leber optic atrophy, shown in some patients to be associated with complex I deficiency (285), was due to a point mutation in mitochondrial DNA in other families (286). Most cases of MERRF and MELAS probably have a similar underlying etiology. When mendelian inheritance, dominant, X-linked or recessive traits underlies a mitochondrial disease, it may be presumed that the defect is in nuclear DNA. Such is thought to be the case in Leigh syndrome due to a cytochrome oxidase deficiency (287). Less phenotypic variability might be expected in mitochondrial diseases due to nuclear DNA errors, although in practice it is not clear if this is, in fact, the case.

The pathogenesis of CNS injury in the mitochondrial diseases is uncertain. Lactic acid accumulation in the brain is toxic to astrocytes and neurons (7,288). In most patients with mitochondrial cytopathy, however, CSF lactate and pyruvate levels are not grossly elevated. Injury in selected areas of the brain probably relates to the local metabolic rate and requirement for oxidative metabolism in particular areas. The brain is so dependent on efficient oxidative metabolism for normal function that it is easy to see at a superficial level how a disorder involving the electron transport chain might result in brain cellular injury.

Ragged red fibers are a common feature of the mitochondrial encephalomyopathies. These muscle fibers, so named because of the irregular red staining appearance with modified Gomori trichrome stain are, however, nonspecific indicators of mitochondrial injury (Figure 3.8). The production of ragged red fibers results from mitochondrial accumulation within the muscle fiber, and this is often within the subsarcolemmal space. Such overproduction of mitochondria is thought to represent an attempt at compensation for inadequate function. Such mitochondria are often abnormally large and contain paracrystalline inclusions. All of these features can be produced in experimental animals by the administration of uncoupling agents such as 2-4 dinitrophenol (289). In addition, the ATPase inhibitor oligomycin, and the complex III inhibitor antimycin A produce swelling and disruption of mitochondria in rat preparations. Mitochondrial structural changes such as ragged red fibers are the morphologic expression of an abnormality in mitochondrial function and may be absent in some patients with mitochondrial cytopathies.

Defects of Electron Transport Complexes

Complex I

Defects of electron transport complex I have been reported in a number of different clinical presentations. Mitochondrial myopathy affecting both children and adults is one common presentation. In the largest reported series of 30 patients, 14 had complex I abnormalities. Half of these patients suffered from myopathy alone, whereas, the other half had evidence of multisystem disease including features of MELAS and MERRF in some patients. Age of presentation ranged from childhood to 47 years (290).

Fatal infantile lactic acidosis has been described in association with severe deficiency of the iron sulfur clusters of complex I (291,292). This patient died at 4 months of age, with increasing lactic acidemia, cardiomyopathy, hepatomegaly, and encephalopathy with hypotonia. Skin fibroblast studies demonstrated selective inhibition of NADH substrate utilization in an infant who died at 13 days of life of overwhelming lactic acidosis. A patient who died at 7 months with encephalopathy, severe lactic acidosis, and cardiomyopathy was found to have reduced complex I activity in liver and muscle mitochondria (293). The defect was also demonstrated in skin fibroblasts. A sister had died at 7 weeks of age of a similar disorder. Two previous siblings had died of lactic acidosis in the neonatal period (293). A 16-year-old girl with encephalomyopathy and hypertrophic cardiomyopathy had decreased complex I activity in heart mitochondria obtained at autopsy (259). Deficiency of complex I subunits and a moderate decrease in complex IV were found in this patient (294). Four patients with the clinical signs of MELAS had very low complex I activity in skeletal muscle mitochondria. Immunoblotting suggested a deficiency of multiple subunits of complex I in these patients (258).

Two patients with juvenile encephalopathy have been described with complex I deficiency. A 3-year-old boy with a clinical picture of Alpers disease (myoclonus, quadriparesis, ataxia, dementia, and spongy degeneration of the cortex with elevated CSF lactate) was found to have complex I deficiency in muscle and liver (295). A child with Leigh syndrome was reported with reduced complex I activity in skeletal muscle supernatants (296).

Leber hereditary optic neuropathy, a clinically heterogeneous disorder ranging in its manifestations from encephalopathy and death in childhood to movement disorder and optic atrophy, was found to be caused by complex I deficiency when measured in platelet mitochondria

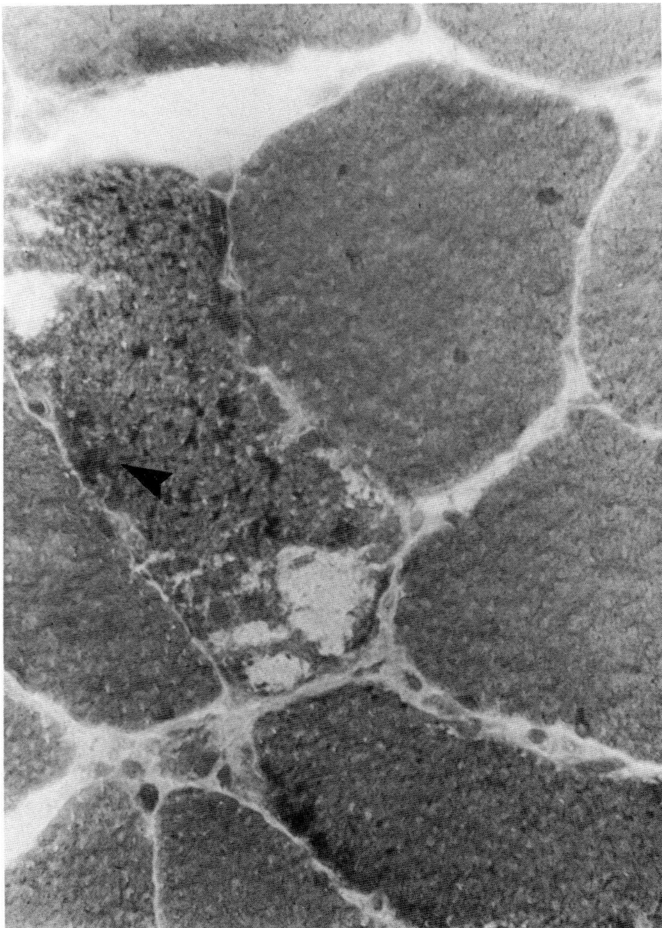

FIGURE 3.8 Transverse section of muscle biopsy showing ragged red fibers in a patient with mitochondrial myopathy. Gomori trichrome stains mitochondrial accumulations (arrow) red. The ragged appearance of these fibers results from disruption of the myofibrillar network. (Original magnification × 600.)

(285). Leber disease has been shown to be maternally inherited, and a point mutation in mitochondrial DNA responsible for encoding complex I has been identified (286), although this defect was not found in the patients reported in the family studied earlier (285). There is considerable interest in the finding of complex I deficiency in Parkinson disease tissues including brain, muscle, and platelet mitochondria. Lowered complex I activity has also been reported in platelet mitochondria from symptomatic Huntington disease patients.

Complex II

Reduced succinate-CoQ reductase (complex II) activity was inferred from autopsy studies of liver and muscle mitochondria from a 20-month-old infant with motor developmental delay, generalized hypotonia, and diffuse muscle weakness. Intellectual development appeared normal. Muscle biopsy showed increased glycogen and lipid with marked mitochondrial abnormalities (297). Two siblings had features of early-onset MERRF characterized by short stature, myoclonic jerks, ataxia, intellectual impairment, and occasional seizures. Onset of symptoms in both children was at 5 1/2 years, and they were evaluated at 7 and 9 years, respectively. Reduced complex II/III activity in the face of normal I/III activity suggested a defect in complex II (272).

Coenzyme Q

Two female siblings aged 12 and 14 years had learning disabilities, progressive generalized muscle weakness, epileptiform EEGs without clinical seizures, and lactic acidemia. The older girl developed cerebellar symptoms and signs of dysarthria, truncal, and limb ataxia, and head tremor at 12 years of age. Isolated activities of electron transport complexes I, II, III, and IV were normal, but activities of complex I-III and II-III, both dependent on coenzyme Q_{10} were low. Direct measurement of muscle coenzyme Q activity was less than 5% of control (298). Decreased coenzyme Q_{10} has been reported in Kearns-Sayre patients with an apparent response to Q supplementation (299).

Complex III

Electron transport complex III abnormalities are manifested with a variety of clinical presentations in both adult and pediatric patients. Six of 30 patients investigated had complex III deficiency presenting as myopathy, whereas 3 had multisystem disease. Ages of presentation ranged from childhood to 33 years (290). One of these patients, a 20-year-old woman, suffered from lifelong ptosis and fatigable muscle weakness. A deficiency of cytochrome c_1 and b was suggested by difference spectra studies of muscle mitochondria. Cytochromes b and c_1 are components of complex III (300). A 17-year-old girl with progressive muscle weak-

ness, mitochondrial myopathy, and lactic acidosis had reduced complex III activity in isolated skeletal muscle mitochondria. Reducible cytochrome b and several other polypeptides of complex III were deficient in this patient (301). In later studies, nuclear magnetic resonance spectroscopy provided evidence of improvement in the phosphocreatine/inorganic phosphate ratio following treatment with menadione and ascorbate (302). Failure of assembly of complex III was proposed in a patient with mitochondrial myopathy and lactic acidosis (283).

In two separate reports, patients with clinical features of MERRF were found to have deficient muscle complex III activity (303,304). In one of these patients, the low complex III activity was due to an absolute reduction of reducible cytochrome b as well as an apparent structural abnormality of cytochrome b (303). A 25-year-old man previously reported with a deficiency of the E_1 component of pyruvate dehydrogenase suffered intermittent episodes of ataxia, tremor, dysarthria, and lactic and pyruvic acidemia. Studies of platelet mitochondria showed decreased complex III activity with an abnormality of myxothiozol binding to cytochrome b (305).

Cytochromes aa_3 were absent, and cytochrome b nearly absent in an infant with familial lactic acidemia, myopathy, and deToni-Fanconi-Debré syndrome. This patient died at 13 weeks of age. Skeletal muscle mitochondria were enlarged with abnormal cristi; the muscle contained increased glycogen and lipid. This defect seemed isolated to voluntary striated muscle, because cytochrome activities were normal in cardiac muscle (306).

Complex IV

Complex IV (cytochrome c oxidase [COX]) is composed of 13 polypeptide subunits in mammals. Subunits I, II, and III are mitochondrially encoded, I and III are associated with prosthetic groups, 2 heme-iron porphyrins, and 2 copper atoms. The 10 smaller subunits of complex IV are encoded by nuclear DNA, synthesized in the cytosol, and transported into the mitochondria. Complex IV defects have been identified in a wide spectrum of human disorders. This subject has been reviewed (307). Different clinical manifestations of complex IV deficiency depend on the amount of residual COX activity and the tissues involved in the individual patient. Clinical phenotypes range from muscle COX deficiency to generalized cytopathy affecting the brain and other organs manifested as Leigh syndrome, MERRF, or mixed mitochondrial encephalomyopathies. In patients with mitochondrial DNA deletions characterized by encephalomyopathy with ophthalmoplegia, COX deficiency due to deficiency of mitochondrially encoded subunits may be found together with other electron transport complex and cytochrome deficiencies.

Fatal infantile lactic acidosis associated with muscle deficiency of COX has now been described in a number of patients (3,308,309). The typical manifestation is hypotonia, generalized weakness, areflexia, and severe lactic acidemia. Some patients have had macroglossia. This disease is usually fatal by 6 months of age. In some patients, generalized amino aciduria is present (3); in others, there is a severe cardiomyopathy (308). In several patients, a spontaneously reversing myopathy with transient severe COX deficiency has been found. These patients presenting in infancy are indistinguishable from those with the fatal form of muscle COX deficiency (310). An infant who died at 18 months had apparent COX deficiency limited to skeletal muscle. The manifestation at 3 months of age was weight loss, hypotonia, external ophthalmoplegia, and severe lactic acidosis. A second cousin, however, died at 5 months of age with weight loss and hepatomegaly, but no systemic acidosis. Liver biopsy in this child showed a proliferation of enlarged mitochondria. Cytochrome b and COX were low in the liver of this child, but kidney mitochondria were normal (311). These two cases demonstrate clinical heterogeneity within a single family suffering from cytopathy due to COX deficiency.

Following the initial description of a patient with Leigh syndrome and muscle COX deficiency (287), a large number of these cases have been described (312–315). In some patients, a deToni-Fanconi-Debré syndrome has accompanied the encephalopathy and muscle disease, confirming the multisystem nature of this cytopathy (316). In three patients, COX deficiencies were demonstrated in muscle, liver, brain platelets, leukocytes, and fibroblasts. In these cases, immunoblotting confirmed a decrease in eight subunits of COX in all three patients (317). Transformed COX-deficient fibroblasts from a child with Leigh syndrome provided evidence for a nuclear DNA-encoded mutation (318).

Other juvenile presentations of COX deficiency include Alpers syndrome (progressive sclerosing poliodystrophy) (319). An infant with features of MELAS syndrome presented at 23 months with a right hemiparesis followed 3 months later by a left hemiparesis. She had progressive psychomotor deterioration with seizures from 5 months of age, microcephaly, and intracranial calcifications. There was elevated CSF lactate. Severe COX deficiency was found in muscle obtained at biopsy (263). Presumably, this patient had a cytopathy with more extensive COX deficiency. Childhood ataxia with psychomotor delay, weakness, and absent deep tendon reflexes were reported in an 8-year-old who had decreased COX activity in muscle, and platelets (320). In Menkes kinky hair disease, cytochrome c oxidase deficiency is due to deficiency of the prosthetic copper group from the holoenzyme (307,321,322).

Adult presentations of COX deficiency are being reported frequently. COX deficiency accompanying other electron transport deficiencies has been demonstrated in a number of patients with Kearns-Sayre syndrome (278,323,324). A cytopathy characterized by hypothyroidism, hypogonadism, growth retardation, muscle weak-

ness and wasting, ophthalmoplegia, cardiac conduction defect, and cerebral atrophy in a 19-year-old man was associated with muscle COX deficiency and deficiency of cytochrome b (325). A 16-year-old girl with psychomotor deterioration from the age of 7 years, hypotonia, bilateral pyramidal and cerebellar signs, lactic acidemia, and epilepsy, had ragged red fibers and diminished COX activity in muscle with normal fibroblast activity (326). A 42-year-old woman with a complex multisystem disorder characterized by external ophthalmoplegia, malabsorption, muscle atrophy, polyneuropathy, leukodystrophy, lactic acidosis, and ragged red fibers, had partial deficiency of COX in muscle and liver mitochondria. The onset of this patient's disorder was at 32 years of age (327). COX deficiency has been reported in two families with MERRF. The COX deficiency may be due to a t-RNA lysine defect in these families. Mixed cytopathies with involvement of COX along with other electron transport complexes and features of MERRF include a 39-year-old man with myoclonus and generalized muscle weakness who had complex II and COX deficiency in muscle and skin fibroblasts (328). A 27-year-old man with muscle weakness and deafness along with peripheral neuropathy, optic atrophy, and cortical, brain stem and cerebellar atrophy had both COX and complex I deficiency in muscle (329). Brain COX deficiency was found in autopsy samples from Huntington disease brain in the caudate nucleus. Other electron transport complexes were normal (330). Reduced COX activity has been reported in platelet mitochondria from Alzheimer disease subjects. These observations raise the possibility that degenerative brain diseases not previously thought to be related to electron transport chain abnormalities may, in fact, be due to such deficiencies.

Complex V

ATP synthase (complex V) utilizes the protein gradient across the matrix mitochondrial membrane to synthesize ATP from adenosine diphosphate (ADP). ATP synthesis through the activity of the electron transport chain is essential for the function of all cells respiring through oxidative metabolism. Thus, a severe deficiency of complex V is unlikely to be compatible with life. Partial deficiency has been described in a Kearns-Sayre patient who, because of mitochondrial DNA deletion, also demonstrated partial deficiency of complex IV and severe deficiency of complex I (278). A 37-year-old woman with a mitochondrial myopathy appeared to have deficiency of mitochondrial ATPase (331). The original patient described by Luft with hypermetabolism caused by loosely coupled oxidative phosphorylation had high endogenous mitochondrial ATPase activity with little increase induced by uncouplers of oxidative phosphorylation (332). A complex V subunit accumulates in ceroid lipofuscinosis. It is likely that other human diseases caused by deficiency or defective regulation of complex V will be identified.

Glutaric Aciduria Type II

Also known as multiple acyl CoA dehydrogenase deficiency, this disorder has been shown in a number of cases to result from a defect of the entry of electrons into the electron transport chain at coenzyme Q. A side pathway different from complex II is responsible for the entry of reducing equivalents from the flavine-containing acyl CoA dehydrogenases responsible for the oxidation of fatty acids and the branched-chain amino acids: valine, leucine, and isoleucine. Entry of electrons into the main electron transport chain is through the activity of electron transfer flavoprotein ubiquinone oxidoreductase (ETF-QO) (See Figure 3.5). Most patients studied with GA II have been found to have a deficiency of electron transfer flavoprotein (ETF), or its dehydrogenase ETF-QO (190). Organic aciduria results from the secondarily impaired activity of multiple CoA dehydrogenases, producing a characteristic pattern of glutaric aciduria with dicarboxylic acids, lactic acid, and 2-hydroxyglutaric acid without the excretion of 3-hydroxyglutaric acid.

Clinical and Neurologic Features

The original description of GA II in 1976 was that of a severe infantile presentation with intractable hypoglycemia and acidosis without ketosis (333). This male infant was tachypneic at 2 hours of age and severely acidotic and hypoglycemic at 16 hours. Despite intravenous glucose and bicarbonate, severe hypoglycemia and acidosis persisted, leading to cardiac arrest, artificial ventilation, and death by 70 hours of age. A number of similar fatal neonatal presentations have been described (334–337). Seizures are common. An acrid odor likened to sweaty feet has been noted in a number of patients (333,334,336). Pallor is usually noted, and the first patient described had a macrocytic anemia (333). Hyperammonemia may be seen (334,336,338). Patients who survive a few weeks develop cardiomegaly and hepatomegaly.

A number of patients with a milder juvenile presentation have been described. One male infant presented at 6 weeks of age with hypoglycemia and hypotonia (339). This infant was managed with a low-fat, low-protein, high-carbohydrate diet and riboflavin supplementation. At 7 months of age, serum and muscle total carnitine levels were reduced with reduced serum-free carnitine. At 10 months, life-threatening episodes of deterioration were treated with carnitine. At 22 months of age, this boy was reportedly mildly retarded with predominant motor delays. Beta-oxidation of fats was impaired in isolated skeletal muscle mitochondria

and skin fibroblasts. A personal case was a 4-year-old boy who presented with a clinical picture of severe athetoid cerebral palsy with severe intellectual retardation. Poor compliance with riboflavin, a low-fat diet, and L-carnitine supplementation contributed to acute decompensation with acidosis and cardiac failure at 5 years of age. Slow recovery was followed by death at the age of 6 years during an episode of gastroenteritis while in Mexico. The brain MRI scan (Figure 3.9) shows a striking pattern of high T2 signal intensity in the basal ganglia. Other cases of juvenile disease with movement disorders and similar MRI changes have been identified, but are not as yet reported (190), although there is one early description of choreoathetosis that may have been due to GA II (187). Patients with milder presentations generally have higher ETF or ETF-QO activity than do neonatal patients (190). An adult presentation of GA II with recurrent episodes of hypoglycemia without ketosis and proximal myopathy in a 19-year-old woman was described (340). Liver biopsy showed severe microvesicular lipid accumulation. Lipid accumulation was also seen in muscle. There was a secondary carnitine deficiency. It is likely that some patients with apparently primary carnitine

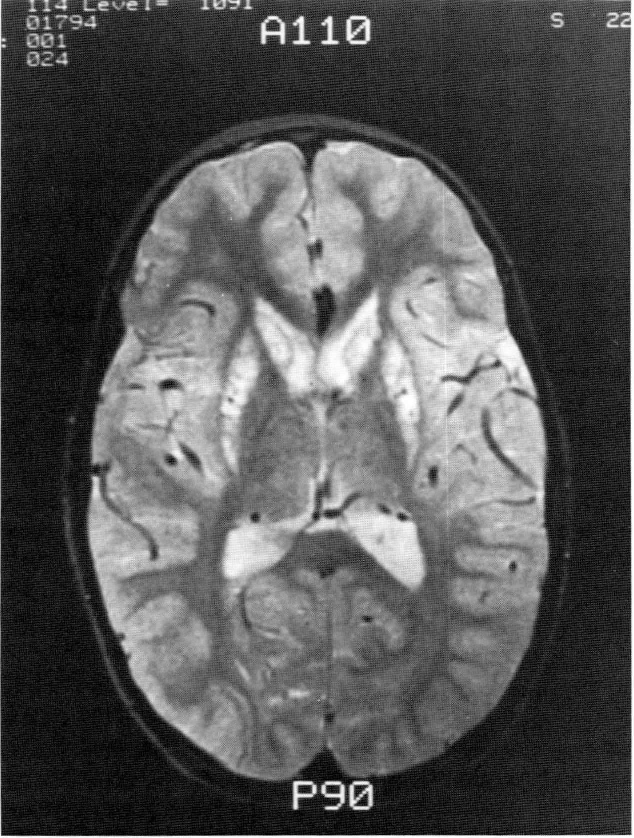

FIGURE 3.9 Glutaric aciduria type II. This T2-weighted MRI brain scan shows symmetrical high signal in the caudate nuclei and putamina. The patient was a 5-year-old boy with "athetoid cerebral palsy."

deficiency actually have milder forms of GA II. Prenatal diagnosis of GA II has been achieved in a number of patients, having first been reported in 1983 (341).

Pathology

Several pathologic reports are available of cases of infantile GA II. An autopsy of a 4-month-old female showed hepatic, renal, and myocardial fat accumulation both intracellular and extracellular. Spinal cord and skeletal muscle were normal (337). Cystic changes in kidney are commonly found (342–344), and are sometimes seen by ultrasound of the fetus (335). Studies of the brain have revealed neuronal migrational abnormalities in some cases with decreased numbers of frontal, temporal, and parietal cortical gyri (344).

Treatment of Electron Transport Complex Deficiency

It is exciting that metabolic defects as fundamental as those in the electron transport chain may respond to treatment. Increasingly, the development and use of effective treatment modalities will play an important part in the management of patients with defects in electron transport complexes. Some therapies in use are quite specific for individual electron transport complex deficiencies, and thus it is important that the exact nature and extent of a patient's deficiency be characterized before the institution of such specific therapies. An example of such therapy is the management of a young woman with muscle complex III deficiency with a combination of menadione (vitamin K_3), and ascorbic acid (302). In this patient, clinical improvement was matched by an improvement in the phosphocreatinine/inorganic phosphate ratio measured by NMR spectroscopy. A theoretic risk of electron shunting maneuvers is the partial bypass of functional components of the electron transport chain.

As early as 1975 with the original description of MELAS (267), steroid treatment was advocated. A patient with MELAS appeared to improve with steroid treatment and repeatedly deteriorated when the steroids were tapered (261). It may be that steroid therapy is not safe in all patients with encephalomyopathies, however, and a deterioration apparently caused by steroid therapy in a patient with Kearns-Sayre disease adds a cautionary note. One of the most promising, apparently safe nonspecific therapies is the use of coenzyme Q_{10}. CoQ is thought to have a stabilizing effect on the inner mitochondrial membrane in which the electron transport chain functions. Additionally, in the case of Kearns-Sayre syndrome, Q levels are low (299). A rare case of familial muscle CoQ deficiency appeared to respond clinically to 50 mg of CoQ_{10} three times daily (298). Treatment with CoQ and succinate has been used in a patient with Complex I deficiency, and MELAS (278). Patients with mitochondrial disorders in general including electron transport chain defects may be secondarily carnitine-deficient as a result of sequestration and excretion of accumulated organic acids as carnitine esters. Carnitine deficiency was identified in one patient with mitochondrial cytopathy and severe lactic acidosis (280). Defects of ETF or ETF dehydrogenase resulting in glutaric aciduria type II are treated with riboflavin and L-carnitine. A low fat diet may also be beneficial. One patient with GA II was treated with methylene blue with temporary success (345).

Secondary Lactic Acidemia

Lactic acid accumulation will occur in any situation in which oxidative metabolism is compromised. Diabetic ketoacidosis and hypoxic/ischemic injury are two common situations in which secondary lactic acidemia is found. A number of inborn errors of metabolism also disrupt mitochondrial metabolism sufficiently to cause secondary lactate accumulation. Glycogen storage diseases (types I and III) form one group, and gluconeogenetic defects another. Patients with the classic organic acid disorders detailed earlier may all present with metabolic acidosis and a high lactic acid masking the true underlying defect. Quantitative urine organic acid analysis is essential as a first step in the evaluation of a patient with lactic acidemia. We believe that a comprehensive approach to the evaluation of the patient with lactic acidemia as detailed in Figure 3.4 is the only certain way to diagnose secondary causes of lactic acidemia, which may masquerade as primary oxidative defects.

4-AMINOBUTYRATE DEFECTS

4-Hydroxybutyric Aciduria

4-Hydroxybutyric aciduria is an unusual inborn error of metabolism in which there is a defect in the metabolic pathway for 4-aminobutyrate (GABA), an important neurotransmitter and the compound that is the source of 4-hydroxybutyric acid, itself of known neuropharmacologic activity.

Clinical and Neurologic Features

4-Hydroxybutyric aciduria has been documented in 11 patients (346). All have had abnormalities of the CNS (347–350). Neurologic features of this disorder vary from seizures, ataxia, and severe mental retardation to hyperactivity with attention deficit, language delay, mild mental retardation, and mild spastic diplegia. Most patients described have been hypotonic in infancy and have displayed both gross motor and language developmental delays. The first four children described had hypotonia with static truncal and appendicular ataxia. Two children presenting at 20 months and 6 years of age respectively, could not walk independently, but two siblings presenting at 9 and 11 years, respectively, were able to walk independently (347). Ocular apraxia was noted in two severely affected children (347). Head size has been reported as decreased, normal, and increased in individual patients (346).

Seizures would be expected to be severe and intractable in a condition generating gamma hydroxybutyric acid. 4-Hydroxybutyric acid in animal studies is ictogenic (351). In the human disease, however, seizures are not universal; those that have occurred have been brief motor generalized seizures, which have been easily controlled in infancy. One patient with marked hyperactivity had a sleep EEG showing poor development of vertex waves, K complexes and spindles, but no ictal phenomena were observed, and there was no history to suggest seizures in this child. A CT brain scan at 20 months of age in an ataxic, hypotonic patient with severe motor developmental delays showed generalized cerebral atrophy (347), but a normal MRI scan was obtained in the hyperactive 9-year-old girl with mild retardation but no seizures.

The neurologic features of 4-hydroxybutyric aciduria appear to include hypotonia, motor and language developmental delay, and mild-to-moderate mental retardation in all patients. Other features, such as seizures, ataxia, and hyperactivity, are found only in some patients.

Biochemical Characteristics

The molecular defect in 4-hydroxybutyric aciduria is in the enzyme succinic semialdehyde dehydrogenase (352). Succinic semialdehyde is the product of the GABA transaminase reaction. The dehydrogenase step provides entry into the oxidative pathway of the citric acid cycle. The enzyme has been studied predominantly in brain where there is considerable activity. It is not expressed in fibroblasts. The observation that permitted the definition of the enzyme defect in this disorder is that the enzyme is active in normal lymphocytes (352–354). It may also be studied in cultured human lymphoblasts (355). A whole cell assay has been developed in which considerably more activity is displayed in both normal cells and those of affected individuals than in cell extracts (346).

There are a number of metabolic consequences of the deficiency of the enzyme. The most immediate is the accumulation of succinic semialdehyde, but concentrations of this compound are not very high in patients because it is promptly converted to 4-hydroxybutyrate, and this is the major metabolic product of the deranged metabolism (356). This compound is further oxidized leading to 3, 4-dihydroxybutyric acid and glycolic acid. Increased amounts of glycine may be found in the urine (349,357), and there may be a dicarboxylic aciduria. Either of these latter findings may serve as alerting signals to seek out the diagnosis.

Chemical documentation of the diagnosis is not easy. Certainly the disorder was discovered by gas chromatographic analysis of the urine (356). The nature of the molecule leads to variant lactone formation under conditions of analysis, however, and the compound can be missed under conditions of organic acid analysis employed in many biochemical genetics laboratories. The availability of a stable isotope dilution internal standard GCMS method (358) has made it apparent that most published values in patients are considerably lower than the true concentrations. In patients, concentrations are higher in CSF than in plasma.

Genetics

4-Hydroxybutyric aciduria is inherited as an autosomal-recessive trait. The initial reports were abundant in consanguinity (348,356,359). Assay of the enzyme in lymphocytes or lymphoblasts yields intermediate levels of activity in heterozygotes (348). Prenatal diagnosis is available by direct GCMS analysis of the amniotic fluid (358): An unaffected fetus has been detected prenatally to date. The enzyme is also active in chorionic villus samples (52), permitting another approach to prenatal diagnosis.

Treatment

Specific effective treatment has not been devised. Seizures tend to be readily controlled with the usual anticonvulsant medications.

REFERENCES

1. Sweetman L. Qualitative and quantitative analysis of organic acids in physiological fluids for diagnosis of the organic acidemias. In: Nyhan WL, ed. Abnormalities in Amino Acid Metabolism in Clinical Medicine. Norwalk, CT: Appleton Century Crofts; 1984:419–453.
2. Lowry OH, Passoneau JV, Hasselberger FX. Effect of ischemia on known substrates and cofactors of the glycolytic pathway in brain. J Biol Chem 1964;239:18–30.
3. DiMauro S, Bonilla E, Zeviani E, et al. Mitochondrial myopathies. Ann Neurol 1985;17:521–538.
4. Haas RH, Stumpf DA. Mitochondrial mechanisms in Reye-like syndromes. Journal of the National Reye's Syndrome Foundation 1981;2:61–69.
5. Hawkins RA, Mans AM. Intermediatry metabolism of carbohydrates and other fuels. In: Lajtha A, ed. Handbook of Neurochemistry Vol. 3, New York: Plenum; 1988:259–294.
6. Wolff JA, Le TP, Haas R, et al. Carnitine reduces fasting ketogenesis in patients with disorders of propionate metabolism. Lancet 1986;1:289–291.
7. Myers RE. Lactic acid accumulation as cause of brain edema

and cerebral necrosis resulting from oxygen deprivation. In: Korobkin R, Guilleminault C, eds. Advances in Perinatal Neurology. Vol. 1. New York: Spectrum; 1979:85–114.

8. Childs B, Nyhan WL, Borden MA, et al. Idiopathic hyperglycinemia and hyperglycinuria, a new disorder of amino acid metabolism. Pediatrics 1961;27:522–538.

9. Nyhan WL, Ando T, Gerritsen T. Hyperglycinemia. In: Nyhan WL, ed. Amino Acid Metabolism and Genetic Variation. New York: McGraw-Hill; 1967:225.

10. Satoh T, Narisawa K, Tazawa Y, et al. Dietary therapy in a girl with propionic acidemia: Supplement with leucine resulted in catch up growth. Tohoku J Exp Med 1983;139:411–415.

11. Wolf B, Hsia YE, Sweetman L, et al. Propionic acidemia: A clinical update. J Pediatr 1981;99:835–846.

12. Wolf B, Paulson EP, Hsia YE. Asymptomatic propionyl CoA carboxylase deficiency in a 13-year-old girl. J Pediatr 1979;95:563–565.

13. Brandt IK, Hsia YE, Clement DH, et al. Propionicacidemia (Ketotic Hyperglycinemia): Dietary treatment resulting in normal growth and development. Pediatrics 1974;53:391–395.

14. Steinman L, Clancy RR, Cann H, et al. The neuropathology of propionic acidemia. Dev Med Child Neurol 1983;25:87–94.

15. Wadlington WB, Kilroy A, Ando T, et al. Hyperglycinemia and propionyl CoA carboxylase deficiency and episodic severe illness without consistent ketosis. J Pediatr 1975;86:707–712.

16. Shuman RM, Leech RW, Scott CR. The neuropathology of the nonketotic and ketotic hyperglycinemias: Three cases. Neurology 1978;28:139–146.

17. Asconape J, Challa VR, Angelo JN. Spongy degeneration of the nervous system associated with propionic acidemia. Acta Neurol Latinoam 1981;27:91–98.

18. Watanabe I, Bingle GJ. Dysmyelination in "quaking" mouse. J Neuropathol Exp Neurol 1972;31:352–369.

19. Coude FX, Sweetman L, Nyhan WL. Inhibition by propionyl-coenzyme A of N-acetylglutamate synthetase in rat liver mitochondria. A possible explanation for hyperammonemia in propionic and methylmalonic acidemia. J Clin Invest 1979;64:1544–1551.

20. Coude FX, Ogier H, Grimber G, et al. Correlation between blood ammonia concentration and organic acid accumulation in isovaleric and propionic acidemia. Pediatrics 1982;69:115–117.

21. Wolf B, Hsia YE, Tanaka K, et al. Correlation between serum propionate and blood ammonia concentrations in propionic acidemia. J Pediatr 1978;93:471–473.

22. Saudubray JM, Coude FX, Ogier H, et al. Hyperammonemia secondary to hereditary organic acidurias: A study of 29 cases. Adv Exp Med Biol 1982;153:135–140.

23. Cavanagh JB, Blakermore WF, Kyu MH. Fibrillary accumulations in oligodendroglial processes of rats subjected to portocaval anastomosis. J Neurol Sci 1971;14:143–152.

24. Parsons-Smith BG, Summerskill WHJ, Dawson AM, et al. The electroencephalograph in liver disease. Lancet 1957;2:867–871.

25. Hsia YE. Inherited hyperammonemic syndromes. Gastroenterology 1974;67:347–374.

26. Kye-Wing C, Pond WG. Biochemical and morphological aspects of mitochondrial swelling in ammonia toxicity (36098). Proc Soc Exp Biol Med 1972;139:150–156.

27. James IM, Dorf G, Hall S, et al. Effect of ornithine alpha ketoglutarate on disturbances of brain metabolism caused by high blood ammonia. Gut 1972;13:551–555.

28. Saheki T, Towatari T, Katunuma N. Effect of ammonia on tricarboxylate utilization in rat liver mitochondria. J Biochem (Tokyo) 1971;70:529–531.

29. Stumpf DA, McAfee J, Parks JK, et al. Propionate inhibition of succinate:CoA ligase (GDP) and the citric acid cycle in mitochondria. Pediatr Res 1980;14:1127–1131.

30. Hayasaka K, Metoki K, Satoh T, et al. Comparison of cytosolic and mitochondrial enzyme alterations in the livers of propionic or methylmalonic acidemia: A reduction of cytochrome oxidase activity. Tohoku J Exp Med 1982;137:329–334.

31. Johnson JW, Ascher P. Glycine potentiates the NMDA response in cultured mouse brain neurons. Nature 1987;325:529–531.

32. Cheema Dhadli S, Leznoff CC, et al. Effect of 2-methylcitrate on citrate metabolism: Implications for the management of patients with propionic acidemia and methylmalonic aciduria. Pediatr Res 1975;9:905–908.

33. Ando T, Rasmussen K, Wright JM, et al. Isolation and identification of methylcitrate, a major metabolic product of propionate in patients with propionic acidemia. J Biol Chem 1972;247:2200–2204.

34. Shafai T, Sweetman L, Weyler W, et al. Propionic acidemia with severe hyperammonemia and defective glycine metabolism. J Pediatr 1978;92:84–86.

35. Hayasaka K, Narisawa K, Satoh T, et al. Glycine cleavage system in ketotic hyperglycinemia: A reduction of H-protein activity. Pediatr Res 1982;16:5–7.

36. Sweetman L, Weyler W, Nyhan WL, et al. Abnormal metabolites of isoleucine in a patient with propionyl-CoA carboxylase deficiency. Biomed Mass Spectrom 1978;5:198–207.

37. Harris DJ, Yang BI, Wolf B, et al. Dysautonomia in an infant with secondary hyperammonemia due to propionyl Coenzyme A carboxylase deficiency. Pediatrics 1980;65:107–110.

38. Cathelineau L, Briand P, Ogier H, et al. Occurrence of hyperammonemia in the course of 17 cases of methylmalonic acidemia. J Pediatr 1981;99:279–280.

39. Hsia YE, Scully KJ, Rosenberg LE. Human propionyl CoA carboxylase: Some properties of the partially purified enzyme in fibroblasts from controls and patients with propionic acidemia. Pediatr Res 1979;13:746–751.

40. Hsia YE, Scully KJ. Propionic acidemia: Diagnosis by enzyme assay in frozen leukocytes. J Pediatr 1973;83:625–628.

41. Hsia YE, Scully KJ, Rosenberg LE. Defective propionate carboxylation in ketotic hyperglycinaemia. Lancet 1969;1:757–758.

42. Gompertz D, Storres CN, Bau DCK, et al. Localization of enzymatic defect in propionic-acidemia. Lancet 1970;1:1140–1143.

43. Hsia YE, Scully KJ, Rosenberg LE. Inherited propionyl CoA carboxylase deficiency in "ketotic hyperglycinemia." J Clin Invest 1971;50:127–130.

44. Ando T, Nyhan WL, Connor JD, et al. The oxidation of glycine and propionic acid in propionic acidemia with ketotic hyperglycinemia. Pediatr Res 1972;6:576–583.

45. Lysiak W, Stepinski J, Angielski S. Inhibition of alpha-oxoglutarate and pyruvate oxidation by alpha-oxoderivatives of leucine and valine in rat tissues. Acta Biochim Pol 1970;17:131–141.

46. Gravel RA, Lam K-F, Scully KJ, et al. Genetic complementa-

tion of propionyl CoA carboxylase deficiency in cultured human fibroblasts. Am J Hum Genet 1977;29:378–388.

47. Kalousek F, Orsulak MD, Rosenberg LR. Absence of cross-reacting material in isolated propionyl CoA carboxylase deficiency: Nature of residual carboxylating activity. Am J Hum Genet 1983;35:409–420.

48. Lamhonwah AM, Barankiewicz TJ, Willard HF, et al. Isolation of cDNA clones coding for the alpha and beta chains of human propionyl CoA carboxylase: Chromosomal assignments and DNA polymorphisms associated with PCCA and PCCB genes. Proc Natl Acad Sci USA 1986;83:4864–4868.

49. Kraus JP, Williamson CL, Firgaira FA, et al. Cloning and screening with nanogram amounts of immunopurified mRNAs: cDNA cloning and chromosomal mapping of cystathionine betasynthase and the beta subunit of propionyl CoA carboxylase. Proc Natl Acad Sci USA 1986;83: 2047–2051.

50. Wolf B, Rosenberg LE. Heterozygote expression in propionyl coenzyme A carboxylase deficiency. Differences between major complementation groups. J Clin Invest 1978;62:931–936.

51. Gompertz D, Goodey PA, Thom H, et al. Prenatal diagnosis and family studies in a case of propionic acidaemia. Clin Genet 1975;8:244–250.

52. Sweetman FR, Gibson KM, Sweetman L, et al. Activity of biotin-dependent and GABA metabolizing enzymes in chorionic villus samples: Potential for 1st trimester prenatal diagnosis. Prenat Diagn 1986;6:187–194.

53. Willard HF, Ambani LM, Hart AC, et al. Rapid prenatal and postnatal detection of inborn errors of propionate, methylmalonate, and cobalamin metabolism. A sensitive assay using cultured cells. Hum Genet 1976;32:277–283.

54. Morrow G III, Revsin B, Mathews C, et al. A simple, rapid method for prenatal detection of defects in propionate metabolism. Clin Genet 1976;10:218–221.

55. Sweetman L, Weyler W, Shafai T, et al. Prenatal diagnosis of propionic acidemia. JAMA 1979;242:1048–1052.

56. Trefz FK, Schmidt H, Tauscher B, et al. Improved prenatal diagnosis of methylmalonic acidemia: Mass fragmentography of methylmalonic acid in amniotic fluid and maternal urine. Eur J Pediatr 1981;137:261–266.

57. Naylor G, Sweetman L, Nyhan WL, et al. Isotope dilution analysis of methylcitric acid in amniotic fluid for the prenatal diagnosis of propionic and methylmalonic acidemia. Clin Chim Acta 1980;107:175–183.

58. Buchanan PD, Kahler SG, Sweetman L, et al. Pitfalls in the prenatal diagnosis of propionic acidemia. Clin Genet 1980;18:177–183.

59. Saudubray JM, Amedee Manesme O, Lavaud J, et al. Emergency treatment of inborn amino errors of amino acid metabolism detected in the neonatal period. Arch Fr Pediatr 1979;36:969–980.

60. Robert MF, Schultz DJ, Wolf B, et al. Treatment of a neonate with propionic acidaemia and severe hyperammonaemia by peritoneal dialysis. Arch Dis Child 1979;54: 962–965.

61. Petrowski S, Nyhan WL, Reznik V, et al. Pharmacologic amino acid acylation in the acute hyperammonemia of propionic acidemia. J Neurogenet 1987;4:87–96.

62. Nyhan WL. Disorders of propionate metabolism. In: Bickel H, Wachtel U, eds. Inherited Diseases of Amino Acid Metabolism. Recent Progress in the Understanding, Recognition and Management. International Symposium in Heidelberg, 1984. Stuttgart/New York: Georg Thieme Verlag Thieme; 1985:363–382.

63. Queen PM, Fernhoff PM, Acosta PB. Protein and essential amino acid requirements in a child with propionic acidemia. J Am Diet Assoc 1981;79:562–565.

64. Queen PM, Acosta PB, Fernhoff PM. The effects of spacing protein intake on nitrogen balance and plasma amino acids in a child with propionic acidemia. J Am Coll Nutr 1982;1:305–308.

65. Chalmers RA, Roe CR, Stacey TE, et al. Urinary excretion of L-carnitine and acylcarnitines by patients with disorders of organic acid metabolism: Evidence for secondary insufficiency of L-carnitine. Pediatr Res 1984;18:1325–1328.

66. Roe CR, Bohan TP. L-Carnitine therapy in propionic-acidaemia. Lancet 1982;1:1411–1412.

67. Di Donato S, Rimoldi M, Garavaglia B, et al. Propionylcarnitine excretion in propionic and methylmalonic acidurias: A cause of carnitine deficiency. Clin Chim Acta 1984; 139:13–21.

68. Millington DS, Roe CR, Maltby DA. Application of high resolution fast atom bombardment and constant B/E ratio linked scanning to the identification and analysis of acylcarnitines in metabolic disease. Biomed Mass Spectrom 1984;11:236–241.

69. Roe CR, Millington DS, Maltby DA, et al. L-carnitine enhances excretion of propionyl coenzyme A as propionylcarnitine in propionic acidemia. J Clin Invest 1984; 73:1785–1788.

70. Matsui SM, Mahoney MJ, Rosenberg LE. The natural history of the inherited methylmalonic acidemias. N Engl J Med 1983;308:857–861.

71. Schuh S, Rosenblatt DS, Cooper BA, et al. Homocystinuria and megaloblastic anemia responsive to vitamin B_{12} therapy. An inborn error of metabolism due to a defect in cobalamin metabolism. N Engl J Med 1984;310:686–690.

72. Rosenblatt DS, Laframboise R, Pichette J, et al. New disorder of vitamin B_{12} metabolism (cobalamin F) presenting as methylmalonic aciduria. Pediatrics 1986;78:51.

73. Yu A, Sweetman L, Nyhan WL. The pathogenetic mechanism of recurrent mucocutaneous candidiasis in a patient with methylmalonic acidemia (MMA). Clin Res 1981; 29:124A.

74. Heidenreich R, Natowicz M, Hainline BE, et al. Acute extrapyramidal syndrome in methylmalonic acidemia: "Metabolic stroke" involving the globus pallidus. J Pediatr 1988;113:1022–1027.

75. Bartholomew DW, Batshaw ML, Allen RH, et al. Therapeutic approaches to cobalamin-C methylmalonic acidemia and homocystinuria. J Pediatr 1988;112:32–39.

76. Robb RM, Dowton SB, Fulton AB, et al. Retinal degeneration in vitamin B_{12} disorder associated with methylmalonic aciduria and sulfur amino acid abnormalities. Am J Ophthalmol 1984;97:691–696.

77. Carmel R, Goodman SI. Abnormal deoxyuridine suppression test in congenital methylmalonic aciduria-homocystinuria without megaloblastic anemia: Divergent biochemical and morphological bone marrow manifestations of disordered cobalamin metabolism in man. Blood 1982; 59:306–311.

78. Carmel R, Watkins D, Goodman SI, et al. Hereditary defect of cobalamin metabolism (cblG mutation) presenting as a neurologic disorder in adulthood. N Engl J Med 1988; 318:1738–1741.

79. Dave P, Curless RG, Steinman L. Cerebellar hemorrhage complicating methylmalonic and propionic acidemia. Arch Neurol 1984;41:1293–1296.

80. Korf B, Wallman JK, Levy HL. Bilateral lucency of the globus pallidus complicating methylmalonic acidemia. Ann Neurol 1986;20:364–366.

81. Lindblad B, Lindblad BS, Olin P, et al. Methylmalonic acidemia. A disorder associated with acidosis, hyperglycinemia, and hyperlactatemia. Acta Paediatr Scand 1968; 57:417–424.

82. Gerbarski SS, Gabrielsen TO, Knake JE, et al. Cerebral CT findings in methylmalonic acid propionic acidemias. AJNR 1983;4:955–957.

83. Bousounis DP. Methylmalonic aciduria resulting in globus pallidus neurosis. Ann Neurol 1988;24:302–303.

84. Adams RD, Lyon G. Neurology of Hereditary Metabolic Diseases of Children. New York:McGraw-Hill; 1982:25–28.

85. Wajner M, Brites EC, Dutra JC, et al. Diminished concentrations of ganglioside N-acetylneuraminic acid (G-NeuAc) in cerebellum of young rats receiving chronic administration of methylmalonic acid. J Neurol Sci 1988;85:233–238.

86. Nyhan WL, Fawcett N, Ando T, et al. Response to dietary therapy in B_{12} unresponsive methylmalonic acidemia. Pediatrics 1973;51:539–548.

87. Morrow G III, Mahoney MJ, Mathews C, et al. Studies of methylmalonyl coenzyme A carbonylmutase activity in methylmalonic acidemia. I. Correlation of clinical, hepatic, and fibroblast data. Pediatr Res 1975;9:641–644.

88. Willard HF, Rosenberg LE. Inherited methylmalonyl CoA mutase apoenzyme deficiency in human fibroblasts. Evidence for allelic heterogeneity, genetic compounds, and codominant expression. J Clin Invest 1980;65:690–698.

89. Kolhouse JF, Utley C, Fenton WA, et al. Immunochemical studies on cultured fibroblasts from patients with inherited methylmalonic acidemia. Proc Natl Acad Sci USA 1981; 78:7737–7741.

90. Ledley FD, Lumetta M, Nguyen PN, et al. Molecular cloning of L-methylmalonyl CoA mutase: Gene transfer and analysis of mut cell lines. Proc Natl Acad Sci USA 1988; 85:3518–3521.

91. Ledley FD, Lumetta MR, Zoghbi HY, et al. Mapping of human methylmalonyl CoA mutase (MUT) locus on chromosome 6. Am J Hum Genet 1988;42:839–846.

92. Mahoney MJ, Rosenberg LE, Mudd SH, et al. Defective metabolism of vitamin B_{12} in fibroblasts from patients with methylmalonic aciduria. Biochem Biophys Res Commun 1971;44:375–381.

93. Rosenberg LE, Lilljeqvist AC, Hsia YE, et al. Vitamin B_{12} dependent methylmalonic aciduria. Defective metabolism in cultured fibroblasts. Biochem Biophys Res Commun 1969;37:607–614.

94. Gravel RA, Mahoney MJ, Ruddle FH, et al. Genetic complementation in heterokaryons of human fibroblasts defective in cobalamin metabolism. Proc Natl Acad Sci USA 1975;72:3181–3185.

95. Willard HF, Mellman IS, Rosenberg LE. Genetic complementation among inherited deficiencies of methylmalonyl CoA mutase activity. Evidence for a new class of human cobalamin mutant. Am J Hum Genet 1978;30:1–13.

96. Fenton WA, Rosenberg LE. The defect in the cbl B class of human methylmalonic acidemia: Deficiency of cob(I)alamin adenosyltransferase activity in extracts of cultured fibroblasts. Biochem Biophys Res Commun 1981;98:283–289.

97. Whelan DT, Ryan E, Spate M, et al. Methylmalonic acidemia: 6 years' clinical experience with two variants unresponsive to vitamin B_{12} therapy. Can Med Assoc J 1979;120:1230–1235.

98. Wolff JA, Strom C, Griswold W, et al. Proximal renal tubular acidosis in methylmalonic acidemia. J Neurogenet 1985;2:31–39.

99. Coulombe JT, Shih VE, Levy HL. Massachusetts metabolic disorders screening program. II methylmalonic aciduria. Pediatrics 1981;67:26–31.

100. Ledley FD, Levy HL, Shih VE, et al. Benign methylmalonic aciduria. N Engl J Med 1984;311:1015–1018.

101. Morrow G, Schwartz RH, Hallock JA, et al. Prenatal detection of methylmalonic acidemia. J Pediatr 1970;77: 120–123.

102. Mahoney MJ, Rosenberg LE, Lindblad B, et al. Prenatal diagnosis of methylmalonic aciduria. Acta Paediatr Scand 1975;64:44–48.

103. Zinn AB, Hine DG, Mahoney MJ, et al. The stable isotope dilution method for measurement of methylmalonic acid: A highly accurate approach to the prenatal diagnosis of methylmalonic acidemia. Pediatr Res 1982;16:740–745.

104. Sweetman L, Naylor G, Ladner T, et al. Prenatal diagnosis of propionic and methylmalonic acidemia by stable isotope dilution analysis of methylcitric and methylmalonic acids in amniotic fluids. In: Schmidt HL, Forstel H, Heinzinger K, eds. Stable Isotopes. Amsterdam: Elsevier Scientific Publishing; 1982,287–293.

105. Ampola MG, Mahoney MJ, Nakamura E, et al. Prenatal therapy of a patient with vitamin B_{12} responsive methylmalonic acidemia. N Engl J Med 1975;293:311–317.

106. Morrow G, Burkel GM. Long-term management of a patient with vitamin B_{12}-responsive methylmalonic acidemia. J Pediatr 1980;96:425–426.

107. Ney DN, Bay C, Saudubray J-M, et al. An evaluation of protein requirements in patients with methylmalonic acidemia. J Inherited Metab Dis 1985;8:132–142.

108. Kelts DG, Ney D, Bay C, et al. Studies on requirements for amino acids in infants with disorders of amino acid metabolism. I. Effect of alanine. Pediatr Res 1985; 19:86–91.

109. Snyderman SE, Sansarico C, Norton P, et al. The use of neomycin in the treatment of methylmalonic acidemia. Pediatrics 1972;50:925–927.

110. Berry GT, Yudkoff M, Segal S. Isovaleric acidemia: Medical and neurodevelopmental effects of long-term therapy. J Pediatr 1988;113:58–64.

111. De Sousa C, Chalmers RA, Stacey TE, et al. The response to L-carnitine and glycine therapy in isovaleric acidaemia. Eur J Pediatr 1986;144:451–456.

112. Hyman DB, Tanaka K. Isovaleryl CoA dehydrogenase activity in isovaleric acidemia fibroblasts using an improved tritium release assay. Pediatr Res 1986;20:59–61.

113. Duran M, Bruinvis L, Ketting D, et al. Isovaleric acidaemia presenting with dwarfism, cataract and congenital abnormalities. J Inherited Metab Dis 1982;5:125–127.

114. Rousson R, Guibaud P. Long-term outcome of organic acidurias: Survey of 105 French cases (1967–1983). J Inherited Metab Dis 1984;7:10–12.

115. Duran M, van Sprang FJ, Drewes JG, et al. Two sisters with isovaleric acidaemia, multiple attacks of ketoacidosis and normal development. Eur J Pediatr 1979;131:205–211.

116. Fischer AQ, Challa VR, Burton BK. Cerebellar hemorrhage complicating isovaleric acidemia: A case report. Neurology 1981;31:746–748.

117. Williams KM, Peden VH, Hillman RE. Isovalericacidemia appearing as diabetic ketoacidosis. Am J Dis Child 1981; 135:1068–1069.

118. Tanaka K, Rosenberg LE. Disorders of branched chain amino and organic acid metabolism. In: Stanbury JB, Wyngaarden JB, Frederickson DS, et al., eds. The Metabolic Basis of Inherited Disease. New York: McGraw-Hill; 1983: 440–447.

119. Wilson WG, Audenaert SM, Squillaro EJ. Hyperammonaemia in a preterm infant with isovaleric acidaemia. J Inherited Metab Dis 1984;7:71.

120. Mendiola J Jr, Robotham JL, Liehr JG, et al. Neonatal lethargy due to isovaleric acidemia and hyperammonemia. Tex Med 1984;80:52–54.

121. Krieger I, Tanaka K. Therapeutic effects of glycine in isovaleric acidemia. Pediatr Res 1976;10:25–29.

122. Ando T, Nyhan WL, Bachmann C, et al. Isovaleric acidemia: Identification of isovalerate, isovalerylglycine and 3-hydroxyisovalerate in urine of a patient previously reported as having butyric and hexanoic acidemia. J Pediatr 1973;82:243–248.

123. Malan C, Neethling AC, Shanley BC, et al. Isovaleric acidaemia in two South African children. S Afr Med J 1977;51:980–983.

124. Newman CG, Wilson BDR, Callaghan P, et al. Neonatal death associated with isovalericacidaemia. Lancet 1967; 2:439–442.

125. Spirer Z, Swirsky-Fein S, Zakut V, et al. Acute neonatal isovaleric acidemia: A report of two cases. Isr J Med Sci 1975;11:1005–1010.

126. Varanasi U, Malino DC. Brain lipids from the porpoise (Delphinus Delphis). Phosphoglycerides rich in isovaleric acid and long-chain iso-acids. BBA 1975;409:304–310.

127. Hird FJR, Weideman MJ. Oxidative phosphorylation accompanying oxidation of short chain fatty acids by rat liver mitochondria. Biochem J 1966;98:378.

128. Bergen BJ, Stumpf DA, Haas R, et al. A mechanism of toxicity of isovaleric acid in rat liver mitochondria. Biochem Med 1982;27:154–160.

129. Coude FX, Grimber G, Parvy P, et al. Role of N-acetylglutamate and acetyl CoA in the inhibition of ureagenesis by isovaleric acid in isolated rat hepatocytes. Biochim Biophys Acta 1983;761:13–16.

130. Clark JB, Land JM. Phenylketonuria and maple syrup urine disease and their association with brain mitochondrial substrate utilization. In: Hommes FA, Van der Berg CJ, eds. Normal and Pathological Development of Energy Metabolism. New York: Academic Press; 1975:177–191.

131. Ando T, Klingberg WG, Ward AN, et al. Isovaleric acidemia presenting with altered metabolism to glycine. Pediatr Res 1971;5:478–486.

132. Tanaka K, Isselbacher KJ. The isolation and identification of N-isovalerylglycine from urine of patients with isovaleric acidemia. J Biol Chem 1967;242:2966–2972.

133. Tanaka K, Orr JC, Isselbacher KJ. Identification of 3-hydroxyisovaleric acid in the urine of a patient with isovaleric acidemia. Biochim Biophys Acta 1968;152:638–641.

134. Truscott RJ, Malegan D, McCairns E, et al. New metabolites in isovaleric acidemia. Clin Chim Acta 1981; 110:187–203.

135. Lehnert W, Niederhof H. 4-Hydroxyisovaleric acid: A new metabolite in isovaleric acidemia. Eur J Pediatr 1981; 136:281–283.

136. Hine DG, Tanaka K. The identification and the excretion pattern of isovaleryl glucuronide in the urine of patients with isovaleric acidemia. Pediatr Res 1984;18:508–512.

137. Rhead WJ, Tanaka K. Demonstration of a specific mitochondrial isovaleryl CoA dehydrogenase deficiency in fibroblasts from patients with isovaleric acidemia. Proc Natl Acad Sci USA 1980;77:580–583.

138. Rhead WJ, Hall CL, Tanaka K. Novel tritium release assays for isovaleryl CoA dehydrogenases. J Biol Chem 1981;256: 1616–1624.

139. Matsubara Y, Kraus JP, Ito M, et al. Molecular cloning, nucleotide sequence, and human chromosome assignment of cDNA encoding rat isovaleryl CoA dehydrogenase. Am J Genet 1987;41:A228.

140. Levy HL, Erickson AM, Lott IT, et al. Isovaleric acidemia. Results of family study and dietary treatment. Pediatrics 1973;52:83–94.

141. Wolff JA, Kelts DG, Algert S, et al. Alanine decreases the protein requirements of infants with inborn errors of amino acid metabolism. J Neurogenet 1985;2:41–49.

142. Cohn RM, Yudkoff M, Rothman R, et al. Isovaleric acidemia: Use of glycine therapy in neonates. N Engl J Med 1978;299:996–999.

143. Yudkoff M, Cohn RM, Puschak R, et al. Glycine therapy in isovaleric acidemia. J Pediatr 1978;92:813–817.

144. Mitchell G, Ogier H, Munnich A, et al. Neurological deterioration and lactic acidemia in biotinidase deficiency. A treatable condition mimicking Leigh's disease. Neuropediatrics 1986;17:129–131.

145. Baumgartner ER, Suormala TU, Wick H, et al. Biotinidase deficiency: A cause of subacute necrotizing encephalomyelopathy (Leigh syndrome). Report of a case with a lethal outcome. Pediatr Res 1989;26 (3):260–266.

146. Wolf B, Grier RE, Allen RJ, et al. Phenotypic variation in biotinidase deficiency. J Pediatr 1983;103:233–237.

147. Sherwood WG, Saunders M, Robinson BH, et al. Lactic acidosis in biotin-responsive multiple carboxylase deficiency caused by holocarboxylase synthetase deficiency of early and late onset. J Pediatr 1982;101:546–550.

148. Packman S, Sweetman L, Baker H, et al. The neonatal form of biotin-responsive multiple carboxylase deficiency. J Pediatr 1981;99:418–420.

149. Sweetman L. Two forms of biotin-responsive multiple carboxylase deficiency. J Inherited Metab Dis 1981;4:53–54.

150. Sweetman L, Nyhan WL, Sakati NA, et al. Organic aciduria in neonatal multiple carboxylase deficiency. J Inherited Metab Dis 1982;5:49–53.

151. Weyler W, Sweetman L, Maggio DC, et al. Deficiency of propionyl CoA carboxylase in a patient with methylcrotonylglycinuria. Clin Chim Acta 1977;76:321.

152. Bartlett K, Gompertz D. Biotin activation of carboxylase activity in cultured fibroblasts from a child with a combined carboxylase defect. Clin Chim Acta 1989;84:399.

153. Burri BJ, Sweetman L, Nyhan WL. Heterogeneity of holocarboxylase synthetase in patients with biotin-responsive multiple carboxylase deficiency. Am J Hum Genet 1985;37:326–337.

154. Burri BJ, Sweetman L, Nyhan WL. Mutant holocarboxylase synthetase: Evidence for the enzyme defect in early infantile biotin-responsive multiple carboxylase deficiency. J Clin Invest 1981;68:1491–1495.

155. Jakobs C, Sweetman L, Nyhan WL, et al. Stable isotope dilution analysis of 3-hydroxyisovaleric acid in amniotic fluid: Contribution to the prenatal diagnosis of inherited disorders of leucine catabolism. J Inherited Metab Dis 1984;7:15–20.

156. Packman S, Cowan MJ, Golbus MS, et al. Prenatal treatment of biotin responsive multiple carboxylase deficiency. Lancet 1982;1:1435–1438.

157. Di Rocco M, Superti-Furga A, Caprino D, et al. Phenotypic variability in biotinidase deficiency [letter]. J Pediatr 1984; 104:964–965.

158. Campana G, Valentini G, Legnaioli MI. Ocular aspects in biotinidase deficiency. Clinical and genetic original studies. Ophthalmol Paediatr Genet 1987;8:125–129.

159. Leonard JV, Daish P, Naughten ER, et al. The management and long-term outcome of organic acidaemias. J Inherited Metab Dis 1984;7:13–17.

160. Cowan MJ, Wara DW, Packman S, et al. Multiple biotin-dependent carboxylase deficiencies associated with defects in T-cell and B-cell immunity. Lancet 1979;2:115–118.

161. Schulz PE, Weiner SP, Belmont JW, et al. Basal ganglia calcifications in a case of biotinidase deficiency. Neurology 1988;38:1326–1328.

162. Fois A, Cioni M, Balestri P, et al. Biotinidase deficiency: Metabolites in CSF. J Inherited Metab Dis 1986;9:284–285.

163. Taitz LS, Leonard JV, Bartlett K. Long-term auditory and visual complications of biotinidase deficiency. Early Hum Dev 1985;11:325–331.

164. Sander JE, Malamud N, Cowan MJ, et al. Intermittent ataxia and immunodeficiency with multiple carboxylase deficiencies: A biotin-responsive disorder. Ann Neurol 1980;8:544–547.

165. Allen RJ, Wolf B, Grier RE. Infantile seizures in biotinidase deficiency. Ann Neurol 1983;14:386.

166. Diamantopoulos N, Painter MJ, Wolf B, et al. Biotinidase deficiency: Accumulation of lactate in the brain and response to physiologic doses of biotin. Neurology 1986;36:1107–1109.

167. Di Rocco M, Supeti-Furga A, Durand P, et al. Different organic acid patterns in urine and in cerebrospinal fluid in a patient with biotinidase deficiency. J Inherited Metab Dis 1984;7:119–120.

168. Bressman S, Fahn S, Eisenberg M, et al. Biotin-responsive encephalopathy with myoclonus, ataxia, and seizures. In: Fahn S ed. Advances in Neurology. New York: Raven Press. 1986;43:119–125.

169. Nyhan WL, Sarati NO. Diagnostic Recognition of Cierke Disease. Philadelphia: Lea and Febiger, 1987:221–237.

170. Suchy SF, McVoy JS, Wolf B. Neurologic symptoms of biotinidase deficiency: Possible explanation. Neurology 1985; 35:1510–1511.

171. Bonjour JP, Bausch J, Suormala T, et al. Detection of biocytin in urine of children with congenital biotinidase deficiency. Int J Vitam Nutr Res 1984;54:223–231.

172. Wolf B, Grier RE, Heard GS. Hearing loss in biotinidase deficiency [letter]. Lancet 1983;2:1365–1366.

173. Wolf B, Grier RE, Allen RJ, et al. Biotinidase deficiency: The enzymatic defect in late-onset multiple carboxylase deficiency. Clin Chim Acta 1983;131:273–281.

174. Gaudry M, Munnich A, Saudubray JM, et al. Deficient liver biotinidase activity in multiple carboxylase deficiency [letter]. Lancet 1983;2:397.

175. Thuy LP, Zielinska B, Zammarchi E, et al. Multiple carboxylase deficiency due to deficiency of biotinidase. J Neurogenet 1986;3:357–363.

176. Heard GS, Secor McVoy JR, Wolf B. A screening method for biotinidase deficiency in newborns. Clin Chem 1984; 30:125–127.

177. Sweetman L, Nyhan WL. Inheritable biotin-treatable disorders and associated phenomena. Annu Rev Nutr 1986; 6:317–343.

178. Middleton B, Bartlett K, Romanos A, et al. 3-Ketothiolase deficiency. Eur J Pediatr 1986;144:586–589.

179. Robinson BH, Sherwood WG, Taylor J, et al. Acetoacetyl CoA thiolase deficiency: A cause of severe ketoacidosis in infancy simulating salicylism. J Pediatr 1979; 95:228–233.

180. Henry CG, Strauss AW, Keating JP, et al. Congestive cardiomyopathy associated with beta-ketothiolase deficiency. J Pediatr 1981;99:754–757.

181. Sabetta G, Bachmann C, Giardini O, et al. Beta-Ketothiolase deficiency with favourable evolution. J Inherited Metab Dis 1987;10:405–406.

182. Schutgens RB, Middleton B, Blij JF, et al. Beta-ketothiolase deficiency in a family confirmed by in vitro enzymatic assays in fibroblasts. Eur J Pediatr 1982;139:39–42.

183. Jakobs C, Sweetman L, Nyhan WL. Hydroxy acid metabolites of branched-chain amino acids in amniotic fluid. Clin Chim Acta 1984;140:157–166.

184. Daum RS, Scriver CR, Mamer OA, et al. An inherited disorder of isoleucine catabolism causing accumulation of a-methylacetoacetate and a-methyl-β-hydroxybutyrate, and intermittent metabolic acidosis. Pediatr Res 1973;7:149.

185. Gompertz D, Saudubray JM, Charpentier C, et al. A defect in isoleucine metabolism associated with a-methyl-β-hydroxybutyric acid and a-methylacetoacetic aciduria: Quantitative in vivo and in vitro studies. Clin Chim Acta 1974;57:269.

186. Goodman SI, Markey SP, Moe PG, et al. Glutaricaciduria; a 'new' disorder of amino acid metabolism. Biochem Med 1975;12:12.

187. Brandt NJ. Progressive choreo-athetosis with glutaric acid uria. Ugeskr Laeger 1980;142:583–584.

188. Dunger DB, Snodgrass GJ. Glutaric aciduria type I presenting with hypoglycaemia. J Inherited Metab Dis 1984; 7:122–124.

189. Yamaguchi S, Orii T, Yasuda K, et al. A case of glutaric aciduria type I with unique abnormalities in the cerebral CT findings. Tohoku J Exp Med 1987;151:293–299.

190. Goodman SI, Frerman FE, Loehr JP. Recent progress in understanding glutaric acidemias. Enzyme 1987;38:76–79.

191. Goodman SI, Norenberg MD. Glutaric acidemia as a cause of striatal necrosis in childhood [letter]. Ann Neurol 1983;13:582–583.

192. Goodman SI, Norenberg MD, Shikes RH, et al. Glutaric aciduria: Biochemical and morphologic considerations. J Pediatr 1977;90:746–750.

193. Stutchfield P, Edwards MA, Gray RG, et al. Glutaric aciduria type I misdiagnosed as Leigh's encephalopathy and cerebral palsy. Dev Med Child Neurol 1985;27:514–521.

194. Hellstrom B. Progressive dystonia and dyskinesia in childhood. A review of some recent advances. Acta Paediatr Scand 1982;71:177–181.

195. Lipkin PH, Roe CR, Goodman SI, et al. A case of glutaric acidemia type I: Effect of riboflavin and carnitine. J Pediatr 1988;112 (1):62–65.

196. Gregersen N, Brandt NJ, Christensen E, et al. Glutaric aciduria: Clinical and laboratory findings in two brothers. J Pediatr 1977;90:740–745.

197. Bennett MJ, Marlow N, Pollitt RJ, et al. Glutaric aciduria type 1: biochemical investigations and postmortem findings. Eur J Pediatr 1986;145:403–405.

198. Leibel RL, Shih VE, Goodman SI, et al. Glutaric acidemia: A metabolic disorder causing progressive choreoathetosis. Neurology 1980;30:1163–1168.

199. Goodman SI, Kohlhoff JG. Glutaric aciduria: Inherited deficiency of glutaryl CoA dehydrogenase activity. Biochem Med 1975;13:138.

200. Brandt NJ, Gregersen N, Christensen E, et al. Treatment of glutaryl CoA dehydrogenase deficiency (glutaric aciduria). Experience with diet, riboflavin, and GABA analogue. J Pediatr 1979;94:669–673.

201. Christensen E, Brandt NJ. Studies on glutaryl CoA dehydrogenase in leucocytes, fibroblasts and amniotic fluid cells. The normal enzyme and the mutant form in patients with glutaric aciduria. Clin Chim Acta 1978;88:267.

202. Jakobs C, Sweetman L, Wadman SK, et al. Prenatal diagnosis of glutaric aciduria type II by direct chemical analysis of dicarboxylic acids in amniotic fluid. Eur J Pediatr 1984;141:153–157.

203. Goodman SI, Gallegos DA, Pullin CJ, et al. Antenatal diagnosis of glutaric acidemia. Am J Hum Genet 1980; 32:695–699.

204. Blass JP, Lonsdale D, Uhlendorf BW, et al. Intermittent ataxia with pyruvate-decarboxylase deficiency. Lancet 1971;1:1302.

205. Sheu KFR, Hu CW, Utter MF. Pyruvate dehydrogenase complex activity in normal and deficient fibroblasts. J Clin Invest 1981;67:1463–1471.

206. Haas RH, Thompson G, Morris B, et al. Pyruvate dehydrogenase activity in osmotically shocked rat brain mitochondria: Stimulation by oxaloacetate. J Neurochem 1988;50(3):673–680.

207. Robinson BH, MacMillan H, Petrova-Benedict R, et al. Variable clinical presentation in patients with defective E1 component of pyruvate dehydrogenase complex. J Pediatr 1987;111:525–533.

208. Leigh D. Subacute necrotizing encephalomyelopathy in an infant. J Neurol Neurosurg Psychiatry 1951;14:216–221.

209. Pincus JH. Subacute necrotising encephalomyelopathy (Leigh's disease): A consideration of clinical features and etiology. Dev Med Child Neurol 1972;14:87–101.

210. Hall K, Gardner-Medwin D. CT scan appearances in Leigh's disease (subacute necrotizing encephalomyelopathy). Neuroradiology 1978;16:48–50.

211. Sheu KFR, Blass JP. Pyruvate dehydrogenase phosphate (PDHb) phosphatase activity in fibroblasts from Leigh's disease. Neurology 1984;34:1187–1191.

212. DeVivo DC, Haymond MW, Obert KA, et al. Defective activation of the pyruvate dehydrogenase complex in subacute necrotizing encephalomyelopathy (Leigh disease). Ann Neurol 1979;6(6):483–494.

213. Robinson BH, Taylor J, Sherwood WG. Deficiency of dihydrolipoyl dehydrogenase (a component of the pyruvate and alpha-ketoglutarate dehydrogenase complexes): A cause of congenital chronic lactic acidosis in infancy. Pediatr Res 1978;11:1198–1202.

214. Munnich A, Saudubray JM, Taylor J, et al. Congenital lactic acidosis, alpha-ketoglutaric aciduria and variant form of maple syrup urine disease due to a single enzyme defect: Dihydrolipoyl dehydrogenase deficiency. Acta Paediatr Scand 1982;71:167–171.

215. Matalon R, Stumpf DA, Michals K, et al. Lipoamide dehydrogenase deficiency with primary lactic acidosis: Favorable response to treatment with oral lipoic acid. J Pediatr 1984;104:65–69.

216. Hommes FA, Polman HA, Reerink JD. Leigh's encephalomyelopathy: An inborn error of gluconeogenesis. Arch Dis Child 1968;43:423.

217. Moosa A, Hughes EA. Proceedings: L-glutamine therapy in Leigh's encephalomyelopathy. Arch Dis Child 1974;49:246.

218. Van Biervliet JP, Duran M, Wadman SK, et al. Leigh's disease with decreased activities of pyruvate carboxylase and pyruvate decarboxylase. J Inherited Metab Dis 1980; 2:15–18.

219. Gilbert EF, Arya S, Chun R. Leigh's necrotizing encephalopathy with pyruvate carboxylase deficiency. Arch Pathol Lab Med 1983;107:162–166.

220. Grover WD, Auerbach VH, Patel MS. Biochemical studies and therapy in subacute necrotizing encephalomyelopathy (Leigh's syndrome). J Pediatr 1979;81:39.

221. Gruskin AB, Patel MS, Linshaw M, et al. Renal function studies and kidney pyruvate carboxylase in subacute necrotizing encephalomyelopathy (Leigh's syndrome). Pediatr Res 1973;7:832–841.

222. Murphy JV, Isohashi F, Weinberg MB, et al. Pyruvate carboxylase deficiency: An alleged biochemical cause of Leigh's disease. Pediatrics 1981;68:401–404.

223. Atkin BM, Utter MF, Weinberg MB. Pyruvate carboxylase and phosphoenol pyruvate carboxykinase activity in leukocytes and fibroblasts from a patient with pyruvate carboxylase deficiency. Pediatr Res 1979;13:38–43.

224. Saudubray JM, Marsac C, Charpentier C, et al. Neonatal congenital lactic acidosis with pyruvate carboxylase deficiency in two siblings. Acta Paediatr Scand 1976;65:717.

225. Coude FX, Ogier H, Marsac C, et al. Secondary citrullinemia with hyperammonemia in four neonatal case of pyruvate carboxylase deficiency. Pediatrics 1981;68:914.

226. Wong LT, Davidson AG, Applegarth DA, et al. Biochemical and histologic pathology in an infant with cross-reacting material (negative) pyruvate carboxylase deficiency. Pediatr Res 1986;20:274–279.

227. Atkin BM, Buist NR, Utter MF, et al. Pyruvate carboxylase deficiency and lactic acidosis in a retarded child without Leigh's disease. Pediatr Res 1979;13:109–116.

228. DeVivo DC, Haymond MW, Leckie MP, et al. The clinical and biochemical implications of pyruvate carboxylase deficiency. J Clin Endocrinol Metab 1977;45:1281–1296.

229. Robinson BH, Oei J, Sherwood WG, et al. The molecular basis for the two different clinical presentations of classical pyruvate carboxylase deficiency. Am J Hum Genet 1984; 36:283–294.

230. Haworth JC, Robinson BH, Perry TL. Lactic acidosis due to pyruvate carboxylase deficiency. J Inherited Metab Dis 1981;4:57.

231. Robinson BH, Oei J, Saudubray JM, et al. The French and North American phenotypes of pyruvate carboxylase deficiency. Correlation with biotin containing protein by 3H-biotin incorporation, 35S-streptavidin labelling and Northern blotting with a cloned cDNA probe. Am J Hum Genet 1987;40:50.

232. Tommasi M, Jouvet Telinge A, Kopp N, et al. Alpers' infantile cerebral poliodystrophy. A case with abnormal hepatic pyruvate carboxylase. Ann Anat Pathol (Paris) 1977;22:337–342.

233. Shank RP, Bennett GS, Freytag SO, et al. Pyruvate carboxylase: An astrocyte-specific enzyme implicated in the replenishment of amino acid neurotransmitter pools. Brain Res 1985;329:364–367.

234. Perry TL, Haworth JC, Robinson BH. Brain amino acid abnormalities in pyruvate carboxylase deficiency. J Inherited Metab Dis 1985;8:63–66.

235. Bardin RE, Taylor BL, Osohashi I. Structural properties of pyruvate carboxylase from chicken liver and other sources. Proc Natl Acad Sci USA 1975;72:4308.

236. Scrutton MC, White MD. Purification and properties of human liver pyruvate carboxylase. Biochem Med 1974; 9:271.

237. Lamhonwah A, Quan F, Gravel RA. Sequence homology around the biotin-binding site of human propionyl CoA carboxylase and pyruvate carboxylase. Arch Biochem Biophys 1987;254:631–636.

238. Freytag SO, Collier KJ. Molecular cloning of a cDNA for human pyruvate carboxylase. J Biol Chem 1984;259:12831–12837.

239. Marsac C, Augerau GL, Feldman G, et al. Prenatal diagnosis of pyruvate carboxylase deficiency. Clin Chim Acta 1982;119:121.

240. Robinson BH, Toon JR, Petrova-Benedict R, et al. Prenatal diagnosis of pyruvate carboxylase deficiency. Prenat Diagn 1985;5:67.

241. Hommes FA, Bendien K, Elema JD, et al. Two cases of phosphoenolpyruvate carboxykinase deficiency. Acta Paediatr Scand 1976;65:233.

242. Robinson BH, Taylor J, Kahler S. Mitochondrial phosphoenolpyruvate carboxykinase deficiency in a child with lactic acidemia, hypotonia and failure to thrive. Am J Hum Genet 1979;31:60A.

243. Clayton PT, Hyland K, Brand M, et al. Mitochondrial phosphoenolpyruvate carboxykinase deficiency. Eur J Pediatr 1986;145:46.

244. Tuboi S, Sato M, Ono H, et al. Mechanism of synthesis and localization of mitochondrial and cytosolic fumarases in rat liver. Adv Enzyme Regul 1986;25:461–484.

245. Zinn AB, Keer DS, Hoppel CL. Fumarase deficiency: A new cause of mitochondrial encephalomyopathy. N Engl J Med 1986; 315.

246. Petrova-Benedict R, Robinson BH, Stacey TE, et al. Deficient fumarase activity in the infant with fumaricacidemia and its distribution between the different forms of the enzyme seen on isoelectric focussing. Am J Hum Genet 1987;40:257.

247. Taylor J, Robinson BH, Sherwood WG. A defect in branched-chain amino acid metabolism in a patient with congenital lactic acidosis due to dihydrolipoyl dehydrogenase deficiency. Pediatr Res 1978;12:60–62.

248. Kohlschutter A, Behbehani A, Langenbeck U, et al. A familial progressive neurodegenerative disease with 2-oxoglutaric aciduria. Eur J Pediatr 1982;138:32–37.

249. Blass JP, Schulman JD, Young DS, et al. An inherited defect affecting the tricarboxylic acid cycle in a patient with congenital lactic acidosis. J Clin Invest 1972;51:1845–1851.

250. Prick MJ, Gabreels FJ, Renier WO, et al. Progressive infantile poliodystrophy (Alpers' disease) with a defect in citric acid cycle activity in liver and fibroblasts. Neuropediatrics 1982;13:108–111.

251. Miyabayashi S, Ito T, Narisawa K, et al. Biochemical study in 28 children with lactic acidosis, in relation to Leigh's encephalomyelopathy. Eur J Pediatr 1985;143:278–283.

252. Robinson BH, Taylor J, Sherwood WG. The genetic heterogeneity of lactic acidosis: Occurrence of recognizable inborn errors of metabolism in a pediatric population with lactic acidosis. Pediatr Res 1980;14:956–962.

253. Shapira Y, Harel S, Russell A. Mitochondrial encephalomyopathies. A group of neuromuscular disorders with defects in oxidative metabolism. Isr J Med Sci 1977;13(2):161–164.

254. Heymans HSA, Schutgens RBH, Tan R, et al. Severe plasmalogen deficiency in tissues of infants without peroxisomes (Zellweger syndrome). Nature 1983;306:69.

255. Matalon R, Michals K, Sebesta D, et al. Aspartoacylase deficiency and N-acetylaspartic aciduria in patients with Canavan disease. Am J Med Genet 1988;29(2):463–471.

256. Rowland LP. Molecular genetics, pseudogenetics, and clinical neurology. Neurology 1983;33:1179–1195.

257. Pavlakis SG, Phillips PC, DiMauro S, et al. Mitochondrial myopathy, encephalopathy, lactic acidosis, and stroke-like episodes: A distinctive clinical syndrome. Ann Neurol 1984;16:481–488.

258. Ichiki T, Tanaka M, Nishikimi M, et al. Deficiency of subunits of Complex I and mitochondrial encephalomyopathy. Ann Neurol 1988;23:287–294.

259. Nishizawa M, Tanaka K, Shinozawa K, et al. A mitochondrial encephalomyopathy with cardiomyopathy. A case revealing a defect of complex I in the respiratory chain. J Neurol Sci 1987;78:189–201.

260. Kuriyama M, Umezaki H, Fukuda Y, et al. Mitochondrial encephalomyopathy with lactate-pyruvate elevation and brain infarctions. Neurology 1984;34:72–77.

261. Skogland RR. Reversible alexia, mitochondrial myopathy and lactic acidemia. Neurology 1979;29:717–720.

262. Driscoll PF, Larsen PD, Gruber AB. MELAS syndrome involving a mother and two children. Arch Neurol 1987;44:971–973.

263. Maertens P, Richardson R, Bastian F, et al. A new type of mitochondrial encephalomyopathy with stroke-like episodes due to cytochrome oxidase deficiency. J Inherited Metab Dis 1988;11:186–188.

264. Allard JC, Tilak S, Carter AP. CT and MR of MELAS syndrome. AJNR 1988;9:1234–1238.

265. Oldfors A, Tulinius M, Holme E, et al. Mitochondrial encephalomyopathy. A variant with heart failure and liver steatosis. Acta Neuropathol (Berl) 1987;74:287–293.

266. Hart ZH, Chang C-H, Perrin EVD, et al. Familial poliodystrophy mitochondrial myopathy and lactic acidemia. Arch Neurol 1977;34:180–185.

267. Shapira Y, Cederbaum SD, Cancilla PA, et al. Familial poliodystrophy, mitochondrial myopathy, and lactic acidemia. Neurology 1975;25:614–621.

268. Gibson KM, Nyhan WL, Jackan T. Inborn errors of GABA metabolism. Bioessays 1986;4:24–26.

269. Tsairis P, Engel W, Kark P. Familial myoclonic epilepsy syndrome associated with skeletal muscle mitochondrial abnormalities. Neurology 1973;23:408.

270. Rosing HS, Hopkins LC, Wallace DC, et al. Maternally inherited mitochondrial myopathy and myoclonic epilepsy. Ann Neurol 1985;17:228–237.

271. Schon EA, Bonilla E, Lombes A, et al. Clinical and biochemical studies on cytochrome oxidase deficiencies. Ann NY Acad Sci 1988;550:348–359.

272. Riggs JE, Schochet SS Jr, Fakadej AV, et al. Mitochondrial encephalomyopathy with decreased succinate-cytochrome c reductase activity. Neurology 1984;34:48–53.

273. Kearns T, Sayre GP. Retinitis pigmentosa, external opthalmoplegia, and complete heart block. Arch Ophthalmol 1958;60:280–289.

274. Berenberg RA, Pellock JM, DiMauro S, et al. Lumping or splitting? "Opthalmoplegia-plus" or Kearns-Sayre syndrome? Ann Neurol 1977;1:37–54.

275. Seigel RS, Seeger JF, Gabrielsen TO, et al. Computed tomography in oculocraniosomatic disease (Kearns-Sayre syndrome). Radiology 1979;130:159–164.

276. Martens ME, Peterson PL, Lee CP, et al. Kearns-Sayre syndrome: Biochemical studies of mitochondrial metabolism. Ann Neurol 1988;24:630–637.

277. Moraes CT, DiMauro S, Zeviani M, et al. Mitochondrial DNA deletions in progressive external opthalmoplegia

and Kearns-Sayre syndrome. N Engl J Med 1989; 320:1293–1299.

278. Shoffner JM, Lott MT, Voljavec AS, et al. Spontaneous Kearns-Sayre/chronic external opthalmoplegia plus syndrome associated with a mitochondrial DNA deletion: A slip-replication model and metabolic therapy. Proc Natl Acad Sci USA 1989;86:7952–7956.

279. Ishitsu T, Miike T, Kitano A, et al. Heterogeneous phenotypes of mitochondrial encephalomyopathy in a single kindred. Neurology 1987;37:1867–1869.

280. Kitano A, Nishiyama S, Miike T, et al. Mitochondrial cytopathy with lactic acidosis, carnitine deficiency and DeToni-Fanconi-Debré syndrome. Brain Dev 1986;8:289–295.

281. Sengers RC, Fischer JC, Trijbels JM, et al. A mitochondrial myopathy with a defective respiratory chain and carnitine deficiency. Eur J Pediatr 1983;140:332–337.

282. Borund O, Torbergsen T, Mathiesen E. Increased lactate in cerebrospinal fluid from 7 siblings in a family with mitochondrial myopathy and cerebellar ataxia. J Inherited Metab Dis 1987;10:400.

283. Darley-Usmar VM, Kennaway NG, Buist NRM, et al. Deficiency in ubiquinone cytochrome c reductase in a patient with mitochondrial myopathy and lactic acidosis. Proc Natl Acad Sci USA 1983;80:5103–5106.

284. DiMauro S, Miranda AF, Sakoda S, et al. Metabolic myopathies. Am J Med Genet 1986;25:635–651.

285. Parker WD Jr, Oley CA, Parks JK. A defect in mitochondrial electron transport activity (NADH- coenzyme Q oxidoreductase) in Leber's hereditary optic atrophy. N Engl J Med 1989;320:1331–1333.

286. Singh G, Lott MT, Wallace DC. A mitochondrial DNA mutation as a cause of Leber's hereditory optic neuropathy. N Engl J Med 1989;320:1300–1305.

287. Willems JL, Monnens LAH, Trijbels JMF, et al. Leigh's encephalomyelopathy in a patient with cytochrome c oxidase deficiency in muscle tissue. Pediatrics 1977;60:850–857.

288. Norenberg MD, Mozes LW, Gregorios JB, et al. Effects of lactic acid on astrocytes in primary culture. J Neuropathol Exp Neurol 1987;46 (2):154–166.

289. Sahgal V, Subramani V, Hughes R, et al. On the pathogenesis of mitochondrial myopathies. An experimental study. Acta Neuropathol (Berl) 1979;46:177–183.

290. Morgan-Hughes JA, Hayes DJ, Cooper M, et al. Mitochondrial myopathies: Deficiencies localized to complex I and complex III of the mitochondrial respiratory chain. Biochem Soc Trans 1985;13:648–650.

291. Moreadith RW, Batshaw ML, Ohnishi T, et al. Deficiency of the iron-sulfur clusters of mitochondrial reduced nicotinamide-adenine dinucleotide-ubiquinone oxidoreductase (Complex I) in an infant with congenital lactic acidosis. J Clin Invest 1984;74:685–697.

292. Moreadith RW, Cleeter MWJ, Ragan CI, et al. Congenital deficiency of two polypeptide subunits of the iron-protein fragment of mitochondrial Complex I. J Clin Invest 1987;79:463–467.

293. Hoppel CL, Kerr DS, Dahms B, et al. Deficiency of the reduced nicotinamide adenine dinucleotide dehydrogenase component of complex I of mitochondrial electron transport. Fatal infantile lactic acidosis and hypermetabolism with skeletal-cardiac myopathy and encephalopathy. J Clin Invest 1987;80:71–77.

294. Tanaka M, Nishikimi M, Suzuki H, et al. Deficiency of subunits in heart mitochondrial NADH-ubiquinone oxidoreductase of a patient with mitochondrial encephalomyopathy and cardiomyopathy. Biochem Biophys Res Commun 1986;140:88–93.

295. Prick MJJ, Gabreels FJM, Renier WO, et al. Progressive infantile poliodystrophy. Association with disturbed pyruvate metabolism in muscle and liver. Arch Neurol 1981;38:767–772.

296. Van Erven PM, Fischer JC, Gabreels FJ, et al. Defect of NADH dehydrogenase in Leigh syndrome [letter]. Acta Neurol Scand 1986;74:167.

297. Angelini C, Battistella PA, Laverda A, et al. Fatal lipid storage with abnormal mitochondria in an infant. Acta Neuropathol Suppl (Berl) 1981;7:221–225.

298. Ogasahara S, Engel AG, Frens D, et al. Muscle coenzyme Q deficiency in familial mitochondrial encephalopathy. Proc Natl Acad Sci USA 1989;86:2379–2382.

299. Ogasahara S, Yorifuji S, Nishikawa Y, et al. Improvement of abnormal pyruvate metabolism and cardiac conduction defect with coenzyme Q_{10} in Kearns-Sayre syndrome. Neurology 1985;35:372–377.

300. Hayes DJ, Lecky BR, Landon DN, et al. A new mitochondrial myopathy. Biochemical studies revealing a deficiency in the cytochrome b-c1 complex (complex III) of the respiratory chain. Brain 1984;107:1165–1177.

301. Kennaway NG, Buist NR, Darley-Usmar VM, et al. Lactic acidosis and mitochondrial myopathy associated with deficiency of several components of complex III of the respiratory chain. Pediatr Res 1984;18:991–999.

302. Eleff S, Kennaway NG, Buist NMR, et al. 31P NMR study of improvement in oxidative phosphorylation by vitamins K3 and C in a patient with a defect in electron transport at complex III in skeletal muscle. Proc Natl Acad Sci USA 1984;81:3529–3533.

303. Morgan-Hughes JA, Hayes DJ, Clark JB, et al. Mitochondrial encephalomyopathies: Biochemical studies in two cases revealing defects in the respiratory chain. Brain 1982;105:553–582.

304. Federico A, Cornelio F, Di Donato S, et al. Mitochondrial encephalo-neuro-myopathy with myoclonus epilepsy, basal nuclei calcification and hyperlactacidemia. Ital J Neurol Sci 1988;9:65–71.

305. Parker WD Jr, Frerman F, Haas R, et al. Myxothiazol resistance in human mitochondria. BBA 1988;936:133–138.

306. Van Biervliet JPGM, Bruinvis L, Ketting D, et al. Hereditary mitochondrial myopathy with lactic acidemia, a DeToni-Fanconi-Debré syndrome, and a defective respiratory chain in voluntary striated muscles. Pediatr Res 1977;II:1088–1093.

307. DiMauro S, Zeviani M, Rizzuto R, et al. Molecular defects in cytochrome oxidase in mitochondrial diseases. J Bioenerg Biomembr 1988;20:353–364.

308. Bresolin N, Zeviani M, Bonilla E, et al. Fatal infantile cytochrome c oxidase deficiency: Decrease of immunologically detectable enzyme in muscle. Neurology;35:802–812.

309. Zeviani M, Van Dyke DH, Servidei S, et al. Myopathy and fatal cardiomyopathy due to cytochrome c oxidase deficiency. Arch Neurol 1986;43:1198–1202.

310. DiMauro S, Nicholson JF, Hays AP, et al. Benign infantile mitochondrial myopathy due to reversible cytochrome c oxidase deficiency. Ann Neurol 1983;14:226–234.

311. Boustany RN, Aprille JR, Halperin J, et al. Mitochondrial cytochrome deficiency presenting as a myopathy with hypotonia, external ophthalmoplegia, and lactic acidosis in an infant and as fatal hepatomegaly in a second cousin. Ann Neurol 1983;14:462–470.

312. DiRocco M, Veneselli E, Ciccone MO, et al. Cytochrome c oxidase deficiency in three patients with Leigh's disease. J Inherited Metab Dis 1988;11:189–192.

313. Miyabayashi S, Narisawa K, Tada K, et al. Two siblings with cytochrome c oxidase deficiency. J Inherited Metab Dis 1983;6:121–122.

314. DiMauro S, Servidei S, Zeviani M, et al. Cytochrome c oxidase deficiency in Leigh syndrome. Ann Neurol 1987;22:498–506.

315. Arts WF, Scholte HR, Loonen MC, et al. Cytochrome c oxidase deficiency in subacute necrotizing encephalomyelopathy. J Neurol Sci 1987;77:103–115.

316. Ogier H, Lombes A, Scholte HR, et al. DeToni-Fanconi-Debré syndrome with Leigh syndrome revealing severe muscle cytochrome c oxidase deficiency. J Pediatr 1988;112:734–739.

317. Miyabayashi S, Ito T, Abukawa D, et al. Immunochemical study in three patients with cytochrome c oxidase deficiency presenting Leigh's encephalomyelopathy. J Inherited Metab Dis 1987;10:289–292.

318. Miranda AF, Ishii S, DiMauro S, et al. Cytochrome c oxidase deficiency in Leigh's syndrome: Genetic evidence for a nuclear DNA-encoded mutation. Neurology 1989;39:697–702.

319. Prick MJ, Gabreels FJ, Trijbels JM, et al. Progressive poliodystrophy (Alpers' disease) with a defect in cytochrome aa3 in muscle: A report of two unrelated patients. Clin Neurol Neurosurg 1983;85:57–70.

320. Angelini C, Bresolin N, Pegolo G, et al. Childhood encephalomyopathy with cytochrome c oxidase deficiency, ataxia, muscle wasting, and mental impairment. Neurology 1986;36:1048–1052.

321. Menkes JH. Kinky hair disease: Twenty five years later. Brain Dev 1988;10:77–79.

322. Maehara M, Ogasawara N, Mizutani N, et al. Cytochrome c oxidase deficiency in Menkes kinky hair disease. Brain Dev 1983;5:533–540.

323. Bresolin N, Moggio M, Bet L, et al. Progressive cytochrome c oxidase deficiency in a case of Kearns-Sayre syndrome: Morphological, immunological, and biochemical studies in muscle biopsies and autopsy tissues. Ann Neurol 1987;21:564–572.

324. Nishikawa Y, Takahashi M, Yorifuji S, et al. Long-term coenzyme Q_{10} therapy for a mitochondrial encephalomyopathy with cytochrome c oxidase deficiency: A ^{31}PNMR study. Neurology 1989;39:399–403.

325. Doriguzzi C, Palmucci L, Mongini T, et al. Endocrine involvement in mitochondrial encephalomyopathy with partial cytochrome c oxidase deficiency. J Neurol Neurosurg Psychiatry 1989;52:122–125.

326. Van Erven PM, Gabreels FJ, Ruitenbeek W, et al. A mitochondrial encephalomyopathy with a partial cytochrome c oxidase deficiency of muscle. J Neurol Neurosurg Psychiatry 1988;51:704–708.

327. Bardosi A, Creutzfeldt W, DiMauro S, et al. Myo-, neuro-, gastrointestinal encephalopathy (MNGIE syndrome) due to partial deficiency of cytochrome-c-oxidase. A new mitochondrial multisystem disorder. Acta Neuropathol (Berl) 1987;74:248–258.

328. Harigaya Y, Shoji M, Okamoto K, et al. A case of mitochondrial encephalomyopathy with myoclonic attacks, hyper-lactic-pyruvic acidemia, and decreased activities of complex II and cytochrome c oxidase. Rinsho Shinkeigaku 1988;28:24–31.

329. Ohnishi A, Nakano S, Hashimoto T, et al. A case of mitochondrial encephalomyopathy with a defect in electron transport at complex I and IV in skeletal muscle showing peripheral neuropathy. Rinsho Shinkeigaku 1988;28:107–111.

330. Brennan WA Jr, Bird ED, Aprille JR. Regional mitochondrial respiratory activity in Huntington's disease brain. J Neurochem 1985;44:1948–1950.

331. Schotland DL, DiMauro S, Bonilla E, et al. Neuromuscular disorder associated with a defect in mitochondrial energy supply. Arch Neurol 1976;33:475–479.

332. Luft R, Ikkos D, Palmieri G, et al. A case of severe hypermetabolism of non thyroid origin with a defect in the maintenance of mitochondrial respiratory control: A correlated clinical, biochemical and morphological study. J Clin Invest 1962;41:1776–1804.

333. Przyrembel H, Wendel U, Becker K, et al. Glutaric aciduria type II: Report on a previously undescribed metabolic disorder. Clin Chim Acta 1976;66:227–239.

334. Coude FX, Ogier H, Charpentier C, et al. Neonatal glutaric aciduria type II: An X-linked recessive inherited disorder. Hum Genet 1981;59:263–265.

335. Gregersen N, Klvraa S, Rasmussen K, et al. Biochemical studies in a patient with defects in the metabolism of acyl CoA and sarcosine: Another possible case of glutaric aciduria type II. J Inherited Metab Dis 1980;3:67–72.

336. Sweetman L, Nyhan WL, Trauner DA, et al. Glutaric aciduria Type II. J Pediatr 1980;96:1020–1026.

337. Bennett MJ, Curnock DA, Engel PC, et al. Glutaric aciduria type II: Biochemical investigation and treatment of a child diagnosed prenatally. J Inherited Metab Dis 1984;7:57–61.

338. Goodman SI, Stene DO, McCabe ERB, et al. Glutaric aciduria type II: Clinical, biochemical, and morphologic considerations. J Pediatr 1982;100:946–950.

339. Mooy PD, Giesberts MA, van Gelderen HH, et al. Glutaric aciduria type II: Multiple defects in isolated muscle mitochondria and deficient beta-oxidation in fibroblasts. J Inherited Metab Dis 1984;7:101–102.

340. Dusheiko G, Kew MC, Joffe BI, et al. Recurrent hypoglycemia associated with glutaric aciduria type II in an adult. N Engl J Med 1979;301:1405–1409.

341. Mitchell G, Saudubray JM, Benoit Y, et al. Antenatal diagnosis of glutaricaciduria type II. Lancet 1983;1:1099.

342. Mitchell G, Saudubray JM, Gubler MC, et al. Congenital anomalies in glutaric aciduria type 2 [letter]. J Pediatr 1984;104:961–962.

343. Harkin JC, Gill WL, Shapira E. Glutaric acidemia type II: Phenotypic findings and ultrastructural studies of brain and kidney. Arch Pathol Lab Med 1986;110:399.

344. Bohm N, Uy J, Kiessling M, et al. Multiple acyl CoA dehydrogenase deficiency (glutaric aciduria type II), congenital polycystic kidneys, and symmetrical warty degeneration of the cerebral cortex in two newborn brothers. II Morphology and pathogenesis. Eur J Pediatr 1982;139:60.

345. Harpey JP, Charpentier C, Coude M. Methylene-blue for riboflavin-unresponsive glutaricaciduria type II. Lancet 1986;1:391.

346. Pattarelli PP, Nyhan WL, Gibson KM. Oxidation of U-14C succinic semialdehyde in cultured human lymphoblasts: Measurement of residual succinic semialdehyde dehydrogenase activity in 11 patients with 4-hydroxybutyric aciduria. Pediatr Res 1988;24:435–460.

347. Rating D, Hanefeld F, Siemes H, et al. 4-Hydroxybutyric aciduria: A new inborn error of metabolism. I. Clinical review. J Inherited Metab Dis 1984;7 Suppl 1:90–92.

348. Gibson KM, Jansen I, Sweetman L, et al. 4-Hydroxybutyric aciduria: A new inborn error of metabolism. III. Enzymology and inheritance. J Inherited Metab Dis 1984;7 Suppl 1:95–96.

349. Haan EA, Brown GK, Mitchell D, et al. Succinic semialdehyde dehydrogenase deficiency—a further case. J Inherited Metab Dis 1985;9:99.

350. Gibson KM, Nyhan WL, Jaeker J. Inborn errors of GABA metabolism. Bioessays 1986;4:24–27.

351. Snead OC. Gamma-hydroxy-butyrate in the monkey. I. Electroencephalographic, behavioural and pharmacokinetic studies. Neurology 1978;28:636–642.

352. Gibson KM, Sweetman L, Nyhan WL, et al. Succinic semialdehyde dehydrogenase deficiency: An inborn error of gamma-aminobutyric acid metabolism. Clin Chim Acta 1983;133:33–42.

353. Gibson KM, Sweetman L, Nyhan WL, et al. Defective succinic semialdehyde dehydrogenase activity in 4-hydroxybutyric aciduria. Eur J Pediatr 1984;142:257–259.

354. Gibson KM, Sweetman L, Nyhan WL, et al. Succinic semialdehyde dehydrogenase deficiency. J Neurogenet 1984;1:213–218.

355. Gibson KM, Sweetman L, Jansen I, et al. Properties of succinic semialdehyde dehydrogenase in cultured human lymphoblasts. J Neurogenet 1985;2:111–122.

356. Jakobs C, Bojasch M, Monch E, et al. Urinary excretion of gamma-hydroxybutyric acid in a patient with neurological abnormalities. The probability of a new inborn error of metabolism. Clin Chim Acta 1981;111:169–178.

357. Roesel RA, Hartlage PL, Carroll JE, et al. 4-Hydroxybutyric aciduria and glycinuria in two siblings. Am J Hum Genet 1987;41:A16.

358. Gibson KM, Aramaki S, Sweetman L, et al. Stable isotope dilution analysis of 4-hydroxybutyric acid: An accurate method for quantification in physiological fluids and the prenatal diagnosis of 4-hydroxybutyric aciduria. Biomed Environ Mass Spectrom 1988;19:89–93.

359. Divry P, Baltassat P, Rolland MO, et al. A new patient with 4-hydroxybutyric aciduria, a possible defect of 4-aminobutyrate metabolism. Clin Chim Acta 1984;129:303–309.

Chapter 4
Abnormalities of Carbohydrate Metabolism

S. Robert Snodgrass

GLUCOSE METABOLISM IN THE NORMAL STATE

Dietary carbohydrates are degraded to monosaccharides in the intestine; glucose, galactose, and fructose are the primary sugars of concern to humans. Galactose and fructose are entirely of dietary origin; lactose in milk is a disaccharide comprised of glucose and galactose, and sucrose is made up of glucose and fructose.

Anaerobic Glycolysis

Life on earth is believed to have developed in an oxygen-free atmosphere (1), and only later, when significant oxygen was present did eukaryotic, mitochondria-containing cells capable of oxidative phosphorylation appear. All cells today retain the enzymatic machinery for anaerobic metabolism of glucose, the so-called glycolytic or Embden-Meyerhof pathway, which leads from glucose to lactic acid. This sequence of 11 enzymatic reactions takes place in the cytoplasm and results in the net production of 2 adenosine triphosphate (ATP) molecules per molecule of glucose metabolized. In contrast, full oxidation of lactate to carbon dioxide and water by the tricarboxylic acid (TCA) or Krebs cycle adds 36 molecules of ATP but requires oxygen and pyruvate entry into the mitochondrion (2). Activation of cells or a change in the functional state of cells is often associated with a change of an enzyme or process from solution to a membrane compartment, or vice versa. For example,

the process of long-term potentiation seems to be associated with translocation of protein kinase C from the cytosol to a membrane compartment within neurons (3).

Heart and skeletal muscle tend to oxidize free fatty acids (FFAs) rather than glucose under most conditions, a preference intensified by starvation. Glucose differs from fatty acids as a fuel because it can provide high-energy phosphate molecules under anaerobic conditions. Muscle oxygen delivery often becomes rate limiting during heavy exercise so that glycolysis becomes the main or only ATP source. White muscle has less oxidative capacity than red muscle, so glycolysis is always more important for those fibers (Figure 4.1). The pathways of glycolysis and glycogen metabolism intersect at glucose-6-phosphate. Three groups of cytosolic enzymes compete for this critical metabolite: the enzymes of the glycolysis, glycogenesis, and pentose phosphate pathways. The latter two pathways siphon off glucose molecules for essential nonenergy-related functions (Figure 4.2).

Flux through the glycolytic pathway is regulated at three main points: the most important regulatory phosphofructokinase (PFK) step, the hexokinase, and glucose transport steps (2). Phosphofructokinase has two ATP-binding sites; the catalytic site binds ATP, which becomes the second phosphate group of fructose-1,6-bisphosphate, while a second allosteric site binds ATP with resultant inhibition of enzyme activity. The ATP concentration of resting muscle is about 5 mM, at which PFK activity is markedly inhibited. As tissue ATP content falls, glycolytic flux greatly

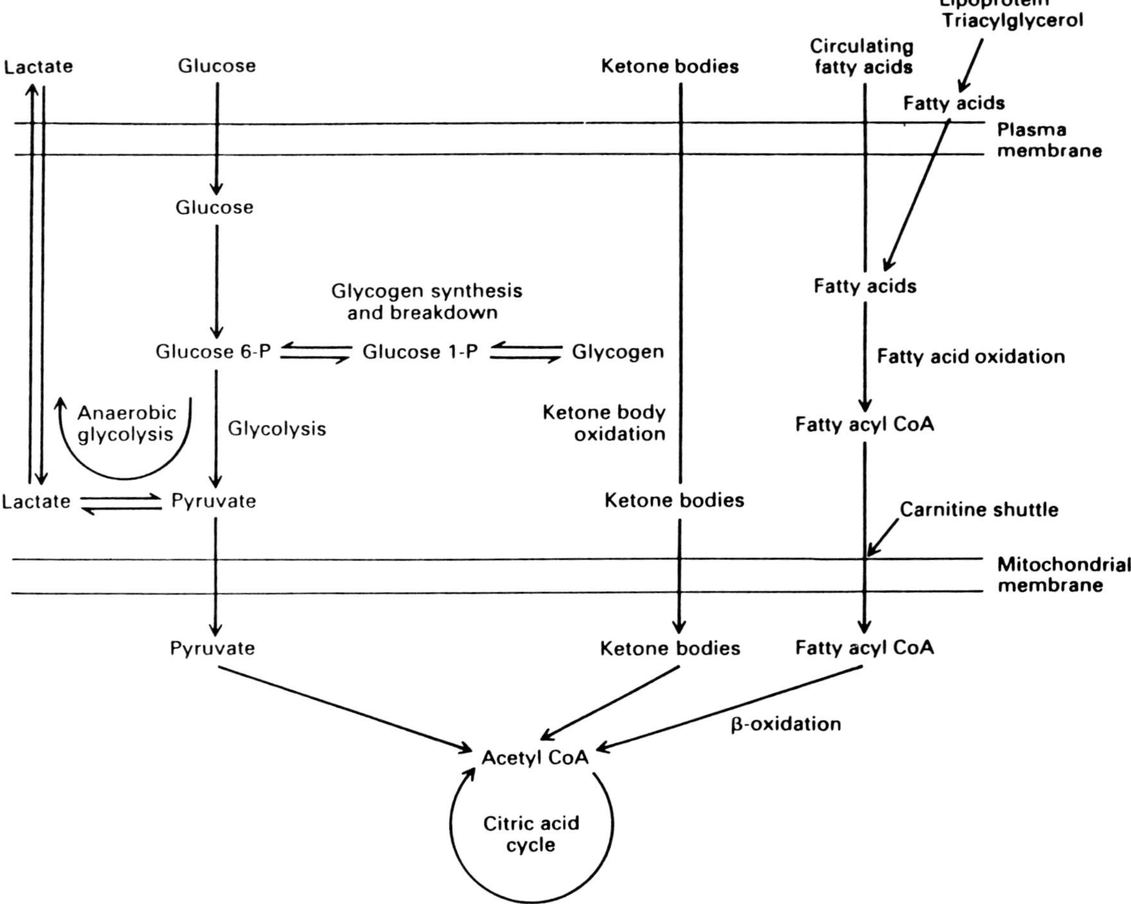

FIGURE 4.1 Energy metabolism in muscle. The diagram shows the major pathways for energy production in skeletal muscle. With the exception of glycolysis, all of the pathways are dependent on oxygen. (With permission from Martin BR. Metabolic regulation: A molecular approach. Oxford: Blackwell Scientific Publications, 1987.)

increases. In the rat heart, anaerobiosis producing a 20% decrease in ATP concentration leads to a ninefold increase in glycolytic flux. The function of the glycolytic enzyme group in muscle is to provide ATP for muscle contraction. In addition to its own less efficient generation of high-energy phosphate groups, glycolysis is the source of pyruvate for the TCA cycle, which is transformed into acetyl CoA by the multienzyme complex within the mitochondrion known as pyruvate dehydrogenase. Inhibition of PFK by ATP is influenced by several regulatory molecules. As ATP content falls, adenosine monophosphate (AMP) increases and acts to reverse the enzyme inhibition by ATP; therefore, the signal produced by the declining ATP concentration is amplified. Inhibition by ATP is also reversed by inorganic phosphate (Pi), fructose-6-phosphate, the enzyme substrate, and by fructose-1,6-bisphosphate, its product. Inhibition by ATP is increased by the citrate ion, which provides a signal of the availability of other ATP sources such as fatty acids or ketone bodies. In starvation, the citrate control promotes lipid oxidation (Figure 4.3).

The regulation of hexokinase is more simple. This enzyme is inhibited by its product, glucose-6-phosphate.

When PFK is inhibited, glucose-6-phosphate concentrations rise quickly and inhibit further glucose phosphorylation. Activation of glycogen synthesis causes a fall in glucose-1-phosphate, then a decrease in glucose-6-phosphate, resulting in increased phosphorylation. Flux from glucose to glycogen can be independently regulated, and glycogen synthesis is generally active in states of low glycolytic activity.

It has been suggested that the glycolytic enzymes float freely in cytoplasmic water and can be considered as independent of one another except for their effects on substrate concentration. Studies using subcellular fractionation led to the categorization of the enzymes of glycolysis and the pentose phosphate pathway as soluble enzymes, because most enzyme activity remained in solution after high-speed centrifugation, which sediments organelles such as mitochondria and microsomes (4). The interaction of clusters of cytosolic enzymes with cellular matrices including the cytoskeleton and the plasma membrane, and organization of localized multienzyme complexes within the cytoplasm are now well established (5). It has been shown that membrane fractions of some cells could catalyze the entire

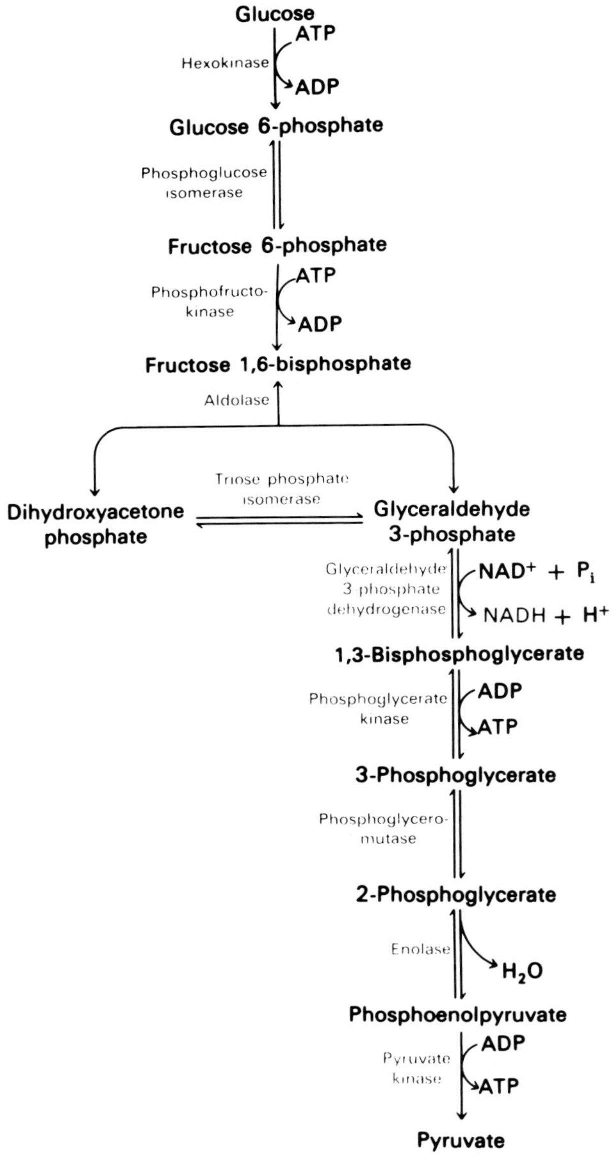

FIGURE 4.2   The glycolytic pathway. (Reprinted with permission from Stryer L. Biochemistry, 3rd ed. New York: W. H. Freeman and Company, 1988.)

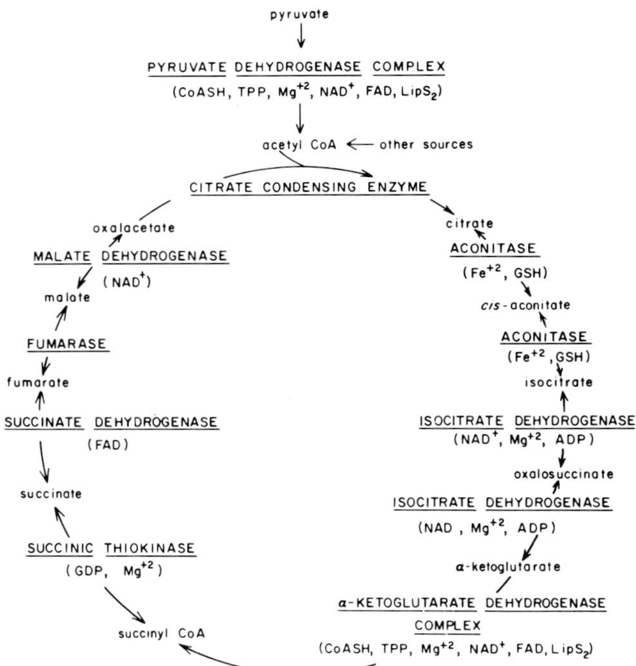

FIGURE 4.3   Enzymes and coenzymes of the Krebs cycle. Cofactors are shown in parentheses below each enzyme. (Reprinted with permission from Montgomery R, Dryer RL, Conway TW, et al. Biochemistry, A Case Oriented Approach. St. Louis: Mosby-Year Book, 1974.)

Karadshen and Ukeda showed that the catalytic properties of PFK were markedly altered by adsorption to cell membranes (8). The enzyme could no longer be inhibited by ATP, implying that it was "frozen" into a new conformation. Mutations that alter the ability of cytosolic enzymes to associate with one another or with structural elements (noncatalytic mutations) may not be evident in standard enzyme assays. Moreover, enzyme studies of human disease material have often neglected protein changes that did not affect the enzyme catalytic site.

If certain groups of enzymes are physically and functionally close to certain patches of membrane, one might expect inhibitors of those enzymes to selectively impair certain membrane functions. This appears to be true for the potassium channels of the guinea pig ventricular myocyte (9). These channels open when local ATP concentration falls below a certain value. Mitochondrial substrates such as pyruvate and glutamate were significantly less able to keep the channels closed than were glycolytic substrates, like fructose-1,6-biphosphate. Even though glycolytic enzymes generate much less ATP than does oxidative phosphorylation, their proximity to certain patches of membrane makes them better able to support membrane function than more distant organelles with theoretical greater energy production. It is likely that some neuronal ion channels are similarly associated with groups of cytosolic enzymes. If the placement of organelles and enzyme clusters within the cell is nonrandom as all evidence suggests, the processes

glycolytic sequence with higher specific activity than that exhibited by the original tissue homogenate (6), suggesting that glycolytic enzymes may be topographically linked to certain membranes. Liver and muscle exhibit distinctive isozymic profiles for at least seven of the glycolytic enzymes. Aldolase, for example, has been found to exist in at least nine separate forms in higher organisms (5). These multiple forms arise from the assembly of polypeptide chains coded by three different genes. They differ in kinetic properties and, more importantly, in their ability to be adsorbed onto various particulate structures within the cell (7). Some aldolase isozymes are selectively released from brain particulate fractions by altering salt concentration or pH or both.

controlling that placement must come under scrutiny as possibly involved in human disease.

Clegg has shown that glycolytic enzymes tend to be associated with structures containing actin filaments such as thin filaments in muscle and microfilaments of the cytoskeleton (10). Calcium ions that promote the polymerization of actin filaments can alter the association between filaments and glycolytic enzymes with consequent effects on energy metabolism (11). Bronstein and Knull proposed that some glycolytic enzymes will not bind to actin filaments unless other enzymes of the glycolytic sequence are also present (12). Ureta has stressed the likely presence of multiple different complexes of isozymes in some tissues, each complex having a different product and without mixing of intermediates between complexes (13).

Transfer of metabolite from one enzyme to another without dissociation into the aqueous phase has been demonstrated for many enzyme pairs within the glycolytic sequence (14). These particular enzymes are present in very high concentrations in muscle and brain, at concentrations similar to those of their substrates in most cases (hexose phosphates and lactate are exceptions owing to their higher concentrations). Therefore, ordinary studies of enzyme kinetics with very dilute enzyme suspensions and enzyme concentrations much less than those of the substrate may fail to predict behavior in vivo (14). In states of renal failure, ischemia, and acidosis, the orderly arrangement of multienzyme complexes may unwind in ways undetectable in broken-cell preparations. Nuclear Magnetic Resonance (NMR) spectroscopy of intact cells is one way to study metabolite concentrations and regulation of cellular metabolism in response to various control signals.

There is no doubt that glycolytic activity is greatly influenced by the concentrations of small molecules and the rates of energy utilization. However, gene expression for the glycolytic enzymes can also be regulated in a coordinate fashion. This would represent a higher or earlier level of control. Webster found that chronic exposure to low oxygen concentration induced increased amounts of mRNA for multiple glycolytic enzymes (15,16). Since the genes for these enzymes are found on unlinked chromosomal loci, it was suggested that trans-acting proteins can bind to common DNA sequences associated with these genes. Mutations in noncoding regions of DNA that regulate transcription would not be detectable either by sequencing the enzyme polypeptide or by measuring its catalytic behavior in dilute solution. Fibroblasts are readily available for study but may be inadequate for studies of transcription regulation because of their limited repertoire of transcription factors.

Glycolysis and Muscle Function

It has been known for decades that muscular contraction consumes high-energy phosphates and that ATPases are found in muscle fibers (17). Fatty acids provide the main fuel for muscle at rest and during light to moderate exercise, but as one progresses to more severe exercise, carbohydrate fuel becomes dominant. Carbohydrate oxidation through the TCA cycle provides much more ATP than does anaerobic glycolysis. Training increases strength and endurance; it increases the mitochondrial content of muscle, muscle blood flow, and has a glycogen-sparing effect (18).

As Ranvier recognized, red and white skeletal muscles differ in structure. Most skeletal muscles are comprised of several different fiber types, and a variety of histochemical procedures have been used to categorize them. Dubowitz and Pearse (1960) proposed that muscle fibers should be categorized on the basis of oxidative enzyme activity (19). A similar classification scheme based upon ATPase activity was introduced by Engel (1962) and has been widely accepted for clinical analysis of muscle biopsies (20). These first schemes were oversimplifications; red fibers, for example, are not necessarily slow (21). Fibers can be classified by their mitochondrial content, mitochondrial enzyme activity, or muscle glycogen content (22). No single classification scheme meets all needs, but Engel's ATPase scheme with various modifications is the most widely used (23). When considering disordered carbohydrate metabolism, it is useful to speak of three basic fiber types: slow (type I fibers in the ATPase schemes), fast red (type IIa fibers), and fast white (type IIb fibers). Each of these types has a different form of myosin, coded by a *different gene* (24).

Kugelberg and Edstrom showed that stimulation of a motor neuron selectively depleted the glycogen of the muscle fibers innervated by that neuron (25). This showed that all the fibers within a single motor unit belonged to one histochemical category. The physiologic properties of motor neurons are determined by motor unit type rather than neuronal size. Alpha motor neurons innervating slow-twitch muscle of rats have higher oxidative capacity than do similarly sized motor neurons supplying fast-twitch muscles (26). The pattern of fiber types can be changed by even modest physiologic alterations. For example, thyroidectomy leads to major changes in fiber type, but only in innervated fibers (27). Adrenergic stimulation of muscles produces different effects in slow and fast muscles (28), and slow-twitch muscles are reported to have more beta-receptors than fast-twitch muscles (29). Several reports indicate that β_2 adrenergic agonists produce skeletal muscle hypertrophy and retard the atrophic effects of denervation (30). Although muscle ATP concentrations are about 5 mM, this store is depleted by a few seconds of vigorous exercise (31). When contractile activity increases, fuel oxidation must also increase. The ratio of oxidation to utilization remains remarkably constant during a variety of conditions. This constancy requires precise regulation of metabolism.

First, enzymes that use ATP as substrate are inhibited by ADP and vice versa. Small decreases in the ATP/ADP ratio produce large increases in the intracellular concentrations of AMP, NH_4^+, and Pi, which release PFK from inhibition.

Oxidation of long-chain fatty acids provides a major share of muscle energy after the first minutes, which are typically carbohydrate-driven (32). In humans all muscle fiber types have similar glycogen content, while lipid stores are greater in the more oxidative fibers (32). If not supplemented by fatty acid oxidation or glucose infusion, muscle glycogen stores decline rapidly as exercise continues. The blockade of FFA release with nicotinic acid causes more rapid glycogen depletion and shorter endurance times (33).

It has been shown that the capacity for prolonged strenuous exercise is closely related to pre-exercise muscle glycogen content (34). For example, the initial glycogen content of the quadriceps muscle predicted the length of time that trained subjects could exercise (35); moreover, muscle glycogen content was much greater after high-carbohydrate diets. This work stimulated the practice of carbohydrate loading by endurance athletes. Earlier studies may have distorted the ability of fat oxidation to support muscle function (36). Eskimo sled dogs eat a high-fat diet and are capable of prolonged arduous exercise, but they do less well on high-carbohydrate diets (37). Cyclists on a high-fat, low-carbohydrate diet for 4 weeks had, as expected, less muscle glycogen prior to exercise; however, their endurance was equal to that of others on ordinary diets (38). Both groups became exhausted at similar muscle glycogen levels. The chronic fat group consumed glycogen more slowly, but when it was depleted, they could no longer oxidize fat. Other studies in humans and rats have demonstrated increased activity of muscle fat oxidizing enzymes, such as carnitine palmityl transferase after weeks on the high-fat diets (39). There is a species difference in that rats generally oxidize fats better than humans. Rats and dogs also have a somewhat different distribution of muscle fiber types than humans, with a greater oxidative profile (40); moreover, the fast-twitch fibers of rats, dogs, and humans are each somewhat different.

Muscle can adapt to high-fat diets, but the process takes weeks rather than days. There may be metabolic diseases in which a high-fat diet, avoiding those fats that promote atherosclerosis, is helpful. Hypoglycemia occurs in some cases of prolonged severe exercise but it is rare in humans. It is known from NMR spectroscopic studies that intracellular pH decreases as the muscle becomes exhausted (41). Exhaustion is associated with increased inosine monophosphate (IMP) and hypoxanthine, small decreases in ATP, and essentially no change in lactate concentrations from those found after several minutes of exercise (42). IMP and hypoxanthine are metabolites produced from adenosine and AMP by the enzyme adenylate deaminase, an enzyme important in purine metabolism. The catalytic properties and regulation of adenylate deaminase should be defined in any comprehensive study of its role in muscle disease.

As long as working muscle is supplied with FFAs, ketone bodies, and oxygen, the basic elements required for ATP production are present. The maximum duration and degree of muscle contraction is then a function of muscle mass and level of training. Although trained athletes have more muscle glycogen, they use less glycogen for the same amount of work and have a lower respiratory quotient (lipids carry more of the metabolic load in muscle). Only muscles that have undergone training show the changes of increased aerobic oxidative capacity. Studies of single human muscle fibers suggest that oxidative muscle fibers (types I and II) are involved in low to medium work loads, with recruitment of fast-twitch glycolytic fibers as the work load increases. Glycolytic or type II fibers break down much more glycogen and produce more lactic acid. Studies of human forearm muscles at high work load with ^{31}P NMR spectroscopy showed two different Pi peaks, suggesting fibers of internal pH 6.9 (oxidative) and 5.9 to 6.4 (glycolytic) (43). Rapid disappearance of the Pi pool at pH 6.9 was interpreted as meaning rapid restoration of ATP and PCr in the oxidative fibers, while recovery was much slower in the glycolytic fibers. Spectroscopic studies comparing the spectra of both forearms suggest that the more active dominant forearm has a different profile of fiber types. While the correlation of fiber type and pH is consistent and fatigued muscles certainly have lower pH values, more recent data suggest that the effect of acidity is indirect and mediated through formation of the intermediate $H_2PO_4^-$ (44). Availability of Pi and the balance between high energy and inorganic phosphates are important considerations.

Glycogen and Glycogenolysis

While nearly all tissues store glycogen, its use varies among tissue types. The liver uses glycogen to buffer blood glucose, and skeletal muscle uses it as an energy reserve to support mechanical work. Glycogen in the liver and adipose tissue falls with fasting, while muscle glycogen is less closely correlated with time of the last meal. Muscle glycogen cannot support blood glucose because the enzyme glucose-6-phosphate is not found in muscle. Various control mechanisms determine the flow of carbohydrate metabolites. When dietary glucose is abundant, the liver takes up glucose and lipid, storing some glucose as glycogen and converting some to fat. If the liver did not take up glucose efficiently, massive increases in blood glucose would cause tissue dehydration and possible death. Coulson calculated that 175 g of glucose present in a sweet would produce a blood glucose level of about 70 mM, or 1260 mg/dL, if there were no liver (45). Glycogen has no fixed molecular weight, is highly branched and hydrated, and is present in almost all cells. In the satiated state, lactate and fructose in addition to glucose are important substrates for glycogen synthesis (2). Much of the glucose-6-phosphate destined for hepatic glycogen is made from three carbon precursors rather than dietary glucose, the indirect pathway (46).

Liver glycogen content exceeds that of any other organ, sometimes reaching 8% to 10% of its mass. Although the hepatocytes are more freely permeable to glucose than most cells, they are not permeable to glucose-6-phosphate, which must be dephosphorylated before leaving the cell (47). Glucokinase rather than the more general hexokinase (2 different enzymes) is responsible for hepatic glucose phosphorylation. However, glucokinase plus hexokinase activity is much less than that of hepatic glucose-6-phosphatase and insufficient to account for observed rates of net glucose uptake. Another enzyme, glucose-6-phosphatase, operating in the synthetic direction, contributes to glucose phosphorylation using pyrophosphate and carbamyl phosphate as phosphoryl donors. The hydrolytic and synthetic capacities of glucose-6-phosphatase are separately regulated (47). Glucose-6-phosphatase differs from other enzymes of the glucogenic pathways in being intimately associated with a membrane system, the endoplasmic reticulum. Arion et al. (48) postulated that translocases were responsible for bringing specific substrates from the cytosol to the catalytic machinery in the endoplasmic reticulum, across the microsomal membrane. These translocases are drug-sensitive (49) and can be deficient in certain glycogen storage diseases (GSDs) (50). Inability to transport glucose-6-phosphate into the microsome or endoplasmic reticulum (ER) is functionally equivalent to a mutation inactivating the enzyme. Such a disease exists, one in which all the features of glucose-6-phosphatase deficiency coexist with normal enzyme activity (51).

The critical step that commits glucose to glycogen synthesis is that of isomerization by the enzyme phosphoglucomutase. The rate-controlling enzymes of glycogen synthesis and breakdown, glycogen synthase and phosphorylase, exist in both active and inactive forms. The intracellular concentration of phosphorylase a, the active form, is the best single indicator of the state of glycogen metabolism. This enzyme also regulates glycogen synthase phosphorylase and, therefore, the rate of glycogen synthesis. Glycogen itself is an important regulator of its own synthesis, acting on glycogen synthetase to inhibit further accumulation and stimulating conversion of phosphorylase into its active form. Glycogen metabolism is regulated by multiple hormones. Glucagon activates glycogen breakdown by cyclic adenosine-3′,5′-monophosphate (AMP)-mediated phosphorylation of the enzyme phosphorylase. The calcium-mobilizing hormones vasopressin, angiotensin II, and alpha-1 adrenergic agonists act to open calcium channels and promote glycogen breakdown, stimulating phosphorylase kinase and inhibiting glycogen synthase (2). Phorbol esters act directly on glycogen synthase but have no effect on phosphorylase (52). Insulin stimulates glycogen synthase and inhibits phosphorylase (Figure 4.4).

Glycogen homeostasis is very different in muscle where energy usage can override extrinsic or hormonal regulation (2). Muscle phosphorylase is activated by three main factors: energy demand as shown by increases in AMP and Pi, decreases in ATP and glucose-6-phosphate; muscle contraction, which acts via Ca^{++}-mediated activation of phosphorylase kinase (one of whose subunits is calmodulin);

and catecholamines, which stimulate cyclic AMP-dependent phosphorylation and activation of phosphorylase kinase. Glycogen synthase can be phosphorylated on multiple sites and exists, therefore, in more than two forms. As more sites are phosphorylated, its activity progressively declines. A single enzyme, protein phosphatase 1, dephosphorylates most of the phosphoproteins involved in glycogen metabolism, although other phosphatases play minor roles (2). Dephosphorylation is regulated by various molecules. For example, the binding of AMP to the active form of phosphorylase a inhibits phosphate removal. Skeletal muscle can synthesize significant amounts of glycogen after exercise in spite of fasting, while the liver must wait for a meal (53). Vigorous exercise produces marked increases in blood lactate, which is reused for gluconeogenesis. Glycogen is repleted faster and to higher levels in oxidative fibers.

The complex regulation of glycogen synthesis and breakdown remains only partially understood; studies of homogenates and perfused livers suggest different mechanisms than studies of intact working heart and skeletal muscle (54). It is now possible to detect and quantify muscle glycogen by natural abundance ^{13}C NMR spectroscopy, wherein no chemical need be infused for labeling. This work, however, requires use of multiple surface coils and a 4.7 Tesla magnet into which subjects insert their limbs (55), allowing the study of glycogen metabolism sequentially in response to exercise, fasting, and glucose, for example, without obtaining muscle biopsies. The study of both ^{13}C and ^{31}P spectra is required for maximum information.

Central Nervous System Glycogen

It is known that brain tissue is dependent on carbohydrate metabolism. Given the genes for glycogen synthesis and breakdown, why are they so weakly expressed in the central nervous system (CNS)? The answer seems to be twofold. Cells swell as glycogen is stored in their cytoplasm. Liver size can safely change with feeding status, but marked swelling of brain cells leads to dire consequences. Moreover, evolution favored strength of limb and swiftness of foot, which benefited from an exquisitely regulated muscle energy supply relatively independent of meals. Exposure to cerebral ischemia typically comes late in life (after reproduction), and there would be no natural selection for resistance to cerebral ischemia. Survival of newborns after difficult births may not have been evolutionarily advantageous as a result of limitations it would impose on a band of hunter-gatherers. Considerable glycogen exists in the newborn brain at birth. Chesler and Himwich (1943) showed that glycogen content decreased with development in phylogenetically old portions of brain, such as cerebellum, medulla, and spinal cord, while increasing with age in cortex and basal ganglia (56). Glycogen is generally not visible in tissue sections because of rapid postmortem hydrolysis, but it can be easily demonstrated in CNS tissue

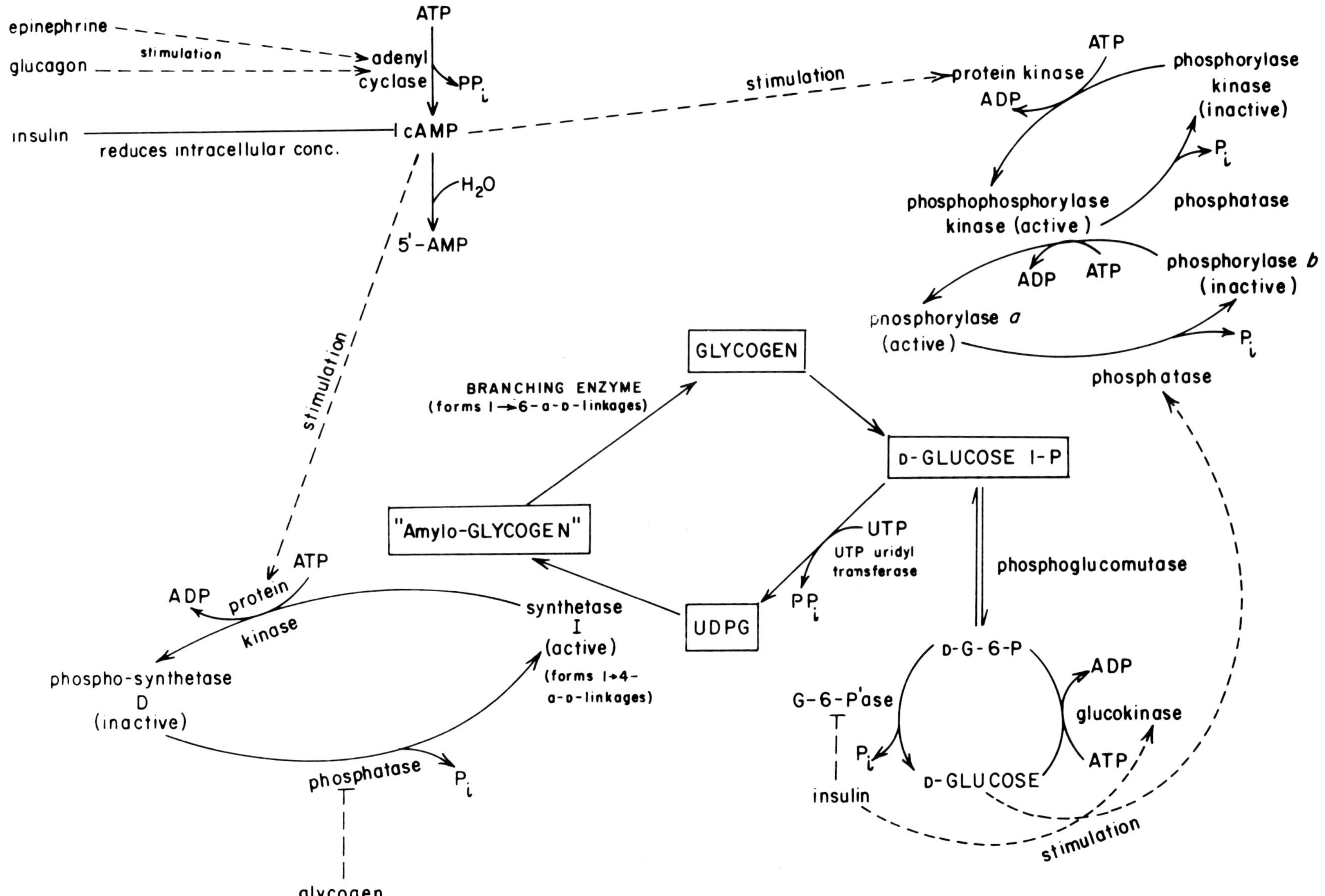

FIGURE 4.4 Regulation of glycogen metabolism. (Reprinted with permission from Montgomery R, Dryer RL, Conway TW, et al. Biochemistry: A Case Oriented Approach, St. Louis: Mosby-Year Book, 1974.)

after perfusion fixation of experimental animals or rapid freezing of surgical specimens.

As in other tissues, the enzymes of glycogen synthesis and degradation in the brain are responsive to various hormones (6). The concentration of enzyme uridine diphosphate glucose (UDPG) pyrophosphorylase needed for glycogen synthesis is high in brain, while glycogen synthase activity is low (57). Many studies using electron microscopy have shown that glycogen is more abundant in glial and ependymal cells than neurons. Microdissection studies of the rodent hippocampus have shown 50% more glycogen in fiber layers than in the pyramidal cell layer or adjacent cerebral cortex (58); however, methodologic problems limit the value of older cerebral glycogen data. Sagar et al. found that brain glycogen content was significantly higher after microwave killing, which more rapidly inactivates cerebral enzymes than after conventional decapitation and brain removal (59). Greatest glycogen content was found in the brain stem, with lowest values in the striatum. Various studies in the older literature had reported increased brain glycogen with anesthesia, but Sagar found no effect of anesthesia with pentobarbital. The duration and depth of anesthesia may be important variables, but the effects of anesthesia on brain glucose utilization are not in doubt. Petroni et al. studied the effects of hypoxia (breathing 5% O_2 for 30 minutes) in the rat, using microwave radiation to avoid postmortem artifacts and found increased brain glucose and lactate without any change in glycogen content at the end of the hypoxic period (60). It is likely that hyperglycemia was the main factor responsible for increasing brain glucose. A decrease in brain glycogen after bilateral carotid occlusion in the gerbil was found with a subsequent overshoot to supranormal values (58). This overshoot coincided with maximal tissue lactate values and was greatest in pyramidal cell and cortical layers, which contain few glial cells. These workers employed rapid freezing, which is preferable to simple decapitation, but probably gives different glycogen values than microwave irradiation.

If postmortem hydrolysis of glycogen were much greater in neurons than glial cells, the idea that glial cells have more glycogen than neurons would be incorrect. Brain glycogen synthase differs in molecular properties from that found in skeletal muscle (61). Studies of immunoreactive glycogen synthase in the dog and rat brain showed that all cell types contain the enzyme, and that forebrain structures such as hippocampus, neocortex, and striatum contained more of the enzyme in spite of their lower glycogen levels (59). Neurons had more of the antigen than glial cells and differences between neuronal types were evident (62). The relative importance of glycogen for neurons and glial cells remains to be determined. In a series of in vitro studies, it was shown that brain glycogen breakdown is influenced by many transmitters and by the extracellular potassium concentration (63). These effects appear to be neuronal rather than glial. They do not prove, however, that glycogen supports any specific neuronal function, but they do suggest that ischemia and depolarization would cause immediate reductions in glycogen content (60). At this time it is not known what would happen if brain glycogen were not stored in response to increased glucose availability or could not be hydrolyzed. Glycogen does not seem to be a significant protective factor in cerebral ischemia. Only one of the known GSDs, acid maltase deficiency or GSD type II, has been proven to affect the brain directly.

Gluconeogenesis and Minor Pathways of Glucose Metabolism

Liver glycogen content is sufficient to sustain blood glucose levels for only a few hours of fasting (2), and fat oxidation is activated unless we eat every few hours. Protein breakdown and conversion of amino acids to glucose is a back-up mechanism, one that is particularly destructive to the growing infant. Gluconeogenesis from lactate, pyruvate, and amino acids, as in the case of hepatic glycogen breakdown, is activated by glucagon, vasopressin, angiotensin II, and catecholamines. Glucagon is the single most important hormone controlling liver glucose metabolism. Most catecholamine effects are mediated by alpha$_1$ receptors.

The gluconeogenesis pathway reverses the glycolytic sequence; however, three glycolytic steps are functionally irreversible, requiring substrate cycles or metabolic bypasses when gluconeogenesis is operative. These bypasses are exquisitely regulated. Starting with pyruvate, the conversion of phosphoenolpyruvate (PEP) to pyruvate + ATP is functionally irreversible (Figure 4.5). The enzyme involved, pyruvate kinase, is closely regulated in the liver but not in muscle, which has no direct role in gluconeogenesis. Pyruvate carboxylase, a biotin-dependent enzyme, and PEP-CK are needed to bypass the effect of pyruvate kinase. The fate of pyruvate lies between pyruvate carboxylase, pyruvate dehydrogenase (which pushes it into the Krebs cycle), transamination to alanine, and lactate dehydrogenase (which produces lactic acid and ATP). The first two reactions occur inside the mitochondrion, indicating that mitochondrial disorders, including interference with pyruvate transport into mitochondria, can impair both energy metabolism and gluconeogenesis. Transamination can occur in the mitochondria or cytosol and results in transfer of an amino group to pyruvate, oxaloacetate, or alpha-ketoglutarate.

Alanine accounts for a much greater proportion of plasma amino acids than amino-acid residues in protein. The difference comes from transamination of pyruvate, making alanine available for transport between different organs. Alanine is also an allosteric inhibitor of pyruvate kinase, acting to shut down entry into the TCA cycle. Alanine and lactate, both derived from pyruvate, are the most important extracellular molecules contributing directly to gluconeogenesis (64). More than half the glucose made in the liver from smaller molecules is used in the brain. The newborn infant has limited liver glycogen; however, gluco-

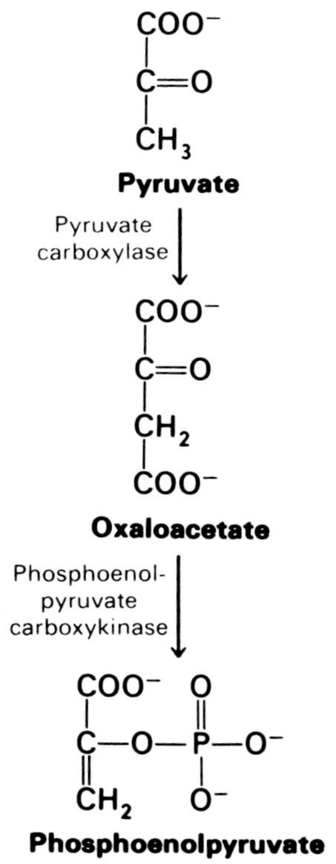

$$COO^-$$
$$C=O$$
$$CH_3$$

Pyruvate

Pyruvate carboxylase

$$COO^-$$
$$C=O$$
$$CH_2$$
$$COO^-$$

Oxaloacetate

Phosphoenol-pyruvate carboxykinase

$$COO^- \quad O$$
$$C-O-P-O^-$$
$$CH_2 \quad O^-$$

Phosphoenolpyruvate

FIGURE 4.5   Phosphoenolpyruvate is formed from pyruvate by way of oxaloacetate. (Reprinted with permission from Stryer L. Biochemistry, 3rd ed. New York: W.H. Freeman and Company, 1988.)

neogenesis increases dramatically on the first day of postnatal life. Much of that increase results from increased activity of the rate-limiting enzyme PEP-CK (65), one of the most rapidly turned over enzymes in the body. Stimuli that increase cyclic AMP-mediated phosphorylation can increase transcription within minutes.

During starvation, hormonal mechanisms lead to fat hydrolysis and export of fatty acids to the liver. Hepatic fatty acid oxidation increases dramatically with marked increases in acetyl CoA content; however, flow through the hepatic TCA cycle is reduced. Concentrations of malate and aspartate decrease, perhaps because of activation of PEP-CK. This enzyme is rapidly induced by glucagon, but the induction is inhibited by glucose or insulin or both. Several chemicals are known to inhibit gluconeogenesis in spite of increased oxidation by tying up acetyl CoA, including lipoamide (66), methylene cyclopropylacetate, a metabolite of hypoglycin (67); and 4-pentenoic acid (68), which closely resembles a major valproic acid metabolite, 4-en-VPA. It is likely that other organic acids, which accumulate in pathologic states or are used for therapeutic purposes, may inhibit gluconeogenesis in similar ways.

All body tissues utilize the glycolytic sequence of reactions; gluconeogenesis is essentially restricted to the liver and kidney. Brain pyruvate carboxylase activity is low compared with most tissues, but it is crucial to gluconeogenesis and appears to be expressed in astrocytes but not in neurons (69). Brain can oxidize fatty acids in small amounts, although it can oxidize ketone bodies derived from hepatic fatty acid oxidation. This is why hypoglycemia is so poorly tolerated. Replenishment of TCA cycle intermediates in nerve endings is thought to depend upon transfer of alpha-ketoglutarate and malate from glia (70).

The pentose phosphate pathway is an alternative pathway for glucose oxidation, which begins with glucose-6-phosphate. Oxidation of glucose-6-phosphate to ribulose-5-phosphate produces two molecules of NADPH. The two oxidative enzymes, glucose-6-phosphate dehydrogenase and 6-phosphogluconate dehydrogenase, are each inhibited by their product, NADPH. Considering that aerobic oxidation of glucose through the TCA cycle produces two molecules of acetyl CoA and that each acetyl CoA molecule requires two molecules of NADPH in order to be incorporated into fatty acids, it is apparent that this pathway must be important in tissues such as brain, which synthesize fatty acids. NADPH can also be generated from the pyruvate/malate cycle (2).

A subsequent nonoxidative segment of the pathway converts various pentose-5-phosphates to fructose-6-phosphate and glyceraldehyde-3-phosphate (Figure 4.6). Because carbon 1 of glucose-6-phosphate is oxidized to CO_2 in the pentose phosphate pathway, the quantitative contribution of this pathway may be estimated by comparing the quantity of labeled CO_2 formed from $^{1\text{-}14}C$-glucose with that formed from $^{6\text{-}14}C$-glucose (71). Various studies suggest that the pentose pathway accounts for less than 10% of brain glucose metabolism in adult rodents or humans. One would predict greater utilization by oligodendrocytes involved in active myelination. Mutations of glucose 6-phosphate dehydrogenase are well-known causes of hemolytic anemia and drug intolerance (72). The symptoms of these diseases are explained by the lack of reducing equivalents needed for drug metabolism. While the pentose pathway accounts for only a small portion of cerebral glucose oxidation, its inhibition by the drug 6-aminonicotinamide produces a severe neurotoxic syndrome (73); elimination of the pathway due to mutation or toxic exposure would probably be lethal.

A less well-known pathway of glucose metabolism begins with the production of sorbitol from glucose by the enzyme aldose reductase (74). This pathway bypasses the control points of hexokinase and PFK, and can rejoin the glycolytic sequence at the step after aldolase. Sorbitol is present in pancreatic cells; brain contains aldose reductase, sorbitol dehydrogenase, and is rich in aldehyde reductase enzymes whose activity is anticonvulsant-sensitive (75).

The accumulation of sorbitol leads to lenticular cataract formation and demyelination of peripheral nerve (76). This pathway, often called the sorbitol or polyol pathway, leads to glycerol synthesis and can utilize ethyl alcohol. It can be involved in fatty-acid accumulation in the liver of alcoholics, and in galactosemia.

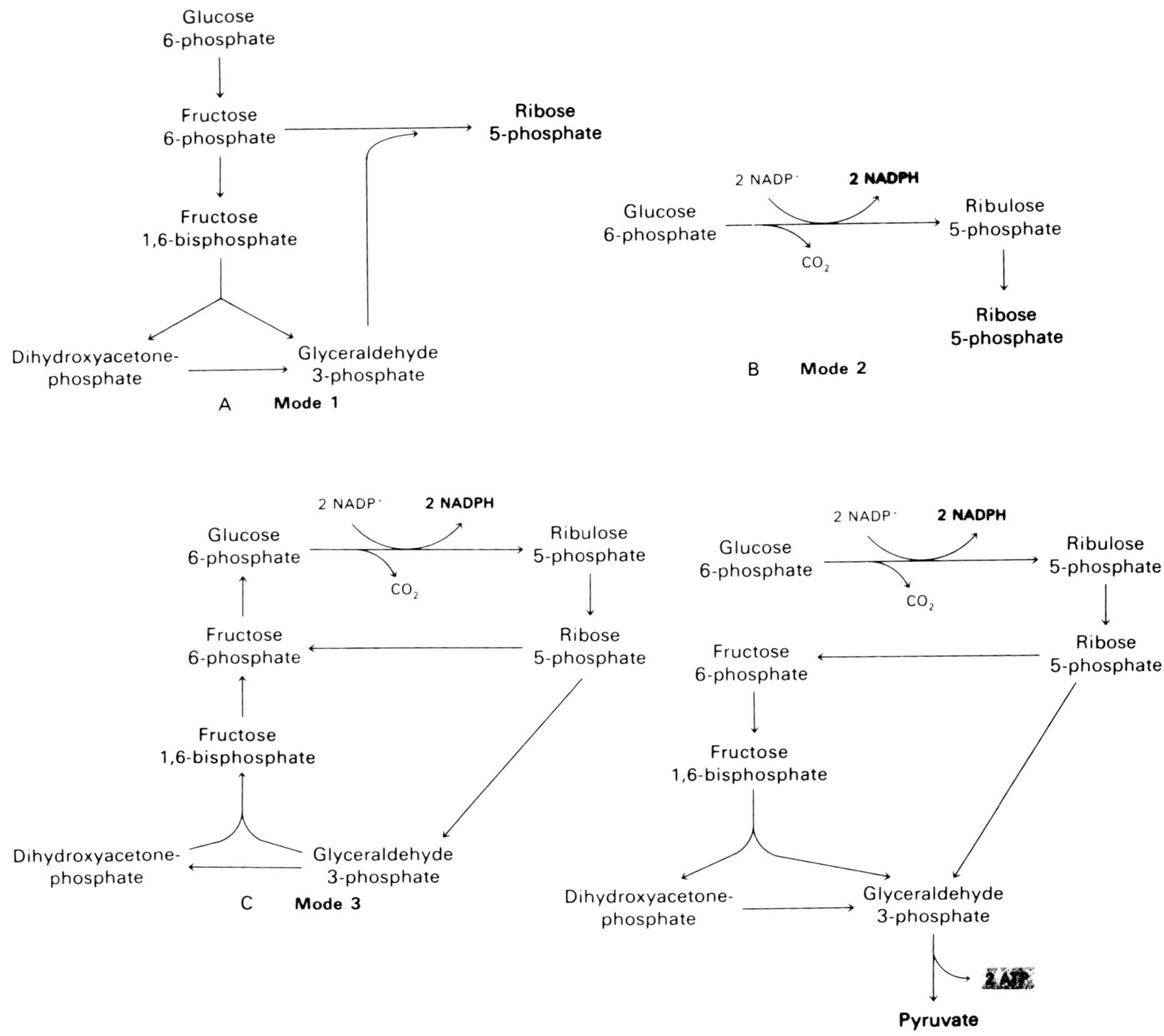

FIGURE 4.6 Four modes of the pentose phosphate pathway. (Reprinted with permission from Stryer L. Biochemistry, 3rd ed. New York: W.H. Freeman and Company, 1988.)

Glucose Transport

Mammalian cells have at least three different glucose transporters: the Na^+-dependent active transporter of kidney and small intestine; the facilitative glucose transporter found in erythrocytes and brain; and the facilitative carrier found in rat liver. Only the first transporter type can increase intracellular glucose concentration to values above those outside the cell, requiring the use of energy from ATP hydrolysis. The functional importance of some kind of blood-brain barrier and blood glucose to brain function has been known since the turn of this century. The mechanism of glucose entry into brain, however, was not known until Crone worked out the kinetics of blood-brain glucose transfer, showing that a saturable mechanism; that is, transport reaches a limit in spite of increasing blood concentrations, was responsible for glucose entry (76,77).

Intracellular brain glucose concentration is very low. Facilitated or nonconcentrative transport of glucose across the blood-brain barrier accounts for about 75% of glucose entry into the dog brain (78). The erythrocyte glucose carrier is a 55-Kd glycoprotein (79). Antibodies produced against it were used to isolate a cDNA clone for the transporter from human hepatoma cells (80). Analysis of the amino-acid sequence predicted from the DNA sequence suggested that the transporter has 12 membrane-spanning helices, a small external domain that is glycosylated and a larger, highly charged cytoplasmic domain (81). Transport is initiated by the binding of glucose to and dissociation of water from hydrogen bonding sites, perhaps formed by the conjunction of helices 7 through 11 into a hydrophilic channel. Subsequently, small changes in protein conformation cause the other end of the channel to open up and allow glucose to diffuse out of the channel at the opposite membrane face. The transporter does not move through the membrane, but it does change conformation depending upon the direction of transport. Because the purified transporter has a Kd or half saturation point for glucose only slightly greater than usual plasma glucose concentrations, small changes in plasma concentration produce large changes of glucose transport into the red cell.

The brain glucose transporter is very similar to that found in the red cell. Antibodies to the human red cell transporter were used to screen a rat brain cDNA bacterial expression library prepared from immunoselected brain RNA. A full-length cDNA clone was isolated with 97.6% identity of amino-acid sequence to the human hepatoma carrier (82). This extraordinary sequence identity across species and between brain and red cell suggests that virtually all regions of the protein are important and have been conserved; that is, mutations anywhere in the molecule are deleterious. Since only a small portion of the molecule directly binds glucose, regulation of the transporter must be vitally important. It is interesting to note that transporter mRNA in an insulin-responsive tissue (adipose tissue) was identical to the transporter message isolated from brain. All present evidence suggests that a single gene codes for this brain transporter and that the same molecule is found in cerebral blood vessels and in membranes of neurons and glial cells (83). The function of this transporter is influenced by the nature of the membrane in which it is embedded (84). Kinetic studies of deoxyglucose transport by dissociated rat brain cells suggest the presence of two somewhat different transporters, possibly differing between neurons and glia (85). One might expect differences in transport kinetics with the same basic gene product if glycosylation of the transporter varied between cell types or at different ages, or if membranes of different cell types differed in their lipid content. It is likely that both mechanisms operate in the CNS. Alternative splicing to generate multiple products from a single transcription unit (86) is also possible, but no supporting evidence, such as differences in message length, has been provided.

At usual blood concentrations, glucose penetration into brain exceeds that of the ketone bodies that can serve as alternative substrates. Although insulin exists in the CNS, its effects on CNS glucose transport are weak and highly variable (87).

The endothelial cells of brain capillaries are especially rich in mitochondria (88). Brain capillaries contain a greater density of glucose transporters than other cortical structures. They transport glucose much faster than they metabolize it and oxidize alternative substrates to a considerable extent (89). These endothelial cells have many features of secretory epithelia. Most of the increased glucose transport capacity of adults as compared to neonates appears to occur in noncapillary cells; namely, neuronal and glial membranes.

Insulin-sensitive tissues have an antigenically unique glucose transporter (90). Such a concept can explain tissue-specific abnormalities in insulin-dependent glucose utilization, as in type II diabetes. A separate insulin-dependent carrier specific to muscle and adipose tissue has been postulated (91), in addition to the three well-established glucose carriers.

Glucose entry into diabetic muscle is decreased in spite of hyperglycemia, whereas circulating FFAs and ketone bodies are markedly increased. Muscle glycolysis is decreased while oxidation of fatty acids and ketone bodies is enhanced. Decreased plasma insulin levels retard the flow of pyruvate into the Krebs cycle, thereby favoring the oxidation of acetyl CoA derived from fatty acids and ketone bodies.

Insulin can markedly increase glucose transport in sensitive tissues and causes the translocation of additional transporters from intracellular storage sites to the plasma membrane. It has been shown that insulin can increase the glucose transport activity of plasma membrane preparations while decreasing that of the Golgi complex (92–94). Although glucose uptake into most tissues does not require ATP, insulin mobilization of transporters is energy-dependent. Insulin may also induce structural or conformational changes in the membrane-bound transporter, altering both transport kinetics and immunoreactivity (95). It is not the only regulator of glucose transport, however. Hypoglycemia and cellular starvation of various types lead to increased numbers of glucose transporters (96) as does malignant transformation with various oncogenes (97). Different stimuli affect glucose transport in different ways; for example, transformation by the oncogene src slows transporter degradation, while glucose starvation and mitogenic stimuli increase synthesis of transporters in fibroblasts (97). Various other agents including concanavalin A and sodium vanadate, increase the V_{max} and translocation of the glucose transporter (98).

Insulin and Insulin-Like Growth Factors in the Central Nervous System

While insulin is well known to stimulate glucose transport into many cell types; it has many other effects (99), including stimulation of membrane Na,K-ATPase, activation of crucial enzymes such as pyruvate dehydrogenase (the entry point into the TCA cycle) and glycogen synthase, and stimulation of DNA synthesis and gene expression in multiple and diverse tissues. There is general agreement that insulin is present in brain at low concentrations, but the exact concentrations found and whether insulin is synthesized by brain tissue are uncertain (100). Plasma insulin can enter brain, probably both by receptor-mediated endocytosis (101) and through circumventricular organs and at the choroid plexus blood-cerebrospinal fluid (CSF) interface (100). Insulin-like growth factors (IGFs) are identified in brain by various radioimmunoassays. Brain has the highest concentration of IGF-II mRNA found in any major organ

(102), whereas, concentrations of IGF-I are very low. IGF-II-like material with various molecular weights has been found in human brain (103).

Small and highly variable effects of insulin infusion on cerebral glucose utilization have been reported over the years. These studies have been confounded by effects of insulin on plasma glucose levels. Namba et al. demonstrated a weak insulin effect on hexose transport in normoglycemic rats, using the nonmetabolized sugar 3-0-methyl glucose (104); moreover, modest but statistically significant effects of insulin on local cerebral glucose utilization in some hypothalamic nuclei are reported (105). Insulin effects on macromolecular synthesis and gene expression in cultured neural tissue are robust, reproducible, and seen with physiologic concentrations of insulin (106). Studies of neurons cultured under serum-free conditions demonstrate that insulin is required for optimal growth of early fetal neurons (107). Brain may lack an enzyme or factor needed to confer insulin sensitivity on the glucose transporter (different posttranslational processing, perhaps), but many other insulin responses are present. Since transport of insulin into the CNS may be rate-limiting, mutations involving insulin transport or receptors may have significant effects on brain development.

Receptor sites for insulin, IGF-I, and IGF-II are found in cultured neural cells and in membrane preparations derived from adult and fetal brain (100). Lowe et al. found that insulin binding was greater in the newborn than the adult brain (108). Other studies suggest that insulin receptors in newborn rats are confined to neurons (109), while IGF-I receptors are found on both neurons and glial cells (110). Brain insulin receptors differ in molecular weight from those of most peripheral tissues, probably because of differences in glycosylation (111). While the precise role of insulin and IGFs in brain is poorly understood, there is good reason to believe that they are important and that insulin may be particularly important in late fetal brain development.

GLUCOSE METABOLISM IN THE DISEASED STATE

Inborn Errors of Carbohydrate Metabolism

Inborn errors of carbohydrate metabolism are much less frequent than diabetes, stroke, and perinatal asphyxia. The glycogen storage diseases (GSD) and galactosemia are the inborn errors of metabolism most commonly encountered.

Glycogen Storage Diseases

The first description of pathologic accumulation of glycogen in the liver and kidney came from Von Gierke (1929) but shortly thereafter Pompe disease, or acid maltase defi-

ciency, was described (112,113). The latter condition was the basis for Hers' concept of lysosomal storage diseases, an important concept in the evolution of medical genetics (114) (Table 4.1).

Central Nervous System

Several GSDs are associated with hypoglycemia as a result of failure of hepatic glycogen breakdown. The hypoglycemia, increased by fasting, can produce cerebral symptoms and some patients with type I GSD have also had strokes and consequent neurologic morbidity. One would not expect glycogen accumulation in the brain of these patients because of the different role of glucose-6-phosphatase in brain. Accumulation of abnormal glycogen within the central nervous system is limited to Pompé disease or type II GSD (113).

Pompé disease has a highly variable phenotype with at least 10 different mutant phenotypes, based on studies of the acid alpha-glucosidase enzyme in cultured fibroblasts (115,116). It is likely that additional mutations will be identified by DNA and RNA studies. Patients with early onset of signs and symptoms have a more profound deficiency of catalytically active mature enzyme. It is likely that enzyme mutations disturb its transport and perhaps its stability in various intracellullar compartments; only a fraction of the mutant enzyme appears to reach the lysosomal compartment. At least four different mutations have been associated with the infantile form of the disease. Fibroblast studies can provide no information about differences in gene expression between various organs.

Affected children have profound hypotonia, relatively normal muscle bulk, cardiomegaly, and congestive heart failure. Electrocardiograms are often striking because of so-called giant QRS complexes. The liver is rarely enlarged until heart failure occurs, and the tongue may or may not be enlarged. Some patients have an abnormality of brain function beyond that expected for a sick infant, manifested by a failure to communicate and interact with the environment. Some patients do not have striking cardiac involvement and may resemble patients with spinal muscular atrophy. Electromyographic studies are remarkable because of pseudomyotonic discharges, and muscle biopsy shows vacuolar changes with PAS-positive material contained within the vacuoles. Most patients will die before the age of 18 months, although some patients with early onset of signs and symptoms progress slowly and survive beyond the age of 20 years. At autopsy, glycogen deposition is evident in heart, liver, kidney, muscle, and CNS. The CNS abnormalities commonly affect motor neurons of the spinal cord and brain stem more than other cell types (117).

Patients with later onset of signs and symptoms may be inappropriately diagnosed as having limb-girdle muscular dystrophy or inflammatory polymyopathy because of increased serum creatine kinase (CK). Weakness of respiratory muscles can be an important cause of morbidity. Four

Table 4.1   Glycogen storage diseases

Type	Clinical Manifestations	Enzyme Defect
Glucose-6-phosphatase deficiency (von Gierke disease, Cori type I)	Enlarged liver and kidneys Hyperlipidemia, hypoglycemia, ketoacidosis Seizures	Glucose-6-phosphate
Infantile acid maltase deficiency (Pompé disease, Cori type II)	Cardiomegaly: death in infancy Progressive hypotonia and weakness; swallowing and respiratory difficulty	Acid maltase
Late infantile maltase deficiency, adult acid maltase deficiency	Atonic anal sphincter Calf muscle hypertrophy Hip weakness (Gowers sign) Slow or regressing motor development, Achilles tendon contractures	Acid maltase
Debrancher deficiency (Forbes limit dextrinosis, Cori type III)	Hepatomegaly Hypoglycemia Late onset weakness Mild growth failure Early, severe weakness with myopathy is rare	Amylo-1,6-glucosidase
Brancher deficiency (Anderson disease, Cori type IV)	Cirrhosis Growth failure Hepatosplenomegaly Hypotonia Muscle wasting in legs Slow motor development Weakness	Amylo-1,4 $\rightarrow$ 1,6 transglucosidase
Myophosphorylase deficiency (McCardle disease, Cori type V)	Atrophy in older patients Myoglobinuria Poor stamina Severe muscle cramps with exercise	Muscle phosphorylase
Hepatophosphorylase deficiency (Hers disease, Cori type VI)	Growth retardation Hepatomegaly Hypoglycemia Mild ketosis	Liver phosphorylase
Phosphorylase kinase deficiency (also deficiency of activation sequence including loss of activity of 3′,5′-AMP dependent kinase in muscle and probably liver)	Marked hepatomegaly, with glycogen storage No hypoglycemia No skeletal muscle disease Normal mental development	Phosphorylase kinase or 3′,5′-AMP dependent kinase
Phosphoglucomutase deficiency	Calf hypertrophy Mild generalized weakness Regression in motor development Toe walking	Phosphoglucomutase
Phosphohexose isomerase deficiency	Late onset of myopathy Muscle cramps Poor stamina	Phosphohexose isomerase
Phosphofructokinase deficiency	Similar to myophosphorylase deficiency	Phosphofructokinase
Glycogen synthetase deficiency	Hypoglycemia Mental retardation Seizures	Glycogen synthetase

*Table modified with permission from: Swaiman KF. Diseases associated with primary abnormalities in carbohydrate and copper metabolism. In: Swaiman KF, ed. Pediatric Neurology, Principles and Practice. St. Louis: C. V. Mosby, 1989:2:992.

patients have been reported with normal alpha-glucosidase (acid maltase) activity in muscle homogenates in spite of demonstrably increased glycogen content and muscle histopathology very typical of GSD type II. These patients had some unusual clinical features including significant cardiomyopathy and mental impairment, neither of which is often observed except in the infantile form of the disease (118).

Isolation of a cDNA for human alpha-glucosidase was reported by Martiniuk et al. (119), demonstrating three different types of mRNA in human patients. Since this enzyme undergoes a complex maturational process with much posttranslational processing (120), molecular analysis of the different mutations must include studies at both the protein and nucleic acid level.

There is no specific treatment at this time for acid maltase deficiency, despite various attempts at enzyme replacement therapy. Some patients have objectively gained in strength from a high-protein diet, apparently because of the utilization of branched-chain amino acids as an alternate energy source for muscle (121). More recently, Dutch workers have demonstrated treatment of cultured myocytes from a patient with typical infantile acid maltase deficiency by targeting the mannose-6-phosphate receptor with alpha-glucosidase enzyme from human urine, which has a high mannose-6-phosphate content. Considerable amounts of a precursor form of alpha-glucosidase are excreted in human urine, suggesting that it is secreted by renal epithelial cells. This enzyme precursor was shown to be incorporated into lysosomes and to increase glycogen clearance (122). Whether this approach is feasible in vivo is not presently known.

A few patients with childhood-onset acid maltase deficiency have been mentally retarded, but the relationship between abnormal energy metabolism and mental defect is unknown. Increased brain glycogen content and peripheral neuropathy can occur in type III GSD, or debrancher deficiency. Occasional patients with GSD type IV, or Andersen disease, have had a phenotype suggestive of spinal muscular atrophy; whereas others, have had extensive glycogen storage in the CNS at autopsy but no corresponding symptoms (123). Seizures and mental retardation occur more frequently in patients with McArdle syndrome (GSD type V, muscle phosphorylase deficiency) than in the general population. Attempts to explain this by exercise-induced hypoglycemia (123) are not convincing. PFK deficiency or GSD type VII is a mild disease generally indistinguishable from McArdle syndrome; however, two patients with this disorder have had major cerebral symptoms (124), probably because of a different mutation with greater impact on cerebral metabolism. Mental retardation and seizures are even more common in phosphoglycerate kinase deficiency (125), a rare X-linked disorder that produces hemolytic anemia, CNS dysfunction, and myopathy. It is one of the five GSDs that has been associated with recurrent myoglobinuria; the others include deficiencies of phos-

phorylase, PFK, phosphoglycerate mutase, and lactate dehydrogenase.

Massive asymptomatic storage of glycogen in astrocytes has been reported in one patient whose phenotype suggested GSD type IV but whose enzyme activity was normal in homogenates of muscle and fibroblasts (126). Very rare unclassified cases of symptomatic CNS glycogen storage have been reported, some without hepatic glycogen storage (127). These may represent as yet undefined diseases.

Muscle Involvement in Glycogen Storage Disease

It is understandable that deficient storage or mobilization of glycogen would impair muscle function, but glycogen utilization is not abnormal in acid maltase deficiency. Since glycogen is greatly hydrated, it occupies a relatively large fraction of the cell, and as stored glycogen increases, cellular organelles are compressed and distorted. Even minimally affected muscle fibers show lysosomal hypertrophy, evident by increased acid phosphatase activity among other things. It is also suggested that lysosomal enzymes may leak from lysosomes and that autophagy stimulated by lysosomal hypertrophy may lead to digestion of normal organelles.

Hyperuricemia is common in GSD type I, and exercise results in excessive degradation of muscle purine nucleotides in glycogenolysis types III, V, and VII (128), associated with increased plasma concentrations of ammonia, inosine, and hypoxanthine. This exercise-induced hyperuricemia can directly produce cell damage. Hypoxanthine, for example, can give rise to oxygen free radicals (129).

While McArdle syndrome is rare, its pathophysiology has provided many insights into muscle function. The first reported case (130) was a 30-year-old man who had pain and weakness with even light exercise as long as he could remember. Although no muscle biopsy was performed, McArdle showed that the patient's muscle failed to produce lactate under ischemic exercise conditions and deduced the presence of a defect of glycogen breakdown. By 1959, the responsible enzyme had been identified. Exercise intolerance often begins in childhood, but cramps are rarely reported until adult life (131). Some patients have myoglobinuria, but seldom before adolescence (132). The human muscle phosphorylase gene has been cloned and studies in 8 unrelated patients have shown an absence of both phosphorylase enzyme activity and mRNA in 5, with 3 patients expressing normal length mRNA in subnormal amounts and without detectable enzyme activity (133). As a group, these patients exhibit a striking "second wind" phenomenon (134). During the first few minutes of submaximal exercise, patients report weakness and fatigue but they are able to continue, and as time passes, the symptoms diminish. These patients have disproportionate increases in cardiac output compared to normal subjects, which further increases muscle blood flow. Electrophysiologic changes probably reflect recruitment of more motor units (135). Glucose infusions will produce a second wind phenomenon in these patients, but they can experience the same phenomenon without exogenous fuel. Trained athletes also experience a second wind phenomenon but only with additional vigorous exercise. The second wind phenomenon exemplifies the body's ability to compensate for a significant metabolic defect; however, the cost to the patient (purine breakdown and cytotoxicity) is not eliminated.

Muscle Cramp Syndromes

Muscle cramps are relatively common complaints and do not necessarily indicate any abnormality. They can occur at rest or during exercise. Cramps related to metabolic diseases are caused by exercise and tend to be proportionate to the degree of that exercise. Most cramps are confined to a single muscle, usually in the legs. During the first decade of life children rarely present to physicians with complaints of excessive fatigability, and some of those who will have these complaints in later life avoid exercise and outdoor play.

Although a patient complains of cramps, fatigue, or pain with exercise and has evidence of a metabolic disorder, one cannot presume that the metabolic disorder is the cause of the patient's symptoms. Many of the histochemical procedures employed to estimate enzyme activity are not quantitative, and more importantly metabolic abnormalities may be asymptomatic. The controversy surrounding myoadenylate deaminase deficiency (MAD) is a case in point. This familial disorder of purine metabolism is relatively common, and is observed in about 2% of muscle biopsies (136). While there is theoretical justification for assuming that it might impair muscle function (137), the majority of MAD-deficient patients are asymptomatic (138).

Denny-Brown suggested that cramps result from hyperexcitability of the terminal or intramuscular portion of motor nerves (139). They appear to be related to fasciculations, repetitive posttetanic muscle discharges, and to be penicillin-induced after discharges of motor nerve terminals (140). These phenomena can all be produced in normal nerve terminals. Fasciculations in patients with motor neuron disorders and disorders of peripheral nerve appear to have the same basis as those seen in normal subjects (141). There is no special relationship between carbohydrate metabolism and muscle cramps occurring at rest. The occurrence of muscle cramps or contracture during ischemic exercise, however, is suspicious of a disorder of glucose or glycogen metabolism. Typically noted in McArdle syndrome, or myophosphorylase deficiency, exercise-induced contracture is also described in deficiencies of debrancher enzyme, lactate dehydrogenase, PFK, and phosphoglycerate kinase. Although some have thought that carnitine palmityltransferase deficiency might be associated with exercise-induced cramps, this is probably not the case,

nor is this observed in acid maltase deficiency (140). Although many people complain of muscle cramps, exercise-induced contracture has a specific association with disorders of the glycolytic or glycogenolytic pathways that provide energy for muscle contraction.

Studies of exercise-induced cramps in patients with McArdle syndrome using ^{31}P NMR spectroscopy (142) show that pain and contracture occur before creatine phosphate stores are exhausted, and at a time of relatively normal tissue ATP concentration. Even mild exercise, however, causes a greater fall of creatine phosphate in these patients than in normal subjects. Given the heterogeneity of fiber types in most muscles and the fact that the NMR signal is averaged over multiple fibers, it is reasonable to assume that ATP concentration in a specific subgroup of fibers can be limiting. Ischemic stimulation of the nerve to the human adductor pollicis muscle provides a test of fatigability that is relatively objective and independent of patient motivation. These studies show that patients with McArdle syndrome and PFK deficiency fatigue more rapidly than normal subjects (143).

Muscle fatigue occurring during aerobic exercise has a different basis, and appears to be more clearly linked to lactate accumulation and decreased pH. Fast-twitch glycolytic fibers (type IIB) produce more lactate than other fiber types and are especially susceptible to fatigue. The rate of development of mechanical fatigue during voluntary exercise correlates closely with the proportion of type II fibers and with lactate accumulation (144). Mechanical fatigue produced by aerobic exercise does not eliminate the contractile response to agents such as caffeine (145) and may involve a defect of excitation-contraction coupling.

Galactosemia

Galactosemia is one of the most common inborn errors of metabolism responsible for mental retardation. In many respects, our concepts and treatment of galactosemia have paralleled those of phenylketonuria. Untreated galactosemia results in severe liver disease, profound mental deficiency, epilepsy, and choreoathetosis. Isselbacher et al. (146) showed that galactose-1-phosphate uridyl transferase activity was deficient in this disorder. Another form of the disease was shown to be due to galactokinase deficiency (147). Galactokinase deficiency produces a milder syndrome with cataracts but no CNS or hepatic pathology; it has been associated with pseudotumor cerebri. Two pathogenic factors are the accumulation of galactitol and galactose-1-phosphate; only galactitol accumulates in galactokinase deficiency. The administration of low galactose diets brought major improvement in the outcome of patients with classic galactosemia (148,149); however, most diet-treated patients exhibit mild and varied neurologic impairment, primarily in the intellectual sphere, and a few patients have more severe neurologic abnormalities. A small number of diet-treated patients with cerebellar and extrapyramidal syndromes have been reported (150,151). The simplest explanation of their less than satisfactory outcome is that they have a different mutation. Kaufman et al. (152) described hypergonadotropic hypogonadism, which develops in the majority of girls homozygous for galactosemia. The obvious conclusion is that some additional treatment or nutrient is needed to optimize gonadal and CNS development in these patients. Male hypogonadism seems to be relatively uncommon. Until the transferase gene is cloned and different mutations can be sorted out, the task of finding the extra factor in addition to a galactose-free diet necessary for optimal neurologic outcome may be very difficult.

Sialidosis

Sialidosis and related syndromes, rare in North America, exhibit a special relationship with disorders resulting from a deficiency of the enzyme galactosidase, the enzyme deficient in GM_1 gangliosidosis (153). Spranger considered this group of patients (1968) to have lipomucopolysaccharidosis (154). Two patients had vacuolated lymphocytes, foam cells in the bone marrow, metachromatic material in their urinary sediment, and progressive impairment of CNS and peripheral nervous system function. In spite of their appearance they had no evidence of abnormal mucopolysaccharide excretion. Within 2 years, Spranger had revised the name of this disorder to mucolipidosis I, as part of a broader scheme to include diseases related to both the mucopolysaccharidoses and the sphingolipidoses (155). Shortly thereafter an increased urinary excretion of sialic acid–containing sugars and deficient activity of $\alpha(2\text{-}6)$-neuraminidase in fibroblasts and leukocytes was identified. This substantiated the case for an inborn error of metabolism by demonstrating intermediate enzyme values in the parents (156–159). A short time later, Lowden and O'Brien (160) categorized patients with sialidosis into two groups (Table 4.2). Further studies soon demonstrated that patients with sialidosis I were generally of normal intelligence, were free of dysmorphic features, and had less severe reduction of enzyme activity than those of the sialidosis II (161). The electrophoretic mobility of multiple lysosomal enzymes was abnormal in patients with sialidosis (162), and was consistent with failure of sialic acid catabolism. Enzyme function was little impaired as judged by in vitro assays of enzyme activity and the absence of accumulation of abnormal metabolites. Some patients who had been classified as GM_1 gangliosidosis because of reduced α-galactosidase activity in leukocytes or fibroblasts were reclassified as having sialidosis, type II (163); these patients are now considered to have galactosialidosis. The clinical features of congenital and infant-onset sialidosis often overlap with those of the much better known GM_1 gangliosidosis.

Neuraminidases (neuraminidase and sialidase are synonymous) are widely distributed in viruses, bacteria, and

Table 4.2   Features of sialidosis subtypes

	Type I	Type II
Dysmorphism	–	+
Skeletal dysplasia	–	+
Mental retardation	– /Mild	Often severe
Survival: >30 years	Usual	Usual early death
Visceromegaly	–	Common
Hydrops or ascites	–	Congenital form
Impaired vision	+	+
Marrow foam cells	@ 50 %	All
Abnormal galactosidase	–	*

*Patients with combined deficiency of both alpha-galactosidase and neuraminidase were formerly classified as type II sialidosis but are now recognized as having galactosialidosis. Modified with permission from Lowden JA, Warner TG. Sialidosis: A review of human neuraminidase deficiency. Am J Hum Genet 1978;31:1–30.

throughout the animal kingdom (164). Sialic acids are found in many glycoproteins and glycolipids; and gangliosides are sialic acid containing glycosphingolipids, generally believed to be located on the outer leaflet of the plasma membrane of mammalian cells. Two different groups of neuraminidases have been distinguished in human fibroblasts on the basis of localization and substrate specificity. Lysosomal neuraminidases act on sialyl linkages in oligosaccharides and glycoproteins, while ganglioside neuraminidases, probably located in the plasma membrane, act only on gangliosides (165). Normal activity of the lysosomal alpha-neuraminidase and increased free sialic acid in cells and body fluids are found in three other sialic acid related disorders: Salla disease, sialuria, and infantile sialic acid storage disease. Just as sialidosis and galactosialidosis had been incorrectly diagnosed as GM_1 gangliosidosis, it is likely that some patients reported as having Niemann-Pick disease actually had infantile sialic acid storage disease. Patients with Salla disease are primarily of Finnish extraction, named from the district in which the disease was first discovered (166). Signs and symptoms of Salla disease are usually evident by 1 year of age and are manifested by coarse facial features, ataxia, and marked psychomotor retardation. As adults, they tend to be severely retarded but can survive into late adulthood. All patients excrete large amounts of free sialic acid in the urine and exhibit lysosomal storage in multiple organs. They have normal sialic acid synthesis and cleavage of exogenous sialic acid containing oligosaccharides; the basic defect is believed to be related to sialic acid transport across the lysosomal membrane (167,168). Fibroblasts from patients with Salla disease have greatly reduced transport of sialic acid out of the cells after loading with a sialic acid precursor. A similar pathophysiology appears to underly the more common nephropathic cystinosis in which the lysosomal cystine transporter is defective because of mutation. The few autopsied cases of Salla disease have shown marked reduction in cerebral white matter, abnormal neuronal storage of lipofuscin, neuronal loss in the nucleus basalis of Meynert and the locus ceruleus, with neurofibrillary tangles in these nuclei and in the neocortex similar to that observed in Alzheimer and Parkinson disease (169).

Rare variants of Salla disease characterized by sialyluria without evidence of tissue storage have variable clinical presentations that have included seizures, visceromegaly, and metabolic acidosis (170). They probably represent different mutations. Still other patients have been reported with sialyluria, vacuolated lymphocytes, increased sialidase in lymphocytes, with normal enzyme activities in fibroblasts (171). Sialic acid storage disease is somewhat more common than the other variants. The infantile form of this disorder is typically characterized by growth failure, severe CNS dysfunction, visceromegaly, anemia, ascites, and foam cells in the bone marrow (172). Some patients with this disorder have evidence of defective sialic acid transport (173). Abnormal proteolytic processing of lysosomal enzymes similar to that seen in I-cell disease has also been reported in patients with infantile sialic acid storage disease (174).

This group of diseases also includes patients with deficiencies of both galactosidase and neuraminidase activity, the so-called galactosialidoses (175). The congenital form presents with ascites or hydrops, while infantile cases have had visceromegaly, coarse facies, and skeletal changes. Patients with a juvenile form may have mild disease similar to that seen in the cherry red spot-myoclonus syndrome, although their angiokeratoses and skeletal abnormalities would not be seen in sialidosis type I (176). Human lysosomal galactosidase and neuraminidase have been shown to be packaged together in the lysosomal membrane, together with a 32-Kd glycoprotein. All cases of galactosialidosis studied have been found to have defects in the 32-Kd protective protein (165). This defect produces an unstable galactosidase which is rapidly degraded, and a neuraminidase molecule lacking enzymatic activity. Therefore, mutations involving the 32-Kd glycoprotein result in secondary loss of activity of the two enzymes packaged together with it. Patients with the early infantile form of galactosialidosis have no mRNA for the glycoprotein, while those with the late infantile form have normal amounts of mRNA and presumably a different mutation (177).

Of seven human disorders of glycoprotein degradation, it is likely that multiple mutations will be found in each case. Mental retardation and dysmorphic features are common in these disorders (Table 4.3). Disorders of sialic acid metabolism, which need not all be hereditary, merit attention beyond that due to their relatively small numbers, because of the special role of sialyl residues in cell-cell and membrane-protein interactions.

Disorders of Lactate and Pyruvate Metabolism

Mitochondria are complex structures with multiple compartments demarcated by membranes; their primary function is to generate energy. The tricarboxylic acid cycle and fatty acid oxidation take place in the mitochondrial

Table 4.3   Human disorders of glycoprotein metabolism

β-Galactoasidase deficiency
α-Fucosidase deficiency
Sialidase deficiencies
α-Mannosidase deficiency
β-Mannosidase deficiency
Defects of galactosialidosis glycoprotein
Aspartylglycosaminidase deficiency

membranes. Mitochondrial diseases, therefore, tend to be expressed in tissues with the greatest aerobic metabolic demands: the brain, heart, and skeletal muscle. Since the activity of TCA cycle enzymes cannot be measured by ordinary spectrophotometric methods in intact mitochondria because of poor permeability of the mitochondrial membranes to the substrates employed (178), the mitochondria must be treated with detergents, sonication, or other disruptive measures. Sumegi and Srere have shown that several dehydrogenases of the citric acid cycle bind to complex I but not to complexes II or III of the respiratory chain (179). NMR studies of the water signal of intact mitochondria show a broad signal, suggesting that water molecules move more slowly and less freely than in cytoplasm (178). If one assumes that all proteins within the mitochondrial matrix have an average molecular weight of 50,000, then protein concentrations would be extremely high, about 15mM. Similarly, intramitochondrial nucleotide concentrations must be very high, although most may be protein bound. Because of these unusual features, the components of the highly viscous mitochondrial matrix space are largely invisible to NMR spectroscopy (180).

The oxidative metabolic processes of the mitochondrion can be summarized by a single equation:

$$3 \text{ ADP} + 3 \text{ Pi} + \text{NADH} + \text{H}^+ + 1/2 \text{ O}_2 =$$
$$3 \text{ ATP} + \text{NAD}^+ + \text{H}_2\text{O} \qquad (180)$$

Note that ADP, Pi, and H^+ all enter the mitochondria by specialized transporters and that the mitochondrion is permeable to NAD^+, but not to NADH. Mitchell's chemiosmotic hypothesis has grown to dominate thinking about mitochondrial function (181). This hypothesis implies that the energy resulting from substrate oxidation is transduced into synthesis of high-energy phosphates (ATP) by a proton-motive force, p, existing across the inner mitochondrial membrane. This proton-motive force has a chemical component or pH gradient, pH, and an electrical component, or membrane potential, related as follows:

$$P = -2.3 \text{ (RT/F) pH} \qquad (182)$$

where R and T are a proportionality constant and temperature, and F is the Faraday. The proton motive force arises from the transfer of hydrogen from substrates to oxygen by a series of alternating hydrogen and electron carriers in the inner mitochondrial membrane. This force causes expulsion of protons into the extramitochondrial compartment. Protons may reenter the mitochondrion via the proton-translocating ATPase (182). Cytosolic ADP enters the mitochondrion by the adenine nucleotide translocase, which also exports mitochondrial ATP, and phosphate ion enters via coupled transport with various ions. In simple terms, the high-energy intermediates of oxidative phosphorylation are protons that move in the opposite direction from the electrons.

Warburg and other early biochemists knew that oxygen reacted directly with a carbon-monoxide sensitive macromolecule and that NADH did not react with this macromolecule. They envisioned a series of electron transporters that connected NADH at one end to oxygen at the other. It was recognized that no respiration occurred if substrates were provided without NAD^+. The oxidative phosphorylation system of eukaryotes is contained within the inner mitochondrial membrane, and about half of the protein of that membrane is associated with enzyme systems involved in oxidative phosphorylation. This mitochondrial system consists of five protein-lipid enzyme complexes, which have been designated complexes I through V. Complexes I through IV plus coenzyme Q or ubiquinone and cytochrome c make up the respiratory chain (183).

More than 60 polypeptides are involved in the respiratory chain, but only about 25% of them are coded by mtDNA. The electron carriers of the respiratory chain are quinoid structures such as flavin mononucleotide (FMN) (oxidized), flavin adenine dinucleotide (FAD) (oxidized), and coenzyme Q, and transition metal complexes (Fe-S clusters, heme, and protein-bound copper). At three stages along the respiratory chain (complexes I, III, and IV), oxidative energy is conserved by proton translocation that drives ATP synthesis. The stoichiometry of this process remains uncertain. Either complex I or II can be the entry point for reducing equivalents produced by the TCA cycle enzymes. Succinic dehydrogenase, an important TCA cycle enzyme, is directly embedded in the inner mitochondrial membrane and an integral part of complex II. Complex I catalyzes the rotenone-sensitive reduction of coenzyme Q analogs by NADH, and is called NADH : ubiquinone oxidoreductase. Obviously, no single antibody or nucleic acid probe can verify the integrity of such a complex assembly of multiple gene products. Its oxidation-reduction function can be studied with ferricyanide or coenzyme Q analogs. Inhibitors that arrest electron transport at various stages are useful in dissecting function in normal and diseased states; for example, antimycin A binds to cytochrome c reductase (complex III), inducing changes in the light absorption of cytochrome b, and mutations within the cytochrome b gene confer resistance to antimycin (184). Substrates acting distally in the respiratory chain can bypass the effects of these inhibitors. In the case of antimycin A-treated mitochondria, cytochrome c can still accept electrons from the soluble enzyme sulfite oxidase or from cytochrome b_5 of the outer mitochondrial membrane (185). Mitochondria of fibroblasts from patients with Zellweger syndrome are especially sensitive to antimycin A (186). It is therefore believed that complex III is abnormal

in these patients, who also lack peroxisomes. If complex I is deficient, pyruvate oxidation is reduced, while that of succinate should be normal.

Similarly, one can study mitochondrial function by measuring oxygen uptake under various specific conditions, as first described by Chance and Williams (187). Under these circumstances, substrate permeability and respiratory chain function are limiting. In stage 4 respiration, little oxygen is consumed because ADP is limiting. The ratio of stage III to stage IV respiration can be used as a measure of respiratory control (182), or coupling of electron transport to ADP phosphorylation. While ADP addition to mitochondria regularly increases respiration and the ratio of $[ATP]/[ADP] \cdot [Pi]$ is a relatively good predictor of respiratory rate, the $NADH/NAD^+$ ratio appears to have powerful effects on mitochondrial respiration, and at times overriding the effects of ADP levels (188). Changes in NADH redox potential, resulting from activation of intramitochondrial dehydrogenase enzymes by increased Ca^{++} entry into mitochondria, may explain the increased respiration that follows increased work of organs like the heart. Brain content of NAD and NADH is substantially lower than that of skeletal muscle (189). This suggests that cerebral mitochondria are less potent ATP generators than those in heart, liver, and skeletal muscle that contain about twice as much NAD and NADH.

Mitochondria are formed by the growth and division of preexisting organelles. Newly synthesized components are added to preformed structures. Mitochondria contain their own separate DNA (mtDNA) and systems for its transcription and translation. The entire mitochondrial genome has been sequenced in many species, including humans, a relatively simple feat because it is small (16,600 base pairs). The mammalian mitochondrial genome is compact, lacks introns, and some of the genes overlap. Ordinarily, mtDNA is identical in all cells of any one organism (190), however, mtDNA codes for less than 10% of mitochondrial proteins. The process of evolution has moved almost all mitochondrial genes into the nucleus, leaving behind a few very hydrophobic proteins, whose transport into the mitochondrion might be especially difficult.

Most mitochondrial proteins, the products of nuclear genes, are made on cytoplasmic polysomes and imported into the mitochondrion. Nucleoside triphosphates are required to keep the proteins in the proper conformation. Protein precursors bind to specific receptors on the mitochondrial surface and are translocated across the mitochondrial membrane(s) to destinations in four compartments: the outer membrane, intermembrane space, inner membrane, and matrix. Many proteins are assembled into large complexes within the mitochondrion. Some of these complexes contain subunits of both cytoplasmic and mitochondrial origin. The cytoplasmic precursors of mitochondrial proteins differ in several ways from the mature mitochondrial proteins. Most have an amino-terminal extension or presequence that is subsequently removed by proteolytic processing (191). Some undergo complex processing in two different sites, the mitochondrial matrix and the intermembrane space (192). Cytosolic cofactors are reported to be essential for the energy-consuming importation of certain proteins into mitochondria (193).

Many of the proteins in the inner mitochondrial membrane are transport proteins. Although poorly understood, mitochondrial transport processes are essential to oxidative metabolism. None of these carriers have been cloned. While small molecules (less than a few thousand daltons molecular weight) pass the outer membrane easily, only those that are lipid soluble or bind to specific transporters pass the inner membrane. Pyruvate transport is limiting under certain conditions and merits special scrutiny from investigators of mitochondrial diseases. Pyruvate exchanges for OH^- or acetoacetate leaving mitochondria. Conditions that promote hepatic ketogenesis, such as glucagon, fatty acid (194), and carnitine treatment, all increase the amount of acetoacetate within the mitochondria and secondarily increase pyruvate entry and oxidation. If the acetoacetate gradient across the mitochondrion is dissipated by adding acetoacetate to hepatocytes, the stimulation of pyruvate oxidation is reversed (194).

Several shuttles are known to play an essential role by moving reducing equivalents from the cytoplasm into the mitochondrion where they can enter the respiratory chain for generation of ATP. NADH cannot itself enter the mitochondrion. The most important of these shuttles, particularly in brain, seems to be the malate-aspartate shuttle. The cytoplasmic $NADH/NAD^+$ ratio is much higher than that within the mitochondrion (195). This shuttle moves malate and glutamate into the mitochondrion in exchange for aspartate and alpha-ketoglutarate, which come out into the cytoplasm (196). Inhibition of the shuttle, for example, caused by inhibition of the enzyme aspartate aminotransferase (197), results in increased lactate/pyruvate ratios, decreased entry of pyruvate into the TCA cycle, and an overall picture similar to that resulting from hypoglycemia. The mitochondrial dicarboxylic acid carrier exchanges aspartate for glutamate in an energy-dependent process (198). Palaiologos et al. postulate that aspartate aminotransferase (AAT), known to be concentrated in glutamate releasing neurons, is also involved in a second shuttle that processes glutamate destined for transmitter use (199). This glutamate is apparently made inside mitochondria and used outside the cell. They further suggest that glutamate is made in the intermembranous space of the mitochondrion from glutamine (by phosphate-activated glutaminase), exchanges with aspartate to cross the inner membrane, and is transaminated by AAT there to alpha-ketoglutarate, which leaves via the ketodicarboxylic acid carrier. Upon reaching the cytoplasm, it is again transaminated by AAT (now cytosolic AAT) to glutamate.

Another shuttle or bypass is the alpha-glycerophosphate shuttle. This simpler process takes dihydroxyacetone phosphate, a glycolytic intermediate, and reduces it to L-glycerol-3-phosphate, which diffuses through the outer mitochondrial membrane to encounter mitochondrial glycerol phosphate dehydrogenase, a flavoprotein accessible at the inner mitochondrial membrane. FAD, the prosthetic group of GPD, is reduced to $FADH_2$ with regeneration of dihydroxyacetone phosphate, which returns to the cytosol. $FADH_2$ can be used to reduce NAD^+ inside the mitochondrion. Therefore, NADH appears inside mitochondria without crossing the mitochondrial membrane. The malate-aspartate and d-glycerophosphate shuttles use intermediate vehicles for the reducing equivalents or hydrogen atoms (malate and dihydroxyacetone phosphate) and both are effectively unidirectional. Each can be inhibited by enzyme inhibitors, and the more complex malate-aspartate shuttle also depends upon two specific transporters, each subject to toxic and genetic lesions. In general, these shuttles and mitochondrial transport systems can only be studied in fresh tissue. The transport properties of liver and heart mitochondria have been extensively studied (200), and though the transport properties of brain and muscle mitochondria are less well characterized, they are thought to be similar.

Mitochondria take up Ca^{++} ions by an energy-dependent process and can be viewed as calcium-storing organelles. However, recent studies utilizing electron probe microanalysis suggest that the role of mitochondria as calcium reservoirs or buffers is less than had been suspected, because their in vivo calcium content is less than formerly believed and is less responsive to physiologic activation (201). The membranes of the sarcoplasmic or endoplasmic reticulum appear to be quantitatively much more important sources of calcium that is mobilized by hormones and other physiologic stimuli like inositol trisphosphate. Although mitochondrial calcium content changes very little when liver or muscle is stimulated, we have learned that mitochondrial Mg^{++} content changes considerably under such conditions, suggesting that the known mitochondrial Mg transporter may be important for mitochondrial responses to physiologic stimuli.

Cytochromes are heme-proteins found in all aerobic organisms, including plants. These electron carriers operate by reduction and reoxidation of their iron components, which alternate between ferrous and ferric states. Although many oxygen-linked enzymes have evolved since the appearance of molecular oxygen in the earth's atmosphere, only one, cytochrome c oxidase (ferrocytochrome-c : oxygen oxidoreductase) couples the reduction of oxygen to water with the production of ATP. Cytochrome c oxidase (COX) occurs in all eukaryotes and in some aerobic bacteria. The basic enzyme mechanism is identical in bacteria, yeasts, and mammals. However, the number of subunits increases dramatically as one ascends the evolutionary scale, going from 2 in prokaryotes to 13 in mammals. The function of the extra subunits found in mammalian COX is not known. They may have regulatory roles, contributing to mitochondrial Ca^{++} transport, protein import into the mitochondrion, and other activities (185). The occurrence of tissue-specific isozymes of COX was first suggested when small differences in molecular weights of its nuclear-coded subunits were identified in liver and heart preparations (202). Subsequent work has demonstrated both tissue and developmentally specific subunits of COX in mammals (203). The first three subunits of COX are coded by mtDNA and do not vary between tissues. Whether the kinetics of cytochrome c oxidation differ significantly between organs is uncertain (203). Since COX is the only protein in the respiratory chain that reacts directly with oxygen, its destruction or inhibition has a devastating effect on cells. There is evidence that nitrous oxide interacts directly with it and that this may be related to certain anesthetic effects (204). The molecular basis of anesthesia remains poorly understood, and only a few anesthetics react with COX.

Mitochondrial cytochrome content can be crudely estimated by spectral analysis in which the difference in light absorption between oxidized and reduced mitochondria are compared. This approach works best with fresh tissues, but it is not quantitative and subject to interference from contaminating hemoglobin, myoglobin, and other macromolecules with similar absorptive profiles (205,206). It can provide the first clues to a cytochrome abnormality, and can be applied to autopsy material. These methods formed the basis for some of the early biochemical studies of mitochondrial myopathies. Currently they should be supplemented by additional more specific methods, such as antibody studies, nucleic acid studies, or 2D-gel electrophoresis.

Coenzyme Q or ubiquinone was first isolated in 1940. The name ubiquinone came from its ubiquity. Shown in 1957 to be a component of the respiratory chain (207), it is a fat-soluble vitamin resembling vitamin K in structure. The number of isoprene units in the side chain varies depending upon the species of origin. Human coenzyme Q has a side chain with 10 isoprene units and is, therefore, called coenzyme Q_{10} or simply CoQ_{10}. The heart, liver, pancreas, and kidney have the highest concentrations of CoQ in the body. It is not limited to mitochondria and is also found in the nucleus and microsomes. Several different CoQ binding proteins have been described, and it is likely that CoQ is always protein bound inside the cell. CoQ seems to have several functions. It has a role in electron transport; namely, CoQ accepts hydrogens from various flavoproteins such as NADH dehydrogenase and succinate dehydrogenase, restoring FMN and FAD to their oxidized forms. It returns to the quinone form after transferring two electrons to the heme iron of cytochromes and releasing two protons that drive ATP synthesis. In this way it regulates the state and activity of NADH dehydrogenase in complex I and other dehydrogenases linked to complex I, as well as the cytochrome b-c_1 complex. Moreover, it prevents the oxidative manifestations of vitamin E deficiency, implying antioxidant ability, and it may function in a more general sense as a "membrane stabilizing agent." CoQ has been used for therapy of many different conditions. Its first therapeutic use was for cardiac ischemia (208) and it has been proposed as a PET scan tracer for myocardial imaging (very little of the positron labeled CoQ reaches the CNS, in spite of its very lipophilic nature) (209). Most reports of CoQ efficacy for treatment of various conditions are anecdotal or refer to in vitro studies whose relevance to human disease is uncertain. It appears to be well tolerated by humans.

Mitochondrial Disease

The first proved mitochondrial disease was described by Luft et al. in 1962 (210), although several disorders subsequently found or suspected to be primary mitochondrial diseases had already been considered. Perhaps the most important was Leigh's report of a 7-month-old infant who died after a rapidly progressive illness (211). Pathologic changes were limited to the CNS and resembled those of Wernicke encephalopathy because of striking vascular proliferation and spongy change with a predilection for a gray matter of the basal ganglia and brain stem. This analysis was further refined by Richter (212) and Dayan (213) who stressed the involvement of gray matter near the aqueduct of Sylvius and floor of the fourth ventricle. Unlike Wernicke disease, the mammillary bodies and white matter were almost always spared. Following Huckabee's 1961 report (214), physicians began to look for lactic acidosis in these patients. While early reports about the anion gap and excess lactate came from adult medicine, they were to have a major impact on concepts of inborn errors of metabolism, most of which become evident in the first years of life. Two major developments in understanding Leigh disease were reported during the next decade: the report of a clinical response to lipoic acid therapy (215), and a concept of a specific inhibitor of the enzyme ATP-thiamine diphosphate phosphoryltransferase (216). Lipoic acid was used because it is a cofactor for pyruvate dehydrogenase, as is thiamine pyrophosphate. It was shown later that the clinical course of patients with Leigh disease and other mitochondrial disorders can markedly fluctuate, making it difficult to be sure of the efficacy of any therapy.

Kearns and Sayre reported two patients with ophthalmoplegia, retinitis pigmentosa, and complete heart block in 1958 (217). One of their patients who had onset of ptosis at 3 years and deafness at 4 years of age, died of heart block at 17 years. There was no suggestion of mitochondrial disease detected at autopsy, although there were myopathic changes of the extraocular muscles and abnormal white matter was mentioned. Engel et al. reported "ragged-red fibers" in muscle biopsies of several patients with oculocraniosomatic neuromuscular disease using a modified Gomori trichrome stain (218). Five of their seven patients had onset of their symptoms in childhood and all had signs and symptoms consistent with the Kearns-Sayre syndrome. None resembled the disorder described by Leigh and Richter. Although only a few percent of the affected fibers showed the ragged-red fiber change, this abnormality was suggestive of some mitochondrial abnormality. Today mitochondrial myopathies are often considered disorders associated with ragged-red fibers (219–225).

Kearns-Sayre syndrome is currently considered to include many patients with cytochrome oxidase deficiency, some patients who have catastrophically deteriorated with corticosteroid therapy (226), and many patients with very slow progression of clinical disease (227). There is an abnormality of white matter evident in magnetic resonance imaging (MRI) head scans. Some patients with this disorder have derived objective benefit from CoQ therapy (228).

Spiro et al. (224–230) reported abnormal cytochrome spectra and possibly abnormal respiratory control in a father and son with CNS and muscle disease. Rowland (231) and DiMauro (232) attempted to correlate biochemical defects with patient symptoms, and pointed to the limitations of an exclusively morphologic approach to mitochondrial diseases. They added two more clinical entities to the group of mitochondrial diseases: mitochondrial myopathy, encephalopathy, lactic acidosis, and stroke-like episodes (MELAS) (233) and myoclonic epilepsy with ragged-red fibers (MERRF) (234). DiMauro et al. suggested that biochemical defects in the mitochondrial disorders could be categorized as defects of substrate utilization, coupling of oxidation and phosphorylation, or respiratory chain defects. Clearly, mitochondrial transport defects form an additional group.

New diagnostic entities with similar clinical pictures to the mitochondrial diseases continue to be defined. Noteworthy among them are the disorders associated with deficiency of the enzyme biotinidase. Many of these patients have intermittent disorders beginning in the 1st years of life with metabolic acidosis, often suggesting the diagnosis of Leigh disease (235), and some patients have increased CSF lactate content (236). However, these diseases usually respond dramatically to therapy with biotin.

The possible mitochondrial basis for some spinocerebellar degenerations is unsettled (237), although abnormalities of pyruvate dehydrogenase (PDHC) and glutamate dehydrogenase have been reported in several forms of spinocerebellar degeneration.

The Concept of Leigh Syndrome

Leigh's only patient died after a very short illness (211), and no extracerebral pathology was found at autopsy or suspected in life. Cerebral pathologic changes were those of a spongiform encephalopathy with striking vascular proliferation. The vascular lesion and its forebrain distribution were reminiscent of Wernicke encephalopathy. Worsley et al. were the first to report lactic acidosis associated with

these pathologic findings (238). Although the pathology remains distinctive, the clinical picture associated with this disorder has been variable. The first chemical abnormalities reported were those of pyruvate carboxylase abnormality (239). Di Mauro et al. suggest, however, that pyruvate carboxylase deficiency cannot be closely linked to Leigh syndrome (240). Neuropathologic changes were similar to those observed in Wernicke disease and led many to seek explanations in thiamine metabolic pathways. Those studies led to the discovery a glycoprotein found in the urine and other body fluids of some patients, which inhibited the brain enzyme responsible for the synthesis of thiamine triphosphate (TTP) (216), as well as in a few cases of striatal necrosis associated with beri-beri (241). The assay for the TTP inhibitor has, however, been questioned (242). Case reports not supported by autopsy data should carry little weight in formulating a mechanism for Leigh syndrome, and the interpretation of some autopsied cases is open to dispute (223). Three of 11 patients with MELAS syndrome have come to autopsy, and there has been no consistent evidence linking it with Leigh syndrome. The MELAS syndrome is a clinical concept and may lack distinctive pathology. Reports, however, link it to abnormalities of complex I (243). If one requires patients with MELAS to have ragged red fibers, most cases of Leigh syndrome will be excluded. Relatively symmetric cerebral softenings consistent with infarction are a hallmark of Leigh syndrome, and they almost always include putaminal lesions. Lactic acidosis and ragged red fibers may be present only during advanced stages of these diseases. Kearns-Sayre syndrome, on the other hand, has a relatively distinctive clinical picture and the diagnosis can often be confidently made during life.

Deficiencies of the PDHC complex have been reported in almost 20 pathologically proved cases of Leigh syndrome (244). Since tissue specific isozymes of PDHC have not been found, the biochemical disorder might affect all tissues, unlike the manisfestations of the clinical illness. The first recognized patient with the disease associated with cytochrome oxidase deficiency by Willems et al. (245) was of interest because the histochemical study of a muscle biopsy was normal, though electron microscopy showed abnormal subsarcolemmal mitochondria. At present, the most common finding in patients with pathologically proved Leigh syndrome is COX deficiency (240), but many cases with PDHC abnormalities have been reported. A few patients are reported to have deficiency of complex I of the respiratory chain (246). These patients should now be studied by the methods of Holt et al. (247), which might provide further evidence of a defect intrinsic to complex I. There is little reason to think of Leigh syndrome as a primary disorder of mtDNA; all proteins of the PDHC complex are coded by nuclear genes, and the three COX subunits, which are coded for by mtDNA, should be equally expressed in all tissues (247). Furthermore, some Leigh cases exhibit autosomal-recessive inheritance. While the pathologically proved Leigh cases, unlike Kearns-Sayre syndrome, have shown little extracerebral pathology, there is an interesting subgroup of Leigh cases with myocardial pathology (248).

The combination of normal light microscopic observations of muscle biopsies and abnormal findings at electron microscopy has been observed in autopsy proved cases of Leigh syndrome (240). This is of note because muscle biopsies are considered important in the evaluation of patients who are suspected of having Leigh syndrome. Adequate study of biopsies from any patient suspected of mitochondrial disease requires light and electron microscopic studies.

In addition to beri-beri and Wernicke disease, Leber disease with extrapyramidal involvement shares important features with Leigh syndrome. A large family reported by Novotny et al. (249) exhibited maternal inheritance and prominent dystonic signs attributed to striatal necrosis; unfortunately, no autopsy material was available. A mitochondrial enzyme abnormality has been reported in Leber disease and the maternal inheritance of Novotny's family points strongly to a mitochondrial disorder (250).

McCandless suggested that all patients with Leigh syndrome were associated with the ATP-TPP phosphoryl transferase inhibitor (251), implying that this was the abnormal gene product responsible for the disease. This view is not widely supported, but could be revived by sequencing the glycoprotein isolated by Cooper and Pincus, cloning the responsible gene and showing that this gene was the cause of Leigh syndrome.

Evaluation and Therapy of Mitochondrial Diseases

Mitochondria rapidly become swollen and distorted after death, reducing the value of postmortem material for biochemical study. On the other hand, DNA is relatively stable postmortem and usually survives fixation in tissue blocks so that it can later be extracted, amplified, and sequenced (252). Mitochondrial function and morphology are often altered by extrinsic disorders. The changes of mitochondrial structure and function found in the kinky hair disease, for example, have been interpreted as secondary to the disturbance of metal transport, since copper ions are essential to the cytochromes, and copper disturbances are also known to disturb the mitochondrial adenine nucleotide translocator (253) that regulates mitochondrial respiration. Only a few studies of mtDNA in human mitochondrial diseases have been done, so far. Holt et al. found several patients with abnormalities of mtDNA coding for subunits of complexes I and III (247).

Because drugs and functional changes, such as mitochondrial swelling, can change enzyme activity and transport, these parameters are less reliable than studies of the protein itself or its DNA coding sequence. When possible, enzyme abnormalities should be confirmed by nucleic acid studies to separate secondary effects from primary gene defects. Until more mitochondrial proteins have been cloned and their nucleic acid sequence is known, we must rely on studies of enzyme activity and metabolite transport for probing many aspects of mitochondrial function. Fortunately, most enzymes can be studied in frozen tissue. Mitochondrial proteins can also be studied electrophoretically.

There must be verification that a mitochondrial defect is present. If resting lactate is normal, investigation of the lactate response to exercise and glucose loading may be useful, and CSF lactate may be elevated when blood lactate is normal. While NMR spectroscopy can provide strong evidence for mitochondrial dysfunction in some cases, biopsy and morphologic study remain important. When the existence of a mitochondrial disorder is established, precise etiologic classification is often needed for genetic and therapeutic purposes. This may require a second muscle biopsy guided by the results of NMR spectroscopy or in vitro studies performed on the first specimen.

When NMR spectroscopy is not available, preliminary classification can be assisted by a sequence of studies on a muscle biopsy specimen, including probes of the respiratory chain, and oxidation of several labeled substrates such as pyruvate, malate, alpha-ketoglutarate, acetate, and long-chain fatty acids. Polarographic studies of mitochondrial respiration and studies of mitochondrial transport will probably be reserved for large laboratories doing many specimens each year. Studies with antibodies, DNA probes, and labeled substrates may be feasible for smaller centers seeing fewer cases.

Although many authors have restricted the term mitochondrial myopathy to patients with ragged red fibers, this can be unwise, for it deflects attention from mitochondrial disturbances not usually associated with ragged red fibers, such as Leigh syndrome. Moreover, it implies that ragged red fibers will be found in all muscle biopsies, which is not true.

Some patients in the Kearns-Sayre syndrome group do well without treatment. Younger relatives in the earlier stages of the illness might, however, be recruited for a controlled trial of CoQ, which seems to be helpful and may prevent progression to a more impaired state. There has been a tendency to think of CoQ, carnitine, and corticosteroids as broad-spectrum drugs that may help any mitochondrial disorder (254–256). CoQ therapy probably has a very limited spectrum of applicability and a quantitatively modest effect. Corticosteroids are hazardous to patients who may have Kearns-Sayre syndrome; moreover, their growth inhibitory effects are significant in the younger child. Controlled separate studies of carnitine and CoQ in selected mitochondrial disorders are needed.

Ideally, one could test a variety of agents in cultured cells from a patient and choose an agent that corrected the biochemical defect. Mitochondrial abnormalities are frequently demonstrable in cultured fibroblasts (257–259). Muscle cells can be grown in culture (260,261), a technique which deserves greater use.

Finally, physicians must be alert for mitochondrial diseases secondary to exogenous toxins. An interesting cause of toxic encephalopathy with a likely mitochondrial basis is the syndrome of encephalopathy due to D-lactic acid produced by intestinal flora (262). A few patients with intestinal bypass surgery (jejunoileostomy) for massive obesity developed D-lactic acidosis and encephalopathy with prominent ataxia. They were shown to have intestinal bacteria that produced the unusual form of lactate, and their symptoms remitted with fasting and intravenous feedings. Accumulation of D-lactic acid would not be recognized by the usual enzymatic assay for L-lactate. As noted by Cross and Callaway, certain forms of hereditary ataxia have been serendipitously found to respond to acetazolamide (263). This agent might influence lactate and pyruvate metabolism or the Na^-/H^+ membrane exchanger mentioned.

Mitochondrial Toxins and Valproic Acid

Among the interesting mitochondrial toxins is MPP^+, the active metabolite of MPTP and recognized cause of Parkinson disease found in improperly made meperidine (264). The great species differences in MPTP sensitivity and the fact that the drug is activated inside by glial cells by monoamine oxidase B, after which its active metabolite is taken up by neurons with dopamine uptake systems (265), will probably hold true for other environmental toxins. MPP^+ is toxic to brain and liver mitochondria and would presumably enter any cell (266). The detailed basis for its mitochondrial toxicity remains uncertain and MPP^+ may have additional extramitochondrial mechanisms of toxicity.

Reye syndrome, now decreasing in incidence, appears to include a toxic component, as evident from the fact that serum from patients with Reye syndrome inhibits mitochondrial function (267). A number of toxins produce states similar to Reye syndrome including hypoglycin, the active principle of the akee fruit, which is responsible for so-called Jamaican vomiting sickness (268).

Valproic acid (VPA), a useful anticonvulsant, may cause a Reye-like mitochondrial toxicity that can be fatal (269). This outcome occurs most frequently in very young children receiving VPA in addition to other enzyme-inducing anticonvulsants like phenobarbital (270). Many VPA metabolites have been identified, some of which may play a special role in hepatotoxicity and are produced in greater amount if phenobarbital is also given (271). Valproate itself has a fundamental tendency to oppose hepatic fatty acid oxidation and ketosis (272). This implies that the drug is particularly hazardous in small children who do not exhibit a ketotic response to fasting. Single doses of VPA produce ultrastructural changes in hepatic mitochondria of rodents. Any circumstance that reduces carbohydrate intake can alter the metabolic balance in young patients receiving VPA, causing mobilization of fat from adipose tissue, steatosis in the liver, and lactic acidosis that can progress to Reye syndrome with hypoglycemia and death. The blood level of valproate is an unreliable guide to this toxic syndrome, since it can occur with usual doses of the drug and therapeutic blood levels. Drug levels will rise as the syndrome progresses because VPA can no longer be metabolized; increased serum lactate will precede this stage, while increases in serum transaminase may not. For the young infant receiving valproate who seems ill and has vomited a few times, a normal lactate and the presence of urinary ketones are reassuring. Unless the child is able to keep down a carbohydrate-containing liquid, the VPA dose should be reduced until the child resumes oral intake. Children who appear more than mildly ill should receive IV glucose, which can often be accomplished without hospitalization.

Panic Disorders

This heterogeneous group of disorders may not belong with mitochondrial disorders, although many are associated with lactate metabolism. If one defines panic attacks as discrete episodes of anxiety accompanied by strong symptoms of autonomic arousal, there is a large group of predominantly female patients, whose symptoms begin in adolescence or young adult life. This category of panic attacks is not absolutely separate from those of hyperventilation syndrome, anxiety neurosis, or neurocirculatory asthenia. In some patients hyperventilation is a secondary component and patients report termination of an attack if they breathe into a paper bag. Pitts and McClure infused sodium lactate into patients with a history of typical panic attacks and found that in 13 of 14 patients typical panic episodes could be provoked, while only 2 of 10 controls experienced panic (273). Dextrose infusions provoked no attacks. The findings have been reproduced many times; isoproterenol infusions also produce panic attacks and it has been theorized that brain norepinephrine systems arising from the locus coeruleus are overactive in these patients.

There is some evidence that patients with panic disorders are more sensitive to caffeine than normal patients (274) as well as to the effects of breathing high concentrations of carbon dioxide (275). Panic attacks induced by sodium lactate, caffeine, or exposure to phobic stimuli rarely produce increased plasma levels of the norepinephrine metabolite, 3-methoxy, 4-hydroxyphenylethylene glycol (MHPG), while panic attacks caused by the alpha-receptor blocker yohimbine are associated with increases in plasma MHPG.

Abnormalities in relatives of these patients are common, but individual family members do not usually have the same symptoms and no simple hereditary mechanism has been evident from family studies. A linkage study of families with panic attacks evaluated 29 genetic markers and found evidence for one significant association (276): namely, mitral valve prolapse, which is known to be disproportionately common in patients with panic disorder. Patients with mitral valve abnormality and panic attacks do not differ, however, in their psychiatric manifestations from others without heart disease (277).

While current categorization of panic disorders leaves much to be desired, the diagnostic label of panic disorder is much better than that of hyperventilation syndrome or chronic anxiety because of the therapeutic options it suggests. Panic attacks clearly respond to drug therapy, and the standard treatment is the administration of imipramine. The antidepressant benzodiazepine alprazolam may be as effective as imipramine (278). Monoamine oxidase (MAO) inhibitors are also effective, but are not standard therapy because of their potential for serious side effects. Patients with panic disorder often require psychotherapy or social measures as well as drug therapy; rarely can one "turn off the problem with a chemical." It is interesting that β-adrenergic blockers, which reduce the symptoms of severe "stage fright" or performance anxiety in relatively normal individuals, are rarely effective in panic disorder (279).

GLUCOSE USE IN EMERGENCY SITUATIONS

Cerebral Anoxia/Ischemia

Global anoxic events in infants and children are more frequent than cerebral ischemia due to stroke, but both categories of disease are important. Brain damage is worsened in each case by glucose provision before or after the event. Hyperglycemia consistently increases brain damage due to ischemia (cardiac arrest or stroke) in animal studies (280). Glucose supplementation prior to the event is most damaging, although few investigators have separately evaluated preischemic and postischemic glucose (281). Many studies of human strokes show that higher blood sugar levels are associated with worse outcome. However, these are observational or correlational studies; no investigator has tried to reduce post stroke glucose and improve outcome.

For children older than 2 years of age without historical or clinical evidence of liver disease, initial treatment with saline solutions is recommended. Blood glucose should be determined and if below 50 mg/dL, glucose-containing solutions should be infused slowly in an attempt to keep blood glucose below 100 mg/dL. Children with possible liver disease or histories suggesting inborn errors of metabolism, such as recurrent episodes of vomiting,

acidosis, or dehydration, should receive glucose containing solutions, attempting to avoid blood glucose levels above 100 mg/dL. If circulatory function is adequate as judged by blood pressure and urine output after 2 hours, the need to restrict glucose is less clear and glucose containing solutions may be used. Hyperglycemia should still be avoided, however, by reducing glucose infusion rate or switching to lactated Ringer's solution. Insulin should not be used. The concomitant use of glucocorticoids, which worsen the effects of cerebral ischemia (282), should be avoided unless there is an overwhelming indication for their use.

Infants beyond the perinatal period are best treated with lactated Ringer's solution if there is no evidence of liver or metabolic disease or prior malnutrition. No recommendation for or against use of glucose-containing solutions in perinatal anoxia and ischemia can be made today because of lack of data. Studies are urgently needed to compare the outcome of groups of newborns who receive extracorporeal membrane oxygenation (ECMO) therapy and are randomized between free glucose replacement (current practice) and restricted glucose replacement (to hold blood glucose level between 50 and 60 mg/dL) during the whole period of ECMO, during which time cerebral hypoxia is virtually inevitable.

Possible VPA toxicity can be suspected by nausea, vomiting, and decreasing alertness. Serum transaminases and other liver function tests will usually but not always be abnormal. Since VPA interferes with mitochondrial function, the absence of acidosis, increased blood lactate, hyperpnea, and other signs of hepatic encephalopathy would suggest that abnormal liver function tests are not due to VPA. Given a sick child with a rising blood lactate, the drug should be stopped and intravenous glucose provided. If the child does not quickly improve or becomes comatose, intravenous L-carnitine should also be given. In another instance, should a physician phone for consultation about a patient on VPA who is sick and vomiting, one should ask for a blood lactate and urine ketones. This *may* result in overreaction (unnecessary test) to viral gastroenteritis, but it will permit one to detect valproate hepatotoxicity at an early stage, when it is more likely to be reversible.

The control of blood sugar may improve the outcome in other disease states. It has been suggested that elevated blood sugar concentrations might reduce the morbidity from bacterial meningitis (283); however, a survey of patients with meningitis suggested no evidence that hyperglycemia altered the prognosis (284). These studies are limited by the fact that blood sugar concentrations may vary greatly and an integrated measure of blood sugar over time is required to provide the needed information. Glycosylation of proteins like albumin that turn over rapidly could provide such an index (285). This could be the first and simplest way to study the relationship between blood sugar and any pathologic process before controlled therapeutic trials.

REFERENCES

1. Kimball JW. Biology, 5th ed. Reading, MA: Addison-Wesley, 1983.
2. Martin BR. Metabolic Regulation, A Molecular Approach. Oxford: Blackwell, 1987.
3. Akers RF, Lovinger DM, Colley PA, et al. Translocation of protein kinase C activity may mediate long-term potentiation. Science 1986;231:587–589.
4. Hogeboom GH. Fractionation of cell components of animal tissues. In: Colowick SP, Kaplan NO, eds. Methods in Enzymology. New York: Academic Press, 1955;1:16–19.
5. Masters CJ. Interactions between soluble enzymes and subcellular structure. CRC Crit Rev Biochem 1981;11:105–143.
6. Green DE, Murer E, Hultin HO, et al. Association of integrated metabolic pathways with membranes. I. Glycolytic enzymes of red blood corpuscle and yeast. Arch Biochem Biophys 1965;112:635–647.
7. Clarke FM, Masters CJ. Reversible and selective adsorption of aldolase isoenzymes in rat brain. Arch Biochem Biophys 1972;153:258–265.
8. Karadshen NS, Ukeda K. Changes in allosteric properties of phosphofructokinase bound to erythrocyte membranes. J Biol Chem 1977;252:7418–7424.
9. Weiss JN, Lamp ST. Glycolysis preferentially inhibits ATP-sensitive K^+ channels in isolated guinea pig myocytes. Science 1987;238:67–69.
10. Clegg JS. Interrelationships between water and cellular metabolism in Artemia cysts. IX Evidence for the organization of soluble cytoplasmic enzymes. Cold Spring Harbor Symp Quant Biol 1981;46:23–37.
11. Nanhua C, Masters C. The influence of calcium ions on the adsorption of glycolytic enzymes to cellular structures. Biochem Int 1987;15:835–842.
12. Bronstein WW, Knull HR. Interaction of muscle glycolytic enzymes with thin filament proteins. Can J Biochem 1981;59:494–499.
13. Ureta T. The role of isozymes in metabolism: A model of metabolic pathways as the basis for the biological role of isozymes. Curr Top Cell Regul 1978;13:233–266.
14. Bernhard SA, Srivastava DK. Functional consequences of the direct transfer of metabolites in muscle glycolysis. Biochem Soc Trans 1986;15:977–981.
15. Clegg JS. Properties and metabolism of the aqueous cytoplasm and its boundaries. Am J Physiol 1984;246:R133–R151.
16. Webster A. Regulation of glycolytic enzyme RNA transcriptional rates by oxygen availability in skeletal muscle cells. Mol Cell Biochem 1987;77:19–28.
17. Engelhard VA, Lyubinova MN. Myosin and adenosinetriphosphatase. Nature 1939;144:668–669.
18. Holloszy JO, Rennie MJ, Hickson RC, et al. Physiological consequences of the biochemical adaptation to endurance exercise. Ann N Y Acad Sci 1977;301:440–450.
19. Dubowitz V, Pearse AGE. A comparative histochemical study of oxidative enzyme and phosphorylase activity in skeletal muscle. Histochemie 1960;2:105–119.
20. Engel WK. The essentiality of histo- and cytochemical studies in the investigation of neuromuscular disease. Neurology 1962;12:778–791.
21. Barnard RJ, Edgerton VR, Furukawa T, et al. Histochemical, biochemical, and contractile properties of red, white, and intermediate fibers. Am J Physiol 1971;220:410–414.
22. Peter JB, Barnard RJ, Edgerton VR, et al. Metabolic profiles of three fiber types of skeletal muscle in guinea pigs and rabbits. Biochemistry 1972;11:2627–2633.
23. Brooke MH, Kaiser KK. Muscle fiber types: How many and what kind? Arch Neurol 1970;23:369–379.
24. Young RB, Moriarity DM, McGee CE. Structural analysis of myosin genes using recombinant DNA techniques. J Anim Sci 1986;63:259–268.
25. Kugelberg E, Edstrom L. Differential histochemical effects of muscle contraction on phosphorylase and glycogen in various types of fibers. Relation to fatigue. J Neurol Neurosurg Psychiatry 1968;31:415–423.
26. Ishihara A, Naitoh H, Araki H, et al. Soma size and oxidative enzyme activity of motoneurones supplying the fast twitch and slow twitch muscles in the rat. Brain Res 1988;446:195–198.
27. Johnson MA, Mastaglia FL, Montgomery A, et al. Changes in myosin light chains in the rat soleus after thyroidectomy. FEBS Lett 1980;110:230–235.
28. Tashiro N. Effects of isoprenaline on contractions of directly stimulated fast and slow skeletal muscles of the guinea pig. Br J Pharmacol 1973;48:121–131.
29. Reddy NB, Oliver KL, Engel WK. Differences in catecholamine-sensitive adenylate cyclase and (β)-adrenergic receptor binding between fast-twitch and slow-twitch skeletal muscle membranes. Life Sci 1979;24:1765–1772.
30. Zeman RJ, Ludemann R, Etlinger JD. Clenbuterol, a (β_2)-agonist, retards atrophy in denervated muscles. Am J Physiol 1987;252:E152–155.
31. Newsholme EA. The regulation of intracellular and extracellular fuel supply during sustained exercise. Ann N Y Acad Sci 1977;301:81–91.
32. Essen B. Intramuscular substrate utilization during prolonged exercise. Ann N Y Acad Sci 1977;301:30–44.
33. Bergstrom JE, Hultman E, Jorfeldt L, et al. Effects of nicotinic acid on physical working capacity and on metabolism of muscle glycogen in man. J Appl Physiol 1969;26:1170–1176.
34. Hermansen L, Hultman E, Saltin B. Muscle glycogen during prolonged severe exercise. Acta Physiol Scand 1967;71:129–139.
35. Bergstrom JE, Hultman E, Saltin B. Diet, muscle glycogen, and physical performance. Acta Physiol Scand 1967;71:140–150.
36. Conlee RK. Muscle glycogen and exercise endurance: a twenty-year perspective. Exercise Sport Sci Rev 1987;15:1–28.
37. Kronfeld DS. Diet and the performance of facing sled dogs. J Am Vet Med Assoc 1973;162:470–473.
38. Phinney SD, Bistrian BR, Evans WJ, et al. The human metabolic response to chronic ketosis without caloric restriction: preservation of submaximal exercise capacity with reduced carbohydrate oxidation. Metabolism 1983;32:769–776.
39. Saltin B, Gollnick PD. Skeletal muscle adaptability: significance for metabolism and performance. In: Peachey LD, Adrian RH, Geiger SR, eds. Handbook of Physiology, section 10: Skeletal Muscle. American Physiological Society, 1983;555–631.

40. Maxwell LC, Barclay JK, Mohrman DE, et al. Physiological characteristics of skeletal muscles of dogs and cats. Am J Physiol 1977;233:C14–C18.

41. Arnold DL, Matthews PM, Radda GK. Metabolic recovery after exercise and the assessment of mitochondrial function in vivo in human skeletal muscle by means of ^{31}P NMR. Magn Reson Med 1984;1:307–315.

42. Norman B, Sollevi A, Kaijser L, et al. ATP breakdown products in human skeletal muscle during prolonged exercise to exhaustion. Clin Physiol 1987;7:503–509.

43. Park JH, Brown RL, Park CR, et al. Functional pools of oxidative and glycolytic fibers in human muscle observed by ^{31}P magnetic resonance spectroscopy during exercise. Proc Natl Acad Sci U S A 1987;84:8976–8980.

44. Wilson JR, McCully KK, Mancini DM, et al. Relationship of muscular fatigue to pH and diprotonated Pi in humans: a ^{31}P-NMR study. J Appl Physiol 1988;64:2333–2339.

45. Coulson RA. Aerobic and anaerobic glycolysis in mammals and reptiles in vivo. Comp Biochem Physiol 1987;87B:207–216.

46. Johnson JL, Bagby GJ. Gluconeogenic pathway in liver and muscle glycogen synthesis after exercise. J Appl Physiol 1988;64:1591–1599.

47. Nordlie RC. Fine tuning of blood glucose concentrations. Trends Biochem Sci 1985;10:70–75.

48. Arion WJ, Wallin BK, Lange AJ, et al. On the involvement of a glucose 6-phosphate transport system in the function of microsomal glucose 6-phosphatase. Mol Cell Biochem 1975;6:75–83.

49. Arion WJ, Lange AJ, Walls HE. Microsomal membrane integrity and the interactions of phlorizin with the glucose 6-phosphatase system. J Biol Chem 1980;255:10387–10395.

50. Lange AJ, Arion WJ, Beaudet AL. Type IB glycogen storage disease is caused by a defect in the glucose 6-phosphate translocase of the microsomal glucose 6-phosphatase system. J Biol Chem 1980;255:8381–8384.

51. Senior B, Loridan L. Studies of liver glycogenoses, with particular reference to the metabolism of intravenously administered glycerol. N Engl J Med 1968;279:959–965.

52. Roach PJ, Goldman P. Modification of glycogen synthase activity in isolated rat hepatocytes by tumor-promoting phorbol esters: evidence for differential regulation of glycogen synthase and phosphorylase. Proc Natl Acad Sci U S A 1983;80:7170–7172.

53. Antwi D, Youn JH, Shargill NS, et al. Regulation of glycogen synthase in muscle and adipose tissue during fasting and refeeding. Am J Physiol 1988;E720–E725.

54. Shulman RG. High resolution NMR in vivo. Trends Biochem Sci 1988;13:37–39.

55. Avison MJ, Rothman DL, Nadel E, et al. Detection of human muscle glycogen by natural abundance ^{13}C NMR. Proc Natl Acad Sci U S A 1988;85:1634–1636.

56. Chesler A, Himwich HE. The glycogen content of various parts of the central nervous system of dogs and cats at different ages. Arch Biochem 1943;2:175–181.

57. Vallejo CG, Marco R, Sebastian J. The glucose 6-phosphate metabolic crossroads in brain: Studies at the enzyme level. Arch Biochem Biophys 1971;147:41–48.

58. Yasumoto Y, Passonneau JV, Feussner G, et al. Metabolic alterations in fiber layers of the CA 1 region of the gerbil hippocampus following short-term ischemia: High energy phosphates, glucose-related metabolites, and amino acids. Metab Brain Dis 1988;3:133–149.

59. Sagar SM, Sharp FR, Swanson RA. The regional distribution of glycogen in rat brain fixed by microwave irradiation. Brain Res 1987;417:172–174.

60. Petroni A, Borghi A, Blasevich M, et al. Effects of hypoxia and recovery on brain eicosanoids and carbohydrate metabolites in rat brain cortex. Brain Res 1987;415:226–232.

61. Inoue N, Iwasa T, Fukunaga K, et al. Phosphorylation and inactivation of brain glycogen synthase by a multifunctional calmodulin-dependent protein kinase. J Neurochem 1987;48:981–988.

62. Inoue E, Matsukado Y, Goto S, et al. Localization of glycogen synthase in brain. J Neurochem 1988;50:400–405.

63. Hof PR, Pascale E, Magistretti PJ. K$^+$ at concentrations reached in the extracellular space during neuronal activity promotes a Ca^{++}-dependent glycogen hydrolysis in mouse cerebral cortex. J Neurosci 1988;8:1922–1928.

64. Kalderon B, Gopher A, Lapidot A. A quantitative analysis of the metabolic pathways of hepatic glucose synthesis in vivo with ^{13}C-labeled substrates. FEBS Lett 1987;213:209–214.

65. Duee PH, Pegorier JP, El Manoubi L, et al. Development of gluconeogenesis from different substrates in newborn rabbit hepatocytes. J Dev Physiol 1986;8:387–394.

66. Blumenthal SA. Inhibition of gluconeogenesis in rat liver by lipoic acid. Biochem J 1984;219:773–780.

67. Bressler R, Corredor C, Brendel K. Hypoglycin and hypoglycin-like compounds. Pharmacol Rev 1969;21:105–130.

68. Billington D, Osmundsen H, Sherratt HSA. Mechanisms of the metabolic disturbances caused by hypoglycin and by pent-4-enoic acid in vivo studies. Biochem Pharmacol 1978;27:2891–2900.

69. Shank RP, Bennett GS, Frewytag SO, et al. Pyruvate carboxylase: an astrocyte-specific enzyme implicated in the replenishment of amino acid neurotransmitter pools. Brain Res 1985;329:364–367.

70. Casazza JP, Veech RL. The interdependence of glycolytic and pentose cycle intermediates in ad libitum fed rats. J Biol Chem 1986;261:690–698.

71. Singh H. Glucose 6-phosphate dehydrogenase deficiency: A preventable cause of mental retardation. Br Med J 1986;292:397–398.

72. Gaitonde MK, Evison E, Evans GM. The rate of utilization of glucose via the hexose monophosphate shunt in brain. J Neurochem 1983;41:1253–1260.

73. Jeffery J, Jornvall H. Enzyme relationships in a sorbitol pathway that bypasses glycolysis and pentose phosphates in glucose metabolism. Proc Natl Acad Sci U S A 1983;80:901–905.

74. Whittle SR, Turner AJ. Anticonvulsants and brain aldehyde metabolism: inhibitory characteristics of ox brain aldehyde reductase. Biochem Pharmacol 1981;30:1191–1196.

75. Gabbay HK, O'Sullivan JB. The sorbitol pathway, enzyme localization and content in normal and diabetic nerve and cord. Diabetes 1968;17:239–243.

76. Crone C. The permeability of brain capillaries to nonelectrolytes. Acta Physiol Scand 1965;64:407–417.

77. Crone C. Facilitated transfer of glucose from blood into brain tissue. J Physiol 1965;181:103–113.

78. Gilboe DD, Betz AL. Kinetics of glucose transport in the isolated dog brain. Am J Physiol 1970;219:774–778.

79. Wheeler TJ, Hinkle PC. The glucose transporter of mammalian cells. Ann Rev Physiol 1985;47:503–517.

80. Mueckler M, Caruso C, Baldwin SA, et al. Sequence and structure of a human glucose transporter. Science 1985;229:941–945.

81. Walmsley AR. The dynamics of the glucose transporter. Trends Biochem Sci 1988;13:226–231.

82. Birnbaum MJ, Haspel HC, Rosen OM. Cloning and characterization of a cDNA encoding the rat brain glucose-transporter protein. Proc Natl Acad Sci U S A 1986; 83:5784–5788.

83. Dick APK, Harik SI. Distribution of the glucose transporter in the mammalian brain. J Neurochem 1986; 46:1406–1411.

84. Cestaro B, Cervato G, Carandente O, et al. Erythrocyte D-glucose transport in reconstituted model membranes of different lipid composition. Biochem Int 1988;16:323–329.

85. Roeder LM, Tildon JT, Williams IB. Transport of 2-deoxy-D-glucose by dissociated brain cells. Brain Res 1985;345: 298–305.

86. Leff SWE, Rosenfeld MG, Evans RM. Complex transcriptional units: diversity in gene expression by alternative RNA processing. Annu Rev Biochem 1986;55:1091–1117.

87. Bachelard HS. Glucose transport and phosphorylation in the control of carbohydrate metabolism in the brain. In: Brierley JB, Meldrum BS, eds. Brain Hypoxia. Spastics International Medical Publications. London: William Heinemann, 1971;251–260.

88. Oldendorf WH, Cornford ME, Brown WJ. The large apparent work capacity of the blood-brain barrier: A study of the mitochondrial content of capillary endothelial cells in brain and other tissues of the rat. Ann Neurol 1977;1:409–417.

89. Betz AL, Goldstein GW. Specialized properties and solute transport in brain capillaries. Annu Rev Physiol 1986; 48:241–250.

90. James DE, Brown R, Navarro J, et al. Insulin-regulatable tissues express a unique insulin-sensitive glucose transport protein. Nature 1988;333:183–185.

91. Elbrink J, Bihler I. Membrane transport: Its relation to cellular metabolic rates. Science 1975;188:1177–1184.

92. Suzuki K, Kono T. Evidence that insulin causes translocation of glucose transport activity to the plasma membrane from an intracellular storage site. Proc Natl Acad Sci U S A 1980; 77:2542–2545.

93. Cushman SW, Wardzala LJ. Potential mechanism of insulin action on glucose transport in the isolated rat adipose cell. Apparent translocation of intracellular transport systems to the plasma membrane. J Biol Chem 1980;255:4758–4762.

94. Sternlicht E, Barnard RJ, Grimditch GK. Mechanism of insulin action on glucose transport in rat skeletal muscle. Am J Physiol 1988;254:E633–E638.

95. Joost HG, Weber TM, Cushman SW. Qualitative and quantitative comparison of glucose transport activity and glucose transporter concentration in plasma membranes from basal and insulin-stimulated rat adipose cells. Biochem J 1988; 249:155–161.

96. Yamada K, Tillotson LG, Isselbacher KJ. Regulation of hexose carriers in chicken embryo fibroblasts: Effect of glucose starvation and role of protein synthesis. J Biol Chem 1983;258:9786–9792.

97. Shawver LK, Olson SA, White MK, et al. Degradation and biosynthesis of the glucose transporter protein in chick embryo fibroblasts transformed by the src oncogene. Mol Cell Biol 1987;7:2112–2118.

98. Simpson IA, Cushman SW. Hormonal regulation of mammalian glucose transport. Annu Rev Biochem 1986; 55:1059–1089.

99. Standaert ML, Pollet RJ. Insulin-glycerolipid mediators and gene expression. FASEB J 1988;2:2453–2461.

100. Baskin DG, Wilcox BJ, Figlewicz DP, et al. Insulin and insulin-like growth factors in the CNS. Trends Neurosci 1988;11:107–111.

101. Duffy K, Pardridge W. Blood-brain barrier transcytosis of insulin in developing rats. Brain Res 1987;420:32–38.

102. Murphy LJ, Bell G, Friesen HG. Tissue distribution of insulin-like growth factor I and II messenger ribonucleic acid in the adult rat. Endocrinology 1987;120:1279–1282.

103. Haselbacher GK, Schwab ME, Pasi A, et al. Insulin-like growth factor II (IGF II) in human brain: Regional distribution of IGF II and of higher molecular mass forms. Proc Natl Acad Sci U S A 1985;82:2153–2157.

104 Namba H, Lucignani G, Nehlig A, et al. Effects of insulin on hexose transport across blood-brain barrier in normoglycemia. Am J Physiol 1987;252:E299–E303.

105. Lucignani G, Namba H, Nehlig A, et al. Effects of insulin on local cerebral glucose utilization in the rat. J Cereb Blood Flow Metab 1987;7:309–314.

106. Clarke DW, Boyd FT, Kappy MS, et al. Insulin stimulates macromolecular synthesis in cultured glial cells from rat brain. Am J Physiol 1985;249:C484–C489.

107. Aizenman Y, Weichsel ME, De Vellis J. Changes in insulin and transferrin requirements of pure brain neuronal cultures during embryonic development. Proc Natl Acad Sci U S A 1986;83:2263–2266.

108. Lowe WL, Boyd FT, Clarke DW, et al. Development of brain insulin receptors: structural and functional studies of insulin receptors from whole brain and primary cell cultures. Endocrinology 1986;119:25–35.

109. Boyd FT, Clarke DW, Mutuer TF, et al. Insulin receptors and insulin modification of norepinephrine uptake in neuronal cultures from rat brain. J Biol Chem 1985; 260:15880–15884.

110. Shemer J, Raizada MK, Masters BA, et al. Insulin-like growth factor I receptors in neuronal and glial cells. J Biol Chem 1987;262:7693–7699.

111. Yoshimasa Y, Seino S, Whittaker J, et al. Insulin-resistant diabetes due to a point mutation that prevents insulin proreceptor processing. Science 1988;240:784–787.

112. Von Gierke E. Hepato-nephro-megalia glykogenia (Glykogenspeicherkrankheit der Leber und Nieren) Beitr Pathol Anat 1929;82:497–513.

113. Pompe JC. Over idiopatische hypertofie van het hart. Ned Tijdschr Geneeskd 1932;76:304–311.

114. Hers HG. Inborn lysosomal diseases. Gastroenterology 1965;48:625–633.

115. Reuser AJJ, Kroos M, Willemsen R, et al. Clinical diversity in Glycogenosis Type II, biosynthesis and in situ localization of acid α-glucosidase in mutant fibroblasts. J Clin Invest 1987;79:1689–1699.

116. Howell RR, Williams JC. The glycogen storage diseases. In: Stanbury JB, Wyngaarden JB, Frederickson DS, et al., eds. The Metabolic Basis of Inherited Disease, 5th ed. New York: McGraw-Hill, 1983;141–166.

117. Gambetti P, DiMauro S, Baker L. Nervous system in Pompe's disease: ultrastructure and biochemistry. J Neuropathol Exp Neurol 1971;30:412–430.

118. Riggs JE, Schochet SS, Gutmann L, et al. Lysosomal glycogen storage disease without acid maltase deficiency. Neurology 1983;33:873–877.

119. Martiniuk F, Mehler M, Pellicer A, et al. Isolation of a cDNA for human acid α-glucosidase and detection of genetic heterogeneity of mRNA in three α-glucosidase-deficient patients. Proc Natl Acad Sci U S A 1986;83:9641–9644.

120. Reuser AJJ, Kroos M, Oude Elferink RPJ, et al. Defects in synthesis, phosphorylation and maturation of acid α-glucosidase. J Biol Chem 1985;260:8336–8342.

121. Isaacs H, Savage N, Badenhorst M, et al. Acid maltase deficiency: A case study and review of the pathophysiological changes and proposed therapeutic measures. J Neurol Neurosurg Psychiat 1986;49:1011–1018.

122. Van Der Ploeg AT, Loonen MCB, Bolhuis PA, et al. Receptor-mediated uptake of acid α-glucosidase corrects lysosomal glycogen storage in cultured skeletal muscle. Pediatr Res 1988;24:90–94.

123. DiMauro S, DeVivo DC. Disorders of glycogen metabolism. Handbook of Neurochemistry 1985;10:1–13.

124. Servidei S, Bonilla E, Diedrich RG, et al. Fatal infantile form of muscle phosphofructokinase deficiency. Neurology 1986; 36:1465–1470.

125. Konrad PN, McCarthy DJ, Mauer AM, et al. Erythrocyte and leukocyte phosphoglycerate kinase deficiency with neurologic disease. J Pediatr 1973;82:456–460.

126. Greene GM, Weldon DC, Ferrans VJ, et al. Juvenile polysaccharidosis with cardioskeletal myopathy. Arch Pathol Lab Med 1987;111:977–982.

127. Resibois-Gregoire A, Dourov N. Electron microscopic study of a case of cerebral glycogenosis. Acta Neuropathol 1966; 6:70–79.

128. Mineo I, Kono K, Hara N, et al. Myogenic hyperuricemia, a common pathophysiological feature of glycogenosis types III, V, and VII. N Engl J Med 1987;317:75–80.

129. Fox IH, Palella TD, Kelley WN. Hyperuricemia: a marker for cell energy crisis. N Engl J Med 1987;317:111–112.

130. McArdle B. Myopathy due to defect in muscle glycogen breakdown. Clin Sci 1951;10:13–35.

131. Sengers RCA, Stadhouders AM, Jaspers HHJ, et al. Muscle phosphorylase deficiency in childhood. Eur J Pediatr 1980; 134:161–170.

132. DiMauro S, Bresolin N. Phosphorylase deficiency. In: Engel AM, Banker BQ, eds. Myology. New York: McGraw-Hill, 1986,2:1585–1601.

133. Gautron S, Daegelen D, Mennecier F, et al. Molecular mechanisms of McArdles's disease (Muscle Glycogen Phosphorylase deficiency), RNA and DNA analyses. J Clin Invest 1987; 79:275–281.

134. Braakhekke JP, De Bruin MI, Stegeman DF, et al. The second wind phenomenon in McArdle's disease. Brain 1986; 109:1087–1101.

135. Pearson CM, Rimer DG, Mommaerts WFHM. A metabolic myopathy due to absence of muscle phosphorylase. Am J Med 1961;30:502–517.

136. Fishbein WN. Myoadenylate deaminase deficiency. Inherited and acquired forms. Biochem Med 1985;33:158–169.

137. Lowenstein JM. Ammonia production in muscle and other tissues: the purine nucleotide cycle. Physiol Rev 1972;52: 382–414.

138. Sinkeler SPT, Joosten EMG, Wevers RA, et al. Myoadenylate deaminase deficiency: a clinical, genetic, and biochemical study in nine families. Muscle Nerve 1988;11:312–317.

139. Denny-Brown DD. Clinical problems in neuromuscular physiology. Am J Med 1953;15:368–390.

140. Layzer RB. Diagnostic implications of clinical fasciculations and cramps. In:Rowland LP, ed. Hum Motor Neuron Diseases. New York: Raven Press, 1982,23–27.

141. Roth G. The origin of fasciculations. Ann Neurol 1982;12: 542–547.

142. Ross BD, Radda GK, Gadian DG, et al. Examination of a case of suspected McArdle's syndrome by ^{31}P nuclear magnetic resonance. N Engl J Med 1981;304:1338–1342.

143. Edwards RHT, Wiles CM. Energy exchange in human skeletal muscle during isometric contraction. Circ Res 1981;48 supp 1:11–19.

144. Tesch P, Sjoden B, Thorstensson A, et al. Muscle fatigue and its relation to lactate accumulation and LDH activity in man. Acta Physiol Scand 1978;103:413–420.

145. Nassar-Gentina V, Passoneau JV, Rapoport SI. Fatigue and metabolism of frog muscle fibers during stimulation and response to caffeine. Am J Physiol 1981;241:C160–C166.

146. Isselbacher KJ, Anderson EP, Kurahashi K, et al. Congenital galactosemia, a single enzymatic block in galactose metabolism. Science 1956;123:635–636.

147. Segal S. Disorders of galactose metabolism. In: Stanbury JB, Wyngaarden JB, Fredrickson DS, et al., eds. The Metabolic Basis of Inherited Disease, 5th ed. New York: McGraw-Hill, 1983,167–191.

148. Donnell GN, Collado M, Koch R. Growth and development of children with galactosemia. J Pediatr 1961;58:836–839.

149. Gitzelmann R, Steinmann B. Galactosemia: How does long term treatment change the outcome? Enzyme 1984;32: 37–46.

150. Lo W, Packman S, Nash S, et al. Curious neurologic sequelae in galactosemia. Pediatrics 1984;73:309–312.

151. Bohles H, Wenzel D, Shin YS. Progressive cerebellar and extrapyramidal motor disturbances in galactosemic twins. Eur J Pediatr 1986;145:413–417.

152. Kaufman FR, Kogut MD, Donnell GN, et al. Hypergonadotropic hypogonadism in female patients with galactosemia. N Engl J Med 1981;304:994–998.

153. O'Brien JS. The gangliosidoses. In: Stanbury JB, Wyngaarden JB, Fredrickson DS, et al., eds. The Metabolic Basis of Inherited Disease, 5th ed. New York: McGraw-Hill, 1983, 945–972.

154. Spranger JW, Weidemann HR, Tolksdorf M, et al. Lipomucopolysaccharidose. Z Kinderheilk 1968;103:285–306.

155. Spranger JW, Weidemann HR. The genetic mucolipidoses. Diagnosis and differential diagnosis. Humangenetik 1970;9: 113–139.

156. Spranger JW, Gehler J, Cantz M. Mucolipidosis I- a sialidosis. Am J Med Genet 1977;1:21–29.

157. Durand P, Gatti R, Cavalieri S, et al. Sialidosis (mucolipidosis I). Helv Paediat Acta 1977;32:391–400.

158. Rapin I, Goldfischer S, Katzman R, et al. The cherry red spot-myoclonus syndrome. Ann Neurol 1978;3:234–242.

159. O'Brien JS. The cherry red spot-myoclonus syndrome: A newly recognized inherited lysosomal storage disease due to acid neuraminidase deficiency. Clin Genet 1978;14:55–60.

160. Lowden JA, O'Brien JS. Sialidosis: A review of human neuraminidase deficiency. Am J Hum Genet 1979;31:1–30.

161. O'Brien JS, Warner TG. Sialidosis: Delineation of subtypes by neuraminidase assay. Clin Genet 1980;17:35–38.

162. Thomas PK, Abrams JD, Swallow D, et al. Sialidosis type 1: Cherry red spot-myoclonus syndrome with sialidase deficiency and altered electrophoretic mobilities of some enzymes known to be glycoproteins. J Neurol Neurosurg Psychiat 1979;42:873–881.

163. Gravel RA, Lowden JA, Callahan JW, et al. Infantile sialidosis: A phenocopy of type 1 G_{M1} gangliosidosis distinguished by genetic complementation and urinary oligosaccharides. Am J Hum Genet 1979;31:669–679.

164. Schauer R. Sialic acids; chemistry, metabolism, and function. Wien: Springer Verlag, 1982.

165. Galjaard H, Willimsen R, Hoogeveen AT, et al. Molecular heterogeneity in human β-galactosidase and neuraminidase deficiency. Enzyme 1987;38:132–143.

166. Aula P, Autio S, Raivio KO, et al. "Salla disease": A new lysosomal storage disorder. Arch Neurol 1979;36:88–99.

167. Renlund M, Tietze F, Ghal WA. Defective sialic acid egress from isolated fibroblast lysosomes of patients with Salla disease. Science 1986;232:759–762.

168. Gahl WA. Disorders of lysosomal membrane transport-cystinosis and Salla disease. Enzyme 1987;38:154–160.

169. Autio-Harmainen H, Oldfors A, Sourander P, et al. Neuropathology of Salla disease. Acta Neuropathol 1988;75:481–490.

170. Wilcken B, Don N, Greenaweay R, et al. Sialuria: A second case. J Inherited Metab Dis 1987;10:97–102.

171. Ylitalo V, Hagberg B, Rapola J, et al. Salla disease variants; sialoylaciduric encephalopathy with increased sialidase activity in two non-Finnish children. Neuropediatrics 1986;17:44–47.

172. Stevenson RE, Lubinsky M, Taylor HA, et al. Sialic acid storage disease with sialuria: Clinical and biochemical features of the severe infantile type. Pediatrics 1983;72:441–449.

173. Renlund M, Kovanen PT, Raivio KO, et al. Studies on the defect underlying the lysosomal storage of sialic acid in Salla disease. J Clin Invest 1986;77:568–574.

174. Hancock LW, Ricketts JP, Hildreth J. Impaired proteolytic processing of lysosomal N-acetyl-α-hexosaminidase in cultured fibroblasts from patients with infantile generalized N-acetylneuraminic acid storage disease. Biochem Biophys Res Commun 1988;152:83–92.

175. Andria G, Strisciuglio P, Pontarelli G, et al. Infantile neuraminidase and β-galactosidase deficiencies with mild clinical course. Perspect Inher Metab Dis 1981;4:379–395.

176. Young ID, Young EP, Mossman J, et al. Neuraminidase deficiency: Case report and review of the phenotype. J Med Genet 1987;24:283–290.

177. Palmeri S, Hoogeveen AT, Verheijen FW, et al. Galactosialidosis: Molecular heterogeneity among distinct clincial phenotypes. Am J Hum Genet 1986;38:137–148.

178. Srere PA, Sumegi B, Sherry AD. Organizational aspects of the citric acid cycle. Biochem Soc Symp 1987;54:173–182.

179. Sumegi B, Srere PA. Complex I binds several mitochondrial NAD-coupled dehydrogenases. J Biol Chem 1984;259:15040–15045.

180. Chance B, Leigh JS, Smith DS, et al. Phosphorus magnetic resonance spectroscopy studies of the role of mitochondria in the disease process. Ann N Y Acad Sci 1986;488:140–153.

181. Mitchell P. Coupling of phosphorylation to electron and hydrogen transfer by a chemiosmotic type of mechanism. Nature 1961;191:144–148.

182. Hansford RG. Control of mitochondrial substrate oxidation. Curr Top Bioenerg 1980;10:217–278.

183. Hatefi Y. The mitochondrial electron transport and oxidative phosphorylation system. Annu Rev Biochem 1985;54:1015–1069.

184. Weiss H. Structure of mitochondrial ubiquinol-cytochrome-c reductase (complex III). Curr Top Bioenerg 1987;15:67–90.

185. Kadenbach B, Kuhn-Nentwig L, Buge U. Evolution of a regulatory enzyme: Cytochrome-c oxidase (complex IV). Curr Top Bioenerg 1987;15:113–161.

186. Kelley RI, Corkey BE. Increased sensitivity of cerebrohepatorenal syndrome fibroblasts to Antimycin A. J Inherited Metab Dis 1983;6:158–163.

187. Chance B, Williams GR. The respiratory chain and oxidative phosphorylation. Adv Enzymol 1956;17:65–134.

188. Balaban RS, Koretsky A, Katz L. NMR investigations of cellular energy metabolism. Ann N Y Acad Sci 1986;508:48–53.

189. Kaplan NO. The role of pyridine nucleotides in regulating cellular metabolism. Curr Top Cell Reg 1985;26:371–381.

190. Avise JC, Lansman RA. Polymorphism of mitochondrial DNA in populations of higher animals. In: Nei M, Koehn RK, eds. Evolution of Genes and Proteins. Sutherland: Sinauer, 1983, 147–164.

191. Pfanner N, Neupert W. Biogenesis of mitochondrial energy transducing complexes. Curr Top Bioenerg 1987;15:178–219.

192. Hartl FU, Ostermann J, Gulard B, et al. Successive translocation into and out of the mitochondrial matrix: targeting of proteins to the intermembrane space by a bipartite signal peptide. Cell 1987;51:1027–1034.

193. Hay R, Bohni P, Gasser S. How mitochondria import proteins. Biochim Biophys Acta 1984;779:65–87.

194. Kummel L. Mitochondrial pyruvate carrier—A possible link between gluconeogenesis and ketogenesis in the liver. Biosci Rep 1987;7:593–597.

195. Williamson DH, Lund P, Krebs HA. The redox state of free nicotinamide-adenine dinculeotide in the cytoplasm and mitochondria of rat liver. Biochem J 1967;103:514–526.

196. Cederbaum AI, Lieber CS, Beattie DS, et al. Characterization of shuttle mechanisms for the transport of reducing equivalents into mitochondria. Arch Biochem Biophys 1973;159:763–781.

197. Cheeseman AJ, Clark JB. Influence of the malate-aspartate shuttle on oxidative metabolism in synaptosomes. J Neurochem 1988;50:1559–1565.

198. Minn A, Gayet J. Kinetic study of glutamate transport in rat brain mitochondria. J Neurochem 1977;29:873–881.

199. Palaiologos G, Hertz L, Schousboe A. Evidence that aspartate aminotransferase activity and ketodicarboxylate carrier function are essential for biosynthesis of transmitter glutamate. J Neurochem 1988;51:317–320.

200. LaNoue KF, Schoolwerth AC. Metabolite transport in mitochondria. Annu Rev Biochem 1979;48:871–922.

201. Somlyo AV, Bond M, Broderick R, et al. Calcium and magnesium movements through sarcoplasmic reticulum, endoplasmic reticulum, and mitochondria. Adv Exp Med Biol 1988;232:221–229.

202. Merle P, Kadenbach B. On the heterogeneity of vertebrate cytochrome c oxidase polypeptide chain composition. Hoppe-Seyler's Z Physiol Chem 1980;361:1257–1259.

203. Kuhn-Nentwig L, Kadenbach B. Isolation and properties of cytochrome c oxidase from rat liver and quantitation of immunological difference between isozymes from various rat tissues. Eur J Biochem 1985;149:147–159.

204. Einarsdottir O, Caughey WS. Interactions of the anesthetic nitrous oxide with bovine heart cytochrome c oxidase. Effects on protein structure, oxidase activity, and other properties. J Biol Chem 1988;263:9199–9205.

205. Bookelman H, Trijbels JMF, Sengers RCA, et al. Measurement of cytochromes in human skeletal muscle mitochondria, isolated from fresh and frozen stored muscle specimens. Biochem Med 1978;366–373.

206. Sherratt HSA, Watmough NJ, Johnson MA, et al. Methods for study of normal and abnormal skeletal muscle mitochondria. Methods Biochem Anal 1987;33:243–335.

207. Crane FL, Hatefi Y, Lester RL, et al. Isolation of a quinone from beef heart mitochondria. Biochim Biophys Acta 1957;25:220–221.

208. Nayler WG. The use of coenzyme Q_{10} to protect ischemic heart muscle. In: Yamamura Y, Folkers K, Ito K, eds. Biomedical and Clinical Aspects of Coenzyme Q, Vol. 2. Amsterdam: Elsevier/North Holland, 1980,409–425.

209. Ishiwata K, Miura Y, Takahashi T, et al. ^{11}C-Coenzyme Q_{10}: A new myocardial imaging tracer for positron emission tomography. Eur J Nucl Med 1985;11:162–165.

210. Luft R, Ikkos D, Palmierei G, et al. A case of severe hypermetabolism of nonthyroid origin with a defect in the maintenance of mitochondrial respiratory control: A correlated clinical, biochemical and morphological study. J Clin Invest 1962;41:1776–1804.

211. Leigh D. Subacute necrotizing encephalomyelopathy in an infant. J Neurol Neurosurg Psychiatry 1951;14:216–221.

212. Richter RB. Infantile subacute necrotizing encephalopathy with predilection for the brain stem. J Neuropath Exp Neurol 1957;16:281–307.

213. Dayan AD, Ockenden BG, Crome L. Necrotizing encephalomyelopathy of Leigh: Neuropathological findings in 8 cases. Arch Dis Child 1970;45:39–848.

214. Huckabee WE. Abnormal resting blood lactate. Am J Med 1961;30:840–848.

215. Clayton BE, Dobbs RH, Patrick AD. Leigh's subacute necrotizing encephalopathy: Clinical and biochemical study, with special reference to therapy with lipoate. Arch Dis Child 1967;42:467–478.

216. Pincus JH, Itokawa Y, Cooper JR. Enzyme inhibiting factor in subacute necrotizing encephalomyelopathy. Neurology 1969;19:841–845.

217. Kearns TP, Sayre GP. Retinitis pigmentosa, external ophthalmoplegia, and complete heart block. Arch Ophthalmol 1958;60:280–289.

218. Olson W, Engel WK, Walsh GO, et al. Oculocraniosomatic neuromuscular disease with "ragged-red fibers." Arch Neurol 1972;26:193–211.

219. Shapira Y, Harel S, Russell A. Mitochondrial encephalomyopathies; A group of neuromuscular disorders with defects in oxidative metabolism. Is J Med Sci 1977;13:161–164.

220. Barbeau A, Butterworth RF, Ngo T, et al. Pyruvate metabolism in Freidreich's ataxia. Can J Neurol Sci 1976;3:379–386.

221. Leone A. Metallothionein gene regulation in Menkes' disease. Horiz Biochem Biophys 1986;8:207–256.

222. Egger J, Lake BD, Wilson J. Mitochondrial cytopathy. A multisystem disorder with ragged-red fibers on muscle biopsy. Arch Dis Child 1981;56:741–752.

223. Crosby TW, Chou SM. "Ragged-red" fibers in Leigh's disease. Neurology 1974;24:49–54.

224. Spiro AJ, Moore CL, Prinea JW, et al. A cytochrome-related inherited disorder of the nervous system and muscle. Arch Neurol 1970;23:103–112.

225. Shapira Y, Cederbaum SD, Cancilla PA, et al. Familial poliodystrophy, mitochondrial myopathy, and lactate acidemia. Neurology 1975;25:614–621.

226. Curless RG, Flynn J, Bachynski B, et al. Fatal metabolic acidosis, hyperglycemia, and coma after steroid therapy for Kearns-Sayre syndrome. Neurology 1986;36:872–873.

227. Petty RKH, Harding AE, Morgan-Hughes JA. The clinical features of mitochondrial myopathy. Brain 1986;109:915–938.

228. Bresolin N, Bet L, Binda A, et al. Clinical and biochemical correlations in mitochondrial myopathies treated with coenzyme Q_{10}. Neurology 1988;38:892–899.

229. Sellinger K, Seitelberger F. Spongy glio-neuronal dystrophy in infancy and childhood. Acta Neuropath 1970;16:125–140.

230. Alpers BJ. Diffuse progressive degeneration of the gray matter of the cerebrum. Arch Neurol Psychiat 1931;25:469–505.

231. Rowland LP, Hays AP, DiMauro S, et al. Diverse clinical disorders associated with morphological abnormalities of mitochondria. In: Scarlato G, Cerri C, eds. Mitochondrial pathology in muscle diseases. Padua: Piccin, 1983;142–158.

232. DiMauro S, Bonilla E, Zeviani M, et al. Mitochondrial myopathies. Ann Neurol 1985;17:521–538.

233. Pavlakis SG, Phillips PC, DiMauro S, et al. Mitochondrial myopathy, encephalopathy, lactic acidosis, and strokelike episodes (MELAS): A distinctive clinical syndrome. Ann Neurol 1984;16:481–488.

234. Fukuhara N, Tokiguchi S, Shirakawa K, et al. Myoclonus epilepsy associated with ragged-red fibers (mitochondrial abnormalities): disease entity or syndrome? Light and electron-microscopic study of two cases and review of the literature. J Neurol Sci 1980;47:117–133.

235. Mitchell G, Ogier H, Munnich A, et al. Neurological deterioration and lactic acidemia in biotinidase deficiency. A treatable condition mimicking Leigh's disease. Neuropediatrics 1986;17:129–131.

236. Diamantopoulos N, Painter MJ, Wolf B, et al. Biotinidase deficiency: Accumulation of lactate in the brain and response to physiologic doses of biotin. Neurology 1986;36:1107–1108.

237. Sheu KFR, Blass JP, Cederbaum JM, et al. Mitochondrial enzymes in hereditary ataxias. Metab Brain Dis 1988;3:151–160.

238. Worsley HE, Brookfield RW, Elwood JS, et al. Lactic acidosis with necrotizing encephalopathy in two sibs. Arch Dis Child 1965;40:492–501.

239. Hommes FA, Polman HA, Reerink JD. Leigh's encephalomyelopathy: an inborn error of gluconeogenesis. Arch Dis Child 1968;43:423–424.

240. DiMauro S, Servidei S, Zeviani M, et al. Cytochrome c oxidase deficiency in Leigh syndrome. Ann Neurol 1987;22:498–507.

241. Wyatt DT, Noetzel MJ, Hillman RE. Infantile beri-beri presenting as subacute necrotizing encephalomyelopathy. J Pediatr 1987;110:888–891.

242. Schrijver J, Dias T, Hommes FA. Studies on ATP thiamine disphosphate phosphotransferase activity in rat brain. Neurochem Res 1978;3:699–709.

243. Ichiki T, Tanaka M, Nishikimi M, et al. Deficiency of subunits of complex I and mitochondrial encephalopathy. Ann Neurol 1988;23:287–294.

244. Miyabayashi S, Ito T, Narisawa K, et al. Biochemical study in 28 children with lactic acidosis, in relation to Leigh's encephalomyelopathy. Eur J Pediatr 1985;143:278–283.

245. Willems JL, Monnens LAH, Trijbels JMF, et al. Leigh's encephalomyelopathy in a patient with cytochrome c oxidase deficiency in muscle tissue. Pediatrics 1977;60:850–857.

246. van Erven PMM, Gabreels FJM, Ruitenbeek W, et al. Mitochondrial encephalomyopathy. Association with an NADH dehydrogenase deficiency. Arch Neurol 1987;44:775–778.

247. Holt LJ, Harding AE, Morgan-Hughes JA. Deletions of muscle mitochondrial DNA in patients with mitochondrial myopathies. Nature 1988;331:717–719.

248. Rutledge JC, Haas JE, Monnat R, et al. Hypertrophic cardiomyopathy is a component of subacute necrotizing encephalomyelopathy. J Pediatr 1982;101:706–710.

249. Novotny EJ, Singh G, Wallace DC, et al. Leber's disease and dystonia: a mitochondrial disease. Neurology 1986;36:1053–1060.

250. Giles RE, Blanc H, Cann HM, et al. Maternal inheritance of human mitochondrial DNA. Proc Natl Acad Sci U S A 1980;77:6715–6719.

251. McCandless DQ. Thiamine deficiency and cerebral energy metabolism. In: McCandless DQ, ed. Cerebral Energy Metabolism and Metabolic Encephalopathy. New York: Plenum Press, 1985,335–351.

252. Impraim CC, Saiki RK, Ehrlich HA, et al. Analysis of DNA extracted from formalin-fixed paraffin-embedded tissues by enzymatic amplification and hybridization with sequence-specific oligonucleotides. Biochem Biophys Res Commun 1987;142:710–716.

253. Davies NT, Lawrence CB. Studies of the effect of copper deficiency on rat liver mitochondria. III Effects on adenine nucleotide translocase. Biochim Biophys Acta 1986;848:294–304.

254. Hayes DJ, Taylor DJ, Hilton-Jones D, et al. A new metabolic myopathy: A malate:aspartate shuttle defect. Biochem Soc Trans 1986;14:1208–1209.

255. Sengers RCA, Bakkeren JAJ, Trijbels JMF. Successful carnitine treatment in a non carnitine deficient lipid storage myopathy. Eur J Pediatr 1980;135:205–209.

256. Arts WFM, Scholte HR, Bogaard JM, et al. NADH-CoQ reductase deficient myopathy: Successful treatment with riboflavin. Lancet 1983;2:581–582.

257. Robinson BH, De Meirleir L, Glerum M, et al. Clinical presentation of mitochondrial respiratory chain defects in NADH-coenzyme Q reductase and cytochrome oxidase: Clues to pathogenesis of Leigh disease. J Pediatr 1987;110:216–222.

258. Rimoldi M, Bottachi E, Rossi L, et al. Cytochrome c oxidase deficiency in muscles of a floppy infant without mitochondrial myopathy. J Neurol 1982;227:201–207.

259. Kerr DS, Berry SA, Lusk MM, et al. A deficiency of both subunits of pyruvate dehydrogenase which is not expressed in fibroblasts. Pediatr Res 1988;24:95–100.

260. Askanas V, Engel WK. A new program for investigation of adult human skeletal muscle grown aneurally in tissue culture. Neurology 1975;25:58–67.

261. Blau HM, Webster C. Isolation and characterization of human muscle cells. Proc Natl Acad Sci U S A 1981;78:5623–5628.

262. Dahlquist NR, Perrault J, Callaway CW, et al. D-Lactic acidosis and encephalopthy after jejunoileostomy: Response to overfeeding and to fasting in humans. Mayo Clin Proc 1984;59:141–145.

263. Cross SA, Callaway CW. D-Lactic acidosis and selected cerebellar ataxias. Mayo Clin Proc 1984;59:202–205.

264. Langston JW, Irwin I, Langston EB, et al. Chronic parkinsonism in humans due to a product of meperidine-analog synthesis. Science 1983;219:979–980.

265. Chiba K, Trevor AJ, Castagnoli N. Active uptake of MPP$^+$, a metabolite of MPTP, by brain synaptosomes. Biochem Biophys Res Commun 1984;128:1229–1232.

266. Nicklas WJ, Youngster SK, Kindt MV, et al. MPTP, MPP$^+$ and mitochondrial function. Life Sci 1987;40:721–729.

267. Tonsgard JH, Getz GH. Effect of Reye's syndrome serum on isolated chinchilla liver mitochondria. J Clin Invest 1985;76:816–825.

268. Tanaka K, Kean EA, Johnson B. Jamaican vomiting sickness: Biochemical investigation of two cases. N Engl J Med 1976;295:461–467.

269. Cotariu D, Zaidman JL. Valproic acid and the liver. Clin Chem 1988;34:890–897.

270. Dreifuss FE, Santilli N, Langer DH, et al. Valproic acid hepatic fatalities. A retrospective review. Neurology 1987;37:379–385.

271. Rettie AE, Rettenmeier AW, Howald WN, et al. Cytochrome P-450-catalyzed formation of ^{4}-VPA, a toxic metabolite of valproic acid. Science 1987;235:890–893.

272. Jezequel AM, Bonazzi P, Novelli G, et al. Early structural and functional changes in liver of rats treated with a single dose of valproic acid. Hepatology 1984;4:1159–1166.

273. Pitts FN, McClure JN. Lactate metabolism in anxiety neurosis. N Engl J Med 1967;277:1331–1336.

274. Boulinger JP, Uhde TW, Wolff EA, et al. Increased sensitivity to caffeine in patients with panic disorders. Arch Gen Psychiatry 1984;41:1067–1071.

275. Woods SW, Charney DS, Goodman WK, et al. Carbon dioxide-induced anxiety: Behavioral, physiologic, and biochemical effects of carbon dioxide in patients with panic disorders and healthy subjects. Arch Gen Psychiatry 1988;45:43–52.

276. Crowe RR, Noyes R, Wilson AF, et al. A linkage study of panic disorder. Arch Gen Psychiatry 1987;44:933–937.

277. Pauls DL, Bucher KD, Crowe RR, et al. A genetic study of panic disorder pedigrees. Am J Hum Genet 1980;40:1065–1069.

278. Rizley R, Kahn RJ, McNair DM, et al. A comparison of alprazolam and imipramine in the treatment of agoraphobia and panic disorder. Psychopharm Bull 1986;22:167–172.

279. Noyes R, Anderson DJ, Clancy J, et al. Diazepam and propranolol in panic disorder and agoraphobia. Arch Gen Psychiatry 1984;41:287–292.

280. Pulsinelli, WA, Waldman, S, Rawlinson, D, et al. Moderate hyperglycemia augments ischemic brain damage: a neuropathologic study in the rat. Neurology 1982;32:1239–1246.

281. Siemkowicz, E, Hyperglycemia in the reperfusion period hampers recovery from cerebral ischemia. Acta Neurol Scand 1981;64:207–216.

282. Sapolsky RM, Pulsinelli WA. Glucocorticoids potentiate ischemic injury to neurons. Science 1985;229:1397–1400.

283. Menkes JH. Improving the outlook in bacterial meningitis. Lancet 1979;3:559–560.

284. Powers WJ. Hyperglycemia is not associated with mortality in bacterial meningitis. Ann Neurol 1983;14:82–83.

285. Bernstein RE. Nonenzymatically glycosylated proteins. Adv Clin Chem 1987;26:1–78.

Chapter 5
The Mucolipidoses

William G. Johnson and
Hiroaki Yoshidome

The mucolipidoses were originally defined as a group of disorders with a variety of findings including: some clinical resemblance to the Hurler syndrome; the storage of acid mucopolysaccharides, sphingolipids, and/or glycolipids in visceral and mesenchymal cells; and storage of abnormal amounts of sphingolipids or glycolipids in neural tissue (1).

The disorders originally in this group were G_{M1}-gangliosidosis, fucosidosis, mannosidosis, juvenile sulfatidosis—Austin type (now known as mucosulfatidosis), mucolipidosis I—lipomucopolysaccharidosis (now known to be a sialidosis type II), mucolipidosis II—I-cell disease, and mucolipidosis III—pseudopolydystrophy. They do not have as much underlying similarity at a biochemical level as the mucopolysaccharidoses, and the term *mucolipidosis* is probably less useful scientifically; however, most of these disorders share an abnormality of oligosaccharide or glycoprotein metabolism. The majority of these disorders have excessive urinary excretion of complex oligosaccharides and/or glycopeptides, which are fragments of more complex structures. This is the basis of a useful diagnostic screening test (urinary thin-layer chromatography for oligosaccharides) and for the French name of this group: *les oligosaccharidoses*. Hence, the name mucolipidosis is still useful as a clinical term for patients with signs and

Table 5.1

Disease	Deficient Enzyme	Gene Locus (chromosome & band #)
Sialidosis	Alpha-L-N-acetylneuraminidase	chromosome 10
Galactosialidosis	Protective protein	chromosome 20
GM_1-Gangliosidosis	Beta-galactosidase	chromosome 3
Mannosidosis	Alpha-mannosidase	chromosome 19 (19p13.2–q12)
Beta-Mannosidosis	Beta-mannosidase	unknown
Fucosidosis	Alpha-L-fucosidase	chromosome 1 (1p34)
Aspartylglycosaminuria	N-aspartyl-beta-glucosaminidase	chromosome 4 (4q21–4qter)
Mucolipidosis II (I-Cell disease) and Mucolipidosis III (pseudo-Hurler polydystrophy)	N-Acetylglucosaminylphosphotransferase	chromosome 4 (q21–q23)
Mucolipidosis IV	? Ganglioside sialidase	unknown
Free Sialic Acid Storage Diseases		
Salla Disease	? transport protein	unknown
Infantile Free Sialic Acid Storage Disease	? transport protein	unknown

symptoms resembling the Hurler phenotype, but who lack excessive mucopolysacchariduria and have excessive oligosacchariduria. The focus of this chapter is lysosomal disorders with a defect in oligosaccharide or glycoprotein metabolism and with oligosacchariduria. Some disorders have been included or excluded somewhat arbitrarily. For example, mucosulfatosis was excluded because it is not known to be a disorder of oligosaccharide or glycoprotein metabolism. Sandhoff disease might reasonably be included because of oligosacchariduria, but was excluded because Tay-Sachs disease lacks oligosacchariduria. The free sialic acid storage diseases have been included because they are lysosomal abnormalities, and sialic acid is an important glycoprotein component (Table 5.1). All of these disorders are inherited as an autosomal-recessive trait (2–11).

SIALIDOSES

Patients in this clinically heterogeneous group of disorders all share a deficiency of glycoprotein sialidase, an alpha-L-neuraminidase or sialidase. There are at least two distinct lysosomal sialidases. One, glycoprotein sialidase, cleaves (alpha 2→3)-linked and (alpha 2→6)-linked sialic acid in polysialogangliosides and glycoproteins. Glycoprotein sialidase is deficient in the sialidoses described below and is conveniently assayed by a variety of substrates including 4MU-alpha-L-neuraminide and neuramin-lactose. The other lysosomal sialidase, monosialoganglioside sialidase, cleaves the (alpha 2→3)-linked sialic acid in monosialoganglioside. Monosialoganglioside sialidase has been reported to be deficient in mucolipidosis IV.

There are three distinct genetic classes of disorders in which glycoprotein sialidase is deficient. In the first, glycoprotein sialidase alone is deficient, the situation in the sialidoses proper, which results from mutations of a structural gene (12) on chromosome 10. In the second, both glycoprotein sialidase and beta-galactosidase (G_{MI}-ganglioside beta-galactosidase) are deficient owing to deficiency of a protective protein, which is required for activity of both enzymes and is coded for by a gene on chromosome 20 (12). This latter group of disorders is referred to as galactosialidosis. In the third type, sialidase and multiple lysosomal enzymes are decreased because of deficient post-translational modification, which is the case in mucolipidosis types II and III.

In these disorders, sialic acid–containing glycoproteins, oligosaccharides, and glycolipids accumulate in tissue, and sialo-oligosaccharides are excreted in urine. The diagnosis is established by the clinical picture, the presence of abnormal sialo-oligosaccharides in the urine, and the demonstration of deficiency of the glycoprotein sialidase in cultured skin fibroblasts, tissue, leukocytes, amniotic fluid cells, or chorionic villus samples.

The true sialidoses, or isolated sialidoses, in which glycoprotein sialidase alone is deficient, have been divided into two groups (3,13): the nondysmorphic group (sialidosis type 1, also known as the cherry-red spot-myoclonus syndrome), and the dysmorphic group (sialidosis type 2, which includes mucolipidosis I).

Sialidosis Type 1 (The Cherry-Red Spot-Myoclonus Syndrome)

In this striking disorder, the onset of myoclonus or decreasing visual acuity characteristically occurs between the ages of 8 and 15 years. Although there appears to be a predilection for Italian patients (3), patients of a variety of backgrounds, including Japanese (14), German (15), and Saudi Arabian (16), have been described.

Patients develop action myoclonus beginning in the limbs, which becomes increasingly debilitating. They may become unable to stand or walk and are ultimately bedridden. Tonic-clonic seizures may occur, and burning pain in the limbs, worse in hot weather, is reminiscent of that occurring in Fabry disease. Intelligence is usually normal, but occasionally may be impaired. Macular cherry-red spots are found at funduscopy, and although the corneas are clear, punctate lens opacities or lamellar cataracts may be seen. Hyperactive tendon reflexes and cerebellar ataxia may be present. Renal impairment is not a feature of this disorder, but severe renal involvement has occurred in two siblings with otherwise typical cherry-red spot-myoclonus syndrome. Coarse facial features, organomegaly, and skeletal dysplasia are not features of this disorder.

The cherry-red spot may disappear during the course of the disease (17). Consequently, the absence of a cherry-red spot is not grounds for excluding this diagnosis.

Neuropathologic examination shows that the brain stem and spinal cord contain swollen PAS-positive neurons. PAS-positive material may also be present in the central nervous system in swollen dendrites of Purkinje cells, in Bergmann glia, capillary endothelia and in macrophages. PAS-positive material may also be seen outside the nervous system, and electron microscopy shows atypical membranous cytoplasmic bodies (15).

The diagnosis of sialidosis type 1 is made by the characteristic clinical picture, finding excessive abnormal sialo-oligosaccharides in urine, and by demonstrating a deficiency of sialidase in cultured skin fibroblasts and leukocytes. Patients do not have mucopolysacchariduria, and the amount of urinary uronic acid excretion is comparable with that of controls (14). Rectal biopsy examination is useful, because the stored material is visible in the ultrastructure of rectal ganglion cells (15).

Although no treatment is available for the underlying disorder, 5-hydroxytryptophan has been reported to result in mild (15) or dramatic (16) improvement of the action myoclonus.

Sialidosis Type 2

Patients with a deficiency of glycoprotein sialidase, without deficiency of beta-galactosidase, and with clinical features of somatic dysmorphism (facial and skeletal) and organomegaly fall into the category of type 2 sialidosis (18,19). A variety of clinical phenotypes with onset at birth, in later childhood, or later have been described.

Congenital Sialidoses

This is the most severe form of sialidosis known and is, in fact, the most severe phenotype of lysosomal disease. Affected neonates are born prematurely and have the clinical appearance of hydrops fetalis. They may be stillborn or may survive 1 to 3 months and perhaps longer. At birth they are plethoric, depressed, hypotonic, with generalized skin edema, ascites, hepatosplenomegaly, puffy face and eyelids, and a prominent telangiectatic skin rash. Seizures may occur, and the neurologic development is arrested. The disorder is uncommon although not rare, and a number of cases have been described (18–23). Two of the four families have been of Jewish background.

Because Rh-incompatibility is largely being prevented, it is no longer the most common cause of hydrops fetalis. Although there are many causes of the hydrops fetalis phenotype, metabolic disorders should always be considered when such patients are seen. Salla and Gaucher disease, galactosialidosis, G_{M1}-gangliosidosis, and mucopolysaccharidosis type VII have all been found to produce this phenotype (21). In addition to the benefit of establishing a diagnosis, these families are at risk for having future affected infants. Prenatal diagnosis is available.

Neuropathologic examination of one patient (22,23) showed zebra bodies in neurons of the spinal cord only. Neurons in the cerebral and cerebellar cortices and autonomic ganglial cells showed only membrane-bound vacuoles, but no membranous cytoplasmic bodies. Vacuolated cells were also found in the periphery; viz, hepatocytes, endothelial and Kupfer cells in the liver, as well as glomerular and tubular epithelial cells in the kidney.

Vacuolated lymphocytes are plentiful on examination of the peripheral blood smear, and vacuolated histiocytes are present in the bone marrow. Foam cells in large numbers are seen in multiple tissues as well as the placenta. Fibroblasts contain numerous vacuoles, and whorled membranous structures are observed at electron microscopy, although they appear normal at light microscopy. The diagnosis is established by the characteristic clinical picture, finding abnormal sialo-oligosaccharides in urine, and demonstrating a deficiency of neuraminidase in cultured skin fibroblasts. Carrier detection and prenatal diagnosis are possible in this disorder. There is some resemblance to patients reported with congenital lipidosis or congenital lipidosis of Norman and Wood (24,25) in whom the biochemical defect was never defined (26).

Severe Infantile Sialidosis

Patients described as having severe infantile sialidosis (27) show many similarities to patients with congenital sialidosis, but they survive into the 2nd year. These patients have congenital ascites, progressive organomegaly, delayed neurologic development, and progressive renal disease in the 2nd year. This phenotype lacks the features present in congenital sialidosis including premature birth, anasarca, skin telangiectasias, vascular abnormalities, optic atrophy, and seizures. Sialidase was markedly decreased and sialic acid content increased in fibroblast sonicates.

It is not clear whether severe infantile sialidosis and congenital sialidosis are different manifestations of the same phenotype or are different phenotypes. The same problem is seen when severe infantile sialidosis is compared with nephrosialidosis.

Nephrosialidosis

Nephrosialidosis was defined in studies that focused on the renal component of this disorder (28,29). These patients appear to have a milder phenotype than that of congenital sialidosis or severe infantile sialidosis. Infants come to medical attention at 4 to 6 months of age because of facial dysmorphism, hernias, heptosplenomegaly, and psychomotor retardation. Late in the clinical course they develop severe progressive renal disease with proteinuria, macular cherry-red spot, and fine corneal opacities observed at slit-lamp examination. The autopsy of one patient at 4 1/2 years of age, showed storage material in renal glomeruli and sympathetic ganglia. This was thought to distinguish nephrosialidosis from other sialidoses; however, the same findings are seen in patients described as having severe infantile sialidosis or congenital sialidosis.

The diagnosis of nephrosialidosis is established by the characteristic clinical picture, finding a large excess of abnormal sialo-oligosaccharides in urine, and demonstrating deficient sialidase in leukocytes and cultured skin fibroblasts.

Mucolipidosis I (Lipomucopolysaccharidosis)

The term mucolipidosis I is used for the forms of sialidosis that may be noted in infancy, but are more slowly progressive and are usually diagnosed in the juvenile period.

This disorder was originally defined clinically, but some suspected cases turned out to be mannosidosis. It was also termed GAL + disease in the earlier literature because beta-galactosidase was elevated; however, the term *mucolipidosis I* is now appropriately applied only to patients with the characteristic phenotype and sialidase deficiency without beta-galactosidase deficiency.

These patients develop normally for the 1st 6 months of life, but motor development slows and mental delay becomes apparent. Somatic abnormalities are observed in the 2nd or 3rd year, but are milder than those found in patients with Hurler syndrome. These include mild coarsening of facial features, short trunk sometimes with spinal deformity, relatively long limbs, mild restriction of joint mobility, and inconsistent hepatosplenomegaly. Impaired hearing, corneal opacity, and macular cherry-red spots are usually seen, and growth disturbance is common. In addition to the ocular abnormalities, neurologic findings include seizures, myoclonic jerks, slowly progressive gait ataxia, cerebellar signs, tremor, hypotonia, muscle wasting, and peripheral neuropathy. Radiographic changes are characteristically those of mild to moderate dysostosis multiplex (8). Kyphoscoliosis and a hypoplastic odontoid have been described.

Ultrastructural studies (30) of cultured skin fibroblasts in sialidosis showed vacuolar inclusions of low electron density similar to those in mannosidosis and the mucopolysaccharidoses. A few myelin-like figures were seen. An unusual type of large round membrane-bound inclusions with many concentrically arranged tubules in a fine reticulogranular matrix was also seen.

Sialic acid content is increased in tissue. In a postmortem study (31), water-soluble bound sialic acid was increased 10- to 17-fold in visceral organs, but only about twofold in the brain. Lipid bound sialic acid was increased up to eightfold in visceral organs, but was not elevated in the brain. The increase in visceral sialic acid resulted from elevated amounts of G_{D3} and probable G_{M4} and L_{M1}. This pattern of accumulation supported the idea that ganglioside accumulation in the sialidoses was a secondary phenomenon, perhaps induced by inhibition of a ganglioside sialidase by substances stored because of the primary sialidase deficiency.

The diagnosis of mucolipidosis I is made by the characteristic clinical picture, finding a large excess of urinary sialo-oligosaccharides, and demonstrating a severe sialidase deficiency without beta-galactosidase deficiency.

GALACTOSIALIDOSIS

This disorder was originally described as the Goldberg syndrome (32) and was observed to have decreased lysosomal beta-galactosidase. It was suspected that this was not the primary enzyme deficiency, however, because there was great variation among various tissues and body fluids in the degree of beta-galactosidase deficiency and because heterozygous carriers did not regularly show a 50% decrease in beta-galactosidase levels. Later, the deficiency of alpha-L-neuraminidase was noted as well in these patients (33), and the designation galactosialidosis was determined (34).

The primary defect in patients with galactosialidoses is deficiency of neither beta-galactosidase nor alpha-L-neuraminidase, but rather of a 32 Kd glycoprotein, referred to as a "protective protein," which is required for full biologic activity of both beta-galactosidase and alpha-L-neuraminidase. This 32 Kd glycoprotein is synthesized as a 452 amino acid precursor molecule (35) that is processed to give the mature protective protein, a heterodimer of 32 Kd and 20 Kd polypeptides joined by disulfide linkages. This protective protein has some sequence homology with proteases (35). Apparently, this protective protein is associated in some way in the lysosome with beta-galactosidase and alpha-L-neuraminidase, and any of its defects affect both enzymes.

Galactosialidosis has also been classified as sialidosis type 2, because somatic abnormalities including coarse facial features and dysostosis multiplex are characteristically found (36). In the true sialidoses, however, glycoprotein sialidase alone is deficient. The sialidoses result from mutations of a structural gene (12) on chromosome 10. In the galactosialidoses, on the other hand, both glycoprotein sialidase and beta-galactosidase (G_{M1}-ganglioside beta-galactosidase) are deficient because of the deficiency of the protective protein, which is coded for by a gene (12) on chromosome 20.

Galactosialidosis shows complementation in fibroblast culture with both mucolipidosis I, in which alpha-L-neuraminidase deficiency is the primary defect, and mucolipidosis II, in which alpha-L-neuraminidase deficiency is secondary, resulting from a defect in processing of multiple lysosomal enzymes (37).

In the true sialidoses, urinary oligosaccharide excretion is increased 50-fold to 500-fold. In galactosialidosis, the increased excretion is more modest, usually three- to fivefold (12). Ultrastructural study of cultured fibroblasts in galactosialidosis show both vacuolar and lamellar inclusions, which are similar to those in G_{M1}-gangliosidosis (30).

A variety of different clinical phenotypes are found (38,39) including a congenital/early-infantile form, a late-infantile form, and a juvenile/adult form. The juvenile/adult form is the most common and has been reported mainly from Japan (36,38). In addition to the various human phenotypes in humans, the disease has been described in sheep (40).

Congenital or Early-Infantile Galactosialidosis

In congenital or early-infantile galactosialidosis, the clinical disease is severe and survival is short. Patients may be premature and stillborn, or they may survive a few weeks to months. These patients may have neonatal ascites, edema, or even anasarca, and present as hydrops fetalis. Besides galactosialidosis, patients with other lysosomal storage diseases may present with congenital ascites or hydrops fetalis including sialidosis (isolated sialidase deficiency), G_{M1}-gangliosidosis, Gaucher and Salla disease (41), as well as Wolman disease, and mucopolysaccharidosis type VII (beta-glucuronidase deficiency). There are a variety of causes for the phenotype of hydrops fetalis, the most common of which has been hematologic. Now that most cases of fetal hydrops due to blood group incompatibility are being prevented, however, cases of nonimmune hydrops are becoming relatively more common. Lysosomal storage disease is a particularly important etiology to consider because of the implications for genetic counseling and prenatal diagnosis.

The prenatal diagnosis for congenital/early-infantile galactosialidosis has been reported (42) and has been carried out by assay of alpha-L-neuraminidase in amniotic fluid cells and chorionic villus samples. Amniotic fluid oligosaccharide concentration is increased, and beta-galactosidase is decreased; considerable residual beta-galactosidase activity may be present, making this assay useful as a confirmatory test (42).

Besides neonatal ascites, patients have psychomotor retardation, coarse facial features, hepatosplenomegaly, dystosis multiplex, and susceptibility to infection (43,44). Macular cherry-red spots, corneal clouding (43), renal involvement (41,45), hypoplastic lungs (41,46), cerebral infarction (41), cardiac septal thickening and cardiomyopathy (45), petechial skin hemorrhage (46), and inguinal hernia may occur.

At electron microscopy (43), membrane-bound vacuoles have been found in Schwann cells, fibroblasts, endothelial cells, lymphocytes, and plasma cells, as well as hepatocytes and renal glomerular and renal tubular cells. Pleomorphic dense bodies and membranous cytoplasmic bodies have been seen in neurons. Generally, these features resemble those of infantile G_{M1}-gangliosidosis.

The diagnosis of congenital or early-infantile galactosialidosis is made by the clinical appearance and course, finding decreased alpha-L-neuraminidase and beta-galactosidase in leukocytes and cultured skin fibroblasts, and a characteristic pattern of oligosaccharide excretion in the urine. Vacuolation of lymphocytes is a useful finding because it increases the index of one's suspicion of the diagnosis.

It is obvious that all patients who appear to have G_{M1}-gangliosidosis based on the clinical picture and decreased beta-galactosidase must also be studied for galactosialidosis, which may be the correct diagnosis in some patients. This group of patients has no detectable alpha-L-neuraminidase activity and about 10% of the normal amount of beta-galactosidase activity. The 85 Kd beta-galactosidase precursor is synthesized, and about 10% of the mature 64 Kd beta-galactosidase protein is present. Neither the 32 Kd protective protein nor its 54 Kd precur-

sor are detectable, however, and this is the primary cause of the disease (38,39).

Late-Infantile Galactosialidosis

A late-infantile form of galactosialodosis has been described in which the presentation is at 6 to 12 months of age, and the clinical picture is milder than that of the severe congenital/early-infantile form (34,47). The clinical features include mild mental defect, macular cherry-red spot, dysmorphic features, and dysostosis multiplex. This category is probably heterogeneous, because a patient (45) has been described with a phenotype intermediate between the severe congenital/early-infantile form and the late-infantile form. This patient had cardiomyopathy and renal enlargement and later developed ascites and generalized edema, but lacked the macular cherry-red spot. Electron microscopic study (48) of a skin biopsy from the case of Andria et al. (34) showed large electron-lucent vacuoles in most cell types. Membranous cytoplasmic bodies were found in Schwann cells.

The diagnosis is established by the patient's clinical appearance and course, finding decreased alpha-L-neuraminidase and beta-galactosidase in leukocytes and cultured skin fibroblasts, and a characteristic pattern of oligosaccharide excretion in the urine.

The biochemical findings in this group (38,39) are notable in that little if any of the 32 Kd protective protein is detected, but synthesis of its 54 Kd precursor is detected. The 85 Kd beta-galactosidase precursor is synthesized, and about 10% of the control amount of mature 64 Kd beta-galactosidase protein and beta-galactosidase activity are found. About 1% to 4% residual alpha-L-neuraminidase activity is present.

Juvenile and Adult Galactosialidosis

This disorder strongly resembles mucolipidosis I except for its later onset, secondary deficiency of beta-galactosidase less severe than that of G_{M1}-gangliosidosis, and an occurrence most commonly found in Japanese patients. These patients commonly develop symptoms and signs in the juvenile or adolescent period (36) with coarsened features, skeletal changes, joint stiffness, and growth disturbances. Corneal clouding, macular cherry-red spot, and hearing loss are common. Neurologic abnormalities include seizures, myoclonus, ataxia, corticospinal tract dysfunction, and peripheral neuropathy. Inguinal hernias and angiokeratoma (49) may be seen, but organomegaly is not a feature. The clinical course is slowly progressive.

The most common clinical findings appear to be coarse facial features, macular cherry-red spot, lumbar vertebral deformity, and vacuolization of lymphocytes. The intelligence is often normal, but mental retardation may be present (37).

The macular cherry-red spot has been reported to disappear during the course of the disease and is not always found. Its absence is no reason to exclude the diagnosis.

The ultrastructure of cultured fibroblasts is abnormal (30), and storage inclusions, varying in size and character, have been observed. Vacuolar inclusions were empty or contained fine reticulogranular or amorphous material. Some inclusions resembled the membranous cytoplasmic bodies of gangliosidosis.

Rectal biopsies have been found to be abnormal in galactosialidosis (50), with axons distended by numerous electron-dense bodies and vesicles containing electron-dense materials. Schwann cells were found to include membranous cytoplasmic bodies, zebra bodies, and membrane-bound vacuoles with reticulogranular material. Fibroblasts, plasma cells, and endothelial cells were distended with numerous membrane-bound vacuoles often containing dispersed reticulogranular materials, globules, or some lamellar profiles.

Sialidase is nearly absent in cultured fibroblasts of patients, and beta-galactosidase is decreased to about 10% of control levels. The lysosomal fraction of sialidase is also nearly absent in blood lymphocytes of patients and is decreased in heterozygotes. However, considerable residual activity of sialidase (20% to 50%) and beta-galactosidase is present in mixed leukocytes in which the lysosomal fraction of sialidase has not been separated (49). Consequently, assay of leukocyte sialidase is not necessarily a reliable procedure in this disorder. The elevation of urinary oligosaccharides (three- to five-times control values) is less than that seen in mucolipidosis I (50- to 500-times control values) where alpha-L-neuraminidase alone is deficient.

The diagnosis is made by the characteristic clinical picture, finding excess sialo-oligosaccharides in urine, a marked deficiency of sialidase in cultured skin fibroblasts, and a deficiency of beta-galactosidase in cells or tissue but not plasma. Finding lymphocytes vacuolization is useful because it is simple to demonstrate and increases the index of suspicion of the disease.

The pattern of deficient enzymes and proteins distinguishes juvenile and adult galactosialidosis from the congenital/severe infantile form and the late-infantile form (38,39). The mature 32 Kd protective protein is not detectable, and its 54 Kd precursor is detected in trace amounts, if at all. No residual alpha-L-neuraminidase is detected. The 85 Kd beta-galactosidase precursor is synthesized. About 10% of the normal amount of mature 64 Kd beta-galactosidase protein and beta-galactosidase enzyme activity is detected.

G_{M1}-GANGLIOSIDOSIS

This group of disorders is characterized by a genetically determined deficiency of G_{M1}-ganglioside beta-galactosi-

dase and the resulting storage of compounds containing a terminal beta-linked galactose moiety. These include G_{M1}-ganglioside, asialo-G_{M1}, keratan sulfate-like oligosaccharides, and glycoproteins. Other beta-galactosidases, such as those cleaving galactosylceramide and lactosylceramide, are not deficient, and those compounds do not accumulate.

The enzyme G_{M1}-ganglioside beta-galactosidase consists of only one kind of subunit and is coded for by a single gene locus. All forms of G_{M1}-gangliosidosis, then, arise from allelic mutations. Patients with galactosialidosis have combined beta-galactosidase deficiency and alpha-L-neuraminidase deficiency. This results from mutations affecting neither the beta-galactosidase nor the alpha-L-neuraminidase structural gene but rather a protein affecting the stability of both.

The structural gene for beta-galactosidase is located on chromosome 3. The enzyme is synthesized as an 85 Kd precursor peptide, which is processed by various steps to a mature 64 Kd enzyme. A protective protein is required for aggregation of monomeric beta-galactosidase into a high molecular weight multimeric form, preventing rapid proteolysis in the lysosome (51).

The clinical syndromes (52,53) of primary beta-galactosidase deficiency (that is, deficiency of G_{M1}-ganglioside beta-galactosidase) have been grouped into five different phenotypes: infantile G_{M1}-gangliosidosis (type 1), late-infantile G_{M1}-gangliosidosis (type 2A), juvenile G_{M1}-gangliosidosis (type 2B), adult G_{M1}-gangliosidosis (type 3), and Morquio syndrome (type B). The first four phenotypes have associated neurologic abnormalities with varying degrees of somatic disease; whereas, Morquio syndrome (type B) has somatic disease without neurologic dysfunction (51).

Morquio syndrome (type B) clinically resembles classic Morquio syndrome, now known as mucopolysaccharidosis (type IVA) or Morquio syndrome (type A). Morquio syndrome (type A) is associated with severe somatic involvement, but without neural involvement. Keratan sulfate but not oligosaccharides is excreted in the urine, and a galactosamine-6-sulfatase is deficient. Despite this distinction, some patients reported as having Morquio syndrome (type B) have had nervous-system involvement (54).

The subtypes of G_{M1}-gangliosidosis can be diagnosed biochemically using urinary oligosaccharides as substrates (52). In addition, the late-infantile form (type 2A) excretes more urinary oligosaccharides than the juvenile form (type 2B). There are a number of genetically different tissue beta-galactosidases in humans. G_{M1}-ganglioside beta-galactosidase is the major form demonstrated by such artificial substrates as 4-methylumbelliferyl-beta-D-galactopyranoside. G_{M1}-ganglioside beta-galactosidase appears to be identical with galactosyl-ceramidase II and lactosyl-ceramidase II (55,56). In addition to the phenotypes discussed in humans G_{M1}-gangliosidosis has been described in cats, dogs, and cattle (57–62).

Infantile G_{M1}-Gangliosidosis

Infantile G_{M1}-gangliosidosis (G_{M1}-gangliosidosis type 1), neurovisceral lipidosis, generalized gangliodosis, or Landing disease) is clinically apparent soon after birth, and its course is more rapid and severe than that of either Tay-Sachs disease or Hurler syndrome. Shortly after birth, these infants are hypotonic and weak, with a poor suck; they gain weight slowly. There is frontal bossing, large low-set ears, and increased distance between the nose and upper lip. They have a facial downy hirsutism, and gingival hypertrophy (especially the maxilla) and macroglossia are constant features. The corneas are usually clear, but a facial corneal haze is usually seen on close examination. About 1/2 of these children develop a macular cherry-red spot, and peripheral edema is usually noted. Psychomotor development is slow, and infants may reach for objects, but do not sit or crawl. Strabismus, horizontal nystagmus, and convulsions appear, accompanied in some cases by an acoustic motor response to sound.

By 6 months of age, hepatomegaly and slight splenomegaly are noted, as well as joint stiffness, thoracolumbar kyphosis, skin thickening, and claw hand deformity. These infants become apathetic and eventually become decerebrate. Frequent respiratory infections or cardiac arrhythmias lead to death before the age of 2 years. The macular cherry-red spot has been observed to disappear during the clinical course of G_{M1}-gangliosidosis, the cherry-red spot-myoclonus syndrome, galactosialidosis, and Niemann-Pick type C disease (17).

Vacuolated lymphocytes and foamy histiocytes are found in the bone marrow, but are less prominent than observed in Niemann-Pick or Gaucher disease. Eosinophilic granulocytes in blood and bone marrow may contain faintly staining greyish blue or pale brown-orange granules, which may assist in diagnosis (63).

After the age of 6 months, characteristic radiographic changes are seen, including beaking of vertebral bodies, swelling of long bones at midshaft, and cloaking of the ribs and long bones with new bone formation. Skull radiographs resemble those in patients with Hurler syndrome and may show J-shaped sella turcica. Computed tomographic (CT) head scans in infantile G_{M1}-gangliosidosis show cerebral atrophy with enlargement of the ventricles and subarachnoid space and hypodensity of the white matter (64,65).

The rectal biopsy is abnormal in patients with infantile G_{M1}-gangliosidosis (50), showing zebra bodies and membrane-bound vacuoles with electron-dense material in Schwann cells. Electron-dense bodies are seen in a few axons. Fibroblasts, plasma cells, and endothelial cells are filled with many membrane-bound vacuoles.

Neurons throughout the central nervous system and the myenteric plexus are markedly ballooned. At electron microscopy, multiple intracellular membranous cytoplasmic bodies consisting of concentric lamellae usually with a granular core are seen. Brain atrophy in older infants is associated with neuronal dropout, demyelination, and gliosis. There are large numbers of foamy histiocytes and vacuolated parenchymal cells found in the viscera, and renal storage occurs, a relatively unusual finding that is also seen in nephrosialidosis. Storage is even seen in Ito cells (66), generally thought to be lysosomally inactive.

Tissue pathology is evident as early as the 2nd trimester. At 24 weeks' gestation (67), foam cells have been found in the viscera and placenta. Central nervous system storage detectable microscopically is confined to the retina and dorsal root ganglia; however brain ganglioside content is increased. At electron microscopy at 22 weeks' gestation (68) membrane-bound vacuoles, occasionally containing stacks of fine fibrils, are seen in large young neurons in the deeper part of the cortical plate, but other cerebral cortical neurons have no storage materials. Similar findings have been recorded in Purkinje cells and spinal cord neurons, the latter of which also contained zebra-like bodies. Lamellar membranous cytoplasmic inclusions are found within retinal ganglion cells (69).

Oligosaccharides and sialo-oligosaccharides (70) are increased in urine and amniotic fluid as measured by thin-layer chromatography, high-performance thin-layer chromatography, or high-performance liquid chromatography (71).

The diagnosis of infantile G_{M1}-gangliosidosis is made by the characteristic clinical picture, finding a large excess of oligosaccharides in urine, and by demonstrating the nearly total deficiency of G_{M1}-ganglioside beta-galactosidase in leukocytes and cultured skin fibroblasts. Detection of heterozygote carriers is possible because they show intermediate levels of enzyme activity, but carrier testing is less reliable than is Tay-Sachs carrier testing. Prenatal diagnosis is made possible by a number of methods, including enzyme assay amniotic fluid cells or chorionic villus sampling (72). The demonstration of abnormal oligosaccharides in amniotic fluid is a useful confirmatory test.

The differential diagnosis includes infantile Gaucher and Niemann-Pick disease, both of which run a similar course and have organomegaly, but do not show the prominent bony abnormalities of infantile G_{M1}-gangliosidosis. Mucolipidosis II—I-cell disease has similar bony changes, but less severe organomegaly. Tay-Sachs disease is manifested later and lacks visceral involvement. Hurler disease has a much more protracted course and less rapidly progressive neurologic signs. Spasticity develops earlier in patients with Krabbe disease than in patients with G_{M1}-gangliosidosis. All of these diagnoses can be made with specific enzyme assays. All patients suspected of having G_{M1}-gangliosidosis should be tested for urinary sialo-oligosaccharides and for sialidase deficiency because patients with galactosialidosis (q.v.) have identical clinical features as well as severe beta-galactosidase deficiency.

Residual beta-galactosidases from infantile G_{M1}-gangliosidosis, adult G_{M1}-gangliosidosis, and Morquio (type B) all have different kinetic and stability properties;

however, genetic complementation studies demonstrate that these disorders all result from mutations of a single structural gene (73). Permanent cell lines from G_{M1}-gangliosidosis retain deficiency of beta-galactosidase (74).

Studies of beta-galactosidase processing have clarified in part how the mutation causes a lack of beta-galactosidase activity. In infantile G_{M1}-gangliosidosis, the 85 Kd precursor of beta-galactosidase is synthesized normally, but more than 90% of the enzyme is subsequently degraded at an early step in posttranslational processing (70). In cultured fibroblasts, the mutation interferes with the phosphorylation of the precursor of beta-galactosidase so that the precursor is secreted instead of being compartmentalized into lysosomes and further processed (75). There is some evidence that processing of the 85 Kd beta-galactosidase precursor involves a higher molecular weight (88 Kd) intermediate form (76).

Late-Infantile and Juvenile G_{M1}-Gangliosidosis

Late-infantile and juvenile G_{M1}-gangliosidosis (type 2) appear to be genetically distinct from the infantile form, although resulting from a mutation at the same locus; this category is probably heterogeneous. Clincial manifestations appear at 1 to 3 years of age and are limited to the nervous system. Developmental delay and muscle weakness may be noted in early infancy. The ocular fundi may be normal or show optic atrophy late in the clinical course of the disease. Corneas are clear, there is no organomegaly, and bony changes are usually absent. The earliest findings are usually gait unsteadiness and ataxia, followed by hypotonia and increased deep tendon reflexes. Speech becomes dysarthric and is ultimately lost. Rapidly progressive dementia, seizures, spastic quadriplegia, and evidence of anterior horn cell disease develop. Patients usually die between 3 and 10 years of age but may survive longer. Radiographic changes are those of severe dysostosis multiplex, but early on there is a resemblance to mucolipidosis II with periosteal cloaking of long bones, expansion of the short bones, and widening of the ribs (8).

This phenotype, type 2 G_{M1}-gangliosidosis, intermediate between infantile (type 1) and adult (type 3) G_{M1}-gangliosidosis, has been further subdivided into type 2A and type 2B G_{M1}-gangliosidosis based on the clinical picture and the amount of urinary oligosaccharide excretion (53). If urinary oligosaccharides were used as substrates, types 1, 2A, 2B, and 3 could be distinguished by the amount of residual enzyme activity (52).

Adult G_{M1}-Gangliosidosis

As in the case of type 2 G_{M1}-gangliosidosis, (type 3) is a heterogeneous category. Some patients have symptoms in childhood but survive into adulthood when the diagnosis was made. Others first became symptomatic as adults in the 3rd or 4th decade. Considerable intrafamilial variability may occur (77).

The more common phenotype is that manifesting with extrapyramidal features (77,78). Dystonia of the neck and the limbs is prominent and facial dystonia and dysarthria may be present. Tremor, rigidity, bradykinesia, and masked facies may lead to the diagnosis of juvenile parkinsonism; however, these patients do not respond to levodopa. Dementia of mild-to-severe degree may be present (79). Increased deep tendon reflexes (77) and spastic quadriparesis (79) may be seen. These patients lack seizures, myoclonus, macular cherry-red spot, cerebellar disturbance, facial dysmorphism, bone or joint abnormalities (though scoliosis may occur), or organomegaly.

CT head scans may show atrophy of the basal ganglia, particularly the head of caudate nucleus (77). Membranous cytoplasmic bodies are found in rectal ganglion cells (78,80), and conjunctival biopsies are abnormal with intracytoplasmic vacuoles (79). Skin biopsies are ultrastructurally abnormal (80), but this procedure is less valuable than rectal biopsy. Pathologic studies demonstrate that neuronal lipid storage is selective and prominent in the basal ganglia. Although organomegaly is not seen, visceral and renal glomerular storage is noted. A characteristic pattern of oligosaccharides is found in urine, but sialo-oligosaccharides are not increased.

Other patients with adult-onset G_{M1}-gangliosidosis have a different phenotype. Members of a single highly inbred family have been reported (81) with severe myoclonus, ataxia, pyramidal signs, as well as mental defect, cataracts, and some degree of corneal clouding. Macular cherry-red spots were present in some but not in others.

The diagnosis of adult G_{M1}-gangliosidosis is made by the characteristic clinical picture, finding severe deficiency of beta-galactosidase in leukocytes and cultured skin fibroblasts without deficiency of other lysosomal enzymes such as sialidase, and the finding of a characteristic pattern of urinary oligosaccharides. Rectal biopsy is a useful confirmatory procedure.

The residual beta-galactosidase activity has abnormal properties. Mutant beta-galactosidase purified from the liver of a patient with adult G_{M1}-gangliosidosis had altered enzyme properties, such as pH optimum, K_M value, substrate specificity, and heat-stability (82). Adult G_{M1}-gangliosidosis can be distinguished from other types of G_{M1}-gangliosidosis enzymatically if urinary oligosaccharides are used as substrates (52).

The processing of beta-galactosidase is abnormal in adult G_{M1}-gangliosidosis (70). The residual beta-galactosidase, 5% to 10% of control levels, consists of the 64 Kd mature enzyme. This has normal catalytic properties but a reduced ability of the monomeric form to aggregate into the high molecular weight multimer (70). In cultured fibroblasts, the mutation interferes with the phosphorylation of the precursor of beta-galactosidase so that the precursor is secreted instead of being compartmentalized into lysosomes and further processed (75).

Morquio Syndrome (Type B)

Patients with this phenotype have onset of signs and symptoms in childhood or adolescence with severe spondyloepiphyseal dysplasia resembling that of classic Morquio syndrome, although milder in degree. In addition, corneal clouding can be present. The intelligence is normal (51) as in classic Morquio syndrome, although mental regression did occur in an atypical family (54) reported with the diagnosis of Morquio syndrome (type B). Patients with Morquio type B are dwarfed, although less severely than patients with classic Morquio syndrome (now Morquio type A). Joint laxity is present in patients with type A but is lacking in patients with type B. Cord compression can complicate both disorders.

Radiographic findings can include generalized platyspondyly, acetabular dysplasia, flattening and fragmentation of femoral heads, and minor dysplastic changes in hand films (51). Excess urinary excretion of both keratan sulfate and oligosaccharides is characteristic. Beta-galactosidase is severely decreased in leukocytes and cultured skin fibroblasts. N-acetylgalactosamine-6-sulfate sulfatase, deficient in Morquio syndrome (type A), is normal in Morquio syndrome (type B).

The diagnosis of Morquio syndrome (type B) is made by the characteristic clinical picture, determining a severe deficiency of beta-galactosidase in leukocytes and cultured skin fibroblasts without deficiency of other lysosomal enzymes such as N-acetylgalactosamine-6-sulfate sulfatase or sialidase, and finding a characteristic pattern of urinary oligosaccharides along with keratan sulfate.

The defect in Morquio syndrome (type B) is allelic to that causing the various phenotypes of G_{M1}-gangliosidosis, but the residual beta-galactosidase has different properties (73). In Morquio syndrome (type B), the mutation does not interfere with the normal processing and does not interfere greatly with intralysosomal aggregation of beta-galactosidase (70,83). The mutation chiefly affects the catabolism of keratan sulfate, accounting for the preponderance of clinical abnormality in the skeleton (83).

MANNOSIDOSIS

The clinical picture of mannosidosis is quite varied, ranging from mild to severe disease. Severely affected patients have been confused with mucolipidosis I. The initial patient with mannnosidosis (84) was tall for his age with large hands and feet, slight hepatosplenomegaly, and mild psychomotor retardation. Later, growth slowed and he developed lumbar kyphosis, rather coarse features, macroglosia, and small cloudy lenticular opacities although the corneas were

clear. Subsequently, he developed mental and motor deterioration, hypotonia and hyperreflexia, and extensor plantar responses. He died in his 5th year during an episode of suspected increased intracranial pressure.

Other patients have had slower progression of the disorder with notable dysmorphism, corneal opacities, and longer survival; whereas, some others have presented primarily with marked mental defect, striking gingival hyperplasia, and have survived into the 3rd decade or longer. Facial dysmorphism, skeletal involvement and organomegaly have been slight in these patients.

More than 70 cases of mannosidosis have been reported (85) with a variable clinical picture. Patients with a severe form of mannosidosis have hepatogmegaly, severe infections, and early death. The more common mild form (86) shows no clinical abnormalities or nonspecific abnormalities during the 1st year of life (psychomotor delay, speech delay, or frequent infections) and only later develops mild to moderate or severe mental defect, coarse facial features, sensorineural hearing loss, ataxia, and dysostosis multiplex. Patients have short stature and may survive into adulthood (86) without hepatomegaly, at least until the age of 41 years (87). Cognitive and language impairment do not correlate well with the amount residual alpha-mannosidase activity measured with an artificial substrate (88). Pancytopenia with antiplatelet and antineutrophil antibodies can occur (89). Destructive synovitis can occur with damage to the ankles (90), knee, or spine (87).

The most notable radiographic finding is a dense thickening of the calvaria; dysostosis multiplex tends to be mild and decreases in prominence with the age of the patient (8). CT head scans can be normal or can show increased subarachnoid spaces and hypodensity of the white matter (65).

Establishing the diagnosis requires a high index of suspicion, finding an excess of abnormal urinary oligosaccharides, and demonstrating decreased alpha-mannosidase in leukocytes and cultured skin fibroblasts. Ultrastructural study of cultured skin fibroblasts (30) in mannosidosis shows vacuolar inclusions containing fine reticulogranular material with low electron density similar to those in sialidosis and the mucopolysaccharidoses.

There are no manifestations of muscle involvement in mannosidosis; however, there may be ultrastructural abnormalities (91) of muscle biopsies. A 32-year-old patient (92) had numerous membrane-bound inclusions in biopsied skeletal muscle as well as interstitial fibroblasts and some endothelial cells. The inclusions were small (0.5 to 5 μm), membrane bound, and contained dark granules as well as electron-lucent spaces. They were not believed to be related to the patient's mild muscle weakness. However, in another patient, with generalized muscle weakness and spastic paraplegia, the muscle pathology may have been related to the weakness (85).

Lectin histochemistry of paraffin-embedded tissue sections can distinguish between alpha- and beta-mannosidosis, fucosidosis, and sialidosis. Mannosidosis tissue showed staining with concanavalin A (Con A), wheat germ agglutinin (WGA), and succinyl-wheat germ agglutinin (S-WGA) (93). Fucosidosis tissue stained with Ulex europous-I UEA-I. Sialidosis tissue stained with WGA but not S-WGA. Beta-mannosidosis did not stain with Con A, WGA, S-WGA, UEA-I, or Arachis hypogea (PNA).

Bone marrow transplant has been attempted as treatment for mannosidosis. A 6-year-old boy survived for 18 weeks after transplant. There was some evidence that the transplant reversed the somatic changes of mannosidosis, but did not affect its storage in the brain (94).

The gene for alpha-mannosidase was found to be on chromosome 19 by means of studies in somatic cell hybrids and is located in the central region (p13→q13) of the chromosome (95). Besides the human disease, mannosidosis occurs in cattle and cats (62,96). Ingestion of swainsonine, an inhibitor of mannosidase, causes a mannosidase-like disorder in cattle, sheep, and horses (97–101).

BETA-MANNOSIDOSIS

Beta-mannosidosis, a condition secondary to deficiency of beta-mannosidase, is unusual because the disease was initially described in goats (102,103) and only later recognized in humans (104–106). The disease in goats differs from that in humans, and is characterized by pendular nystagmus, ataxia, dysmorphism, the inability to stand, and marked intention tremor (107,108). The disorder is present at birth. A major element of the neuropathology is a defect of myelin, perhaps due to an oligodendrocytic defect (109) and in addition, there are axonal abnormalities with axonal spheroids. In the peripheral nervous system, there are vacuolated Schwann cells and axonal spheroids (110). Characteristic lysosomal storage vacuoles are seen in all tissues in most cell types.

In humans the disorder is manifested by mental retardation, angiokeratoma, and tortuosity of conjunctival vessels (104). Hearing loss has been reported in some but not all patients (104,105,106). One of the patients (105) had dysmorphic features and a deficiency of heparin sulfamidase, the enzyme deficient in Sanfilippo syndrome type A, in addition to deficiency of beta-mannosidase. The other patients did not show dysmorphic features.

Beta-mannosidase in humans is measurable in plasma (111), where it varies with age (but not, as in goats, with sex), leukocytes, fibroblasts, and urine (112) and is deficient in all of these in beta-mannosidosis. Interestingly, beta-mannosidase activity in human fibroblasts is ten times as high as in goat fibroblasts (113). Oligosacchariduria is present (104–106) and is easily detected by thin layer chromatography. However, the disaccharide mannosyl-beta-(1→4)-N-acetylglucosamine requires a special solvent system in order to distinguish it from lactose (106).

The diagnosis of beta-mannosidosis is established by demonstrating the characteristic oligosacchariduria and the

enzyme defect in blood and fibroblasts. Heterozygotes can be detected (111), and the prenatal diagnosis of the disease could presumably be detected in humans as has been done in goats (114).

Lectin histochemistry of paraffin-embedded tissue sections can distinguish between alpha- and beta-mannosidosis, fucosidosis, and sialidosis (93). Alpha-mannosidosis tissue showed staining with Con A, WGA, and S-WGA. Beta-mannosidosis did not stain with Con A, WGA, S-WGA, UEA-I, or PNA.

FUCOSIDOSIS

Patients with fucosidosis differ greatly in the type of clinical involvement as well as the severity of their illness. Some patients (type I) present with severe, progressive neurologic disorder; whereas, others with milder disease (type II) resemble patients with the Hurler phenotype. Some patients have survived into the 2nd, 3rd, or 4th decade; however, they usually become symptomatic in childhood. Some authors refer to the adult patients as type II, whereas others recognize a type III (115). Types I and II may appear in the same family (116,117).

Severely affected infants (type I) develop symptoms and signs in the 1st year of life manifested by psychomotor retardation, hypotonia and then hypertonia, and later in the disease course, spasticity, tremor, and mental deterioration leading to loss of contact with their environment (115,116,118). They have thick skin, sweat excessively, and may lose gall bladder function. They have only mild facial coarsening and organomegaly, and cardiac enlargement may occur. Radiographic bone changes have been described. Some patients die at 4 to 5 years of age.

Other patients (type II) have onset of symptoms in the 2nd year of life with more markedly coarsened facial features and greater resemblance to the Hurler syndrome (115–117). These patients also deteriorate mentally and die around 5 years of age.

Some patients (117) with infantile or juvenile onset have a milder course with coarsened facial features, skin changes resembling the angiokeratoma of Fabry disease, skeletal abnormalities, and dwarfing, and may survive into the 3rd decade. Angiokeratoma is characteristic of patients with longer survival. Besides Fabry disease and fucosidosis, angiokeratoma corporis diffusum also occurs in sialidosis, and in at least one patient without a defined lysosomal disease (119).

Radiographic changes are similar to those of a mild dysostosis multiplex, but are most marked in the pelvis, the hips, and the spine (8). These findings are not in themselves diagnostic, but should point the way to more specific studies (120).

Rectal biopsy has been found to contain three kinds of inclusions in vascular endothelial cells: clear vacuoles, dark vacuoles, and mixed vacuoles. Clear vacuoles and dark vacuoles appeared to contain fucosyl-oligosaccharides, and the presence of these two types together is considered pathognomonic of fucosidosis (117). Lectin histochemistry of paraffin-embedded tissue sections can distinguish between alpha- and beta-mannosidosis, fucosidosis, and sialidosis. Fucosidosis tissue stained with UEA-I, whereas the others did not (93).

The diagnosis of fucosidosis requires a high index of suspicion because of the diverse clinical pictures. All of these phenotypes have deficiency of the lysosomal enzyme alpha-L-fucosidase. Fucose residues form part of the structure of oligosaccharides, glycoproteins, and glycolipids including "fucogangliosides." Urinary oligosaccharides are increased in characteristic pattern (115).

The diagnosis is made by finding a large excess of abnormal oligosaccharides in urine and demonstrating severely decreased alpha-L-fucosidase in serum, leukocytes, and cultured skin fibroblasts. It is important to realize that 6% to 11% of the normal population have a polymorphism (121) in which serum alpha-L-fucosidase but not leukocyte alpha-L-fucosidase is severely decreased; residual activity from both sources is heat-labile. Residual fucosidase in occasional or unusual patients may be 60% of control values but with heat-labile enzyme (118). Therefore, it is important to carry out thin-layer chromatography for oligosaccharides, for these patients will be otherwise missed. On the other hand, a false-positive diagnosis of fucosidosis was made in a patient with pseudohypoparathyroidism because the serum and fibroblast alpha-fucosidase activity was about 10% of control values (122).

Fucosidase is synthesized as a 53 Kd precursor which is processed to a 50 Kd mature form (123). Eleven patients with severe fucosidase deficiency usually synthesized no precursor, but 2 patients synthesized precursor that was not processed, and one synthesized small amounts of cross-reacting material (123).

Human fucosidase appears to be coded by a single locus on chromosome 1; the gene has been cloned (124). Two restriction fragment length polymorphisms have allowed demonstration of genetic linkage between fucosidosis and its structural gene (125). Molecular analysis of the gene in patients with fucosidosis from two families has demonstrated an abnormal banding pattern after restriction endonuclease from *Escherichia coli* (Eco R1) digestion (126) in one case. In one family, deletion of an Eco R1 site in exon 7 of the fucosidase structural gene has been found (116).

Fucosidosis has been found in dogs (127). Attempted treatment with bone marrow transplants in canine fucosidosis had no beneficial clinical effect (128); however, cloned human complementary DNA encoding for human alpha-L-fucosidase has been successfully inserted into canine hemtopoietic cells using retroviral vectors, and this model may become useful for assessing the effectiveness of gene therapy (128).

ASPARTYLGLYCOSAMINURIA

This disorder occurs almost solely in Finland, where at least 138 patients have been described in a population of 4.5 million (129,130). It is inherited as an autosomal recessive trait. Patients are normal until 1 to 5 years of age, when they develop progressive somatic and mental changes (129). Progressive coarsening of facial features is noted with depressed nasal bridge, anteverted nostrils, broad nose, broad face, and rosy cheeks. Skeletal changes include thickening of the skull, cranial asymmetry, short neck, and thoracic or lumbar scoliosis. Psychomotor development is delayed. Diarrhea, frequent respiratory infections, and cutaneous manifestations may be seen. Intellectual deterioration leading to severe mental defect occurs in the adult, and episodic hyperactivity, psychotic behavior, speech defects, and seizures may occur.

Patients excrete in their urine large amounts of aspartylglucosamine [2-acetamido-1-(beta'-L-aspartamido)-1,2-dideoxyglucose] and more complex compounds containing this moiety (129,131). This results from a deficiency of the lysosomal enzyme N-aspartyl-beta-glucosaminidase, an amidase that cleaves aspartylglucosamine. This bond constitutes the linkage region between the protein portion and saccharide portion of one class of glycoproteins and of keratan sulfate.

Diagnosis is established by the characteristic clinical and genetic features, finding of aspartylglucosamine in urine, and demonstrating a deficiency of N-aspartyl-beta-glucosaminidase. Aspartylglucosamine is easily detected with thin-layer chromatography of urine for oligosaccharides or by the amino acid analyzer (131). N-aspartyl-beta-glucosaminidase deficiency can be demonstrated most satisfactorily in cultured skin fibroblasts although the deficiency is also found in plasma, seminal fluid, and tissue. Aspartylglucosaminuria has been demonstrated in amniotic fluid (132), fetal urine.

N-ACETYLGLUCOSAMINYLPHOSPHOTRANSFERASE DEFICIENCIES

Mucolipidosis II—I-cell disease and mucolipidosis III—pseudo-Hurler polydystrophy are biochemically similar because they both result from genetically determined deficiency of the enzyme N-acetyl-glucosaminylphosphotransferase. They are different from the disorders discussed thus far, however, because multiple lysosomal hydrolase enzymes, which are themselves substrates for the phosphotransferase are also abnormal and deficient in these disorders. However, it is not the protein portions of the enzymes that are abnormal; rather, the enzymes lack a recognition marker that allows their uptake into the cell.

The lysosomal hydrolase enzymes are themselves glycoproteins containing sialic acid, N-acetylated hexosamines, and a variety of sugars, including phosphorylated mannose, bound to the enzyme protein. This saccharide portion, especially the phosphorylated mannose, appears to be the recognition marker that allows the newly synthesized lysosomal enzymes to be correctly packaged into lysosomes, attached to the cell surface or secreted outside the cell.

In mucolipidosis II and III, a phosphate is missing from a mannose moiety, and the lysosomal enzyme is consequently secreted into the extracellular space rather than packaged into lysosomes. The basic defect, a deficiency of a transferase enzyme (UPD-N-acetylglucosamine:lysosomal-enzyme-precursor N-acetylglucosamine-1-phosphate transferase, or N-acetylglucosaminylphosphotransferase), is related to post-translational modification of these proteins. This enzyme is present in the Golgi structures and is required for the formation of the mannose-6-phosphate residue on the oligosaccharide chain of enzyme as a recognition marker for sorting lysosomal enzymes. There are three complementation groups for deficiencies of N-acetyl-glucosaminyl phosphotransferase. These disorders are inherited as an autosomal recessive trait.

Mucolipidosis II—I-Cell Disease

Patients with I-cell disease are abnormal at birth or shortly thereafter. The name *I-cell disease* derives from the coarse granular inclusions that are seen in patients' cultured fibroblasts, which were called *inclusion-cells* or *I-cells.* Nonimmune hydrops fetalis is the most severe presentation for I-cell disease. These patients resemble the phenotype of sialidosis or galactosialidosis presenting with fetal hydrops. I-cell disease with fetal hydrops may become symptomatic in utero. Fetal ascites, scalp edema, placental thickening, and increased amniotic fluid volume have been noted at 24 (menstrual) weeks (133). Delivery may be premature and survival is short. Patients have generalized edema, pleural effusion, ascites, and hepatosplenomegaly (133).

I-cell disease usually manifests in the neonatal period and has a slowly progressive course leading to death around 4 to 6 years of age (134–136). The chief clinical features are the early cessation of growth, psychomotor retardation, and dysmorphism. Motor development tends to be more severely affected than mental development (135). Patients develop markedly coarsened facial features, severe dysostosis multiplex and restricted joint mobility, dwarfism, and severe mental defect. Corneas are usually, but not always, clear, although clouding is often visible by slit lamp. There is marked gingival hyperplasia, hoarse voice, thickened indurated skin, hirsutism, thoracic deformity, hernias, and congenital hip dislocation. Kyphoscoliosis, gibbus, and enlargement of liver and less frequently spleen are often noted. Cardiac involvement includes progressive hypertrophic cardiomyopathy and valvular heart disease and is often the cause of death. A bout of pneumonia can exacerbate congestive heart failure leading to death. Clinical features resembling those of mucolipidosis II have been noted in patients (137) with partial trisomy 3q(3q25→qter).

Radiographic changes involve multiple bony structures and include generalized dysostosis multiplex, osteopenia, periosteal new bone formation, punctuate calcifications, and oar-shaped rib deformities (134,136,138). The radiographic changes of severe dysostosis multiplex are seen in the 1st year of life. Neonatal periosteal cloaking of the long bones, demineralization with foci of metaphyseal destruction, and pathologic fractures may be seen (8). There is considerable resemblance to the picture of congenital lues. Radiographic changes have been noted as early as 19 weeks' gestation (138).

The most characteristic histologic feature of mucolipidosis II is the intracytoplasmic storage in fibroblasts of membrane-bound vacuoles with fibrillo-granular contents and smaller inclusions with concentric ring-like profiles in endothelial cells. Only in older patients are heterogeneous cell inclusions with osmiophilic lamellar profiles found (139).

Ultrastructural studies of cultured skin fibroblasts in I-cell disease show a variety of inclusion types; viz, vacuolar, lamellar, amorphous, or mixed (30). Cells in skin containing multiple vacuoles include fibroblasts, histiocyte-like cells, eccrine secretory cells, and Schwann cells (140). These vacuoles contained sparse reticulo-floccular and vesicular material. Multivesicular, electron-dense, membrane-bound inclusions were seen in dermal capillaries; epidermis and pilosebaceous appendages were normal. Cultured skin fibroblasts contained prominent inclusions that were acid phosphatase-positive indicating lysosomal origin (140).

The diagnosis of mucolipidosis II is made by the characteristic clinical picture, finding a large excess of sialo-oligosaccharides in the urine, demonstrating deficiencies of multiple lysosomal enzymes in cultured skin fibroblasts with elevated levels of these enzymes in plasma, and demonstrating a deficiency of N-acetylglucosaminylphosphotransferase (the primary defect). Enzymes deficient in cultured skin fibroblasts but elevated in plasma include: beta-galactosidase, hexosaminidase, beta-glucurondidase, alpha-galactosidase, and sulfatase A. Acid phosphatase and beta-glucosidase (glucocerebrosidase) are not deficient. Acid phosphatase is not elevated in plasma. In brain and visceral organs, only beta-galactosidase is consistently deficient. A useful screening test is the determination of two- to threefold elevation of hexosaminidase in serum. Heterozygous carriers have been detected (141) for complementation group A.

Ultrastructural studies of lysosomal acid phosphatase localization in I-cell fibroblasts (142) showed that the enzyme was present in the same subcellular organelles as in controls, but always associated with membranous structures. It was suggested that the association of acid phosphatase with membranes might explain the normal enzyme activity found in I-cell fibroblasts. Studies of glucocerebrosidase, the second lysosomal enzyme not decreased in I-cell fibroblasts, were found (143) not to require oligosaccharide phosphorylation, a step essential for transport of soluble lysosomal enzymes to the lysosomes in fibroblasts.

Biochemical heterogeneity in I-cell disease has been identified (144), based on the fact that I-cell fibroblasts from some patients showed significant increase of intracellular lysosomal hydrolase activities after growth in 88 mmol/L sucrose-supplemented medium for 2 weeks, whereas some other lines did not. It is possible that different mutations of the N-acetylglucosaminyl phosphotransferase are identified in this way.

There is likely to be locus genetic heterogeneity for deficiencies of N-acetylglucosaminylphosphotransferase (mucolipidosis II and III) because of the finding of multiple complementation groups. This suggests that the enzyme may have multiple genetically distinct subunits. Three complementation groups were described (141,145,146) for N-acetylglucosaminylphosphotransferase: A, B, and C. If this is true, then at least three different gene loci participate in determining N-acetylglucosaminylphosphotransferase activity. The largest group is group A, which encompasses all cases of mucolipidosis II and many cases of mucolipidosis III. There are occasional instances of complementation within group A, which are regarded as suggesting intragenic heterogeneity. The other 2 groups consist entirely of less common variants of mucolipidosis III. The properties of the mutationally altered enzyme differ between complementation groups A and C. In group A, low enzyme activity is due to a low maximum velocity. The Michaelis-Menton constants for the substrates UDP-Glc-NAc and alpha-methylmannoside are in the normal range (141). The presence of multiple complementation groups has been interpreted to mean that the N-acetylglucosaminylphosphotransferase enzyme consists of multiple subunits. The defect in group A may be a catalytic subunit that is absent or defective, whereas a recognition subunit may be altered or defective in another complementation group (145).

Further evidence for heterogeneity of disorders with deficiency of N-acetylglucosaminylphosphotransferase is the finding (146) that the mutant enzyme in complementation group A is smaller than the normal enzyme, whereas the mutant enzyme from complementation group C is larger than the normal enzyme.

Mucolipidosis III—Pseudo-Hurler Polydystrophy

This disorder is milder and has a later onset than mucolipidosis II, but both diseases have deficiencies of multiple lysosomal hydrolases, and in both, lysosomal hydrolases lack a specific recognition marker. The basic cause is a deficiency in the processing enzyme N-acetylglucosaminylphosphotransferase, the same enzyme that is deficient in mucolipidosis II, but the defect in mucolipidosis III is milder than that in mucolipidosis II.

Patients with mucolipidosis III usually notice onset of progressive skeletal symptoms at 2 to 4 years of age. Pro-

gressive stiffness of the hands result in a claw hand deformity and progressive stiffness at the shoulder leads to inability to raise the arms above the head. Marked dwarfism, mildly coarsened facial features, short neck, and mild-to-moderate mental retardation become evident. Radiographic changes of dysostosis multiplex of variable degree become evident (8), and claw hand deformities tend to be severe. The combination of paddle-shaped ribs with narrowing of the vertebral ends, peculiar vertebral changes, and severe pelvic changes with hypoplastic iliac bodies, and abnormalities of the proximal femora are rather specific for this disorder. Corneas appear clear, but slit-lamp examination may show fine corneal opacities. Cardiac murmurs related to aortic or mitral valves are commonly heard. Bilateral carpal tunnel syndrome is a feature. Progression of the disease primarily occurs during childhood and patients have prolonged survival into the 4th decade or longer. Interestingly, males seem to be more severely affected than females, though inheritance is by an autosomal-recessive trait. The diagnosis is similar to that of mucolipidosis II. Distinction between the two disorders is determined on clinical grounds.

The basic defect is N-acetylglucosaminylphosphotransferase, as described earlier. Patients with mucolipidosis III may belong to complementation groups A, B, or C, whereas those with mucolipidosis II are all in complementation group A. There is some evidence that among patients with mucolipidosis III, alteration of the N-acetylglucosaminylphosphotransferase from group C patients affects the recognition site for the protein portion of lysosomal enzymes; whereas, group A patients have mutations giving rise to temperature-sensitive enzyme (147).

MUCOLIPIDOSIS IV

This disorder is characterized (148) by severe psychomotor retardation associated with corneal clouding, but without organomegaly or skeletal deformities. These patients come to medical attention because of the appearance of corneal clouding in the neonatal period or as early as 6 weeks of age. The corneal opacity may become static and even improve. About 1/2 of the reported infants have been from Ashkenazim families. Mild retardation is noted early on, but this progresses and results in a severe mental and motor defect in adolescence; the oldest patients reached the 3rd decade (149,150). Other findings may include optic atrophy, retinopathy (151), hypotonia, and truncal ataxia; however, seizures do not occur. Facial dysmorphism, organomegaly, and bony changes are not features of this disease.

Numerous vacuolated, lipid-laden, weakly PAS-positive histiocytic cells are found in the bone marrow. In brain widespread storage of autofluorescent, PAS-positive, Sudan B positive granular material was present in neurons and glial cells, most of which were not enlarged. A milder clinical variant has been described (152) in which excessive urinary oligosaccharide was found.

Brain, liver, conjunctiva, skin, cultured skin fibroblasts, and amniotic fluid cells have been found to have ultrastructural abnormalities which include vacuoles and membranous cytoplasmic bodies. Biochemical studies have shown accumulation of gangliosides, phospholipids (153), sulfated mucopolysaccharide and hyaluronic acid (a nonsulfated mucopolysaccharide), and an unknown lipid (151). Excess oligosaccharides have not been found in urine. However, G_{M_3} and G_{D_3} gangliosides have been found to accumulate in cultured skin fibroblasts. Soluble ganglioside sialidase has been reported to be deficient. This may be the basic defect, because partial deficiency has been demonstrated in heterozygotes, or this may be a secondary finding (148,150,154). There is some evidence that the catabolism of gangliosides is impaired (155). Because of the biochemical findings, the name *sialolipidosis* was suggested for this disorder (149). The diagnosis is established by the characteristic clinical, ultrastructural, and biochemical findings.

Although skeletal muscle is not symptomatically involved in mucolipidosis IV, PAS-positive inclusions are seen in almost all muscle fibers by light and electron microscopy, in which lamellar bodies are seen (91).

FREE SIALIC ACID STORAGE DISEASES

Two diseases have been associated with the storage of free sialic acid and appearance of excessive amounts of sialic acid in the urine. The first is Salla disease, initially described by Aual et al. (156). The second is infantile free sialic acid storage disease (157). These disorders are inherited as an autosomal-recessive trait and appear to affect the transport of sialic acid across the lysosomal membrane.

Salla Disease

Although this disorder has very early onset, it is compatible with prolonged survival. Patients have been described between the ages of 2 and 64 years (158). The chief clinical features include a severe, early onset of psychomotor retardation, speech impairment, ataxia, athetosis, spasticity, and rigidity. Slow motor development is noted in the 1st year of life, and occasionally nystagmus transiently is noted during the 1st year of life. By the age of 2 years, a definite delay in speech development is noted. All patients have ataxia, spasticity, or rigidity (158). Psychomotor development continues slowly for the 1st 2 decades of life, but then a slow deterioration commonly supervenes. Most, but not all patients learn to walk and most patients learn to speak single words or short sentences. Some patients have seizures, usually absence in type, but occasionally generalized tonic-clonic convulsions occur (158). Other common

findings include short stature, exotropia, hypertelorism, and thickened calvaria. Facial features are normal or show mild coarsening, and there is no organomegaly.

Vacuolated lymphocytes are seen on peripheral smear, and clear round vacuoles are seen seen in fibrocytes, Schwann cells, and eccrine sweat gland duct cells by light microscopy of semi-thin sections. At electron microscopy, these are seen to be electron-lucent lysosomes, which are usually empty and without distinguishing characteristics for Salla disease.

The diagnosis is made by the characteristic clinical picture, the presence of elevated amounts of free sialic acid in urine by assay or by thin-layer chromatography (130,158,159). Urinary free sialic acid is increased five- to tenfold compared with controls (160). Electron microscopy of biopsy material, such as skin, is a useful confirmatory test. The basic defect seems to be defective sialic acid egress from lysosomes (161), a finding that suggests that a carrier-mediated transport system exists by which sialic acid exits from the lysosome. Salla disease fibroblasts accumulate 10 to 30 times the normal amount of free sialic acid (160). Nearly all patients are of Finnish origin (158), and many of the early cases originated from the Salla region of northern Finland. Some apparently nonFinnish cases have been reported (162,163).

Infantile Free Sialic Acid Storage Disease

Patients with infantile free sialic acid storage disease are more severely affected, surviving only a few years. These patients have infantile hepatosplenomegaly and marked bony involvement (157).

The ultrastructural findings are similar to those of Salla disease (157). Urinary free sialic acid concentration is increased to a greater extent than in Salla disease (20- to 200-fold). As in Salla disease, the egress of sialic acid from lysosomes is impaired, perhaps because of a defect in carrier-mediated transport system for this substance (164). Fibroblasts from patients with infantile free sialic acid storage disease accumulate up to 200 times the normal amount of free sialic acid (160).

The diagnosis is based on the characteristic clinical picture and the finding of elevated urine free sialic acid by thin-layer chromatographic screening. Electron microscopy of biopsy material, such as skin, is a useful confirmatory test.

ACKNOWLEDGMENTS

The authors are grateful to the Parkinson's Disease Foundation, the Muscular Dystrophy Association, the Schultz Foundation, the American Parkinson's Disease Association, and NIH grants NS-15281 and NS-11766 for support.

REFERENCES

1. Spranger JW, Wiedmann HR. The genetic mucolipidoses. Diagnosis and differential diagnosis. Humangenet 1970;9:113–139.
2. Van Hoof F. Mucopolysaccharidoses and mucolipidoses. J Clin Pathol Suppl (R Coll Pathol) 1974;8:64–93.
3. Lowden JA, O'Brien JS. Sialidosis: A review of human neuraminidase deficiency. Am J Hum Genet 1979;31:1–18.
4. Cantz M. Sialidosis. Chemistry, metabolism and function. In: Schauer, ed. Sialic Acids. Vienna: Springer, 1982:306–320.
5. Durand P, O'Brien JS. Genetic Errors of Glycoprotein Metabolism. New York: Springer-Verlag, 1982.
6. Warner TG, O'Brien JS. Genetic defects in glycoprotein metabolism. Annu Rev Genet 1983;17:395–441.
7. Kornfeld S, Sly WS. Lysosomal storage defects. Hosp Pract [Off] 1985;20:71–5, 78–82.
8. Eggli KD, Dorst JP. The mucopolysaccharidoses and related conditions. Semin Roentgenol 1986;21:275–294.
9. Johnson WG. Lysosomal Disorders. I. Lipidoses; II. Leukodystrophies; III. Mucopolysaccharidoses; IV. Mucolipidoses. In: Rudolph AM, ed. Pediatrics. Norwalk: Appleton & Lange, 1987:1725–1732.
10. Beaudet AL, Thomas GH. Disorders of glycoprotein degradation: Mannosidosis, fucosidosis, sialidosis, and aspartylglycosamininuria. In: Scriver CR, Beaudet AL, Sly WS, eds. The Metabolic Basis of Inherited Disease. New York: McGraw-Hill, 1989:1603–1621.
11. Johnson WG. Lysosomal diseases. In: Rowland LP, ed. Merritt's Textbook of Neurology. Philadelphia: Lea & Febiger, 1989:500–527.
12. Mueller OT, Henry WM, Haley LL, et al. Sialidosis and galactosialidosis: Chromosomal assignment of two genes associated with neuraminidase-deficiency disorders. Proc Natl Acad Sci USA 1986;83:1817–1821.
13. O'Brien JS, Warner TG. Sialidosis: Delineation of subtypes by neuraminidase assay. Clin Genet 1980;17:35–38.
14. Kitagawa T, Owada M, Sakiyama T, et al. Cherry-red spot—myoclonus syndrome in a Japanese family. J Inherited Metab Dis 1982;5:75–76.
15. Harzer K, Cantz M, Sewell AC, et al. Normomorphic sialidosis in two female adults with severe neurologic disease and without sialyl oligosacchariduria. Hum Genet 1986;74:209–214.
16. Gascon G, Wallenberg B, Daif AK, et al. Successful treatment of cherry-red spot-myoclonus syndrome with 5-hydroxytryptophan. Ann Neurol 1988;24:453–455.
17. Kivlin JD, Sanborn GE, Myers GG. The cherry-red spot in Tay-Sachs and other storage diseases. Ann Neurol 1985;17:356–360.
18. Johnson WG, Thomas GH, Miranda AF, et al. Congenital sialidosis, a new form of alpha-L-neuraminidase deficiency—its possible relation to hydrops fetalis (abstract). Neurology 1980;30:377.
19. Johnson WG, Thomas GH, Miranda AF, et al. Prenatal diagnosis in two pregnancies at risk for congenital sialidosis (abstract). Ann Neurol 1980;8:216.
20. Laver J, Fried K, Beer SI, et al. Infantile lethal neuraminidase deficiency (sialidosis). Clin Genet 1983;23:97–101.
21. Beck M, Bender SW, Reiter HL, et al. Neuraminidase deficiency presenting a non-immune hydrops fetalis. Eur J Pediatr 1984;143:135–139.
22. Yamano T, Shimada M, Matsuzaki K, et al. Pathological study on a severe sialidosis (alpha-neuraminidase deficiency). Acta Neuropathol (Berl) 1986;71:278–284.
23. Matsuzaki K, Matsumoto Y, Yoshihara W, et al. A case of infantile sialidosis associated with congenital chylous ascites. No To Hattatsu 1987;19:249–253.
24. Norman RM, Wood N. A congenital form of amaurotic family idiocy. J Neurol Neurosurg Psychiatry 1941;4:175–190.
25. Brown NJ, Corner BD, Dodgson MCH. A second case in the same family of congenital familial cerebral lipoidosis resembling amaurotic family idiocy. Arch Dis Child 1954;29:48–54.
26. Hagberg B, Hultqvist G, Ohman R, et al. Congenital amaurotic idioicy. Acta Paediatr Scand 1965;54:116–130.
27. Aylsworth AS, Thomas GH, Hood JL, et al. A severe infantile sialidosis: Clinical, biochemical, and microscopic features. J Pediatr 1980;96:662–668.
28. Maroteaux P, Humbel R, Strecker G, et al. Un nouveau type de sialidose avec atteinte renale: La nephrosialidose. I. Etude clinique, radiologique et nosoligique. Arch Fr Pediatr 1978;35:819–829.
29. Le Sec G, Stanescu R, Lyon G. Un nouveau type de sialidose avec atteinte renale: La nephrosialidose. II. Etude anatomique. Arch Fr Pediatr 1978;35:830–844.
30. Takahashi K, Naito M, Suzuki Y. Genetic mucopolysaccharidoses, mannosidosis, sialidosis, galactosialidosis, and I-cell disease. Ultrastructural analysis of cultured fibroblasts. Acta Pathol Jpn 1987;37:385–400.
31. Ulrich Bott B, Klem B, Kaiser R, et al. Lysosomal sialidase deficiency: Increased ganglioside content in autopsy tissues of a sialidosis patient. Enzyme 1987;38:262–266.
32. Goldberg MF, Cotlier E, Fichenscher LG, et al. Macular cherry-red spot, corneal clouding, and beta-galactosidase deficiency: Clinical biochemical, and electron microscopic study of a new autosomal recessive storage disease. Arch Intern Med 1971;128:387–398.
33. Wenger DA, Tarby TJ, Wharton C. Macular cherry-red spots and myoclonus with dementia: Coexistent neuraminidase and beta-galactosidase deficiencies. Biochem Biophys Res Commun 1978;82:589–595.
34. Andria G, Strisciuglio P, Pontarelli G, et al. Infantile neuraminidase and beta-galactosidase deficiencies (galactosialidosis) with mild clinical courses. In: Tettamanti G, Durand P, DiDonato S, eds. Sialidase and Sialidoses. Milan: Edi. Ermes, 1981:379–395.
35. Galjart NJ, Gillemans N, Harris A, et al. Expression of cDNA encoding the human "protective protein" associated with lysosomal beta-galactosidase and neuraminidase: homology to yeast proteases. Cell 1988;54:755–764.
36. Matsuo T, Egawa I, Okada S, et al. Sialidosis type 2 in Japan. Clinical study in two siblings' cases and review of literature. J Neurol Sci 1983;58:45–55.
37. Strisciuglio P, Creek KE, Sky WS. Complementation, cross correction, and drug correction studies of combined beta-galactosidase neuraminidase deficiency in human fibroblasts. Pediatr Res 1984;18:167–171.
38. Palmeri S, Hoogeveen AT, Verheijen FW, et al. Galactosialidosis: Molecular heterogeneity among distinct clinical phenotypes. Am J Hum Genet 1986;38:137–148.

39. Galjaard H, Willemsen R, Hoogeveen AT, et al. Molecular heterogeneity in human beta-galactosidase and neuraminidase deficiency. Enzyme 1987;38:132–143.

40. Ahern Rindell AJ, Prieur DJ, Murnane RD, et al. Inherited lysosomal storage disease associated with deficiencies of beta-galactosidase and alpha-neuraminidase in sheep. Am J Med Genet 1988;31:39–56.

41. Gillan JE, Lowden JA, Gaskin K, et al. Congenital ascites as a presenting sign of lysosomal storage disease. J Pediatr 1984;104:225–231.

42. Sewell AC, Pontz BF. Prenatal diagnosis of galactosialidosis. Prenat Diagn 1988;8:151–155.

43. Yamano T, Shimada M, Sugino H, et al. Ultrastructural study on a severe infantile sialidosis (beta-galactosidase-alpha-neuraminidase deficiency). Neuropediatrics 1985;16:109–112.

44. Okada S, Sugino H, Kato T, et al. A severe infantile sialidosis (beta-galactosidase-alpha-neuraminidase deficiency) mimicking G_{M1}-gangliosidosis type 1. Eur J Pediatr 1983;140:295–298.

45. Sewell AC, Pontz BF, Weitzel D, et al. Clinical heterogeneity in infantile galactosialidosis. Eur J Pediatr 1987;146:528–531.

46. Daneman A, Stringer D, Reilly BJ. Neonatal ascites due to lysosomal storage disease. Radiology 1983;149:463–467.

47. Tada H, Miyake S, Yamada M, et al. A case of galactosialidosis discovered with external strabismus and cherry-red spots in late infancy. No To Hattatsu 1988;20:69–73.

48. Ceuterick C, Martin JJ. Diagnostic role of skin or conjunctival biopsies in neurological disorders. An update. J Neurol Sci 1984;65:179–191.

49. Tsuji S, Yamada T, Ariga T, et al. Carrier detection of sialidosis with partial beta-galactosidase deficiency by the assay of lysosomal sialidase in lymphocytes. Ann Neurol 1984;15:181–183.

50. Yamano T, Shimada M, Okada S, et al. Ultrastructural study of biopsy specimens of rectal mucosa. Its use in neuronal storage diseases. Arch Pathol Lab Med 1982;106:673–677.

51. Beck M, Petersen EM, Spranger J, et al. Morquio's disease type B (beta-galactosidase deficiency) in three siblings. S Afr Med J 1987;72:704–707.

52. Takahashi Y, Orii T. Diagnosis of subtypes of G_{M1}-gangliosidosis in vitro and in vivo—Using urinary oligosaccharides as substrates. Clin Chim Acta 1989;179:219–228.

53. Takahashi Y, Orii T. Severity of G_{M1}-gangliosidosis and urinary oligosaccharide excretion. Clin Chim Acta 1989;179:153–162.

54. Giugliani R, Jackson M, Skinner SJ, et al. Progressive mental regression in siblings with Morquio disease type B (mucopolysaccharidosis IV B). Clin Genet 1987;32:313–325.

55. Kobayashi T, Shinnoh N, Goto I, et al. Hydrolysis of galactosylceramide is catalyzed by two genetically distinct acid beta-galactosidases. J Biol Chem 1985;260:14982–14987.

56. Goda S, Kobayashi T, Goto I. Hydrolysis of galactosylsphingosine and lactosylsphingosine by beta-galactosidases in human brain and cultured fibroblasts. Biochim Biophys Acta 1987;920:259–265.

57. Byrne MC, Ledeen RW. Regional variation of brain gangliosides in feline G_{M1}-gangliosidosis. Exp Neurol 1983;81:210–225.

58. Wood PA, McBride MR, Baker HJ, et al. Fluorescence polarization analysis, lipid composition, and Na^+, K^+-ATPase kinetics of synaptosomal membranes in feline G_{M1} and G_{M2} gangliosidosis. J Neurochem 1985;44:947–956.

59. Alroy J, Ucci AA, Goyal V, et al. Lectin histochemistry of glycolipid storage diseases on frozen and paraffin-embedded tissue sections. J Histochem Cytochem 1986;34:501–505.

60. Koenig ML, Jope RS, Baker HJ, et al. Reduced Ca^{2+} flux in synaptosomes from cats with G_{M1}-gangliosidosis. Brain Res 1987;424:169–176.

61. Walkley SU. Further studies on ectopic dendrite growth and other geometrical distortions of neurons in feline G_{M1}-gangliosidosis. Neuroscience 1987;21:313–331.

62. Castagnaro M, Alroy J, Ucci AA, et al. Lectin histochemistry and ultrastructure of feline kidneys from six different storage diseases. Virchows Arch [B] 1987;54:16–26.

63. Gitzelmann R, Spycher MA, Adank S, et al. Anomalous eosinophil granulocytes in blood and bone marrow: a diagnostic marker for infantile G_{M1}-gangliosidosis? Eur J Pediatr 1985;144:82–84.

64. Curless RG. Computed tomography of G_{M1}-gangliosidosis. J Pediatr 1984;105:964–966.

65. Wende S, Ludwig B, Kishikawa T, et al. The value of CT in diagnosis and prognosis of different inborn neurodegenerative disorders in childhood. J Neurol 1984;231:57–70.

66. Elleder M. Ito cells in lysosomal storage disorders. An ultrastructural study. Virchows Arch [B] 1984;46:13–19.

67. Bieber FR, Mortimer G, Kolodny EH, et al. Pathologic findings in fetal G_{M1}-gangliosidosis. Arch Neurol 1986;43:736–738.

68. Yamano T, Shimada M, Okada S, et al. Ultrastructural study on nervous system of fetus with G_{M1}-gangliosidosis type 1. Acta Neuropathol (Berl) 1983;61:15–20.

69. Cogan DG, Kuwabara T, Kolodny E, et al. Gangliosidoses and the fetal retina. Ophthalmology 1984;91:508–512.

70. Hoogeveen AT, Graham Kawashima H, d'Azzo A, et al. Processing of human beta-galactosidase in G_{M1}-gangliosidosis and Morquio B syndrome. J Biol Chem 1984;259:1974–1977.

71. Warner TG, Robertson AD, Mock AK, et al. Prenatal diagnosis of G_{M1}-gangliosidosis by detection of galactosyl-oligosaccharides in amniotic fluid with high-performance liquid chromatography. Am J Hum Genet 1983;35:1034–1041.

72. Gatti R, Lombardo C, Filocamo M, et al. Comparative study of 15 lysosomal enzymes in chorionic villi and cultured amniotic fluid cells. Early prenatal diagnosis in seven pregnancies at risk for lysosomal storage disease. Prenat Diagn 1985;5:329–336.

73. Mutch T, Naoi M, Takahashi A, et al. Atypical adult G_{M1}-gangliosidosis: biochemical comparison with other forms of primary beta-galactosidase deficiency. Neurology 1986;36:1237–1241.

74. Momoi T, Furuya T, Suzuki Y, et al. In vitro establishment of human fibroblasts of lysosomal diseases, G_{M1}-gangliosidosis and Sandhoff disease, by transformation with origin-minus SV40 DNA. Biosci Rep 1985;5:267–273.

75. Hoogeveen At, Reuser AJ, Kroos M, et al. G_{M1}-gangliosidosis. Defective recognition site on beta-galactosidase precursor. J Biol Chem 1986;261:5702–5704.

76. Nanba E, Tsuji A, Omura K, et al. G_{M1}-gangliosidosis: Abnormalities in biosynthesis and early processing of beta-galactosidase in fibroblasts. Biochem Biophys Res Commun 1988;152:794–800.

77. Nakano T, Ikeda S, Kondo K, et al. Adult G_{M1}-gangliosidosis: clinical patterns and rectal biopsy. Neurology 1985;35:875–880.

78. Ushiyama M, Ikeda S, Nakayama J, et al. Type III (chronic) G_{M1}-gangliosidosis. Histochemical and ultrastructural studies of rectal biopsy. J Neurol Sci 1985;71:209–223.

79. Guazzi GC, DAmore I, Van Hoof F, et al. Type 3 (chronic) G_{M1}-gangliosidosis presenting as infanto-choreo-athetotic dementia, without epilepsy, in three sisters. Neurology 1988;38:1124–1127.

80. Ikeda S, Ushiyama M, Nakano T, et al. Ultrastructural findings of rectal and skin biopsies in adult G_{M1}-gangliosidosis. Acta Pathol Jpn 1986;36:1823–1831.

81. Mutch T, Sobue I, Naoi M, et al. A family with beta-galactosidase deficiency: Three adults with atypical clinical patterns. Neurology 1986;36:54–59.

82. Mutch T, Naoi M, Nagatsu T, et al. Purification and characterization of human liver beta-galactosidase from a patient with the adult form of G_{M1}-gangliosidosis and a normal control. Biochim Biophys Acta 1988;964:244–253.

83. Van der Horst GT, Kleijer WJ, Hoogeveen AT, et al. Morquio B syndrome: A primary defect in beta-galactosidase. Am J Med Genet 1983;16:261–275.

84. Öckerman P.A. A generalized storage disorder resembling Hurler's-syndrome. Lancet 1967;2:239–241.

85. Kawai H, Nishino H, Nishida Y, et al. Skeletal muscle pathology of mannosidosis in two siblings with spastic paraplegia. Acta Neuropathol (Berl) 1985;68:201–204.

86. Autio S, Louhimo T, Helenius M. The clinical course of mannosidosis. Ann Clin Res 1982;14:93–97.

87. Patton MA, Barnes IC, Young ID, et al. Mannosidosis in two brothers: Prolonged survival in the severe phenotype. Clin Genet 1982;22:284–289.

88. Noll RB, Kulkarni R, Netzloff ML. Follow-up of language and cognitive development in patients with mannosidosis. Arch Neurol 1986;43:157–159.

89. Press OW, Fingert H, Lott IT, et al. Pancytopenia in mannosidosis. Arch Intern Med 1983;143:1266–1268.

90. Weiss SW, Kelly WD. Bilateral destructive synovitis associated with alpha mannosidase deficiency. Am J Surg Pathol 1983;7:487–494.

91. Carpenter S, Karpati G. Lysosomal storage in human skeletal muscle. Hum Pathol 1986;17:683–703.

92. Halperin JJ, Landis DM, Weinstein LA, et al. Communicating hydrocephalus and lysosomal inclusions in mannosidosis. Arch Neurol 1984;41:777–779.

93. Alroy J, Orgad U, Ucci AA, et al. Identification of glycoprotein storage diseases by lectins: A new diagnostic method. J Histochem Cytochem 1984;32:1280–1284.

94. Will A, Cooper A, Hatton C, et al. Bone marrow transplantation in the treatment of alpha-mannosidosis. Arch Dis Child 1987;62:1044–1049.

95. Shaw DJ, Brook JD, Meredith AL, et al. Gene mapping and chromosome 19. J Med Genet 1986;23:2–10.

96. Warren CD, Alroy J, Bugge B, et al. Oligosaccharides from placenta: Early diagnosis of feline mannosidosis. FEBS Lett 1986;195:247–252.

97. Walkley SU, James LF. Locoweed-induced neuronal storage disease characterized by meganeurite formation. Brain Res 1984;324:145–150.

98. Cenci di Bello I, Dorling P, Winchester B. The storage products in genetic and swainsonine-induced human mannosidosis. Biochem J 1983;215:693–696.

99. Tulsiani DR, Touster O. Swainsonine, a potent mannosidase inhibitor, elevates rat liver and brain lysosomal alpha-D-mannosidase, decreases Golgi alpha-D-mannosidase II, and increases the plasma levels of several acid hydrolases. Arch Biochem Biophys 1983;224:594–600.

100. Walkley SU, Siegel DA, Wurzelmann S. Ectopic dendritogenesis and associated synapse formation in swainsonine-induced neuronal storage disease. J Neurosci 1988;8:445–457.

101. Walkley SU, Wurzelmann S, Siegel DA. Ectopic axon hillock-associated neurite growth is maintained in metabolically reversed swainsonine-induced neuronal storage disease. Brain Res 1987;410:89–96.

102. Jones MZ, Dawson G. Caprine beta-mannosidosis. J Biol Chem 1981;256:5185–5188.

103. Jones MZ, Laine RA. Caprine oligosaccharide storage disease. J Biol Chem 1981;256:5181–5184.

104. Cooper A, Sardharwalla IB, Roberts MM. Human beta-mannosidase deficiency. N Engl J Med 1986;315:1231.

105. Wenger DA, Sujansky E, Fennessey PV, et al. Human beta-mannosidase deficiency. N Engl J Med 1986;315:1201–1205.

106. Dorland L, Duran M, Hoefnagels FE, et al. Beta-mannosidosis in two brothers with hearing loss. J Inherited Metab Dis 1988;11:255–258.

107. Jones MZ, Cunningham JG, Dade AW, et al. Caprine beta-mannosidosis. In: Desnick RF, Patterson DF, Scarpelli DG, eds. Animal Models of Inherited Metabolic Diseases. New York: Liss, 1982:165–176.

108. Jones MZ, Cunningham JG, Dade AW, et al. Caprine beta-mannosidosis: Clinical and pathological features. J Neuropathol Exp Neurol 1983;42:268–285.

109. Lovell KL, Jones MZ. Axonal and myelin lesions in beta-mannosidosis: ultrastructural characteristics. Acta Neuropathol (Berl) 1985;65:293–299.

110. Malachowski JA, Jones MZ. Beta-mannosidosis: lesions of the distal peripheral nervous system. Acta Neuropathol (Berl) 1983;61:95–100.

111. Cooper A, Hatton C, Sardharwalla IB. Acid beta-mannosidase of human plasma: Influence of age and sex on enzyme activity. J Inherited Metab Dis 1987;10:229–233.

112. Cooper A, Hatton C, Thornley M, et al. Human beta-mannosidase deficiency: Biochemical findings in plasma, fibroblasts, white cells and urine. J Inherited Metab Dis 1988;11:17–29.

113. Panday RS, van Diggelen OP, Kleijer WJ, et al. Beta-Mannosidase in human leukocytes and fibroblasts. J Inherited Metab Dis 1984;7:155–156.

114. Jones MZ, Rathke EJ, Cavanagh K, et al. Beta-mannosidosis: Prenatal biochemical and morphological characteristics. J Inherited Metab Dis 1984;7:80–85.

115. Christomanou H, Beyer D. Absence of alpha-fucosidase activity in two sisters showing a different phenotype. Eur J Pediatr 1983;140:27–29.

116. Willems PJ, Garcia CA, De Smedt MC, et al. Intrafamilial variability in fucosidosis. Clin Genet 1988;34:7–14.

117. Ikeda S, Kondo, Oguchi K, et al. Adult fucosidosis: Histochemical and ultrastructural studies of rectal mucosa biopsy. Neurology 1984;34:451–456.

118. Blitzer MG, Sutton M, Miller JB, et al. A thermolabile variant of alpha-L-fucosidase—clinical and laboratory findings. Am J Med Genet 1985;20:535–539.

119. Holmes RC, Fensom AH, McKee P, et al. Angiokeratoma corporis diffusum in a patient with normal enzyme activities. J Am Acad Dermatol 1984;10:384–387.

120. Lee FA, Donnell GN. Radiographic features of fucosidosis. Pediatr Radiol 1977;5:204–208.

121. DiCioccio RA, Barlow JJ, Matta KL. Specific activity of alpha-L-fucosidase in sera with phenotypes of either low, intermediate, or high total enzyme activity and in a fucosidosis serum. Biochem Genet 1986;24:115–130.

122. Sewell AC, Gehler J, Docktor G. Low fibroblast fucosidase activity: False-positive diagnosis of fucosidosis in a patient with pseudohypoparathyroidism. J Inherited Metab Dis 1987;10:197–198.

123. Johnson K, Dawson G. Molecular defect in processing alpha-fucosidase in fucosidosis. Biochem Biophys Res Commun 1985;133:90–97.

124. Fukushima H, de Wet JR, O'Brien JS. Molecular cloning of a cDNA for human alpha-L-fucosidase. Proc Natl Acad Sci USA 1985;82:1262–1265.

125. Darby JK, Willems RJ, Nakashima P, et al. Restriction analysis of the structural alpha-L-fucosidase gene and its linkage to fucosidosis. Am J Hum Genet 1988;43:749–755.

126. O'Brien JS, Willems PJ, Fukushima H, et al. Molecular biology of the alpha-L-fucosidase gene and fucosidosis. Enzyme 1987;38:45–53.

127. Barker C, Dell A, Rogers M, et al. Canine alpha-L-fucosidase in relation to the enzymic defect and storage products in canine fucosidosis. Biochem J 1988;254:861–868.

128. Taylor RM, Farrow BR, Stewart GJ, et al. The clinical effects of lysosomal enzyme replacement by bone marrow transplantation after total lymphoid irradiation on neurologic disease in fucosidase deficient dogs. Transplant Proc 1988;20:89–93.

129. Aula P, Autio S, Raivio KO, et al. Aspartylglucosaminuria. In: Durand P, O'Brien JS, eds. Genetic Errors of Glycoprotein Metabolism. New York: Springer-Verlag, 1982:123–152.

130. Aula P, Renlund M, Raivio KO, et al. Screening of inherited oligosaccharidurias among mentally retarded patients in northern Finland. J Ment Defic Res 1986;30:365–368.

131. Rudy JL. Aspartylglycosaminuria diagnosed by routine urine amino acid assay. Clin Chem 1988;34:2164.

132. Monoen I, Kaartinen V, Mononen T. Amniotic fluid glycoasparagines in fetal aspartylglycosaminuria. J Inherited Metab Dis 1988;11:194–198.

133. Schulz R, Vogt J, Voss W, et al. Mucolipidosis type II (I-cell disease) with unusually severe heart involvement. Monatsschr Kinderheilkd 1987;135:708–711.

134. Whelan DT, Chang PL, Cockshott PW. Mucolipidosis II. The clinical, radiological and biochemical features in three cases. Clin Genet 1983;24:90–96.

135. Okada S, Owada M, Sakiyama T, et al. I-cell disease: Clinical studies of 21 Japanese cases. Clin Genet 1985;28:207–215.

136. Kamiya M, Tada T, Kuhara H, et al. I-cell disease. A case report and review of the literature. Acta Pathol Jpn 1986;36:1679–1692.

137. Anneren G, Gustavson KH. Partial trisomy 3q (3q25→qter) syndrome in two siblings. Acta Paediatr Scand 1984;73:281–284.

138. Babcock DS, Bove KE, Hug G, et al. Fetal mucolipidosis II (I-cell disease): Radiologic and pathologic correlation. Pediatr Radiol 1986;16:32–39.

139. Martin JJ, Leroy JG, van Eygen M, et al. I-cell disease. A further report on its pathology. Acta Neuropathol (Berl) 1984;64:234–242.

140. Endo H, Miyazaki T, Asano S, et al. Ultrastructural studies of the skin and cultured fibroblasts in I-cell disease. J Cutan Pathol 1987;14:309–317.

141. Mueller OT, Little LE, Miller AL, et al. I-cell disease and pseudo-Hurler polydystrophy: Heterozygote detection and characteristics of the altered N-acetylglucosaminylphosphotransferase in genetic variants. Clin Chim Acta 1985;150:175–183.

142. Parenti G, Willemsen R, Hoogeveen AT, et al. Immunocytochemical localization of lysosomal acid phosphatase in normal and "I-cell" fibroblasts. Eur J Cell Biol 1987;43:121–127.

143. Aerts JM, Schram AW, Strijland A, et al. Glucocerebrosidase, a lysosomal enzyme that does not undergo oligosaccharide phosphorylation. Biochim Biophys Acta 1988;964:303–308.

144. Okada S, Inui K, Furukawa M, et al. Biochemical heterogeneity in I-cell disease. Sucrose-loading test classifies two distinct subtypes. Enzyme 1987;38:267–272.

145. Ben Yoseph Y, Pack BA, Mitchell DA, et al. Characterization of the mutant N-acetylglucosaminylphosphotransferase in I-cell disease and pseudo-Hurler polydystrophy: Complementation analysis and kinetic studies. Enzyme 1986;35:106–116.

146. Ben Yoseph Y, Potier M, Mitchell DA, et al. Altered molecular size of N-acetylglucosamine 1-phosphotransferase in I-cell disease and pseudo-Hurler polydystrophy. Biochem J 1987;248:697–701.

147. Little LE, Mueller OT, Honey NK, et al. Heterogeneity of N-acetylglucosamine 1-phosphotransferase within mucolipidosis III. J Biol Chem 1986;261:733–738.

148. Amir N, Zlotogora J, Bach G. Mucolipidosis type IV: Clinical spectrum and natural history. Pediatrics 1987;79:953–959.

149. Caimi L, Tettamanti G, Berra B, et al. Mucolipidosis IV, a sialolipidosis due to ganglioside sialidase deficiency. J Inherited Metab Dis 1982;5:218–224.

150. Riedel KG, Zwaan J, Kenyon KR, et al. Ocular abnormalities in mucolipidosis IV. Am J Ophthalmol 1985;99:125–136.

151. Goebel HH, Kohlschutter A, Lenard HG. Morphologic and chemical biopsy findings in mucolipidosis IV. Clin Neuropathol 1982;1:73–82.

152. Lake BD, Milla PJ, Taylor DS, et al. A mild variant of mucolipidosis type 4 (ML4). Birth Defects 1982;18:391–404.

153. Bargal R, Bach G. Phospholipids accumulation in mucolipidosis IV cultured fibroblasts. J Inherited Metab Dis 1988;11:144–150.

154. Zeigler M, Bach G. Ganglioside sialidase distribution in mucolipidosis type IV cultured fibroblasts. Arch Biochem Biophys 1985;241:602–607.

155. Zeigler M, Bach G. Internalization of exogenous gangliosides in cultured skin fibroblasts for the diagnosis of mucolipidosis IV. Clin Chim Acta 1986;157:183–189.

156. Aula P, Autio S, Raivio KO, et al. Salla disease. A new lysosomal storage disorder. Arch Neurol 1979;36:88–94.

157. Tondeur M, Libert J, Vamos E, et al. Infantile form of sialic acid storage disorder: clinical, ultrastructural, and biochemical studies in two siblings. Eur J Pediatr 1982;139:142–147.

158. Renlund M, Aula P, Raivio KO, et al. Salla disease: A new lysosomal storage disorder with disturbed sialic acid metabolism. Neurology 1983;33:57–66.

159. Renlund M. Clinical and laboratory diagnosis of Salla disease in infancy and childhood. J Pediatr 1984;104:232–236.

160. Gahl WA. Disorders of lysosomal membrane transport—cystinosis and Salla disease. Enzyme 1987;38:154–160.

161. Renlund M, Tietze F, Gahl WA. Defective sialic acid egress from isolated fibroblast lysosomes of patients with Salla disease. Science 1986;232:759–762.

162. Ylitalo V, Hagberg B, Rapola J, et al. Salla disease variants. Sialoylaciduric encephalopathy with increased sialidase activity in two non-Finnish children. Neuropediatrics 1986;17:44–47.

163. Baumkotter K, Cantz M, Mendla K, et al. N-Acetylneuraminic acid storage disease. Hum Genet 1985;71:155–159.

164. Tietze F, Renlund M, Harper G, et al. Characteristics of lysosomal free sialic acid transport, defective in infantile free sialic acid storage disease. Am J Hum Genet 1986;39:A21–A21.

Chapter 6
Disorders of Lipid Metabolism

Roscoe O. Brady

The disorders of lipid metabolism considered in this chapter consist of the heritable metabolic conditions called sphingolipidoses. Each of these diseases is characterized by the accumulation of a member of the class of lipids known as sphingolipids. The long-chain amino alcohol sphingosine [$CH_3-(CH_2)_{12}-CH=CH-CH(OH)-CH(NH_2)-CH_2OH$] is a constant portion of the structure of the accumulating substances. A long-chain fatty acid is linked by an amide bond to the nitrogen atom on carbon 2 of sphingosine in all of these lipids forming a chemical unit called ceramide. In each of the 10 known sphingolipid storage disorders except Farber disease, in which ceramide itself is the major accumulating substance, various sugars or phosphocholine are linked to carbon atom 1 of the sphingosine moiety of ceramide. Each of these disorders is characterized by insufficient activity of a specific hydrolytic enzyme that initiates the catabolism of the stored lipid. Abbreviated structures of the accumulating lipids, their immediate precursors, and the sites of enzymatic deficiencies are indicated in Figures 6.1 and 6.2. The accumulating lipids arise from normal turnover of cells and, in particular, from cell membranes where sphingolipids are major components. Knowledge of the enzymatic lesions in the sphingolipidoses has led to the development of important practical tests for the diagnosis of patients; the identification of heterozygous carriers; and the prenatal detection of these disorders. Present investigations are centered mainly on identifying the mutations that have occurred in the genes of the involved enzymes and the development of therapy for patients with these conditions.

Because this text is concerned with pediatric patients with nervous system damage, descriptions of some of the subtypes of sphingolipid storage disorders like Gaucher disease type 1 and Niemann-Pick disease type B, in which there is no apparent involvement of the central or peripheral nervous systems, have not been included in this presentation. For simplicity, I have chosen to indicate in a temporal format when the clinical manifestations of lipid storage disorders occur. As a further diagnostic aid, patients have been subdivided into those with hepatosplenomegaly along with nervous system involvement and other forms in which organomegaly is not apparent.

DISORDERS WITH ORGANOMEGALY MANIFESTING EARLY IN INFANCY

Niemann-Pick Type A (Classic Infantile) Disease

The principal manifestations of this disorder are hepatosplenomegaly, foam cells in the bone marrow, and delay or arrest of mental and motor development (Figure 6.3). Vision becomes progressively impaired. Some patients have a cherry-red spot in the macula, but it is not a constant feature and is not specific for this condition. Foamy histiocytes that are said to have a mulberry appearance are present in marrow biopsy specimens or aspirates. The lungs frequently become diffusely infiltrated. These patients have a progressively downhill neurologic course characterized by

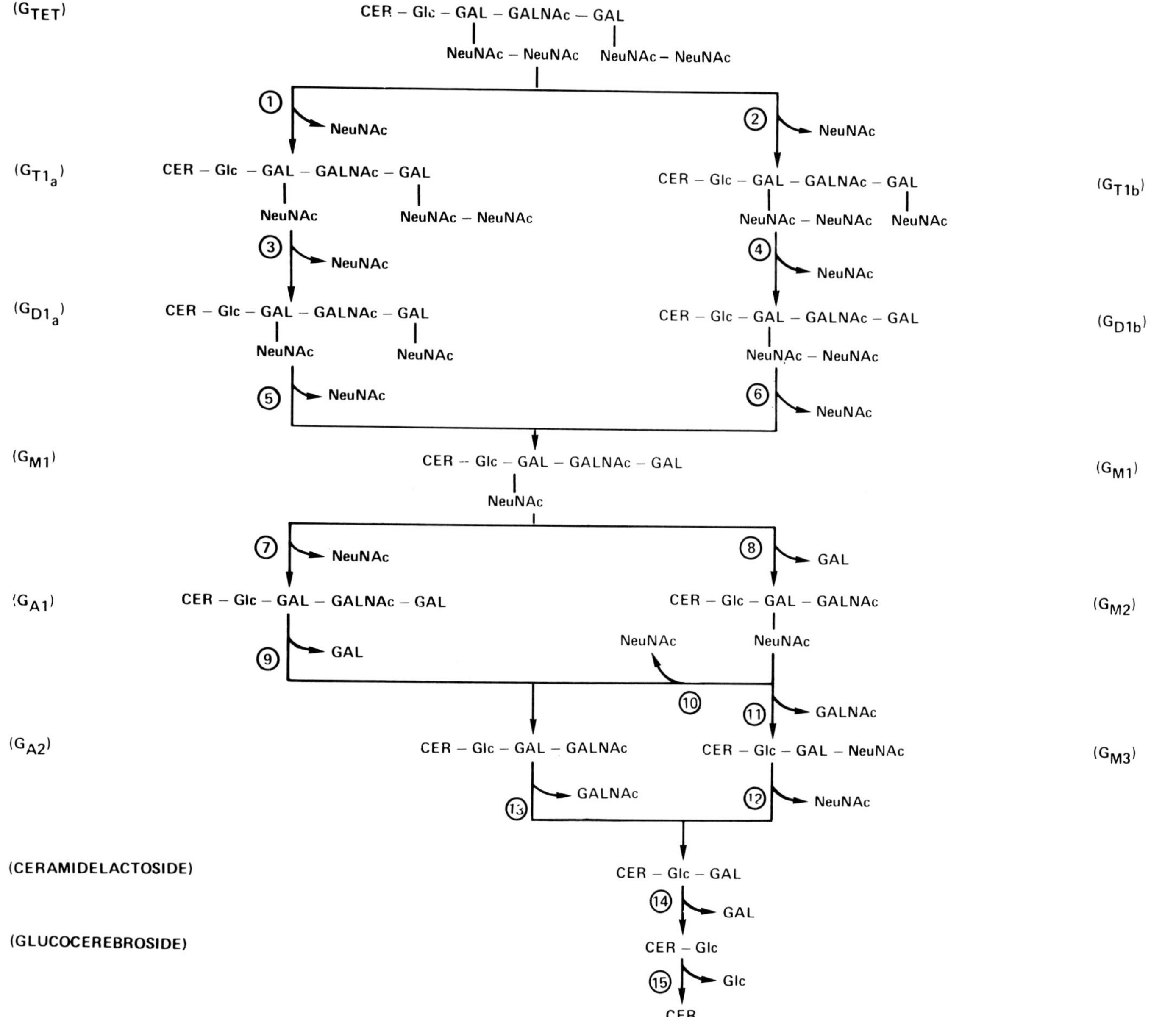

FIGURE 6.1 Pathways of ganglioside catabolism. Sphingolipid designations in parentheses are according to Svennerholm (1). CER = ceramide; Glc = glucose; GAL = galactose; GALNAc = N-acetylgalactosamine; NeuNAc = N-acetylneuraminic acid (sialic acid). The numbers within circles indicate reactions catalyzed by sphingolipid hydrolases.

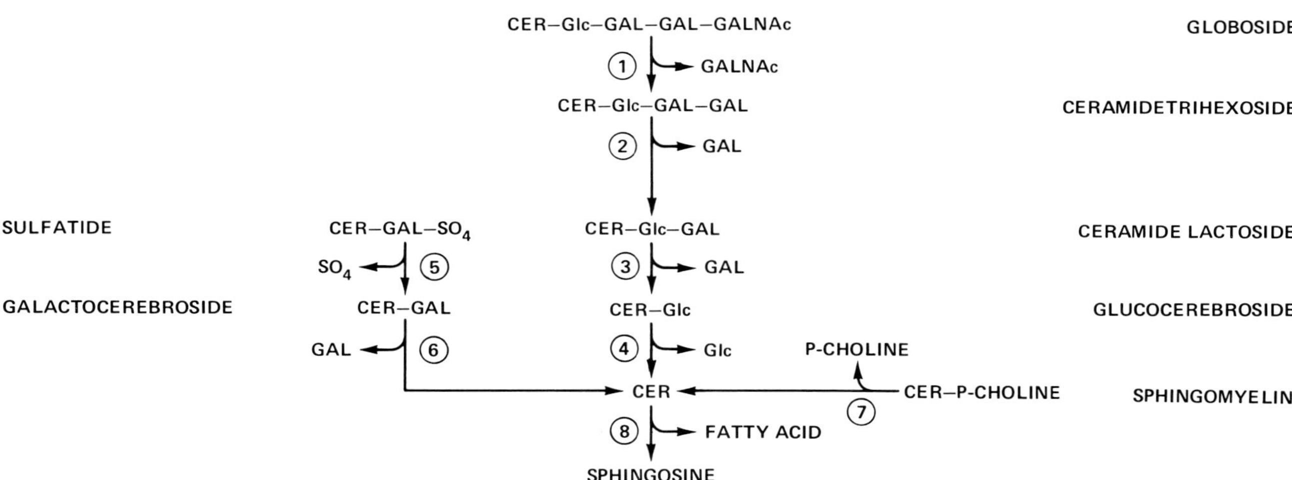

FIGURE 6.2 Pathways involved in the catabolism of neutral sphingoglycolipids (center); sulfoglycolipid (sulfatide) (left); and phosphosphingolipid (sphingomyelin) (right). Abbreviations are the same as in Figure 6.1. P-choline = phosphocholine. The numbers within circles indicate reactions catalyzed by sphingolipid hydrolases.

hypotonicity and flaccidity. Many, but certainly not all, of these patients are of Ashkenazic Jewish ancestry.

There is a large accumulation of sphingomyelin in the liver, spleen, lungs, lymph nodes, and adrenal medulla in these infants as a result of a drastic reduction in the activity of the enzyme sphingomyelinase (See Figure 6.2, Reaction 7). Along with sphingomyelin in these tissues, there is frequently an increased quantity of unesterified cholesterol as well as bis(monoacylglycerol) phosphate (Figure 6.4). The latter lipid is believed to be a characteristic component of lysosomal membranes (2,3). Less dramatic increases of other sphingolipids also occur (4).

The diagnosis of Niemann-Pick type A disease should be suspected when there is an early appearance of hepatosplenomegaly, delay in mental development, and the presence of foam cells in the bone marrow. Accurate confirmatory tests are available using radioactive sphingomyelin or the chromogenic analog of sphingomyelin, 2-N-hexadecanoylamino-4-nitrophenylphosphocholine to assay sphingomyelinase activity (5). The latter substrate is particularly useful because it is water-soluble and does not require radioisotope counting equipment. Leukocytes or cultured skin fibroblasts are most frequently used as source material, although biopsy specimens of organs such as the liver have also been used.

No specific therapy is available for Niemann-Pick type A disease. Small quantities of sphingomyelinase have been isolated from several human tissues and urine, but no enzyme replacement trials have been undertaken. One

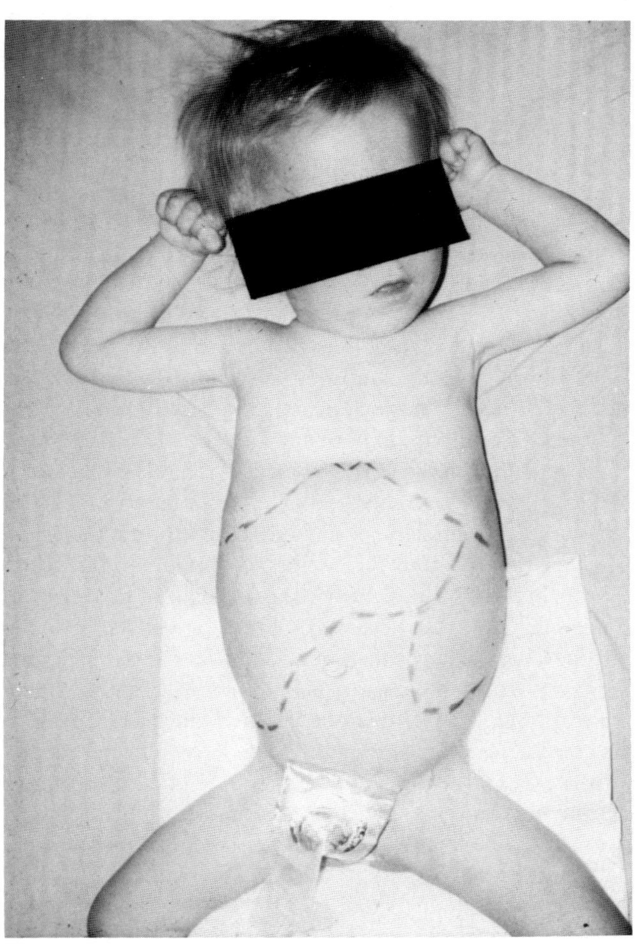

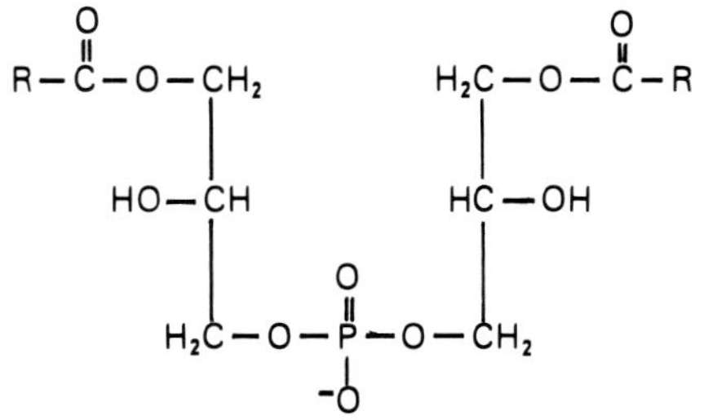

FIGURE 6.3 Patient with Niemann-Pick type A disease.

$$R-\overset{\overset{\text{O}}{\|}}{C}-O-CH_2 \qquad H_2C-O-\overset{\overset{\text{O}}{\|}}{C}-R$$
$$HO-CH \qquad\qquad HC-OH$$
$$H_2C-O-\overset{\overset{\text{O}}{\|}}{\underset{\underset{\text{O}}{|}}{P}}-O-CH_2$$

FIGURE 6.4 Structure of bis(monoacylglycerol) phosphate that accumulates in parenchymal organs of patients with Niemann-Pick disease.

patient received a liver transplantation that was said to have provided some benefit, but the survival of the recipient was not prolonged (6). A report of benefit in a patient with Niemann-Pick type B (nonneuronopathic) disease from subcutaneous implantation of chorionic membrane has appeared (7); the lack of success of such an approach in patients with mucopolysaccharidoses (8,9), however, makes one skeptical of the applicability of this strategy, especially when the central nervous system (CNS) is involved. Another approach under consideration is bone marrow transplantation, which has been reported to be effective in Niemann-Pick type B disease (10). Attempts have been made to alleviate a number of neurogenetic disorders by this approach. Except for some possible indication of benefit in metachromatic leukodystrophy (11), however, and a questionable effect on psychometric performance in Gaucher type 3 disease (12) (vide infra), little, if any, convincing evidence has been forthcoming of effectiveness of bone marrow transplantation for patients with sphingolipid storage disorders that involve the nervous system.

The gene for sphingomyelinase has been localized on human chromosome 11 by analysis of somatic cell hybrids (13). Reports are beginning to appear concerning the molecular mutations in this disorder, and the gene has been cloned.

Generalized (G_{m1}) Gangliosidosis

A second disorder of sphingolipid metabolism characterized by early onset of hepatosplenomegaly, foam cells in the bone marrow, and mental retardation is generalized gangliosidosis. This disorder is also called G_{m1}-gangliosidosis because the principal accumulating lipid in this condition is ganglioside G_{m1} (See Figure 6.1). About half of these patients have a cherry-red spot in the macula. These infants are hypotonic, have coarse facies, and nonpitting edema of the extremities. Skeletal deformations may cause kyphoscoliosis. The patients may exhibit macroglossia and hirsutism. Vacuolated lymphocytes have been reported in the blood of these infants.

The disorder is caused by a dramatic deficiency of the beta-galactosidase that catalyzes the initial step in the catabolism of G_{m1} (See Figure 6.1, Reaction 8). Excessive quantities of G_{m1} appear in the brain and in the liver. Lesser increases occur in other organs. The reduction of beta-galactosidase activity also provides an explanation for the accumulation of galactose-terminated glycoproteins that occurs in these patients. In addition, there is a marked increase in the quantity of oligosaccharides in the urine.

The diagnosis of G_{m1}-gangliosidosis may be readily confirmed by measuring beta-galactosidase activity in leukocytes, cultured skin fibroblasts, or specimens of other tissues. The fluorogenic compound 4-methylumbelliferyl-β-*D*-galactopyranoside and the chromogenic substrate

p-nitrophenyl-β-*D*-galactopyranoside are generally used for these assays.

There is no specific treatment for this disorder. Although beta-galactosidase has been isolated from human placenta and various bovine tissues (14), no reports of enzyme-replacement trials have appeared. The gene for human beta-galactosidase has been localized on the small arm of chromosome 3, and a portion of the gene has been cloned (15). Gene replacement has not yet been attempted.

Gaucher Disease Type 2 (Acute Neuronopathic)

Hepatosplenomegaly may be apparent soon after birth in patients with this disorder. The majority of these patients are brought to pediatricians' attention between the 3rd and 6th months of life, however. The abdomen may be greatly protruding because of enlargement of the spleen and liver. There are also a number of signs of CNS damage, including difficulty in sucking and swallowing, neck rigidity with retroflexion, and other indications of retarded psychomotor development. Cranial nerves may be affected, causing strabismus, facial weakness, and dysphagia. Hypertonicity and hyperactive reflexes give way to flaccidity and unresponsiveness. Some of these infants have seizures. These patients generally die between the 1st and 2nd year from complications like pneumonia.

In contrast with the high frequency of the occurrence of Gaucher type 1 disease, in which the CNS is not involved. Gaucher type 2 disease is a rarely encountered disorder. There is no ethnic predilection for Gaucher type 2 disease; whereas, Gaucher type 1 disease is the predominant genetic disorder in individuals of Ashkenazic Jewish ancestry.

Both forms of Gaucher disease are caused by insufficient glucocerebrosidase activity (See Figure 6.1, Reaction 15; Figure 6.2, Reaction 4). Note that these are not separate enzymes, but the metabolic schemes are drawn separately to reflect the various lipid precursors of the accumulating glucocerebroside. There appears to be less residual glucocerebrosidase activity in patients with Gaucher type 2 than in those with type 1 (16,17). The deficit leads to the accumulation of glucocerebroside in most organs resulting in organomegaly and damage and loss of neurons in the brain. It is generally presumed that the accumulating glucocerebroside in the CNS arises from the turnover of gangliosides (See Figure 6.1) that occurs at a rapid rate in the neonatal period. Glucocerebroside that accumulates in parenchymal organs most likely arises from the turnover of cell membrane sphingolipids. Most of the stored glucocerebroside in the spleen and liver is thought to be derived from erythrocytorrhexis and leukocytorrhexis (18). Brain damage may be augmented by the accumulation of significant, but lesser, amounts of glycosylsphingosine (glucopsychosine) (19). Rather than being produced by a catabolic reaction, this compound appears to arise from the transfer of glucose to sphingosine from uridine diphosphoglucose (UDP-glucose). The hydrolysis of glucosylsphingosine is catalyzed by glucocerebrosidase, but the reaction with psychosine is much less rapid than that with glucocerebroside (20). A detailed discussion of the biology of Gaucher disease is available (21).

Gaucher type 2 disease can usually be suspected from the signs and symptoms listed. There are characteristic "crumpled silk" foam cells in the bone marrow, and serum acid phosphatase is usually above normal. The diagnosis can be readily confirmed by measuring glucocerebrosidase activity in leukocytes, cultured skin fibroblasts, or in tissue biopsy specimens (22). The fluorogenic analog 4-methylumbelliferyl-β-D-glucopyranoside is used most frequently. However, the chromogenic analog 2-hexadecanoyl-amino-4-nitrophenyl-β-D-glucopyranoside has also been used successfully (23, 24).

Molecular Biology

The gene for glucocerebrosidase is on the long arm of chromosome 1 in the region q21-q23 (25), and has been cloned by several groups (26–28). A point mutation resulting in a single base substitution has been described in Gaucher type 2 disease (29). This mutation causes a change in the amino-acid sequence at position 444 of glucocerebrosidase, whereby a molecule of proline is substituted for the normal leucine at this position. This mutation was claimed to be specific for Gaucher type 2 disease; however, later studies disproved this contention. The same mutation also occurs in Jewish patients with Gaucher disease who do not have CNS damage (Gaucher type 1 disease) (30). Furthermore, a different base substitution was identified in cloned complementary DNA derived from another patient with Gaucher type 2 disease. The mutation in the latter case was a change of the amino acid from proline to arginine at position 415 (30). Because of the large variability in clinical presentations, particularly of Gaucher type 1 disease, it is anticipated that a considerable number of point mutations will be discovered in the glucocerebrosidase gene. It remains to be determined whether the majority of deleterious mutations occurs near the catalytic site that is near the carboxy terminus of the enzyme that includes amino-acid residues 429–465 (31).

It is of more than theoretical interest to identify the alterations in the gene for metabolic storage disorders like Gaucher and other diseases. One of the principal advantages of the acquisition of this information is the possibility for additional diagnostic procedures, particularly with regard to improved ability to detect heterozygotes. There are two principal approaches to this goal. The first is the identification of restriction fragment length polymorphisms (RFLPs). Here, the DNA derived from cells such as lymphocytes or cultured skin fibroblasts is isolated and treated with enzymes that cut the DNA into characteristic fragments that can be identified on polyacrylamide gels. If a specific mutation has occurred, changing the bases of the DNA so that the restriction enzymes can no longer react at

certain sites of the DNA, a change in the pattern will be seen. The change(s) may be indicative of the particular mutation that is associated with patient phenotypes. These changes would be helpful in assessing the presence of the mutation in the gene for glucocerebrosidase (and other enzymes in other conditions) on one of the carrier's chromosomes. In the case of affected individuals, except for the X-linked disorder, Fabry disease, in which only the mother need be a carrier to have an affected (hemizygous) son, the RFLP would be seen on both of the chromosomes if both parents have the same allelic mutation. Clearly, patients exist in whom more than a single mutation has occurred (genetic compounds). Investigation of RFLPs may still be helpful in the latter situation.

Another potentially helpful diagnostic procedure may result from identification of the specific base change that has occurred in affected individuals. In this instance, one can construct labeled oligonucleotide probes that will react (hybridize) with DNA specimens only if they contain the mutation. The hybridization can be detected by radioautography or more recently developed chromogenic procedures. This technology is used extensively to diagnose patients and carriers with certain forms of beta-thalassemia in which specific mutations have been demonstrated. Such nucleotide hybridization can also provide for carrier detection.

Treatment

There has been no report of successful treatment for patients with Gaucher type 2 disease. Although enzyme replacement is very effective for Gaucher type 1 disease (32) and the human glucocerebrosidase gene has been cloned, replacing these factors appears to be extraordinarily formidable in conditions like Gaucher type 2 disease in which the CNS is so extensively involved. In like manner, it is uncertain whether bone marrow transplantation will be beneficial. This latter approach is discussed further in the section on Gaucher type 3 disease because several patients with Gaucher disease with CNS damage appearing after infancy have received a bone marrow transplant.

DISORDERS MANIFESTING BETWEEN 3 AND 6 MONTHS OF AGE WITH MINIMAL OR MODERATE ORGANOMEGALY

Sandhoff Disease (the O-Variant Form of Tay-Sachs Disease)

Infants with this condition exhibit many of the clinical features of the more common classic (B-variant) form of Tay-Sachs disease (vide infra). Patients with the O-variant form are generally considered to have a slightly earlier onset of signs and symptoms associated with this disorder than do patients with the B-variant form. O-variant infants may have a normal appearance in the very early months. Developmental milestones including sitting and crawling are not met or lost. The patients exhibit a startle reaction to sharp sounds, and they have a cherry-red spot in the macula. Progression of mental deterioration is characterized by inattention to the environment, loss of vision, hypotonicity, and seizures. The liver may be slightly enlarged, but splenomegaly is rare. Neurons in the CNS are filled with multilamellated membranous cytoplasmic bodies, and vacuolated histiocytes occur in the liver. In contrast with classic B-variant Tay-Sachs disease, a disorder of unusually high frequency in infants of Ashkenazic Jewish extraction, Sandhoff disease is panethnic. By and large, patients with Sandhoff disease expire considerably earlier than do infants with conventional Tay-Sachs disease.

The enzymatic defect in Sandhoff disease is a total lack of hexosaminidase activity in the patient's tissues. Human tissues, leukocytes, and serum contain two isozymes of hexosaminidase termed *hexosaminidase A (Hex A)* and *hexosaminidase B (Hex B)*. Hex A is composed of separate polypeptide chains called alpha and beta. Beta-chain fragments may not be completely identical and have been termed β_a and β_b. Thus, Hex A is considered to have the composition $\alpha\beta_a\beta_b$. Hex B is generally represented as $2(\beta_a\beta_b)$. The gene for the alpha chain is on chromosome 15, whereas the gene for the beta chain is on chromosome 5. Hex A is necessary for the enzymatic cleavage of the terminal molecule of N-acetylgalactosamine from ganglioside G_{m2} (See Figure 6.1, Reaction 11). A smaller, heat-stable protein called an *activator* or *cohydrolase* is also required for this reaction (33). This cohydrolase is believed to function as a carrier protein that transfers membrane-bound ganglioside G_{m2} to Hex A for enzymatic cleavage of N-acetylgalactosamine (Figure 6.5). Mutations of the gene for the beta-chain(s) have occurred in Sandhoff disease; therefore, neither functional Hex A nor Hex B is present. A small amount of Hex S (α, α), a catalytically ineffective molecule as far as ganglioside G_{m2} catabolism is concerned, is usually present in tissues from these patients. Because of the absence of normal Hex A there is a great accumulation of ganglioside G_{m2} in the brain of these infants. Increased amounts of ganglioside G_{m2} also occur in the liver, and to a lesser extent, in other organs. In addition, there is some evidence that deacylated ganglioside G_{m2} (lyso-G_{m2}) may be present in the brains of these patients and may contribute to neuronal damage (34).

Moreover, because of the complete absence of hexosaminidase activity, other substances that have terminal amino sugar residues accumulate in addition to ganglioside G_{m2} in patients with Sandhoff disease. Among these materials is an extraordinarily large accumulation of asialo-G_{m2} (gangliotriaosylceramide) in the brain (34). The reason for the elevated level of this substance is that an enzyme is present in both normal and Sandhoff patients' brains that can initiate the catabolism of ganglioside G_{m2} by the hydrolytic cleavage of N-acetylneuraminic acid, a molecule that is co-terminal with N-acetylgalactosamine in ganglioside G_{m2} (Figure 6.1, Reaction 10). This neuraminidase

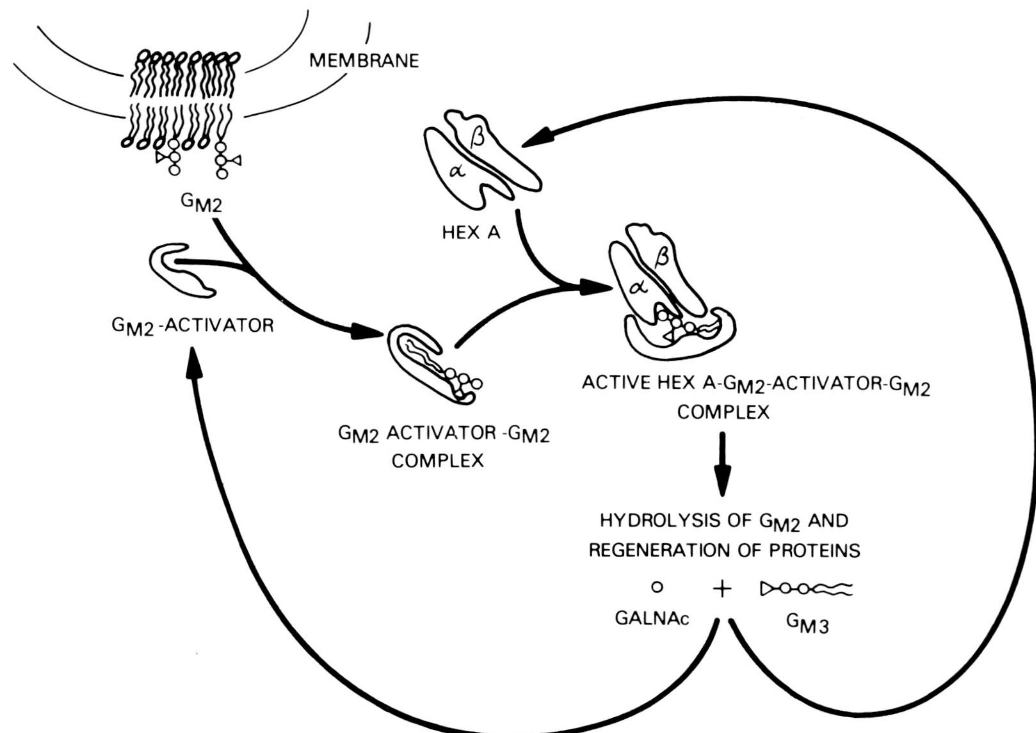

FIGURE 6.5   Schematic diagram of the enzymatic hydrolysis of ganglioside G_{m2} involving both Hex A and Hex B along with the heat-stable cofactor. GALNAc = N-acetylgalactosamine. Modified with permission from Neuropediatrics 1984;15 Suppl:85–92. (33)

(sialidase) is active normally in Sandoff and Tay-Sachs disease (35), and it can therefore catalyze the formation of asialo-G_{m2}. Hex B can catalyze the hydrolysis of asialo-G_{m2}, but the absence of this enzyme in patients with Sandhoff disease results in the accumulation of asialo-G_{m2} in the nervous system. The accumulation of asialo-G_{m2} in addition to ganglioside G_{m2}, may well augment and accelerate pathogenetic mechanisms in this disorder.

Another consequence of the total absence of hexosaminidase activity is the accumulation of globoside (See Figure 6.2) in parenchymal organs and, to a lesser extent, in the brain (34). One of the sources of globoside is erythrocytorrhexis because it is the major neutral glycolipid of red blood cell membranes. It must be catabolized when senescent erythrocytes are removed from the circulation. Hex B can initiate the catabolism of globoside (Figure 6.2, Reaction 1), and the lack of this enzyme results in a moderate elevation of this material in the blood and a much greater accumulation in organs such as the liver in patients with Sandhoff disease.

The diagnosis of Sandhoff disease is fairly straightforward. Total hexosaminidase activity is drastically reduced in the serum and in all of the patient's tissues. This activity is conveniently measured using 4-methylumbelliferyl-β-D-N-acetylglucosaminide as substrate (21). The fluorogenic N-acetylgalactosaminide derivative can also be used for this determination. However, it is not required because of the low stringency of substrate specificity of Hex A and Hex B. The galactosaminyl derivative is considerably more expensive than the N-acetylglucosaminide. Chromogenic substrates such as p-nitrophenyl-β-D-N-acetylglucosamine or p-nitrophenyl-β-D-N-acetylgalactosamine can also be used.

Therapeutic Considerations

Although no specific therapy is currently available for this disorder, some noteworthy observations were made in an investigation of the effect of infusing Hex A into a patient with this condition (36). Hex A was partially purified (6000-fold enrichment) from human urine. When the enzyme was injected intravenously into a 1-year-old girl with Sandhoff disease, it was cleared from the blood with surprising rapidity. Most of the enzyme became localized in the recipient's liver. None of the injected enzyme reached the brain. It was discovered that the amount of globoside (See Figure 6.2) in the circulation had decreased by 43% within 4 hours after infusion of Hex A. This observation indicated, for the first time, that administration of an exogenous enzyme could reduce the amount of an accumulated sphingolipid. It is part of the rationale for current investigations of enzyme replacement as specific therapy for patients with sphingolipid storage disorders.

The delivery of Hex A to the brain has been investigated extensively in experimental animals. A detectable amount of Hex A reaches the CNS when the blood-brain barrier (BBB) is temporarily modified by intracarotid infusion of hyperosmolar sugar solutions (37). However, a maximum of 1% of the intra-arterially injected Hex A reached the substance of the brain even after the BBB was modified by this procedure. Therefore, enzyme-replacement trials in humans have been precluded by the inability to deliver therapeutically realistic quantities of Hex A to the CNS. Intra-arterial infusion of protamine sulfate has been reported to alter the BBB temporarily in rabbits (38). Whether this technique will permit the delivery of larger quantities of Hex A to the brain of patients with Sandhoff disease and other metabolic disorders that involve the CNS remains to be determined.

Farber Disease (Lipogranulomatosis)

Signs of this rarely encountered sphingolipid storage disorder include hoarseness, swollen, painful joints, and nodules over affected joints and pressure points. These manifestations are accompanied by progressive aphonia, swallowing and feeding difficulties, and vomiting. The patients may be febrile as a result of pulmonary involvement. The skin, joints, larynx, and lungs are infiltrated with granulomatous material. Related accumulations also occur in neurons. Hepatomegaly may be present, but it is not a universal finding in this disorder.

The enzymatic lesion in Farber lipogranulomatosis is a deficiency of ceramidase (See Figure 6.2, Reaction 8) (39). This enzymatic reaction must be assayed under highly acidic conditions in order to demonstrate this defect. The pathogenesis of this disorder is not completely understood. Increased quantities of glycolipids and complexes of polysaccharides and of polypeptides also appear in patients' organs. Moderate accumulations of substances like glycolipids, which are not immediately involved in the deficient catabolic reaction, occur in many of the sphingolipid storage disorders. It seems particularly difficult, however, to understand the accumulation of the various nonlipid substances in Farber disease. Perhaps the excess of ceramide inhibits a plethora of lysosomal catabolic processes.

The diagnosis of Farber disease is usually confirmed by measuring ceramidase activity in extracts of cultured skin fibroblasts. Radioactive ceramide is used most frequently for this assay. No specific therapy trials have been reported.

DISORDERS WITH ONSET BETWEEN 3 AND 6 MONTHS WITHOUT ORGANOMEGALY

Tay-Sachs Disease

This disorder is probably the most frequently encountered, and certainly the most widely publicized, sphingolipid storage disorder of infancy prior to the introduction of prenatal monitoring. Patients with this condition appear normal for the first 3 to 6 months of life. After this period they begin to fail to meet neurodevelopmental milestones. The infants become listless, fail to sit up on schedule, and develop a startle reaction to sharp noises. Although they initially appear to interact with parents and environment, they gradually become detached. They become difficult to feed, lose muscle tone, and become paralyzed. Eventually they become blind, deaf, and hypertonic, and they have convulsions.

In addition to the progressive neurologic deterioration, a cardinal sign of Tay-Sachs disease is the presence of a cherry-red spot in the macula. Actually, this is the normal macular color. Neurons in the surrounding area have become distended with lipid causing compression of the retinal vessels and blanching of the region. Macrocephaly is frequently noted during the 2nd year. Many of these children are said to have an unusually fair complexion. These patients generally die from pneumonia between the 3rd and 4th year, although some may live longer.

The major accumulating lipid in the brain of patients with Tay-Sachs disease is ganglioside G_{m2} (See Figure 6.1). This accumulation is caused by insufficient activity of Hex A that catalyzes the hydrolytic cleavage of N-acetylgalactosamine from ganglioside G_{m2} (See Figure 6.1, Reaction 11) (40,41). This, the classic form of Tay-Sachs disease, is caused by deleterious mutations in the gene for the alpha-polypeptide of Hex A. As discussed in the section on Sandhoff disease, in order to enzymatically cleave N-acetylgalactosamine from ganglioside G_{m2}, Hex A containing functional alpha- and beta-polypeptide-chains is required as well as a heat-stable "activator." The activity of Hex B (beta-chains only), measured by chromogenic or fluorogenic substrates, is greatly enhanced over normal in the brains of patients with this form of Tay-Sachs disease. Because Hex B is present, and it is even more than normally active, this condition is known as the B-variant form of Tay-Sachs disease.

The diagnosis is generally made by differentially assaying Hex A and B activities with the fluorogenic substrate 4-methylumbelliferyl-β-D-N-acetylglucosamine as substrate. Total hexosaminidase activity is determined in an aliquot of serum or tissue extract. Conventionally, a separate aliquot is heated at 49°C or 50°C for 2 to 3 hours to inactivate Hex A (41). Hex B is stable under these conditions and, therefore, the hexosaminidase activity that remains after heating is attributed to Hex B. This value for Hex B is subtracted from total hexosaminidase activity to indicate the level of Hex A, which is greatly reduced from normal in this form of Tay-Sachs disease. Other methods have been developed to distinguish Hex A from Hex B including separation of these isozymes on small ion-exchange columns. The most recent diagnostic advance, however, is the use of the sulfated, fluorogenic substrate 4-methylumbelliferyl-6-sulpho-2-acetamido-2-deoxy-β-D-glucopyranoside. Hex A is catalytically much more active with this material than is Hex B, thereby providing a one-step diagnostic assay procedure (42–45).

Carrier detection of Tay-Sachs disease is a well-established procedure using serum, leukocytes, and cultured skin fibroblasts (46). The prenatal diagnosis of this disorder has been available for 2 decades by assaying Hex A activity directly in the amniotic fluid or in extracts of cultured amniocytes (46). More recently, prenatal diagnosis has been performed using chorionic villus biopsies (47). The use of the sulfated derivative of 4-methylumbelliferone with chorionic villus specimens has been reported (48,49).

Molecular Biology

Deleterious mutations have occurred in the gene coding for the alpha-chain in this form of Tay-Sachs disease rendering Hex A catalytically defective. Full-length genomic clones for both the alpha-polypeptide and beta-polypeptide have been obtained. The mutations in the alpha-polypeptide-chain gene may be expressed in several ways: in some instances, the alpha-chains are not translated from messenger RNA; mutant alpha-chains may be insoluble; alpha-chains may be labile and proteolytically destroyed; mutated alpha-chains may not associate with beta-chains; alpha-chains may not mature from the normal larger precursor gene product (50). Specific mutations and defects in alpha-polypeptide chains have been identified. An example of this phenomenon is the deletion of a large portion of the alpha-chain gene in French-Canadian patients with Tay-Sachs disease (51). Another mutation has been detected that resulted from a single base change in the alpha-chain gene causing a change of amino acids at position 178 from arginine to histidine (52). In contrast with the suspected susceptible loci near the carboxylic acid end of glucocerebrosidase in patients with Gaucher disease, the latter mutation in Tay-Sachs disease is about 90 amino acids from the amino terminus of mature hexosaminidase. This mutation does not result in reduced catalytic hexosaminidase activity when measured with fluorogenic or chromogenic substrates. The enzyme is not effective, however, with ganglioside G_{m2} or with 4-methylumbelliferyl-N-acetylglucosamine-6-sulfate.

A number of laboratories are actively searching for a (the) specific mutation that is believed to have occurred in the majority of Tay-Sachs patients of Ashkenazic Jewish ancestry. One possibility that has been reported is a substitution of a guanine by a cytidine in intron 12 of the gene for Hex A (53). Because introns are noncoding regions of the gene, this change would not be expected to cause a single amino-acid alteration in the final enzyme. Rather, it is expected that a defective splice site between exons (coding portions) of the messenger RNA leads to decreased stability of the messenger RNA. Unexpectedly, this mutation in exon 12 does not seem to be the single cause of the expression of Tay-Sachs disease even in this population at high risk. One cell line examined by the Toronto group had the G to C substitution mutation on only one chromosome, indicating that this patient was a genetic compound and that there appears to be at least one additional allelic mutation in that, and probably other, patients with Tay-Sachs disease.

No specific therapy is available. Considerations of enzyme replacement discussed in the section on Sandhoff disease are equally applicable to this form of Tay-Sachs disease.

AB-Variant of Tay-Sachs Disease

Still another clinical form of Tay-Sachs disease is characterized by the presence of both Hex A and Hex B activities when these enzymes are assayed with 4-methylumbelliferyl-N-acetylglucosaminide or p-nitrophenyl-β-D-N-acetylglucosaminide (54,55). These patients differ from patients with classic (B-variant) Tay-Sachs disease in that there is no predilection for Jewish ancestry. They do not have the cherry-red spot in their maculas. The clinical course is milder with longer preservation of alertness and vision and little, if any, optic atrophy. As in patients with the other variant forms of Tay-Sachs disease, however, these patients are also unable to catabolize ganglioside G_{m2} (56). Conzelmann and Sandhoff showed that these patients lack a functional activator protein that is required along with Hex A for the hydrolysis of ganglioside G_{m2} (57,58). I have not found a report concerning the usefulness of 4-methylumbelliferyl-6-sulpho-2-acetamido-2-deoxy-β-D-glucopyranoside as a substrate for the diagnosis of this form of Tay-Sachs disease. The gene for the human G_{m2} activator protein is on chromosome 5 (59).

Krabbe Disease (Globoid Cell Leukodystrophy)

The clinical manifestation in these patients may begin insidiously between 3 and 6 months of age with vague signs and symptoms of irritability, hyperesthesia, and some delays of psychomotor development. Tonic seizures, extensor rigidity, hyperthermia of unknown cause, deafness, and progression of motor difficulties follow. Involvement of peripheral nerves occurs, but varies in severity. Other, but variable, signs include ichthyosis, infantile obesity, weight loss, and ammoniacal breath. The optic nerves may be atrophic, and the pupils react sluggishly to light. The clinical course is characterized by progressive deterioration accompanied by flaccidity, decreased deep tendon reflexes, and blindness. Patients with the infantile form usually die during the first few years of life. In some instances, the disorder becomes apparent later in infancy. Although rare, patients with adult onset do occur whose initial manifestations are weakness, abnormal gait, and spasticity. There is no organomegaly associated with this disorder.

Cerebrospinal fluid protein is frequently increased. There is generalized atrophy of the brain by computed tomography (CT) with significant white matter disease. Magnetic resonance imaging (MRI) may be superior to CT for revealing the extent of white matter involvement (Figure 6.6). There is a severe lack of myelin, astrogliosis, and nests of "globoid cells" in perivascular regions of the white matter. Globoid cells may contain several nuclei, and they react positively with periodic acid-Schiff stain for carbohydrate.

The metabolic defect in Krabbe disease is a deficiency of the enzyme galactocerebroside-beta-galactosidase (See Figure 6.2, Reaction 6). Because of the extensive demyelination, there is generally no net accumulation of galactocerebroside in the brain. A contributing factor to the pathogenesis of Krabbe disease is considered to be the occurrence of psychosine (galactosylsphingosine; galactocerebroside without the long-chain fatty acid) in the brains of these patients, which has been reported to be increased more than 100-fold in this disorder (60). Psychosine has been demonstrated to be highly toxic to nerve cells. Its accumulation is ascribed to its formation from sphingosine

FIGURE 6.6 T-2 weighted magnetic resonance image of the brain of a patient with the late-onset form of Krabbe disease showing increased intensity in the white matter of the parieto-occipital region.

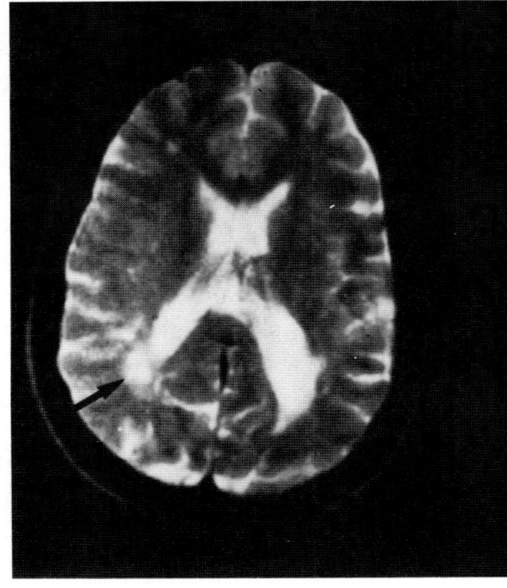
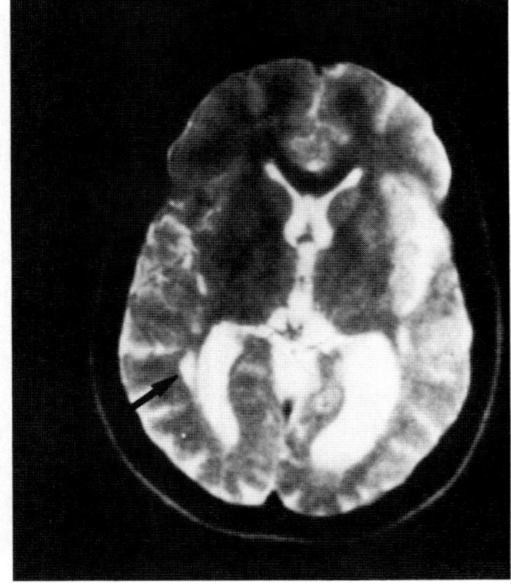

and uridine diphosphategalactose (UDP-galactose). This reaction has been demonstrated repeatedly in experimental animals. The catabolism of psychosine is catalyzed by galactocerebroside-beta-galactosidase, albeit at a much reduced rate than that with galactocerebroside. The severe deficiency of the galactocerebroside-beta-galactosidase in patients with Krabbe disease is believed to be responsible for the accumulation of psychosine.

Enzymatic tests are available to confirm the diagnosis of this disorder. Radioactively labeled galactocerebroside is most frequently employed because there are other beta-galactosidases in human tissues whose presence precludes the use of simple chromogenic or fluorogenic substrates for this assay. Chromogenic (61) and fluorogenic (62) substrates have been synthesized. However, the ease of producing radioactive galactocerebroside-[^{3}H] labeled in the galactose portion of the molecule with the enzyme galactose oxidase and the specificity provided through the use of this substrate has led to its general use for the detection of homozygotes and heterozygotes.

There is no specific treatment for Krabbe disease. Several laboratories have examined the effect of bone marrow transplantation in a murine model, the twitcher mouse (63–66). The basis for this approach is the presumption that the cells that form the globoid bodies arise from the bone marrow, and a low, but significant increase in galactocerebroside-β-galactosidase activity has been reported in the CNS following bone marrow transplantation. Bone marrow transplantation did not cure these animals, however, and its value in humans with Krabbe disease is not established.

DISORDERS WITH ONSET BETWEEN 6 MONTHS AND 2 YEARS OF AGE WITHOUT ORGANOMEGALY

Metachromatic Leukodystrophy (Infantile Form)

This disorder is one of the more common metabolic abnormalities encountered by pediatricians and pediatric neurologists. The principal manifestations are ataxia accompanied by hypotonicity and diminished deep tendon reflexes. Spasticity eventually ensues. Intellectual deterioration progresses at a variable rate. Speech is gradually lost. The optic nerve atrophies, and the macula may become gray in appearance; signs of decerebrate posturing may follow. There may be evidence of gallbladder dysfunction. Nerve-conduction velocity in peripheral nerves is frequently slowed, and this finding is important in the differential diagnosis. CT shows hypolucent white matter (Figure 6.7). Cerebrospinal fluid protein is usually increased. Granules that stain brownish yellow with cresyl violet dye (metachromasia) are frequently present in the urine.

One of the major features of metachromatic leukodystrophy is the occurrence of lipid metachromatic droplets in

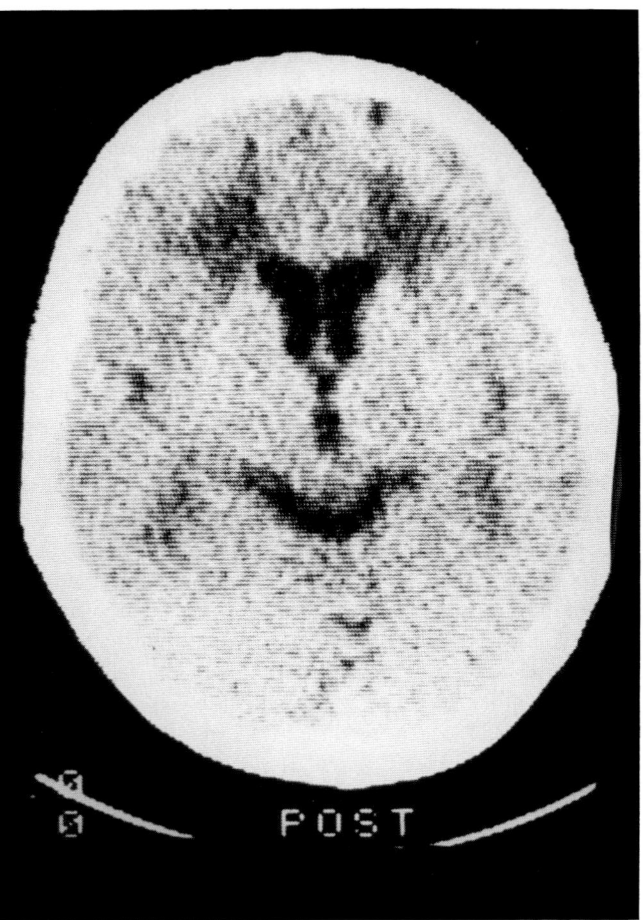

FIGURE 6.7   Computed tomography of the brain of a patient with metachromatic leukodystrophy showing attenuation of the white matter in the region of the anterior horns of the ventricles.

peripheral nerve biopsy specimens. The urinary excretion of the sphingolipid called sulfatide (See Figure 6.2) is increased in patients with this disorder. This lipid also accumulates in the central and peripheral nervous system, gallbladder, kidneys, and pancreas. The disorder is caused by a profound deficiency of the enzyme arylsulfatase A (See Figure 6.2, Reaction 5). Enzymatic activity is conveniently measured with ortho- or para-nitrophenyl or 4-methylumbelliferyl sulfate esters. Reduced arylsulfatase A activity in leukocytes, cultured skin fibroblasts, or urine substantiates the diagnosis. Homozygotes and heterozygotes can be detected with white blood cells or fibroblasts as source material for enzyme assay. Prenatal diagnosis is available using cultured amniocytes, and the use of chorionic villus biopsy is under investigation.

The hydrolysis of sulfatide requires the presence of an auxiliary protein (activator) in addition to arylsulfatase A (67). A few patients have been described that lack the activator protein rather than the enzyme itself. In this circumstance, it is necessary to use labeled sulfatide as substrate for enzyme assays to confirm the diagnosis. The activator protein for the enzymatic hydrolysis of sulfatide appears to be the same as that which participates in the hydrolysis of ganglioside G_{m1} and ceramidetrihexoside that accumulate in generalized (G_{m1}) gangliosidosis and Fabry disease, respectively (68). If this is so, and if the activator protein is the same, why then is its absence (or inactivity) manifested as metachromatic leukodystrophy rather than a diverse clinical presentation representative of all of these conditions? It is conceivable that a specific mutation has occurred in the gene for the activator that alters its amino-acid sequence so that it does not interact with sulfatide but can still assist in the catabolism of ganglioside G_{m1} and ceramidetrihexoside. Although this explanation may be valid, it is wanting if there are cases in which there is no transcription of the gene, if unstable messenger RNA is synthesized, or if a rapidly degraded activator is formed, as has been shown to be the result of mutations in many sphingolipid storage disorders.

A number of enzyme-replacement trials have been attempted in metachromatic leukodystrophy including intrathecal, intracisternal, and intracerebral injection of partially purified arylsulfatase A. Despite the demonstrated ability to correct the metabolic block in metachromatic leukodystrophy in skin fibroblasts derived from these patients through enzyme supplementation in tissue culture (69,70), none of the procedures cited produced a beneficial clinical effect. Some suggestion of benefit has been reported following bone marrow transplantation (11,71), although this has by no means been consistently observed (72,73). Because of the many hazards associated with bone marrow replacement, much substantiation must be provided before clinicians can recommend this procedure with confidence as a therapeutic measure for metachromatic leukodystrophy.

Generalized (G_{m1}) Gangliosidosis Type 2 (Juvenile Form)

There are a number of differences between the clinical manifestations of the phenotypes of generalized (G_{m1}) gangliosidosis that have been classified as type 1 (infantile) and type 2 (juvenile) forms. The onset of psychomotor difficulties is later in type 2 than in type 1. Clinical signs of the disorder progress at a somewhat slower rate. Extensive bone involvement is usually not seen, but there may be beaking of the lumbar vertebrae. Hepatosplenomegaly is usually not observed. Patients with type 2 generalized (G_{m1}) gangliosidosis present initially with ataxia, dysarthria, and weakness. These children eventually become blind, but again, later in life than the patients with type 1. I am not aware of a report of a cherry-red spot in the macula of these patients. Affected individuals may live as long as 10 years. Foamy histiocytes are present in the bone marrow, and lymphocytes are vacuolated. As in type 1 generalized (G_{m1}) gangliosidosis, there is a profound deficiency of ganglioside G_{m1} beta-galactosidase activity in the tissues of the patients

with type 2. However, slightly greater residual beta-galactosidase activity may be present in type 2 patients than in type 1 patients. It is not yet known whether this phenomenon is responsible for the pathologic differences, but such a relationship seems likely. Although beta-galactosidases have been isolated from several mammalian and human tissues, no specific treatment for this condition exists presumably because of the inability to deliver sufficient quantities of any enzyme to the nervous system at the present time. A feline analog of the human disorder has been identified, and a breeding colony has been established (74). Proper exploitation of this model may facilitate the development of therapy for humans.

ONSET BETWEEN 2 YEARS AND ADOLESCENCE WITH ORGANOMEGALY

Gaucher Type 3 Disease (Juvenile Form)

The initial signs and symptoms of this form of Gaucher disease vary considerably from early in life to the preteen years. In many of these patients, the first finding is enlargement of the spleen with a lesser degree of hepatomegaly. Gaucher cells are present in the bone marrow, and thrombocytopenia is a usual feature. Painful bone crises occur with variable frequency. Looping movements of the eyes occur with voluntary horizontal movement. Some investigators consider this sign characteristic of this form of Gaucher disease. Electroencephalographic (EEG) abnormalities may appear fairly early. Myoclonic seizures develop that may be difficult to control. Signs of brain deterioration usually begin with difficulties in performance at school. Incoordination, spasticity, and progressive mental impairment lead to loss of ambulation and confinement to bed. Patients may live a number of years after the onset of CNS damage, and the course of the clinical progression is not necessarily identical in affected siblings.

Clinicians associated with the Developmental and Metabolic Neurology Branch have proposed that there may be subtypes of this form of Gaucher disease (75). Patients in the second phenotype exhibit early, massive hepatosplenomegaly. Splenectomy has usually been required because of severe thrombocytopenia. Liver enlargement progresses rapidly and is accompanied by portal hypertension with dilated veins on the surface of the abdomen and esophageal varices that may rupture and require cauterization to arrest hemorrhaging. Extensive bone damage is also usually seen in these patients. These individuals may have a questionable or only mild degree of horizontal looping movements of the eyes, and the EEG may be normal. They generally die from hepatic failure without exhibiting the extensive brain involvement that characterizes the patient with conventional Gaucher type 3 disease.

Both of these forms of Gaucher disease are characterized by diminished glucocerebrosidase activity in all of the patients' tissues. To date, therapy has been symptomatic and includes splenectomy, cautery of esophageal varices, and use of sodium valproate for the myoclonic seizures. It is not apparent whether these patients will respond to enzyme-replacement therapy. In a sense, it may be anticipated that they may, because much of the accumulated glucocerebroside in the brain appears to reside in phagocytic cells in the Virchow-Robin spaces. It remains to be determined whether these cells will take up exogenous glucocerebrosidase and whether the stored glucocerebroside will be cleared and lead to reversal of the CNS damage.

The possibility that such patients may respond to bone marrow transplantation has been raised by two reports concerning this procedure in patients with Gaucher type 3 disease. In the first case, glucocerebrosidase activity in the donor-derived leukocytes that appeared in the blood was normal. Plasma glucocerebroside gradually declined to normal values, and the Gaucher cells gradually disappeared from the bone marrow (76). The patient never regained his ability to produce platelets, however, and he died from an overwhelming infection 13 months following the procedure. The second possibility of benefit from bone marrow transplantation stems from the report of a favorable response in a patient with a genetic isolate of Gaucher disease known as the Norrbottnian form (12). CNS damage appears to be the rule in these patients. It is not clear whether the recipient's mental status improved or, judging from psychometric testing, continued to decline (77). Thus, it is not possible to judge the effect of bone marrow transplantation on brain function in patients with Gaucher type 3 disease at this time.

Niemann-Pick Types C and D Disease

Major advances have occurred concerning our knowledge of the clinical aspects, pathogenetic mechanisms, and counseling for patients classified as having Niemann-Pick types C and D disease. This classification was proposed by Crocker in 1961 to include patients with organomegaly, mental deterioration, and a modest accumulation of sphingomyelin in the liver (78). Niemann-Pick type D disease was considered to be a subgroup of French ancestry residing in Nova Scotia with basically the same clinical presentation. The nosology of this condition was perennially hampered by the inconstant reduction of sphingomyelinase activity in patient-derived materials like leukocytes and cultured skin fibroblasts (5,79), the hallmark of Niemann-Pick types A (neuronopathic) and B (nonneuronopathic) disease. Furthermore, somatic cell hybridization indicated that the gene mutation was different in Niemann-Pick type C disease from that in Niemann-Pick types A and B (80). More recent progress has led to the identification of abnormalities of intracellular cholesterol processing in Niemann-Pick type C (81–83) and in type D disease (84). These findings and the important clinical implications of these discoveries are summarized in this section.

For many years, Niemann-Pick types C and D disease were considered to be unusual forms of the conventional Niemann-Pick A phenotype with considerable chronologic and other differences in their clinical manifestations. These variants have also been called juvenile dystonic lipidosis; DAF syndrome (down gaze paresis ataxia, foam cells in the bone marrow); and supranuclear vertical gaze palsy with sea-blue histiocytosis. The onset of signs and symptoms varies greatly. Hepatosplenomegaly, foam cells (sea-blue histiocytes) (Figure 6.8), cholestatic jaundice, inanition,

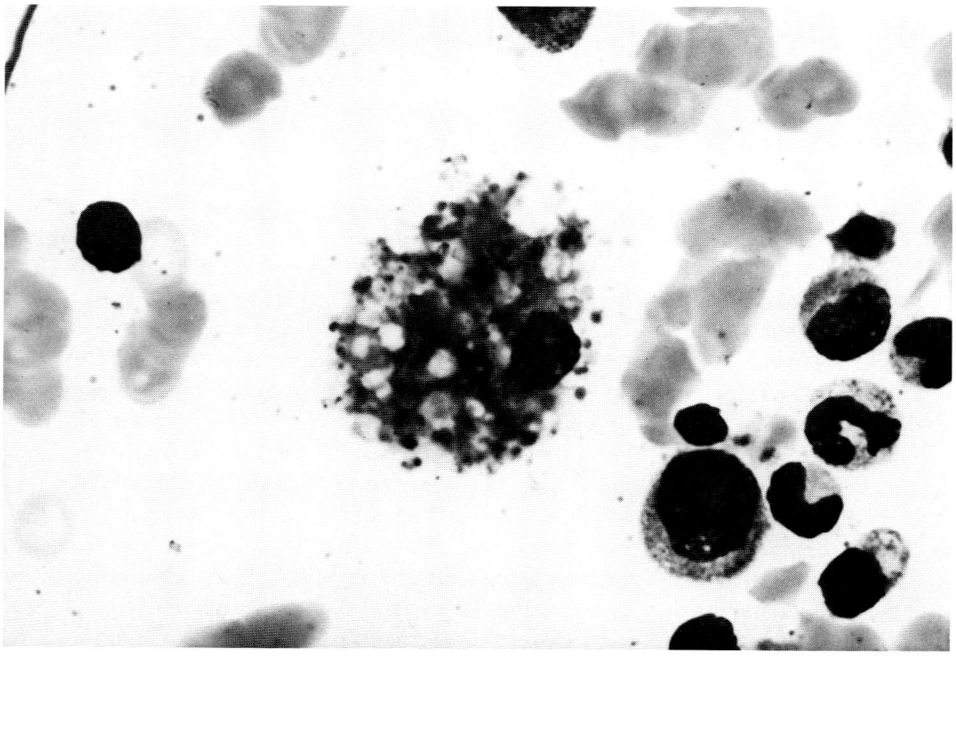

FIGURE 6.8 Sea-blue histiocyte in the bone marrow of a patient with Niemann-Pick type C disease. Reproduced with permission from Johnson WG. Neurogenetic Disease. In: Neurologic Clinics. Philadelphia: WB Saunders, 1989;1:80.

and profound psychomotor deterioration occasionally appear in early infancy. Neonatal giant-cell hepatitis may be found on pathologic examination of the liver. In these patients, death occurs in the early years.

The majority of patients with Niemann-Pick types C and D disease show evidence of the disorder at a later time. The onset may vary from late infancy to early adulthood (Figure 6.9). Splenomegaly with variable hepatomegaly usually occurs before the development of neurologic deficits, but these signs are not invariably observed. The liver cells are enlarged and have a foamy appearance (Figure 6.10). A characteristic of the disorder is the presence of vertical supranuclear gaze paresis (Figure 6.11), although this finding may be absent early in the course. This delay seems particularly true of patients with onset in the early adult years. The vertical gaze paresis may first appear as a loss of downward or upward volitional saccades. As the disease progresses, there is usually total loss of volitional vertical movements. Slow vertical pursuit may be present when vertical saccadic movement is greatly impaired. Horizontal saccadic eye movements may eventually become somewhat affected. Reflex eye movements remain functional in the late stage of the disease.

As patients age, learning impairment becomes increasingly apparent, although memory for past events may persist. Typically, a major presenting complaint is diminished school performance, even in remedial classes. Dementia progresses and eventually becomes apparent in all patients. Patients also have behavioral disturbances that may include delusions and hallucinations.

Other prominent features of Niemann-Pick type C disease are dystonia and progressively worsening ataxia. Parents of patients often remark that the child's gait seems clumsy. Cerebellar involvement is indicated early by diminished ability to perform tandem walking. Eventually, there is profound gait ataxia, and the patients must be supported or be confined to a wheelchair (Figure 6.12). Many of the patients with Niemann-Pick type C disease have severe, mixed seizures that respond poorly to antiepileptic medication. Sodium valproate has produced the best results in our patients.

Involvement of the pyramidal and extrapyramidal tracts is common in Niemann-Pick type C disease. Dystonia and choreoathetosis may appear subtly or is present in a profound degree. Patients become dysarthric. Some patients with Niemann-Pick type C disease become blind late in the disease. The peripheral nervous system is usually not affected in this disorder. There are no distinctive radiographic findings associated with this disorder. CT scans of the brain range from normal to atrophic changes, which may be focal or global in their distribution. MRI provides little additional diagnostic assistance. Aspiration pneumonia is a frequent complication leading to death in these patients.

Numerous reports have appeared concerning the presence of foam cells or sea-blue histiocytes (or both) in the

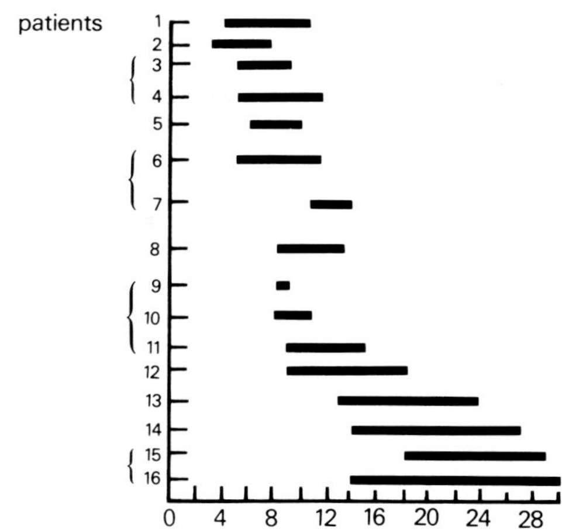

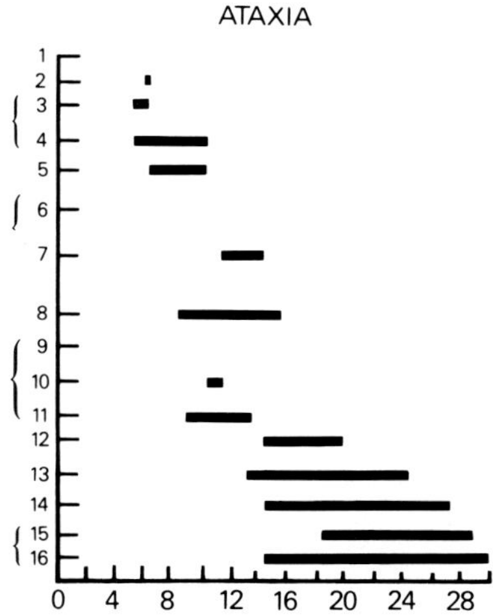

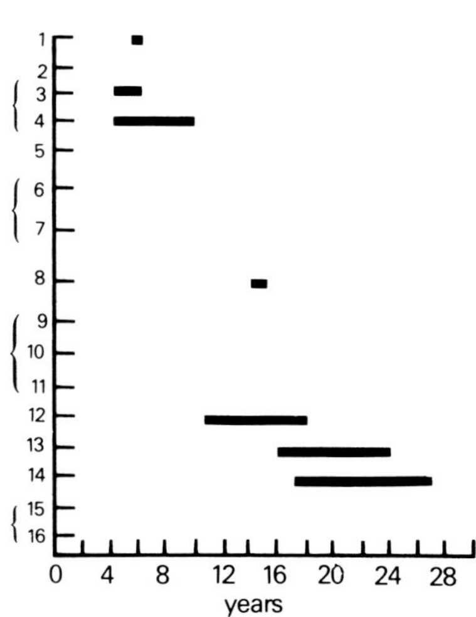

FIGURE 6.9 Chronology of onset of major clinical manifestations in Niemann-Pick types C and D disease.

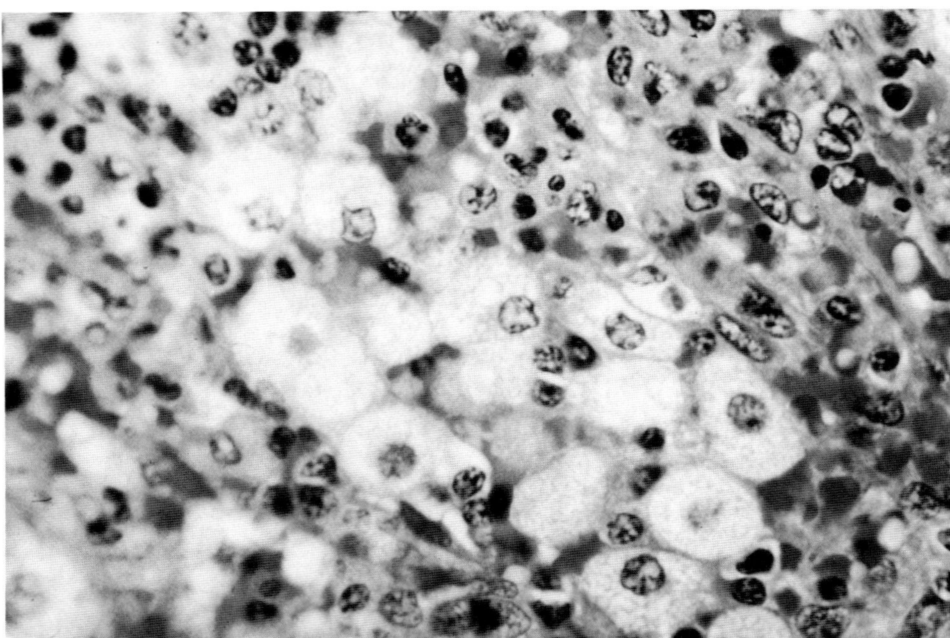

FIGURE 6.10   Foam cells in the spleen of patients with Niemann-Pick type C disease.

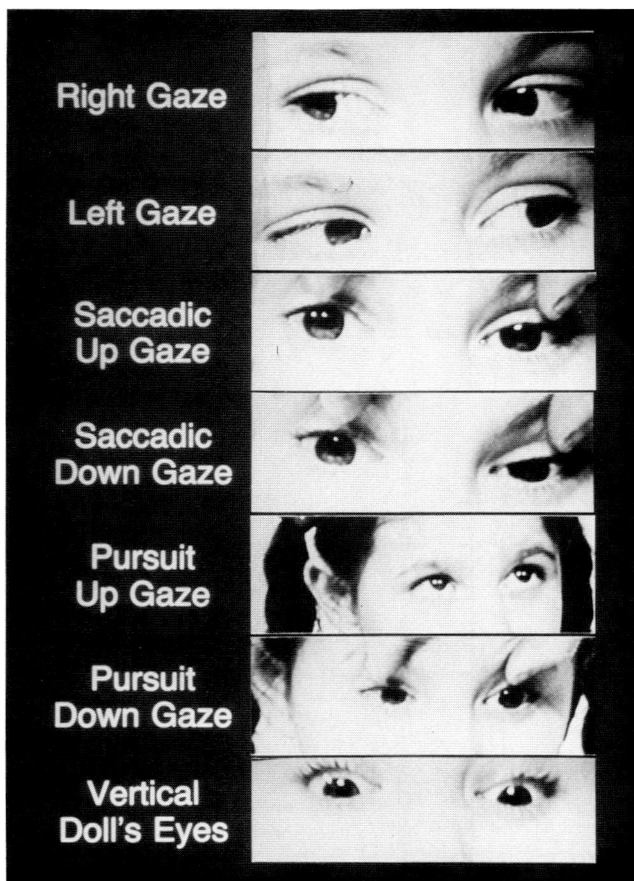

FIGURE 6.11   Restriction of vertical eye movements in a patient with Niemann-Pick type C disease. Reproduced with permission from Johnson WG. Neurogenetic Disease. In: Neurologic Clinics. Philadelphia: WB Saunders, 1989;1:78.

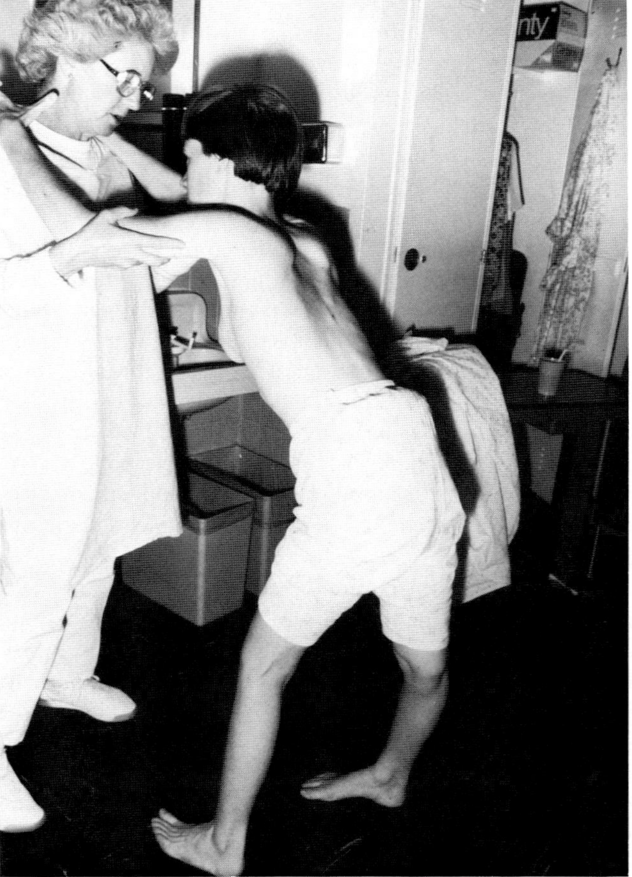

FIGURE 6.12   Dystonic posturing in a patient with Niemann-Pick type C disease. Reproduced with permission from Johnson WG. Neurogenetic Disease. In: Neurologic Clinics. Philadelphia: WB Saunders, 1989;1:79.

bone marrow of patients, many of whom can probably now be confirmed as having Niemann-Pick type C disease. The identification of such cells is not pathognomonic of Niemann-Pick type C disease, however, and conversely, the absence of such cells from bone marrow specimens does not exclude the diagnosis. Lipid-laden cells are present in the spleen as well as the liver in patients with this disorder. Lysosomes in both of these types of cells may be engorged with multilamellar inclusion bodies. Cells in the skin and muscles have also been reported to show similar pathologic changes. Neurons in deep cortical layers of the brain, pallidum, thalamus, red nucleus, and substantia nigra may also show histologic evidence of lipid storage. The type 2 Golgi cells in the inner granular layer of the cerebellum are preferentially involved. Atrophy and loss of myelin may be observed, particularly in the optic tracts.

Because of the inconsistent accumulation of sphingomyelin and the prominence of the elevated free cholesterol in the organs of Niemann-Pick types C and D disease, it was postulated a number of years ago that the condition was not primarily due to decreased sphingomyelinase activity, but should more properly be considered a cholesterol storage disorder (85). Another basis for this deduction was the variable, and at most a partial, reduction, of sphingomyelinase activity in cultured skin fibroblasts derived from patients with Niemann-Pick type C disease. The proposed abnormality of a defect in cholesterol disposition has been amply substantiated in investigations in both Niemann-Pick type C and in type D disease as well as in a murine analog of the human disorder (86). There is a specific block in the intracellular esterification of exogenously derived cholesterol in cultured cells obtained from patients and from the animal model. Importantly, this abnormal cholesterol processing is not associated with a deficiency of the enzyme that catalyzes the transfer of long-chain fatty acids to cholesterol to form cholesterol esters [acyl-CoA:cholesterol O-acyltransferase] (ACAT). Investigations with cultured skin fibroblasts derived from patients with Niemann-Pick types C and D disease revealed that cells from both patients and the murine mutant exhibited abnormal cellular homeostatic responses to cholesterol that include delayed down-regulation of low-density lipoprotein (LDL) receptors through which LDL-bound plasma cholesterol is endocytosed; delayed down-regulation of hydroxymethylglutaryl coenzyme A reductase, a major regulatory step in cholesterol formation; and delay in the up-regulation of ACAT that catalyzes the esterification of free cholesterol intracellularly (82). These abnormalities of cellular homeostatic responses to the uptake of cholesterol by cells result in excessive intracellular accumulation of unesterified cholesterol and a block in the further intracellular translocation of exogenously derived cholesterol (83).

Although the precise site and molecular defect are yet to be identified in Niemann-Pick types C and D disease, much important benefit has been derived from these investigations. Defective esterification of exogenously derived cholesterol in cultured skin fibroblasts is now the most conclusive evidence for the diagnosis of Niemann-Pick type C disease (87). Furthermore, this assay permits the identification of heterozygous carriers of the disorder, and it has been used successfully for the prenatal diagnosis of Niemann-Pick type C disease.

Because the primary underlying mutation has not yet been identified, treatment for Niemann-Pick type C disease must be on an empirical basis. Cellular damage, including that in the CNS (88), appears to be the result of improper intracellular disposition of cholesterol that has entered the cells largely via the LDL-receptor pathway. Several procedures have been initiated to try to reduce the cholesterol overload in these cells. One approach is the use of a diet low in cholesterol; it is not yet possible to state with certainty, however, that this strategy has provided measurable benefit. Other procedures include the administration of nicotinic acid and techniques such as plasmapheresis or passing plasma over an immunoaffinity column that binds LDL (89). Other forms of treatment like administration of cholestyramine or lovastatin (or both) have also been considered. A potential major drawback of the use of these agents, however, is their demonstrated ability to up-regulate LDL receptors on cell membranes. This cellular response could increase the amount of LDL-derived cholesterol taken into cells and could conceivably be detrimental to patients with Niemann-Pick types C and D disease. Despite the limitations regarding currently available therapy, one must always anticipate that the discovery of the molecular defect in Niemann-Pick types C and D disease will ultimately lead to the development of effective remedial measures.

ONSET BETWEEN 2 YEARS AND ADOLESCENCE. CENTRAL AND PERIPHERAL NERVOUS SYSTEM INVOLVEMENT WITHOUT ORGANOMEGALY

Juvenile Metachromatic Leukodystrophy

Patients with metachromatic leukodystrophy who present later than those with the classic signs in infancy have been identified in a number of genetic clinics. The initial symptoms in these children may appear at about 3 years of age or even later. Usually, the first indications of this pathologic state are deterioration of school performance and emotional disturbances. These signs are generally followed by ataxia. Later, postural abnormalities, hypertonic muscles, nystagmus, and intention tremor frequently occur. The prognosis is a lengthy downhill course leading to complete dependence on external care and support.

CT brain scan alterations were reported in two patients with late-onset metachromatic leukodystrophy (90). The ventricles were widened, and white matter hypodensities were initially seen adjacent to the frontal horns as in the infantile form (Figure 6.7). These changes progressed to moderate central and cortical atrophy. MRI revealed more extensive white matter involvement than did CT.

As in the classic infantile form of the disorder, the metabolic defect is a reduction in arylsulfatase A activity resulting in an accumulation of sulfatide. It has been suggested that patients with later onset of clinical manifestations have somewhat more residual arylsulfatase A activity than have those with the infantile form, although this assertion remains to be documented more conclusively. An activator-deficient patient has also been reported with this form of metachromatic leukodystrophy (91). It has been reported that the residual arylsulfatase A protein in their tissues is less stable than is normal arylsulfatase A (92). This observation led to a therapeutic attempt in a patient with the protease inhibitor leupeptin. There was no significant improvement in his clinical status. The patient suffered temporarily from a clotting defect, which is not surprising in view of the extensive proteolytic reactions involved in the clotting cascade. Thus, at this time, no established therapy is yet available. If beneficial effects from bone marrow transplantation that were asserted in a patient with the conventional form of this disorder are substantiated, it is certain that this procedure will be tried in patients with the juvenile form of metachromatic leukodystrophy.

ONSET BETWEEN 2 YEARS AND ADOLESCENCE. CENTRAL NERVOUS SYSTEM INVOLVEMENT WITHOUT ORGANOMEGALY

Mucolipidosis IV

This is a rare disorder characterized by mental retardation and corneal clouding. Another, possibly more accurate, name for this condition is ganglioside sialidosis, because at least a partial deficiency of sialidase activity that is associated with ganglioside catabolism has been reported in cultured skin fibroblasts derived from such patients (93). This defect would be expected to lead to the accumulation of gangliosides like G_{D1b} (Figure 6.1, Reaction 4) and G_{D1a} (Figure 6.1, Reaction 5). Bach and co-workers moved that they believed they were able to identify heterozygotes based on assays of neuraminidase activity. Although increased quantities of ganglioside have been reported in patients' cells, there was even a larger accumulation of such mucopolysaccharides as dermatan sulfate and heparan sulfate (94). These conceptual difficulties have been discussed previously (95). There has still been no satisfactory resolution of these findings or convincing explanation of the pathogenesis of this disorder.

ONSET BETWEEN 2 YEARS AND ADOLESCENCE. PERIPHERAL NERVOUS SYSTEM INVOLVEMENT WITHOUT ORGANOMEGALY

Fabry Disease

All of the above documented sphingolipid storage disorders are autosomal recessive conditions. Fabry disease is the exception, because the gene for the involved enzyme ceramidetrihexosidase (alpha-galactosidase A) is on the X-chromosome. Hence, only the female need be a carrier to produce an affected male child. Half of her sons will have the disorder, and half of her daughters will be carriers. It should be noted that some of the heterozygotes have some clinical manifestations of the condition. This expressivity is believed to be caused by variable inactivation of one of the X-chromosomes in females (Lyon hypothesis). Overt clinical signs in females usually do not occur in childhood, however, and therefore this situation is rarely, if ever, encountered by pediatricians.

On the other hand, many of the hemizygous (affected) males do show evidence of the disorder in their early years. The initial signs are usually painful, burning sensations in their hands and feet. These acroparesthesias are worse with heat and with exercise, frequently causing the boys to stop their activity until the pain resides. The boys may feel weak and fatigued with these episodes. One of the hallmarks of the disorder is the absence of sweating, which seems likely to contribute to the worsening of these difficulties in summer. Impairment of autonomic function (96) and pathologic aspects of the peripheral neuropathy in these patients are discussed in detail elsewhere (97,98). A number of these boys have gastrointestinal difficulties, often manifesting as frequent, uncontrollable bowel movements. The basis of the gastrointestinal difficulties in Fabry disease has been attributed to lipid deposition in neurons of the submucous and myenteric plexes of the large and small intestines as well as the intestinal mucosa (99). It should be stressed that the majority of the young men brought to pediatricians with the acroparesthesias of Fabry disease have been misdiagnosed in the past. Frequently the pains are dismissed as a mild anxiety or psychoneurotic syndrome. Great personal and family distress occurs in this situation if the basis of the problem is not identified correctly.

Males with Fabry disease often have reddish purple maculopapular lesions on the skin, which may be difficult to detect in some young individuals because of their scarcity. The region of the umbilicus and the scrotum in particular should be examined for these angiokeratomata. These patients usually have corneal opacification and tortuosity of retinal blood vessels. Vision is not affected. In time, the glomeruli and tubules of the kidney become laden with the sphingolipid ceramide trihexoside because of insufficient activity of the alpha-galactosidase required for the catabolism of this substance (99) (See Figure 6.2, Reaction

2). Much of the accumulating lipid is probably derived from erythrocytorrhexis in which ceramidetrihexoside itself is a known component of the red blood cell stroma. A quantitatively more important source is globoside, which is the immediate catabolic precursor of ceramidetrihexoside. Globoside is the major sphingoglycolipid of erythrocyte stroma.

A persistent unresolved aspect of the pathogenesis of Fabry disease concerns the lack of splenomegaly or hepatomegaly in this disorder compared with the extensive involvement of these organs in Gaucher disease and Niemann-Pick disease. If the accumulating ceramidetrihexoside is indeed primarily derived from sphingolipids of erythrocyte stroma, and if erythrocytorrhexis occurs primarily in macrophages including the Kupffer cells in the liver, one wonders how the spleen and liver escape enlargement. Two possibilities may be thought of in this context. The first is that the slowly accumulating ceramidetrihexoside in these organs manages to diffuse out of and away from macrophages. Although intercellular movement of certain phospholipids has been demonstrated, it has been much more difficult to show this phenomenon with sphingolipids. On the other hand, evidence suggests that there was long-term displacement of a nonmetabolizable analog of glucocerebroside from Kupffer cells, possibly exiting from the liver via the bile (100).

Another possibility that should be considered is that lipids with a terminal alpha-galactoside do not cause the plethora of pathologic responses seen with a glucose-terminal sphingolipid (101). Specific experimentation directed toward assessing this possibility seems to indicate that ceramidetrihexoside was, in fact, less cytotoxic than glucocerebroside to cultured macrophages (101).

Affected males may have a mild to moderate proteinuria. In the absence of a satisfactory alternative explanation, Fabry disease should be considered in the differential diagnosis of young males with albuminuria. The kidney involvement progresses to eventual renal shutdown, and hemodialysis or kidney transplantation is usually required. In addition, there is premature atherosclerosis of the blood vessels that is attended by premature myocardial infarction and stroke.

The diagnosis of Fabry disease may be readily confirmed by measuring alpha-galactosidase A activity in extracts of leukocytes or cultured skin fibroblasts (22,102). Prior to the development of these enzymatic assays, kidney biopsy was frequently used as a diagnostic procedure.

The gene for ceramidetrihexosidase has been cloned (103), and mutations that have occurred in various pedigrees of patients with Fabry disease have been investigated (104). As in Tay-Sachs disease, a varied picture has emerged concerning the enzyme alterations. In one case, the synthesis, stability, and immunologic cross-reactivity of the catalytically defective enzyme were similar to normal. In another, no cross-reacting protein could be detected. In a third, maturation of the nascent protein by carbohydrate addition, and possibly proteolytic cleavage, was retarded. In two others, the protein was synthesized, but it was rapidly degraded after incorporation into lysosomes. This wide range of differences should probably not be too surprising, because it is estimated that approximately 1/3 of the mutations in X-linked recessive disorders occur spontaneously. Knowledge of the mutations has led to the development of procedures for the molecular diagnosis of some patients and carriers of Fabry disease (105).

The treatment of patients with Fabry disease is mainly symptomatic at this time. Carbamazepine is often used for the relief of the acroparesthesias, occasionally in conjunction with amitriptyline. Phenytoin has also been reported to be of some help. We have used metoclopramide with notable success for the management of gastrointestinal difficulties in patients with Fabry disease.

Specific treatment for Fabry disease has taken several routes. One of the more unusual is the engraftment of fetal liver cells (106). Other, more conventional, therapy directed toward reducing the amount of ceramidetrihexoside has been attempted by repeated plasmaphereses without significant clinical benefit (107). The effect of intravenous infusion of partially purified ceramidetrihexosidase obtained from human placenta (108), plasma, and human spleen tissue (109) has been examined. The exogenous enzyme reduced the quantity of ceramidetrihexoside in the plasma for a period of time, but so far, no clinical improvement has been reported from this form of therapy. An investigation is under way to target the exogenous enzyme to the specific cells in which ceramidetrihexoside accumulates. It is hoped that this strategy, which has proved successful in enzyme-replacement therapy in Gaucher type 1 (nonneuronopathic) disease (32) will be effective in Fabry disease as well.

CONCLUDING REMARKS

There are currently many accurate, time-tested ways to diagnose patients with sphingolipid storage disorders, procedures to identify heterozygotes, and methods to provide an antenatal diagnosis when fetuses are at risk for these conditions. These techniques are available in many medical centers. Counseling services, national referral centers, and network and peer-support groups have been established to assist families in which children with these disorders occur. Several critical aspects concerning sphingolipid storage disorders that involve the nervous system remain to be pursued. One of these is to determine the etiologic basis of the faulty cholesterol processing in Niemann-Pick types C and D disease. When this information is available, we expect to be able to conceptualize an effective remedy for these patients. Meanwhile, indirect therapeutic measures are being explored to limit the cellular cholesterol burden and neuronal damage.

The next few years will certainly bring forth expanded knowledge concerning the gene mutations in many of the sphingolipid storage disorders. Specific alterations in the genes for glucocerebrosidase and for hexosaminidase have been identified in Gaucher disease and Tay-Sachs disease, respectively. Abnormalities of enzyme production, processing, glycosylation, and stability have been demonstrated in many instances in which the specific gene change or deletion has not been identified as exemplified in Fabry disease. It is hoped that this information can be exploited for patients' benefit. Perhaps agents will be discovered that can influence protein processing and lead to stabilization of some of the mutant enzymes. Other factors may be developed to increase the lysosomal targeting of mutated proteins should their delivery to this requisite site for catalytic activity be altered.

Much current research emphasis is directed toward formulating and examining various strategies for the treatment of sphingolipid storage disorders. It is not apparent at this time when effective measures will be developed that will permit delivery of realistic quantities of exogenous enzymes to cells in the nervous system. It is conceivable that a technique may eventually be developed that will permit enzymes to traverse the BBB without harm to the recipient. If this occurs, an important corollary concern is whether such a method will be applicable to patients with peripheral nervous system involvement.

Finally, everyone involved in the management of patients with metabolic disorders characterized by nervous system damage has an acute and continuing interest in the ongoing investigations concerning the effect of bone marrow transplantation on the course of these illnesses. There are many important implications in the publications indicating possible neurologic benefit in patients with metachromatic leukodystrophy (11) and in the mucopolysaccharidoses (110).

Additional impetus for further work along this line has come from studies with an animal analogue of Hurler disease in which reduction of mucopolysaccharides in the brain and cerebrospinal fluid has been observed following bone marrow transplantation (111). It should be remembered that there are many differences between the cell biology of sphingolipidoses and the mucopolysaccharidoses. In particular, it has been possible to demonstrate metabolic cooperativity (correction) between certain enzymatically deficient mammalian fibroblasts when they are grown in contact with normal fibroblasts (112). This correction, which is presumed to be mediated by transfer of the missing enzyme from the control cells to the deficient cells, has been difficult to show in the sphingolipidoses. It is therefore believed that intercellular transfer of sphingolipid hydrolases is not a major biologic phenomenon.

One possible exception to this situation are the comparatively large amounts of Hex A and Hex B that are present in normal human serum. Even in this situation, these enzymes probably do not gain access to the brain (36). For these reasons, there is considerable uncertainty regarding the eventual effectiveness of bone marrow replacement for many of the sphingolipid storage disorders, particularly those that involve neurons in the central and peripheral nervous systems.

REFERENCES

1. Svennerholm L. IUPAC-IUB Commission on Biochemical Nomenclature. Eur J Biochem 1977; 79:11–21.
2. Wherrett JR, Huterer S. Enrichment of bis-(monoacylglyceryl) phosphate in lysosomes from rat liver. J Biol Chem 1972; 247:4114–4120.
3. Stremmel W, Debuch H. Bis(monoacylglycerin)phosphosaure - ein marker-lipid sekundarer lysosomen. Hoppe-Seyler's Z Physiol Chem 1976; 357:803–810.
4. Brady RO. Sphingomyelin lipidosis: Niemann-Pick disease. In: Stanbury JB, Wyngaarden JB, Fredrickson DS, et al., eds. The Metabolic Basis of Inherited Disease, 5th ed. New York: McGraw-Hill, 1983, 842–856.
5. Gal AE, Brady RO, Hibbert SR, et al. A practical chromogenic procedure for the detection of homozygotes and heterozygous carriers of Niemann-Pick disease. N Engl J Med 1975; 293:632–636.
6. Daloze P, Delvin EE, Glorieux FH, et al. Replacement therapy for inherited enzyme deficiency: Liver orthotopic transplantation in Niemann-Pick disease Type A. Am J Med Genet 1977; 1:229–235.
7. Scaggiante B, Pineschi A, Sustersich M, et al. Successful therapy of Niemann-Pick disease by implantation of human amniotic membrane. Transplantation 1987; 44:59–61.
8. Tylki-Szymanska A, Maciejko D, Kidawa M, et al. Amniotic tissue transplantation as a trial of treatment in some lysosomal storage diseases. J Inherited Metab Dis 1985; 8: 101–104.
9. Yeager AM, Singer HS, Buck JR, et al. A therapeutic trial of amniotic epithelial implantation in patients with lysosomal storage diseases. Am J Med Genet, 1985; 22:347–355.
10. Vellodi A, Hobbs JR, O'Donnell NM, et al. Treatment of Niemann-Pick disease type B by allogeneic bone marrow transplantation. Br Med J 1987; 295:1375–1376.
11. Krivit W, Lipton ME, Lockman LA, et al. Prevention of deterioration in metachromatic leukodystrophy by bone marrow transplantation. Am J Med Sci 1987; 294:80–85.
12. Erikson A. Gaucher's disease - Norbottnian type (III). Neuropaediatric and neurobiological aspects of clinical patterns and treatment. Acta Paediatr Scand (Suppl) 1986; 326: 1–42.
13. da Veiga Pereira L, Desnick RJ, Adler DA, et al. Regional assignment of the human acid sphingomyelinase gene (SMPD1) by PCR analysis of somatic cell hybrids and in situ hybridization to 11p15.1—p15.4. Genomics 1991; 9:229–234.
14. Distler JJ, Jourdian GW. Isolation of β-galactosidase from bovine testicular tissue. Methods Enzymol 1978; 50C: 514–520.
15. O'Brien JS, de Wet J, Fukushima H, et al. Cloning of lysosomal genes. In: Barranger JA, Brady RO, eds. Molecular Basis

of Lysosomal Storage Disorders. Orlando: Academic Press, 1984, 387–403.

16. Brady RO, Kanfer JN, Bradley RM, et al. Demonstration of a deficiency of glucocerebroside-cleaving enzyme in Gaucher's disease. J Clin Invest 1966; 45:1112–1115.

17. Svennerholm L, Hakansson G, Mansson JE, et al. Chemical differentiation of the Gaucher subtypes. In: Desnick RJ, Gatt S, Grabowski GA, eds. Gaucher disease: A Century of Delineation and Research. New York: Alan R Liss, 1982, 231–252.

18. Kattlove HE, Williams JC, Gaynor E, et al. Gaucher cells in chronic myelocytic leukemia: An acquired abnormality. Blood 1969; 33:379–390.

19. Nilsson O, Svennerholm L. Accumulation of glucosylceramide and glucosylsphingosine (psychosine) in cerebrum and cerebellum in infantile and juvenile Gaucher's disease. J Neurochem 1982; 39:709–718.

20. Pentchev PG, Brady RO, Hibbert SR, et al. Isolation and characterization of glucocerebrosidase from human placental tissue. J Biol Chem 1973; 248:5256–5261.

21. Glew RH, Basu A, LaMarco KL, et al. Biology of disease. Mammalian glucocerebrosidase: Implications for Gaucher's disease. Lab Invest 1988; 58:5–15.

22. Suzuki K. Enzymatic diagnosis of sphingolipidoses. Methods Enzymol 1987; 138:727–762.

23. Gal AE, Pentchev PG, Fash FJ. A novel chromogenic substrate for assaying glucocerebrosidase activity. Proc Soc Exp Biol Med 1976; 153:363–366.

24. Barns RJ, Clague AE. An improved procedure for diagnosis of Gaucher disease using cultured skin fibroblasts and the chromogenic substrate, 2-hexadecanoylamino-4-nitrophenyl-β-D-glucopyranoside. Clin Chim Acta 1982; 120: 57–63.

25. Barneveld RA, Keijzer W, Tegelaers FPW, et al. Assignment of the gene coding for human β-glucocerebrosidase to the region q21-31 of chrosome 1 using monoclonal antibodies. Hum Genet 1983; 64:227–231.

26. Ginns EI, Choudary PV, Martin BM, et al. Isolation of cDNA clones for human β-glucocerebrosidase. Biochem Biophys Res Commun 1984; 123:574–580.

27. Sorge J, West C, Westwood B, et al. Molecular cloning and nucleotide sequence of human glucocerebrosidase cDNA. Proc Natl Acad Sci USA 1985; 82:72–93.

28. Reiner O, Wilder S, Givol D, et al. Efficient in vitro and in vivo expression of human glucocerebrosidase cDNA. DNA 1987; 6:101–108.

29. Tsuji S, Choudary PV, Martin B, et al. A mutation in the human glucocerebrosidase gene in neuronopathic Gaucher's disease. N Engl J Med 1987; 316:570–579.

30. Horowitz, M. Personal communication, 1987.

31. Dinur T, Oisecki KM, Legler G, et al. Human acid β-glucocerebrosidase: Isolation and amino acid sequence of a peptide containing the catalytic site. Proc Natl Acad Sci USA 1986; 83:1660–1664.

32. Barton NW, Brady RO, Dambrosia OM, et al. Replacement therapy for inherited enzyme deficiency-macrophage-targeted glucocerebrosidase for Gaucher's disease. N Engl J Med 1991; 324:1464–1470.

33. Sandhoff K, Conzelmann E. The biochemical basis of gangliosidoses. Neuropediatrics 1984; 15 Suppl:85–92.

34. Rosengren B, Mansson JE, Svennerholm L. Composition of gangliosides and neutral glycosphingolipids of brain in classical Tay-Sachs disease and Sandhoff disease: More lyso-G_{M2} in Sandhoff disease. J Neurochem 1987; 49:834–840.

35. Tallman JF, Johnson WG, Brady RO. The metabolism of Tay-Sachs ganglioside: Catabolic studies with lysosomal enzymes from normal and Tay-Sachs brain tissue. J Clin Invest 1972; 51:2339–2345.

36. Johnson WG, Desnick RJ, Long DM, et al. Intravenous injection of purified hexosaminidase A into a patient with Tay-Sachs disease. In: Desnick RJ, Bernlohr RW, Krivit W, eds. Enzyme Therapy in Genetic Diseases. Birth Defects Original Article Series, Baltimore: Williams and Williams, 1973; IX: 109–119.

37. Neuwelt EA, Barranger JA, Pagel MA, et al. Delivery of active hexosaminidase across the blood brain barrier in rats. Neurology 1984; 34:1012–1019.

38. Strausbaugh LJ. Intracarotid infusions of protamine sulfate disrupt the blood-brain barrier of rabbits. Brain Res 1987; 409:221–226.

39. Moser HW, Chen WW. Ceramidase deficiency: Farber's lipogranulomatosis. In: Stanbury JB, Wyngaarden JB, Fredrickson DS, et al., eds. The Metabolic Basis of Inherited Disease; 5th ed. New York: McGraw-Hill, 1983, 820–830.

40. Okada S, O'Brien JS. Tay-Sachs disease: Generalized absence of a beta-D-N-acetylhexosaminidase component. Science 1969; 165:698–700.

41. Kolodny EH, Brady RO, Volk BW. Demonstration of an alteration of ganglioside metabolism in Tay-Sachs disease. Biochem Biophys Res Commun 1969; 37:526–531.

42. Kresse H, Fuchs W, Glossl J, et al. Liberation of N-acetylglucosamine-6-sulfate by human β-N-acetylhexosaminidase A. J Biol Chem 1981; 256:12926–12932.

43. Bayleran J, Hechtman P, Saray W. Synthesis of 4-methylumbelliferyl-β-D-N-acetylglucosamine-6-sulfate and its use in the classification of G_{M2} gangliosidosis genotypes. Clin Chim Acta 1984; 143:73–89.

44. Ben-Yoseph Y, Reid JE, Shapiro B, et al. Diagnosis and carrier detection of Tay-Sachs disease: Direct determination of hexosaminidase A using 4-methylumbelliferyl derivatives of β-N-acetylglucosamine-6-sulfate and β-N-acetylgalactosamine-6-sulfate. Am J Hum Genet 1985; 37:733–748.

45. Inui K, Yutaka T, Okada S, et al. Hexosaminidase A activity in skin fibroblasts from various types of G_{M2} gangliosidosis using a fluorogenic sulphated substrate. J Inherit Metab Dis 1985; 8:149–150.

46. O'Brien JS. The gangliosidoses. In: Stanbury JB, Wyngaarden JB, Fredrickson DS, et al., eds. The Metabolic Basis of Inherited Disease; 5th ed. New York: McGraw-Hill, 1983; 945–969.

47. Grebner E, Jackson LG. Prenatal diagnosis for Tay-Sachs disease using chorionic villus sampling. Prenatal diagnosis 1985; 5:313–320.

48. Inui K, Wenger DA, Furukawa M, et al. Prenatal diagnosis of G_{M2} gangliosidoses using a fluorogenic sulfated substrate. Clin Chim Acta 1986; 154:145–150.

49. Grebner EE, Wenger DA. Use of 4-methylumbelliferyl-6-sulpho-2-acetamido-2-deoxy-β-D-glucopyranoside for prenatal diagnosis of Tay-Sachs disease using chorionic villi. Prenatal Diag 1987; 7:419–423.

50. Neufeld EF, d'Azzo A, Proia RL. Defective synthesis or maturation of the α-chain of β-hexosaminidase in classic and variant forms of Tay-Sachs disease. In: Barranger JA, Brady RO, eds. Molecular Basis of Lysosomal Storage Disorders. Orlando: Academic Press, 1984, 251–256.

51. Myerowitz R, Hogikyan ND. A deletion involving Alu sequences in the beta-hexosaminidase alpha-chain of French Canadians with Tay-Sachs disease. J Biol Chem 1987; 262: 15396–15399.

52. Ohno K, Suzuki K. Mutation in G_{M2}-gangliosidosis B1 variant. J Neurochem 1988; 50:316–318.

53. Arpaia E, Dumbrille-Ross, A, Maler T, et al. Identification of an altered splice site in Ashkenazi Tay-Sachs disease. Nature 1988; 333:85–86.

54. Cogan DG, Kuwabara T, Kolodny EH. A variant of Tay-Sachs disease. XIInd Concilium of Ophthalmology. 1974; 700–701.

55. Cogan DG. Gangliosidosis AB. Neuro-ophthalmology 1984; 4:65–68.

56. Sandhoff K, Harzer K, Wassle W, et al. Enzyme alterations and lipid storage in three variants of Tay-Sachs disease. J Neurochem 1971; 18:2469–2489.

57. Conzelmann E, Sandhoff K. AB variant of infantile G_{M2} gangliosidosis: Deficiency of a factor necessary for stimulation of hexosaminidase A-catalyzed degradation of ganglioside G_{M2} and glycolipid G_{A2}. Proc Natl Acad Sci USA 1975; 75:3979–3983.

58. Conzelmann E, Sandhoff K. Activator proteins for lysosomal glycolipid hydrolysis. Methods Biochem Analysis 1987; 32:1–23.

59. Burg J, Conzelmann E, Sandhoff K, et al. Mapping of the gene coding for the human G_{M2} activator protein to chromosome 5. Ann Hum Genet 1985; 49:41–45.

60. Svennerholm L, Vanier MT, Mansson JE. Krabbe disease: A galactosylsphingosine (psychosine) lipidosis. J Lipid Res 1980; 21:53–64.

61. Gal AE, Brady RO, Pentchev PG, et al. A practical chromogenic procedure for the diagnosis of Krabbe's disease. Clin Chim Acta 1977; 77:53–59.

62. Vidershian GYA, Kozlova IK, Ilina GS. Novel fluorogenic substrate for human galactocerebroside-β-galactosidase. Biokhimiya 1985; 50:1665–1667.

63. Yeager AM, Brennan S, Tiffany C, et al. Prolonged survival and remyelination after hematopoietic cell transplantation in the twitcher mouse. Science 1984; 225:1052–1054.

64. Ichioka T, Kishimoto Y, Brennan S, et al. Hematopoietic cells transplantation in murine globoid cell leukodystrophy (the twitcher mouse): Effects on levels of galactosylceramidase, psychosine, and galactocerebrosides. Proc Natl Acad Sci USA 1987; 84:4259–4263.

65. Hoogerbrugge PM, Suzuki K, Suzuki K, et al. Donor-derived cells in the central nervous system of twitcher mice after bone marrow transplantation. Science 1988;239: 1035–1038.

66. Hoogerbrugge PM, Poorthuis BJHM, Romme AdE, et al. Effect of bone marrow transplantation on enzyme levels and clinical course in the neurologically affected twitcher mouse. J Clin Invest 1988; 81:1790–1794.

67. Li SC, Kihara H, Serizawa S, et al. Activator protein required for the enzymatic hydrolysis of cerebroside sulfate. J Biol Chem 1985; 260:1867–1871.

68. Vogel A, Furst W, Abo-Hashish MA, et al. Identity of the activator proteins for the enzymatic hydrolysis of sulfatide, ganglioside G_{M1}, and globotriaosylceramide. Arch Biochem Biophys 1987; 259:627–638.

69. Porter NT, Fluharty AL, Kihara H. Correction of abnormal cerebroside sulfate metabolism in cultured metachromatic leukodystrophy fibroblasts. Science 1971; 172:1263–1265.

70. Weismann VN, Rossi EE, Hershkowitz NN. Treatment of metachromatic leukodystrophy fibroblasts by enzyme replacement. N Engl J Med 1971; 204:672–673.

71. Krivit W, Whitley CB. Bone marrow transplantation for genetic diseases. N Engl J Med 1987; 316:1085–1087.

72. Bayever E, Ladisch M, Phillippart M, et al. Bone marrow transplantation for metachromatic leukodystrophy. Lancet 1985; 1:471–473.

73. Ladisch S, Bayever E, Phillippart M, et al. Biochemical findings after bone marrow transplantation for metachromatic leukodystrophy. In: Krivit W, ed. Birth Defects: March of Dimes Original Article Series. New York: Alan R. Liss, 1986; 22:7–24.

74. Walkley SU, Wurzelmann S, Purpura D. Ultrastructure of neurites and meganeurites of cortical pyramidal neurons in feline gangliosidosis as revealed by the combined Golgi-EM technique. Brain Res 1981; 211:393–398.

75. Filling-Katz MR, Barton NW, Katz NN. Gaucher's disease. In: Gold DH, Weingeist TA, eds. The Eye in Systemic Disease. Philadelphia: JB Lippincott, 1990; 365–368.

76. Rappeport JM, Ginns EI. Bone-marrow transplantation in severe Gaucher's disease. N Engl J Med 1984; 311:84–88.

77. Svennerholm, L. Personal communication, 1991.

78. Crocker AC. The cerebral defect in Tay-Sachs disease and Niemann-Pick disease. J Neurochem 1961; 7:69–80.

79. Besley GTN. Sphingomyelinase defect in Niemann-Pick disease type C fibroblasts. FEBS Lett 1977; 80:71–74.

80. Besley GTN, Hoogeboom AJM, Hoogeveen A, et al. Somatic cell hybridisation studies showing different gene mutations in Niemann-Pick variants. Hum Genet 1980; 54:409–412.

81. Pentchev PG, Comly ME, Kruth HS, et al. A defect in cholesterol esterification in Niemann-Pick disease (type C) patients. Proc Natl Acad Sci USA 1985; 82:8247–8251.

82. Pentchev PG, Comly ME, Kruth HS, et al. Group C Niemann-Pick disease: Faulty regulation of low-density lipoprotein uptake and cholesterol storage in cultured fibroblasts. FASEB J 1987; 1:40–45.

83. Sokol J, Blanchette-Mackie EJ, Kruth HS, et al. Type C Niemann-Pick disease: Lysosomal accumulation and defective intracellular mobilization of LDL-cholesterol. J Biol Chem 1988; 263:3411–3417.

84. Butler JdeB, Comly ME, Kruth HS, et al. Niemann-Pick variant disorders: Comparison of errors of cellular cholesterol homeostasis in group-D and group-C fibroblasts. Proc Natl Acad Sci USA 1987; 84:556–560.

85. Brady RO. Sphingomyelin lipidosis: Niemann-Pick disease. In: Stanbury JB, Wyngaarden JB, Fredrickson, DS, Goldstein JL, Brown MS, eds. The Metabolic Basis of Inherited Disease; 5th ed. New York: McGraw-Hill, 1983, 831–841.

86. Pentchev PG, Boothe AD, Kruth HS, et al. A genetic storage disorder in Balb/C mice with a metabolic block in esterification of exogenous cholesterol. J Biol Chem 1984; 259:5784–5791.

87. Vanier MT, Wenger DA, Comly ME, et al. Niemann-Pick disease group C: Clinical variability and diagnosis based on defective cholesterol esterification. Clin Genet 1988; 33:331–348.

88. Patel SC, Suresh S, Weintroub H, et al. Impaired cholesterol esterification in primary brain cultures of the lysosomal cholesterol storage disorder (LCSD) mouse mutant. Biochem Biophys Res Commun 1987; 143:233–240.

89. Hombach V, Borberg H, Gadzkowski A, et al. Regression of coronary sclerosis in familial hypercholesterolemia IIa by specific LDL apheresis. Dtsch Med Wochenschr 1986; 111:1709–1715.

90. Reider-Grosswasser I, Bornstein N. CT and MRI in late-onset metachromatic leukodystrophy. Acta Neurol Scand 1987; 75:64–69.

91. Inui K, Emmett M, Wenger DA. Immunological evidence for deficiency in an activator protein for sulfatide sulfatase in a variant form of metachromatic leukodystrophy. Proc Natl Acad Sci USA 1983; 80:3074–3077.

92. Von Figura K, Steckel F, Conary J, et al. Heterogeneity in late-onset metachromatic leukodystrophy. Effect of inhibitors of cysteine proteinases. Am J Hum Genet 1986; 39: 371–382.

93. Bach G, Zeigler M, Schaap T, et al. Mucolipidosis type IV: Ganglioside sialidase deficiency. Biochem Biophys Res Commun 1979; 90:1341–1347.

94. Hahn LC, Ben-Joseph Y, Nadler HL. Glycoprotein and ganglioside alpha-neuraminidases in sialidosis and mucolipidoses. Am J Hum Genet 1980; 32:41A.

95. Brady RO. Inherited metabolic storage disorders. Annu Rev Neurosci 1982; 5:33–56.

96. Cable WJL, Kolodny EH, Adams RD. Fabry disease: Impaired autonomic function. Neurology 1982; 32: 498–502.

97. Brady RO. Fabry's disease. In: Dyck PJ, Thomas PK, Lambert EH, et al., eds. Peripheral Neuropathy II. Philadelphia: WB Saunders, 1984, 1717–1727.

98. Case records of the Massachusetts General Hospital. N Engl J Med 1984; 311:106–114.

99. Brady RO, Gal AE, Bradley RM, et al. Enzymatic defect in Fabry's disease. Ceramidetrihexosidase deficiency. N Engl J Med 1967; 276:1163–1167.

100. Tokoro T, Gal AE, Gallo LL, et al. Studies of the pathogenesis of Gaucher's disease: Tissue distribution and biliary excretion of ^{14}C-L-glucosylceramide in rats. J Lipid Res 1987; 28:968–972.

101. Gery I, Zigler JS Jr, Brady RO, et al. Selective effects of glucocerebroside (Gaucher's storage material) on macrophage cultures. J Clin Invest 1981; 68:1182–1189.

102. Mayes JS, Scheerer JB, Sifers RN, et al. Differential assay for lysosomal alpha-galactosidases in human tissues and its application to Fabry's disease. Clin Chim Acta 1981; 112:247–251.

103. Bishop DF, Calhoun DH, Bernstein HS, et al. Human alpha-galactosidase A: Nucleotide sequence of a cDNA clone encoding the mature enzyme. Proc Natl Acad Sci USA 1986; 83:4859–4863.

104. Lemansky P, Bishop DF, Desnick RJ, et al. Synthesis and processing of alpha-galactosidase A in human fibroblasts. Evidence for different mutations in Fabry disease. J Biol Chem 1987; 262:2062–2065.

105. Desnick RJ, Bernstein HS, Astrin KH, et al. Fabry disease: Molecular diagnosis of hemizygotes and heterozygotes. Enzyme 1987; 38:54–64.

106. Touraine JL, Malik MC, Perrot H, et al. Maladie de Fabry: Deux malades ameliores par la greffe de cellules de foie foetal. Nouv Presse Med 1979; 8:1499–1503.

107. Moser HW, Braine H, Pyeritz RE, et al. Therapeutic trial of plasmapheresis in Refsum disease and in Fabry disease. Birth Defects: Original Article Series. Baltimore: Williams and Wilkins, 1980, Volume XVI: 491–497.

108. Brady RO, Tallman JF, Johnson WG, et al. Replacement therapy for inherited enzyme deficiency: Use of purified ceramidetrihexosidase in Fabry's disease. N Engl J Med 1973; 289:9–14.

109. Desnick RJ, Dean KJ, Grabowski GA, et al. Enzyme therapy XVII: Metabolic and immunologic evaluation of α-galactosidase A replacement in Fabry disease. In: Desnick RJ, ed. Enzyme therapy in Genetic Diseases: 2. New York: Alan R. Liss, 1980, 393–413.

110. Hobbs JR. Correction of 34 genetic diseases by displacement bone marrow transplantation. Plasma Therapy Transfus Technol 1985; 6:221–226.

111. Shull RM, Hastings NE, Selcer RR, et al. Bone marrow transplantation in canine mucopolysaccharidosis I. J Clin Invest 1987; 79:435–442.

112. Subak-Sharpe H, Burk RR, Pitts JD. Metabolic co-operation between biochemically marked mammalian cells in tissue culture. J Cell Sci 1969; 4:353–367.

Chapter 7
Disorders of Trace Element Metabolism

Warren D. Grover

Trace elements are cations present in microgram or picogram quantities in body fluids and tissues and are components of a number of metalloenzymes and chemical reactions important in multiple essential functions, ranging from transfer of genetic information and somatic growth to activation of cellular and humoral molecules (1–4). Currently, there are 15 minerals identified as trace elements; iron, copper, zinc, magnesium, cobalt, molybdenum, selenium, chromium, and iodine are required for homeostasis in humans. Abnormalities of metabolism are caused by deficient intake (parenteral alimentation), defective absorption from the gastrointestinal tract (GI) (acrodermatitis enteropathy), abnormalities in transport or storage (Wilson disease), or in cell membrane kinetics and intracellular binding—Menkes steely hair syndrome (MSHS). The role of a number of trace elements in central nervous system (CNS) disease has been cited, but only in defects of copper metabolism, Wilson disease, and MSHS can abnormalities of brain function be specifically related to trace metals.

The measurement of trace elements is critical in documenting disease states and can be accomplished by atomic absorption spectrophotometry, plasma emission spectroscopy, neutron activation (5), mass spectrograph proton-induced x-ray emission (6), and laser microprobe mass analysis (7). Atomic absorption spectrometry is the procedure of choice for measuring single elements in fluids and tissues. The ubiquitous nature of small quantities of the many trace elements requires assiduous techniques in collecting specimens and performing the assay, and most investigators rely on research laboratories rather than commercial facilities for those assays.

DISORDERS OF COPPER METABOLISM

Copper (Cu) is an element necessary for a number of neuronal functions, ranging from energy production by electron transfer chain to the synthesis of norepinephrine. Metalloenzymes requiring copper include ceruloplasmin, cytochrome oxidase, dopamine betahydroxylase, superoxide dismutase, tyrosinase, and lysyl oxidase (8,9). The ontogenesis of copper begins in the third trimester as the fetus acquires the element in large amounts with primary storage in the liver (10). At term, serum copper concentrations are 30% of adult values (11); however, the newborn liver contains 5 to 10 times greater copper concentration than in the adult organ (10). The adult copper level, approximating 0.78 μM/g dry weight (wt) (50 μg/g dry wt), is reached after the third month of age (12). In the newborn liver, copper is localized in cytoplasmic granules resembling lysosomes; however, in the adult, copper is concentrated in cytosolic binding sites (13).

Changes of anabolism in infancy are initiated with absorption of dietary copper by a process assumed to be energy dependent (14). The metal is transported to the liver by the terminal amino acid of albumin before chelation to ceruloplasmin, utilization for hepatic metabolism, or excretion by the biliary system (15). Studies with intravenous administration of ^{64}Cu or ^{67}Cu in older patients have documented two peaks of incorporation into ceruloplasmin at 2 and 48 hours, respectively.

Copper is transported to body organs by ligand formation with ceruloplasmin, albumin, or amino acids. The trace element is also bound to red blood cells. The kinetics of binding indicate that only albumin or amino acids provide copper for cell intake (16). In mammals, transport across the cell membrane is energy dependent and utilizes carrier molecules (8). Intracellular copper is chelated to specific sulhydryl containing proteins, metallothioneins, as well as metalloenzymes, mitochondrial protein, and cytosolic binding sites (17).

Wilson Disease

Wilson disease (18), hepatolenticular degeneration, is caused by an abnormality of copper metabolism, producing a deposition of the element in many body organs including the liver, brain, eye, kidney, bone, parathyroid gland, and pancreas. Treatment with chelating agents reverses the deposition of copper and improves organ function.

Pathophysiology

The precise metabolic defect in Wilson disease has not been defined, but available data suggest there is a failure of mobilization of copper from the newborn liver associated with defective biliary excretion and decreased incorporation into ceruloplasmin (12). Postulated mechanisms include an abnormality of the lysosomal binding of copper resulting in decreased availability to biliary and ceruloplasmin compartments (19), failure to form a copper-low molecular compound essential for biliary excretion with decreased absorption of copper from the small intestine (15), and deficiency of a specific protein carrier for copper or an enzyme necessary for incorporation of copper into proteins (20). Because of low serum levels of ceruloplasmin, an increase in diffusable copper occurs, although the total serum copper value is usually lower than normal values. The continued hepatic deposition of dietary copper and the failure to mobilize copper from intracellular compartments result in a shift from cytosolic to lysosomal binding sites and a release of copper into the blood with entry into other organs. No abnormality of the amino-acid composition of ceruloplasmin has been demonstrated. Cellular components cited as damaged by excessive copper deposition in humans and experimental animals include mitochondria, lysosomes, peroxisomes, microtubules, nuclear DNA, and glutathione (17). The evolution of pathophysiologic processes has been defined by Deiss et al. (21), describing the relationship of the hepatic and tissue copper (Table 7.1).

Although a genetically determined multisystem defect in intracellular binding of copper has been postulated in Wilson disease, there is no abnormality of intracellular copper distribution observed when brain tissue of affected patients is compared to normal brain homogenates (22). In addition, hepatic transplantation results in resolution of neurologic signs and symptoms (23), indicating that Wilson disease is caused by chronic exposure to elevated serum concentrations of copper rather than a multiorgan avidity for copper.

Clinical Presentation

The major clinical features of Wilson disease are caused by copper deposition in liver and brain. Toxicity of other organ systems, including blood (hemolytic anemia), renal (tubular acidosis), and endocrine (hypoparathyroidism), may produce initial manifestations. Approximately 25% of patients will present with dysfunction of two or more systems (24).

The signs and symptoms of liver dysfunction are the presenting manifestations in 42% of patients with Wilson disease, usually occurring before evidence of neurologic disease, and rarely before the age of 6 years (24). Any acute or chronic abnormality of liver function in a child over the age of 4 years, without documented etiology by serologic testing or toxicologic study, should be considered as Wilson disease until that diagnosis has been excluded. Lethargy and anorexia (70%), jaundice (56%), and abdominal pain are early manifestations of the disease (25).

Table 7.1   Ontogeny of Wilson disease

Stage	Hepatic Disease	Neurologic Disease	Kayser-Fleischer Ring	Blood *Ceruloplasm	Copper	Urine Copper	Radiocopper@
I Hepatic Copper Accumulation	Asymptomatic: may have ↑ transaminase values	0	0	↓	N or ↓	↑ or N	N/A
II Systemic Cupremia Hepatic Failure	Impaired function → failure	0	0 → +	↓	↓	↑	Impaired incorporation ^{67}Cu into ceruloplasm
Cerebral Copper Accumulation Hemolytic Anemia Nephropathy							
III Neurologic Dysfunction	Asymptomatic → impaired function	+	+	↓	↓	↑	Impaired incorporation ^{67}Cu into ceruloplasm
IV Chelation Therapy	Improved → normal (weeks)	Improved → normal (months)	0 → +	↓	↓	↑	Impaired incorporation ^{67}Cu into ceruloplasm

Modified from Deiss et al. (21)
* ↓ in 90%–95% Patients
  0 = Absent
  + = Present
N/A = Not Available

Other clinical and laboratory evidence of liver disease ranges from elevated serum transaminase levels in the asymptomatic homozygote, to symptoms and signs suggesting acute viral hepatitis with recovery, chronic active hepatitis, or cirrhosis with hepatosplenomegaly and esophageal varices. Acute liver failure with encephalopathy and GI bleeding caused by Wilson disease may be the presenting manifestations in adolescents (12).

Abnormal neurologic signs and behavioral manifestations are initial features of Wilson disease in 44% of patients, and defective motor function may range from progressive spastic diparesis to any variety of dyskinesias (24). The typical syndrome consists of the ingravescent onset of dysarthria, sialorrhea, motor clumsiness, and dysgraphia in patients from 8 to 10 years of age. Psychologic testing usually documents that cognitive abilities are within the normal range but with a discrepancy between verbal and performance intelligence quotients (IQs), an attentional deficit, and defective self-image.

A gradual progression of abnormal motor function to wing-beating tremor, slurred speech, saccadic ocular motility, and a fixity of facial expression (pseudosclerosis form), occurs over a period 5 to 10 years after onset of symptoms and signs. In other patients, dystonic posturing and a persistent facile smile with open mouth are admixed with a rapid distal tremor that may evolve to repetitive focal myoclonus (progressive lenticular degeneration form) (26).

Patients with Wilson disease may present with abnormal behavior ranging from an attentional deficit syndrome and adjustment reactions in children and adolescents, to psychosis and dementia in young adults. Completion of a careful neurologic history and examination are required to determine subtle signs and symptoms not otherwise detailed by the history of a patient with school failure or psychotic behavior (18).

Inspection of the patient with Wilson disease may reveal hypermelanotic macules of nail lunulae, but only detection of copper deposition in Descemet membrane of the cornea, the Kayser-Fleischer ring, establishes excessive storage (Figure 7.1). This ocular abnormality usually requires a slit lamp examination for its detection and may not be present in patients with copper storage confined only to the liver. The Kayser-Fleischer ring has also been identified in other hepatopathies, including biliary cirrhosis, Indian childhood cirrhosis, and newborns with cholestatic jaundice (27). Other ocular signs include (sunflower) cataracts (28), which are caused by copper deposition.

Diagnosis

The diagnosis of Wilson disease is established by measuring serum copper and ceruloplasmin levels, urine excretion of copper and, when indicated, hepatic copper content and copper kinetics by ^{64}Cu or ^{67}Cu uptake.

Stage I of the disease involves hepatic copper accumulation (Table 7.1). The serum ceruloplasmin levels are low,

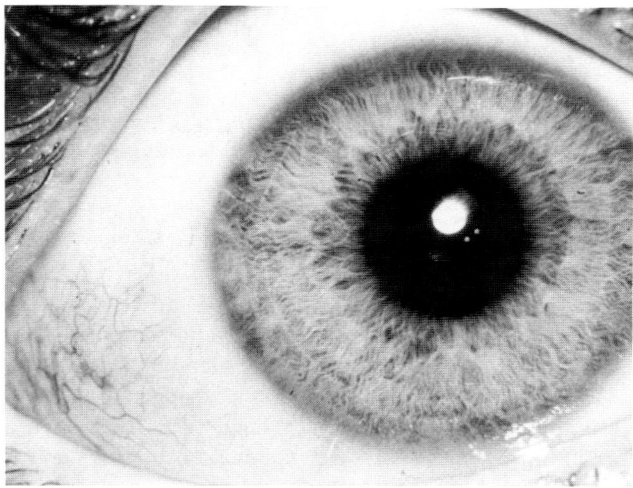

FIGURE 7.1   Characteristic Kayser-Fleischer ring in an 11-year-old boy with Wilson Disease. (Courtesy of Dr. Bruce O. Berg, University of California Medical Center, San Francisco).

< 0.13 μM/L (< 20 mg/dL; n: 0.99 to 3.31 μM/L) in 90% of patients. The serum concentrations of total copper (N: 14.1 to 29.8 μM/L: 90 to 190 μg/dL) is variable, but the unbound fraction is increased. The urine excretion of copper may not be increased (N: 16 μM/24 hr: < 100 μg/L/24 hr). The hepatic copper content is always greater than 3.87 μM/g dry wt: < 250 μg/g/dry wt. (N: 0.78 μM/g dry wt.: < 50 μg/g dry wt).

In stage II and later stages, serum ceruloplasmin values are decreased and urine excretion of copper is consistently > 1.6 μM/L (>100 μg/24 hr). Hepatic copper content may decrease with copper mobilization but always exceeds (3.87 μM/L: 250 μg/g dry wt)(29).

The measurement of copper kinetics by ^{64}Cu or ^{67}Cu isotope techniques documents decreased biliary excretion and the failure of incorporation of ^{67}Cu into ceruloplasmin 48 hours after administration, which is pathognomonic of Wilson disease (30).

The finding that fibroblasts from patients with Wilson disease demonstrate increased uptake of copper when grown in media containing copper has not been duplicated by other investigators (31).

Differential Diagnosis

In any progressive movement disorder, abnormality of muscle tone, or psychiatric abnormality beginning in mid-childhood years without defined etiology, Wilson disease should be considered as possible until biochemical tests of copper metabolism are obtained. For patients with symptoms and signs of hepatopathy or neurologic dysfunction, the presence of Kayser-Fleischer ring is highly suggestive of Wilson disease. Abnormal serum ceruloplasmin and copper levels as well as the concurrence of renal disease, hemolysis, arthralgias, and endocrinopathies, differentiate

Wilson disease from neurologic system degenerations, leukodystrophies, neuronal storage diseases, and disorders of amino-acid metabolism.

Neurophysiologic and Neuroimaging Studies

Electroencephalograms (EEG) of asymptomatic patients are usually normal. Generalized or complex partial seizures, however, may occur in Wilson disease and are related to neuronal deposition of copper or to metabolic encephalopathy induced by hepatic dysfunction (32). No specific abnormalities of evoked potentials have been described in these patients.

Computed tomographic (CT) head scans are usually normal in patients without neurologic signs but may reveal low density changes in the thalamocapsular regions or lentiform nuclei as well as ventricular dilation, reflecting cortical atrophy in untreated patients with chronic disease (33). Magnetic resonance imaging (MRI) of young adults receiving chelation therapy demonstrates abnormal T2 weighted images correlating anatomy with dyskinesia in the following manner: dystonia-putamen, bradykinesia-putamen, and dysarthria-caudate and putamen. Generalized brain atrophy and ventricular dilation are common (34).

Pathology

The hepatic pathology of Wilson disease has been described by various investigators (35,36). Changes of gross anatomy of the brain include putamenal atrophy caused by hepatic failure, even in patients without neurologic signs. Microscopic examination of the putamen reveals decreased large and small neurons and myelinated fibers with reactive glial changes. Characteristic glial cells include Opalski and Alzheimer types I and II cells. The changes of the caudate and globus pallidus are less severe than those noted in the putamen; the substantia nigra is usually normal. Focal demyelination and spongiform changes are present in the cortex with a frontal lobe prominence.

Genetics

The genetic defect in Wilson disease occurs in 1 in 200 to 1 in 400 of the general population, and the disease incidence approximates 1 in 200,000. Males and females are equally affected. Based on the evaluation of an esterase linkage in a specific pedigree, a mutation on chromosome 13 has been suggested (37). Other investigators have postulated that an abnormal controller gene rather than a structural mutation produces the defect in copper metabolism (12).

The asymptomatic siblings and parents of patients, as well as relatives with suggestive symptoms, should be studied to exclude the presymptomatic state. Low ceruloplasmin levels usually represent a carrier state (38), and documentation of urine copper excretion and the hepatic copper content is mandatory before initiating life-long therapy.

Therapy

Since the documentation of copper intoxication as the cause of Wilson disease in 1948 (39), investigators have attempted to remove copper by chelating agents. The successful use of penicillamine by Walshe in 1956 provides the basis for current therapy (40). The development of triethylene tetramine dihydrochloride (trientine) in 1985 has provided a second therapeutic agent (41,42). Administration of zinc to block copper absorption in the GI tract has achieved a decrease in copper stores in patients with Wilson disease (43). For the 2% of patients with hepatic failure attributable to Wilson disease, plasmapheresis and liver transplantation should be considered since a response to chelation therapy does not occur (23).

The chelation of copper by D-penicillamine achieves removal of copper from tissues to restore organ function over a period of weeks (neurologic symptoms) to months (hepatic signs) (14). The hepatic copper concentration should be measured before instituting life-long chelation therapy. In children under 10 years of age, the initial dose of D-penicillamine of 500 mg/day may be increased to 0.75 to 1 g/day. Older children and adolescents should receive between 1 to 2 g/day. The dose should be titrated to achieve a urine excretion of 2 mg copper per day for the first 12 months and 1 mg copper per day after that time. Because penicillamine acts as a pyridoxine antagonist, pyridoxine administered at a dose of 25 to 50 mg/day, should be considered as supplemental therapy. Although many patients also receive a low copper diet, the value of this diet is uncertain.

Complications of penicillamine therapy include death from a fatal hepatopathy occurring with noncompliance, hypersensitivity reactions to the medication with urticaria, neutropenia and thrombocytopenia, nephrosis, myasthenia gravis, systemic lupus erythematosis (SLE), a chronic dermal state, elastosis perforans serpiginosa, and the depletion of zinc.

Sternlieb et al. (44) have described the rapid onset of a fatal hepatopathy in 8 of 11 patients, about 2 1/2 years after therapy was discontinued. No acquired hepatic dysfunction was observed in patients with continued therapy.

Acute hematologic and hypersensitivity reactions with bone marrow suppression usually occur at the onset of treatment, and improvement is rapid after discontinuation of the drug. Reinstitution of small doses (25 mg), gradually increasing to the standard dosage with concomitant use of steroids and antihistamines, induces tolerance. Nephrosis (45), SLE (46), and myasthenia gravis (47) may be noted in older patients with immune dysfunction. A decrease in the dose of penicillamine or substitution of another agent results in improvement.

Elastosis perforans serpiginosa is a disfiguring dermal state caused by penicillamine that persists for the duration of therapy. Since penicillamine chelates zinc, its depletion may reach symptomatic levels. Administration of oral supplemental zinc corrects the deficiency.

Because penicillamine alters collagen linkage, the agent was considered a possible teratogen; however, clinical experience to date has not defined a significant embryopathy in infants of mothers who received the drug (48).

Other Agents

Triethylene tetramine dihydrochloride has been available only since 1985, but it appears to induce cupruresis in a dosage comparable to that of penicillamine (42). It is second only to penicillamine as the treating drug of choice; the mechanisms of action are uncertain. Mild anemia appears to be the only significant side effect.

Zinc depletes total body concentrations of copper by forming a ligand with intestinal metallothioneins (43). Zinc is as effective in preventing fatal hepatic disease in patients with Wilson disease, as shown in an animal model of Bedlington terriers.

The development of fulminant hepatic failure in patients with Wilson disease indicates the need for a more rapid removal of copper than can be achieved by chelation therapy. Plasmapheresis is effective in removing large amounts of copper, as well as other factors producing hepatic coma (49). In patients with irreversible hepatic damage, liver transplantation has been demonstrated to be life-saving. CNS abnormalities gradually improve over a period of weeks (14).

Menkes Steely Hair Syndrome

Menkes et al. (50) described a disease involving copper metabolism after evaluating a family with five male siblings who had steely hair, seizures, spasticity, and who died at an early age. Subsequent analyses of brain lipids suggested a defect in fatty acid metabolism (51). French et al. (52) documented an abnormality in electron transport at the level of cytochrome A1 + A2 in brain, liver, and muscle. Because of changes in the wool and systemic vasculature in copper deficient sheep, analagous to abnormalities noted in patients with steely hair, Danks (53) examined copper metabolism in these patients and documented defective absorption from the GI tract and decreased hepatic and serum levels. Goka et al. (54) found elevated copper concentrations in fibroblasts obtained from patients with the steely hair syndrome; and Heydorn et al. (55) measured copper levels in affected fetuses, determining there was decreased copper concentrations in liver but increased concentrations in all other organs.

The neurodegenerative disorder, inherited as an X-linked recessive trait, involves mutliple organ systems and has been variously named, including kinky hair syndrome, tri-chopoliodystrophy, and X-linked copper malabsorption syndrome. The term *MSHS* denoted the neurologic features, the hair abnormality, and the defect in copper metabolism (56).

Pathophysiology

Available data document the cause of abnormal levels of copper in organs and body fluids as a tissue-specific defect in the formation of intracellular copper ligands, occurring during organogenesis. Concentrations of copper in the brain are decreased in the cerebral cortex and basal ganglia when fetal data are compared to postmortem findings (56,57). The concentrations of copper and ceruloplasmin in cord blood are within the normal range, but the physiologic increase in blood-copper concentrations at 2 months of age does not occur (11,58). The hepatic copper levels are 10 to 20 times lower than control specimens (57), and there is defective absorption from the GI tract as determined by radioisotope techniques (59) and electron microscopy of the small bowel wall (60). No abnormality in systemic transport of copper has been documented; concentrations of ceruloplasmin increase with therapy to increase the serum copper level, and the amino-acid profile of ceruloplasmin is comparable to control specimens (59).

At the cellular level, abnormal copper sequestration has been documented in fibroblasts of patients utilizing elemental and radiocopper (61). Examinations of cell homogenates from patients or from the animal model, the brindled mouse, have indicated either an increase in the membrane-bound component or the cytosolic fraction, depending on techniques (59,62). The decreased function of cuproenzymes (cytochrome oxidase, lysyl oxidase, dopamine betahydroxylase (DBH), superoxide dismutase, tyrosinase, ceruloplasmin) reflects an abnormality in intracellular compartmentalization of copper. An increase in metallothioneins, a metal-binding protein with abundant cysteine appears related to increased intracellular copper levels rather than defective gene control according to data obtained from a mouse model (63).

Impairment of brain function and structure in this disease may be caused by abnormal kinetics of DBH (63), lysyl oxidase (64), cytochrome oxidase (65), or abnormalities in lipid components of myelin resulting from decreased long-chain fatty acid concentrations and desaturation of other fatty acids (66). Decreased concentrations of norepinephrine and increased concentrations of dopamine have been documented in the cerebrospinal fluid (CSF) of patients with MSHS (64). Although studies of animals suggest a relationship of norepinephrine levels to seizures (67), no clinical correlation of frequency of convulsions and CSF norepinephrine levels has been noted in nine patients (Tables 7.2, 7.3).

Abnormalities of lysyl oxidase activity cause defective collagen formation producing angiodysplasia with abnormal vascular structures, permeability, and neovascularization,

Table 7.2   MSHS clinical and laboratory data*

Patient	Birth Date	Initial Examination	Current Status	Neurologic Findings at Onset	Facial Features	Radiologic Findings		CT[1]	EEG	Family History
						Osseous	Bladder Diverticuli			
1	2–13–73	2 mos	E- 15 mos	Seizures	+	+	+	NA	Spike wave	+
2	5–29–73	3 days	A- 14 yrs	Hypotonia	+	+	+	+	Mild slowing	+
3	8–29–74	3 years	E- 10 yrs	Seizures	+	+	+	+	Spike wave	−
4	5–29–75	1 day	E- 3 mos	Hypotonia Spasticity	+	+	+	NA	Spike wave	+
5	5–2–82	2 mos	E- 6 mos	Seizures	+	+	+	+	Spike wave	+
6	11–10–82	9 mos	A- 5 yrs	Seizures	+	+	+	+ +	Spike wave	−
7	11–3–83	8 mos	A- 4 yrs	Seizures	+	+	−	+	Spike wave	−
8	2–10–85	8 mos	A- 3 yrs	Hypotonia Spasticity	+	+	−	+	Spike wave	−
9	6–14–86	5 mos	A- 18 mos	Seizures	+	+	+	+	Spike wave	−
10	5–29–87	5 mos	A- 8 mos	Seizures	+	+	+	+	Spike wave	−

* − Serial Examinations of 10 patients at St. Christopher's Hospital for Children
E = Expired
A = Alive
NA = Not Available
Osseous = Wormian Bones and/or Metaphyseal Spurring

[1]CT + = cerebral atrophy and angiodysplasia
  + + = cerebral atrophy, angiodysplasia, and subdural effusion

Table 7.3   MSHS clinical and laboratory data*

Patient	Copper Metabolism			Catecholamine Metabolism		
	Blood Level Onset µmol/L	Metabolism Therapy	Blood Level on Therapy µmol/L	Dopamine	Norepinephrine	Therapy (DOPS)
1	0.18	Oral chelate	1.1	NA	NA	0
2	0.39	IV → Oral chelate DOPS*	0.93	↑	↓	+
3	1.72	Oral chelate	1.72	N	N	0
4	0.39	Oral chelate	1.01	NA	NA	0
5	0.19	Oral chelate DOPS*	0.93	↑	↓	+
6	0.36	Oral chelate DOPS*	0.96	↑	↓	+
7	0.25	Oral chelate	1.00	N	N	0
8	0.38	Oral chelate	0.69	N	N	0
9	0.31	Oral chelate	0.95	↑	↓	0
10	0.19	Oral chelate	0.69	N	N	0

*DOPS-DL- Threo 3,4-dihydroxyphenylserine

as well as defective bone structure. It is probable that abnormal vascular structures are critical in formation of subdural effusion noted in one of our patients (Table 7.2, patient 6). The demonstration of normal vessel structures by angiography in our patient at 6 weeks of age (Table 7.2, patient 2) and the documentation of abnormal vessels by the same procedure at 5 years of age, indicate that angiodysgenesis occurs during the course of the disease. The bony abnormalities are characterized by metaphyseal spurring and osteopenia. These changes can mimic scurvy or fractures caused by trauma.

Abnormal mitochrondrial function and cytochrome oxidase deficiency decreases energy production and may impair the function of many organs, including the peripheral and central nervous systems.

Clinical Presentation

The concurrence of abnormal hair, suggestive facial features, and marked hypotonia, the most common clinical findings in the perinatal period, suggest the diagnosis of MSHS to the astute examiner. The facial characteristics include a rounded countenance with depressed nasal bridge and a prominent philtrum. Hypotonia is present in proximal and distal musculature. The abnormality of hair is usually, but not always, present and may effect both scalp and body hair. The hair is pale (decreased melanin), tortuous (abnormal keratin), and may entangle in small knots. Microscopy easily identifies the structural changes of pili torti, monilethrix, and trichorrhexis nodosa; fluorescent microscopy reveals a defective hair shaft. Hypothermia, osseous deformities (talipes equinovarus), and icterus commonly occur (57).

After the neonatal period, seizures, usually infantile spasms, are noted and are associated with persistent or periodic hypothermia, hyperreflexia and failure to achieve motor abilities, adaptive skills, and language. Seizures do not usually respond to administration of standard anticonvulsant drugs or to treatment with adrenocorticotropic hormone (ACTH). We have demonstrated, however, improved seizure control in 3 of 6 patients (Table 7.2, patients 3,5,6) receiving antiepileptic drugs and supplemental copper. One patient receiving parenteral and later oral copper supplements from 3 weeks of age has not developed seizures by 14 years of age (Table 7.2, patient 2).

Progressive bulbar dysfunction precedes a persistent vegetative state that is noted in the majority of patients by the age of 1 year. Only one patient has been able to sit alone, and none have developed language. Abnormalities of other organ systems include large bladder diverticuli, producing urinary stasis, and repeated urinary tract infections (UTIs). Gastroesophageal reflux may cause pneumonitis, and 2 of 10 patients (Table 7.2, patients 2,6) have required gastrostomy and fundoplication. Three patients required laryngoscopy and bronchoscopy, and a tracheostomy was required in one patient (Table 7.2, patient 2). The ages of death in 4 of 10 patients have ranged from 6 months to 10 years. The oldest patient in our series is 14 years of age.

The clinical manifestations of the MSHS are homogeneous in our patient population, but genetic heterogeneity is suggested by the report of one male patient (68) with an ataxic gait but normal cognitive abilities. Several female patients with clinical and biochemical features of MSHS have X-chromosome translocations (69). Our data also document variations in the DBH activity in 4 of 8 patients (Table 7.3).

Diagnosis

The diagnosis of MSHS in the infant or child is established by documenting low serum or hepatic copper concentrations in the presence of typical clinical manifestations of the disease. The serum concentrations in untreated patients are always below 0.78 μM/L (50 μg/dL). Low blood levels of ceruloplasmin, less than 0.67 μM/L (10 mg/dL), reflect decreased copper concentrations. Measurements of copper in hepatic tissue may be necessary to establish the diagnosis during the physiologic nadir of the serum copper levels (11). Hepatic copper concentrations are less than 0.31 μM/ g dry wt (20 μg/g dry wt), when measured from birth to 2 months of age. An elevated muscle copper concentration measured in one patient at 5 months of age was documented in MSHS (70). A marked increase in fibroblast content of elemental copper or [67]Cu has been noted in all patients with the disease; the assay is available in only selected laboratories (61).

The radiologic examinations and neuroimaging studies show findings suggestive of the diagnosis. Skull radiographs may demonstrate wormian bones, and radiographs of long bones document metaphyseal fractures or spurring that can mimic the findings observed in child abuse or scurvy (56). Angiodysplasia can be demonstrated on CT, MRI, and digital subtraction angiography, or angiograms performed by direct arterial puncture. Serial CT or MRI studies may demonstrate emerging subdural effusions and progressive cerebral atrophy (71). Voiding cystourethrograms or ultrasound examinations frequently document bladder diverticuli (72).

Pathology

The consistent neuropathologic features of MSHS include nerve cell loss and gliosis in the cerebral cortex, cerebellum, and thalamus; there is generalized reduction in myelinated axons. The abnormal arborization of Purkinje cells with swelling of the dendrites is unique. Defects in cortical lamination are consistent with an abnormality in cell migration occurring during the 6th fetal month (73).

Mitochondrial changes of enlarged tubulovesiculated crista, swelling, dense body formation, and occasional accumulation of glycogen have been noted throughout the brain (74). The abnormalities are more apparent in Purkinje cells, neurons of the molecular and granular layers of the cerebellum, cerebral cortex, globus pallidus, and lateral thalamus than in myelinated axons of white matter.

Genetics

The gene frequency for MSHS is unknown, but the estimated disease incidence is 1 in 90,000 to 100,000. By comparative gene mapping, the most likely locus for the gene of MSHS is band q13 on the long arm of the human X chromosome (37). Current data suggest that abnormal accumulation of copper may be caused by defective regulation of metallothionein production by abnormal functioning of the gene on the X chromosome (75,76) contrasts with data from the brindled mouse (62).

Detection of the carrier state is possible by noting the hair abnormality, measuring placental copper content of female newborns, or by documenting elemental copper or [67]Cu uptake in fibroblasts. Pili torti has been identified in 49% of obligate carriers (77). Horn (78) has successfully demonstrated levels of copper consistent with the carrier state in 9 of 18 female fetuses by study of the placental copper content and tissue culture studies. Copper uptake of fibroblasts from females at risk has revealed a significant overlap between heterozygotes and normal homozygotes. Measuring the copper uptake of specific clones produces a more reliable method of heterozygote identification but is not generally available (79). The copper uptake by fibroblasts from amniotic fluid and increased copper content of chorionic villus reliably identify affected fetuses.

The availability of mutants of the mottled mouse, an animal model with defective intracellular compartmentalization of copper of undetermined similarity to MSHS, has permitted detailed study of metabolism. Useful data in determining the pathophysiology of MSHS (58) have been provided by the measurement of hepatocyte and fibroblast copper values and kinetics; the relationship of metallothionein production to copper levels; the analysis of brain lipids; and the histologic and ultrastructural changes of origin.

Therapy

Treatment of the disorder has included supportive care, efforts to increase copper concentrations in liver, brain, and blood by administration of supplemental copper, and attempts to increase low levels of norepinephrine in the CSF and blood.

Supportive care has focused on treatment of seizures with drugs. With the exception of patients treated with supplemental copper and medication, the response to therapy is incomplete. Infantile spasms are usually not controlled by ACTH therapy. Generalized tonic-clonic and complex partial seizures usually occur later in life. Only 1 of 10 patients in our series has not developed seizures by 14 years of age (See Table 7.2).

The treatment of repeated UTIs, the careful manipulation to avoid fractures of long bones, and the attention directed to nutrition and dysphagia, at times requiring gastrostomy and fundoplication, improve the status of the patient. Vitamin C may be helpful in improving bone integrity (80). Intravenous (IV) access becomes increasingly difficult and usually necessitates catheter placement when parenteral fluids are required. A proclivity to hypothalamic dysfunction and hypothermia requires consideration during any required anesthesia. Serial neurologic evaluations and CT are necessary for early detection of subdural effusions.

Supplemental Copper

Decreased copper concentrations of liver, brain, and blood have suggested an approach to therapy. The improvement in oxidative metabolism in muscle of a patient receiving IV copper salts (57) and the demonstration of increased lysyl oxidase activity in fibroblasts of the brindled mouse after increasing copper levels in the media (81), support the use of copper supplements. Our data in two patients demonstrate that IV administration of copper acetate or sulfate achieves normal levels of serum, CSF, hepatic copper, as well as ceruloplasmin (82). Copper chelated to nitrilotriacetate or histidine was administered by mouth to 10 patients. An increase in serum concentrations of copper to twice baseline values was noted, but not to the normal range (57). Inconsistent elevations of CSF, copper, and hepatic concentrations were documented. No reversal in the neurologic signs has been noted, however, although observations suggest there is improved seizure control and modification of rapid deterioration. No untoward effects of IV copper salts or oral copper chelates have been observed.

Investigators have administered substrates of lysyl oxidase and DBH in an attempt to improve function. A decrease in fractures was noted in one patient receiving vitamin C (80). DL- Threo 3,4-dihydroxyphenylserine (DOPS), an unnatural precursor of norepinephrine metabolized to norepinephrine by a nonspecific L-amino acid oxidase, was administered to three patients (83). An increase in plasma norepinephrine concentrations was noted, but there was no consistent change in CSF norepinephrine levels, and only negligible increases in urinary vanillylmandelic acid (84) were observed. No improvement in function was documented.

REFERENCES

 1. Garnica AD, Chan W, Rennert OM. Trace elements in development and disease. Major problems in pediatrics. Philadelphia: WB Saunders, 1986; 16(2):51–119.
 2. Danks DM. Inborn errors of trace element metabolism. Clin endocrinol metab 1985; 14(3):591–615.
 3. Hambridge MK. Disorders of mineral metabolism. Clin Gastroenterol 1982; 11(1):87–117.
 4. Garnica AD, Chan W-Y, Rennert OM. Trace metals in genetic disease: A review. Trace Elem Med 1985; 2(2): 47–58.
 5. Smallwood RA, Williams HA, Rosenoer VM, et al. Liver-copper levels in liver disease. Studies using neutron activation analysis. Lancet 1968; 2:1310–1313.
 6. Spieker C, Heck D, Zidek W, et al. Application of proton-induced-x-ray emission (PIXE) to the determination of trace elements in biological samples. Trace Elem Med 1986; 3(2): 87–89.
 7. Schmidt PF. Localization of trace elements with laser microprobe mass analyzer (LAMMA). Trace Elem Med 1984; 1:13–26.
 8. Evans GW. Copper homeostasis in the mammalian system. Physiol Rev 1973; 53(3):525–570.
 9. Walshe JM. The physiology of copper in man and its relation to Wilson's Disease. Brain 1967; 90:149–176.
10. Widdowson EM, Chan H, Harrison GE, et al. Accumulation of Cu, Zn, Cr, Co in the human liver before birth. Biol Neonate 1972; 20:360–367.
11. Henkin RI, Schulman JD, Schulman CB, et al. Changes in total, nondiffusable and diffusable plasma zinc and copper during infancy. J Pediatr 1987; 82(5):831–837.
12. Epstein O, Sherlock S. Is Wilson's disease caused by a controller gene mutation resulting in perpetuation of the fetal mode of copper metabolism in childhood? Lancet 1981; 1:303–305.

13. Goldfisher S. The localization of copper in the pericanalicular granules (lysosomes) of liver in Wilson's disease (hepatolenticular degeneration). Am J Pathol 1985; 46:977–983.

14. Danks DM. Hereditary disorders of copper metabolism in Wilson's disease and Menkes' disease. In: Stanbury JB, Wyngaarden JD, Frederickson D, et al., eds. The Metabolic Basis of Inherited Diseases, ed 5. New York: McGraw-Hill, 1983; 1251–1268.

15. Owen CA. Copper and hepatic function. Ciba Foundation Symposium 79: Biological Roles of Copper. Amsterdam: Exerpta Medica, 1980: 267.

16. Peters T Jr. Serum albumin: Recent progress in understanding of its structure and biosynthesis. Clin Chem 1977; 23(1):5–12.

17. Scheinberg HI, Sternlieb I. Wilson's Disease. In: Smith LHJ, ed. Major Problems in Internal Medicine. Philadelphia: WB Saunders, 1984; 29–31.

18. Wilson SAK. Progressive lenticular degeneration: A familial nervous disease associated with cirrhosis of the liver. Brain 1912; 34:295–507.

19. Sternlieb I, Van den Hamer CJA, Merrell AG, et al. Lysosomal defect of hepatic copper excretion in Wilson's disease (hepatolenticular degeneration). Gastroenterology 1973; 64(1):99–105.

20. Sass-Kortsak A. Hepatolenticular degeneration (Kinnier-Wilson) disease. In: Schweigh H, ed. Handbook der Inneren Medizin. Berlin: Springer 1974; 8:627–666.

21. Deiss A, Lynch RE, Lee GR, et al. Long-term therapy of Wilson's disease. Ann Intern Med 1971; 75:57–65.

22. Porter H. Copper proteins in brain and liver in normal subjects and in cases of Wilson's disease. In: Bregsma D, Scheinberg IH, Sternlieb I, eds. Wilson's Disease, Birth Defects. Original Article Series, Vol IV. New York: The National Foundation-March of Dimes, 1968: 23–28.

23. Starzl TE, Iwatsuki S, Van Thiel DH, et al. Evolution of liver transplantation. Hepatology 1982; 2:614–636.

24. Sternlieb I, Scheinberg IH. Wilson's Disease. In: Wright R, Aberti KGM, Karran S, et al, eds. Liver and Biliary Disease: Pathophysiology, Diagnosis, Management. London: WB Saunders 1979; 774–804.

25. Mazer H, Ede HJ, Mowat AP, et al. Wilson's disease: Clinical presentation and the use of prognostic index. Gut 1986; 27(11):1377–1381.

26. Brown DD. Hepatolenticular degeneration. N Engl J Med 1968; 278:352–359.

27. Smith LHJ, ed. Major Problems in Internal Medicine. Philadelphia: WB Saunders, 1984; 86–92.

28. Dunn LL, Annable WL, Kliegman RM. Pigmented corneal rings in neonates with liver disease. J Pediatr 1987; 110(5):771–776.

29. Smith LHJ, ed. Major Problems in Internal Medicine. Philadelphia: WB Saunders, 1984; 93–98.

30. Sternlieb I, Scheinberg IH. The role of radiocopper in the diagnosis of Wilson's disease. Gastroenterology 1979; 77:138–142.

31. Chan W, Cushing W, Coffman MA, et al. Genetic expression of Wilson's Disease in cell culture: A diagnostic marker. Science 1980; 208:299–300.

32. Hansotia P, Harris R, Kennedy J. EEG changes in Wilson's disease. Clin Neurophysiol 1969; 27:523–528.

33. Selekler K, Kansu T, Zileli T. Computed tomography in Wilson's disease. Arch Neurol 1981; 38:727–728.

34. Starosta-Rubinstein S, Young AB, Kluin K, et al. Clinical assessment of 31 patients with Wilson's disease. Correlation with structural changes on magnetic resonance imaging. Arch Neurol 1987; 44:365–370.

35. Smith LHJ, ed. Major Problems in Internal Medicine. Philadelphia: WB Saunders, 1984; 38–63.

36. Martin JP. Wilson's disease. In: Vinken PJ, Bruyn GW, eds. Handbook of clinical neurology. New York: Elsevier, 1968; 6:267–278.

37. McKusick V. The Morbid Anatomy of the Human Genome. Medicine 1987; 66:237–296.

38. Sternlieb I, Scheinberg HI. Prevention of Wilson's Disease in asymptomatic patients. N Engl J Med 1968; 278:352–359.

39. Cumings JM. The copper and iron content of brain and liver in the normal and in hepato-lenticular degeneration. Brain 1948; 71:410–415.

40. Walshe JM. Wilson's disease. New oral therapy. Lancet 1956; 1:25–26.

41. Walshe JM. Treatment of Wilson's disease with trientine (triethylene tetramine) dihydrochloride. Lancet 1982; 1:643–647.

42. Scheinberg IH, Jaffe ME, Sternlieb I. The use of trientine in preventing the effects of interrupting penicillamine therapy in Wilson's disease. N Engl J Med 1987; 317(4):209–213.

43. Van Callie-Bertrand M, Degenhart HJ, Visser HK, et al. Oral zinc sulfate for Wilson's disease. Arch Dis Child 1985; 60:656–659.

44. Sternlieb I. Personal communication. 1985.

45. Crawhall JC. Proteinuria in d-penicillamine-treated arthritis. J Rheumatol 1981; 8:161–163.

46. Walshe JM. Penicillamine and the SLE syndrome. J Rheumatol 1981; 8:155–160.

47. Kuncl RW, Pestronk A, Drachman DB, et al. The pathophysiology of penicillamine-induced myasthenia gravis. Ann Neurol 1986; 20:740–744.

48. Scheinberg IH, Sternlieb I. Pregnancy in penicillamine-treated patients with Wilson's disease. N Engl J Med 1975; 293:1300–1302.

49. Riviello JJ Jr, Halligan GE, Widzer SJ, et al. The value of plasmapheresis in hepatic encephalopathy. Ann Neurol 1986; 20(3):442.

50. Menkes JH, Alter M, Steigleder GK, et al. A sex linked recessive disorder with retardation growth of peculiar hair, and focal cerebellar degeneration. Pediatrics 1962; 29:764–779.

51. O'Brien JS, Sampson EL. Kinky hair disease. II. Biochemical studies. J Neuropath Exp Neurol 1966; 25:523–530.

52. French JH, Sherard ES, Lubell H, et al. Trichopoliodystrophy. I. Report of a case and biochemical studies. Arch Neurol 1972; 26:229–244.

53. Danks DM, Campbell PE, Stevens JB, et al. Menkes' kinky hair syndrome. An inherited defect in copper absorption with widespread effects. Pediatrics 1972; 50:188–201.

54. Goka TJ, Stevenson RE, Heffer PM, et al. Menkes disease: A biochemical abnormality in cultured human fibroblasts. Proc Natl Acad Sci 1976; 73:604–606.

55. Heydorn K, Dansgaard E, Horn N, et al. Extra-hepatic storage of copper. A male fetus suspected of Menkes' Disease. Hum Genet 1975; 29:171–175.

56. Grover WD, Johnson WC, Henkin RI. Clinical and biochemical aspects of Trichopoliodystrophy. Ann Neurol 1978; 5(1):65–71.

57. Danks DM. Of mice and men, metals and mutations. J Med Genet 1986; 23:99–106.

58. Mallet B, Aquaron R. Isolation and purification of ceruloplasm in oculocutaneous albinism, Menkes' disease, Wilson's disease and pregnant women. Clin Chem Acta 1983; 132(3):245–246.

59. Beratis N, Price P, LaBadie G, et al. ^{64}Cu metabolism in Menkes and normal cultured skin fibroblasts. Pediatr Res 1978; 12:699–702.
60. Horn N, Jensen OA. Menkes Syndrome: Subcellular distribution of copper determined by an ultrastructural histochemical technique. Ultrastruct Pathol 1980; 1:237–242.
61. Gregoriadis G, Sourkes TL. Intracellular distribution of copper in the liver of the rat. Can J Biochem 1967; 45:1841–1851.
62. Packman S, Palmiter R, Karim M, et al. Metallothionein messenger RNA regulation in the mottled mouse and Menkes kinky hair syndrome. J Clin Invest 1987; 79(5):1338–1342.
63. Grover WD, Henkin RI, Schwartz M, et al. A defect in catecholamine metabolism in kinky hair disease. Ann Neurol 1982; 12:263–266.
64. Royce PM, Camakaris J, Danks DM. Decreased lysyloxidase activity in skin fibroblasts from patients with Menkes's syndrome. J Biochem 1980; 192:579–586.
65. Maehara M, Ogasawara N, Mizutani N, et al. Cytochrome c oxidase deficiency in Menkes kinky hair disease. Brain Dev 1983; 5(6):533–540.
66. Blackett PR, Lee BM, Donaldson DL, et al. Studies of lipids, lipoproteins, and apolipoproteins in Menkes's disease. Pediatr Res 1984; 18(9):864–870.
67. Feller DJ, O'Dell BL. Dopamine and norepinephrine in discrete areas of copper-deficient rat brain. J Neurochem 1980; 34:1259–1263.
68. Procopis P, Camakaris J, Danks DM. A mild form of Menkes' Syndrome. J Pediatr 1981; 98:96–99.
69. Kapur S, Higgins JV, Delp K, et al. Menkes syndrome in a female with x-autosome translocation. Am J Hum Genet 1986; 39(3) Suppl:193.
70. Tonnesen T, Muller-Schauenburg G, Damsgaard E, et al. Copper measurement in a muscle biopsy. A possible method for postmortem diagnosis of Menkes disease. Clin Genet 1986; 29(3):258–261.
71. Faerber EN, Grover WD, DeFillipp G, et al. Cerebral MRI of Menkes kinky hair syndrome. Am J Radiol 1989; 10:190–192.
72. Harke TH, Capitanio MA, Grover WD, et al. Bladder diverticuli and Menkes Syndrome. Radiology 1977; 124(2):459–461.
73. Troost D, van Rossum A, Straks W, et al. Menkes kinky hair disease. II. A clinicopathological report of three cases. Brain Dev 1986; 4(2):115–126.
74. Yoshimara N, Kudo H. Mitochondrial abnormalities in Menkes Kinky Hair Disease (MKHD). Electron-microscopic study of the brain from an autopsy case. Acta Neuropathol 1983; 59(4):295–303.
75. McKusick V. The Morbid Anatomy of the Human Genome. Medicine 1987; 66:237–296.
76. Schmidt CJ, Dean HH, McBride WO. Chromosomal location of human metallothioneine gene: Implications for Menkes' Disease. Science 1984; 224:1104–1106.
77. Moore CM, Howell RR. Ectodermal manifestations in Menkes' syndrome. Clin Genet 1985; 28(6):532–540.
78. Horn N. Menkes X-linked disease: Prenatal diagnosis of hemizygous males and heterozygous females. Prenat Diagn 1981; 1:107–120.
79. Horn N. Menkes X-linked disease: Heterozygous phenotype in uncloned fibroblast cultures. J Med Genet 1980; 17(4):257–261.
80. Vek Y, Marazaki O, Hanai T. Menkes disease: Is vitamin C treatment effective? Brain Dev 1985; 7(5):519–522.
81. Royce PM, Camakaris J, Mann JR, et al. Copper metabolism in the mottled mouse mutants. The effect of copper therapy on lysyl oxidase activity in brindled (Mobr) mice. Biochem J 1982; 202(22):369–371.
82. Grover WD, Scrutton MC. Copper infusion therapy in trichopoliodystrophy. J Pediatr 1975; 86(2):216–220.
83. Grover WD, Hobdell E, Pellechia P, et al. Catecholamine replacement therapy in steely hair disease. Ann Neurol 1984; 16(5):413.
84. Hoeldtke RD, Cavanuagh ST, Hughes JD, et al. Catecholamine metabolism in steely hair disease. Pediatr Neurol. 1988; 4:23–26.

Chapter 8
Abnormalities of Purine and Pyrimidine Metabolism

Theodore Page and William L. Nyhan

Eleven well-documented defects are known in the synthesis, interconversion, and catabolism of purine and pyrimidine compounds. Many of these are associated with neurologic abnormalities. In several, presentations of varying severity have been described, and these are likely to be related to varying amounts of residual enzyme activity. Only in the Lesch-Nyhan syndrome is the phenotype distinctive enough to be diagnostic; in the others the hypertonicity/hypotonicity and delayed motor development encountered give little indication of the enzyme defect.

The role of purine and pyrimidine compounds in human metabolism is varied. These compounds are required not only for nucleic acid production (DNA and RNA), but also as energy transducers (adenosine triphosphate [ATP] and guanosine triphosphate [GTP]), mediators of hormone action (cyclic AMP), and neuromodulators (adenosine and guanosine). The clinical manifestations of patients with disorders of purine and pyrimidine metabolism are similarly varied.

BIOCHEMICAL PATHWAYS

Purine and pyrimidine nucleotides are synthesized in humans by both de novo and salvage pathways (Figures 8.1 to 8.4). Purine compounds are degraded ultimately to uric acid, which is excreted in the urine. Pyrimidine compounds are degraded to intermediary metabolites, which enter the citric acid cycle. The steady state concentrations of purine and pyrimidine nucleotides are controlled by their respective rates of synthesis, salvage, and catabolism.

Purine salvage is catalyzed by the enzymes adenine phosphoribosyltransferase (APRT) (1), adenosine kinase (2), and hypoxanthine guanine phosphoribosyltransferase (HPRT) (3). Pyrimidine salvage is catalyzed by uridine (4), cytidine (4), and thymidine kinases (5), and by orotate phosphoribosyltransferase (OPRT) (6). The normal substrate for OPRT is orotate, but the enzyme also converts uracil to uridine monophosphate at a low rate. The major route of pyrimidine salvage is via the nucleoside kinases. Deoxycytidine kinase phosphorylates various purine and pyrimidine deoxynucleosides. These purine and pyrimidine salvage pathways are controlled for the most part by the availability of substrates for the particular enzymes. HPRT and APRT are also inhibited by their products (7).

The rates of purine and pyrimidine catabolism are similarly controlled by substrate availability. Purine mononucleotides are converted to their respective nucleosides by a purine-specific 5′nucleotidase (8). Adenosine deaminase converts adenosine and deoxyadenosine to inosine and deoxyinosine, respectively (9). Inosine and guanosine, as well as their 2′deoxy analogs, are converted to their respective bases and the appropriate pentose-1-phosphate by purine nucleoside phosphorylase (10). These purine bases are ultimately oxidized to uric acid.

Pyrimidine mononucleotides are similarly converted to their respective nucleosides by a pyrimidine-specific 5′nucleotidase (11). Cytidine is converted to uridine by cytidine deaminase (12). Uridine and thymidine are converted to their respective bases by specific pyrimidine nucleoside phosphorylases (13,14). After reduction to their dihydro analogs, these compounds are ultimately converted to coenzyme A derivatives and enter the citric acid cycle. Purine and pyrimidine nucleotide concentrations are largely regulated through de novo synthesis. Purines are synthesized de novo by a 10-step pathway that is regulated

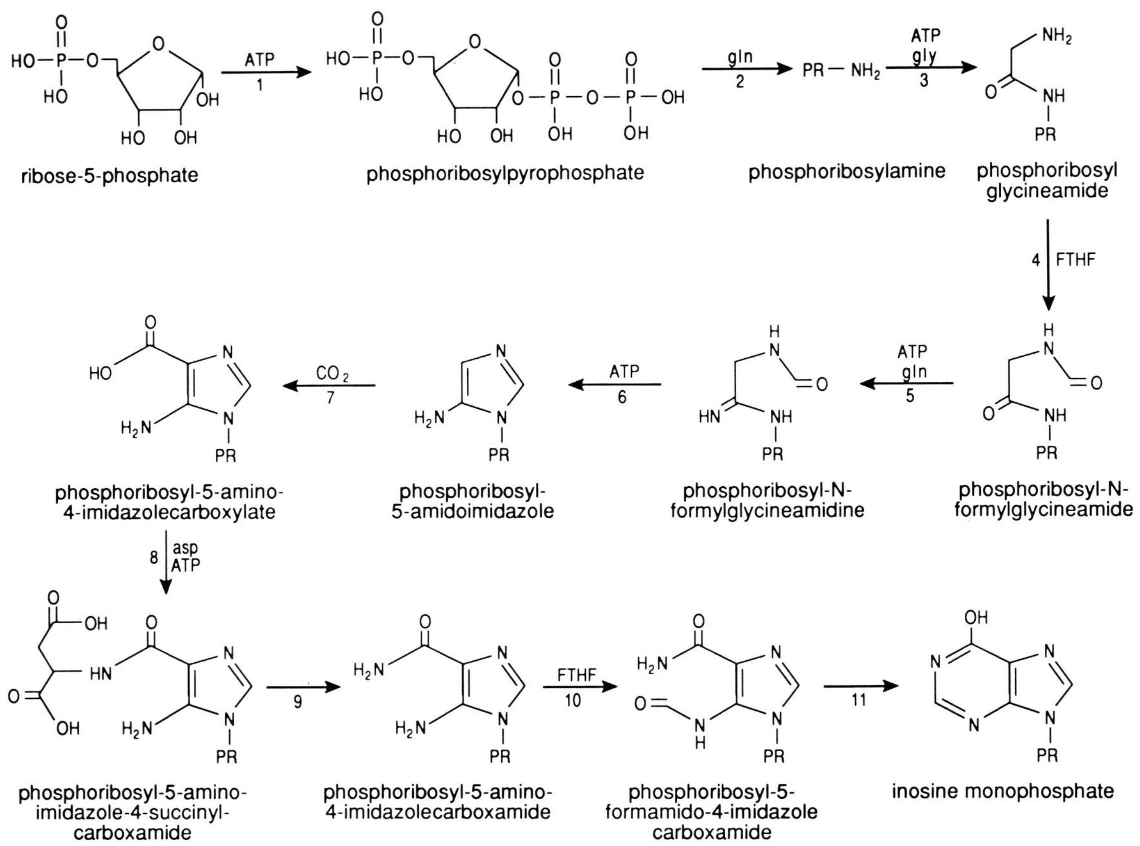

FIGURE 8.1 De novo purine synthesis. The enzymes are 1-PRPP synthetase; 2-PRPP amidotransferase; 3-phosphoribosylglycine-amide synthetase; 4-phosphoribosylglycineamide formyltransfer-ase; 5-phosphoribosylformylglycineamidine synthetase; 6-phos-phoribosylaminoimidazole synthetase; 7-phosphoribosylaminoim-idazole carboxylase; 8-phosphoribosylaminoimidazolesuccinyl-carboxamide synthetase; 9-adenylosuccinate lyase; 10-phosphori-bosylaminoimidazolecarboxamide transformylase; 11-inosinicase. The abbreviations are: asp-aspartic acid; ATP-adenosine triphos-phate; FTHF-formyltetrahydrofolate; gln-glutamine; gly-glycine.

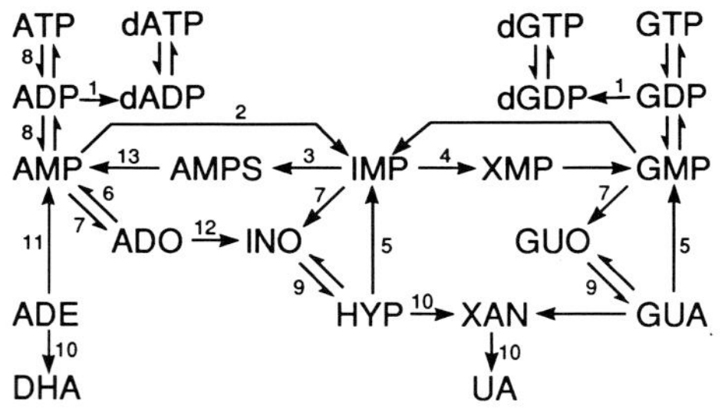

FIGURE 8.2 The major reactions of purine metabolism. The enzymes are 1-ribonucleotide reductase; 2-adenylate deaminase; 3-adenylosuccinate synthetase; 4-inosine monophosphate dehy-drogenase; 5-hypoxanthine-guanine phosphoribosyltransferase; 6-adenosine kinase; 7-5′nucleotidase; 8-adenylate kinase; 9-purine nucleoside phosphorylase; 10-xanthine oxidase; 11-adenine phos-phoribosyltransferase; 12-adenosine deaminase; 13-adenylosucci-nate lyase. The abbreviations are: ADE-adenine; ADO-adenosine; AMP,ADP,ATP-adenosine mono-, di-, and triphosphate; AMPS-adenylosuccinate; dADP,dATP-deoxyadeosine di- and triphos-phate; dGDP,dGTP-deoxyguanosine di- and triphosphate; DHA-dihydroxyadenine; GMP,GDP,GTP-guanosine mono-, di- and triphosphate; GUA-guanine; GUO-guanosine; HYP-hypoxan-thine; IMP-inosine monophosphate; INO-inosine; UA-uric acid; XAN-xanthine; XMP-xanthosine monophosphate.

at several points. The synthesis of the starting compound 5′phosphoribosyl-1-pyrophosphate (PRPP), catalyzed by PRPP synthetase, is inhibited by purine nucleotides, espe-cially adenosine diphosphate (ADP), ATP, and GTP (15). The synthesis of phosphoribosylamine by PRPP ami-dotransferase is the first committed step of de novo purine synthesis. This reaction is inhibited by AMP and guanosine monophosphate (GMP) (16). The branch point at inosine monophosphate (IMP) is regulated by the availability of GTP; this triphosphate is a substrate for adenylosuccinate synthetase (17), the committed step of adenine nucleotide synthesis, and an inhibitor of IMP dehydrogenase (18), the committed step of guanine nucleotide synthesis. These two reactions are also inhibited by their product nucleotides AMP and GMP, respectively (17,19) (Figure 8.2).

The initial reaction of de novo pyrimidine synthesis, the synthesis of carbamyl phosphate by carbamyl phosphate synthetase II (CPS II), is inhibited by uridine triphosphate (UTP) and stimulated by PRPP (20,21); CPS I, which is thought to be primarily a urea cycle enzyme, shows no such regulation (Figure 8.3). A secondary point of regulation is at OPRT; the K_m of this enzyme for orotic acid is approxi-

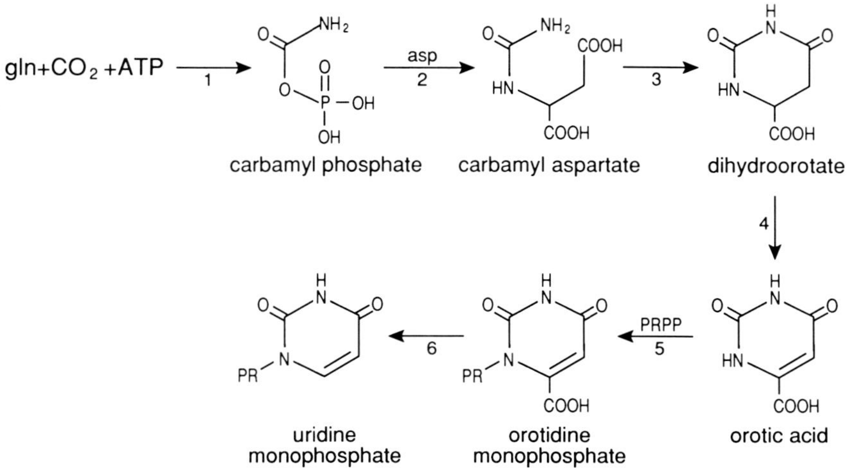

FIGURE 8.3 De novo pyrimidine synthesis. The enzymes are 1-carbamyl phosphate synthetase II; 2-aspartate transcarbamylase; 3-dihydroorotase; 4-dihydroorotate dehydrogenase; 5-orotate phosphoribosyltransferase; 6-orotidine monophosphate decarboxylase. The abbreviations are: asp-aspartic acid; ATP-adenosine triphosphate; gln-glutamine; PRPP-phosphoribosyl pyrophosphate.

mately 10 times the physiologic concentration, so the availability of PRPP also affects the rate of de novo pyrimidine synthesis (22) (Figure 8.4). Since both the salvage and de novo production of purine nucleotides are also regulated by the availability of PRPP, the synthesis of purine and pyrimidine nucleotides are coordinated. Coordination may also occur through the availability of ATP; this triphosphate activates CPS II and inhibits purine synthesis (23).

An enzyme defect in the synthesis, interconversion, or catabolism of purines or pyrimidines does not always affect the intracellular, plasma, and urinary concentrations of these compounds in a predictable way. For example, a deficiency of pyrimidine 5′nucleotidase causes the expected intracellular increase in pyrimidine nucleotides, whereas deficiency of adenine phosphoribosyltransferase does not seem to cause a deficiency of adenine nucleotides.

In several disorders, notably HPRT deficiency, there are syndromes of varying severity that are related to varying degrees of enzyme activity. The correlation of enzyme activity with the severity of the accompanying clinical syndrome can be demonstrated by assay of the relevant enzyme in intact cells (24,25). Since mutant enzymes are often unstable and may denature upon cell lysis, assays that use cell lysates as an enzyme source often underestimate the true in vivo enzyme activity.

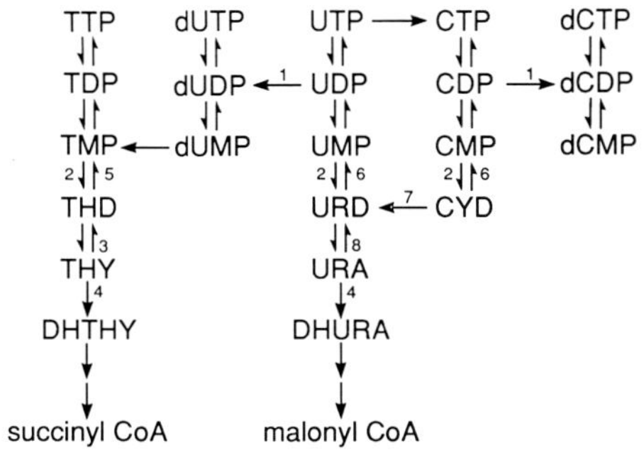

CLINICAL DISORDERS IN PURINE AND PYRIMIDINE METABOLISM

Hypoxanthine-Guanine Phosphoribosyltransferase Deficiency

The most common and best studied disorder of purine and pyrimidine metabolism is the deficiency of HPRT. This enzyme is responsible for the conversion of hypoxanthine and guanine to their corresponding 5′ribonucleotides. Usually the deficiency is complete and results in the Lesch-Nyhan syndrome (26–28). The cardinal features of this syndrome are mental retardation, spasticity, choreoathetosis, hyperuricemia, and compulsive self-injurious behavior (29,30). Milder variants of the syndrome in which the enzyme deficiency is not complete are also known (24). The HPRT gene is on the X chromosome, and the HPRT deficiency syndromes are inherited as X-linked recessive traits (28). The frequency of HPRT defects is estimated at 1 in 100,000 to 1 in 380,000 (31,32).

Lesch-Nyhan patients are normal at birth and develop normally for the first 6 months of life. The first manifestation of the disease is often the occurrence of uric acid crystals, resembling orange sand, in the diaper. Hyperuricemia is severe enough that hematuria and urinary tract stones may occur; older patients may have uric acid tophi and gouty arthritis in the absence of treatment. Delayed neurologic development becomes evident within the 1st year. Infants fail to develop or lose the ability to sit up unsupported and are unable to stand or walk. All patients eventu-

FIGURE 8.4 The major reactions of pyrimidine metabolism. The enzymes are 1-ribonucleotide reductase; 2-pyrimidine 5′nucleotidase; 3-thymidine phosphorylase; 4-dihydropyrimidine dehydrogenase; 5-thymidine kinase; 6-uridine kinase; 7-cytidine deaminase; 8-uridine phosphorylase. The abbreviations are: CMP,CDP,CTP-cytidine mono-, di- and triphosphate; CYD-cytidine; dCMP,dCDP,dCTP-deoxycytidine mono-, di- and triphosphate; DHTHY-dihydrothymidine; DHURA-dihydrouracil; dUMP,dUDP,dUTP-deoxyuridine mono-, di- and triphosphate; THD-thymidine; THY-thymine; TMP,TDP,TTP-thymidine mono-, di- and triphosphate; UMP,UDP,UTP-uridine mono-, di- and triphosphate; URA-uracil; URD-uridine.

ally become hypertonic, and have increased deep tendon reflexes. Ankle clonus and extensor plantar responses are common. The strong muscle pull may cause dislocation of the hips. There are dystonic, athetoid, and choreic movements, as well as dysarthric speech, and dysphagia, which may cause inanition. In addition, all patients have recurrent vomiting. In at least three instances, it has been associated with esophagitis complicated by a stricture in one patient, major bleeding in another, and severe anemia in two of the three. The vomiting becomes incorporated into the abnormal behavior so that at least some of it appears semi-voluntary. Mental development is retarded; intelligence quotients (IQs) usually range from 40 to 70 (28).

The most distinctive aspect of Lesch-Nyhan syndrome is the compulsive self-mutilative behavior (30). Though self-injury may occur in other disorders, the behavior seen in Lesch-Nyhan syndrome is unique and diagnostically useful. It often begins with the eruption of teeth and takes the form of destructive biting of the lips and fingers to the extent that there is actual loss of tissue. Patients are easily identified by the loss of tissue around the mouth and mutilation of the fingers (Figures 8.5 and 8.6). This is in contrast to the callus

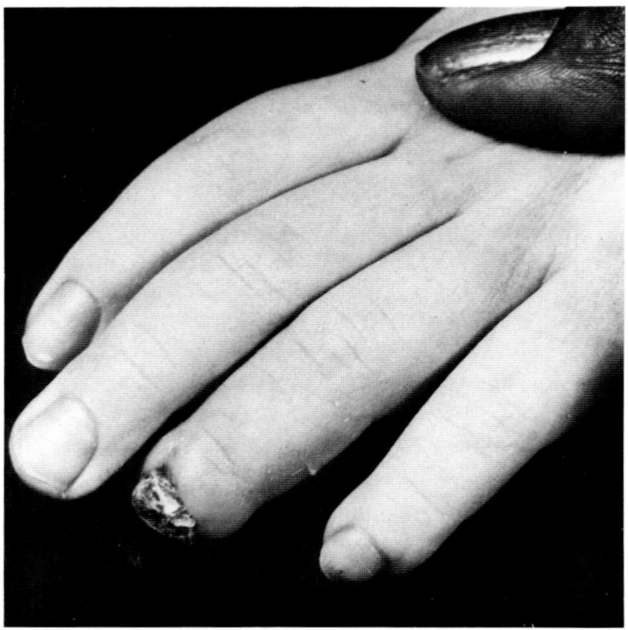

FIGURE 8.6   Partial amputation of a finger. (Reprinted with permission from Nyhan WL. A disorder of uric acid metabolism and cerebral function in children. Arthritis Rheum 1965;8:659–664.)

or swelling that results from the hitting, picking, or banging on parts of the body observed in patients with other types of self-injurious behavior; these patients rarely have actual loss of tissue. Patients with Lesch-Nyhan syndrome do not have a neuropathy that could make them insensitive to pain, for they scream in pain when they bite themselves. They are aggressive to others, they use language aggressively, and they may hit or kick other persons.

In all HPRT deficiency syndromes there is overproduction of purines and hyperuricemia (28,29). Serum urate is usually above 5 mg/dL and is often in the vicinity of 10 mg/dL. The daily excretion of uric acid is 3 to 4 times that of normal children of comparable size. Expressed in relation to creatinine, Lesch-Nyhan patients excrete 3 to 4 mg uric acid/mg creatinine; normal control values are less than 1 mg uric acid/mg creatinine.

Patients with partial HPRT deficiency are known in which some or all of the symptoms of Lesch-Nyhan syndrome are absent (24,28). If HPRT activity is measured in intact cultured fibroblasts, patients with the complete Lesch-Nyhan syndrome have 1.4% or less of the normal HPRT activity. Patients with 1.4% to 1.6% of the normal HPRT activity have normal intelligence, but otherwise manifest all the Lesch-Nyhan symptoms and signs. In the range of 1.6% to 8%, patients have normal intelligence and do not show self-mutilation, but the neurologic manifestations and hyperuricemia of Lesch-Nyhan patients are present. With 8% to 60% of the normal HPRT activity, patients have hyperuricemia and its consequences as their only clinical manifestations. Other combinations of symptoms, such as self-mutilation without neurologic symptoms, have not been associated with HPRT deficiency.

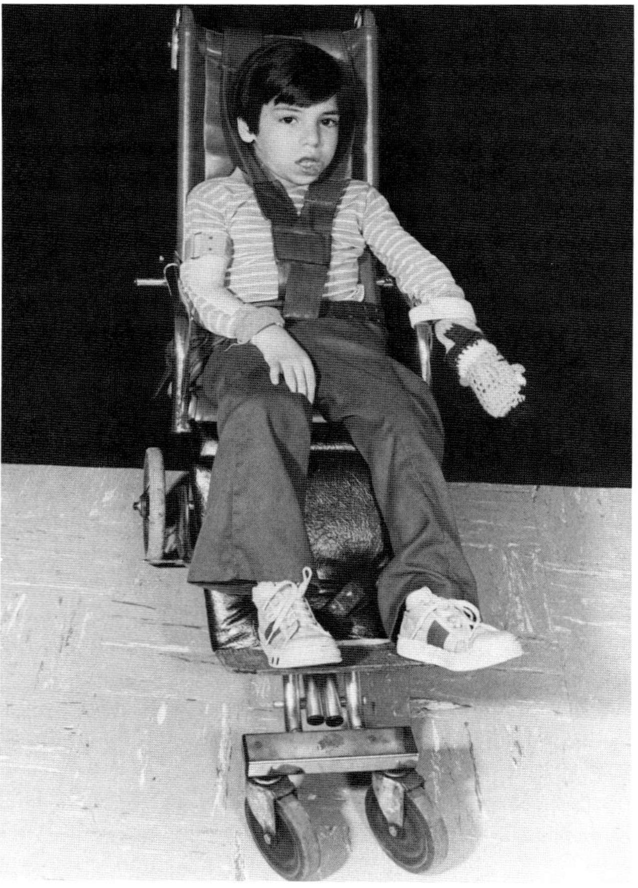

FIGURE 8.5   Patient with the Lesch-Nyhan disease. The self-mutilation around the mouth is evident, as well as the classic position restrained in a wheelchair. He had an elbow restraint on one arm and a mitten on the other hand.

The symptoms of HPRT deficiency that are related to uric acid overproduction are readily explained by the excessive purine synthesis. This is caused by underutilization of PRPP, which is the starting material for de novo purine synthesis. The origin of the neurologic and behavioral manifestations is unknown. Aberrant neurotransmitter metabolism is almost certainly involved and the evidence points to a dopaminergic abnormality (28,33). However, there is no obvious connection between the metabolism of purines and that of dopamine and serotonin. High concentrations of uric acid or hypoxanthine and excessive purine synthesis are thought not to be responsible for the observed abnormalities since their occurrence in other genetic disorders, or in partial HPRT deficiency, is not necessarily accompanied by neurologic dysfunction.

A presumptive diagnosis of the Lesch-Nyhan syndrome can usually be made on the basis of the phenotype. The combination of self-mutilation with loss of tissue around the mouth, choreoathetosis, and spasticity is almost certainly Lesch-Nyhan syndrome. In the case of partial HPRT deficiency, the neurologic symptoms may appear without self-mutilation or mental retardation (24). Hyperuricemia and increased uric acid excretion are seen in all patients with HPRT deficiency.

A definitive diagnosis requires the assay of HPRT enzyme activity. Red blood cells are most convenient for this purpose; cultured skin fibroblasts, lymphocytes, or hair roots can also be used (28). In assays in which HPRT activity is measured in cell lysates, Lesch-Nyhan patients have less than 1% of the normal enzyme activity. In the usual erythrocyte assay the activity is most often indistinguishable from zero. Patients with partial HPRT deficiency may have from 0% to 60% of the normal activity in these assays, and the apparent enzyme activity does not necessarily correlate with severity of the patient's symptoms. Since clinical phenotypes do not vary within a pedigree, a finding of HPRT deficiency by one of these assays indicates a prognosis similar to that of an affected relative. However, in a presymptomatic infant with no affected relatives, the more accurate intact cell assay may be required to determine the prognosis.

A number of techniques are available for the detection of carriers of HPRT deficiency. Since the HPRT gene is on the X chromosome, female heterozygotes are mosaics in whom there are two populations of cells. These two cell populations cannot be detected in erythrocytes and leukocytes: mothers of Lesch-Nyhan patients have only HPRT$^+$ blood cells, presumably because of selection against HPRT$^-$ cells (34). This selection is less complete for carriers of partial HPRT deficiency (35). The growth of cultured skin fibroblasts from a possible heterozygote in media containing 6-thioguanine or 8-azaguanine will select for HPRT$^-$ cells (36); any cell growth is thus an indication of heterozygosity. However, the cells of some Lesch-Nyhan patients retain enough HPRT activity that they are not selected by these antimetabolites (37). It is therefore necessary to confirm cell selection with the proband's cells before attempting heterozygote detection in this way. The ability of individual cultured fibroblasts to incorporate ^{3}H hypoxanthine into nucleotides has also been used to detect heterozygotes (38). After incubation with the radiolabeled precursor, the two populations are apparent as dark and light cells. The current technique of choice for heterozygote detection is the hair root assay (39,40). Embryonic development of hair follicles is largely clonal so that each follicle expresses only one of the two X chromosomes. Heterozygotes can be detected by assaying HPRT in a number of individual hair roots. In many cases, heterozygotes may also be detected by restriction fragment length polymorphisms (RFLP) (41). A large number of probes for the X chromosome are now available including the HPRT gene itself. RFLP analysis may make it possible to detect the origin of a mutation as well as the type of alteration in the gene which is responsible for the abnormal enzyme. With the advent of polymerase chain reaction (PCR) technology, gene sequencing is also possible.

Prenatal diagnosis has been performed on amniocytes (42) and chorionic villus cells (41). Amniocytes can be assayed by cell lysis, as with red blood cells, or by the intact cell method. When assaying HPRT in chorionic villus cells, care must be taken to control the activity of 5′nucleotidase, which is high enough to catabolize all the IMP produced by HPRT, making normal cells appear to be HPRT-deficient. Prenatal diagnosis has also been performed by RFLP analysis (41).

Renal failure caused by urate deposition has been the most common cause of death in the untreated patient. Allopurinol is highly effective in the management of those aspects of the disease that are caused by uric acid overproduction. Oral administration of allopurinol at doses of 200 to 500 mg daily greatly reduces uric acid concentrations and effectively prevents tophi, gouty arthritis, and nephropathy. Urate calculi dissolve but xanthine calculi may also occur. Allopurinol has no effect on the behavioral or neurologic manifestations of the disease; to date there is no satisfactory treatment known for these manifestations.

The most effective day-to-day management of Lesch-Nyhan patients is aimed at preventing self-mutilation while, at the same time, allowing some degree of freedom. Self-mutilation can be prevented with elbow splints or by securing the patient's hands. Removing teeth is also effective in managing the biting behavior. Behavioral modification techniques that are effective in extinguishing other types of self-injurious behavior are not effective in Lesch-Nyhan syndrome. This is particularly true of aversion methods. In general, anything that causes patient anxiety leads to a worsening of self-mutilation.

Adenine Phosphoribosyltransferase Deficiency

The only significant pathway for the metabolism of adenine is conversion to AMP, catalyzed by adenine phosphoribosyltransferase (APRT) (1). The consequence of a deficiency of this enzyme is the accumulation of adenine, which is oxidized to 2,8-dihydroxyadenine (43,44). This compound may cause renal calculi and nephropathy. Neurologic abnormalities have not been attributed to APRT deficiency. This enzyme deficiency is transmitted as an autosomal recessive trait, and the gene frequency, at approximately 1 in 100, is more common than the occurrence of the disease would suggest.

The severity of 2,8-dihydroxyadenine accumulation seen in APRT deficiency is highly variable (44,45). Nephropathy may occur as early as the first year of life or late in adulthood. Some homozygotes are completely asymptomatic. Infants typically present in the first 2 years with colic, urinary tract infection, hematuria, or renal failure. The radiolucent stones are often incorrectly identified as uric acid (46). Similarly, the dihydroxyadeninuria may be mistaken for uricosuria when colorimetric tests are employed (44,46). Heterozygotes rarely have symptoms.

Excretion of adenine and 2,8-dihydroxyadenine is 1 to 3 mg/kg/day (44–46). Uric acid concentrations are not decreased. APRT occurs in most tissues and is conveniently assayed in erythrocytes or cultured fibroblasts. Prenatal diagnosis with chorionic villus cells has been reported (47). Homozygotes have virtually zero activity, and heterozygotes show the expected intermediate activity (44,48).

The treatment of APRT deficiency has employed low purine diets, high fluid intake, and the administration of allopurinol to reduce the formation of 2,8-dihydroxyadenine (44,49). The solubility of this metabolite is not altered within the physiologic pH range so alkali therapy is not beneficial (44). The prognosis depends on the degree of renal damage at the onset of therapy.

The frequency of APRT mutations is estimated at 0.41% to 1.1% (44,50). The fact that homozygotes may be asymptomatic or incorrectly diagnosed may help to explain the rarity of reported cases.

Adenosine Deaminase Deficiency

The deamination of adenosine to inosine, catalyzed by adenosine deaminase (ADA) (9) is the most significant pathway for the catabolism of adenosine. ADA deficiency, inherited as an autosomal recessive trait, leads to severe combined immunodeficiency (51,52). The gene is relatively rare, and approximately 100 patients have been reported.

In ADA deficiency the immune defect is present at birth or soon thereafter; both humoral and cellular immunity are defective (51–53). Initially the skin, gastrointestinal tract, and respiratory system are involved; candidiasis, diarrhea, and pneumonia are common findings. Immunoglobulins are decreased and lymphocyte response to phytohemagglutinin stimulation is deficient or absent.

Physical growth and development are delayed in these patients. They have distinctive radiographic features that may include cupping and enlargement of the anterior rib ends, pelvic dysplasia, reduced acetabular angles, and platyspondylia (51–53). The thymic shadow is absent, and at autopsy the thymus is found to be small and poorly differentiated. Severe osteoporosis may be present, and there may be compression fractures of the vertebrae (53).

In view of the nature of the disease, patients may have neurologic manifestations that are the result of infectious diseases. Some patients have been described in whom neurologic abnormalities appeared to be fundamental to the phenotype (54,55). One patient was described in whom a rapid tremor of the trunk and extremities was associated with intermittent dystonic posturing (55). Another patient presented at 3 months of age with head lag, increased muscle tone, athetoid movements, dystonic posturing, and absent deep tendon reflexes (54). The finding that symptoms improved during enzyme therapy suggested a relationship to ADA deficiency (54,55).

The deamination of adenosine to inosine, which is catalyzed by ADA, is the major route of adenosine metabolism. This enzyme also catalyzes the conversion of deoxyadenosine to deoxyinosine. The cytotoxicity of adenosine and deoxyadenosine has been related to at least three mechanisms. In the absence of ADA activity, adenosine and deoxyadenosine accumulate, resulting in an accumulation of ATP and deoxyATP (dATP). Excessive ATP inhibits PRPP synthetase; the main consequence of this inhibition seems to be decreased pyrimidine synthesis and accumulation of orotic acid (56). Excessive dATP inhibits ribonucleotide reductase, leading to decreased production of the deoxynucleotides necessary for DNA synthesis, especially deoxyCTP (57). Finally, adenosine itself inhibits S-adenosylhomocysteine (SAH) hydrolase; SAH is a product of methylation reactions which utilize S-adenosylmethionine, so these reactions are inhibited (58).

The occurrence of severe combined immunodeficiency, along with the characteristic radiographic features already noted, is strongly suggestive of ADA deficiency. Enzyme assay is required for definitive diagnosis. The enzyme is easily assayed in erythrocytes, lymphocytes, and cultured fibroblasts. As with HPRT deficiency, assay of ADA activity in intact erythrocytes reveals the severity of the disease to be related to the degree of the enzyme deficiency (25). Most patients also have elevated levels of the ADA substrates, adenosine and deoxyadenosine, in their serum and urine (51–53). Heterozygotes have intermediate levels of ADA activity; there is some overlap of activity between normal individuals and heterozygotes, so that carrier detection by erythrocyte ADA assay is only about 90% accurate (59). The ADA activity measured in cultured fibroblasts is too variable to be used for carrier detection (60). Prenatal diagnosis of affected fetuses has been accomplished with cultured amniocytes and chorionic villus cells (47,60,61).

The treatment of choice for ADA deficiency is bone marrow transplantation from a histocompatible donor (62,63). Several patients have achieved permanent immune restoration from such treatment. Transplantation of fetal thymus or liver has been successful in some patients (64). Enzyme replacement therapy by erythrocyte transfusion has proved beneficial, especially if there is residual enzyme activity (65). Irradiated packed red cells and polyethylene glycol immobilized enzyme have been utilized for enzyme replacement (54,55,66). In two cases, enzyme replacement therapy eliminated an ADA-deficient patient's neurologic symptoms (54,55). Metabolic replacement therapy with deoxycytidine has not been successful (65).

Purine Nucleoside Phosphorylase Deficiency

Purine nucleoside phosphorylase (PNP) catalyzes the reversible phosphorylytic cleavage of inosine and guanosine to their corresponding purine bases and ribose-1-phosphate; deoxyinosine and deoxyguanosine are also substrates (10). Approximately 20 patients with PNP deficiency have been described. The clinical picture is that of immunodeficiency (51,53,67). This disorder appears to be a rare autosomal recessive trait.

PNP deficiency is characterized by deficient cellular immunity (51,53,67). Humoral immunity may be normal. Patients usually present early in life with viral infections. Examination shows they are lymphopenic, and their lymphocyte response to phytohemagglutinin is deficient. The thymic shadow is absent in x-rays. Immunoglobulin levels may be normal.

In some patients hypotonia, spastic tetraparesis, and developmental delay have been described (68,69). These neurologic manifestations have been more prominent than the immunodeficiency. As in the case of HPRT deficiency, it appears that neurologic findings are confined to patients with the most severe enzyme deficiencies (25,68,69).

As might be expected from the nature of the deficiency, PNP-deficient patients are hypouricemic and hypouricosuric (51,53,67). Purines are excreted as the PNP substrates inosine and guanosine, and total purine excretion is increased. Inosine and guanosine, which are normally undetectable in the serum and urine, may reach concentrations of 10 to 100 μM in the serum and 1 to 1 to 4 mM/24 hours in the urine.

The immunodeficiency is thought to arise from the cytotoxicity of deoxyGTP (dGTP). This deoxynucleotide has been found to inhibit the reduction of cytidine diphosphate (CDP) to deoxyCDP (57). Partial protection by deoxycytidine from dGTP toxicity has been demonstrated in T cells in vitro (70). The greater toxicity of dGTP for T cells than B cells is consistent with the ability of T cells to accumulate greater amounts of this nucleotide in vitro (71).

The etiology of the neurologic features of the disease is unknown. Since PNP is the only enzyme that produces hypoxanthine and guanine from their respective nucleosides, it has been suggested that PNP deficiency is functionally equivalent to HPRT deficiency in the sense that substrates for the latter enzyme would be lacking (68,69). The spasticity seen in PNP deficiency is similar to that of HPRT deficiency, but choreoathetosis, mental retardation, and self-mutilative behavior are not associated with PNP deficiency.

Deficient T cell immunity combined with hypouricemia is strongly suggestive of PNP deficiency. The enzyme can be assayed in erythrocytes, lymphocytes, and cultured fibroblasts. The disorder can be diagnosed prenatally in amniocytes or chorionic villus cells (47,72). Heterozygotes have intermediate activity. It has been shown that the activity of the enzyme in intact erythrocytes is more closely correlated with the severity of the symptoms than the activity measured in lysates (25).

The immune dysfunction accompanying PNP deficiency may be less severe than that seen in ADA deficiency, and some patients have done reasonably well with no specific therapy. However, a number of patients have died of the disease. Bone marrow transplantation from a histocompatible donor is the definitive treatment (63). Enzyme replacement therapy with irradiated erythrocytes has resulted in improved immune function in most patients reported (73). Metabolic therapy with deoxycytidine has not proved beneficial (74). No therapy has been successful in alleviating the neurologic features of the disease.

Adenylate Deaminase Deficiency

The deamination of AMP to IMP is catalyzed by adenylate deaminase (AMPDA). Though the enzyme occurs in most cell types, this reaction appears to be of greatest significance in skeletal muscle in which AMPDA activity is more than 100-fold higher than elsewhere (75). A deficiency of the enzyme in muscle is accompanied by post exercise fatigue and pain (76,77); it is inherited as an autosomal recessive trait. Because of the difficulty of muscle biopsy and the fact that homozygotes may be asymptomatic, the gene frequency is difficult to estimate. More than 100 patients have been diagnosed.

The clinical expression and age of onset of adenylate deaminase deficiency are highly variable (76,77). The disorder is typically characterized by fatigue, cramps, and pain in muscles following exercise. Muscle weakness occurs in about 25% of the patients. Muscle wasting has not been reported. Serum activity of creatine kinase is elevated in half the patients, and about half of patients have electromyographic abnormalities. The age of onset varies from 1 to 70 years with the median age of 22 years. Some persons with the deficiency are completely asymptomatic, whereas several hours of rest may be required in others following even mild activity. A much more severe presentation, which includes hypotonia, visual failure, mental retardation, and developmental delay, has been reported in at least 11 families in Finland (78). Assuming the same genetic event was responsible for this group of patients, it is possible that the neurologic syndrome is closely linked to, but not a direct consequence of, adenylate deaminase deficiency.

The pathogenesis of the postexercise muscle fatigue has been postulated to be straightforward (76–77). After exercise, AMPDA-deficient patients require a longer time to restore resting levels of muscle ATP. During exercise ATP is rapidly converted to AMP. In normal muscle this AMP is cycled between IMP and AMP. Each turn of the cycle produces 1 molecule of fumarate. This cycling also protects AMP from hydrolysis. After the cessation of exercise, the remaining IMP is converted to AMP, and the accumulated fumarate is oxidized by the citric acid cycle, providing energy to convert the AMP to ATP. In the adenylate deaminase-deficient muscle, no fumarate is produced during exercise. In addition, the large pool of AMP produced from ATP is subject to hydrolysis by 5′nucleotidase. In patients with this disorder, adenosine increases in the muscle during exercise (79). After the cessation of exercise, there may be a deficiency of both AMP available for conversion to ATP and of fumarate to provide the energy for this conversion.

The diagnosis of myoadenylate deaminase deficiency requires muscle biopsy. The absence of an increase in venous NH_3 following ischemic exercise of the forearm is a useful screening test (80). The few heterozygotes who have been studied have had approximately one half the normal myoadenylate deaminase activity (76). The limiting of expression of the enzyme to muscle has militated against prenatal diagnosis; ultimately it should be possible through DNA techniques.

Treatment of the disorder is focused on limiting vigorous exercise. Some success has been reported with ribose, but the mechanism of the therapeutic effect is unclear (76). A complete deficiency of erythrocyte adenylate deaminase has been described in individuals who are completely asymptomatic (81).

Xanthine Oxidase Deficiency

Xanthine oxidase catalyzes the oxidation of hypoxanthine to xanthine, and of xanthine to uric acid; xanthinuria results from a deficiency of this enzyme. This disorder is characterized by the excretion of purines as xanthine rather than uric acid, and urinary tract calculi (53,82). Deposition of xanthine crystals in muscle tissue has been encountered in patients with myopathy and muscle cramps. It is inherited as an autosomal recessive trait. The prevalence of the disease has been estimated at 1 in 45,000 (82).

The majority of patients with xanthine oxidase deficiency are asymptomatic and are discovered incidentally because of hypouricemia. Others have presented with xanthine stones. These may produce hematuria, renal colic, infection, hydronephrosis, and renal failure, although most patients have had a relatively benign course. Symptoms referrable to muscle have been associated with the deposi-

tion of xanthine crystals in muscle in approximately four pedigrees. Some of these patients have presented with myopathy, and others have had cramps or tightness of leg muscles after walking. In a rare related disorder, xanthinuria is the consequence of a primary defect in molybdenum metabolism (83,84). The activities of the two molybdenum-containing enzymes xanthine oxidase and sulfite oxidase are severely deficient. The neurologic features, which include mental retardation, seizures, and cerebral atrophy, are thought to be due to sulfite oxidase deficiency.

In the absence of xanthine oxidase activity, hypoxanthine is not converted to xanthine, and xanthine is not converted to uric acid. Xanthine is also produced by the deamination of guanine. Since hypoxanthine is efficiently salvaged in the presence of normal activity of HPRT, the purine that is excreted in xanthine oxidase deficiency is predominantly xanthine. Xanthine is even less soluble than uric acid and is thus more likely to form stones in the urinary tract (85).

The diagnosis of hereditary xanthinuria is suspected because of hypouricemia. The serum concentration of uric acid is usually less than 1 mg/dL. Examination of the urine reveals a similar major reduction in the excretion of uric acid. Oxypurine excretion, which is normally 4 to 8 mg/day, is increased to 50 to 500 mg/day (82). Xanthine oxidase is not appreciably expressed in erythocytes, leukocytes, or cultured fibroblasts. The enzyme may be assayed in biopsied liver or intestine.

The aim of management is the prevention of xanthine stones. High fluid intake is the only reliable measure. Alkalinization is not helpful. A patient with combined deficiency of xanthine oxidase and sulfite oxidase was treated with 300 to 500 μg/day ammonium molybdate (86). Xanthine and sulfite excretion became normal and the neurologic symptoms improved.

Adenylosuccinate Lyase Deficiency

The enzyme adenylosuccinate lyase is unique in purine metabolism in that it catalyzes two very different reactions (87). Both of these reactions involve the conversion of aspartate to fumarate with the donation of an amino group. One of these reactions is the conversion of phosphoribosyl aminoimidazolesuccinylcarboxamide (SAICAMP) to phosphoribosyl aminoimidazolecarboxamide (AICAMP), the eighth step of de novo purine synthesis. The other is the conversion of adenylosuccinate to AMP. Patients reported with deficient activity of this enzyme have had a syndrome of psychomotor delay and autistic behavior (88). The defect is rare and current evidence is consistent with autosomal recessive inheritance. Eight patients have been studied.

Patients appear normal at birth but psychomotor retardation becomes evident within the 1st year. Seizures developed in 5 of 8 patients. Three patients displayed autistic behavior, including lack of eye contact and repetitive stereotypic movements. Surveys of populations of autistic children are not turning up examples of this disorder, and behavior of this sort is common in severely retarded individuals. Growth retardation was noted in two patients. Magnetic resonance imaging (MRI) brain scans in four patients did not show findings consistent with leukodystrophy, but the cerebellum was decreased in size.

A distinctive feature of this disorder is the appearance of the unusual compounds succinyladenosine (SADO) and aminoimidazolesuccinylcarboxamide riboside (SAICAR) in the serum, urine, and cerebrospinal fluid (CSF) (88,89); these are the dephosphorylated substrates for the deficient enzyme. The combined concentration of these two compounds may reach 200 μM in CSF and 10μM in plasma. Excretion of succinylpurines is 2 to 5 mg/mg creatinine. Adenylosuccinate lyase was deficient in all tissues studied, but the deficiency appears to be most severe in the kidney and liver. Activities are in the range of 0% to 60% of control values (88).

The etiology of the neurologic symptoms is not known, but it is thought to be due to toxicity of the succinylpurine compounds rather than to the lack of purine nucleotides. Therapeutic trials with adenine, intended to restore a possible deficiency of adenine nucleotides, were of no benefit.

Adenylosuccinate lyase deficiency can be screened for with the Bratton-Marshall reaction, which can be applied to dried urine on filter paper. Confirmation is made by finding of SADO and SAICAR in the serum, urine, or CSF. The enzyme is usually assayed by following the conversion of adenylosuccinate to AMP spectrophotometrically. The enzyme deficiency may not be prominent in cultured fibroblasts or erythrocytes of all patients.

Phosphoribosylpyrophosphate Synthetase Abnormalities

The production of phosphoribosylpyrophosphate (PRPP) is catalyzed by PRPP synthetase in an important step in the regulation of both purine and pyrimidine metabolism. A small number of patients have been described in which PRPP synthetase activity is greater than normal (53,90,91) and resulting in purine overproduction. Some patients have had neurologic abnormalities, especially deafness. The gene for PRPP synthetase is located on the X chromosome and heterozygous females may also have symptoms. The defect is rare: Only about 20 patients have been reported.

In most patients, symptoms attributable to uric acid overproduction are the only known manifestations (92) and include renal colic, hematuria, crystalluria, and renal stones. Plasma concentrations of uric acid usually range from 8 to 12 mg/dL, and urate excretion is on the order of 2 to 3 mg/mg creatinine (92,93). Gouty arthritis has been noted in older patients (53).

In two families in which PRPP synthetase superactivity has been documented, there have also been neurologic fea-

tures (90,93), hearing loss, hypotonia, and developmental delay. One of these patients had bilateral epicanthus, slight ptosis, low-set ears, a high arched palate, and left-convergent strabismus (90). Another patient had dysplastic teeth and absence of lacrimal glands (93). The mothers of these two patients had some degree of hearing loss as well as hyperuricemia (90,93).

One apparent case of PRPP synthetase deficiency has been reported (94). The patient was severely retarded and suffered convulsions. He had megaloblastic anemia similar to that seen in orotic aciduria, as well as increased excretion of orotic acid and decreased excretion of uric acid. The concentration of PRPP was approximately 50% of normal in the patient's erythrocytes, and PRPP synthetase activity was less than 10% of normal.

An overproduction of purines is the expected consequence of PRPP synthetase superactivity. Intracellular concentrations of PRPP are elevated in cultured fibroblasts of patients with PRPP synthetase superactivity (95). Three types of enzyme defects have been shown to result in excessive PRPP synthetase activity: increased maximum velocity; decreased sensitivity to the inhibitors ATP, ADP, and GTP; and increased affinity (that is, decreased K_m) for the substrates (96). Some mutant enzymes have more than one of these characteristics (95,96). The mutant enzymes often show decreased stability as well.

PRPP synthetase occurs in most tissues, including erythrocytes, leukocytes, and cultured fibroblasts. However, because of the combination of increased activity and decreased stability, several patients were initially thought to have normal activity in their erythrocytes. The enzyme is best studied in cultured fibroblasts or lymphoblasts. Since there are several possible causes for increased activity, detection of this type of defect may require a detailed kinetic study of the enzyme including affinity for substrates, inhibition by nucleotides, and activation by phosphate.

The symptoms attributable to uric acid can be successfully treated with allopurinol. A low-purine diet was reported to be helpful in one case (90). There is no specific treatment for the neurologic manifestations.

Orotate Phosphoribosyltransferase and Orotidine Monophosphate Decarboxylase Deficiency (Orotic Aciduria)

Orotic acid is converted to uridine monophosphate (UMP) in a sequence of two reactions catalyzed by orotate phosphoribosyltransferase (OPRT) and ortidine monophosphate decarboxylase (ODC) (6,20). Hereditary orotic aciduria is unique in that both enzyme activities are absent (23,53). The result is reduced de novo synthesis of pyrimidine nucleotides and accumulation of orotic acid. Patients are characterized by growth retardation and megaloblastic anemia (23,53). Approximately 12 patients have been reported. An autosomal recessive mode of inheritance appears likely.

Patients with hereditary orotic aciduria appear normal at birth, but present at a few months of age with anemia, lethargy, failure to thrive, and developmental delay. Motor retardation is sometimes seen (97). Hematologic abnormalities are a consistent finding and include leukopenia with hypochromic anemia and megaloblastic changes in the bone marrow.

All patients excrete large amounts of orotic acid; this excretion can reach more than 1 g/day (23). Crystalluria is usually apparent and may be accompanied by hematuria and ureteral obstruction (53).

The pathogenesis of this disorder is straightforward. In most cases both OPRT and ODC are deficient; in one patient only ODC activity was found to be absent (98). The substrates orotic acid and PRPP are underutilized, and production of pyrimidine nucleotides is deficient. Patients excrete orotic acid, and the excess PRPP gives rise to increased purine production, which may result in hyperuricemia. Pyrimidine nucleotide deficiency is apparently responsible for the hematological abnormalities.

The activities of OPRT and ODC are most conveniently measured in erythrocytes, leukocytes, or cultured fibroblasts. Excretion of orotic acid is a useful screening test, but enzyme assays are required for a definitive diagnosis. Heterozygotes also show increased excretion of orotic acid together with 40% to 60% of the normal enzyme activity (23); the activity in homozygotes is less than 5% of normal (23,53,97).

Hereditary orotic aciduria is successfully managed by oral uridine replacement (23,53,97). Feedback regulation of the pathway of de novo pyrimidine synthesis leads to greatly reduced production of orotic acid. The hematologic features of the disease resolve completely, and growth and development may become normal. However, patients with impaired mental development prior to treatment remain mentally retarded.

Dihydropyrimidine Dehydrogenase Deficiency

The pyrimidine bases thymine and uracil are converted to their dihydro forms as the first step of their catabolism. This reversible dehydrogenation is catalyzed by dihydropyrimidine dehydrogenase (DPD). A deficiency of this enzyme has been described in at least six pedigrees and is associated with a variety of neurologic abnormalities as well as the excretion of thymine and uracil (99–101). It is inherited as an autosomal recessive trait. The frequency of the mutation is very rare.

Patients with DPD deficiency are normal at birth and develop normally for 1 year or more. Most of the patients have presented in early childhood with developmental delay and seizures. In one patient, deep tendon reflexes were exaggerated (99). Two patients exhibited only autistic behavior. In two patients mental development was retarded, but in others intelligence was thought to be normal (99–101).

One patient remained asymptomatic until the age of 40 years when she was treated with 5-fluorouracil for a breast carcinoma. She developed severe neurologic dysfunction, including loss of speech and memory, and inability to move her extremities. MRI brain scans were consistent with demyelination. Thymine-uraciluria was noted and the activity of DPD in her circulating blood cells was undetectable. Flurouracil was withdrawn and her neurologic function returned to normal within 4 months. A subsequent MRI scan showed remyelination of the previously affected areas (102).

The excretion of thymine and uracil by patients with DPD deficiency may be as much as 0.6 mg/mg creatinine, which is nearly 1000 times normal (100). Elevation of these compounds in the serum may reach 100-fold, to the range of 20 to 25 μM. The unusual metabolite 5-hydroxymethyluracil is also present in the urine.

The pathogenesis of the neurologic symptoms of DPD deficiency is poorly understood at present. These symptoms are probably related to elevated amounts of uracil and thymine in the cerebrospinal fluid. No specific treatment for these symptoms is known.

DPD deficiency is detected on the basis of the greatly increased concentrations of thymine and uracil in the serum or urine. Deficient DPD activity is documented in the erythrocytes, leukocytes, or cultured fibroblasts. DPD activity in the leukocytes of patients is on the order of 0% to 5% of normal (100). The activities of obligate heterozygotes is 30% to 80% of normal (99).

Pyrimidine 5′Nucleotidase Deficiency

Purine and pyrimidine nucleotides are converted to their corresponding bases by nucleotidases, which are specific for one or the other type of nucleotide (11). Thus, in pyrimidine 5′nucleotidase deficiency, hydrolysis of purine nucleotides is normal. Deficiency of this enzyme is associated with severe hemolytic anemia (103–107). The defect has been described in at least 30 pedigrees and inheritance appears to be an autosomal recessive trait. The frequency of the defect is rare.

Patients present in early childhood with jaundice and hemolytic anemia (103–105). One patient was also reported to have hypotonia and developmental delay at 1 year of age (105). Hemoglobin is typically 5 to 10 g/dL and reticulocytosis may be as high as 45%. The anemia is nonspherocytic and there is prominent basophilic stippling. Erythrocyte nucleotide levels are 3 to 6 times normal and analysis reveals the nucleotide content to be 80% pyrimidines (105). Pyrimidine 5′nucleotidase activity is 3% to 15% of normal; considering the high concentration of reticulocytes, which are known to have higher activity of this enzyme, the deficiency is probably greater. Heterozygotes have approximately half the normal activity when compared to subjects with reticulocytosis, but overlap with normal subjects.

The inhibition of glucose-6-phosphate dehydrogenase (G6PD) by high concentrations of pyrimidine nucleotides is believed to be responsible for the hemolysis (106). At present, no therapy other than blood transfusions have been successful.

With the predominance of pyrimidine nucleotides, a simple screening assay is provided by measuring the ultraviolet absorption maximum of deproteinized erythrocytes (104). In pyrimidine 5'nucleotidase-deficient patients, it is shifted from the normal wavelength of 256 to 257 nm to 266 to 270 nm. The high concentration of nucleotides in the erythrocytes makes it possible to diagnose this disorder by nuclear magnetic resonance spectrometry (107). The diagnosis is confirmed by assay of the enzyme in erythrocytes.

A syndrome very similar to hereditary pyrimidine 5'nucleotidase deficiency may result from chronic low-level lead poisoning (108). The enzyme of such patients may be found to be severely deficient during a hemolytic crisis. With the clearing of lead from the system, the anemia resolves, and nucleotidase levels return to normal.

Other Defects of Purine and Pyrimidine Metabolism

One pedigree has been reported in which a deficiency of erythrocyte adenylate kinase was accompanied by hemolytic anemia (109). Two brothers had severe anemia with reticulocytosis and chronic hyperbilirubinemia. Hemoglobin was between 3.7 and 8.6 g/100 mL and reticulocytosis varied from 2.3% to 34%. They had 4% to 10% of the normal adenylate kinase activity and no detectable G6PD activity. The sister of these brothers had 0.5% to 4% of the normal adenylate kinase activity and normal G6PD activity. Upon examination she was found to be mildly anemic; hemoglobin was 8.5% to 9%, but she was in good health.

A syndrome of hyperuricemia, ataxia, and deafness has been described in a single kindred in which five members had hyperuricemia, renal insufficiency, ataxia, and sensorineural deafness (110). At least one member of the kindred had ataxia and deafness without hyperuricemia, and another had ataxia only. Thus, the neurologic abnormalities and the metabolic abnormality may be determined by different genes segregating in this family. The concentration of uric acid in the serum ranged from 7.8 to 10.6 mg/dL. Urate creatinine ratios in urine were 0.3 and 0.96. Erythrocyte activity of HPRT and APRT were measured in 22 members of the kindred, and all were normal.

Encephalopathy and self-mutilation with uric acid accumulation and normal HPRT has been described in a single patient, a twin whose brother had died at birth (111). There were younger twins in the sibship, one of whom had psychomotor retardation, and the other the habit of beating his head against walls. The patient had retarded psychomotor development. Convulsions developed at the age of 3 years, and self-mutilative behavior began at 3 to 4 years. By the age of 14 years all but the stubs of four fingers had been amputated. He also violently bit the inside of his mouth and the lips. On neurologic examination he had choreoathetoid movements, and hypesthesia was noted in the right arm. Pneumoencephalography showed cerebral cortical atrophy. The concentration of uric acid in the blood was 6 mg/dL, and there was increased excretion of urinary urate levels over 900 mg/24 hrs. The activity of HPRT in the erythrocyte was normal.

There has been one report of cytidine deaminase deficiency accompanied by immunodeficiency and hypotonia in a single pedigree (112). The proband was anemic and had deficient T and B cell function. Three previous children had died before 6 months of age from infections and seizures. The activities of ADA, PNP, and other enzymes of purine and pyrimidine metabolism were normal. Cytidine deaminase activity in the patient's leukocytes was approximately 15% of normal. The parents, who were first cousins, had intermediate levels of cytidine deaminase activity.

There are several reports of a deficiency of purine ecto-5'nucleotidase of lymphocytes in association with various types of immunodeficiency, including hypogammaglobulinemia with selective IgA deficiency (113), common agammaglobulinemia (114), and X-linked agammaglobulinemia (113). However, in no case was a mutant enzyme identified and there is no abnormal accumulation of metabolites as seen in deficiencies of pyrimidine 5'nucleotidase, ADA, or PNP. It is likely that the decreased enzyme activity reported was the result of the predominance of lymphocytes of a particular subtype or at a particular stage of development, in which low activity of purine ecto-5'nucleotidase is characteristic rather than a true genetic defect.

REFERENCES

1. Srivastava SK, Beutler E. Purification and kinetic studies of adenine phosphoribosyltransferase from human erythrocytes. Arch Biochem Biophys 1971; 142:426–434.
2. Lindberg B, Klenow H, Hansen K. Some properties of partially purified mammalian adenosine kinase. J Biol Chem 1967; 242:350–356.
3. Krenitsky TA, Papaioannou R. Human hypoxanthine phosphoribosyltransferase II. Kinetics and chemical modification. J Biol Chem 1969; 244:1271–1277.
4. Skold O. Uridine kinase from Ehrlich ascites tumor: Purification and properties. J Biol Chem 1960; 235: 3273–3279.

5. Klemperer HC, Haynes GR. Thymidine kinase in rat liver during development. Biochem J 1968; 103:541–546.

6. Canellakis ES. Pyrimidine metabolism. II. Enzymatic pathways of uracil anabolism. J Biol Chem 1957; 227:329–338.

7. Henderson JF. Kinetic properties of hypoxanthine-guanine phosphoribosyltransferase. Fed Proc 1968; 27:1053–1054.

8. Itoh R, Mitsui A, Tsushima K. Properties of 5′-nucleotidase from hepatic tissue of higher animals. J Biochem 1968; 63:165–169.

9. Schrader WP, Stacy AR, Pollara B. Purification of human erythrocyte adenosine deaminase by affinity column chromatography. J Biol Chem 1976; 251:4026–4032.

10. Kim BK, Cha S, Parks RE Jr. Purine nucleoside phosphorylase from human erythrocytes. I. Purification and properties. J Biol Chem 1968; 243:1763–1770.

11. Paglia DE, Valentine WN. Characteristics of a pyrimidine-specific 5′nucleotidase in human erythrocytes. J Biol Chem 1975; 250:7973–7979.

12. Tomchick R, Saslaw LD, Waravdekar VS. Mouse kidney cytidine deaminase: Purification and properties. J Biol Chem 1968; 243:2534–2537.

13. Kit S. Nucleotides and nucleic acids. In: Greenberg DM, ed. Metabolic Pathways, 3rd ed. New York: Academic Press, 1970, Vol. IV, p 69.

14. Friedkin M, Roberts D. The enzymatic synthesis of nucleosides. I. Thymidine phosphorylase in mammalian tissue. J Biol Chem 1954; 207:245.

15. Hershko A, Rain A, Mager J. Regulation of the synthesis of 5-phosphoribosyl-1-pyrophosphate in intact red blood cells and in cell-free preparations. Biochim Biophys Acta 1969; 184:64–76.

16. Holmes EW, McDonald JA, McCord JM, et al. Human glutamine phosphoribosylpyrophosphate amidotransferase-kinetic and regulatory properties. J Biol Chem 1973; 248:144–150.

17. Van Der Weyden MB, Kelley WN. Human adenylosuccinic synthetase. Partial purification, kinetic and regulatory properties of the enzyme from placenta. J Biol Chem 1974; 249:7242–7281.

18. Holmes EW, Pehlke DM, Kelley WN. The role of human inosinic acid dehydrogenase in the control of purine biosynthesis de novo. Biochim Biophys Acta 1974; 364:209–217.

19. Mager J, Magasanik B. Guanosine-5′-phosphate reductase and its role in the interconversion of purine nucleotides. J Biol Chem 1960; 235:1474–1478.

20. Shambaugh GE. Pyrimidine biosynthesis. Am J Clin Nutr 1979; 32:1290–1297.

21. Tatibana M, Shigesada K. Control of pyrimidine biosynthesis in mammalian tissues. V. Regulation of glutamine-dependent carbamyl phosphate synthetase: Activation by 5-phosphoribosyl 1-pyrophosphate and inhibition by uridine triphosphate. J Biochem 1972; 72:549–560.

22. Shoaf WT, Jones ME. Uridylic acid synthesis in Ehrlich ascites carcinoma: Properties, subcellular distribution, and nature of enzyme complexes of the six biosynthetic enzymes. Biochemistry 1973; 12:4039–4051.

23. Kelley WN. Hereditary orotic aciduria. In: Stanbury JB, Wyngaarden JB, Fredrickson DS, Goldstein JL, Brown MS, eds. The Metabolic Basis of Inherited Disease. New York: McGraw-Hill, 1981, 1202–1226.

24. Page T, Bakay B, Nissinen E, et al. Hypoxanthine-guanine phosphoribosyltransferase variants: Correlation of clinical phenotype with enzyme activity. J Inher Metab Dis 1981; 4:203–206.

25. Fairbanks LD, Simmonds HA, Webster DR. Usefulness of intact erythrocyte studies in the diagnosis of inherited purine and pyrimidine defects. In: Nyhan WL, Thompson LF, Watts RWE, eds. Purine and Pyrimidine Metabolism in Man V. Part A: Clinical Aspects Including Molecular Genetics. New York: Plenum Publishing Corp. 1986, 101–107.

26. Lesch M, Nyhan WL. A familial disorder of uric acid metabolism and central nervous system function. Am J Med 1964; 36:561–570.

27. Seegmiller JE, Rosenbloom FM, Kelley WN. Enzyme defect associated with a sex-linked human neurological disorder and excessive purine synthesis. Science 1967; 155:1682–1684.

28. Kelley WN, Wyngaarden JB. Syndromes associated with hypoxanthine-guanine phosphoribosyltransferase deficiency. In: Stanbury JB, Wyngaarden JB, Fredickson DS, et al., eds. The Metabolic Basis of Inherited Disease. New York: McGraw-Hill, 1981, 1251–1268.

29. Nyhan WL. The Lesch-Nyhan syndrome. Ann Rev Med 1973; 24:41–60.

30. Nyhan WL. Behavior in the Lesch-Nyhan syndrome. J Autism Child Schizo 1976; 6:235–251.

31. Nyhan WL. Lesch-Nyhan syndrome. In: Vinken PJ, Bruyn GW, eds. Handbook of Clinical Neurology, Vol. 42. New York: North Holland, 1981:146–147.

32. Crawhall JC, Kelley WN. Diagnosis and treatment of the Lesch-Nyhan syndrome. Pediatr Res 1972; 6:504–513.

33. Lloyd KG, Hornykiewicz O, Davidson L, et al. Biochemical evidence of dysfunction of brain neurotransmitters in the Lesch-Nyhan syndrome. N Engl J Med 1981; 305: 1106–1111.

34. Emmerson BT, Wyngaarden JB. Purine metabolism in heterozygous carriers of hypoxanthine-guanine phosphoribosyltransferase deficiency. Science 1969; 166:1533–1535.

35. McKearan RO, Howell A, Andrews TM, et al. Observations on the growth in vitro of myeloid progenitor cells and fibroblasts from hemizygotes and heterozygotes for "complete" and "partial" HGPRT deficiency, and their relevance to the pathogenesis of brain damage in the Lesch-Nyhan syndrome. J Neurol Sci 1974; 22:183–187.

36. Migeon BR. X-linked hypoxanthine-guanine phosphoribosyltransferase deficiency: Detection of heterozygotes by selective medium. Biochem Genet 1970; 4:377–383.

37. Page TM, Broock RL, Nyhan WL, et al. Use of selective media for distinguishing variant forms of hypoxanthine phosphoribosyl transferase. Clin Chim Acta 1986; 154:195–202.

38. Rosenbloom FM, Kelley WN, Henderson JF, et al. Lyon hypothesis and X-linked disease. Lancet 1967; 2:305–306.

39. Gartler SM, Scott RC, Goldstein JL, et al. Lesch-Nyhan syndrome: Rapid detection of heterozygotes by the use of hair follicles. Science 1971; 172:572–574.

40. Page T, Bakay B, Nyhan WL. An improved procedure for detection of hypoxanthine-guanine phosphoribosyl transferase heterozygotes. Clin Chem 1982; 28:1181–1184.

41. Gibbs DA, McFadyen IR, Crawford MA, et al. First trimester prenatal diagnosis of Lesch-Nyhan syndrome. Lancet 1984; 2:1180–1183.

42. Boyle JA, Raivio KO. Lesch-Nyhan syndrome: Preventive control by prenatal diagnosis. Science 1970; 169:688–689.

43. Kamatani K, Yamanaka H, Nobori T, et al. Common altered characteristics of mutant enzymes from patients with Japanese type APRT deficiency. In: Nyhan WL, Thompson LF, Watts RWE, eds. Purine and Pyrimidine Metabolism in

Man V, Part A: Clinical Aspects Including Molecular Genetics. New York: Plenum Publishing Corp., 1986, 39–46.

44. Simmonds HA, Van Acker KJ. Adenine phosphoribosyltransferase deficiency: 2,8-dihydroxyadenine lithiasis. In: Stanbury JB, Wyngaarden JB, Fredrickson DS, et al., eds. The Metabolic Basis of Inherited Disease. New York: McGraw-Hill, 1981, 1144–1156.

45. Simmonds HA, Barratt TM, Webster DR, et al. Spectrum of 2,8-dihydroxyadenine urolithiasis in complete APRT deficiency, In: Rapado A, Watts, RWE, De Bruyn CHMM, eds. Purine Metabolism in Man III. New York: Plenum Press, 1980, 337–341.

46. Simmonds HA, Potter DF, Sahota A, et al. Adenine phosphoribosyltransferase deficiency presenting with supposed uric acid stones; pitfalls of diagnosis. J Royal Soc Med 1978; 71:791–795.

47. Durandy A, Peter MO, Freycon F, et al. Early prenatal diagnosis of inherited severe immunodeficiencies linked to enzyme deficiencies. J Pediatr 1987; 111(4):595–598.

48. Barratt TM, Simmonds HA, Cameron JS, et al. Complete deficiency of adenine phosphoribosyltransferase. A third case presenting as renal stones in a young child. Arch Dis Child 1979; 54:25–31.

49. Debray H, Cartier P, Temstet A, et al. Child's urinary lithiasis revealing a complete deficit in adenine phosphoribosyltransferase. Pediatr Res 1976; 1:762–766.

50. Johnson LA, Gordon RB, Emmerson BT. Adenine phosphoribosyltransferase: A simple spectrophotometric assay and the incidence of mutation in the normal population. Biochem Genet 1977; 15:256–272.

51. Kredich NM, Hershfield MS. Immunodeficiency diseases caused by adenosine deaminase deficiency and purine nucleoside phosphorylase deficiency. In: Stanbury JB, Wyngaarden, Fredrickson DS, et al. eds. The Metabolic Basis of Inherited Disease. New York: McGraw-Hill, 1981, 1157–1183.

52. Morgan G, Levinsky RJ, Hugh-Jones K, et al. Heterogeneity of biochemical, clinical and immunological parameters in severe combined immunodeficiency due to adenosine deaminase deficiency. Clin Exp Immunol 1987; 70(3):491–499.

53. Nyhan WL. Disorders of purine and pyrimidine metabolism. In: Kelley VC, ed. Practice of Pediatrics, Vol. 6. Philadelphia: Harper & Row, 1982, 1–18.

54. Hirschhorn R, Papageorgiou PS, Kesarwala HH, et al. Amelioration of neurologic abnormalities after "enzyme replacement" in adenosine deaminase deficiency. N Engl J Med 1980;303:377–380.

55. Polmar SH, Stern RC, Schwartz AL, et al. Enzyme replacement therapy for adenosine deaminase deficiency and severe combined immunodeficiency. N Engl J Med 1976; 295:1337–1343.

56. Fox IH, Burk L, Planet A, et al. Pyrimidine nucleotide biosynthesis: A study of normal and purine enzyme-deficient cells. J Biol Chem 1978; 253:6794–6800.

57. Thelander L, Reichard P. Reduction of ribonucleosides. Ann Rev Biochem 1979; 48:133–158.

58. Kredich NM, Martin DW Jr. Role of S-adenosylhomocysteine in adenosine-mediated toxicity in cultured mouse T-lymphoma cells. Cell 1977; 12:931–938.

59. Scott CR, Chen SH, Giblett ER. Detection of the carrier state in combined immunodeficiency disease associated with adenosine deaminase deficiency. J Clin Invest 1974; 53:1194–1196.

60. Chen SH, Scott CR, Swedberg DR. Heterogeneity for adenosine deaminase deficiency: Expression of the enzyme in cultured skin fibroblasts and amniotic fluid cells. Am J Hum Genet 1975; 27:46–52.

61. Aitken DA, Gilmore DH, Frew CA, et al. Early prenatal investigation of a pregnancy at risk of adenosine deaminase deficiency using chorionic villi. J Med Genet 1987; 23(1):52–54.

62. Chen SH, Ochs HD, Scott CR, et al. Adenosine deaminase deficiency: Disappearance of adenine deoxynucleotides from a patient's erythrocytes after successful marrow transplantation. J Clin Invest 1978; 62:1386–1389.

63. Markert ML, Hershfield MS, Schiff RI, et al. Adenosine deaminase and purine nucleoside phosphorylase deficiencies: Evaluation of therapeutic interventions in eight patients. J Clin Immunol 1987; 7(5):389–399.

64. Hong R, Schulte-Wissermann H, Horowitz S, et al. Cultured thymic epithelium in severe combined immunodeficiency. Transplant Proc 1978; 10:201–202.

65. Polmar SH. Enzyme replacement and other biochemical approaches to the therapy of adenosine deaminase deficiency. In: Elliot K, Whelan J, eds. Enzyme Defects and Immune Dysfunction. Ciba Foundation Symposium 68. New York: Exerpta Medica, 1979; pp 213–216.

66. Beauchamp C, Daddona PE, Menapace DP. Properties of a novel PEG derivative of calf adenosine deaminase. In: De Bruyn CHMM, Simmonds HA, Muller MM, eds. Purine Metabolism in Man-IV. New York: Plenum Press 1984; 47–52.

67. Giblett ER, Ammann AJ, Wara DW, et al. Nucleoside-phosphorylase deficiency in a child with severely defective T-cell immunity and normal B-cell immunity. Lancet 1975; 1:1010–1013.

68. Simmonds HA, Fairbanks LD, Morris GS, et al. Erythrocyte GTP depletion in PNP deficiency presenting with haemolytic anaemia and hypouricaemia. In: Nyhan WL, Thompson LF, Watts RWE, eds. Purine and Pyrimidine Metabolism in Man V, Part A: Clinical Aspects Including Molecular Genetics. New York: Plenum Publishing Corp. 1986, 481–486.

69. Simmonds HA, Fairbanks LD, Morris GS, et al. Central nervous system dysfunction and erythrocyte guanosine triphosphate depletion in purine nucleoside phosphorylase deficiency. Arch Dis Child 1987; 62:385–391.

70. Theiss JC, Morris NR, Fischer GA. Pyrimidine nucleotide metabolism in L5178Y murine leukemia cells: Deoxycytidine protection from deoxyguanosine toxicity. Cancer Biochem Biophys 1976; 1:211–215.

71. Ullman B, Gudas LJ, Clift SM, et al. Isolation and characterization of purine-nucleoside phosphorylase-deficient T-lymphoma cells and secondary mutants with altered ribonucleotide reductase: Genetic model for immunodeficiency disease. Proc Natl Acad Sci USA 1979; 76:1074–1078.

72. Carapella De Luca E, Stagagno M, Dionisi Vici C, et al. Prenatal exclusion of purine nucleoside phosphorylase deficiency. Eur J Pediatr 1986; 145(1–2):51–53.

73. Rich KC, Mejias E, Fox IH. Purine nucleoside phosphorylase deficiency: Improved metabolic and immunologic function with erythrocyte transfusions. N Engl J Med 1980; 303:973–977.

74. Zegers BJM, Stoop JW, Staal GEJ, et al. An approach to the restoration of T cell function in a purine nucleoside phosphorylase deficient patient. In: Elliot K, Whelan J, eds. Enzyme Defects and Immune Dysfunction. Ciba Foundation Symposium 68. New York: Exerpta Medica, 1979, 231–238.

75. Lowenstein JM. Ammonia production in muscle and other tissues: The purine nucleotide cycle. Physiol Rev 1972; 52:382–414.

76. Goebel HH, Bardosi A. Myoadenylate deaminase deficiency. Klin Wochenschr 1987; 65(21):1023–1033.

77. Swain JL, Sabina RL, Holmes EW. Myoadenylate deaminase deficiency. In: Stanbury JB, Wyngaarden JB, Fredrickson DS, et al., eds. The Metabolic Basis of Inherited Disease. New York: McGraw-Hill, 1981, 1184–1191.

78. Raivio KO, Santavuori P, Somer H. Metabolism of AMP in muscle extracts from patients with deficient activity of myoadenylate deaminase. In: De Bruyn CHMM, Simmonds HA, Mullter M, eds. Purine Metabolism in Man IV. New York: Plenum Press 1984, 431–435.

79. Sabina RL, Swain JL, Patten BM, et al. Disruption of the purine nucleotide cycle: A potential explanation for muscle dysfunction in myoadenylate deaminase deficiency. J Clin Invest 1980; 66:1419–1423.

80. Valen PA, Nakayama DA, Veum JA, et al. Myadenylate deaminase deficiency: Diagnosis by forearm ischemic exercise testing. In: Nyhan WL, Thompson LF, Watts RWE, eds. Purine and Pyrimidine Metabolism in Man V, Part B: Basic Science Aspects. New York: Plenum Publishing Corp., 1986, 525–528.

81. Ogasawara N, Goto H, Yamada Y, et al. Deficiency of erythrocyte type isozyme of AMP deaminase in human. In: Nyhan WL, Thompson LF, Watts RWE, eds. Purine and Pyrimidine Metabolism in Man V, Part A: Clinical Aspects Including Molecular Genetics. New York: Plenum Publishing Corp., 1986, 123–127.

82. Holmes EW, Wyngaarden JB. Hereditary xanthinuria. In: Stanbury JB, Wyngaarden JB, Fredrickson DS, et al. eds. The Metabolic Basis of Inherited Disease. New York: McGraw-Hill, 1981, 1192–1201.

83. Duran M, Beemer FA, Heiden CVD, et al. Combined deficiency of xanthine oxidase and sulfite oxidase: A defect of molybdenum metabolism or transport. J Inherited Metab Dis 1978; 1:175–178.

84. Roesel RA, Bowyer F, Blankenship PR, et al. Combined xanthine and sulphite oxidase defect due to a deficiency of molybdenum cofactor. J Inherited Metab Dis 1986; 9(4):343–347.

85. Klinenberg JR, Goldfinger SF, Seegmiller JD. The effectiveness of a xanthine oxidase inhibitor allopurinol in the treatment of gout. Ann Intern Med 1965; 62:639–647.

86. Abumrad NN, Schneider AJ, Steel DR, et al. Acquired molybdenum deficiency. Clin Res 1979; 27:774A.

87. Lowy BA, Ben-Zion D. Adenylosuccinase activity in human and rabbit erythrocyte lysates. J Biol Chem 1970; 245: 3043–3046.

88. Jaeken J, Van den Berghe G. An infantile autistic syndrome characterised by the presence of succinylpurines in body fluids. Lancet 1984; 2:1058–1061.

89. Van den Berghe G, Jaeken J. Adenylosuccinase deficiency. In: Nyhan WL, Thompson LF, Watts RWE, eds. Purine and Pyrimidine Metabolism in Man V. Part A: Clinical Aspects Including Molecular Genetics. New York: Plenum, 1986, 27–33.

90. Simmonds HA, Webster DR, Lingam S, et al. An inborn error of purine metabolism, deafness and neurodevelopmental abnormality. Neuropediatrics 1985; 16:106–108.

91. Becker MA, Losman MJ, Rosenberg AL, et al. Phosphoribosylpyrophosphate synthetase superactivity: A study of five patients with catalytic defects in the enzyme. Arthritis Rheum 1986; 29(7):880–888.

92. Becker MA, Meyer LJ, Wood AW, et al. Purine overproduction in man associated with increased phosphoribosylpyrophosphate synthetase activity. Science 1973; 179: 1123–1126.

93. Nyhan WL, James JA, Teberg AJ, et al. A new disorder of purine metabolism with behavioral manifestations. J Pediatr 1969; 74(1):20–27.

94. Wada Y, Nishimura Y, Tanabu M, et al. Hypouricemic, mentally retarded infant with a defect of 5-phosphoribosyl-1-pyrophosphate synthetase of erythrocytes. Tohoku J Exp Med 1974; 113:149–157.

95. Becker MA, Raivio KO, Bakay B, et al. Variant human phosphoribosylpyrophosphate synthetase altered in regulatory and catalytic functions. J Clin Invest 1980; 65: 109–120.

96. Becker MA, Losman MJ, Simmonds HA. Inherited phosphoribosylpyrophosphate synthetase superactivity due to aberrant inhibitor and activator responsiveness. In: Nyhan WL, Thompson LF, Watts RWE, eds. Purine and Pyrimidine Metabolism in Man V. Part A: Clinical Aspects Including Molecular Genetics. New York: Plenum Publishing Corp. 1986, 59–66.

97. Becroft DMO, Phillips LI. Hereditary orotic aciduria and megaloblastic anaemia: A second case, with response to uridine. Brit Med J 1965; 1:547.

98. Fox RM, Wood MJ, Royse-Smith D, et al. Hereditary orotic aciduria: Types I and II. Am J Med 1973; 55:791–798.

99. Berger R, Stoker-deVries, Wadman SK, et al. Dihydropyrimidine dehydrogenase deficiency leading to thymine-uraciluria. An inborn error of pyrimidine metabolism. Clin Chim Acta 1984; 141:227–234.

100. Bakkeren JAJM, De Abreau RA, Sengers RCA, et al. Elevated urine, blood and cerebrospinal fluid levels of uracil and thymine in a child with dihydrothymine dehydrogenase deficiency. Clin Chim Acta 1984; 140:247–256.

101. De Abreau RA, Bakkeren JAJM, Braakhekke J, et al. Dihydrothymine dehydrogenase deficiency in a family, leading to elevated levels of uracil and thymine. In: Nyhan WL, Thompson LF, Watts RWE, eds. Purine and Pyrimidine Metabolism in Man V. Part A: Clinical Aspects Including Molecular Genetics. New York: Plenum Publishing Corp. 1986, 77–80.

102. Diasio RB, Beavers TL, Carpenter JT. Familial deficiency of dihydropyrimidine dehydrogenase. Biochemical basis for familial pyrimidinemia and severe 5-fluorouracil-induced toxicity. J Clin Invest 1988; 81(1):47–51.

103. Valentine WN, Fink K, Paglia DE, et al. Hereditary hemolytic anemia with human erythrocyte pyrimidine 5′-Nucleotidase deficiency. J Clin Invest 1974; 54:866–879.

104. Torrance JD, Karabus CD, Shinier M, et al. Haemolytic anaemia due to erythrocyte pyrimidine 5′-nucleotidase deficiency. S Afr Med J 1977; 52:671–673.

105. Harley EH, Berman P. Diagnostic and therapeutic approaches in pyrimidine 5′-Nucleotidase deficiency. In: De Bruyn CHMM, Simmonds HA, Muller MM, eds. Purine Metabolism in Man-IV. New York: Plenum Press 1984; 103–108.

106. Tomoda A, Noble NA, Lachant NA, et al. Hemolytic anemia in hereditary 5′nucleotidase deficiency: nucleotide inhibition of glucose-6-phosphate dehydrogenase and the pentose phosphate shunt. Blood 1982; 60:1212–1218.

107. Kagimoto T, Shirono K, Higaki T, et al. Detection of pyrimidine 5′nucleotidase deficiency using ^{1}H- or ^{31}P-nuclear magnetic resonance. Experientia 1986; 42(1):69–72.

108. Valentine WN, Paglia DE, Fink K, et al. Lead poisoning: association with hemolytic anemia, basophilic stippling, erythrocyte pyrimidine 5'Nucleotidase deficiency, and intraerythrocytic accumulation of pyrimidines. J Clin Invest 1976; 58:926–932.

109. Szeinberg A, Kahana D, Gavendo S, et al. Hereditary deficiency of adenylate kinase in red blood cells. Acta Haematol 1969; 42:111–126.

110. Rosenberg AL, Bergstom L, Troost T, et al. Hyperuricemia and neurological deficits. N Engl J Med 1970; 282: 992–997.

111. Champanier JP, Etienne JC, Gougeon J, et al. Encephalopathie avec automutilations chez un jumeau active HGPRT normale hyperuricosurie sans hyperuricemia majeure. A propos des limites du syndrome de Lesch-Nyhan. Rev Neuropsychiatr Infant Hyg Ment Enfance 1972; 20: 777–784.

112. Perignon J-L, Le Deist F, Arenzana-Seisdedos F, et al. Cytidine deaminase deficiency in a child with combined immunodeficiency: More than a coincidence? In: Nyhan WL, Thompson LF, Watts RWE, eds. Purine and Pyrimidine Metabolism in Man V, Part A: Clinical Aspects Including Molecular Genetics. New York: Plenum Publishing Corp. 1986, 129–135.

113. Webster ADB, Matamoros N. Lymphocyte purine metabolism—Significance of 5'nucleotidase deficiency: A review. J Royal Soc Med 1979; 72:266–269.

114. Johnson SM, Asherton GL, Watts RWE, et al. Lymphocyte purine 5'nucleotidase deficiency in primary hypogammaglobulinaemia. Lancet 1977; 1:168–170.

Part II

Neurologic Manifestations of Infective Processes

Chapter 9
Bacterial Infections of the Nervous System

Russell D. Snyder

BACTERIAL MENINGITIS IN INFANTS AND CHILDREN

Bacterial meningitis is a major cause of acquired neurologic disease in infancy and childhood. Additional importance is derived from the fact that early diagnosis and appropriate intervention usually have a favorable influence on outcome. Before the era of antibiotics, bacterial meningitis was almost uniformly fatal. Unfortunately, even with optimal contemporary management, significant neurologic sequelae are found and mortality remains high (1). Children are more likely than adults to have neurologic sequelae from bacterial meningitis.

The epidemiology of bacterial meningitis reflects differences in incidence and severity in various nations and communities. In one community in the United States (US) the incidence rate is about 10 per 100,000 person years. The rate for children under 5 years of age is 87 per 100,000 person years, and for those over 5 years the rate is 2.2 per 100,000 patient years. In the age group under 5 years, the estimated incidence of *Haemophilus influenzae* type b meningitis is 51 to 77 cases per 100,000 children per year. The attack rate peaks between 6 and 12 months of age and declines thereafter. Only 25% of the cases occur after 2 years of age (2).

Bacterial meningitis is more frequent in winter months, except for *H. influenzae* type b which peaks in spring and fall. Risk factors for *H. influenzae* type b meningitis include male sex, black race, native American heritage, household crowding, and attendance at day care centers (3,4). It is the most frequent causative agent of bacterial meningitis of childhood beyond the neonatal period followed by *Neisseria meningitidis* and *Streptococcus pneumoniae*. When *H. influenzae* meningitis develops in infants and children it is almost always type b. Beyond 10 years of age, *N. meningitidis* and *S. pneumoniae* become more common, but *H. influenzae* continues to occur (5). A recent apparent decline in cases of bacterial meningitis in infancy and childhood has been noted. This may be related to the increased use of immunization against *H. influenzae* and a trend to give the immunization at younger ages. Other possibilities for the decline include the requirement by day-care centers for *H. influenzae* immunization and the use of third generation cephalosporins, which are effective against *H. influenzae*, by pediatricians and generalists in the treatment of routine respiratory infections.

Some understanding of the pathogenesis, management, and sequelae of bacterial meningitis is appropriate for all physicians whose practice includes infants and children, but especially for those in primary care positions with responsibility for early recognition of meningitis and institution of initial treatment (6–9).

Pathology

Gross pathologic examination of the brain in bacterial meningitis shows exudate accumulated within the subarachnoid space over the brain, in the sulci, and

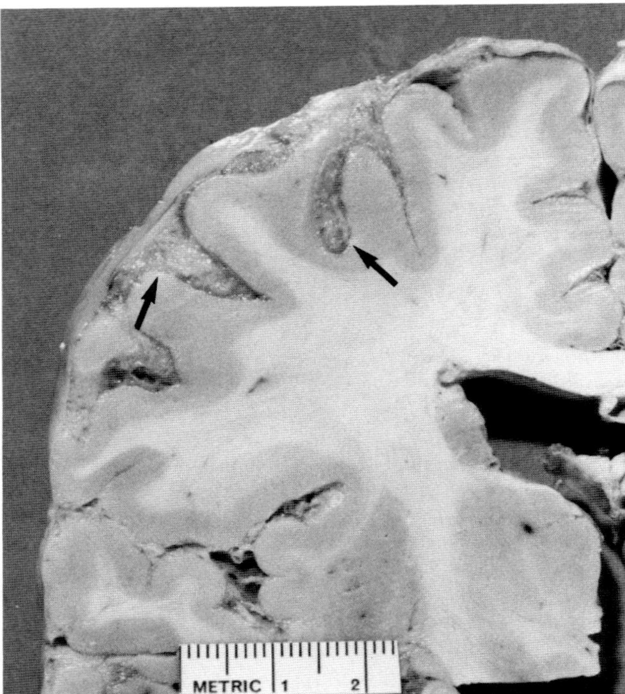

FIGURE 9.1 Coronal section of brain of young child with pneumococcal meningitis: subarachnoid spaces are filled with thick purulent exudate. (Courtesy of Dr. R. L. Davis, University of California Medical Center, San Francisco.)

sometimes around the spinal cord (Figure 9.1). Exudate also accumulates in the basilar cisterns, the perivascular spaces, around blood vessels passing through the subarachnoid space, and about the perineural sheaths of cranial nerves. The exudate consists of polymorphonuclear leukocytes with lesser numbers of lymphocytes and macrophages (Figure 9.2). Bacteria can be found free in the exudate and within the cells of the exudate. By 2 to 3 weeks of illness, the composition of the exudate changes to mononuclear

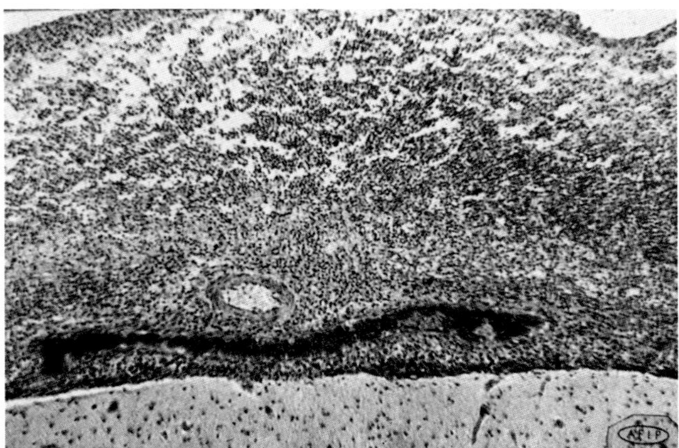

FIGURE 9.2 Section of cortex and leptomeninges in purulent meningitis, showing massive subarachnoidal accumulation of polymorphonuclear leucocytes. (Courtesy of Dr. R. L. Davis, University of California Medical Center, San Francisco.)

cells, primarily macrophages. Fibrosis begins and strands of collagen are found in thickened and inflamed leptomeninges (10).

Although the major gross pathologic impact is within the subarachnoid space, careful examination reveals more widespread involvement. The superficial cortex is swollen with venous congestion. Inflammation is present in varying degrees in the superficial brain parenchyma, usually without the presence of organisms and may be present within the ventricles. Pyknotic changes are found in cortical neurons as well as areas of pallor in cortex and white matter which are attributed to infarcts secondary to inflammatory and obliterative vasculitis of arteries and veins. The inflammatory cell infiltrate may involve the vessel walls with elevation of the endothelium and narrowing of the vessel or actual occlusion. Segmental narrowing of major intracranial arteries has been demonstrated by angiography. The areas of infarction are bland or hemorrhagic. Pathologic abnormalities are more intense in the neonate.

Investigation of the leptomeninges of older children and adults with the scanning electron microscope has modified traditional concepts of the structure of the leptomeninges. The perivascular spaces (Virchow-Robin spaces) do not appear to be continuous with the subarachnoid space. Rather, there is a subpial space which is in continuity with the perivascular space but is separate from the subarachnoid space (11). In bacterial meningitis, leukocytes and macrophages enter this subpial and perivascular space from the subarachnoid space, are in approximation to vessels entering and leaving the brain, and thus may interfere with function of those vessels. The clinical signs and symptoms of meningitis, including seizures, may be present with minimal pathologic alteration, especially in fulminant cases.

Pathogenesis

Factors contributing to the pathogenesis of bacterial meningitis include the status of host defense mechanisms, virulence of the organism, inflammation of the meninges, obstruction of subarachnoid pathways, interference with vessels entering and leaving the brain, irritation of brain parenchyma by toxic products of bacteria and leukocytes (12), anoxia, shock, fever, dehydration, seizures, pH disturbances, and electrolyte imbalance (13,14). Organisms from the nose may enter the cerebrospinal fluid (CSF) by spread along the olfactory nerve fibers and through the cribriform plate, though this is not the usual method for acquiring meningitis. Entry of organisms may also occur through other contiguous structures, by a foreign body in trauma or surgery of the nervous system, or through a CSF shunting device. However, the most common mechanism is hematogenous spread through the choroid plexus or through other parts of the blood-brain barrier (BBB) to the subarachnoid pathways.

Meningitis is found in a significant percentage of cases of sepsis and even in occult bacteremia (15). An infecting organism must possess virulence factors such as capsular polysaccharide, enzymes, and toxins which permit invasion of the host's central nervous system (CNS) and passage through the BBB. The septicemic phase explains the frequency with which blood cultures recover the organism. The usual sequence of infection is host mucosal colonization, systemic invasion with bacteremia, intravascular survival and multiplication, penetration of the BBB through the choroid plexus, appearance of organisms in the CSF, and then the development of pachymeningitis (16,17). The precise mechanism by which pathogens cross the intact BBB has yet to be explained (18). Morphologically, an opening of the tight junctions between vascular endothelial cells and an increase in endothelial pinocytotic vesicles has been found in experimental meningitis (19). *H. influenzae* efficiently replicates in the blood, but the CSF will support growth of most meningeal pathogens. When meningitis becomes established, polymorphonuclear cells migrate from the blood into the CSF, and the meninges become inflamed with a polymorphonuclear infiltrate. In experimental meningitis, CSF lactate is increased and the concentration of high-energy phosphates is decreased (20). It is curious that, except in unusual circumstances, meningitis can be produced experimentally in animals only by direct inoculation of the CNS.

The loss of BBB efficiency during bacterial meningitis has the advantage of providing easier access for antibiotics and higher antibiotic levels in the infected area. When the BBB is injured, immunoglobulins and complement pass from the blood into the CSF. IgG, IgM, and IgA are also produced by the meninges during infection (21). Recovery from bacterial meningitis involves antibody production, cell-mediated immunity, and complement (22). Complement deficiency has not been identified in sporadic bacterial meningitis (23). Fever may be a natural defense mechanism of advantage to the host (24).

The organisms commonly found in bacterial meningitis all produce a capsular polysaccharide which confers virulence and increases the resistance of the organisms to phagocytosis, thus increasing the ability of these organisms to survive (25). Capsular polysaccharide appears to function in immunogenicity, production of inflammatory effects within the CNS, and the response of CNS defense mechanisms. Type-specific anticapsular antibody, which acts with components of complement, may be missing or inefficient in infants and young children. This lack of active antibody may be associated with the inability to immunize young children with purified capsular polysaccharide. Other noncapsular antigens probably also play a role in virulence and immunity. Antigenic similarity has been demonstrated between brain components and some of the bacteria that cause meningitis (26). A genetic predisposition has been described, but the precise mechanism is unknown (27).

An important aspect in the pathogenesis of the clinical findings in bacterial meningitis is inflammation and vasculitis. All vessels entering and leaving the brain must pass through the subarachnoid space. When the subarachnoid space is inflamed, vasculitis with relative hypoxia and the possiblity of thrombosis becomes a problem (28). Cerebral blood flow is decreased and vascular resistance is increased, enhancing susceptibility to ischemia and infarction (29). Reduced blood flow may lead to cerebral damage even before administration of antibiotics (30). The usual compensatory mechanisms for increased intracranial pressure are disturbed; a cerebral edema results in further compromise of cerebral circulation (31). The permanent neurologic deficits after some attacks of meningitis are related to inflammation and subsequent vasculitis with infarction or necrosis.

Cerebral edema contributes to the pathogenesis of the clinical problems in bacterial meningitis, and is a combination of its principal forms: viz, vasogenic, cytotoxic, and interstitial (32). Vasogenic edema is associated with ischemia, vessel necrosis, and altered vessel permeability, perhaps because of toxicity from leukocyte or bacterial products. Cytotoxic edema may be secondary to products from polymorphonuclear cells, especially arachidonic acid, which interfere with membrane function (33). Interstitial edema of the white matter is secondary to interference with CSF circulation and the accompanying increased CSF pressure. The presence of bacteria and leukocytes in the CSF impairs resorption of fluid by the arachnoid villi. These mechanisms result in increased brain water content. The early increase in intracranial pressure, which is often the presenting sign of meningitis, may not have precisely the same mechanism as the more serious increased pressure and brain edema which develops later (34,35). Some antibiotics facilitate the release of endotoxin and cytokines by rapid lysis of the cell wall of gram-negative organisms. This may enhance undesirable inflammation and brain edema, primarily in the subcortical white matter, suggesting vasogenic brain edema. Endotoxin probably damages the endothelium of brain capillaries with subsequent vascular leakage (36–37a).

Clinical Features

There is commonly a history of preceding upper respiratory or gastrointestinal infection with accompanying chills, fever, coryza, cough, anorexia, vomiting, or diarrhea. This preceding infection may have no distinguishing features from a routine self-limited childhood febrile illness. It may be difficult to determine when the lethargy and irritability which is seen in many of these childhood infections becomes a finding of meningitis. An upper respiratory or gastrointestinal infection never evolves into meningitis at a precise moment. Sepsis frequently accompanies meningitis and the signs and symptoms of sepsis and septic shock may mask those of meningitis. Experience in the diagnosis of illnesses of children and a high degree of suspicion of meningitis is of utmost importance. One study from Finland emphasized the difficulty in establishing an early diagnosis of bacterial meningitis (38), pointing out that the correct diagnosis of meningitis was established on first medical examination in only 58% of 130 childhood cases.

The initial neurologic signs and symptoms of bacterial meningitis are associated with leptomeningeal inflammation and increased intracranial pressure. Onset of clinical findings may be gradual over several days or abrupt over several hours. Fever is usually noted except in small infants or debilitated children. An alteration of consciousness is present and may be manifested as depressed consciousness or irritability. Fullness of the fontanel, stiff neck or other signs of meningeal irritation, seizures, and headache help to differentiate meningitis from usual childhood infections (Table 9.1).

The diagnosis of meningitis is not always readily apparent. The seizures which herald meningitis may be indistinguishable from simple febrile seizures. Signs of meningeal irritation are not always present, especially in the child under 1 year of age, and focal neurologic signs are unusual at onset. The complaint of headache is rare under 3 years of age.

Bacterial meningitis should always be a major diagnostic consideration when a febrile child develops neurologic symptoms and/or signs such as a seizure, significant alteration of consciousness, or a full fontanel. In most clinical situations, that diagnostic consideration should be followed by immediate lumbar puncture (LP).

The presence of petechiae or purpuric skin lesions in a febrile child suggest bacterial septicemia (39). These lesions are especially common in *Neisseria meningococcus* meningitis, developing in approximately 30% of cases, but are occasionally seen in infections from other organisms. A maculopapular eruption similar to that seen in viral illness can also develop. Skin lesions appear within the first several days of onset but may develop much more rapidly with fulminant illness. The lesions are produced either by direct cutaneous embolization of organisms or by a cutaneous arteritis.

Meningeal signs other than nuchal rigidity may be present, especially in older children. Kernig sign, or straight-leg raising sign, is obtained in the supine position by flexing the thigh on the chest with the knee flexed and then straightening the knee. In the presence of meningeal irritation, resistance and pain are elicited. Brudzinski sign is obtained by passive flexion of the neck which results in reflex flexion of the legs (40). Opisthotonus in meningitis is probably a manifestation of severe nuchal rigidity.

Retinal hemorrhages and papilledema are unusual findings in children with bacterial meningitis. Retinal hemorrhage suggests head trauma, and the presence of papilledema suggests other causes for increased intracranial pressure such as neoplasm or abscess. Athetosis, chorea, and hemiballismus have been noted in meningitis and may have a sudden onset, sometimes being mistaken for seizures (41). Ataxia has also been reported (42).

"Spinal meningitis" is a term which has been used to describe bacterial meningitis. The CSF obtained by lumbar puncture (LP) usually contains bacteria as well as other abnormalities suggesting that the CSF surrounding the spinal cord is involved in the infectious process. However, clinical spinal signs are surprisingly rare. When there are clinical findings of spinal abnormality, they appear to be related to cord infarction or necrosis (43,44).

Otitis media commonly accompanies bacterial meningitis and is often produced by the same organism which caused the meningitis, although direct spread from the ear to the meninges is unlikely. Arthritis can precede or follow *H. influenzae, N. meningitidis,* and *S. aureus* meningitis, commonly affecting the elbow and knee joints. Arthritis may confuse the examiner by mimicking a monoparesis. Thirty percent of patients with *H. influenzae* type b septic arthritis have concurrent meningitis (45). Two percent of the patients with *H. influenzae* meningitis have arthritis which may be septic, immune complex arthritis, reaction to drugs, or hemarthrosis (46). Orbital cellulitis and pericarditis may also be found in association with *H. influenzae* meningitis.

Included in the differential diagnosis of bacterial meningitis are simple febrile seizure, severe nonneurologic infection, head trauma, subdural hematoma, subarachnoid hemorrhage, viral CNS infection, brain abscess, septicemia, acquired immunodeficiency syndrome (AIDS) with opportunistic infection, metabolic derangement, Reye syndrome, poisoning, intoxication, and neoplastic meningitis. In addition, unusual infecting agents such as fungus, rickettsia, or tuberculosis (TB) must be considered even when the onset of the illness is sudden. Every child with meningitis should have a skin test for TB if an organism is not immediately identified (Table 9.2).

Table 9.1 Symptoms and signs of bacterial meningitis in infants and children

Coryza, cough
Anorexia, vomiting, diarrhea
Depressed consciousness, irritability
Fever seizures
Full fontanel
Stiff neck
Headache
Focal neurologic deficits

Table 9.2 Differential diagnosis of bacterial meningitis

Febrile seizure
Sepsis
Head trauma
Viral CNS infection
Fungal CNS infection
Brain abscess
Intoxication
Metabolic derangement
Reye syndrome

Complications may develop during the acute illness and include increased intracranial pressure, seizures, extra-axial fluid collections, shock, respiratory failure, electrolyte imbalance, the syndrome of inappropriate secretion of antidiuretic hormone (SIADH), brain infarction or necrosis, ventriculomegaly, and involvement of various cranial nerves. Disseminated intravascular coagulation, subdural empyema, and brain abscess may also occur but are less frequent (Table 9.3). Stabilzation of the pulmonary and cardiovascular systems is an extremely important aspect of management for these complications can be a major threat to favorable outcome. The persistence of fever 4 to 6 days after institution of antibiotics is probably not a complication in a patient whose clinical course is otherwise uneventful.

Ideally, childhood bacterial meningitis should be managed at a medical facility with a pediatric intensive care unit and noninvasive neuroimaging diagnostic capability. The circumstances of the individual case do not always permit achievement of this ideal. Computed tomography (CT) or magnetic resonance imaging (MRI) should be obtained in patients with an unfavorable clinical course even without signs of increased intracranial pressure. Clinical signs suggesting the need for neuroimaging include prolonged depressed consciousness, persistent full fontanel or other signs of persistent increased intracranial pressure, prolonged fever, focal neurologic deficits, apnea, and seizures (47). Additional indications are failure to display anticipated clinical improvement or sudden unexplained clinical deterioration (Table 9.4).

Several childhood illnesses predispose to the development of bacterial meningitis, including sickle cell anemia and other hemoglobinopathies, immunodeficiency, and malignancy, particularly when they involve the reticuloendothelial system.

Lumbar Puncture

The lumbar puncture (LP) is an integral part of the initial evaluation of patients suspected of having bacterial meningitis. The performance of LP engenders a certain amount of risk (48); however, the risk is small in infants and children and should not mitigate against its completion in appropriate circumstances. A small-bore spinal needle should be

Table 9.3   Complications of bacterial meningitis

Increased intracranial pressure
Sepsis and shock
Respiratory failure
Seizures
Extra-axial fluid collections
Infarction or necrosis
Ventricular enlargement
Inappropriate secretion of anti-diuretic hormone (ADH)
Cranial nerve deficits
Disseminated intravascular coagulation (DIC)

Table 9.4   Indications for brain imaging

Persistent increased intracranial pressure
Persistent lethargy
Persistent fever
Persistent seizures
Focal neurological deficits
Any unfavorable clinical course

used (49) and only the minimal amount of CSF necessary for appropriate studies should be removed. The quantity of CSF necessary for laboratory examination will vary with laboratory requirements and the clinical situation.

If intracranial pressure is significantly elevated or a diagnosis such as subdural hematoma, brain abscess, or other intracranial mass lesion is seriously considered, completion of CT or MRI head scans may be appropriate prior to the initial LP to assist in determining the nature and degree of increased intracranial pressure. The shift of midline structures, obliteration of CSF pathways, or a unilateral dilated temporal horn suggest incipient cerebral herniation, and constitute a relative contraindication to LP (50). Performance of neuroimaging prior to LP has been more common in adult patients than in children (51). Cerebellar tonsillar herniation can produce a stiff neck indistinguishable from the nuchal rigidity of meningitis. Kernig and Brudzinski signs are believed to suggest an inflammatory process of the lumbar roots and theca and, consequently, these signs should not be present when stiff neck is caused by tonsillar herniation (52) although exceptions occur. If blood cultures are obtained immediately, and if initial antibiotics appropriate for suspected organisms are administered, the delay associated with performing a CT or MRI head scan prior to LP will not result in the loss of therapeutic effectiveness. A short period of antibiotic therapy prior to LP is unlikely to produce significant changes of CSF findings or in the ability to culture the organism (53). When imaging cannot be expeditiously obtained, immediate empirical treatment with appropriate antibiotics may be indicated along with indefinite delay of LP. Prior administration of mannitol or a similar osmotic agent can enhance the safety of LP.

The theoretic possibility exists that performance of an LP in a child with bacteremia will produce bacterial meningitis (54). An increase in the incidence of bacterial meningitis has been noted in infants receiving repeated lumbar punctures for the management of posthemorrhagic hydrocephalus (55). On further analysis, however, it would appear that the risk of producing meningitis by LP in a child with bacteremia is insignificant and does not constitute a contraindication to the procedure (56,57). LP should not be performed through an area of infected skin or subcutaneous infection. If a hypocoagulable state is present, that state can be corrected with administration of appropriate blood products prior to performance of the LP.

If the patient is quiet, as commonly found in meningitis with depressed level of consciousness, the CSF pressure should be obtained at the time of the LP. Sedation may be appropriate for the struggling child in order to perform a successful LP which includes measurement of CSF pressure. A brief period of sedation will not adversely affect the clinical outcome and may significantly enhance the accuracy of findings on LP.

Early in meningitis the CSF may be completely normal only to become abnormal within hours. If the CSF is normal in a child suspected to have meningitis and that suspicion persists, repeat LP is appropriate (58,59).

Controversy surrounds the frequency with which LP should be repeated following the initial abnormal examination. LP should not be repeated unless the findings on LP will modify the management of the patient. With an unfavorable clinical course, repeat LP may be indicated for repeat smear, culture, and pressure measurement. Pleocytosis, elevated protein concentration, and hypoglychorrachia persist in cerebrospinal fluid for days or weeks even in patients who respond favorably. A persistent CSF pleocytosis of more than 60 cells/mm³ is not unusual (60); hence, the return of CSF to normal is not an appropriate end point for treatment. The continued improvement in CSF parameters is to be expected, however, but perhaps an LP should be performed at the end of antibiotic treatment. The terminal LP is of little value in determining if adequate antimicrobial therapy has been administered (61), but the results are useful for comparison if the clinical course is infavorable after discontinuation of antibiotics and yet another LP becomes indicated. Such late clinical deterioration is most unusual (62). A significantly traumatic LP is of value only for culture. Calculation of the red cell/white cell ratio and comparison with the red cell/white cell ratio for whole blood is seldom a valid exercise.

When a death occurs shortly after an LP, the question arises whether the LP was a contributing factor to the outcome. This circumstance usually develops when the patient was desperately ill from the meningitis and its complications. It is seldom possible to determine if LP was responsible in any way; however, caution must always be exercised in performing an LP in a child with meningitis and signs of significant increased intracranial pressure (63).

Cerebrospinal Fluid

Although clinical signs and symptoms may suggest the presence of bacterial meningitis, the diagnosis is firmly established by examination of the CSF. Typical CSF findings include elevated pressure, cloudy fluid, polymorphonuclear pleocytosis, low glucose and elevated protein concentrations, and positive smear and culture for bacteria (Table 9.5).

The finding at LP of cloudy fluid under increased pressure is in itself almost diagnostic of bacterial meningitis. Standard laboratory tests are always indicated: smear for Gram stain, bacterial culture and sensitivities, cell count

Table 9.5   CSF examination

Routine tests
Gram stain
Bacterial culture and sensitivities
Cell count and differential
Glucose and protein
Latex particle agglutination

Special tests
Culture for TB, fungus, and virus
Counterimmunoelectrophoresis
Limulus lysate
Cryptococcus antigen
Serology
India ink
Coccidioidomycosis antibody

and differential (Wright stain), glucose, and protein. Smear for Gram stain remains an excellent diagnostic test even though newer methods to establish an etiologic diagnosis are available; it is of increased value when cytocentrifugation is used. Three milliliters or less of CSF is usually sufficient for testing. Cultures for TB and fungi, India ink preparations, and antibody studies are indicated in selected cases. Blood cultures are essential in every case because the blood may yield an organism when CSF culture is negative. Blood cultures are positive in 80% of cases of *H. influenzae* or *S. pneumoniae* meningitis, and 90 percent of *N. meningitidis* meningitis (64). At least two or three blood cultures should be obtained on each case of suspected meningitis. Cultures of the nose and throat are seldom helpful in identifying the infecting organism.

The cell count on initial CSF examination usually ranges from 500 to 10,000 cells/mm³ with predominantly polymorphonuclear cells. A CSF polymorphonuclear pleocytosis can be noted early in viral meningitis, but total cell counts are seldom as high as in bacterial meningitis. A predominance of lymphocytes or only a minimal cellular response is a confusing early finding in some cases of bacterial meningitis, especially when prior treatment with antibiotics has been undertaken. Care must always be exercised in attributing CSF lymphocytosis to viral meningitis (65). Similar care must be exercised in excluding bacterial meningitis because of an absent or minimal CSF cellular response (66). Several polymorphonuclear cells in CSF are not necessarily abnormal, contrary to usual perceptions (67); this is especially true in the neonate. When clinicians are uncertain about the significance of several polymorphonuclear cells in CSF, it is best to initiate treatment with antibiotics appropriate for bacterial meningitis. A repeat CSF examination at a later time frequently provides clarification of the problem (68).

Damage to intracranial vascular structures produced by meningitis can result in subarachnoid bleeding and the presence of red blood cells in the CSF; however, red blood cells are seldom the predominant cell type. Subarachnoid hemorrhage, when present for several hours, produces a leukocytosis because of irritation. A traumatic LP must always be considered when bloody CSF is obtained.

The normal CSF glucose concentration in patients beyond the neonatal period is usually greater than 40 mg/dL. In meningitis, however, the CSF glucose is low, usually below 20 mg/dL, and is sometimes not detectable. Low CSF glucose concentration represents defective glucose transport across the BBB or increased brain utilization of glucose (69). Common clinical practice dictates that simultaneous blood glucose is obtained and the ratio between blood and CSF glucose concentrations determined. However, blood glucose fluctuates widely and the administration of intravenous (IV) glucose may further complicate the picture. Since CSF glucose is a reflection of blood glucose and lags behind the changes in blood glucose, the blood glucose value should be obtained prior to performance of the CSF examination when attempting to determine a ratio. The absolute value of CSF glucose is probably the parameter of diagnostic importance unless a concomitant condition exists leading to hyper- or hypoglycemia. Low CSF glucose is occasionally found in neurologic infections other than bacterial meningitis, such as viral CNS infection, TB, or fungus infection and in subarachnoid hemorrhage, or meningeal neoplasm. The CSF protein concentration is variably elevated in bacterial meningitis, but there is no elevation of CSF immunoglobins.

Treatment with low-dose antibiotics prior to establishing the diagnosis of bacterial meningitis may diminish the intensity of both clinical symptomatology and CSF changes, making the diagnosis more difficult. The alterations of CSF may resemble the CSF findings in viral meningitis (70). There may be fewer polymorphonuclear leukocytes, less depression of glucose, less elevation of protein, and more difficulty in obtaining a positive Gram stain and culture (71); however, low-dose antibiotic treatment will rarely normalize the cerebrospinal fluid. Some special tests of the CSF such as latex agglutination usually remain positive in spite of partial treatment. Seizures per se do not produce a significant change in CSF cell count, glucose, or protein concentration (72).

The culture of bacteria requires 24 to 72 hours, but additional studies are available that provide more rapid determination of the bacteria involved and guide initial antibiotic therapy. These studies include counterimmunoelectrophoresis (CIE), latex particle agglutination, and limulus lysate assay; they become important when the initial Gram stain is not diagnostic and decisions must be made regarding appropriate antibiotics. CIE distinguishes between capsular polysaccharide of *H. influenzae*, *N. meningitidis*, group B streptococcus, and *S. pneumoniae*, providing rapid etiologic diagnosis, but CIE lacks sensitivity with a high proportion of false negatives. The test is most successful when performed on CSF or urine although serum can be used. Latex particle agglutination is more sensitive than counterimmunoelectrophoresis, especially for *H. influenzae* and *N. meningitidis* and can also identify

S. pneumoniae and group B streptococcus. Latex particle agglutination can be performed on CSF, serum or urine, requires only a small quantity of fluid, and provides results in about 30 minutes. It is especially helpful in the diagnosis of *H. influenzae* meningitis. The test is simple to perform and highly sensitive; it may remain positive even after sterilization of the CSF. Limulus lysate assay of CSF is useful in detecting gram-negative bacterial meningitis, but it is a nonspecific test and does not discriminate among the types of gram-negative organisms (73). When only a single test is performed, latex particle agglutination is appropriate.

Determination of CSF C-reactive protein (CRP) is technically more difficult to perform than serum CRP, and it may only reflect the serum values (74). The role of CSF lactate in diagnosis of bacterial meningitis is not clear. CSF lactate above 2.2 mmol/mL is indicative of a bacterial etiology; however, a variety of conditions other than meningitis are also associated with elevated CSF lactate, including hypoxia and hemorrhage. It is not known where the lactate originates (75). CSF ferritin has recently been reported to be of value in distinguishing viral from bacterial meningitis (76).

The laboratory examinations of most immediate value in determining that an acute CNS infection is bacterial and in identifying etiologic agent include: a positive CSF Gram stain, depressed CSF glucose concentration, positive latex particle agglutination, and elevated serum C-reactive protein. However, the total clinical picture remains important in the decision to treat with antibiotics.

Blood Tests

Routine hematologic studies in bacterial meningitis usually reveal an elevated white blood cell count with a left shift. The white blood cell count may be low when the infection is overwhelming. The hemoglobin is usually normal but in chronic infections may be low. The serum sodium is also frequently low, especially in patients with inappropriate secretion of antidiuretic hormone.

CRP is a nonspecific test for bacterial meningitis and bacterial infections in general (77), and assay is easily performed on serum without requiring elaborate laboratory equipment. Most febrile children with serum CRP greater than 2 mg/dL have bacterial infections, but the test will not be positive until an inflammatory response has developed. Partially treated bacterial meningitis may suppress this inflammatory response. Bacterial meningitis produces levels of CRP much above 2 mg/dL (78). In uncomplicated cases, CRP falls to normal in 1 to 2 days. If a secondary rise develops or if the level remains elevated, the possibility of persistent meningeal infection of extrameningeal bacterial complications, should be considered. CRP is not as reliable in neonates (79), but is one of the best nonspecific indicators that an infection is bacterial and not viral (80). Tissue necrosis will raise the CRP.

Antibiotic Therapy

Aggressive antibiotic therapy is appropriate early in the course of bacterial meningitis and has a favorable influence on outcome in most cases. Antibiotic management has become more complex because of the development of new cephalosporins, the development of resistant organisms, the continued accumulation of new information regarding pharmacokinetics and drug interactions, and the frequent changes in antibiotic recommendations. Antibiotic management should undergo constant analysis during the course of treatment. Appropriate sources should be consulted for assistance in antibiotic management (Table 9.6) (81–85).

Antibiotic penetration into the nervous sytem is dependent on multiple factors including: lipid solubility, ionization at a given pH, serum protein binding, physicochemical characteristics, and molecular weight. Factors relating to the nervous system itself include the integrity of the BBB, cerebral blood flow, uptake and metabolism by various neural structures, and rates of efflux from brain or CSF. Low molecular weight and good lipid solubility, as in the case of chloramphenicol, result in favorable CNS penetration. Beta lactams, such as the penicillins and cephalosporins, have high molecular weights and are actively pumped out of the CSF by a transport system in the choroid plexus. Part of the increased effectiveness of beta lactams during inflammation may result from impairment of this transport system. Some of the newer cephalosporins such as cefotaxime and ceftriaxone have a decreased affinity for this transport system, prolonging their time in the CSF (86).

The integrity of the BBB remains the most important determinant of access to the CNS for most drugs. The breakdown of the BBB with inflammation appears to enhance the effectiveness of antibiotics but large systemic doses are necessary. As recovery progresses, the BBB becomes more resistant to passage of the antibiotic, suggesting that dosage should not be reduced late in the course of therapy. Elevated protein concentration in infected CSF could decrease antibiotic activity by protein binding. Potential antagonism between antibiotics needs to be considered. Most current forms of chemotherapy for meningitis target the cell wall (87). Cytokines released during bacterial lysis are highly inflammatory, and antibiotic therapy may actually transiently enhance inflammation.

It is customary to divide the antibiotic treatment of meningitis into two treatment phases. The initial treatment phase is the period of time prior to establishing a definitive diagnosis. During the initial treatment phase when an organism has not been identified, antibiotics should be administered that are appropriate for the suspected organism. The suspected organism is determined to a large extent by the patient's age. The initial phase may be brief or last several days, depending upon the clinical situation and the outcome of laboratory evaluations. Broad-spectrum

Table 9.6 Antibiotics for bacterial meningitis*

Hemophilus influenzae
Ampicillin
Chloramphenicol
Cefuroxime
Ceftriaxone
Cefotaxime

Streptococcus pneumoniae
Penicillin
Chloramphenicol
Cefotaxime
Ceftriaxone
Cefuroxime
Vancomycin

Neisseria meningitidis
Penicillin G
Chloramphenicol
Cefuroxime
Ceftriaxone

Gram-negative bacillary meningitis
Cefotaxime
Ceftazidime
Ceftriaxone
Amikacin

Staphylococcus
Nafcillin
Cefuroxime
Vancomycin
Rifampin

Tuberculosis
Isoniazid
Rifampin
Ethambutol
Streptomycin
Corticosteroids

Neonatal
Ampicillin
Gentamicin
Tobramycin
Vancomycin
Amikacin
Kanamycin
Ceftriaxone
Cefotaxime
Ceftazidime
Penicillin

*See text. Recommendations change frequently. (Check for current recommendations.)

antibiotics such as ampicillin plus chloramphenicol, or ampicillin plus a second or third generation cephalosporin, or a second or third generation cephalosporin alone are preferred during the initial treatment phase. Ceftriaxone, cefotaxime, or cefuroxime may have some merit for initial single antibiotic therapy (88). If the clinical setting or Gram stain leads to the suspicion that an enteric gram-negative organism is involved, the addition of an aminoglycoside or administration of a third generation cephalosporin should be considered.

If, after the initial LP, transport of the patient to a tertiary medical care facility is planned, antibiotics appropriate to the clinical situation should be started immediately. Transfer should not result in delay in the institution of antibiotic therapy. It is also usually advisable to send an aliquot of CSF with the patient for analysis at the tertiary medical care facility.

In the second phase of antibiotic treatment when the organism has been identified by culture of CSF or blood or by one of the special tests, and sensitivities are available, antibiotic therapy can be modifed as necessary; treatment should be as specific as possible. The use of tube dilution studies may be required to help with antibiotic selection. In vitro testing does not always accurately predict the effectiveness of a particular antibiotic (89). Approximately 1% of all cases of meningitis are caused by more than one bacterial species (90).

Meningitis can develop from common childhood illnesses such as upper respiratory or gastrointestinal infections. Children with meningitis are often placed on antibiotics for these illnesses prior to the development of symptoms and signs of bacterial meningitis, and antibiotics are not administered in dosages adequate to eradicate the meningitis. Treatment with low-dose antibiotics prior to the diagnosis of bacterial meningitis can diminish the intensity of both clinical symptomatology and CSF changes, making the diagnosis more difficult. If there is any doubt regarding the diagnosis of meningitis, it is advisable to institute aggressive treatment with antibiotics appropriate for bacterial meningitis. Most cases of partially treated bacterial meningitis when given appropriate antibiotic treatment have a favorable outcome (91).

Any known allergy to medication should be considered before deciding on specific antibiotic treatment. For most older antibiotics frequent IV administration is appropriate, usually by a slow bolus every 4 to 6 hours. The newer cephalosporins may only require dosages every 8 to 12 hours. Care must be exercised with chloramphenicol or an aminoglycoside when hypotension is present because of diminished hepatic and renal function with poor antibiotic clearance and enhanced toxicity. The final dosages of chloramphenicol or an aminoglycoside should be guided by monitoring of serum concentration to ensure therapeutic efficacy and prevent toxicity. The usual duration of antibiotic treatment is 10 to 14 days, although 7 days may be just as effective for infants and children beyond the neonatal period (92). When meningitis is caused by enteric organisms or TB, the course of treatment is longer. Antibiotic therapy should probably not be prolonged in a child with persistent fever who has otherwise displayed a favorable clinical response and who does not have an obvious cause for persistent fever. In one series of patients the cause for persistent fever was not found in 39% of patients, and in 13% the fever was present for longer than 10 days (93).

The organisms producing meningitis in infants and children vary with patient age, from one time to another, and in different geographic regions. Firm rules for treatment cannot be established and only therapeutic guidelines can be presented. During the first month of life *Escherichia coli*, *Listeria monocytogenes,* and group B streptococcus are common causative organisms; *Proteus, Pseudomonas* species, *S. pneumoniae,* and other less common organisms are also found. Between 3 months and 6 years of age *H. influenzae* is the common causative organism, but *S. pneumoniae* and *N. meningitidis* are also found. These three organisms are present at about the same incidence until adolescence when *N. meningitidis* predominates. Following open head trauma and neurosurgical procedures *Staphylococcus epidermidis, Staphylococcus aureus,* and gram-negative bacilli are the usual offending organisms. Gram-negative bacilli, especially *L. monocytogenes,* are also cultured in immunosuppressed patients.

Haemophilus influenzae Meningitis

Ampicillin has been the traditional treatment of *H. influenzae* meningitis, but strains have appeared which produce beta-lactamase, a substance that interferes with the antibiotic effectiveness of ampicillin, various penicillins, and certain cephalosporins. Resistant strains now constitute approximately 25% of *H. influenzae* in the US. Because of these resistant strains it has been customary to add chloramphenicol to the initial treatment regimen and to continue chloramphenicol until antibiotic sensitivities are available. Serum chloramphenicol levels should be obtained, especially in infants. Peak chloramphenicol concentrations between 15 and 25 μg/mL are usually considered safe, but toxic serum levels can easily develop in critically ill children. To obtain peak chloramphenicol levels blood should be sampled 1 hour after an intravenous dose and 2 hours after an oral dose. Variable drug interactions are noted between chloramphenicol and anticonvulsants necessitating determination of blood levels when these agents are administered concurrently (94). Strains of *H. influenzae* resistant to chloramphenicol are appearing.

Ceftriaxone, cefotaxime, and cefuroxime are cephalosporins which are relatively resistant to beta-lactamase and play an important place as adjunct or sole therapy in the management of central nervous system infections with *H. influenzae.* These cephalosporins may be equally useful against the unusual strains of *H. influenzae* that are resistant to both ampicillin and chloramphenicol. Ceftriaxone can be administered IV or IM, it provides adequate serum concentrations with twice-daily dose, and appears effective as the sole antibiotic in meningitis with *H. influenzae* as well as *S. pneumonia,* and *N. meningococcus* (95). The advantages of single-drug therapy with ceftriaxone include less risk of drug toxicity, and effectiveness against resistant strains of *H. influenzae,* particularly when administered intramuscularly; however, delay in CSF sterilization has been noted with ceftriaxone as sole antibiotic therapy (96). Ampicillin and chloramphenicol continue to remain important antibiotics for treatment of *H. influenzae* meningitis (97).

Streptococcus pneunomiae Meningitis

S. pneumoniae causes a severe meningitis in infants and children, and permanent neurologic sequelae are frequent. The organism usually retains sensitivity to crystalline penicillin G, but resistant and tolerant strains have been noted. Chloramphenicol, cefotaxime, ceftriaxone, cefuroxime, and vancomycin are used in selected situations. As in the case of *H. influenzae,* ceftriaxone can be used as the sole antibiotic with the advantages noted previously.

Neisseria meningitidis Meningitis

N. meningitis meningitis is usually a disease affecting children and young adults. The onset and progression of symptoms are rapid, necessitating prompt intervention. Recommended antibiotic treatment is the administration of crystalline penicillin G. Chloramphenicol, ceftriaxone, and cefuroxime can be utilized in selected situations.

Gram-Negative Bacillary Meningitis

Gram-negative bacillary meningitis is usually associated with sepsis, head trauma, or neurosurgical manipulation. *Klebsiella* and *Pseudomonas* are the common infecting organisms. Antibiotic treatment is unsatisfactory, and intrathecal or intraventricular administration of antibiotics is often necessary. Amikacin or a cephalosporin such as cefotaxime, ceftazidime, or ceftriaxone are indicated.

Staphylococcus aureus and *Staphylococcous epidermidis* Meningitis

Staphylococcus aureus causes meningitis in connection with neurosurgical procedures, parameningeal infection, or brain abscess. There is no completely satisfactory antibiotic treatment available. Nafcillin plus an aminoglycoside is recommended, and Vancomycin has been used. Cephalosporins such as cefuroxime may have a place in the management of *S. aureus* meningitis.

The infection rate after ventricular shunting varies from 2% to 20% and is frequently caused by *S. epidermidis,* resulting in a combination of ventriculitis and meningitis. Shunt removal along with administration of antibiotics

may be necessary to effect a cure (98). Systemic and intraventricular antibiotics are frequently indicated for shunt-related infections (99). Vancomycin with rifampin may have a place in shunt infections with resistant *Staphylococcus* species.

Nontraditional Therapeutic Approaches

Since much of the mortality and morbidity of bacterial meningitis is related to the effects of inflammation, measures which reduce inflammation may be beneficial. In this regard, the place of corticosteroids has remained uncertain even after many years of use, although use of dexamethasone 0.15 mg/kg every 6 hours for 4 days starting before or after antibiotics appears to diminish hearing loss and perhaps improve overall outcome (99a,99b). Recent studies have suggested that nonsteroidal anti-inflammatory agents may be useful (100).

Traditional treatment measures are available for the management of increased intracranial pressure. Whether very early and extremely aggressive application of these measures would improve outcome is unknown. The therapeutic role of continuous intracranial pressure monitoring and barbiturate coma is uncertain.

Other untested therapeutic modalities which may hold promise include calcium channel blockers to reduce vasospasm (101), inhibition of the cyclooxygenase system to reduce cerebral edema, superoxide dismutase to reduce damage from products of leukocyte destruction, monoclonal antibodies to block bacterial products which lead to inflammation (102), and glutamate antagonists to reduce neuronal damage from ischemia (103). Anticoagulants such as salicylates may have a role in the management of vasculitis. Perhaps antibiotics should be developed which do not produce rapid lysis of the bacterial cell wall and, thus, less enhancement of inflammation.

Complications

Seizures

Seizures can be the presenting symptom or later complication of bacterial meningitis. They have been reported as a presenting symptom in 6% of cases (104), although the incidence may be higher. Seizures can be partial or generalized, and develop sometime during the course of acute meningitis in 20% to 50% of cases. They occur most frequently 1 to 3 days after the onset of neurologic signs and usually cease 1 to 3 days later, perhaps irrespective of treatment. Early generalized seizures do not appear to have a negative influence on outcome; however, severe or prolonged seizures may increase damage to an already compromised nervous system.

The etiology of seizures in childhood bacterial meningitis is not known. They can be secondary to toxic products of bacteria or leukocytes, or may result from inflammation, vasculitis, cortical irritation, fever, electrolyte disturbance, an immune process, or some other unrecognized process (Table 9.7). Seizure occurrence does not necessarily indicate a failure of antibiotic treatment or the presence of an extra-axial fluid collection. Ventricular widening and parenchymal infarction or necrosis as observed at CT are associated with seizures (105). The electroencephalogram (EEG) may be normal, show generalized or focal epileptiform abnormalities, focal slowing, or only background slowing.

Although seizures are frequently self-limited, vigorous treatment by standard methods of anticonvulsant administration remains appropriate in an attempt to prevent additional brain injury from increased energy requirements of brain tissue during a seizure and seizure-related hypoxia. The intense sustained activity of neurons during a seizure increases metabolic demand which may only be met with difficulty in meningitis.

Adequate ventilation should be ensured and ventilator support may be indicated, especially in status epilepticus. Parenteral phenobarbital, phenytoin, and diazepam are useful when administered individually or in combination, but phenobarbital is the commonly used anticonvulsant in this situation. The initial dose of phenobarbital is 5 to 15 mg/kg, administered slowly by IV. Phenytoin is the agent of choice for some physicians and may be administered as an initial dose of 10 to 20 mg/kg IV, no faster than 50 mg/min. Cardiac function should be monitored during an injection of phenytoin, discontinuing the injection at any sign of bradycardia, dysrhythmia, or hypotension. Phenytoin has the advantage of causing less sedation than phenobarbital. When needed, diazepam can be administered IV in a dose of 0.3 mg/kg up to a maximum of 10 mg. Lorazepam is also effective (106). The IV dose of lorazepam is 0.05 to 0.1 mg/kg up to a maximum of 4 mg administered no more rapidly than 2 mg/min. If the seizure disorder is not severe and the patient is awake, oral anticonvulsants may suffice.

Sedation, pancuronium bromide, or vercuronium bromide may be required to ensure satisfactory ventilator function. Induced paralysis will mask the motor manifestations of a seizure without affecting the electrographic manifestations. Infants or children who are paralyzed for ventilator management and have not had a clinical seizure should have periodic electroencephalograms to determine if epileptiform activity is present. Appropriate management should be directed to electrographic epileptiform activity.

Seizures are rare after recovery from meningitis, with an incidence of 3% to 7% (107,108,108a). Usually the self-limited seizure disorders present during the first several days after onset of bacterial meningitis may not be an indication for prolonged anticonvulsant therapy. If seizures are easily controlled and cease within several days of their onset, the subsequent clinical course of the illness is benign, severe neurologic deficits are not present, and an EEG obtained near the end of the course of antibiotics is relatively free of epileptiform activity, discontinuation of anticonvulsant therapy (perhaps with tapering) should be considered. A prolonged course of anticonvulsants is usually avoided; however, if seizures recur after the acute illness, anticonvulsants can be restarted. It is unknown if early or continuous treatment with anticonvulsants has an impact on the development of chronic seizures.

Increased Intracranial Pressure

The presence of a full fontanel, a prominent feature of bacterial meningitis in patients with open fontanels, is a reflection of increased intracranial pressure. In the uncomplicated case the full fontanel disappears within several days and an uneventful recovery ensues. The pathogenesis of this initial increased intracranial pressure is not clear, although interference with resorption of CSF over the convexities and subsequent communicating hydrocephalus is the most likely cause.

When intracranial pressure is persistently elevated, there is concern for potential cerebral herniation and other forms of brain dysfunction. Etiologies other than hydrocephalus should be considered such as cerebral edema, large extra-axial fluid collections, or abscess.

In some unfortunate cases, early increased intracranial pressure rapidly becomes malignant instead of resolving, leading to compromise of blood flow (109), cerebral edema, and brain herniation. This situation is manifested by progressive clinical deterioration with seizures and severe obtundation (110). Pupils may become sluggish or unresponsive to light, dilated, and in midposition. Other signs include decorticate/decerebrate posturing, abnormal respiratory patterns, bradycardia, elevated blood pressure, and irregular vital signs. Ventilator support may be necessary. CT or MRI head scans should be obtained to exclude the possibility of an extra-axial fluid collection, but in this situation, imaging usually reveals diffuse cerebral edema. The pathogenesis of this malignant increased intracranial pressure is unknown but may represent a vicious cycle with reduced tissue perfusion leading to increased tissue damage and augmenting vasogenic and cytotoxic edema. LP should be approached with caution in patients with severe increased intracranial pressure.

Overhydration with intravenous fluids may predispose to cerebral edema. Common practice dictates that fluids should be restricted in an attempt to minimize development of cerebral edema. If the blood pressure is not low and serum sodium is not elevated, it is customary to administer 2/3 of calculated daily maintenance fluid intravenously

Table 9.7 Causes of seizures in bacterial meningitis

Inflammation
Toxins
Vasculitis
Fever
Electrolyte disturbance

during the first several days of illness. The fluid is usually administered as 1/4 to 1/3 normal saline in 5% dextrose. Although fluid restriction has theoretical advantages, many patients are dehydrated upon arrival at a medical facility. Fluid restriction may maintain the dehydrated state, encourage intracranial vascular sludging and thrombosis, and predispose to hypotension. In bacterial meningitis, it is perhaps advisable to maintain a state of fluid balance which is as close to physiologic as possible, allowing neither overhydration nor dehydration to develop (111).

At least 20% of children with bacterial meningitis become hyponatremic, usually early in the course of the illness. In some cases the problem is related to excessive fluid administration, but it may also be due to SIADH (112). In either situation the symptoms are those of water intoxication with restlessness, irritability, lethargy, seizures, and depressed consciousness. With SIADH the serum sodium is low, the serum hypo-osmolar, the urine excessively concentrated, and the body weight increases. SIADH may contribute to development of cerebral edema. Treatment for either excessive fluid administration or inappropriate release of antidiuretic hormone is restriction of fluid intake to approximately 100 mL/m²/24 hours. Rapid correction of severe hyponatremia should probably be avoided because of the risk of inducing lesions in white matter (113).

Management of symptomatic increased intracranial pressure is aimed at maintaining cerebral perfusion and preventing brain herniation. The head and chest should be elevated to approximately 30°. Tracheal intubation and controlled hyperventilation may be necessary, and the pCO₂ should be maintained at 25 to 30 mm Hg. Sedation or a neuromuscular blocking agent such as pancuronium bromide or vercuronium bromide may be necessary to enhance controlled ventilation. Mannitol can be administered in the dose of 0.25 to 0.5 g/kg IV over a period of 20 to 30 minutes. This dose can be repeated every two to four hours as necessary. Subsequent mannitol administration may not produce a response as favorable as the initial dose. Mannitol has been effective in reducing CSF pressure in the experimental animal (114). Hypotension and shock frequently accompany increased intracranial pressure and are more common than the Cushing effect with hypertension. Appropriate measures to restore blood pressure should be instituted.

The use of corticosteroids in bacterial meningitis has been shown in older studies to have dubious benefit (115,116), although their use is now being reconsidered. More recent studies have suggested that the use of dexamethasone reduces duration of hospitalization (117), and it is often administered because of the desperate nature of the clinical situation. The recommended dose of dexamethasone is 10 to 12 mg/m²/day IV in four divided doses (118). Corticosteroids have the potential to stabilize the BBB and reduce inflammation. These effects could result in reduced antibiotic penetration into the CSF and less efficient CSF sterilization, although this does not appear to be a significant clinical problem. Decrease in the degree of inflammation could have a salutary effect.

The appropriate indications for an intracranial pressure recording device or ventricular drain in the management of increased intracranial pressure in bacterial meningitis is not clear (119). The insertion of a foreign body into an infected cavity is always a concern, since the devices are known to cause ventriculitis and meningitis themselves (120).

The value of pentobarbital-induced coma to reduce cerebral metabolic demand and cerebral blood flow has not been established. Barbiturates have a protective effect on neurons subjected to ischemia but may also produce significant myocardial depression (121). An aggressive approach to increased intracranial pressure should be considered by clinicians caring for infants and children with bacterial meningitis.

Ventricular Enlargement

Ventricular enlargement leads to the presumption of increased intraventricular pressure and the potential for brain herniation. In the early stages of bacterial meningitis in children, the intracranial pressure is usually increased as manifested by the full fontanel in infants. Indeed, the full fontanel is a clinical feature of bacterial meningitis which often leads to the correct diagnosis.

Persistent ventricular enlargement after the first several days of illness may indicate increased intraventricular pressure; however, this finding may be a reflection of loss of brain parenchyma and could be termed acute "atrophy" or hydrocephalus ex vacuo. This may be a peculiar property of the brain of the infant and young child. Similar acute atrophy is seen in newborns with a variety of other CNS insults. The ability of MRI to demonstrate the characteristic transependymal resorption of increased pressure hydrocephalus suggests this study may be helpful in differentiating increased pressure hydrocephalus from parenchymal atrophy.

Impaired resorption of CSF over the hemispheric convexities may result in increased intraventricular pressure and communicating hycrocephalus in some late-onset cases. Ventricular enlargement is frequently transient (122). When neurosurgical intervention is being considered, caution must be exercised to determine if elevated pressure is indeed present and persistent. The question is usually resolved by continued observation and repeat neuroimaging. A period of observation often eliminates the necessity for surgical intervention. Early surgical intervention is probably seldom indicated (123).

If during the stage of active infection, ventricular enlargement is sufficiently severe and persistent that surgical intervention is necessary, ventricular drainage to an external collection device should probably be undertaken initally to avoid the danger of shunting infected fluid into a body cavity. Ventricular size will not necessarily be reduced by surgical drainage (Figure 9.3). Surgical procedures should be

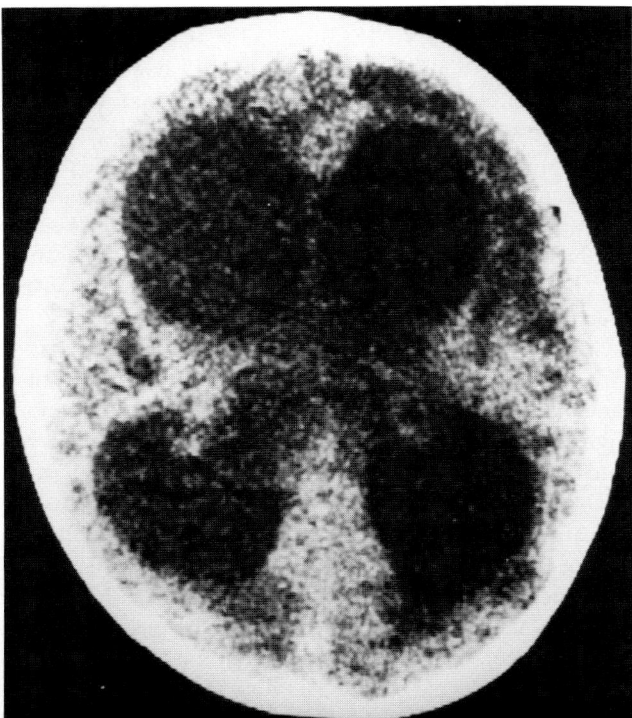

FIGURE 9.3   CT head scan without contrast in an 11-month-old infant with *H. influenzae* meningitis. There is marked ventricular enlargement with left frontal infarction post-shunting. The patient had severe neurologic impairment.

limited to patients who show ventricular enlargement and persistent signs of increased intracranial pressure such as full fontanel, abnormally increasing head circumference, depressed consciousness, vomiting, or elevated intraventricular pressure by direct measurement.

Extra-Axial Fluid Collections

The subdural space is a potential intracranial space situated between the arachnoid and dura. In normal physiologic states the space probably does not exist, at least in the adult (124). For reasons that are not clear, fluid may accumulate in the region of this potential space in children with bacterial meningitis. The fluid collection is more commonly found in younger ages and is usually recognized during the first week of illness by a persistent full fontanel. The fluid containing polymorphonuclear cells is found over the hemispheric convexities, especially the frontal regions, and may be bilateral. It is serosanguineous, sterile, and of high protein content.

Symptoms and signs attributed to these fluid collections include persistent fever, full fontanel, seizures, vomiting, and focal neurologic signs. Similar findings may also be observed, however, in meningitis without fluid collections. Extra-axial fluid collections have been found in 34% of children with bacterial meningitis (125), but they are

unusual in neonatal meningitis and *N. meningococcus* meningitis.

The pathogenesis is unknown. Inflammation in adjacent areas could produce increased vascular permeability in a potential space with loss of albumin-rich fluid and onset of a fluid collection. Alternatively, a collection may be

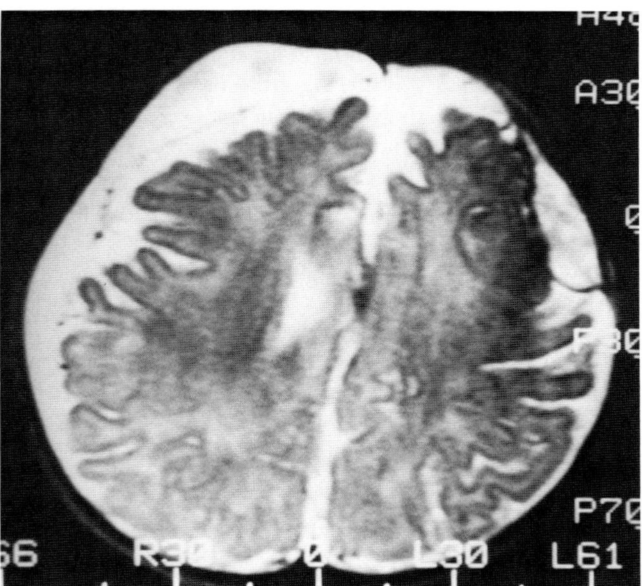

A

B

FIGURE 9.4   A: MRI head scan (intermediate weighted) of a 5-month-old infant with *H. influenzae* meningitis 1 month after onset of symptoms. There is brain atrophy with frontal extra-axial fluid collections, suggesting two compartments on the right. No increased head circumference or neurologic deficits were noted. **B:** CT head scan without contrast of same patient four months later. There is persistence of extra-axial fluid collections with probable frontal atrophy. Patient is asymptomatic with normal head circumference.

caused by the same factors which cause the vasogenic and interstitial edema in brain parenchyma acting outwards instead of inwards.

With time the collection will follow one of several courses: it will resolve; it will continue to accumulate and act as a mass; it will organize into a fibrin network or become surrounded by a membrane; it will remain as an asymptomatic extra-axial space (Figure 9.4); or it will become an empyema. The first course is by far the most common. When the collection is liquid, as is usually the case initially, it can be recovered in part by needle aspiration through the lateral aspect of an open fontanel.

The precise anatomic localization of this fluid is sometimes uncertain. The common analogy with areas of blood accumulation in adult head trauma may not be valid and the physician should probably remain noncommittal, referring to this space as an extra-axial space. Needle aspiration alone cannot determine if recovered fluid is from a subdural space or a widened subarachnoid space. An extra-axial fluid collection may represent subdural fluid, loculated CSF, overproduction of CSF, widening of the subarachnoid space in response to the inflammation or to loss of brain mass.

Computed tomography of the head has resulted in a major improvement in understanding and management of extra-axial fluid collections. MRI provides improved sensi-

tivity and may replace CT in all but the most acute clinical situations (Figure 9.5). The availability of high-resolution, low-Tesla MRI will increase the ease with which MRI can be obtained in critically ill patients. Abnormalities of CT head scans are associated with an unfavorable outcome (126), and a similar association can be anticipated with MRI abnormalities. When an unfavorable outcome occurs in patients with an extra-axial fluid collection, it is possible that both the unfavorable outcome and the fluid collection are independent expressions of the same severe initial infection (127).

Clinically significant extra-axial fluid collections observed at neuroimaging are much less frequent than anticipated from experience prior to the advent of imaging (Figure 9.6). Cortical enhancement beneath an extra-axial fluid collection is not necessarily an indication of subdural empyema, as reported earlier (128), but is presumed to indicate cerebritis and may also indicate meningeal inflammation or brain infarction. Most fluid collections resolve spontaneously over a period of weeks to months (Figure 9.7), but a slight increase in the space between the brain and inner table may persist indefinitely.

Repeat imaging is useful in following the evolution of these abnormalities (129) and determining the need for subsequent intervention. Surgical intervention is required when the intracranial pressure is persistently increased secondary to the mass effect, a major shift in intracranial structures has developed and there is concern for impending brain herniation, the fluid collection is infected, or

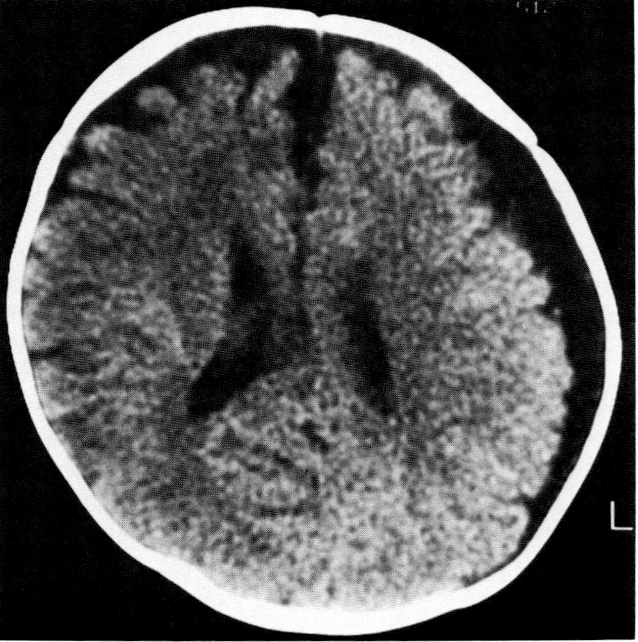

FIGURE 9.5 An MRI head scan (T2 weighted images) of a 2-month-old infant with *S. pneumoniae* meningitis. There is excessive extra-axial space with widened subarachnoid pathways, showing the ability of the MRI to effectively demonstrate extra-axial fluid collections.

FIGURE 9.6 A CT head scan of a 5-month-old infant with *S. pneumoniae* meningitis. Note the excessive extra-axial fluid collections, greater on left than right with mild shift of midline structures to the right. The patient had no clinical symptoms or signs from fluid collections.

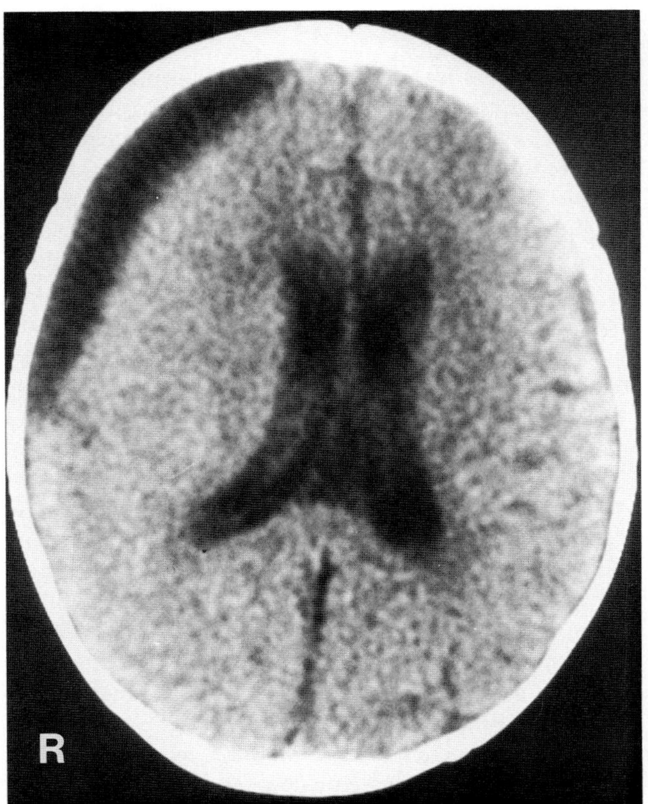

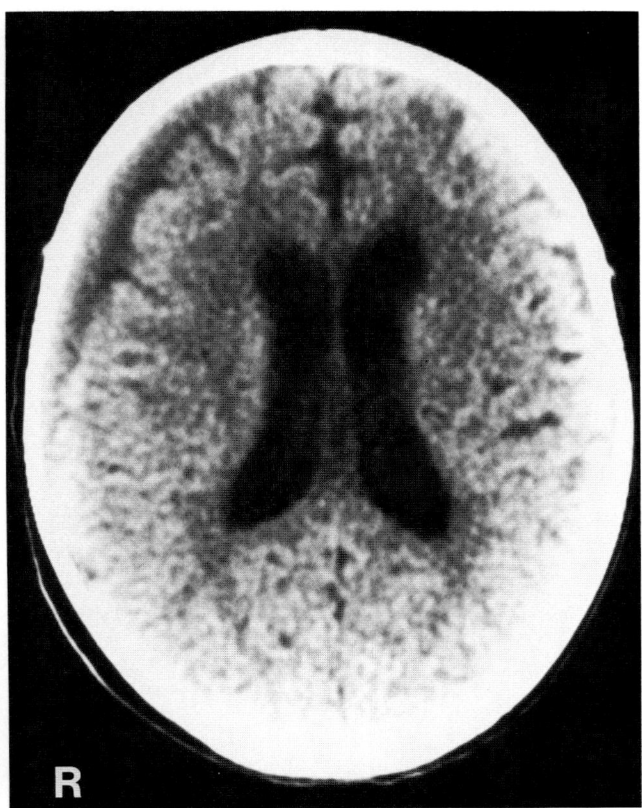

A   B

FIGURE 9.7   A: A CT head scan without contrast in a 6-month-old infant with *H. influenzae* meningitis. Note the right extra-axial fluid collection with shift of midline structures to the left. No intervention undertaken for removal of fluid. **B:** A CT head scan of same patient 1 month later. There is partial resolution of fluid collection and the patient was asymptomatic.

significant symptoms are present which could be attributed to the collection. Initial intervention when the fontanel is open consists of introducing a subdural needle into the fluid-filled space followed by removal of an appropriate quantity of fluid. If there are bilateral fluid collections, both sides can be tapped. The removal of large quantities of fluid can result in unwanted and potentially dangerous shifts of intracranial structures as well as loss of protein. The tap can be repeated as necessary, recognizing the risk of producing intracranial bleeding or infection. Unfortunately, removal of extra-axial fluid seldom changes symptomatology. If, after repeated tapping, CT or MRI head scans reveal progressive increase in the size of the fluid collection or the symptoms persist, continuous external drainage or shunting of the space should be considered. An infected collection of fluid needs immediate drainage. It is believed by some that the tap itself increases fluid formation, although no specific relationship has been established.

The contribution of small extra-axial fluid collections to an unfavorable clinical state or to neurologic sequelae may be minimal. Extra-axial fluid collections are usually benign, and appear to be an intrinsic part of many cases of meningitis. They produce no unique clinical symptoms, can be followed by imaging, resolve spontaneously with time, and usually require no intervention.

Brain Infarction and Necrosis

Focal areas of brain infarction and necrosis have been observed in pathologic studies of children dying of meningitis and in brain biopsies (130). There is extensive inflammation around cerebral vessels and vascular lesions are arterial or venous in origin; they may be multiple and, though usually bland, may be hemorrhagic. These lesions are relatively common in survivors, especially those who had severe illness and persisting deficits. Cortical enhancement on contrasted CT suggests cerebritis or infarction (Figure 9.8), and the development of discrete low-density lesions in the hemispheres indicates infarction.

Discrete cerebral lesions are associated with seizures, hemiparesis, irritability, lethargy, delayed recovery, and ventricular widening. Additional associated abnormalities such as extra-axial fluid collections are often found at neuroimaging. Areas of ischemic necrosis can be confused with brain abscess on imaging (131). Imaging performed late in the course of the acute illness or after the acute illness has the highest yield.

There is no specific treatment known for brain infarction and necrosis. Proper hydration, prevention of hypoxia and shock, control of seizures, and prevention of increased intracranial pressure are appropriate preventive measures

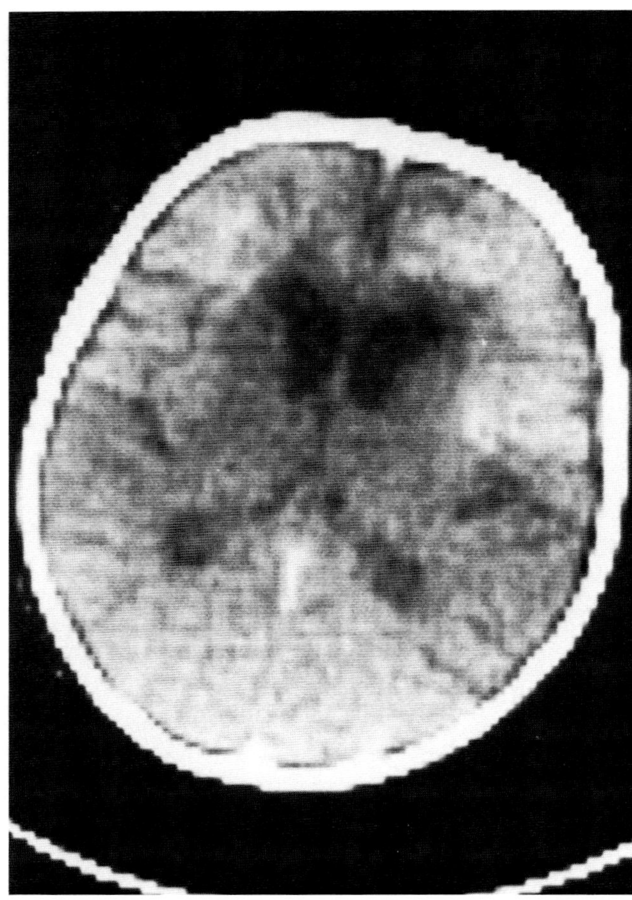

FIGURE 9.8 A CT head scan with contrast of 5-month-old infant with *H. influenzae* meningitis. There is enhancement of frontal and parietal lobes suggesting cerebritis or infarction.

and help to preserve adequate cerebral perfusion. The development of effective prevention and management of vasculitis is essential to achieve improvement in the outcome of bacterial meningitis.

Many of the permanent deficits after meningitis, such as mental retardation and static encephalopathy, appear related to the development of brain infarction and necrosis during the acute illness. Bacterial meningitis is a leading cause of stroke in infants and children.

Cranial Nerve Involvement

As the cranial nerves pass through the subarachnoid space they are intimately involved with the inflammatory process of bacterial meningitis. Cranial nerve function can be compromised by direct effect of toxic products on axons, infarction of the nerves secondary to inflammation and adhesions, or by stretching, secondary to increased intracranial pressure. The eighth nerve is most commonly affected, frequently resulting in permanent deafness. The oculomotor nerves are the next most commonly involved, and may result in ocular palsies that are usually revers-

ible. Other cranial nerves may also be affected, though less frequently.

About 10% of cases of bacterial meningitis in childhood are complicated by clinical deafness (132). In some patients, a conductive hearing loss associated with a middle ear infection accompanies the meningitis. More commonly, however, there is a sensorineural hearing loss found in both ears during the meningitis and related to inner ear infection through the cochlear aqueduct, or to inflammation about the eighth nerve in its subarachnoid course. The cochlear aqueduct passes from the leptomeninges to the base of the cochlea and serves as a passage for bacteria into the inner ear (133). Pathologic examination of the inner ear in fatal cases of meningitis has revealed infection, occlusion of vessels, and toxic neural changes.

The duration of symptoms before institution of antibiotic therapy does not correlate with the development of hearing loss (134) which can be detected in the first 48 hours of illness. This early loss is not necessarily permanent and recovery is usually maximal by the end of the first 2 weeks. Major deficits may persist. Brain stem auditory-evoked potentials are an effective method of detecting auditory abnormalities, especially in very young infants (135,136). Prior to or shortly after discharge a young child with bacterial meningitis should have an evaluation of brain stem auditory-evoked responses and an older child should have audiometry. When hearing loss is found, follow up and early intervention by a team knowledgeable in the management of this problem in infants and children is appropriate. Electronic cochlear stimulation may have a place in management.

Disseminated Intravascular Coagulation

The presence of abnormal bleeding or shock in a child with bacterial meningitis, especially with a gram-negative organism, suggests sepsis. Septic shock is a life-threatening complication, and disseminated intravascular coagulation (DIC) sometimes develops in this setting. In DIC rapid consumption of fibrinogen is found with the formation of fibrin thrombi. Purpuric skin lesions in meningitis suggest that a coagulopathy is present (Figure 9.9); similar lesions are found in other organs.

The diagnosis of DIC should be confirmed with appropriate laboratory studies which include the findings of thrombocytopenia, hypofibrinogenemia, circulating fibrin split products, abnormal prothrombin and partial thromboplastin times, and decreased levels of certain other coagulation factors (137). DIC can develop in bacterial meningitis from any organism but is especially common in *N. meningococcus* meningitis which may present as a fulminate disease with shock and purpura.

The purpuric skin lesions in *N. meningococcus* meningitis are not necessarily DIC and can occur from emboli or organisms. Embolic skin lesions initially have a yellowish-white center and organisms are found on Gram stain of

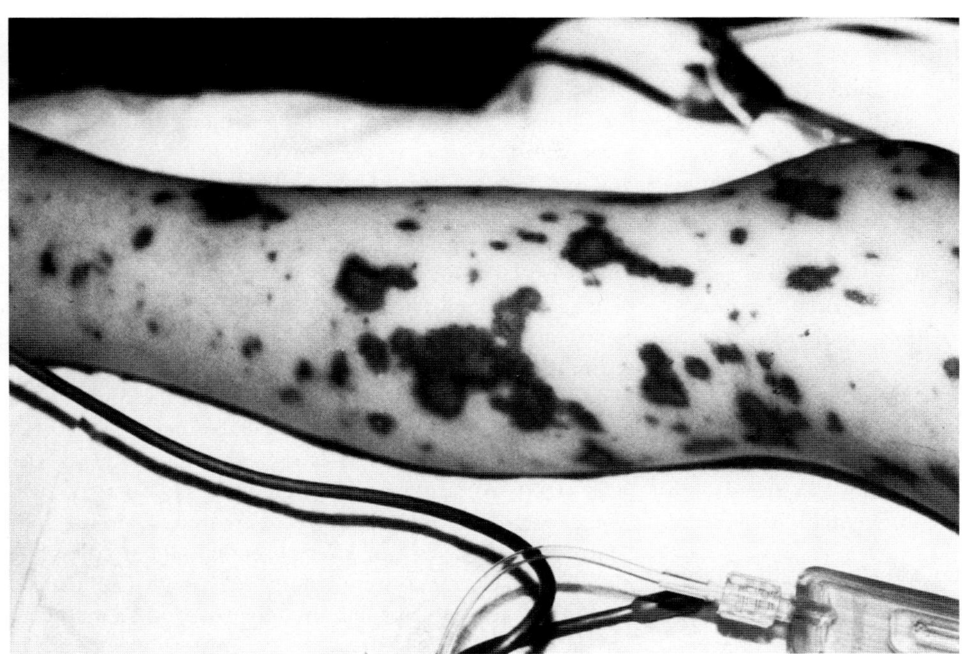

FIGURE 9.9 Purpuric skin lesions in a 4-year-old patient with *H. meningococcus* meningitis. (Courtesy of Dr. Robert Greenberg.)

scrapings from the lesions. The distinction between embolic lesions and those secondary to a coagulopathy may be important in management.

The Waterhouse-Friderichsen syndrome is characterized by adrenal hemorrhage associated with DIC. The presenting clinical feature is the sudden onset of septic shock. The adrenal hemorrhage seldom causes a clinical hypoadrenal state and is not in itself an indication for steroid replacement.

The management of DIC is controversial. Steroids do not appear beneficial and some recommended therapies such as heparin have the potential to cause harm. Treatment of the underlying infection is probably the most successful method for correction of DIC. Blood products should be administered to correct coagulation abnormalities. Other abnormalities of the coagulation system that are found in meningitis and sepsis include thrombocytopenia, purpura fulminans, and symmetrical peripheral gangrene.

Recurrent Meningitis

H. influenzae type b meningitis does not always confer lasting immunity. Certain individuals are at higher risk for a second attack than healthy persons are at risk for a first attack, suggesting a genetic predisposition (138). *H. influenzae* type b meningitis is more common in children with HLA-B12 histocompatibility antigen (139), and certain racial groups such as the Navajo Indian have a very high incidence of meningitis from *H. influenzae* type b.

The possibility of a cranial or spinal defect allowing communication to the external environment, parameningeal focus of infection, immunologic abnormality or genetic predisposition must be considered. The cranial or spinal defect can be acquired or developmental. Acquired defects include fractures of cranial bones such as those of the paranasal sinuses or ear region and may be associated with CSF rhinorrhea or otorrhea. Developmental defects include meningomyelocele, dermal sinus, or neuroenteric cyst.

In addition to the usual investigations for bacterial meningitis, other studies must be considered such as skull and sinus radiographs, CT with bone windows, MRI, intrathecal radioisotope tracer examination of CSF, looking for a site of external leakage, and an immunologic evaluation. Direct coronal thin-section CT is an effective method for detecting small osseous defects (140). If an anatomical defect is uncovered, surgical correction is usually indicated although some minor posttraumatic fistulae resolve spontaneously. Conditions other than bacterial CNS infections may cause recurrent meningitis, including Behçet syndrome, sarcoidosis, and Mollaret meningitis.

Prophylaxis

In certain specific circumstances bacterial meningitis may be a contagious disease with presumed transmission occurring by colonization of the nasopharynx with invasive strains. Outbreaks of *N. meningitidis* meningitis have been found among military recruits and other groups of people living in crowded conditions. Rifampin is recommended as prophylaxis for close contacts of an index case. Close contacts include family members, school contacts, and those in health care facilities. The dose of rifampin is 20 mg/kg (maximum 600 mg/dose) orally once daily for four days.

Invasive *H. influenzae* type b has occasionally been transmitted to family contacts and in day care centers.

Although no immunologic defect has been demonstrated, a genetic susceptibility to the organism with impaired antibody response could explain spread to family contacts. The use of antibiotic prophylaxis against invasive *H. influenzae* and the persons who should receive prophylaxis is an area of controversy (141,142,143). The current recommendation is administration of rifampin to adults and children of households exposed to *H. influenzae* meningitis and to those under 4 years of age exposed in day care centers (144). If prophylaxis is undertaken, children who have been immunized against *H. influenzae* should also receive rifampin (145).

Rifampin is recommended for an index case of *H. influenzae* meningitis to eradicate persistent nasopharyngeal colonization after conventional treatment of the meningitis (146). Rifampin should not be administered while the child is receiving chloramphenicol because of possible drug interference (147).

Passive immunization of susceptible, exposed children with high-titer anti-*Haemophilus influenzae* type b antibody immunoglobulin is possible (148). Recommendations regarding prophylaxis may change with time. Appropriate sources should be consulted.

Immunization

Despite the advances of modern therapy, neurologic sequelae following bacterial meningitis are not uncommon. This discouraging fact has stimulated efforts to prevent the disease by developing vaccines for immunization. A capsular polysaccharide vaccine is available against *N. meningitidis*. Use of the vaccine is appropriate in military recruits and during epidemics, but the vaccine does not appear effective in the prevention of disease once an individual is exposed.

Another capsular polysaccharide vaccine is available against pneumococcus, but the effectiveness of this vaccine in preventing *S. pneumoniae* meningitis is uncertain. The vaccine is recommended only for children who are at increased risk for serious disease should they become infected (149).

A vaccine effective against *H. influenzae* type b is also available, containing type b capsular polysaccharide, which accounts for most cases of meningitis with *H. influenzae*. The vaccine combats meningitis by preventing bacteremia (150). The vaccine can be administered at 2 months of age. The vaccine appears less effective in siblings of children who have had *H. influenzae* meningitis, suggesting that these children have a genetic impairment of antibody response (151). Immunization will not prevent respiratory infection with unencapsulated *H. influenzae,* but these organisms do not cause meningitis. The vaccine appears safe (152,153), but a question remains regarding the degree of vaccine efficacy and the possibility of increased severity of meningitis in vaccine failures (154). The risk of *H. influenzae* disease may actually be increased during the week immediately following immunization (155).

Prognosis

Despite advances in diagnosis and management the outlook for childhood bacterial meningitis remains unfavorable for some cases. Mortality rates for *H. influenzae* range from 4.5% to 14% (156), and when all forms of bacteria causing meningitis are included the mortality rates are higher. Mortality rates have not changed appreciably in the past 30 years (157). Meningitis remains a major cause of acquired neurologic disability in childhood and deficits range from minor and transient problems to lifelong incapacitating disabilities.

Infection with *S. pneumoniae* produces the highest incidence of neurologic sequelae. Detectable deficits are found in 28% of survivors beyond the neonatal period (158–160). An unfavorable outcome is associated with young age, delay in institution of treatment, coma, focal neurologic signs, seizures after onset, SIADH at admission, high CSF bacterial concentration (161), high CSF concentration of bacterial capsular antigen (162), and a malignant clinical course. The degree of CSF protein elevation and decrease of CSF glucose are, in general, associated with unfavorable outcome (163). The duration of illness prior to onset of neurologic signs and symptoms, however, seems to have little bearing on prognosis.

Although the majority of children recover without sequelae, mental retardation, motor impairment, hemiparesis, seizures, hydrocephalus, deafness, blindness, hyperactivity, and learning disabilities are among the problems that may develop (163a). Some children may appear normal but have minor difficulties in academic, motor, and social function (164). In a prospective study of 194 children with bacterial meningitis, 39% had neurologic abnormalities at the time of hospital discharge. Two years later only 9% had detectable deficits. This and other studies suggest cautious optimism about outcome (165). Recovery from spinal cord involvement, however, is poor (166).

Neurologic sequelae appear to result from ischemic damage, inflammation, necrosis, and the development of adhesions. Chronic drug-resistant complex partial seizures after meningitis have been reported, associated with mesial temporal sclerosis. Relief from seizures has been achieved in some patients following anterior temporal lobectomy (167). Further improvement in outcome will probably require improved methods of prevention of meningitis and management of complications, especially inflammation.

NEONATAL BACTERIAL MENINGITIS

Because of high morbidity and mortality, bacterial meningitis in the immediate postnatal period is of major significance. Factors predisposing to neonatal bacterial meningitis include maternal infection, prolonged rupture of maternal membranes, prolonged labor, obstetrical trauma, and fetal distress (168). The incidence of neonatal bacterial meningitis may be decreasing (169).

Pathology

The neonatal period is an active time for brain development, and meningitis during this period may result in disorganization of neural development with abnormal synaptogenesis, abnormal dendritic arborization, and aberrant myelination (170). Ventriculitis and vasculitis are more prominent findings in neonatal meningitis than in meningitis at later ages. Infarction, ventricular enlargement, vascular thrombosis, and multicystic encephalomalacia are found (171–173) but extra-axial fluid collections are infrequent. In some cases the ventricular enlargement represents hydrocephalus ex vacuo, secondary to loss of brain parenchyma rather than increased intraventricular pressure similar to some cases of intraventricular hemorrhage in the newborn. In neonatal meningitis bacteria can invade brain parenchyma and form abscesses, a distinctly unusual finding in the infant and older child.

Pathogenesis

The very young brain is easily invaded by bacteria, and the younger the brain, the more destructive is the infection. If there is no abnormal communication with the external environment, such as a meningomyelocele, meningitis is almost always preceded by and associated with sepsis.

Neonatal bacterial meningitis is usually acquired after rupture of maternal membranes and during the course of labor and delivery. Ventilators, aerosols, and indwelling vascular catheters increase the risk of sepsis and subsequent meningitis in predisposed infants (174). The onset of symptomatic meningitis from organisms acquired after delivery is usually not before 48 hours of age.

The neonate has certain defects in resistance and immune function which increase the risk of bacterial infection, including impaired nonspecific immunity with imperfect leukocyte chemotaxis, phagocytosis, and bacteriocidal activity. IgM antibodies, which are important in defense against gram-negative organisms, are not transferred across the placenta although the neonate has the ability to manufacture them. IgA antibodies, which are abundant in mucosal surfaces and may offer some protection against infection, are also not transferred. A relative deficiency of complement can develop (175,176).

Clinical Features

The typical clinical signs of meningitis are not present in the neonate, and only nonspecific findings of sepsis may be present. Nuchal rigidity is rarely found and fever and a full fontanel may be absent. Seizures, however, are more common at onset of illness in newborns, developing in about 40% of cases, perhaps reflecting the delay in establishing the diagnosis. Because of the high incidence of brain infarction and necrosis in neonatal meningitis, hemiparesis may be present. CT has proven useful in detection of cerebral

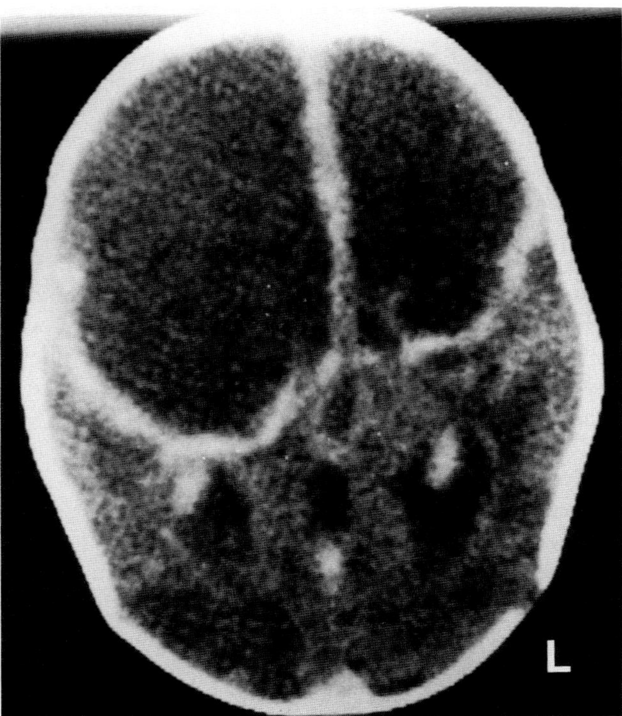

FIGURE 9.10 A CT head scan with contrast of neonate with *E. coli* meningitis. There is severe destruction of brain parenchyma with marked ventricular widening and shift of midline structures to the left.

infarction (177), ventricular enlargement, and other abnormalities (Figure 9.10).

Two clinical forms of neonatal meningitis have been described as early and late onset. The mean age at onset in the early form is 1.4 days and the infection appears related to maternal sepsis or organisms residing in the birth canal. The late form has an onset of symptoms after the first week of life and may also be acquired from the mother but is usually related to contaminated equipment or infected medical personnel (178). The early form is described as showing signs of sepsis, and the late form shows signs of meningitis including seizures.

Bacterial meningitis should be considered in any newborn with irritability, apnea, seizures, a tendency to opisthotonus, poor feeding, emesis, temperature instability, hypotonia, hypertonia, shock, poor perfusion of the extremities, jaundice, or any evidence of sepsis (Table 9.8).

Table 9.8 Signs and symptoms of bacterial meningitis in the neonate

Irritability
Apnea
Full fontanel
Seizures
Opisthotonus
Poor feeding
Temperature instability
Abnormal muscle tone
Sepsis

Lumbar Puncture

The lumbar puncture (LP) is indicated whenever there is a suspicion of meningitis and is part of the routine workup of suspected sepsis at many institutions. Only a limited volume of CSF should be removed from a small neonate. Severe cardiopulmonary disease constitutes a relative contraindication to LP because of the risk of cardiopulmonary compromise during positioning for the procedure. CSF pressure in a normal neonate is lower than in older children (179), and its determination seldom contributes to management of the newborn. Occasionally neonatalogists will give antibiotics in dosages effective against meningitis to a neonate with sepsis without performing an LP.

Cerebrospinal Fluid

Normal CSF parameters for prematures and newborns are not identical to those of older children and adults. Blood-tinged CSF may be found in the infant after an uncomplicated vaginal delivery, and is presumably related to intracranial trauma. Up to 32 WBC/mm^3 with up to 60% polymorphonuclear leukocytes (180) have been found in the CSF of normal newborns; however, it is unusual for more than several polymorphonuclear cells to be present. The number of cells gradually decreases during the first several months of life. Protein concentration as high as 150 mg/dL has been found in the CSF of normal newborns and premature infants, but it gradually decreases during the first several months of life. Small newborns frequently have low concentrations of blood glucose and, consequently, a low CSF glucose (181). Because there is such a wide range of normal CSF findings, the CSF parameters may not be as useful as in older infants and children.

Counterimmunoelectrophoresis and latex agglutination can detect antigens of certain bacteria. However, with the exception of group B streptococcus, these procedures test for pathogens which are not commonly found in the newborn. Limulus lysate assay has been useful for detection of gram-negative organisms in newborns (182).

Antibiotics

The bacteria which predominate in neonatal meningitis are from the mother's vaginal or perineal flora and include *E. coli*, particularly strains with the K1 capsular polysaccharide, group B streptococcus, and *L. monocytogenes*. *Proteus* species, *Pseudomonas* species, and *Streptococcus pneumoniae* are also found.

Initial antibiotic therapy includes ampicillin and an aminoglycoside or with ampicillin and ceftazidime, ceftriaxone or cefotaxime. The aminoglycosides used include gentamicin, amikacin, vancomycin, tobramycin, and kanamycin. While receiving an aminoglycoside, blood levels of the drug should be monitored to ensure attainment of therapeutic concentrations and to prevent ototoxicity and nephrotoxicity. Penicillin G or ampicillin is appropriate for group B streptococcus and ampicillin for *L. monocytogenes*. Ceftriaxone has a broad spectrum of effectiveness, penetrates well into the CSF, and appears safe and well tolerated in the neonate, but it is not effective against Pseudomonas species (183). Resistant organisms may become a problem when cephalosporins are used routinely (184). Cephalosporins must be used in combination with ampicillin or penicillin when given for initial therapy before a specific bacterial etiology is established, because cephalosporins have poor activity against group B streptococcus and *L. monocytogenes*. The use of chloramphenicol requires extreme care in neonates because of the risk of the gray syndrome and blood levels of the drug should be monitored. Chloramphenicol is antagonistic to third generation cephalosporins (185). Antibiotic therapy should be continued for 2 weeks if the infection is gram-positive and for 3 weeks in gram-negative.

The intrathecal administration of aminoglycoside does not appear to be of value in gram-negative meningitis, although it is often performed because of presumed greater effectiveness against concomitant ventriculitis (186). Intraventricular therapy may be appropriate in selected patients with ventriculitis (187).

Recommendations for antibiotics in treating neonatal meningitis vary and change frequently, and new antibiotics are constantly being introduced. Resistant strains develop, drug interactions occur, and neonatal pharmacokinetics differ from those of older children. Appropriate sources should be consulted and antibiotic management constantly monitored.

Prognosis

Morbidity and mortality are high in neonatal meningitis, and the outcome is related to prematurity, age of onset, delay in diagnosis, type of organism, and severity of symptoms (188). In a review of group B streptococcus meningitis during the first 6 months of life, 27% of patients died (189). Significant and permanent deficits are found in many survivors (190). Although deafness may be less a common sequela in survivors of neonatal meningitis than in older infants and children, all survivors should have a hearing evaluation. The use of newer antibiotics has not provided improved prognosis beyond that which can be attributed to improved general management of sick newborns.

UNUSUAL INFECTIONS OF THE NERVOUS SYSTEM IN INFANTS AND CHILDREN

Tuberculosis

The incidence of tuberculous meningitis reflects the prevalence of tuberculosis (TB) in the community, which is related to socioeconomic and hygienic conditions. TB meningitis is rare before the age of 3 months but the incidence is highest during the first 5 years of life. A decline in the incidence of childhood TB meningitis has been reported (191), but the overall incidence can be anticipated to increase because of the rising incidence of TB as an opportunistic infection in AIDS (192,193).

Pathology

The major insult of TB meningitis is to the basal meninges, although extensive meningitis about the hemispheric convexities and arachnoiditis around the spinal cord can develop. Involvement of the brain and spinal parenchyma can be encountered. A thick exudate surrounds vessels and cranial nerves and has been characterized as an inflammatory caseous leptomeningitis (194). The exudate contains lymphocytes, histiocytes, and giant cells, and infecting organisms may be present. Inflammatory vasculitis with thrombosis is a prominent feature. Cerebral infarcts are probably more common in tuberculous meningitis than in other forms of bacterial meningitis, and hydrocephalus is secondary to obliteration of subarachnoid pathways, especially if the disease was present for a prolonged time. Isolated tuberculomas develop within the meninges and may occur within or adjacent to the CNS parenchyma. They are likely to be infratentorial in children (195).

Pathogenesis

The hematogenous spread of TB develops from a primary focus, usually in the lung. Direct hematogenous spread to the nervous system, however, is unlikely during the primary infection except in the very young. After the stage of bacteremia, a caseous focus develops in the subarachnoid space, the brain or spinal cord. Months to years later a discharge of organisms occurs with the development of meningitis or invasion of brain parenchyma. Symptoms of meningitis or of intracranial mass then appear. The accompanying inflammation may be in part an immune reaction (196,197).

Clinical Features

TB meningitis is usually considered a chronic meningitis although an acute onset is present in about one-half of affected children. Untreated TB meningitis in children leads to death in an average duration of 20 days (198). The initial symptoms are vague and characterized by several weeks of generally poor health, malaise, anorexia, low-grade fever, nausea, vomiting, abdominal pain, and headache followed by alteration of consciousness, irritability, and apathy. Nuchal rigidity is not always present. In some cases, gastrointestinal symptoms are more prominent than neurologic symptoms. Cranial nerve deficits, either unilateral or bilateral, develop because of the basilar meningitis (199). The sixth nerve is the most frequently involved, and eighth nerve involvement can lead to deafness. The third, fourth, and second nerves may also be affected. Tuberculous lesions may be found in the choroid of the eye. The organizing exudate leads to obstruction of CSF flow and hydrocephalus, and tremor and movement disorders have been noted (200). As the disease progresses, the patient develops increasing depression of consciousness, convulsions, and major neurologic deficits. The differential diagnosis of this subacute or chronic meningitis includes viral CNS infection, partially treated bacterial meningitis, fungus infection, parameningeal infection, carcinomatous meningitis, sarcoid, and lymphoma.

The EEG shows slowing, but epileptiform features can be present. CT head scan findings are similar to those of bacterial meningitis and may show thickening and enhancement of the basal meninges or the presence of a tuberculoma (201). Similar changes are observed on MRI. Angiography may reveal constricted vessels about the base of the brain (202).

Intracranial tuberculomas, at one time the most common cause of posterior fossa tumor in childhood, have become rare in the US but not elsewhere (203). TB osteomyelitis can involve the spine, especially the vertebral bodies in the lower thoracic region. Collapse of the disc space and development of a paravertebral abscess can lead to cord compression and dysfunction. Spinal block may develop because of involvement of the spinal leptomeninges and subarachnoid space. Myelography, CT, or MRI of the spine is indicated in a child with suspected TB and neurologic signs suggesting cord involvement.

Most children with TB meningitis have radiographic evidence of pulmonary TB (204), but a normal chest radiograph does not exclude TB of the nervous system. A negative tuberculin skin test also does not exclude the presence of TB meningitis.

Cerebrospinal Fluid

At lumbar puncture, the opening CSF pressure may be elevated. The CSF seldom contains more than 500 cells/mm^3, the majority of which are lymphocytes except early in the disease when polymorphonuclear cells may predominate (205); eosinophils may be found. The protein concentration is elevated but rarely above 500 mg/dL, and the glucose concentration may be slightly decreased. Decreased concentration of chloride is nonspecific and has no diagnostic significance. Acid-fast bacilli can be demonstrated in CSF by smear, and tubercle bacilli can be isolated. Smears and cultures are not positive in all patients. If the clinical setting suggests TB of the nervous system and no organism is found, search for the tubercle bacilli should be continued.

A latex particle agglutination test has been developed for rapid detection of mycobacteria plasma membrane antigen in the CSF but has not yet achieved wide acceptance (206). The radioactive bromide partition test, although a rather complex test, has good reliability for the differentiation of tuberculosis from other causes of meningitis; it remains positive for up to 5 months after the initiation of treatment (207). Gas chromatography/mass spectrometry can identify tuberculostearic acid, a structural component of *Mycobacterium tuberculosis,* in the CSF in patients with tuberculous meningitis but not in controls. This test has been positive in suspected cases where the diagnosis could not be established by other means (208). An enzyme-linked immunosorbent assay (ELISA) of spinal fluid shows promise (209). CSF lactic acid and adenosine deaminase may be elevated, at least in adults (210). Repeated examinations of the CSF are often necessary to establish the diagnosis.

Treatment

Isoniazid and rifampin are the mainstays of treatment for TB meningitis, and therapy with antituberculosis chemotherapy should be continued for at least 9 months and perhaps longer. In severely ill patients ethambutol or streptomycin is added, at least for the first several months. Modifications of treatment are required when resistant organisms are found. Therapeutic response will usually be noted within 2 weeks (211).

Delay in the institution of treatment increases morbidity and mortality (212), and this creates added problems when the diagnosis of TB of the nervous system is uncertain. It is usually appropriate to start empirical therapy for TB in these circumstances. If recovery is rapid, and steroids have not been administered, tuberculosis of the nervous system is unlikely, and the discontinuation of therapy should be considered.

Clinical deterioration with cerebral edema has been noted within a few days of starting antituberculosis medication and is thought to be due to an unusual hypersensitivity reaction to the massive release of tuberculoproteins into the CSF (213). The use of corticosteroids to reduce the morbidity from inflammation, exudate, fibroblastic proliferation, and vasculitis remains controversial. Prednisone is often administered in the dose of 1 to 3 mg/kg/day for 2 to 3 weeks followed by gradual tapering of the dosage (214,215). When steroids are used in TB, there is risk of interfering with effectiveness of antituberculosis drugs, producing disseminated tuberculosis, suppressing the immune response, and producing a false sense of well-being. However, steroids may be of value in some patients, especially those who undergo clinical deterioration in spite of antituberculosis treatment and those with cerebral edema or spinal block. Pyridoxine has been added to the treatment regimen in adults to prevent the peripheral neuropathy which is sometimes induced by isoniazid. Pyridoxine does not appear necessary in the treatment of infants and children.

Tuberculomas unresponsive to antituberculosis chemotherapy may need surgical excision, and surgical shunting procedures are sometimes required in hydrocephalus.

Microsurgery to lyse adhesions around the optic nerves may improve failing vision.

Prognosis

The mortality rate varies from 1% to 20%. Major sequelae include hydrocephalus, which is common, and visual and auditory impairment that are secondary to direct involvement of cranial nerves. Hemiparesis, mental retardation, and seizures can occur, and involvement of the hypothalamus and basal cisterns can result in endocrinopathies such as diabetes insipidus, growth retardation, sexual precocity, and obesity (216). Brain atrophy is a late sequela. Spontaneous recovery from tuberculous meningitis has been reported (217,218).

Chronic Meningitis

Chronic meningitis is defined as the symptoms and signs of meningitis that persist for 4 weeks or longer. The symptoms may be more subtle than discerned in the acute illness, and only headache, fever, and mild alteration of consciousness may be present. Signs of meningeal irritation are inconsistent. As the condition progresses, there are more profound alterations in consciousness, with apathy, failure to thrive, seizures, cranial nerve deficits, and focal CNS findings.

Although TB, syphilis, and leptospirosis are caused by bacteria that can produce a meningitis of long duration, chronic meningitis is commonly not bacterial in origin. Additional differential diagnositc considerations include fungal infections such as cryptococcus, smoldering viral encephalitis or meningitis, partially treated bacterial meningitis, neoplasm involving the meninges, slow virus infection, sarcoidosis, Behçet syndrome, Vogt-Koyanagi-Harada syndrome, rickettsial infections, and idiopathic chronic meningitis. The clinical features and the usual CSF parameters do not reliably differentiate one form of infection from the other. A CSF lymphocytic pleocytosis is more likely to be present than a polymorphonuclear response.

Opportunistic chronic infections of the nervous system complicating AIDS in children have not been common (219). The neurologic picture of AIDS in children has been that of a progressive encephalopathy secondary to the HIV virus itself (See Chapter 26).

Childhood brucellosis can also produce a chronic meningitis (220). The organism is acquired from contact with animals or unpasteurized dairy products; however, the disease is seldom seen in the US. CNS involvement is secondary to systemic illness with chronic meningitis as the presenting CNS manifestation. Inflammation of the retina or optic nerve may complicate the clinical illness. Calcification of the basal ganglia has been noted in cerebral brucellosis in adults (221). The organism is difficult to culture and the diagnosis is usually established by a rise in antibodies to

Brucella species. Treatment is with tetracycline, rifampin, or streptomycin, or the combination of trimethoprim and sulfamethoxazole.

Special culture methods of the CSF as well as special immunologic studies may be rewarding in describing the course of chronic meningitis. Meningeal biopsy for culture and microscopic examination or biopsy of extraneural tissues such as lymph nodes, liver, bone marrow, or lung may be the only method by which the diagnosis can be established. If a specific etiologic diagnosis cannot be established in a case of chronic meningitis, a trial of antituberculosis therapy may be indicated. In selected cases of chronic meningitis, a trial of steroids should be considered (222).

Closed Head Trauma

Increasing drowsiness and fever after closed head injury suggests the possibility of posttraumatic meningitis (223). It usually develops shortly after the trauma but in some cases can be delayed for several months. A skull fracture and dural tear with a sinus-CSF fistula can be presumed but is not always demonstrated. When infection develops it usually takes the form of meningitis or brain abscess.

CSF rhinorrhea or otorrhea after a head injury suggests violation of the dura and the possibility of posttraumatic meningitis. Pneumocephalus is of similar significance. Most CSF leaks resolve spontaneously without development of CNS infection, but the persistence of CSF leakage requires surgical repair of the dura. Failure to perform adequate surgical correction can lead to recurrent attacks of meningitis.

The most common organism implicated in posttraumatic meningitis is *S. pneumoniae*. If a CSF leak develops after head trauma in an otherwise asymptomatic individual, treatment with penicillin is frequently recommended, although the benefit of such prophylaxis has not been demonstrated (224). When an antibiotic is used, it should be continued for at least 1 week after cessation of CSF leakage.

Leprosy

Leprosy (Hansen disease), a major health problem in many parts of the world (225), is caused by the acid-fast bacillus *Mycobacterium leprae*. Air travel and immigration from endemic areas increase the likelihood that physicians in the US and all parts of the world will encounter the condition (226). Children appear to be more susceptible than adults and there is a genetic role in patient susceptibility. Although the disease is systemic, the major clinical features involve the skin and peripheral nerves. The organism is acquired from the environment with humans serving as the reservoir, but other, nonhuman reservoirs may exist (227). The incubation period varies from several months to several years, and it is believed that the disease is the most common cause of peripheral nerve disorders in the world (228). The immune system plays an important part in the course of the disease with reported abnormalities of lymphocytes, T cells, and immunoglobulins (229,230).

The cardinal symptom of leprosy is a loss of sensory perception, and local areas of anesthesia develop before other symptoms of the disease are apparent. There is an early impairment of pain and temperature perception, and painless injury or infection can lead to mutilation and disfigurement. Leprosy is a chronic disease with occasional acute episodes, and patients complain of paresthesias or pain as the disease progresses. The disease begins in the Schwann cell, and ultimately, all patients have a peripheral neuropathy. Motor and sensory nerve conduction velocities are slow in the involved as well as uninvolved nerves (231).

There are two forms of lesions in the disease: lepromatous and tuberculoid. The lepromatous form is characterized by diffuse or focal lesions of skin and mucous membranes, especially of the cooler parts of the body. The lesions may not be anesthetic, but there is sensory loss in the hands and feet, and thickening of facial skin results in leonine facies. An associated progressive symmetric peripheral neuropathy is a late finding. Pathologic examination of peripheral nerves shows loss of axons and myelin with swelling of Schwann cells that contain the organisms. These patients have low resistance to leprosy. The lepromin skin test is negative.

Tuberculoid leprosy is the more common form of leprosy in children. Small, plaque-like, anesthetic cutaneous lesions are noted, and sensory loss can be detected early. The peripheral nerves are enlarged, especially the greater auricular nerve, and are affected in an asymmetric fasion with anesthesia of involved areas. Granulomas are found in nerves which do not contain organisms. Tuberculoid leprosy is more slowly progressive than lepromatous leprosy, is less disfiguring, and has a more favorable prognosis. Affected individuals have an associated high resistance to leprosy. The lepromin skin test is positive. Transplacental transmission may occur.

Although the organism can be stained, it cannot be cultured using traditional media. Examination of smears from skin or mucous membrane lesions for acid-fast bacilli is important in diagnosis. The organism infects the footpads of mice in a characteristic fashion.

Leprosy is treated by administration of dapsone (a sulfone), clofazimine (a bacteriostatic riminophenazine dye), and rifampin. Multidrug therapy (MDT) is usually recommended because there are resistant strains of the organism. Treatment can arrest disease progression and sometimes cure, though severe reactions have been noted at onset of therapy. The effectiveness of therapy, which is continued for several years, can be assessed by the disappearance of organisms from skin smears (232). Early therapy significantly improves prognosis. Vaccines are in the developmental stage.

Leprosy is a chronic disease, punctuated by occasional acute episodes. In untreated patients, mutilation, because of anesthesia, is common. Early treatment significantly improves the prognosis.

Mycoplasma pneumonia Infections

Mycoplasma pneumoniae is an organism that produces pulmonary infections of low communicability. These infections can be associated with neurologic disease in children (233,234,235). Neurologic symptoms appear 3 to 23 days after onset of pulmonary disease, are manifested as a remote effect of the infection, and may be autoimmune or related to a neurotoxin. There is a wide spectrum of neurologic symptoms, which may be the major clinical manifestations of the disease. They include the signs and symptoms of meningitis, cerebritis, subacute encephalopathy, transverse myelitis, and radiculitis of cranial or spinal nerve roots. An ascending paralysis similar to the Guillain-Barré syndrome may develop. An associated pulmonary infection with *M. pneumoniae* is commonly found. The infection with *M. pneumoniae* may not be clinically apparent and the role of this organism in neurologic disease is often underestimated.

Successful culture of the organism requires experienced laboratory personnel and recognition of the organism's prolonged incubation period. The CSF shows a mononuclear pleocytosis with normal glucose and elevated protein concentrations; patients with polyneuropathy may have a similar picture to Guillain-Barré syndrome, with albumino-cytologic dissociation. The organism is rarely isolated from CSF. Serum agglutinins are elevated and a rise in serum complement fixation titer establishes the diagnosis.

Antimicrobial therapy with erythromycin or tetracycline (236) is recommended, but though it improves the neurologic aspects of the illness, recovery from the neurologic manifestations is prolonged and permanent deficits are common. Treatment directed towards autoimmune neurologic disease, such as plasmapheresis, may have a place in management.

Brain Abscess

Whereas bacterial meningitis presents as an acute, sometimes fulminating disease, the presentation of bacterial brain abscess, in contrast, is seldom acute and dramatic, and historical and clinical findings are vague. Brain abscesses are found in children in association with cyanotic congenital heart disease, neurosurgical procedures, and penetrating head trauma. They also may develop in association with a contiguous focus of infection, an immunosuppressed state, or in chronic pulmonary disease (237). It is possible that bacterial brain abscesses will be seen as a complication of AIDS in children. The association of brain abscess with bacterial meningitis is rare except in the neonate, and finding a brain abscess as a complication of meningitis after the neonatal period suggests the abscess preceded the development of meningitis.

Pathology

Brain abscesses occur as the result of hematogenous or direct local spread of the organism. An abscess of hematogenous origin is localized at the juncture of the gray and white matter and is initially manifested as a cerebritis which may persist for several weeks. There is surrounding edema which may increase the mass effect. The cerebritis phase is followed by formation of the abscess, a capsule of inflammatory granulation tissue which develops around the infected area. The subacute onset of significant symptoms including headache, confusion, depressed consciousness, seizures, papilledema, and focal neurologic signs suggests brain abscess. In one large series of children with brain abscesses, papilledema was not found in any patient under the age of 2 years, but was apparent in 50% of the older patients (238). Temperature elevation is minimal, intermittent, or absent, and seizures may be focal or generalized. Nuchal rigidity may be found. Findings on neurologic examination are not necessarily localizing. MRI or radionuclide brain scan are appropriate tests during the stage of cerebritis.

Enhanced CT or MRI head scans (239) are the definitive diagnostic tests for brain abscess, showing a characteristic capsular ring (Figure 9.11). The EEG may be normal, but usually shows focal abnormalities in the region of the abscess, with slowing, spikes, periodic lateralized epileptiform discharges (PLEDs), or a diffusely slow pattern.

The brain abscess behaves as an expanding intracranial mass lesion and can obstruct CSF flow, produce hydrocephalus, or lead to cerebral herniation. Multiple abscesses can develop. The differential diagnosis includes neoplasm, hematoma, and focal encephalitis such as that caused by *Herpes simplex*. Although brain abscess is commonly an indolent infection, it can cause a neurologic emergency with rapid clinical deterioration, cerebral edema, and herniation.

Lumbar puncture should be avoided because of the increased risk of cerebral herniation secondary to elevated intracranial pressure. However the diagnosis of brain abscess is not made by LP. If difficulty is encountered in establishing the diagnosis and imaging does not suggest increased intracranial pressure or displacement of intracranial contents, cautious LP can be considered.

The CSF is usually under increased pressure with a mild lymphocytic or polymorphonuclear pleocytosis, elevation of protein, normal or slightly low glucose concentrations, and failure to culture an organism. Gram stain is usually negative and organisms are seldom cultured. The CSF findings are not diagnostic.

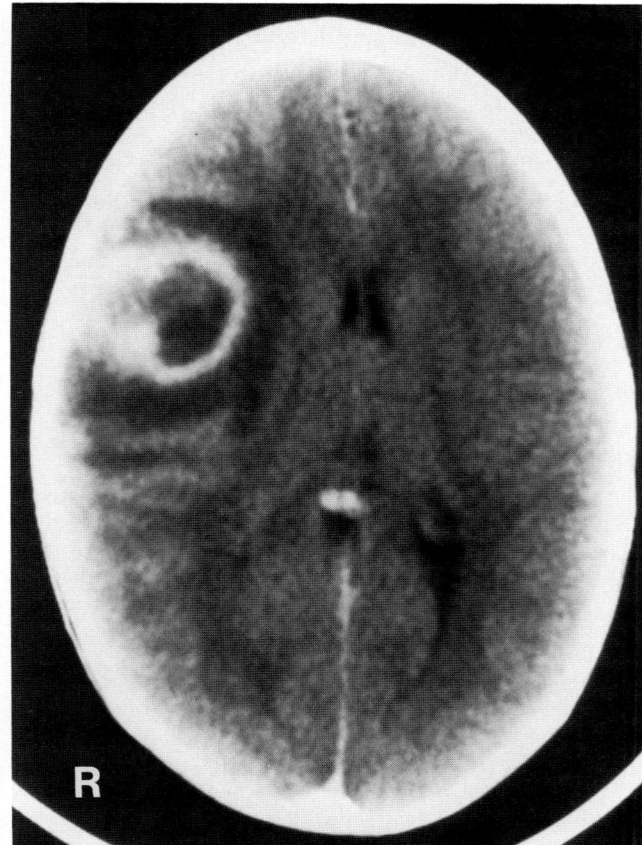

FIGURE 9.11   A CT head scan with contrast of 12-month-old infant who had recurrent vomiting and left partial motor seizures 6 days after right otitis media. Right hemispheric abscess noted with shift of midline structures to the left. Isolated organism was anaerobic beta-hemolytic streptococcus.

Treatment

Anaerobic bacteria account for 70% of brain abscesses, and multiple organisms may be found. Streptococcus species, Straphylococcus species, and *Bacteroides fragilis* are common bacteria in abscesses. Prior to identification of the organism, antibiotics should be administered which are appropriate for the suspected cause of infection. Antibiotics such as penicillin or cefotaxime can be used empirically. Surgical drainage or excision is then usually appropriate; it provides an opportunity to culture the organism(s) and promotes healing. Controversy exists regarding the most appropriate method of surgical approach (240).

Brain abscesses have been cured by antibiotics alone without surgical drainage (241,242). Medical management should be considered at a stage of cerebritis, if there are multiple abscesses, if the abscess is located in a critical area, or when the patient has a severe underlying systemic disease. The course of antibiotic therapy should be 6 to 8 weeks. Shorter durations of therapy have been associated with relapse or the development of new daughter abscesses.

Serial CT or MRI head scans can be used to determine effect of medical therapy (243).

Increased intracranial pressure should be managed by hyperventilation, osmotic agents such as mannitol, steroids such as dexamethasone, and surgical drainage. The administration of dexamethasone, 10 to 12 $mg/m^2/day$ IV every 6 hours frequently produces a dramatic lowering of intracranial pressure. Morbidity and mortality rates, although improving, remain high (244).

Prognosis

Because of the difficulty in diagnosis and management, the mortality is significant, and sequelae are frequent. However, with the advent of neuroimaging and development of newer antibiotics, the outlook for patients with brain abscess is improving (245). Chronic seizure disorders are common after abscesses (246).

Subdural Empyema

Subdural empyema is a collection of pus in the potential space between the dura and the arachnoid. The precise anatomic location of this collection is seldom known and the infection may be in a loculated area of CSF. In children this infection is a rare complication of bacterial meningitis; the empyema contains the same organism that causes the meningitis. Subdural empyema may also develop by spread of infection from contiguous structures, as a complication of a neurosurgical procedure, or as a complication of tapping an extra-axial fluid collection.

Symptoms of subdural empyema include fever, headache, stiff neck, lethargy, vomiting, seizures, papilledema, and focal neurologic signs. Clinical deterioration is usually rapid with the development of an enlarging mass lesion, cerebral edema, increased intracranial pressure, and brain herniation. Lumbar puncture is contraindicated. Brain imaging shows an elliptically shaped collection of fluid between the skull and brain, which, on repeat imaging, may show rapid enlargement and producing reaction in the underlying brain substance. Antibiotic therapy appropriate for the suspected organism combined with surgical drainage is imperative (247).

Epidural Abscess

The collection of pus may be present between the dura and the overlying bone and consititute an epidural abscess. These infections are found with spread from contiguous structures, as complications of neurosurgical procedures, or coexisting with subdural abscesses. Spinal epidural abscesses appear to be hematogenous in origin. Symptoms include fever, overlying pain, and focal neurologic deficits. The organisms causing epidural abscesses are the same as those causing brain abscess. Imaging usually shows a lenticular collection of fluid between the bone and the CNS. Lumbar puncture is contraindicated (248). Treatment consists of antibiotics, surgical drainage, and management of increased intracranial pressure.

Plague Meningitis

Pasteurella pestis can cause meningitis in children (249). A history of exposure to wild rodents and other signs of plague, usually the bubonic form, accompany the meningitis. The meninges are unlikely to be the primary site of infection. The CSF findings are typical for bacterial meningitis, and *P. pestis* is recovered on culture. Streptomycin has been the treatment of choice although other aminoglycides are used when IV administration is necessary. The addition of chloramphenicol may be indicated. Tetracyclines or sulfa preparations are used for prophylaxis. With early recognition and prompt antibiotic treatment, the course is usually benign.

REFERENCES

1. McCracken GH. Management of bacterial meningitis: Current status and future prospects. Am J Med 1984;76 Suppl 5A:215–223.
2. Skoch MG, Walling AD. Meningitis: Describing the community health problem. Am J Public Health 1985;75:550–552.
3. Cochi SL, Fleming DW, Hightower AW, et al. Primary invasive *Haemophilus influenzae* type b disease: A population-based assessment of risk factors. J Pediatr 1986;108:887–896.
4. Broome CV. Epidemiology of *Haemophilus influenzae* type b infections in the United States. Pediatr Infect Dis J 1987;779–782.
5. Tarr PI, Peter G. Demographic factors in the epidemiology of *Hemophilus influenzae* meningitis in young children. J Pediatr 1978;92:884–888.
6. Bell WE, McCormick WF. Neurologic Infections in Children, 2nd edition. Philadelphia: Saunders, 1981.
7. Swartz MN, Dodge PR. Bacterial meningitis—a review of selected aspects. N Engl J Med 1965;272:725–731, 779–787,842–848,898–902,954–960,1003–1010.
8. Klein JO, Feigin RD, McCracken GH. Report of the task force on diagnosis and management of meningitis. Pediatrics 1986;78(Suppl):956–982.
9. Snyder RD. Bacterial infections of the nervous system. In: Swaiman KF. Pediatric Neurology: Principles and Practice. St. Louis: Mosby, 1988;447–473.
10. Bell WE, McCormick WF. Neurologic Infections in Children, 2nd edition. Philadelphia: Saunders, 1981;27–40.
11. Hutchings M, Weller RO. Anatomical relationships of the pia mater to cerebral blood vessels in man. J Neurosurg 1986;65:316–325.
12. Fishman RA, Sligar K, Hake RB. Effects of leukocytes on brain metabolism in granulocytic brain edeam. Ann Neurol 1977;2:89–94.
13. Kroll JS, Moxon ER. Bacterial meningitis in children. In: Asbury AK, McKhann GM, McDonald WI, eds. Diseases of the nervous system. Philadelphia: Saunders, 1986;2: 1375–1383.
14. Tauber MG, Brooks-Fournier RA, Sande MA. Experimental models of CNS infections. Neurol Clinics 1986;4:249–264.
15. Klein JO. The febrile child and occult bacteremia. N Engl J Med 1987;317:1219–1220.
16. Sheld WM. Bacterial meningitis in the patient at risk: Intrinsic risk factors and host defense mechanisms. Am J Med 1984;76 (Suppl 5A):193–207.
17. Kroll JS, Moxon ER. Acute bacterial meningitis. In: Kennedy PGE, Johnson RT, eds. Infections of the Nervous System. London: Butterworth, 1987;3–22.
18. Quagliarello VJ, Scheld WM. Review: Recent advances in the pathogenesis and pathophysiology of bacterial meningitis. Am J Med Sci 1986;292:306–309.
19. Scheld WM. Morphofunctional alterations of the blood-brain barrier during experimental meningitis. Am J Med Sci 1986;292:306–309.
20. Lindquist L, Wibon R, Lundbergh P, et al. Experimental meningitis in the rat. II. Cerebral energy metabolism in relation to increased cerebrospinal fluid concentrations of lactate. Acta Neurol Scand 1987;75:405–409.
21. Maida E, Horvatits E. Cerebrospinal fluid alterations in bacterial meningitis. Eur Neurol 1986;25:110–116.
22. Greenlee JE. Anatomic considerations in central nervous system infections. In: Mandell GR, Douglas RG, Bennett JE, eds. Principals and Practice of Infectious Diseases, 2nd edition. New York: John Wiley & Sons, 1985;551–560.
23. Rasmussen JM, Brandslund I, Teisner B, et al. Screening for complement deficiencies in unselected patients with meningitis. Clin Exp Immunol 1987;68:437–445.
24. Sande MA, Sande ER, Woolwine JD, et al. The influence of fever on the development of experimental *Streptococcus pneumoniae* meningitis. J Infect Dis 1987;156:849–850.
25. Moxon ER. Virulence genes and prevention of *Haemophilus influenzae* infections. Arch Dis Child 1985;60:1193–1196.
26. Finne J, Leinonen M, Makela PH. Antigenic similarities between brain components and bacteria causing meningitis. Lancet 1983;2:355–357.
27. Petersen GM, Silimperi DR, Rotter JI, et al. Genetic factors in *Haemophilus influenzae* type b disease susceptibility and antibody acquision. J Pediatr 1987;110:228–233.
28. Igarashi M, Gilmartin RC, Gerald B, et al. Cerebral arteritis and bacterial meningitis. Arch Neurol 1984;41:531–535.
29. Smith AL, Scheifele D, Daum R, et al. Cerebral blood flow in experimental *Haemophilus influenzae* b meningitis. Pediatr Infect Dis J 1987;6:1159.
30. Smith AL. Pathogenesis of *Haemophilus influenzae* meningitis. Pediatr Infect Dis J 1987;6:783–786.
31. Dacey RG, Scheld WM, Winn HR, et al. Bacterial meningitis. Selected aspects of cerebrospinal fluid pathophysiology. In: Wood JH, ed. Neurobiology of Cerebrospinal Fluid. New York: Plenum, 1983;2:727–738.
32. Syrogiannopoulos GA, Olsen KD, Reisch JS, et al. Dexamethasone in the treatment of experimental *H. influenzae* type b meningitis. J Infect Dis 1987;155:213–219.
33. Chan PH, Fishman RA, Caronna J, et al. Induction of brain edema following intracerebral injection of arachidonic acid. Ann Neurol 1983;13:625–632.
34. Fishman RA. Brain edema. N Engl J Med 1975;293: 706–711.

35. Paulson OB, Brodersen P, Hansen EL, et al. Regional cerebral blood flow, cerebral metabolic rate for oxygen and cerebrospinal fluid acid-base variables in patients with acute meningitis and with acute encephalitis. Acta Med Scand 1974;196:191–198.

36. Tauber MG, Shibl AM, Hackbarth CJ, et al. Antibiotic therapy, endotoxin concentration in cerebrospinal fluid, and brain edema in experimental *Escherichia coli* meningitis in rabbits. J Infect Dis 1986;156:456–462.

37. Toumanen E. Molecular mechanisms of inflammation in experimental pneumococcal meningitis. Pediatr Infect Dis J 1987;6:1146–1149.

37a. Tunkel AR, Wispelwey B, Scheld WM: Bacterial meningitis: Recent advances in pathophysiology and treatment. Ann Int Med 1990;112:610–623.

38. Valmari P. Primary diagnosis in a life-threatening childhood infection. A nationwide study on bacterial meningitis. Ann Clin Res 1985;17:310–315.

39. Silverman RA. Cutaneous manifestations of neurologic infections in children. Neurol Clin 1987;5:459–482.

40. Verghese A, Gallemore G. Kernig's and Brudzinski's signs revisited. Rev Infect Dis 1987;9:1187–1192.

41. Burstein L, Breningstall GN. Movement disorders in bacterial meningitis. J Pediatr 1986;109:260–264.

42. Schwartz JF. Ataxia in bacterial meningitis. Neurology 1972;22:1071–1074.

43. Haupt HM, Kurlinski JP, Barnett NK, et al. Infarction of the spinal cord as a complication of pneumococcal meningitis. J Neurosurg 1981;55:121–123.

44. Tal Y, Crichton U, Dunn HG, et al. Spinal cord damage: A rare complication of purulent meningitis. Acta Paediatr Scand 1980;69:471–474.

45. Rothbart HA, Glode MP. *Haemophilus influenzae* type b septic arthritis in children: Report of 23 cases. Pediatrics 1985;75:254–259.

46. Likitnukul S, McCracken GH, Nelson JD. Arthritis in children with bacterial meningitis. Am J Dis Child 1986;140:424–427.

47. Stovring J, Snyder RD. Computed tomography in childhood bacterial meningitis. J Pediatr 1980;96:820–823.

48. Richards PG, Towu-Aghantse E. Dangers of lumbar puncture. Brit Med J 1986;292:605–606.

49. Byers RK. To tap or not to tap. Pediatrics 1973;52:462–463.

50. Gower DJ, Baker AL, Bell WO, et al. Contraindications to lumbar puncture as defined by computed cranial tomography. J Neurol Neurosurg Psychiatry 1987;50:1071–1074.

51. Bryan CS. Promptness of antibiotic therapy in acute bacterial meningitis. Ann Emerg Med 1986;15:544–547.

52. Gledhill RF. Dangers of lumbar puncture. Brit Med J 1986;292:1134.

53. Kaplan SL, Smith EO, Wills C, et al. Association between preadmission oral antibiotic therapy and cerebrospinal fluid findings and sequelae caused by *Haemophilus influenzae* type b meningitis. Pediatr Infect Dis J 1986;5:626–632.

54. Teele DW, Dashefsky B, Rakusan T, et al. Meningitis after lumbar puncture in children with bacteremia. N Engl J Med 1981;305:1079–1081.

55. Smith KM, Deddish RB, Ogata ES. Meningitis associated with serial lumbar punctures and post-hemorrhagic hydrocephalus. J Pediatr 1986;109:1057–1060.

56. Shapiro ED, Aaron NH, Wald ER, et al. Risk factors for development of bacterial meningitis among children with occult bacteremia. J Pediatr 1986;109:15–19.

57. McLellan D, Giebink GS. Perspectives on occult bacteremia in children. J Pediatr 1986;109:1–8.

58. Feigin RD, Shackelford PG. Value of repeat lumbar puncture in the differential diagnosis of meningitis. N Engl J Med 1973;289:571–574.

59. Polk DB, Steele RW. Bacterial meningitis presenting with normal cerebrospinal fluid. Pediatr Infect Dis J 1987;6:1040–1042.

60. Chartrand SA, Cho CT. Persistent pleocytosis in bacterial meningitis. J Pediatr 1976;88:424–426.

61. Durack DT, Spanos A. End-of-treatment spinal tap in bacterial meningitis. Is it worthwhile? JAMA 1982;248:75–78.

62. Powell KR, Hendley JO, Gadomski A, et al. Acute illness in the 2 weeks after hospitalization for bacterial meningitis. Pediatrics 1987;80:342–343.

63. Benjamin CM, Newton RW, Clarke MA. Risk factors for death from meningitis. Brit Med J 1988;296:220.

64. Bohr V, Rasmussen N, Hansen B, et al. 875 cases of bacterial meningitis: Diagnostic procedures and the impact of preadmission antibiotic therapy. J Infect 1983;7:193–202.

65. Powers WJ. Cerebrospinal fluid lymphocytosis in acute bacterial meningitis Am J Med 1985;79:216–220.

66. Olson LC, Portnoy JM. Normal cerebrospinal fluid values. Pediatrics 1985;76:1024.

67. Cory MJ. Normal cerebrospinal fluid values. Pediatrics 1985;76:1023–1024.

68. Onorato IM, Wormser GP, Nicholas P. "Normal" CSF in bacterial meningitis. JAMA 1980;244:1469–1471.

69. Menkes JH. The causes for low spinal fluid sugar in bacterial meningitis—Another look. Pediatrics 1969;44:1–3.

70. Quaade F, Krislensen KP. Purulent meningitis: A review of 658 cases. Acta Med Scand 1962;171:543–550.

71. Converse GM, Gwaltney JM, Strassburg DA, et al. Alternation of cerebrospinal fluid findings by partial treatment of bacterial meningitis. J Pediatr 1973;83:220–225.

72. Portnoy JM, Olsen LC. Normal cerebrospinal fluid values in children: Another look. Pediatrics 1985;75:484–487.

73. Martin WJ. Rapid and reliable techniques for the laboratory detection of bacterial meningitis. Am J Med 1983;75 Suppl 1B:119–123.

74. Gray BM, Simmons DR, Mason H, et al. Quantitative levels of C-reactive protein in cerebrospinal fluid in patients with bacterial meningitis and other conditions. J Pediatr 1986;108:665–670.

75. Jordan GW, Statland B, Halsted C. CSF lactate in diseases of the CNS. Arch Intern Med 1983;143:85–87.

76. Campbell DR, Skikne BS, Cook JD. Cerebrospinal fluid ferritin levels in screening for meningism. Arch Neurol 1986;43:1257–1260.

77. Clarke D, Cost K. Use of serum C-reactive protein in differentiating septic from aseptic meningitis in children. J Pediatr 1983;102:718–720.

78. Peltola HO. C-reactive protein for rapid monitoring of infections of the nervous system. Lancet 1982;1:980–982.

79. Philip AGS, Baker CJ. Cerebrospinal fluid C-reactive protein in neonatal meningitis. J Pediatr 1983;102:715–717.

80. Eiden J, Yolken RH. C-reactive protein and Limulus amebocyte lysate assay in diagnosis of bacterial meningitis. J Pediatr 1986;108:423–426.

81. Stutman HR, Marks MI. Therapy for bacterial meningitis: Which drugs, and for how long? J Pediatr 1987;110:812–814.

82. Eichenwald HF. Bacterial meningitis: Is there a "best" antimicrobial therapy? Eur J Pediatr 1987;146:216–220.

83. Peter G, Giebink GS, Hall CB, et al., eds. Report of the committee on infectious diseases, twelfth edition. Elk Grove: American Academy of Pediatrics, 1986:169–174,244–247, 277–282.

84. Nelson JD. Emerging role of cephalosporins in bacterial meningitis. Am J Med 1985;79 Suppl 2A:47–51.

85. Overturf GD, Hoeprich PD. Bacterial meningitis. In: Hoeprich PD, ed. Infectious Diseases. Philadelphia: Harper and Row, 1983;1035–1052.

86. Kelly HW. Personal communication, 1987.

87. Donowitz GR, Mandell GL. Beta-lactam antibiotics. N Engl J Med 1988;318:419–426.

88. Overturf, GD. Pyogenic bacterial infections of the CNS. Neurol Clin 1986;4:69–90.

89. McGee ZA. Bacterial meningitis: Current status and directions for the future—an overview. In: Sande MA, Smith AL, Root RK, eds. Bacterial Meningitis. New York: Churchill Livingston, 1985;253–264.

90. Downs NJ, Hodges GR, Taylor SA. Mixed bacterial meningitis. Rev Infect Dis 1987;9:693–703.

91. Dalton HP, Allison MJ. Modification of laboratory results by partial treatment of bacterial meningitis. Am J Clin Path 1968;49:410–413.

92. Jadavji T, Bigger WD, Gold R, et al. Sequelae of acute bacterial meningitis in children treated for seven days. Pediatrics 1986;78:21–25.

93. Lin T-Y, Nelson J, McCracken GH. Fever during treatment for bacterial meningitis. Pediatr Infect Dis J 1984;3:319–322.

94. Smith AL, Weber A. Pharmacology of chloramphenicol. Pediatr Clin North Amer 1983;30:209–236.

95. Yogev R, Shulman ST, Chadwick EG, et al. Once daily ceftriaxone for central nervous system infections and other serious pediatric infections. Pediatr Infect Dis J 1986;5: 298–303.

96. Jacobs RF, Wright MW, Deskin RL, et al. Delayed sterilization of *Haemophilus influenzae* type b meningitis with twice-daily ceftriaxone. JAMA 1988;259:392–394.

97. Marks WA, Stutman HR, Marks MI, et al. Cefuroxime versus ampicillin plus chloramphenicol in childhood bacterial meningitis: A multicenter randomized controlled trial. J Pediatr 1986;109:123–130.

98. Odio C, McCracken GH, Nelson JD. CSF shunt infections in pediatrics. A seven-year experience. Am J Dis Child 1984; 138:1103–1108.

99. Bayston R, Hart CA, Barnicoat M. Intraventricular vancomycin in the treatment of ventriculitis associated with cerebrospinal fluid shunting and drainage. J Neurol Neurosurg Psychiat 1987;50:1419–1423.

99a. Lebel MH, Freij BJ, Syrogiannopoulos GA, et al. Dexamethasone therapy for bacterial meningitis: Results of two double-blind, placebo-controlled trials. N Engl J Med 1988;319:964–971.

99b. Odio CM, Faingezicht L, Paris M, et al. The beneficial effects of early dexamethasone administration in infants and children with bacterial meningitis. N Engl J Med 1991; 324:1525–1531.

100. Tuomanen E, Hengstler B, Rich R, et al. Nonsteroidal antiinflammatory agents in the therapy for experimental pneumococcal meningitis. J Infect Dis 1987;155:985–990.

101. Gelmers HJ, Gorter K, de Weerdt CJ, et al. A controlled trial of nimodipine in acute ischemic stroke. N Engl J Med 1988; 318:203–207.

102. Sande MA, Scheld WM, McCracken GH, et al. Report of a workshop: Pathophysiology of bacterial meningitis—implications for new management strategies. Pediatr Infect Dis J 1987;6:1145,1167–1171.

103. Kochhar A, Zivin JA, Lyden PD, et al. Glutamate antagonist therapy reduces neurologic deficits produced by focal central nervous system ischemia. Arch Neurol 1988;45:148–153.

104. Valmari P, Peltola H, Ruuskanen O, et al. Childhood bacterial meningitis: Initial symptoms and signs related to age, and reasons for consulting a physician. Eur J Pediatr 1987; 146:515–518.

105. Snyder RD. Seizures in childhood bacterial meningitis. Ann Neurol 1984;16:395–396.

106. Crawford TO, Mitchell WG, Snodgrass SR. Lorazepam in childhood status epilepticus and serial seizures: Effectiveness and tachyphylaxis. Neurology 1987;37:190–195.

107. Jadavji T, Biggar WD, Gold R, et al. Sequelae of acute bacterial meningitis in children treated for seven days. Pediatrics 1986;78:21–25.

108. Rosman NP, Peterson DB, Kaye EM, et al. Seizures in bacterial meningitis: Prevalence, patterns, pathogenesis, and prognosis. Pediatr Neurol 1985;1:278–285.

108a. Pomeroy SL, Holmes SJ, Dodge PR, et al. Seizures and other neurologic sequelae of bacterial meningitis in children. N Engl J Med 1990;323:1651–1657.

109. McMenamin JB, Volpe JJ. Bacterial meningitis in infancy: Effects on intracranial pressure and cerebral blood flow velocity. Neurology 1984;34:500–504.

110. Horwitz SJ, Boxerbaum B, O'Bell J. Cerebral herniation in bacterial meningitis. Ann Neurol 1980;7:524–528.

111. Prince AS, Neu HC. Fluid management in *Haemophilus influenzae* meningitis. Infection 1980;8:5–7.

112. Kaplan SL, Feigin RD. The syndrome of inappropriate secretion of antidiuretic hormone in children with bacterial meningitis. J Pediatr 1978;92:758–761.

113. Dickoff DJ, Raps M, Yahr MD. Striatal syndrome following hyponatremia and its rapid correction. Arch Neurol 1988; 45:112–114.

114. Syrogiannopoulos GA, Olsen KD, McCracken GH. Mannitol treatment in experimental *Haemophilus influenzae* type b meningitis. Pediatr Res 1987;22:118–122.

115. DeLemos RA, Haggerty RJ. Corticosteroids as an adjunct to treatment of acute bacterial meningitis. Pediatrics 1969;44: 30–34.

116. Belsey MA, Hoffpauir CW, Smith MMD. Dexamethasone in the treatment of acute bacterial meningitis: The effect of study design on the interpretation of results. Pediatrics 1969;44:503–513.

117. McCracken GH. Use of dexamethasone for treatment of bacterial meningitis in infants and children. Pediatr Infect Dis J 1987;6:1159–1160.

118. Kaplan SL, Fishman MA. Supportive therapy for bacterial meningitis. Pediatr Infect Dis J 1987;6:670–677.

119. Mickell JJ, Reigel DH, Cook DR, et al. Intracranial pressure: Monitoring and normalization therapy in children. Pediatrics 1977;59:606–613.

120. Aucoin PJ, Kotilainen HR, Gantz NM, et al. Intracranial pressure monitors. Epidemiologic study of risk factors and infections. Am J Med 1986;80:369–376.

121. Dacey RG. Monitoring and treating increased intracranial pressure. Pediatr Infect Dis J 1987;6:1161–1163.

122. Cabral DA, Flodmark O, Farrell K, et al. Prospective study of computed tomography in acute bacterial meningitis. J Pediatr 1987;111:201–205.

123. Snyder RD. Ventriculomegaly in childhood bacterial meningitis. Neuropediatrics 1984;15:136–138.

124. Schachenmayr W, Friede RL. The origin of subdural neomembranes. I. Fine structure of the dura-arachnoid interface in man. Am J Pathol 1978;92:53–68.

125. Benson P, Nyhan WL, Shimuzu H. The prognosis of subdural effusions complicating pyogenic meningitis. J Pediatr 1960;57:670–683.

126. Packer RJ, Bilaniuk LT, Zimmerman RA. CT parenchymal abnormalities in bacterial meningitis: Clinical significance. J Comput Assist Tomogr 1982;6:1064–1068.

127. Syrogiannopoulos GA, Nelson JD, McCracken GH. Subdural collections of fluid in acute bacterial meningitis: A review of 136 cases. Pediatr Infect Dis J 1986;5:343–352.

128. Curless RG. Subdural empyema in infant meningitis: Diagnosis, therapy, and prognosis. Child Nerv Sys 1985; 1:211–214.

129. Bodino J, Lylyk P, Del Valle M, et al. Computed tomography in purulent meningitis. Am J Dis Child 1982;136: 495–501.

130. Snyder RD, Stovring J, Cushing AH, et al. Cerebral infarction in childhood bacterial meningitis. J Neurol Neurosurg Psychiatry 1981;44:581–585.

131. Tavora L, Antunes JL. Brain abscesses and ischemic necrotic lesions during early childhood. Neurosurgery 1987;21: 923–927.

132. Dodge PR. Sequelae of bacterial meningitis. Pediatr Infect Dis J 1986;5:618–620.

133. Ruben RJ. Diseases of the inner ear and sensorineural deafness. In: Bluestone DC, Stool SE, eds. Pediatric Otolaryngology. Philadelphia: WB Saunders Co., 1983;595.

134. Dodge PR, Davis H, Feigin RD, et al. Prospective evaluation of hearing impairment as a sequela of acute bacterial meningitis. N Engl J Med 1984;311:869–874.

135. MacDonald JT, Feinstein S. Hearing loss following *Hemophilus influenzae* meningitis in infancy. Diagnosis by evoked response audiometry. Arch Neurol 1984;41:1058–1059.

136. Ozdamar O, Kraus N. Auditory brainstem response in infants recovering from bacterial meningitis. Neurologic assessment. Arch Neurol 1983;40:499–502.

137. McCabe WR, Tredwell TL, DeMaria A. Pathophysiology of bacteremia. Am J Med 1983;75 Suppl 1B:7–18.

138. Granoff DM, McKinney T, Boies EG, et al. *Haemophilus influenzae* type b disease in an Amish population: Studies of the effects of genetic factors, immunization, and rifampin prophylaxis on the course of an outbreak. Pediatrics 1986; 77:289–295.

139. Tejani A, Mahadevan R, Dobias B. Occurrence of HLA types in *H. influenzae* type b disease. Tissue Antigens 1981; 17:205–211.

140. Steele RW, McConnell JR, Jacobs RF, et al. Recurrent bacterial meningitis: Coronal thin-section cranial computed tomography to delineate anatomic defects. Pediatrics 1985; 76:950–953.

141. Osterholm MT, Pierson LM, White KE, et al. The risk of subsequent transmission of *Hemophilus influenzae* type b disease among children in day care. Results of a two-year statewide prospective survillance and contact survey. N Engl J Med 1987;316:1–5.

142. Murphy TV, Clements JF, Breedlove JA, et al. Risk of subsequent disease among day-care contacts of patients with systemic *Hemophilus influenzae* type b disease. N Engl J Med 1987;316:5–10.

143. Broome CV, Mortimer EA, Katz SL, et al. Use of chemoprophylaxis to prevent the spread of *Hemophilus influenzae* b in day-care facilities. N Engl J Med 1987;316:1226–1229.

144. Peter G, Giebink GS, Hall CB, et al. Report of the committee on infectious diseases, twentieth edition. Elk Grove: American Academy of Pediatrics 1986;171–173.

145. Dashefsky B, Wald E, Li K. Management of contacts of children in day care with invasive *Haemophilus influenzae* type b disease. Pediatrics 1986;78:939–941.

146. Li KI, Wald ER. Use of rifampin in *Haemophilus influenzae* type b infections. Am J Dis Child 1986;140:381–385.

147. Kelly HW, Couch RC, Davis RL, et al. Interaction of chloramphenicol and ripfampin. J Pediatr, 1988;112:817–820.

148. Peter G. Treatment and prevention of *Haemophilus influenzae* type b meningitis. Pediatr Infect Dis J 1987;6:787–790.

149. Brunell PA, Bass JW, Daum RS, et al. Recommendations for using pneumococcal vaccine in children. Pediatrics 1985; 75:1153–1157.

150. Peltola H, Kayhty H, Virtanen M, et al. Prevention of *Hemophilus influenzae* type b bacteremic infections with the capsular polysaccharide vaccine. N Engl J Med 1984;310: 1561–1566.

151. Granoff DM, Squires JE, Munson RS, et al. Siblings of patients with *Haemophilus* meningitis have impaired anticapsular antibody responses to *Haemophilus* vaccine. J Pediatr 1983;103:185–191.

152. Black SB, Shinefield HR. b-CAPSA I *Haemophilus influenzae*, type b, capsular polysaccharide vaccine safety. Pediatrics 1987;79:321–325.

153. FDA worship on *Haemophilus* b polysaccharide vaccine—a preliminary report. MMWR 1987;36:529–531.

154. Daum RS, Osterholm MT, Granoff DM. Failure of vaccination with *Haemophilus influenzae* vaccine. N Engl J Med 1987;317:115.

155. Granoff DM, Osterholm MT. Safety and efficacy of *Haemophilus influenzae* type b polysaccharide vaccine. Pediatrics 1987;80:590–592.

156. Schlech WF, Ward JI, Band JD, et al. Bacterial meningitis in the United States, 1978 through 1981. The national bacterial meningitis surveillance study. JAMA 1985;253: 1749–1754.

157. Katz SL, Mortimer EA. Proceedings of a roundtable: *Haemophilus influenzae* type b: The disease and its prevention. Pediatr Infect Dis J 1987;6:773–774.

158. Sell SH. Long term sequelae of bacterial meningitis in children. Pediatr Inf Dis J 1983;2:90–93.

159. Sproles ET, Azerrad J, Williamson C, et al. Meningitis due to *Hemophilus influenzae*: Long-term sequelae. J Pediatr 1969; 75:782–788.

160. Granoff DM, Squires JE. Hemophilus meningitis: New developments in epidemiology, treatment and prognosis. Sem Neurol 1982;2:151–165.

161. Feldman WE. Relation of concentration of bacteria and bacterial antigen in cerebrospinal fluid to prognosis in patients with bacterial meningitis. N Engl J Med 1977;296: 433–435.

162. Feigin RD, Stechenberg BW, Chang MJ, et al. Prospective evaluation of treatment of *Haemophilus influenzae* meningitis. J Pediatr 1976;88:542–548.

163. Laxer RM, Marks MI. Pneumococcal meningitis in children. Am J Dis Child 1977;131:850–853.

163a. Taylor HG, Mills EL, Ciampi A, et al. The sequelae of *Haemophilus influenzae* meningitis in school-age children. N Engl J Med 1990;323:1657–1663.

164. Sell SH. *Haemophilus influenzae* type b meningitis: Manifestations and long term sequelae. Pediatr Infect Dis J 1987;6:775–778.

165. Taylor HG, Michaels RH, Mazur PM, et al. Intellectual, neuropsychological, and achievement outcomes in children six to eight years after recovery from *Haemophilus influenzae* meningitis. Pediatrics 1984;74:198–205.

166. Seay AR. Spinal cord dysfunction complicating bacterial meningitis. Arch Neurol 1984;41:545–546.

167. Ounsted C, Glaser GH, Lindsay J, et al. Focal epilepsy with mesial temporal sclerosis after acute meningitis. Arch Neurol 1985;42:1058–1060.

168. Berman RH, Banker BQ. Neonatal meningitis: A clinical and pathological study of 29 cases. Pediatrics 1966;38:6–24.

169. Bennhagen R, Svenningsen NW, Bekassy AN. Changing pattern of neonatal meningitis in Sweden. A comparative study 1976 vs. 1983. Scand J Infect Dis 1987;19:587–593.

170. Averill DR, Moxon ER, Smith AL. Effects of *Hemophilus influenzae* meningitis in infant rats on neuronal growth and synaptogenesis. Exp Neurol 1976;50:337–345.

171. Friede RL. Cerebral infarcts complicating neonatal leptomeningitis. Acute and residual lesions. Acta Neuropathol (Berl) 1973;23:245–253.

172. Gilles FH, Jammes JL, Berenberg W. Neonatal meningitis. The ventricle as a bacterial reservoir. Arch Neurol 1977;34:560–562.

173. Brown LW, Zimmerman RA, Bilaniuk LT. Polycystic brain disease complicating neonatal meningitis: Documentation of evolution by computed tomography. J Pediatr 1979;94:757–759.

174. Volpe JJ. Neurology of the Newborn, 2nd edition. Philadelphia: Saunders, 1987;599.

175. Wilson CB. Immunologic basis for increased susceptibility of the neonate to infection. J Pediatr 1986;108:1–12.

176. Meade RH. Bacterial meningitis in the neonatal infant. Med Clin North Am 1985;69:257–267.

177. Ment LR, Ehrenkranz RA, Duncan CC. Bacterial meningitis as an etiology of perinatal cerebral infarction. Pediatr Neurol 1986;2:276–279.

178. Albritton WL, Wiggins GL, Feeley JC: Neonatal listeriosis: Distribution of serotypes in relation to age at onset of disease. J Pediatr 1976;88:481.

179. Kaiser AM, Whitelaw AGL. Normal cerebrospinal fluid pressure in the newborn. Neuropediatrics 1986;17:100–102.

180. Otila E. Studies on the cerebrospinal fluid in premature infants. Acta Paediatr 1948;35 (Suppl 8):1–100.

181. Sarff LD, Platt LH, McCracken GH. Cerebrospinal fluid evaluation in neonates: Comparison of high-risk infants with and without meningitis. J Pediatr 1976;88:473–477.

182. Dyson D, Cassady G. Use of limulus lysate for detecting gram-negative neonatal meningitis. Pediatrics 1976;58:105–109.

183. Mulhall A, de Louvois J, James J. Pharmacokinetics and safety of ceftriaxone in the neonate. Eur J Pediatr 1985;144:379–382.

184. Bryan CS, John JF, Pai S, et al. Gentamicin vs cefotaxime for therapy of neonatal sepsis. Relationship to drug resistance. Am J Dis Child 1985;139:1086–1089.

185. Isaacs D, Wilkinson AR. Antibiotic use in the neonatal unit. Arch Dis Child 1987;62:204–208.

186. McCracken GH, Mize SG. A controlled study of intrathecal antibiotic therapy in gram-negative enteric meningitis of infancy. J Pediatr 1976;89:66–72.

187. Lee EL, Robinson MJ, Thoug ML, et al. Intraventricular chemotherapy in neonatal meningitis. J Pediatr 1977;91:991–995.

188. Haslam RHA. Neurological complications of neonatal bacterial meningitis. Int Pediatr 1987;2:100–108.

189. Wald ER, Bergman I, Taylor HG, et al. Long-term outcome of group B streptococcal meningitis. Pediatrics 1986;77:217–221.

190. Karan S. Purulent meningitis in the newborn. Childs Nerv Syst 1986;2:26–31.

191. Klein NC, Damsker B, Hirschman SZ. Mycobacterial meningitis. Retrospective analysis from 1970 to 1983. Am J Med 1985;79:29–34.

192. Ogawa SK, Smith MA, Brennessel DJ, et al. Tuberculous meningitis in an urban medical center. Medicine 1987;66:317–326.

193. Sunderam G, McDonald RJ, Maniatis T, et al. Tuberculois as a manifestation of the acquired immunodeficiency syndrome (AIDS). JAMA 1986;256:362–366.

194. Dastur DK, Lalitha VS. The many facets of neurotuberculosis—An epitome of neuropathology. In: Zimmerman HM, ed. Progress in Neuropathology, Vol. 2. New York: Grune and Stratton, 1972;351–408.

195. Bell WE, McCormick WF. Neurologic Infections in Children. Saunders: Philadelphia, 1981;188–209.

196. Kocen RS. Tuberculosis of the nervous system. In: Kennedy PGE, Johnson RT, eds. Infections of the Nervous System. London: Butterworth, 1987;25–26.

197. Molavi A, LeFrock JL. Tuberculous meningitis. Med Clin North Am 1985;69:315–331.

198. Lincoln EM, Sewell EM. Tuberculosis in Children. New York: McGraw-Hill, 1963;161–183.

199. Lincoln E, Sordillo SVR, Davies PA. Tuberculous meningitis in children: A review of 167 untreated and 74 treated patients with special reference to early diagnosis. J Pediatr 1960;57:807–823.

200. Udani PM, Parekh UC, Dastur KD. Neurological and related syndromes in CNS tuberculosis: Clinical features and pathogenesis. J Neurol Sci 1971;14:341–357.

201. Trautmann M, Kluge W, Otto H-S, et al. Computed tomography in CNS tuberculosis. Eur Neurol 1986;25:91–97.

202. Mathew NT, Abraham J, Chandy J. Cerebral angiographic features in tuberculous meningitis. Neurology 1970;20:1015–1023.

203. Anderson JM, Macmillan JJ. Intracranial tuberculoma—An increasing problem in Britain. J Neurol Neurosurg Psychiatry 1975;38:194–210.

204. Zarabi M, Sane S, Girdany BR. The chest roentgenogram in the early diagnosis of tuberculous meningitis in children. Am J Dis Child 1971;121:389–392.

205. Stockstill MT, Kauffman CA. Comparison of cryptococcal and tuberculous meningitis. Arch Neurol 1983;40:81–85.

206. Krambovitis E, McIllmurry MB, Lock PE, et al. Rapid diagnosis of tuberculous meningitis by latex particle agglutination. Lancet 1984;2:1229–1231.

207. Coovadia YM, Dawood A, Ellis ME, et al. Evaluation of adenosine deaminase activity and antibody to *Mycobacterium tuberculosis* antigen 5 in cerebrospinal fluid and the radioactive bromide partition test for the early diagnosis of tuberculosis meningitis. Arch Dis Child 1986;61:428–435.

208. French GL, Chan CY, Cheung SW, et al. Diagnosis of tuberculous meningitis by detection of tuberculostearic acid in cerebrospinal fluid. Lancet 1987;2:117–119.

209. Prabhakar S, Oommen A. ELISA using mycobacterial antigens as a diagnostic aid for tuberculous meningitis. J Neurol Sci 1987;78:203–212.

210. Ribera E, Martinez-Vazquea JM, Ocana I, et al. Activity of adenosine deaminase in cerebrospinal fluid for the diagnosis and follow-up of tuberculous meningitis in adults. J Infect Dis 1987;155:603–607.

211. Van Scoy RE, Wilkowske CJ. Antituberculous agents. Mayo Clin Proc 1987;62:1129–1136.

212. Fallon RJ, Kennedy DH. Treatment and prognosis in tuberculous meningitis. J Infect 1981;3:39–44.

213. Udani PM, Parekh UC, Dastur DK. Neurological and related syndromes in CNS tuberculosis. Clinical features and pathogenesis. J Neurol Sci 1971;14:341–357.

214. Escobar JA, Belsey MA, Duenas A, et al. Mortality from tuberculous meningitis reduced by steroid therapy. Pediatrics 1975;56:1050–1055.

215. O'Toole RD, Thornton GF, Mukherjee MK, et al. Dexamethasone in tuberculous meningitis: Relationship of cerebrospinal fluid effects to therapeutic efficacy. Ann Int Med 1969;70:39–48.

216. Smith AL. Tuberculous meningitis in childhood. Med J Aust 1975;1:57–60.

217. Emond RTD, McKendrick GDW. Tuberculosis as a cause of transient aseptic meningitis. Lancet 1973;2:234–236.

218. Bell WE, McCormick WF. Neurologic Infections in Children, 2nd ed. Philadelphia: W.B. Saunders, 1981: 610–628.

219. Epstein LG, Sharer LR, Oleske JM, et al. Neurologic manifestations of human immunodeficiency virus infection in children. Pediatrics 1986;78:678–687.

220. Swick HM. Brucella meningoencephalitis in childhood. Neuropediatrics 1981;12:330–336.

221. Mousa AM, Muhtaseb RR, Reddy A, et al. The high rate of prevalence of CT detected basal ganglia calcification in neuropsychiatric (CNS) brucellosis. Acta Neurol Scand 1987; 76:448–456.

222. Anderson NE, Willoughby EW. Chronic meningitis without predisposing illness - a review of 83 cases. Quart J Med 1987;63:283–295.

223. Lau YL, Kenna AP. Post-traumatic meningitis in children. Injury 1986;17:407–409.

224. Hirschmann JV. Bacterial meningitis following closed cranial trauma. In: Sande MA, Smith AL, Root RK, eds. Bacterial Meningitis. New York: Churchill-Livingston 1985; 95–103.

225. Jopling WH. Handbook of Leprosy, 3rd ed. London: Heinemann, 1984;1–145.

226. Younger B, Michaud REM, Fisher M. Leprosy. Our southwest Asian refugee experience. Arch Dermatol 1982; 118:981–984.

227. Thomas DA, Mines JS, Thomas DC, et al. Armadillo exposure among Mexican-born patients with lepromatous leprosy. J Infect Dis 1987;156:990–992.

228. Dastur DK. Leprosy. In: Vinken PJ, Bruyn GW, eds. Handbook of Clinical Neurology. Amsterdam: North-Holland Publishing 1978;33:421–468.

229. Levis WR, Meeker HC, Schuller-Levis GB, et al. Serodiagnosis of Leprosy: Relationship between antibiotics to Mycobacterium leprae phenolic glycolipid I and protein antigens. J Clin Microbiol 1986;24:917–921.

230. Ashmalla L. Immunologic aspects of leprosy. Int J Dermatol 1986;25:452–455.

231. Ponnighaus JM, Fine PEM, Bliss L. Certainty levels in the diagnosis of leprosy. Int J Leprosy 1987;55:454–462.

232. Meyers WM. Leprosy. In: Feigin RD, Cherry JD, eds. Textbook of Pediatric Infectious Diseases, 2nd ed. Philadelphia: W.B. Saunders, 1987, 1172–1190.

233. Clyde WA. Neurologic syndromes and mycoplasmal infections. Arch Neurol 1980;37:65–66.

234. Cassell GH, Cole BC. Mycoplasmas as agents of human disease. N Eng J Med 1981;304:80–89.

235. Carstensen H, Nilsson KO. Neurological complications associated with mycoplasma pneumoniae in children. Neuropediatrics 1987;18:57–58.

236. Cherry JD. Mycoplasma and ureaplasma infections. In: Feigin RD, Cherry JD, eds. Textbook of Pediatric Infectious Disease, 2nd ed. Philadelphia: W.B. Saunders 1987; 1896–1924.

237. Fisher EG, Schwachman H, Wepsic JG. Brain abscess and cystic fibrosis. J Pediatr 1979;95:385–388.

238. Jadavji T, Humphreys RP, Prober CG. Brain abscesses in infants and children. Pediatr Infect Dis J 1985;4:394–398.

239. Schroth G, Kretzschmar K, Gawehn J, et al. Advantage of magnetic resonance imaging in the diagnosis of cerebral infections. Neuroradiol 1987;29:120–126.

240. Taylor JC. The case for excision in the treatment of brain abscess. Br J Neurosurg 1987;1:173–178.

241. Weisberg LA. Nonsurgical management of focal intracranial infection. Neurology 1981;31:575–580.

242. Berg B, Franklin G, Cuneo R, et al. Non-surgical cure of brain abscess: Early diagnosis and follow-up with computerized tomography. Ann Neurol 1978;3:474–478.

243. Ferriero DM, Derechin M, Edwards MSB, et al. Outcome of brain abscess treatment in children: Reduced morbidity with neuroimaging, Pediatr Neurol 1987;3:148–152.

244. Fischer EG, McLennan JE, Suzuki Y. Cerebral abscess in children. Am J Dis Child. 1981;135:746–749.

245. Editorial: Treatment of brain abscess. Lancet 1988;1: 219–220.

246. Hedge AS, Venkataramana NK, Das BS. Brain abscess in children. Child Nerv Syst 1986;2:90–92.

247. Miller ES, Dias PS, Uttley D. Management of subdural empyema: a series of 24 cases. J Neurol Neurosurg Psychiatry 1987;50:1415–1418.

248. Benson CA, Harris AA. Acute neurologic infections. Med Clin North Am 1986;70:978–1011.

249. Martin AR, Hurtado FP, Plessala RA, et al. Plaque meningitis: A report of three cases in children and review of the problem. Pediatrics 1967;40:610–616.

Chapter 10
Viral Infections

James F. Bale, Jr.

Viral infections of the nervous system, potentially life-threatening disorders, affect thousands of children annually throughout the world. Numerous viruses can directly infect the brain or spinal cord, and many others induce neurologic dysfunction through immunologically mediated mechanisms.

Advances in virologic methods, particularly those employing monoclonal antibodies or nucleic-acid detection, enable physicians to identify etiologic agents more expeditiously and economically. Moreover, these molecular techniques have greatly enhanced our understanding of the pathogenesis of many virus-induced neurologic disorders. Although vaccines have reduced the incidence of certain viral disorders, relatively few viral infections can currently be treated with specific antiviral chemotherapy.

VIROLOGY AND EPIDEMIOLOGY

Virology

Numerous viruses have been associated with childhood neurologic disorders (1,2,3). In the arthopod-borne group alone, many different virus species cause neurologic illness. Whether neurologic disease will occur during a viral infection depends on host immune factors and the neurovirulence of the etiologic agent (4).

To infect cells and produce progeny, viruses, obligate intracellular parasites, undergo a complex series of events including: adsorption or attachment of the virus to the cell membrane; penetration of the cell and virus uncoating; replication of viral nucleic acid and production of viral proteins; virus assembly; and release of mature virus particles, or virions (5).

Adsorption of viruses to neural cells depends on virus contact with the host cell and attachment to specific receptors on the cell surface. These receptors, usually glycoproteins, are variably present on cells of the nervous system. This variation in receptor sites contributes to what Richard Johnson has termed the *selective vulnerability* of neural cells to virus infection (4).

After attachment, viruses enter the cell cytoplasm via phagocytosis, fusion of the virus envelope with the cell membrane, or direct release of genomic material. Viruses then use host-cell synthetic activities to produce virus-specific nucleic acids and proteins. Replicative strategies vary among viruses and depend in part on whether the virus contains DNA or RNA (5).

In permissive cells, the final steps in the production of progeny virus are those of assembly and release of mature virions. Certain viruses are assembled in the cell cytoplasm, whereas assembly of others occurs in the nucleus or at the nuclear membrane (5). Ultimately, release of virions from host cells results from lysis of infected cells or budding of virus particles from intact cell membranes.

In nonpermissive cells, virus progeny are not produced. Such cells may undergo latent infections, in which viruses are present in a nonreplicating state. Episodically, these viruses may reactivate, release infectious virus, and induce overt illness. Herpes simplex viruses (HSV), for example, can latently infect neural ganglia and cause recurrent mucocutaneous lesions or neurologic disease.

Epidemiology

Viruses that cause neurologic disease exhibit considerable variation in their geographic distribution (1,2). Some, like the herpesviruses, occur worldwide; whereas, others, like the arthropod-borne viruses (historically grouped as the arboviruses), are restricted to specific countries or continents. Such variation among the arboviruses is attributable in large measure to the geographic range of insect vectors (mosquitoes, ticks, and flies). The epidemiology of several viral agents, notably polio, measles, and rubella viruses, has been altered dramatically by vaccination programs. Infections with these viruses remain important pathogens in many third-world nations, but are now uncommon in the United States and other developed countries.

Viruses also display seasonal variation (1,2,3). Nearly all infections with the arboviruses occur during the summer months, when insect vectors are most active. In temperate climates, like most of North America, enteroviral infections peak in summer and late fall, whereas mumps is more common in late winter and spring. Lymphocytic choriomeningitis virus, an arenavirus that chronically infects rodents, usually causes human illness during winter. By contrast, infections with members of the herpesvirus group show little, if any, seasonal variation.

Host factors, age, and immune status, are important determinants of the epidemiology of virus-induced neurologic disorders. In general, young children between the ages of 6 months and 5 years display greatest susceptibility to infection with many different viral pathogens. Children with congenital immunodeficiency syndromes, the acquired immunodeficiency syndrome (AIDS), or chemotherapy-induced immunosuppression are also at considerable risk for severe or persistent viral infections of the central nervous system (CNS).

PATHOGENESIS AND PATHOLOGY

Pathogenesis

Most viruses that infect the nervous system reach neural tissues by hematogenous spread (6). Primary replication of the virus occurs at the site of inoculation, such as the skin and subcutaneous tissues in arboviral infections, lymph nodes of the gastrointestinal tract in enteroviral infections, or nasopharyngeal lymphoid tissues in infections with several different agents. In susceptible hosts, viremia ensues, and virions are disseminated to other organs. Secondary virus replication in these tissues induces organ-system dysfunction and amplifies viremia.

Certain viral pathogens reach the CNS via neural routes. In experimental rabies, the rabies virus first replicates in muscle and infects muscle spindles (7). The virus then enters peripheral nerve endings and travels via axons retro-

grade to neurons in the spinal cord. Infection subsequently spreads to other neurons of the spinal cord and brain.

The neural route also appears to have an important role in HSV type 1 encephalitis. The studies of Baringer and Swoveland and those of Cook and co-workers demonstrated that neural ganglia harbor latent HSV (8–10). Based on these observations, Davis and Johnson postulated that HSV can reactivate in trigeminal ganglia and travel retrograde via the trigeminal nerve to the middle and anterior fossae of the cerebrum (11).

Viruses induce neurologic dysfunction by direct infection of neural cells or by immunologically mediated mechanisms (3,6). Direct infection and replication of viruses within neural cells cause cell death or disruption of critical cellular functions. Replication of HSV or rabies virus in neurons, for example, results in widespread neuronal dysfunction.

Host immunity to virus infection consists of local factors and humoral and cell-mediated immune responses (1,12). Local factors that inhibit viral invasion include the skin, the pH, and secretory immunoglobulins. In many instances, virus replication is limited to cells at the site of inoculation. In the case of the CNS, however, the blood-brain barrier does not restrict entry of viruses (1).

Antibodies of the immunoglobulin (Ig) M class usually appear within 2 weeks after primary infection; whereas, IgG antibodies can be detected within 2 to 6 weeks of infection. Levels of IgG usually peak approximately 8 weeks after infection. Cell-mediated immune responses, as measured by lymphocyte blastogenic responses to mitogens or viral antigens, tend to parallel or lag slightly behind the humoral responses. Antibody and cell-mediated responses act in concert to neutralize viral pathogens, either in the blood stream or at cellular foci of infection. These responses depend greatly on the individual host, however.

Certain neurologic disorders appear to be mediated through these host immune responses (13). Examples include disseminated encephalomyelitis, an illness that can complicate systemic infections with the measles virus (14) or respiratory viruses, and the Guillain-Barré syndrome (GBS) (15), a disorder that has been linked to infection with several different viruses. These illnesses, particularly disseminated encephalomyelitis, resemble experimental allergic encephalomyelitis, a disease mediated in part by lymphocytes sensitized to neural tissues (16).

Pathology

Local inflammatory responses to viral infection consist principally of mononuclear leukocytes, lymphocytes, and macrophages. Polymorphonuclear leukocytes may also appear, particularly during the acute stages of infection. In meningitis, cellular infiltration occurs in the meninges or the cortex superficially via the Virchow-Robin spaces, whereas deep-brain parenchyma is involved in encephalitis

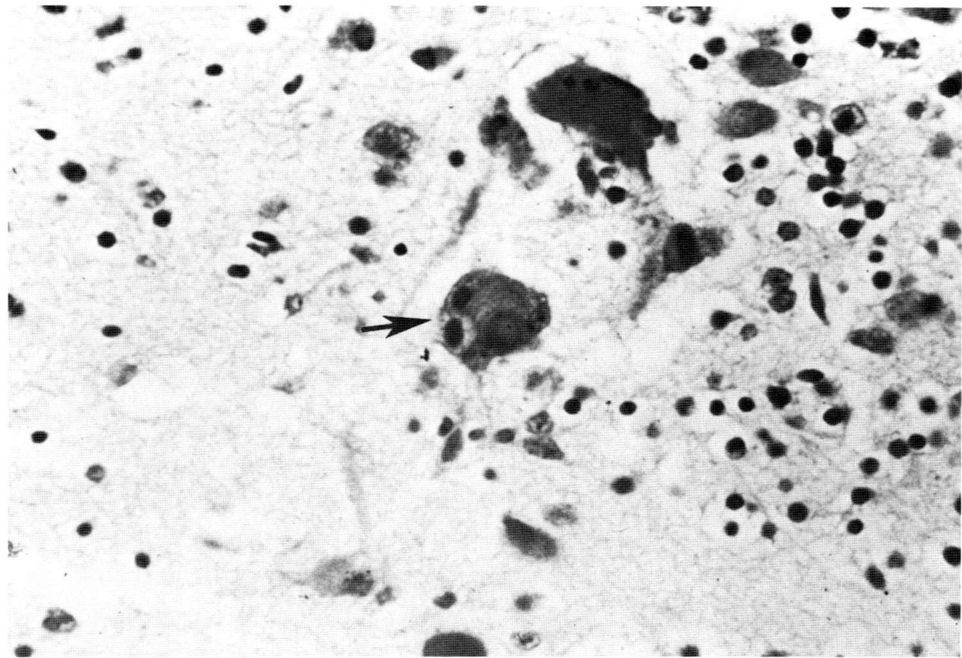

FIGURE 10.1 Brain tissue from an infant with symptomatic congenital cytomegalovirus infection. An enlarged neuron (arrow) contains nuclear and cytoplasmic inclusions.

(1,2). In myelitis and GBS, the pathologic changes are usually restricted to the spinal cord and peripheral nerve, respectively.

If the child dies during the acute stages of viral encephalitis, the brain may be normal or display nonspecific changes like cerebral edema (2). More often, however, lymphocytes invade the leptomeninges, and the brain exhibits mononuclear infiltration, necrosis, microglial proliferation, and infarction (1,2). Perivascular cuffing, vessels surrounded by mononuclear cells, and microglial nodules, foci of inflammation and necrosis, are typical features. These changes may be diffuse, as in the equine encephalitides, or localized, as in HSV encephalitis.

The characteristic pathologic features of encephalomyelitis, presumed to be immunologically mediated, consist of multifocal perivascular demyelination and perivascular cuffing (1,2,13). Necrosis and microglial proliferation are generally absent. In myelitis the cord can be edematous and inflamed or normal; whereas, the typical pathologic findings in GBS are mononuclear inflammation, demyelination, and if severe, secondary axonal degeneration (15).

In congenital viral infections the pathologic abnormalities range from mild meningoencephalitis to severe necrotizing encephalitis (1,2). Microcephaly and polymicrogyria may be features of rubella or cytomegalovirus (CMV) infections. Calcifications can involve the periventricular areas in CMV infection or the basal ganglia in human immunodeficiency virus (HIV) infection. Several viruses, including CMV, HSV, the varicella-zoster virus (VZV), and Venezuelan equine encephalitis virus, can induce severe cerebral necrosis, causing diffuse cystic encephalomalacia.

Several viruses produce inclusion bodies in neural tissues (1,2). Inclusion bodies represent accumulations of virus nucleic acid or proteins in the nucleus or cytoplasm (or both) of infected cells and provide important histopathologic clues regarding viral etiology (Figure 10.1). Inclusions are commonly found in herpesvirus infections, rabies, progressive multifocal leukoencephalopathy, and subacute sclerosing panencephalitis, a degenerative disorder associated with measles virus infection.

DIAGNOSIS

Clinical

The clinical features of virus-induced neurologic disorders reflect several factors. Important elements include the immune responses of the virus-infected host and the tropism and virulence of the specific viral pathogen (3). Although considerable etiologic overlap exists, certain viruses tend to induce specific clinical syndromes. The nonpolio enteroviruses and lymphocytic choriomeningitis virus, for example, usually cause aseptic meningitis but rarely produce encephalitis. Other viruses, notably the herpesviruses, can be associated with several different clinical syndromes, including encephalitis, aseptic meningitis, transverse myelitis, and GBS (Table 10.1).

Patients with acute aseptic meningitis usually have fever, headache, vomiting, meningeal signs, and cerebrospinal fluid (CSF) pleocytosis (2). Seizures, papilledema, or focal neurologic signs are absent. Although the severity of the acute illness varies considerably, most patients with aseptic meningitis have a brief, self-limited disorder.

Table 10.1   Potential viral pathogens in neurologic disorders

	Meningitis	Neurologic Syndrome Encephalitis	Myelitis
V I R U S	Coxsackievirus Echovirus Mumps virus Herpes simplex viruses Epstein-Barr virus Varicella-zoster virus Lymphocytic choriomeningitis virus Adenovirus Poliovirus St. Louis encephalitis virus California encephalitis virus (LaCrosse) Human immunodeficiency virus	Herpes simplex viruses Equine encephalitis viruses St. Louis encephalitis virus California encephalitis virus (LaCrosse) Varicella-zoster virus Epstein-Barr virus Rabies virus Powassan virus Colorado tick fever virus Polioviruses Enterovirus 71 Echoviruses Cytomegalovirus Human immunodeficiency virus Japanese encephalitis virus Other arboviruses	Echovirus Rubella virus Influenza viruses Mumps virus Epstein-Barr virus Herpes simplex viruses Varicella-zoster virus Coxsackie viruses Polioviruses Echoviruses Other enteroviruses Human lymphotrophic viruses
	Guillain-Barré Syndrome	Cerebellar Ataxia	Congenital Infection
V I R U S	Coxsackieviruses Echoviruses Other enteroviruses Rubella virus Influenza virus Cytomegalovirus Adenoviruses Mumps virus Epstein-Barr virus Rabies virus	Varicella-zoster virus Epstein-Barr virus Rubella virus Influenza viruses Coxsackieviruses Echoviruses Measles virus Mumps virus Polioviruses	Cytomegalovirus Rubella virus Herpes simplex viruses Varicella-zoster virus Human immunodeficiency virus Lymphocytic choriomeningitis virus Poliovirus Hepatitis B virus

By contrast, viral encephalitis can be a severe, life-threatening illness. Children with encephalitis have headaches, altered alertness, seizures, and/or focal deficits in association with signs of aseptic meningitis (1,2). Altered consciousness, a prominent feature of encephalitis, reflects infection or inflammation of brain parenchyma or increased intracranial pressure (or both). Severe cases can be associated with spastic or flaccid coma, cranial nerve paralysis, hypothalamic dysfunction, and death.

Viral-induced myelitis begins relatively abruptly, with lower extremity weakness, sensory loss, and bladder and bowel dysfunction (2). Children first experience pain in the chest, back, or abdomen, and motor and sensory loss ensues shortly thereafter. In the majority of children with acute myelitis, a sensory level can be identified between the T5 and T10 dermatomes. The CSF often shows a lymphocytic pleocytosis and increased protein concentration. Approximately 2/3 of children with myelitis recover completely.

Children with GBS usually have an ascending paralysis that begins in the legs. Sensory complaints or objective sensory loss can occur, but are less frequent than in myelitis. Approximately 30% of children with GBS have facial nerve paresis, and autonomic nervous system dysfunction can also occur. The CSF shows an increased protein content, maximum 3 to 6 weeks after onset, and few cells. Children can be affected by variants of GBS. The most common of these, the Miller-Fisher variant, is characterized by ataxia, areflexia, and ophthalmoplegia. Most children with GBS or variants recover completely.

Meningitis and encephalitis usually occur in association with other signs of acute viral infection, such as fever or involvement of systemic organs. By contrast, signs of systemic infection may be absent in patients with transverse myelitis or GBS. These disorders and several other post-infectious disorders, such as disseminated encephalomyelitis and Bell palsy, usually occur temporally remote from the inciting viral infection.

Patients with suspected viral-induced neurologic disorders require neurodiagnostic tests, such as CSF examination, electroencephalography (EEG), electromyography, or a neuroimaging study. Studies are selected on the basis of the patient's clinical syndrome. CSF examination may be sufficient to establish the diagnosis of aseptic meningitis; whereas, a CSF examination and electromyography are essential in patients with GBS. By contrast, patients with suspected viral encephalitis require an extensive evaluation that includes CSF studies, EEG, and computed tomography (CT) or magnetic resonance imaging (MRI) of the head, particularly when HSV encephalitis is suspected. Patients with suspected myelopathy require spinal MRI or contrast myelography with or without CT to exclude a surgically remediable lesion.

Laboratory

Isolation of a viral pathogen from neural tissues or body fluids remains the most specific method by which to identify the etiologic agent (17). Certain viral pathogens require sophisticated isolation procedures or do not grow well in tissue culture, however. For these viruses, serologic methods assume greater importance. Other useful adjunctive tests include electron microscopy, immunocytochemistry, and nucleic-acid hybridization (1,18).

The tissues and fluids chosen for virus isolation depend considerably on the suspected pathogen (Table 10.2), (1,17). Enteroviruses can be readily cultured from feces or cerebrospinal fluid; whereas, diagnosis of HSV or JC polyomavirus infections usually require culture or microscopic examination of brain tissue. Several viruses can be recovered from whole blood or circulating leukocytes. When the etiologic agent is uncertain, specimens submitted for virus isolation should include: throat washing or saliva, feces or rectal swab, whole blood, urine, and CSF (1). Despite appropriate studies, however, an etiologic agent cannot be identified in 25% to 50% of children with serious CNS disorders of presumed viral etiology (3).

Several methods can be used to detect viral antibodies in serum. These methods vary in their sensitivity, specificity, and complexity. In disorders suspected to be virus induced, two serum samples should be collected, an acute serum obtained early in the illness, and a convalescent serum collected 4 to 6 weeks later.

Serologic tests typically detect antibodies of two classes, IgM and IgG. Detection of virus-specific IgM, seroconversion (negative serology followed by virus-positive serology), or a fourfold or greater rise in IgG antibody titer strongly support recent infection with a specific viral pathogen. False-negative results can occur, particularly in infants or immunocompromised patients. False-positive results can result from cross-reacting antibodies or nonspecific reactivation of a latent virus.

The etiologic agent can also be established by detecting viral antigens in autopsy or biopsy tissues. Immunofluorescence, for example, is the diagnostic method of choice for rabies encephalitis. These immunocytochemical methods, although generally less sensitive than virus isolation, allow rapid and specific identification of the viral pathogens.

Molecular techniques, such as the polymerase chain reaction (PCR) or nucleic-acid hybridization, represent the most technologically advanced methods for identification of viral pathogens (19,20). Hybridization methods use radioactive or non-isotopically labeled virus DNA or RNA as probes for virus-specific genomic material. PCR employs small DNA fragments to amplify minute quantities of virus genes. These techniques can be applied to tissues, body fluids, or nucleic acid harvested from cells or tissues.

The CSF in children with viral meningitis or encephalitis usually shows a lymphocytic pleocytosis, modest protein elevation, and a normal glucose content. Early in the course of the illness, polymorphonuclear leukocytes frequently predominate. Some viral infections, such as HSV or mumps virus meningoencephalitis, are associated with mild hypoglycorrhacchia (1,2). The CSF in patients with myelitis may be similar to that of viral meningitis or be normal. By contrast, the CSF in GBS charateristically shows moderate-to-high protein concentration and few leukocytes.

Other nonmicrobiologic tests occasionally provide important clues regarding the etiologic agent. For example, patients with Epstein-Barr virus or CMV infections commonly have atypical lymphocytes in the peripheral circulation or elevated levels of the serum transaminases. Infants with congenital viral infections often exhibit thrombocytopenia, elevated serum bilirubin concentrations, and elevated serum transaminases.

Table 10.2 Specimens for virus diagnosis

Agent	Specimen
Adenoviruses	respiratory secretions, urine, feces
Arboviruses[1]	blood, brain tissue
Enteroviruses	feces, CSF, oral secretions
Influenza virus	oral secretions
Herpesviruses	
CMV	urine, saliva, blood leukocytes
EBV[1]	oral secretions
HSV 1 or 2	mucocutaneous lesions, CSF[2], brain tissue
VZV	cutaneous lesions, CSF, brain tissue
Measles virus	oral secretions
Mumps virus	urine
Retroviruses[1]	blood, CSF
Rubella virus	CSF, urine, oral secretions
JC polyomavirus	brain tissue
CJD	brain tissue

[1] diagnosis usually established serologically.
[2] rarely positive in postnatal encephalitis; occasionally in aseptic meningitis.

TREATMENT

Relatively few virus-induced neurologic disorders can be treated with specific antiviral chemotherapy. In most virus-induced illnesses, treatment consists of supportive care and management of secondary complications (2,21). Specific treatment strategies depend on the type and severity of the individual patient's neurologic illness.

Children with aseptic meningitis or mild encephalitis typically have a self-limited illness. Such patients can be treated with bed rest, nonaspirin analgesia, oral fluids as tolerated, and close observation. Potential complications include seizures, which can be treated with phenobarbital, phenytoin, or benzodiazepines, and increased intracranial pressure (ICP), which may respond to fluid restriction or osmotic diuretics.

Children with moderate or severe encephalitis require hospitalization in an environment that can provide careful monitoring of neurologic and cardiorespiratory functions.

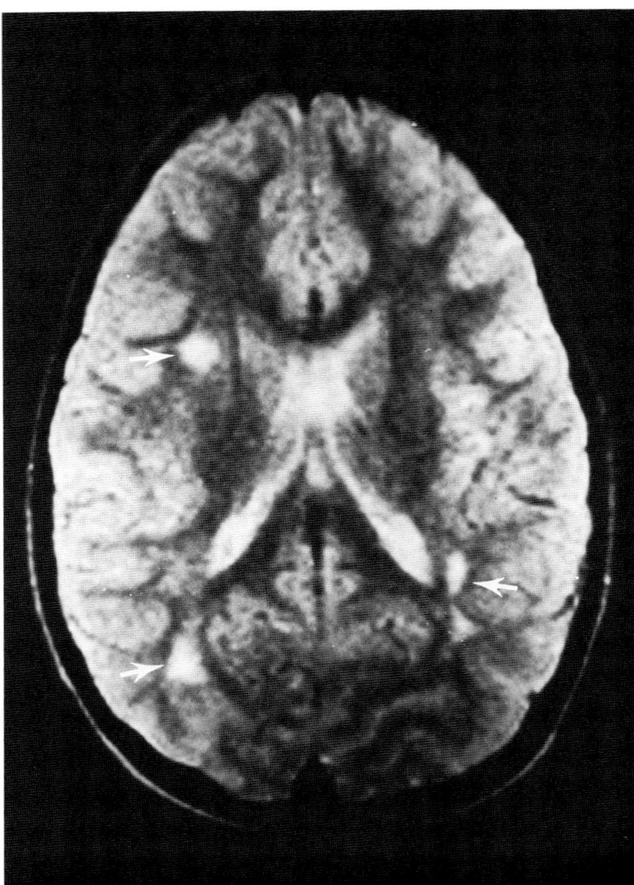

FIGURE 10.2   An MRI study of a 5-year-old child with disseminated encephalomyelitis. The scan shows multiple lesions in the white matter (arrows).

The child's level of alertness, vital signs, and fluid and electrolyte status should be assessed frequently. Seizures, a common complication of encephalitis, result from many causes, including toxic encephalopathy, hypoxemia, cerebral vasculitis, and hyponatremia (2). Because seizures will increase the metabolic demands of the CNS, they should be treated aggressively with intravenous anticonvulsants.

Many patients with severe encephalitis will have elevated ICP. High levels of ICP, as indicated by rapid deterioration, unresponsiveness, flexor or extensor posturing, and pupillary abnormalities, require emergent therapy. This can include: fluid restriction to approximately 2/3 maintenance; administration of osmotic diuretics, such as mannitol; and hyperventilation to maintain the partial pressure of carbon dioxide at approximately 25 to 30 mm Hg. In the comatose patient, an ICP monitor may be needed.

Children with proved or suspected HSV encephalitis require therapy with acyclovir, a purine analogue that inhibits HSV replication (22). Because HSV is rarely isolated from CSF, blood, or other body fluids of patients other than neonates, brain biopsy remains the definitive procedure to confirm HSV infection. The decision to pursue brain biopsy, an issue of considerable debate, should be based on several factors, including the probability of HSV disease, the skill and experience of the neurosurgeon, and the clinical status of the patient (23–25).

Some children with postinfectious encephalomyelitis may respond to corticosteroid therapy (26). This disorder, associated with multifocal neurologic signs, abnormal CSF, and white-matter lesions observed on MRI studies (27), can be difficult to distinguish clinically from acute encephalitis (Figure 10.2). In some instances, the response to corticosteroids will be dramatically evident within 48 to 72 hours.

In children with transverse myelitis or GBS, therapy is directed toward maintaining respiratory function and preventing complications of prolonged bed rest. Patients with GBS can deteriorate rapidly and require ventilatory support. In such patients, pulmonary function should be monitored frequently. Although the therapeutic roles for plasma exchange or intravenous immunoglobulin in GBS are still being investigated, these strategies should be considered in children with rapid deterioration, particularly if intubation and mechanical ventilation are anticipated (28).

SPECIFIC VIRAL PATHOGENS

Arthropod-Borne Viruses

The term, arbovirus or *ar*thopod *bo*rne-virus, has been used to categorize numerous RNA viruses transmitted to humans by mosquitoes, ticks, or biting flies. Current virologic taxonomy divides these agents into several families, including Togaviridae (alphaviruses), Flaviviridae, Bunyaviridae, and Reoviridae. In the United States, eastern equine encephalitis virus (an alphavirus), western equine encephalitis virus (an alphavirus), St. Louis encephalitis virus (a flavivirus), and the California group encephalitis viruses (bunyaviruses) account for several hundred cases of encephalitis annually (Table 10.3). These viruses typically cause encephalitis in the summer months when vectors are most abundant.

Table 10.3   Arboviruses in the United States: 1965–1985[1]

Years	SLE	WEE	EEE	California[2]	Other[3]	Total
1956–1960	933	258	61	—	0	1,262
1961–1965	842	336	14	102	0	1,294
1966–1970	400	107	22	339	3	872
1971–1975	1,964	158	18	369	29	2,538
1976–1980	694	48	17	409	2	1,170
1981–1985	123	38	31	442	0	634
Total	4,956	945	163	1,661	34	7,770

[1] Adapted from Centers for Disease Control. Arboviral infections of the Central Nervous System. MMWR 1986;4:25–32. Includes all ages.
[2] Not reported prior to 1963.
[3] Includes Venezuelan Equine Virus and Powassan Virus Encephalitis.

Western Equine Encephalitis Virus

The western equine encephalitis (WEE) virus causes sporadic disease in horses and occasional illness in humans. Between 1956 and 1985 in the United States, 945 human cases of WEE were reported to the Centers for Disease Control (29). The majority of WEE cases occurs in the western or in the great plains states, an epidemiologic feature that reflects the distribution of the principal vector, the *Culex tarsalis* mosquito.

WEE virus is maintained through a natural cycle of infection between the Culex mosquitoes and wild birds. Small mammals can be infected and serve to amplify WEE virus, whereas horses and humans are dead-end hosts (30). Infected humans infrequently develop clinical symptoms, and in children, the ratio of inapparent to apparent infections may be as high as 50:1. Most cases of WEE encephalitis in the United States are reported between May and October (29).

After an incubation period of 5 to 15 days, WEE begins with headache, malaise, low-grade fever, vomiting, and neck stiffness (31,32). Irritability, lethargy, hallucinations, and convulsions develop as the illness progresses. Patients exhibit diffuse neurologic signs with increased tone, hyperactive deep tendon reflexes, and extensor plantar responses. WEE virus can also infect the fetus via transplacental passage (33). Such infants, presumably infected near term during maternal viremia, have neurologic illnesses (lethargy, dehydration, bulging fontanel) within the 1st week of life.

The CSF shows a lymphocytic pleocytosis, mild protein elevation, and normal or slightly depressed glucose content (31). The EEG usually reveals diffuse slowing, but can have focal features. Although WEE virus can occasionally be detected in body fluids or tissues, the diagnosis of WEE is usually established by serologic methods and not by virus isolation (34). Antibodies to the WEE virus can be detected by complement fixation or hemagglutination inhibition assays. The diagnosis can be made rapidly using antibody capture enzyme immunoassay, which detects IgM antibodies in serum or CSF (35).

Most patients with WEE recover without sequelae. In large epidemics, like a 1941 outbreak in Manitoba affecting more than 500 patients, mortality has averaged less than 15% (36). Nonetheless, infants or young children are often affected adversely by WEE. Earnest and co-workers observed neurologic sequelae, consisting of seizures, paralysis, and intellectual retardation, in approximately 60% of children who had WEE before the age of 2 years (37).

Eastern Equine Encephalitis

The eastern equine encephalitis (EEE) virus, a rare cause of encephalitis among children in the United States, accounted for only 163 cases of encephalitis reported to the Centers for Disease Control between 1956 and 1985 (See Table 10.3) (29). The EEE virus is maintained throughout the eastern United States in an enzootic cycle that involves birds and *Culiseta melanura* mosquitoes. *Cosquillettidia* and *Aedes* mosquito species transmit EEE virus to horses and humans.

Outbreaks of EEE occur in the eastern and southeastern United States in areas near swamps, lakes, and ponds, and have been preceded by above-normal rainfall (38). EEE usually appears in horses before human disease occurs (39). The number of inapparent cases of human EEE virus infection, as with other arboviruses, far exceeds the number of symptomatic cases.

EEE typically begins abruptly, wtih high fever (38.5° to 41° C), lethargy, vomiting, and convulsions (40). Patients may also have focal neurologic signs and nonpitting edema of the face or hands (1,2). Many patients, particularly young children, progress rapidly to coma within 24 to 48 hours, and death often occurs. Occasional patients have a milder illness with malaise, headache, stiff neck, and somnolence.

The CSF findings consist of an elevated protein content, normal glucose content, and pleocytosis, often with polymorphonuclear predominance (41). The diagnosis of EEE can be confirmed by virus isolation or by detection of serologic responses to the virus. Assays employing IgM antibody capture can be used to rapidly identify patients with EEE (35).

EEE has typically been associated with high mortality and morbidity rates. In the 1938 Massachusetts outbreak that affected at least 34 humans, 65% died and nearly all survivors had neurologic sequelae (41). Children accounted for approximately 70% of cases (40). In subsequent sporadic cases, outcome has been variable (42), but for cases seen in the United States since 1955, mortality averages 50%. Because no effective antiviral therapy currently exists for EEE, treatment consists of supportive care. Seizures and increased intracranial pressure, common complications of EEE, should be managed aggressively with anticonvulsants, fluid restriction, and osmotic diuretic therapy.

St. Louis Encephalitis Virus

St. Louis encephalitis (SLE) virus, the most common cause of arboviral encephalitis in the United States, has accounted for more than 5,000 cases of encephalitis since 1956 (See Table 10.3) (29). In 1975 alone, more than 2,000 cases were reported to the Centers for Disease Control (43). This epidemic affected the eastern 2/3 of the United States, with cases reported in 29 states, from Arizona to New York. Eight states—Illinois, Ohio, Indiana, Mississippi, Michigan, Tennessee, Kentucky, and Alabama—each reported more than 50 cases in 1975.

Unlike other arboviruses, SLE virus often affects humans in urban or suburban environments (44). The SLE virus, maintained in the wild by a cycle that involves birds and mosquitoes, is transmitted to humans by several mosquito species, including *Culex tarsalis, Culex pipiens, Culex quinquefasciatus*, and *Culex nigripalpus* (44). Horses or other mammals do not participate in transmission or serve as hosts for SLE virus.

The number of inapparent SLE virus infections far exceeds the number of symptomatic cases. In an SLE outbreak in Mesa County, Colorado, for example, 4% of Grand Junction, Colorado, residents had serologic evidence of infection; whereas, the attack rate was only 33.5/100,000 population, or approximately 0.03% (29).

In symptomatic cases, SLE begins abruptly with headache, vomiting, and fever (43–45). Neurologic symptoms, which can appear within several hours, consist of somnolence, meningeal irritation, or seizures. Fever remains high for approximately 3 days. In most patients, the disease lasts 1 to 2 weeks, although there is considerable variability in the duration and severity of symptoms. Some patients have only nonspecific complaints of nausea, vomiting, or headache, and signs of aseptic meningitis. Others have a fulminant, fatal illness. In the 1975 epidemic, 62% of symptomatic individuals had encephalitis, and 15% had meningitis (43).

Laboratory studies in SLE reveal nonspecific increases in the peripheral white-blood-cell count and alterations in the CSF profile (46). These consist of a lymphocytic pleocytosis and mild elevation in the protein content, usually in the range of 50 to 100 mg/dL. Virologic diagnosis can be established by detecting serologic responses to the SLE virus using complement fixation or hemagglutination inhibition methods. The diagnosis of SLE can be made rapidly using antibody capture immunoassays, a technique that can detect SLE virus-specific IgM in sera within 3 days in 70% of patients (47).

In SLE epidemics since 1933, the mortality rate has ranged from 8% to 20% (43,44). Most survivors recover completely, although approximately 10% have sequelae consisting of seizures, speech or motor disturbances, or intellectual deficits (48). In contrast to EEE or WEE, in which morbidity and mortality are increased in children, adults tend to be more severely affected by SLE. As with other arboviral encephalitides, therapy consists principally of supportive care and management of complications.

California Encephalitis Viruses

Since 1963, the California group of encephalitis viruses, members of the bunyavirus family, have caused approximately 1,700 reported cases of encephalitis in the United States (29). The vast majority of these are attributable to the LaCrosse strain, a virus endemic to the upper midwest (49). This virus was first isolated from the brain tissue of a four-year-old girl who had fatal meningoencephalitis in LaCrosse, Wisconsin, in 1960 (50). In endemic areas, the incidence rates for LaCrosse virus encephalitis approach those of *Haemophilus influenzae* meningitis, which range from 35 to 40/100,000 children under 5 years of age (51).

The LaCrosse virus is transmitted to humans by the *Aedes triseriatus* mosquito, a species that inhabits tree holes in the midwest. The virus spreads venereally between mosquitoes and is maintained in the wild by transovarial transmission and overwintering of the LaCrosse virus in mosquito eggs (52). Chipmunks, squirrels, and rabbits serve as natural hosts for the *A. triseriatus* mosquito. Seroepidemiologic studies indicate that 11% to 18% of residents in endemic areas possess antibody to the LaCrosse virus, an observation that indicates that infections are frequently inapparent (53).

The typical case of California encephalitis occurs during the summer in a child younger than the age of 15 years (54–56). Boys comprise approximately 2/3 of the cases. Affected children often live adjacent to forested areas or enter the forest for recreational purposes. Initial symptoms include fever, vomiting, abdominal pain, or headache. Neurologic abnormalities, which consist of lethargy, seizures, or focal signs, appear within 48 to 72 hours. More than 50% of children with California encephalitis have seizures, and focal findings are present in approximately 25% (54,55). Some patients only have signs of aseptic meningitis. In typical cases, neurologic symptoms last 3 to 7 days.

The laboratory findings in California encephalitis include a peripheral leukocytosis and CSF alterations. The latter consist of a lymphocytic pleocytosis, ranging from 10 to 1000 cells/mm^3, and modest elevations in the protein content, rarely exceeding 100 mg/dL (54,55). The EEG often shows diffuse slowing, although focal abnormalities can be seen. Virologic diagnosis is established through serologic studies, using complement fixation, hemagglutination-inhibition, or immunofluorescence antibody assays. Although the virus can be grown in tissue culture or suckling mice, it is rarely isolated from infected children. Rapid diagnosis can be make by detecting virus-specific IgM in serum or CSF (57).

The great majority of children with California encephalitis survive without neurologic sequelae. Some children have irritability and headache, which can last several months. Long-term neurologic sequelae, such as seizures, behavioral changes, or intellectual deficits, occur in fewer than 20% of survivors (54–56,58).

Other Arboviruses

Several additional encephalitic illnesses of children are attributable to arthropod-borne viruses. In North America these include Colorado tick fever, caused by a tick-borne orbivirus; Powassan encephalitis, caused by a tick-borne flavivirus; and Venezuelan equine encephalitis, caused by a mosquito-borne alphavirus. As a group, these disorders account for rare, sporadic cases of childhood encephalitis (29). By contrast, Japanese encephalitis virus, a mosquito-borne flavivirus, causes numerous cases of encephalitis in endemic areas of Asia (1,59).

Colorado tick fever, transmitted to humans by the wood tick *Dermacentor andersoni,* causes encephalitis, meningitis, and hemorrhagic diathesis (60). Most cases occur in the Rocky Mountain states during the months of March through June. The severe form of the disorder is characterized by high fever, severe headache, stiff neck, somnolence, myalgias, and petechial rash involving the trunk, extremities, and face. Patients typically exhibit a peripheral leukopenia and may have CSF pleocytosis. In most instances, patients recover without sequelae (60).

Powassan virus, first isolated from humans in 1956, occasionally causes encephalitis in Ontario and the northeastern United States (61). Like Colorado tick fever, the virus is transmitted to humans by *D. andersoni* ticks. Woodland animals, such as squirrels, woodchucks, and foxes, presumably serve as natural hosts for the virus. Powassan virus encephalitis begins with prodromal symptoms of sore throat, somnolence, headache, and vomiting. Fever and convulsions occur abruptly, and some children exhibit focal neurologic deficits (61). Outcome has been variable, ranging from death to complete recovery.

Venezuelan equine encephalitis (VEE) virus, an important cause of encephalitis in Central and South America, has occasionally infected humans in the United States (62). Several mosquito species, including the *Culex* and *Aedes* genera, can transmit VEE virus to humans. Clinical symptoms vary from a mild influenza-like illness to severe, fulminant encephalitis. Fever, headache, malaise, and myalgia commonly occur. Most patients with VEE survive without neurologic sequelae. By contrast, fetal infection with VEE virus has produced severe fatal encephaloclastic lesions ranging from cystic encephalomalacia to hydranencephaly (63).

Japanese encephalitis (JE) virus infects humans in a large geographic region that extends from southeast Asia to Siberia (1,59), and children account for the majority of cases. JE can begin with an influenza-like prodrome that may evolve to a more severe illness with headache, meningeal signs and altered consciousness. Children may have a fulminant, fatal disorder with vomiting, coma, and convulsions (64). Mortality ranges from 10% to 40% (65), and approximately 30% of survivors have neurologic sequelae.

Picornaviruses

The Picornaviridae, a family of small RNA viruses, currently comprise two genera, the enteroviruses and the rhinoviruses (66). The rhinoviruses primarily produce upper-respiratory-tract illnesses; whereas, the enteroviruses, consisting of the polioviruses, coxsackieviruses, and echoviruses, cause respiratory or gastrointestinal disorders and can affect the nervous system. The most notable neurologic complication, epidemic poliomyelitis caused by the polioviruses, has been eradicated by vaccination programs in the United States and many other regions of the world (66–69).

The enteroviruses, ingested orally, undergo primary replication in the tonsils and cervical and mesenteric lymph nodes. This induces a transient viremia that leads to infection of several organs, including the CNS. Most infections do not progress, such that the number of inapparent enterovirus infections greatly exceeds that of symptomatic cases.

Polioviruses

The three poliovirus serotypes, 1, 2, and 3, occur worldwide and are transmitted among humans by direct contact with infected feces or oropharnygeal secretions. The viruses spread rapidly in families with young children, a common source of infection. In temperate climates poliovirus infections are usually observed in April through October (68).

Prior to widespread vaccination programs, humans in regions with high population density or poor sanitation were typically infected with the polioviruses by the age of 5 years. By contrast, humans in regions with high socioeconomic standards were not infected until late childhood, adolescence or even, adulthood. Consequently, the incidence of paralytic disease during the U.S. epidemics of the 1950s was highest among children 5 to 10 years of age (70).

With the advent of the inactivated virus vaccine (Salk vaccine) in the mid-1950s, the epidemiology of paralytic poliovirus infections changed dramatically (66–69). Prior to 1950, 10,000 to 20,000 cases of paralytic polio occurred annually in the United States. Within 5 years of the widespread use of the Salk vaccine, the incidence of polio declined to fewer than 1,000 cases per year. The live attenuated poliovirus vaccine (Sabin vaccine), licensed in 1961, brought further declines in the incidence of paralytic polio.

Currently, fewer than 25 cases of polio are reported annually in the United States. The majority of these represent vaccine-related cases or restricted outbreaks among unimmunized individuals (67,69). In other regions of the world, however, paralytic polio remains an important neurologic disorder (71). For example, more than 20,000 cases of poliomyelitis were reported in 1981 among ten countries in Southeast Asia.

The incubation period for poliovirus ranges from 1 to 3 weeks. Symptomatic infections begin with nonspecific complaints of sore throat, fever, and abdominal pain, which reflect viremia. In abortive infections, these symptoms resolve within 5 days, and patients recover completely (70).

The neurologic complications of poliovirus infections consist of aseptic meningitis (nonparalytic polio), poliomyelitis, bulbar polio, and encephalitis. The most frequent serious complication, poliomyelitis, typically begins after systemic symptoms have resolved, and is heralded by headache, vomiting, meningeal signs, renewed fever, and muscle pain (70). Flaccid paralysis, usually asymmetric, appears within 1 to 2 days and can be variable in distribution and severity (2). The neurologic findings, most severe in the legs, evolve to those of a lower motor neuron lesion, with fasciculations, loss of deep tendon reflexes, and eventually, muscle atrophy. Quadriplegia can also occur (72). Most paralytic disease results from infection with poliovirus type 1.

Bulbar polio represents infection of the motor cranial nerves of the medulla, typically the 9th through 11th nerves (73). Affected patients cannot swallow and develop hoarseness or airway obstruction. Neurons of the reticular formation can also be involved, leading to cardiorespiratory disturbances. Less commonly, the 5th through 7th or 12th cranial nerves can be affected. Patients with encephalitis, an uncommon complication, may exhibit seizures and coma. Other unusual neurologic manifestations of poliovirus infection include transverse myelitis (74) and cerebellar ataxia (75).

Because no effective antiviral therapy is available for poliovirus infections, treatment consists of supportive care. Morbidity and mortality depend on the site of greatest pathology. Mortality has been highest in patients with bulbar polio or polioencephalitis (76). Paralytic disease can develop in children with underlying immunodeficiency disorders who receive live oral polio vaccines (77,78), emphasizing that live vaccines should be avoided in such patients.

Coxsackieviruses

Coxsackieviruses, like other enteroviruses, are distributed worldwide and spread among humans by contact with virus-infected feces (79). These viruses, divided into groups A and B, commonly produce human illness during the summer or early fall in temperate climates. The 23 antigenic types of coxsackievirus A infrequently cause serious human disease. By contrast, coxsackievirus B, comprising six antigenic types, can produce life-threatening illnesses through involvement of the heart, CNS, or other organs (80).

The human diseases associated with coxsackievirus infections vary greatly, ranging from minor, transient febrile illnesses to severe disseminated infections involving multiple organs. Common clinical syndromes include pharyngitis, herpangina, pleurodynia, gastroenteritis, sepsis-like illness in the neonate, and the hand, foot, and mouth syndrome. The latter, a disorder characterized by ulcerative lesions of the mouth and vesicular rash of the palms and soles, is typically associated with coxsackieviruses A16, A5, and A10 (81).

Several neurologic conditions have been associated with infections with various coxsackievirus serotypes, including A2, A4, A7, A9, A10, and B1–B6 (82–86). Some disorders, like aseptic meningitis or polio-like syndromes, result from direct viral invasion of neural tissues; whereas, others, such as GBS or acute cerebellar ataxia, are presumably due to immunopathologic mechanisms. Acute childhood hemi-

plegia has been attributed to an infectious vasculitis, associated with coxsackievirus A9 infection (84).

Aseptic meningitis is the most common neurologic complication of coxsackievirus infections (1,2,87). Typical features include fever, headache, photophobia, nausea, vomiting, and stiff neck. Pharyngitis, abdominal pain, myalgias, or rash may also be present. Rarely, patients may have signs of inappropriate antidiuretic hormone secretion (88).

Other neurologic syndromes attributed to coxsackievirus infections include meningoencephalitis, acute cerebellar ataxia (89), acute hemiplegia (84), transverse myelitis, opsoclonus-myoclonus (85), and polio-like disease (86). The polio-like syndrome caused by coxsackieviruses mimics the clinical picture of classic paralytic poliomyelitis. Children have headache, fever, meningeal signs, and asymmetrical, flaccid paralysis, but permanent disability occurs less commonly than with the polioviruses (2).

Children with coxsackievirus aseptic meningitis usually recover without sequelae (82). By contrast, meningoencephalitis, a relatively rare complication, can be life threatening in neonates or in patients with immunodeficiency disorders (90). The outcome for other coxsackievirus-induced neurologic disorders is highly variable. Sells and colleagues observed definite neurologic sequelae in three of 19 (16%) children surviving childhood enteroviral infections of the CNS (91). By contrast, Bergman and coworkers observed no long-term neurologic sequelae among survivors of infantile enteroviral menengitis (92).

Echoviruses

The echoviruses, or *e*nteric *c*ytopathic *h*uman *o*rphan viruses, comprise 31 antigenic types and are distributed worldwide (83). Echoviruses infect humans via the fecal-oral route or less commonly, by respiratory spread. As with other enteroviruses, echovirus epidemics in temperate climates are most frequent in late summer or fall.

Most echovirus-induced illnesses are relatively mild. Clinical symptoms associated with such infections can include cough, sore throat, vomiting, diarrhea, abdominal pain, and rash (93). These symptoms usually last less than 1 week and resolve without sequelae. In neonates, however, echovirus infections can produce disseminated, sepsis-like infection with fever, meningitis, encephalitis, gastroenteritis, and hepatitis (94). Most infants recover without long-term sequelae.

The neurologic syndromes attributed to echovirus infections in childhood parallel those associated with the coxsackieviruses and include acute cerebellar ataxia (95), GBS (96), myelitis (97), and meningitis. Aseptic meningitis, the most common neurologic complication, is usually caused by echoviruses 4, 6, 9, and 30 (98–100). Typical clinical features include fever, headache, vomiting, photophobia, signs of meningeal irritation, and other systemic signs of echovirus infections, like pharyngitis or gastrointestinal complaints. Approximately 10% of patients with echovirus meningitis have rash, either maculopapular or petechial (100). The majority of patients recover uneventfully (92,101).

Patients with underlying immunodeficiency disorders, particularly those with agammaglobulinemia, can develop a persistent, fatal meningoencephalitis due to echovirus infection (102–104). Such patients usually have a dermatomyositis-like illness, and encephalopathy, sensorineural hearing loss, cranial neuropathies or hydrocephalus can occur. Several different echovirus types, including 5, 9, 19, 24, 30, 33, have been isolated from patients with this disorder (102–104). Therapy with intravenous or intraventricular gammaglobulin containing high titers of anti-echovirus antibodies has occasionally been effective (104).

Other Enteroviruses

Recent enteroviral isolates are categorized according to a numerical system beginning with enterovirus 68. At least two of these, enterovirus 70 (EV70) and enterovirus 71 (EV71), have been associated with severe CNS illnesses (105,106). Patients with EV70 infections can develop a polio-like illness in association with acute hemorrhagic conjunctivitis. To date, most affected patients have been adults.

First identified in 1974, EV71 produces a varied spectrum of illness ranging from hand, foot, and mouth disease to neurologic disorders, consisting of meningitis, encephalitis, and polio-like paralysis (107). EV71 has been isolated from patients in several regions of the world, including North America. In a 1975 outbreak in Bulgaria, 21% of patients developed paralytic disease. Fatal encephalitis has been reported sporadically.

Laboratory Diagnosis

The CSF findings in CNS enterovirus infections consist of a lymphocytic pleocytosis and modest elevations in the protein concentration (98). During the early phase of the illness, the CSF may contain numerous neutrophils, but this typically shifts to a lymphocyte predominance. CSF white-blood-cell counts range from less than 10/mm^3 to more than 1,000/mm^3. The protein concentration is normal in almost 50% of patients and rarely exceeds 150 mg/dL. In approximately 20% of patients, the glucose concentration of the CSF is less than 50% of the serum glucose (98).

Enterovirus infection can be confirmed by recovering virus or by detecting serologic responses to the virus. These viruses can be isolated from blood, CSF, oropharyngeal secretions, or feces. In sporadic cases of fatal encephalitis, enteroviruses have also been isolated from brain tissues. Because asymptomatic children frequently shed enteroviruses, isolation of these viruses from feces may only establish a presumptive etiologic role. Infected patients will shed enteroviruses in feces for several weeks.

Rubella Virus

Rubella virus, now classified as a nonarthropod-borne togavirus, was first isolated from humans in 1962 (108). Prior to the development of a vaccine, epidemics commonly occurred in winter and spring in 7 to 9 year cycles. In the last major U.S. pandemic, approximately 13,000,000 persons were infected with the rubella virus.

Rubella virus spreads among humans by the respiratory route. In nonimmunized regions, rubella usually affects children between the ages of 5 to 10 years. In immunized populations, rubella tends to occur at an older age, and occasional outbreaks in the United States have been reported on college campuses and among the military. Despite vaccination programs, as many as 20% of the young adult population in the United States remain susceptible to rubella (109,110).

The incubation period averages 14 to 21 days. Infected individuals develop low-grade fever, malaise, cough, and conjunctivitis, although these features are highly variable. Children typically have suboccipital or posterior auricular lymphadenopathy (111). Within 5 days, an erythematous, maculopapular rash begins on the face and spreads to the trunk and extremities; it can be pruritic in older patients. Rash is absent in 25% to 50% of infected individuals, however. In the majority of patients, rubella subsides within 5 days.

Systemic complications of rubella virus infection include joint involvement and thrombocytopenia (112,113). Arthralgia and arthritis, infrequent in prepubertal children, usually involve the fingers, knees, and wrists and can last up to 1 month. Thrombocytopenia begins after the exanthem, and although thrombocytopenia may persist for several days or weeks, it usually resolves without additional complications.

Rubella virus can affect the nervous system in acquired or congenital infections. Encephalitis, a rare event, occurs in approximately 1 of every 5,000 cases of rubella. Prior to the availability of a vaccine, nearly 1% of the infants born to women who were pregnant during a rubella epidemic had congenital rubella syndrome. With the advent of the rubella vaccine, the incidence of encephalitis and rubella embryopathy declined dramatically (114).

Encephalitis during acquired rubella infections can precede the rash, but usually occurs within the 1st week after onset of the exanthem (112,115,116). Affected children experience headache, vomiting, and altered consciousness; seizures and coma then ensue. Occasional children have ataxia or signs compatible with transverse myelitis (117). The CSF usually shows a lymphocytic pleocytosis, usually less than 100 cells/mm^3, and normal or increased protein concentration.

Other neurologic syndromes linked to acquired rubella virus infections include optic neuritis and GBS (117,118). Although most children with CNS complications recover completely, deaths have been described. Because rubella virus has rarely been recovered from neural tissues, it is not known whether these disorders represent direct virus invasion or immunopathologically mediated events.

Rubella embryopathy, first described by Gregg in 1941 (119), results from fetal infection during maternal viremia. During the last major rubella epidemic in the United States, approximately 30,000 infants were affected by congenital rubella virus infection. The risk to the fetus is greatest during the 1st trimester, when there is a 30% to 50% chance that maternal infection will damage the fetus. After the 4th month, the risk of rubella embryopathy declines to 10% or less (120).

The most frequent signs of rubella embryopathy are cataracts, deafness, and patent ductus arteriosus (120). However, rubella virus can damage numerous organs, causing microphthalmia, chorioretinitis, hepatosplenomegaly, thrombocytopenia, jaundice, rash, osteopathy, several congenital heart lesions, and intrauterine growth retardation (121). Approximately 25% of infected infants have neurologic signs at birth, consisting of lethargy, hypotonia, a full fontanel, and microcephaly. The CSF contains a lymphocytic pleocytosis and an elevated protein concentration.

The survivors of congenital rubella virus infection have a high incidence of long-term neurologic complications, including seizures, mental retardation, visual loss, and sensorineural hearing loss (122–124). The incidence of microcephaly and mental retardation ranges from 25% to 40%; whereas, sensorineural deafness may be found in as many as 75% of surviving children.

Progressive rubella panencephalitis, a disorder that resembles subacute sclerosing panencephalitis (SSPE), was first reported in 1975, and very few patients have been described (125–127). Nearly all cases have occurred in children who had rubella virus embryopathy. These patients had signs of congenital rubella virus infection as neonates, but remained stable until late childhood or adolescence when they deteriorated. Seizures, myoclonus, ataxia, and corticospinal tract signs then developed insidiously over a period of several years. The outcome is often fatal.

The diagnosis of rubella virus infections can be suspected on the basis of the clinical features of acquired or congenital diseases. In acquired illnesses, rubella virus can be isolated from nasal or throat secretions for as long as 2 weeks after the onset of the rash. In congenital infections, rubella virus can be isolated from many different sites, including the nasopharynx, throat, urine, and CSF. Congenitally infected infants can shed rubella virus in urine for a year or more. Rubella virus infections can also be diagnosed by detecting rubella-specific IgM antibody or fourfold or greater changes in IgG antibodies to rubella.

Myxoviruses

The RNA-containing myxovirus group includes the orthomyxoviruses; influenza A, B, and C viruses; and the paramyxoviruses, a heterogeneous family that includes the parainfluenza, mumps, measles, canine distemper, and respiratory syncytial viruses. Of these viruses, influenza, mumps, and measles can induce neurologic disorders in children.

Influenza Viruses

Types A and B influenza viruses cause the vast majority of human influenzal infections (128). Theses viruses occur worldwide, usually in periodic epidemics every 2 to 4 years for type A viruses and 3 to 6 years for type B viruses. In temperate climates, localized outbreaks of influenza occur annually during the winter months. Among children, the attack rate and ratio of symptomatic to silent infections are often high (129). Type A influenza viruses undergo frequent antigenic changes (130,131), a feature that accounts for the epidemic nature of influenzal disease.

Influenza viruses spread among humans via the respiratory route. Symptomatic infections begin abruptly after an incubation period of approximately 48 hours. Patients develop headache, chills, fever, anorexia, fatique, and myalgias of the back and limbs; conjunctivitis or photophobia (or both) may also accur. Fever, typically 38.4° C or higher, usually peaks within 24 hours and can last up to 5 days. As systemic symptoms resolve, respiratory symptoms, consisting of tachypnea, cough, and coryza, predominate (129). The total duration of illness averages approximately 9 days.

Neurologic disorders attributed to influenzal infections include encephalitis (132,133), febrile seizures (134), transverse myelitis, GBS (135), and Reye syndrome (136). Encephalitis, an exceedingly rare event, usually accompanies respiratory symptoms. Clinical features include headache, vomiting, seizures, and somnolence or coma. The CSF is usually normal. In studies of influenza-virus-infected children who required hospitalization, febrile convulsions occurred in as many as 40% (134).

The diagnosis of influenza can be confirmed by isolating virus from respiratory secretions or detecting serologic responses. Because asymptomatic shedding of influenza viruses is uncommon, isolation of influenza virus establishes its etiologic role. Influenza viruses have rarely been isolated from neural tissues, and perivenous demyelination, a feature of postinfectious encephalomyelitis, has been observed in fatal cases. This suggests that influenzal encephalitis is the result of immunologically mediated processes rather than direct viral invasion.

Because influenza epidemics can be associated with considerable morbidity and mortality, annual vaccination has been recommended for patients in several high-risk categories (137). These include children with congenital heart disease, chronic pulmonary conditions like bronchopulmonary dysplasia or cystic fibrosis, chronic renal disease, or patients with immunocompromising conditions. Amantadine hydrochloride can be effective either prophylactically or therapeutically against influenza A infections (138). In children between the ages of 1 and 9 years, the recommended daily dose ranges from 4 to 8 mg/kg.

Measles Virus

Despite the development of an effective vaccine, measles remains an important worldwide public health concern (139). As recently as the 1970s, it was estimated that measles accounted for as many as 1% of all deaths worldwide (140). Vaccination programs in the United States and many other nations have dramatically reduced the number of measles cases. In the pre-vaccine era in the United states, 300,000 to 800,000 cases of measles were reported annually to the Centers for Disease Control. By the 1980s, this number had fallen to fewer than 10,000 cases annually (141).

Measles virus, a highly contagious agent, spreads by contact with droplets from the respiratory tract of individuals who are in the catarrhal prodromal period. After an incubation period of 8 to 12 days, infected persons experience fever (38° to 40° C), malaise, cough, coryza, and conjunctivitis. Within 1 to 2 days, Koplik spots (whitish dots on the buccal mucosa adjacent to the lower molars) appear.

After another 1 to 2 days, an erythematous, maculopapular rash begins on the face and spreads to involve the trunk and extremities. The exanthem lasts approximately 5 days, making the total duration of the usual illness 7 to 10 days. Severe, often fatal measles virus infections with giant-cell pneumonia can develop in immunocompromised patients (142,143).

Of the neurologic complications of measles, acute encephalomyelitis is the most frequent, occuring in approximately 1 of every 1,000 cases of measles (14,144–147). Neurologic symptoms usually begin 2 to 5 days after the onset of the rash and consist of irritability, seizures, and altered consciousness. Cerebellar pathways and spinal cord can also be affected, leading to ataxia, extremity paralysis, and disturbances of bladder and bowel function. Many patients improve within 3 to 4 days. In others, however, the illness progresses, causing increased ICP, focal neurologic signs, and death.

The diagnosis of measles encephalomyelitis can be made clinically in most cases. The CSF findings consist of a modest lymphocytic pleocytosis and an increased protein content (144). The virus can be isolated from respiratory secretions, but is rarely detected in the CSF or neural tissues. Current evidence indicates that measles encephalomyelitis results from immunologically mediated events rather than from direct virus invasion of the CNS. Measles virus antibody is not synthesized intrathecally, and antigens cannot be detected in neural tissues (14,148).

The mortality of measles encephalomyelitis ranges from 10% to 15%, and the incidence of neurologic sequelae averages 20% (144,146,147). Sequelae include ataxia, mental retardation, behavioral changes, seizures, and spastic paraparesis (144,147,149).

Measles virus also causes a rare progressive neurodegenerative disorder, SSPE (139,150). SSPE occurs worldwide, usually in children between the ages of 5 and 14 years (151,152). SSPE has been described in infants as young as 1 year and adults as old as 30 years, however. In the United States, the mean annual incidence of SSPE between 1960 and 1976 was 3.5 per 10 million persons younger than 20 years of age (152). The risk of SSPE has been reduced substantially by measles vaccination (153).

Approximately 50% of individuals with SSPE have natural measles before the age of 2 years. The interval between measles infection and the onset of SSPE averages 6 years. Males are affected two to three times more often than females, and in the United States, the incidence of SSPE is higher among children in rural areas (152).

The clinical features of SSPE conform to relatively distinct stages (154). The disorder begins insiduously with changes in behavior and intellectual decline, which are often attributed to psychiatric causes. Incoordination and myoclonus, consisting of sudden flexion of the extremities, trunk, or head, then ensue. Tonic-clonic seizures may also occur.

As SSPE progresses, myoclonus becomes more frequent, and affected patients show further decline in speech, coordination, and mentation. Extrapyramidal movements may be present. Finally, the patient becomes debilitated with severe dementia, quadriparesis, and autonomic instability (1).

Approximately 50% of patients with SSPE have visual-system abnormalities consisting of chorioretinitis, optic atrophy, or cortical blindness (155). In occasional patients, SSPE begins abruptly with seizures, focal deficits, or increased intracranial pressure. In such patients, death can occur within 2 months (156,157).

The CSF in SSPE has a normal protein content and contains no cells. The CSF immunoglobulin level is usually elevated, reflecting intrathecal synthesis of measles antibodies, and oligoclonal IgG bands are usually present. The EEG often shows a burst-suppression pattern, a finding that can precede the development of myoclonus or other seizure activity. As the disease progresses, background activity becomes severely depressed. CT or MRI reveal progressive cerebral, cerebellar, or brainstem atrophy (158).

Despite trials with several antiviral agents, there remains no effective therapy for SSPE. Some investigators have suggested that isoprinosine, in doses of 100 mg/k/day, may modify the natural course of SSPE (159,160). In most instances, SSPE causes death within 1 to 3 years, although a small percentage of patients have transient remissions and survive for as long as 10 years (161–163).

Other neurologic disorders attributed to measles virus infection include cerebellar ataxia, peripheral neuropathy, and optic neuritis (144–147). Occasional patients with immunodeficiency disorders have developed a fatal neurodegenerative disorder after wild measles infection (164–166). Such patients have seizures, hypotonia, and coma, and usually die within several weeks.

Mumps Virus

The epidemiology of mumps virus infection, like that of rubella and measles viruses, has been altered dramatically by vaccine (3). In the pre-vaccine era in the United States, mumps occurred annually in late winter or early spring with cyclic epidemics every 2 to 3 years. The incidence rate in the United States declined from 100 to 250 cases per 100,000 population annually before 1967, the year of vaccine licensure, to fewer than two cases per 100,000 in 1985 (167).

Mumps virus is transmitted via contact with droplets of saliva or respiratory secretions. Prior to vaccination programs, infections were most frequent in children between the ages of 5 and 9 years. By adulthood, the majority of urban inhabitants possessed neutralizing antibody to the mumps virus; however, as many as 30% of infections were asymptomatic (168).

After an incubation period of 14 to 25 days, infected persons develop fever (as high as 40° C), anorexia, headache, and malaise. Shortly thereafter, parotitis becomes evident with earache, tenderness, and parotid-gland enlargement that obscures the mandibular angle. The submandibular or sublingual glands may occasionally be involved.

Most patients have a benign illness that resolves within 5 to 10 days. Mumps has several potential systemic complications, however, including oophoritis, epididymitis-orchitis, pancreatitis, hepatitis, arthritis, mastitis, and thyroiditis (169). Of these, epididymitis-orchitis affects approximately 25% of post-pubertal men with mumps (170).

Mumps virus infections frequently have neurologic complications (3,171–174). Aseptic meningitis occurs in as many as 10% of infected individuals (174), and CSF pleocytosis is identified in approximately 50% (175). Encephalitis occurs in fewer than 1%. Because of its high incidence, however, mumps virus infection accounted for as many as 30% of etiologically confirmed cases of viral encephalitis in the United States before 1968.

Typical clinical features of mumps virus aseptic meningitis include headache, fever, vomiting, and meningeal signs (174). Patients with encephalitis exhibit signs of meningitis and evidence of cerebral involvement, such as seizures, coma, and focal neurologic deficits (172). In rare instances, signs compatible with myelitis may be present. Although the majority of patients with either meningitis or encephalitis recover completely, residual deficits, consisting of hemiplegia, optic atrophy, and sensorineural hearing loss, have occasionally been observed (172,176).

The CSF in mumps virus infections usually shows a lymphocytic pleocytosis (usually between 50 and 300/mm³), a normal or slightly elevated protein concentration (typically less than 100 mg/dL), and a normal glucose concentration. Hypoglycorrhachia of less than 40 mg/dL has been observed in as many as 30% of patients. Pleocytosis can persist for several weeks.

Other neurologic complications attributed to mumps virus infection include cerebellar ataxia (177), GBS (178), and poliomyelitis-like disorder (179). Transient or permanent hearing loss can also occur (176). Aqueductal stenosis and obstructive hydrocephalus have been linked to mumps virus infections in humans and experimental animals (180–182).

In typical cases, the clinical features of parotitis establish the probable diagnosis of mumps virus infection. Mumps virus can be isolated from the saliva or urine for up to 2 weeks after infection and from CSF or blood during the 1st week. Infection can also be confirmed by measuring serologic responses to the mumps virus, using complement fixation, hemagglutination-inhibition, or neutralization tests (17).

Rabies Virus

Rabies virus, an RNA-containing virus, is maintained in animal reservoirs throughout much of the world. Notable exceptions are the continent of Australia and certain island land masses, such as New Zealand, the British Isles, and Japan (1). In the United States, vaccination programs have substantially reduced the prevalence of rabies in domestic dogs and cats (183).

Numerous wild animals, including the wolf, coyote, fox, skunk, and racoon, act as reservoirs for the rabies virus (1,184). Certain domesticated animals, such as the horse, sheep, and cow, can also be infected with the rabies virus and pose potential risks for human contacts. Rodents and lagomorphs (rabbits, hares, pikas) can be infected with the rabies virus, but no cases of human rabies have been attributed to contact with these animals. In rare instances, rabies has been acquired by laboratory exposure or through corneal transplantation (185,186).

Among human rabies cases in citizens of the United States or its territories from 1960 to 1979, approximately 50% were caused by contact with rabid cats or dogs (187). The majority of these exposures occurred outside the United States, however. Of cases acquired within the United States, rabies infection was linked to bats, skunks, and foxes. A substantial number of human rabies cases in the United States lack a history of exposure to rabies (188).

The World Health Organization receives reports of several hundred fatal cases of rabies per year, but these figures probably underestimate the incidence of rabies. In the United States, the number of humans rabies cases has declined from approximately 25 per year before 1950 to fewer than five cases annually (187). Nearly half of these human rabies cases occurred in individuals younger than 20 years of age.

The reported incubation period for human rabies varies from as short as 10 days to as long as a year or more (7). Most cases of rabies, however, begin within 20 to 60 days of contact with the rabid animal. In some cases, no history of animal encounter can be obtained. Prodromal symptoms consist of fever, malaise, sore throat, headache, and chest or abdominal pain. Pain or parasthesias (or both) occur at the site of the animal bite in approximately 50% of patients (187,189).

Over the next few days, patients with rabies become agitated, develop sialorrhea, and have difficulty drinking and handling oral secretions (189). Spasms of the pharynx and larnyx induced by swallowing and tactile stimuli lead to hydrophobia. These involuntary spasms can affect the diaphragm and accessory respiratory muscles and may lead to respiratory arrest and death.

As rabies progresses, patients become less responsive, incontinent, and eventually lapse into deep coma. Seizures may occur. Depending on the intensity of supportive care, coma can last several weeks before death ensues.

In a minority of patients with rabies, usually adults, the virus causes an ascending paralysis similar to GBS (190). Rabies may be overlooked in such cases unless a history of animal exposure is elicited. Patients with paralytic rabies complain of pain or parasthesias at the site of exposure and have motor weakness typically involving all extremities. In approximately half of these patients, the disease also affects bulbar musculature. Few patients have agitation or hydrophobia.

Rabies cannot be diagnosed by routine neurodiagnostic studies. The CSF frequently shows a lymphocytic pleocytosis, modest elevation of the protein concentration (ranging from 50 to 200 mg/dL), and a normal glucose concentration (187–189). The CT head scan is normal, whereas the EEG can be normal or show diffuse slowing.

The diagnosis of rabies relies predominantly on the historical and clinical features. The diagnosis can be supported by serologic methods and confirmed by isolation of the rabies virus or identification of rabies antigens in biopsy or autopsy tissues. Rabies antibodies can be detected in human sera by day 15 of clinical illness (187) using rapid fluorescent focus inhibition or immunoadherence hemagglutination tests. Rabies virus isolates can be typed by the CDC using monoclonal antibodies to determine the probable origin of the virus (188).

There remains no specific antiviral therapy for human rabies infections, and patients with rabies require intensive support of respiratory and cardiovascular functions. Despite such therapy, the prognosis is grim. Among the 38 patients reviewed by the Centers for Disease Control in 1984, only two survived (187,191). Both had received rabies virus vaccine prior to the onset of their illness. Because the rabies virus can be present in saliva, urine, and other body fluids, patients with suspected or proven rabies should be maintained in strict isolation.

Prevention of rabies in exposed humans requires adherence to guidelines recommended by the Center for Disease Control (Table 10.4) Regardless of the vaccination status of the animal or the human, exposed persons should receive post-exposure prophylaxis *unless* the animal is proved negative for rabies by either tissue examination or quarantine. Current human diploid cell rabies vaccines are effective and less toxic than previous vaccines (192–194).

Adenoviruses

The adenoviruses, a family of DNA viruses commonly associated with acute respiratory-tract illness and kerato-conjunctivitis (195,196), occasionally produce neurologic disorders. Adenoviruses occur worldwide and show winter-spring predominance in temperate climates (197). Although these viruses typically infect children younger than the age of 5 years, epidemics have been observed in adults, particularly among the military.

The adenoviruses are transmitted via aerosolized droplets, the fecal-oral route, or by direct contamination.

Table 10.4 Rabies postexposure prophylaxis[1]

Animal Species	Condition of the Animal	Treatment of Exposed Persons
Dog, cat	Healthy—can be observed	None, unless rabies develops in the animal
	Rabid, or suspected to be rabid	RIG, HDCV
	Unknown	Consult local public health officials
Skunk, bat, fox, racoon, coyote	Regard as rabid unless proved negative by laboratory test	RIG, HDCV
Livestock, rodents		Consult local public health officials

[1] Adapted from Anderson LJ, Nicholson KG, Tauxe RV, et al. Human Rabies in the United States, 1960 to 1979: Epidemiology, diagnosis and prevention. Ann Intern Med. 1984;100:728–735, and CDC. Human rabies—California, 1987. MMWR 1988; 37:305–308.
RIG = Rabies immune globulin.
HDCV = Human diploid cell rabies vaccine.

Keratoconjunctivitis often results from contact with fomites or environmental objects like swimming pools. Of the more than 35 serotypes, types 1 through 7 produce most childhood adenoviral respiratory-tract illnesses (195).

Encephalitis and aseptic meningitis have occasionally been attributed to adenoviral infections. The first recognized cases were reported in 1956, when five children developed neurologic symptoms during a French epidemic of adenoviral respiratory disease (198). In one of these children, adenovirus type 7 was isolated from brain tissue. Subsequently, other cases have been described, usually in otherwise healthy children younger than 5 years of age (199–202).

Patients have low-grade fever, sore throat, rhinorrhea, cough, and conjunctivitis. Neurologic features consist of stiff neck, somnolence, seizures, or coma, and usually last less than 1 week. The CSF may be normal or show a lymphocytic pleocytosis and mildly elevated protein content. The EEG can be diffusely slow. Many children have perihilar or interstitial infiltrates on chest radiographs. Occasional patients have had elevated serum transaminase levels.

Some children with neurologic symptoms have disseminated encephalomyelitis (26), an immunologically mediated disorder, rather than direct invasion of brain tissue by adenoviruses. Neurologic signs in this disorder are usually multifocal and begin after the child has recovered from the acute respiratory illness. Laboratory findings may include an elevated peripheral white-blood-cell count, an elevated erythrocyte sedimentation rate, and abnormal CSF-cell count and chemistries. MRI in disseminated encephalomyelitis can reveal scattered white-matter lesions that may involve cerebrum, cerebellum, and brainstem (27). Children with this disorder may respond favorably to corticosteroid therapy (26).

The diagnosis of CNS adenoviral infection can be established by isolating adenoviruses from CSF or brain tissue and supported by identifying seroconversion or rises in antibody titers to adenoviral serotypes. To date, types 2, 3, 5, 6, 7, and 32 have been isolated from the CSF or brain tissues of patients with neurologic illness, and type 12 has been implicated by recovery from the oropharynx or feces (199–204).

Because there are currently no specific antiviral agents for adenoviral infections, treatment consists of supportive care. In the majority of patients, adenoviral encephalitis or meningitis is a self-limited illness. Although fatalities have been reported, children who survive adenoviral encephalitis usually recover without long-term neurologic sequelae.

Herpesviruses

The herpesviruses, a family of enveloped DNA viruses, include CMV, the Epstein-Barr virus (EBV), HSV types 1 and 2, VZV, and human herpesvirus type 6. Each of these viruses can establish latent infections of humans and be reactivated to produce clinical illness. CMV and EBV tend to be lymphotrophic in their biologic behavior, whereas HSV and VZV are neurotrophic viruses. With respect to the nervous system, the herpesviruses have been associated with several disorders, including encephalitis, meningitis, myelitis, Bell palsy, GBS, and postinfectious encephalomyelitis.

Cytomegalovirus

CMV infection occurs worldwide (205,206). Between 0.5% and 2.5% of all newborns in the western world excrete CMV at birth, making CMV the most common congenital viral infection (207). Moreover, the majority of adults possess antibody to CMV, evidence of prior infection, by the 5th decade (206). Individuals who live in developing nations or in areas with high population density acquire CMV at an early age. Certain groups, such as pregnant women, homosexual men, and children in day care, have relatively high rates of CMV excretion.

CMV infection is usually acquired by close personal contact (208). In infected persons, the virus can be isolated from urine, saliva, blood, tears, semen or cervical secretions, and breast milk. Because CMV can be present in semen or cervical secretions, CMV remains an important sexually transmitted disease. Blood transfusions from seropositive donors are also a potential source of infection among susceptible persons.

Several studies during the 1980s demonstrated that children in large group day care centers have extremely high rates of CMV excretion (209–211). Such children can transmit CMV to other susceptible children and to their parents or caretakers. CMV excretion rates have been highest among the toddler-aged children, a group who are highly mobile and have poor hygiene.

With respect to the nervous system, several clinical syndromes have been attributed to CMV infection (212). These include meningoencephalitis, aseptic meningitis, infantile spasms, GBS, and several ocular disorders, including chorioretinitis. The neurologic complications of CMV infection are most severe in infants who acquire CMV transplacentally or in patients with altered host defense mechanisms, such as those with AIDS.

Congenital cytomegalic inclusion disease (CID), the most widely recognized complication of CMV infection, occurs in approximately 10% of the infants who acquire CMV in utero (205,208,213). The clinical spectrum of CID ranges from severe disseminated disease to isolated involvement of the CNS. Typical systemic features include jaundice, hepatosplenomegaly, petechiae, microcephaly, chorioretinitis, and pneumonitis.

Infants with symptomatic congenital CMV infections usually have laboratory features consisting of thrombocytopenia, anemia, elevated serum transaminases, and hyperbilirubinemia. CT head scans in such infants reveal a variety of abnormalities, ranging from mild cortical atrophy to severe cystic encephalomalacia (214). Approximately 25% to 50% of infants with CID have periventricular calcifications, a feature that reflects the predilection of CMV to infect cells of the subependymal regions.

The majority of children who survive CID have long-term disabilities consisting of developmental retardation, visual loss, sensorineural hearing loss, and seizures (212). In one longitudinal study, 61% had intellectual or developmental impairment, 35% had seizures, spasticity or hemiparesis, 30% had hearing loss, and 22% had ocular abnormalities (213). Microcephaly, chorioretinitis, and neurologic abnormalities in the 1st year of life strongly correlate with adverse intellectual outcome (215).

Approximately 10% to 15% of infants with asymptomatic congenital CMV infections will later exhibit sensorineural hearing loss. This hearing loss occurs as an isolated finding, unaccompanied by chorioretinitis, microcephaly, or other features of CID, and has been attributed to direct infection of the inner ear. Although there were early reports that silent CMV infections were associated with mild degrees of mental retardation, this association has not been confirmed by subsequent longitudinal studies (216,217).

Although the majority of acquired infections are asymptomatic, CMV causes an infections mononucleosis syndrome, similar in its laboratory and clinical features to EBV-induced mononucleosis. CMV infections acquired in childhood rarely cause neurologic disease. CMV has been implicated, however, in some cases of infantile spasms (218). In adults, CMV has a strong epidemiologic association with GBS (219), but this has not been established for childhood GBS. Children with underlying immunodeficiency disorders, including AIDS, are at risk for severe, acquired CMV infections (220).

The diagnosis of CMV infection can be confirmed by detecting CMV in body fluids (212). Urine, saliva, and buffy coat leukocytes contain the greatest amounts of infectious virus. Although the CSF in children with CMV meningoencephalitis will show a lymphocytic pleocytosis and an elevated protein concentration, CMV is infrequently isolated from the CSF (221). A serologic diagnosis of CMV infection can be made by detecting CMV-specific IgM antibody or a fourfold or greater rise in IgG antibodies to CMV. Molecular techniques can be used to detect CMV antigens or DNA in tissues and body fluids (20,222).

Therapy for most CMV infections currently consists of supportive care. Patients with CMV retinitis, particularly in association with AIDS, will show improvement during therapy with ganciclovir, a purine analogue similar to acyclovir (223). Ganciclovir therapy has shown variable efficacy in other serious, acquired CMV infections, however. The role of ganciclovir in treating infants with congenital CMV infections is currently under investigation.

Epstein-Barr Virus

Infection with EBV, the cause of infectious mononucleosis, occurs worldwide without seasonal variation (224–226). Like CMV, EBV infections tend to be acquired early in life in underdeveloped countries or in tropical regions. In the United States and western Europe, approximately 50% of children possess antibody to EBV by the age of 5 years (224). The incidence of infectious mononucleosis in the United States, approximately 45 cases/1000 individuals (227), is highest among children younger than 5 years of age, adolescents, and young adults.

EBV infections are acquired by exposure to infected humans, presumably through contact with oral or respiratory secretions (223). EBV can be cultured from the oral secretions of approximately 10% of healthy adults and from greater numbers of patients who are immunosuppressed. Less frequently, EBV can be acquired via blood transfusion. The incubation period for infectious mononucleosis averages approximately 40 days. In patients with infectious mononucleosis, EBV can persist in the oropharynx for up to 18 months (228).

Several neurologic syndromes, affecting the central or peripheral nervous system, have been reported in association with EBV infection (224,225,228–231). These include myelitis, aseptic meningitis, encephalitis, GBS, brachial plexopathy, optic neuritis, acute hemiplegia (230,232), and cerebellar ataxia (233–235). In addition, EBV has been linked with acute daily headaches in young adults (236), and in rare instances, to childhood chorea. Several patients with isolated cranial neuropathies (237,238), particularly involving the seventh cranial nerve (Bell palsy), have also been reported. The estimated incidence of neurologic complications during primary EBV infection ranges from less than 1% to nearly 10% (231).

Meningoencephalitis, the most common acute neurologic complication of infectious mononucleosis, often accompanies other symptoms of acute EBV infection, such as myalgias, fever, chills, sore throat, anorexia, and fatigue (225). Lymphadenopathy, splenomegaly, and facial swelling are common physical signs. In some patients, however, the systemic signs of infectious mononucleosis can be minimal.

The clinical features of EBV meningoencephalitis include fever, headache, mild meningeal signs, diplopia, and altered sensorium. Seizures, including status epilepticus, can occur (239,240). Occasional patients experience the "Alice in Wonderland syndrome" or metamorphopsia, an altered perception of size relationships (235). Focal deficits, which mimic HSV encephalitis, have also been observed (241).

Patients with acute EBV infections often have a biphasic pattern of leukopenia and thrombocytopenia followed by an atypical lymphocytosis (226). Serum transaminases are elevated in most patients. CSF findings during EBV meningoencephalitis include lymphocytic pleocytosis and mild elevation of protein content. CT head scans are usually normal, whereas an MRI scan in one patient showed abnormal signals bitemporally (242).

Although EBV can be isolated from oropharyngeal secretions and rarely, CSF (243), the necessary culture techniques are not routinely available in most clinical laboratories. At present, the diagnosis of EBV infection is made serologically. Most laboratories use commercial rapid slide tests to detect heterophil antibody in serum (225), and the majority of children older than 2 years of age will have a positive test during acute infection. In younger patients or in atypical cases, serologies for antibodies to EBV antigens, the viral capsid antigen (VCA), the early antigen (EA), and EBV nuclear antigen (EBNA), should be obtained. Acute EBV infection can be established by detecting heterophil antibody or IgM antibody to VCA (244). By contrast, detecting antibodies to EBNA, a late-appearing antibody, suggest remote EBV infection.

Treatment of EBV infections consist principally of supportive care. Certain antiviral agents, such as acyclovir, inhibit EBV replication in vitro, but their efficacy in human infections has not been established. Corticosteroids can relieve upper-airway obstruction caused by EBV and may be of benefit in patients with EBV-induced disseminated encephalomyelitis. The overall mortality rate for EBV meningoencephalitis is less than 1%, and most patients recover without sequelae.

Herpes Simplex Viruses

HSV has two antigenic types, HSV type 1 (HSV-1) and HSV type 2 (HSV-2), which exhibit approximately 50% homology in their DNA sequences. HSV-1, usually transmitted via oral secretions, generally causes oral mucocutaneous lesions and sporadic cases of encephalitis; whereas, HSV-2, a sexually transmitted virus, typically causes genital lesions and neonatal infection (245). Both viruses establish latent infections in neural ganglia and produce recurrent mucocutaneous disease.

Primary infection with HSV-1, an endemic disorder, occurs commonly in young children between the ages of 6 months and 4 years (246). Among patients with gingivostomatitis studied by Juretic, boys and girls were affected equally, and there was no seasonal variation (247). Approximately 25% of these cases were linked to contact with other children or adults with HSV infections. Children with poor hygiene or in areas with high population density acquire HSV-1 at an early age. In such conditions, almost all adults possess antibody to HSV-1 (246).

By contrast, HSV-2 causes primary genital infection in young adults, with the highest incidence in the 3rd decade (246). Men and women are affected equally. The prevalence of HSV-2 infection varies considerably, as high as 22% in some studies (248). Rates of infection depend on age, socioeconomic factors, race, and sexual activities.

HSV-1 encephalitis, the most common nonepidemic form of encephalitis in humans, typically begins with non-specific complaints of malaise, headache, vomiting, and low-grade fever (241,249–252). After a variable interval, ranging from several hours to a few days, neurologic signs appear. These consist of seizures, altered mental status, memory loss, or focal deficits, such as hemiparesis or aphasia. HSV encephalitis, particularly in its early stages, can mimic a psychiatric disorder. In severe or untreated cases, patients lapse into deep coma, often with signs of uncal herniation. Death may occur within 1 to 2 weeks after onset of the illness.

HSV-1 encephalitis can complicate primary or reactivated HSV-1 infections, and reinfection with new HSV-1 strains also occurs. Because the virus latently infects trigeminal ganglia, it has been postulated that some cases of HSV-1 encephalitis represent retrograde neural transmission of HSV-1 (9,11). Focal signs reflect the predilection of HSV-1 to infect the orbitofrontal and mesiotemporal areas of the cerebral cortex.

Patients with suspected HSV-1 encephalitis require emergent evaluation with EEG, neuroimaging studies, and CSF examination (249). The EEG will often reveal focal hemispheric slowing or periodic lateralizing epileptiform discharges (253). CT head scans may detect unilateral low density lesions of the temporal lobe, but these changes may not be evident in the early stages of the disorder (254). T2-weighted MRI images frequently reveal areas of increased signal in the mesial temporal lobe (255).

In one large series, 80% of patients with biopsy-proved HSV-1 encephalitis had abnormal EEG's, and 60% had abnormal CT scans (249,251). Recent reports indicate that MRI is more sensitive than CT (255). The CSF findings consist of a lymphocytic pleocytosis, increased protein content, and in some cases, erythrocytes and xanthochromia (256).

The diagnosis of HSV-1 encephalitis can be confirmed only by brain biopsy (257,258). The CSF rarely contains HSV-1 (259), and recovery of HSV-1 from other sites, such as the oropharynx, can represent nonspecific reactivation of HSV-1. When obtained, brain tissues should be processed for virus isolation by tissue culture, the most sensitive and specific method for diagnosing HSV encephalitis (257). Histopathologic studies, particularly electron microscopy and immunocytochemistry, are important adjunctive tests. Although patients exhibit antibody responses to HSV-1, detection of antibody in CSF or serum has not been a reliable diagnostic method in the acute stages of HSV-1 encephalitis (256).

Currently, therapy with acyclovir, 30 mg/kg/day given intravenously in three divided doses, should be initiated as soon as the diagnosis of HSV-1 encephalitis is strongly considered (22). In proved or highly-suspected cases, therapy is continued for 10 days. Potential complications of acyclovir therapy include mild nephrotoxicity or rarely, tremors or convulsions. Despite antiviral chemotherapy, some patients have adverse outcomes, including death or severe neurologic sequelae (22). Age (younger than 30 years) and absence of coma are favorable prognostic factors.

Whether brain biopsy should be done or therapy initiated empirically has become a vigorously debated issue as less toxic anti-HSV drugs have been developed (23–25, 260). Many continue to recommend biopsy, because certain CNS disorders, like infections with other agents, can mimic HSV-1 encephalitis. The decision to obtain a biopsy should consider such factors as the local surgical experience, the clinical probability of HSV-1 encephalitis, and the toxicity of currently recommended antiviral agents.

In neonates, HSV can cause severe, necrotizing encephalitis (261–263) (Figure 10.3). Because infection is acquired via the maternal genital tract, the vast majority of cases are caused by HSV-2. Rarely, infants acquire HSV transplacentally and exhibit microcephaly, chorioretinitis, and skin lesions (264,265). Neonatal HSV encephalitis may occur as an isolated finding or be associated with disseminated, sepsis-like infection (261). Initial clinical features include lethargy, low-grade fever, poor feeding, apnea, and in some infants, herpetiform skin lesions. Seizures occur in nearly all infants. As the disease progresses, many infants develop shock and signs of disseminated intravascular coagulopathy.

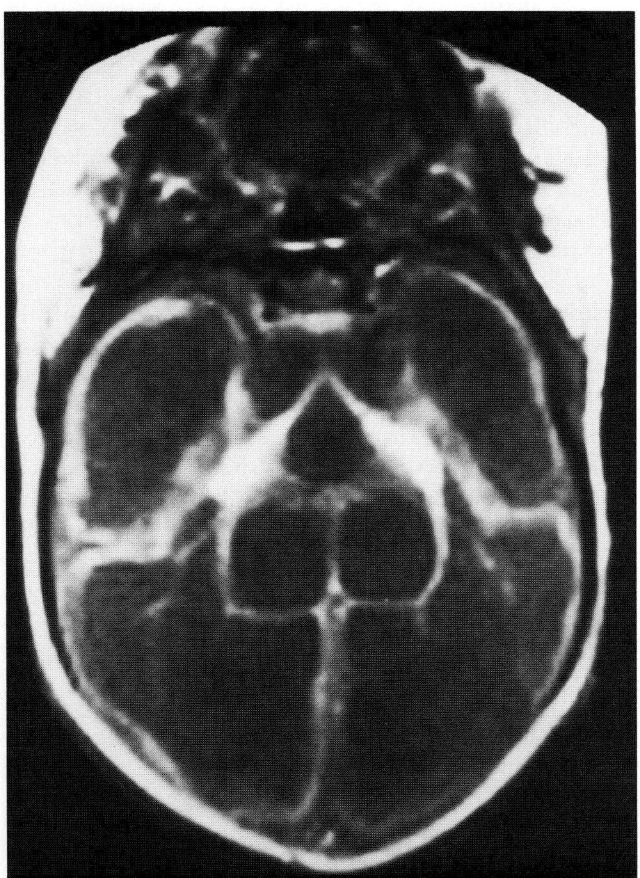

FIGURE 10.3 An MRI study from a neonate with HSV-2 encephalitis. The scan reveals near-complete loss of brain parenchyma and multiple fluid-filled cavities, consistent with multicystic encephalomalacia.

Infants with HSV encephalitis may have CSF abnormalities that consist of a lymphocytic pleocytosis and protein elevation (263). Many infants also have thrombocytopenia, depletion of liver-derived clotting factors, and elevations in the serum transaminases, a feature that reflects a propensity of HSV-2 to involve the liver. The EEG shows focal or diffuse abnormalities (266), whereas the CT scan is usually normal in the acute stages. In contrast to HSV-1 encephalitis, in which virus is rarely isolated from body fluids or tissues other than the brain, HSV-2 can often be recovered from CSF, blood, the oropharynx, or skin lesions (261–263). In some cases, however, brain biopsy has been necessary to confirm the diagnosis of neonatal HSV-2 encephalitis (263).

Therapy of neonatal HSV infections currently consists of acyclovir (30 mg/kg/day) divided in three doses, for 10 days (267). Occasional patients may require more prolonged therapy. Despite antiviral therapy, many infants with CNS HSV-2 disease die or have neurologic disabilities (261–263,268). As is the case with HSV-1 encephalitis occurring in children or adults, early therapy with acyclovir improves outcome.

HSV-1 and HSV-2 have been associated with several additional neurologic disorders. These include myelitis (269), aseptic meningitis (270), and Bell palsy (271). In most instances these diseases represent self-limited disorders and may not require antiviral therapy. Severe, fatal HSV infections can develop, however, in patients with underlying disorders that affect cell-mediated immunity (272,273).

Varicella-Zoster Virus

VZV, the causative agent of chickenpox and shingles, has been associated with several childhood neurologic disorders (3,274–279). These include meningoencephalitis, myelitis, GBS, acute cerebellar ataxia, Bell plasy, and Reye syndrome. Certain disorders, such as meningoencephalitis, presumably result from direct VZV replication in neural tissues; whereas, others such as acute cerebellar ataxia may be immunologically mediated.

Primary VZV infection, chickenpox or varicella, typically affects young children. In the United States, approximately 85% of cases occur in children younger than 10 years of age, with the peak incidence between the ages of 5 and 9 years (277). VZV infections occur frequently in winter and spring and result from contact with the respiratory secretions of an infected human. Persons with chickenpox are contagious for approximately 4 days prior to and 5 days after onset of the typical vesicular rash. The incubation period ranges from 10 to 20 days, although most cases begin 12 to 14 days after exposure.

Rash, the first clinical manifestation of varicella, usually starts on the head or trunk and spreads centrifugally (2). The rash evolves rapidly from erythematous macules to delicate vesicles surrounded by a red areola which appear in crops over a period of 2 to 5 days. Malaise and low-grade fever often accompany the rash. In immunocompetent children, the illness lasts approximately 5 to 7 days, and complications are rare. Newborns or immunosuppressed children are at risk for severe disseminated infections involving the lung, liver, and CNS (278–280).

Acute CNS complications of varicella consist of encephalitis, aseptic meningitis, cerebellar ataxia, and myelitis (274–276,281,282), affecting approximately 0.3% of children with chickenpox. In typical cases of varicella encephalitis, headache, vomiting, and lethargy begin approximately 5 to 7 days after the onset of the rash. Seizures and focal signs, such as aphasia or hemiparesis, occur commonly. Forty percent of the patients described by Johnson and Milbourn had seizures (276). In occasional patients, the clinical features reflect increased intracranial pressure and consist of coma, pupillary abnormalities, spasticity, hyperactive deep tendon reflexes, and extensor plantar responses (281,282).

Approximately half of the children with VZV-induced neurologic disease have acute cerebellar ataxia (276,282). This syndrome, characterized by irritability, vomiting, ataxia, slurred speech, nystagmus, and meningeal signs, also tends to occur within 10 days of onset of the rash. Occasional patients have transverse myelitis or an asymmetric flaccid paralysis that resembles poliomyelitis (276). Stroke has also been reported after childhood varicella infections (283).

Shingles or zoster, the clinical syndrome associated with reactivated VZV infection, occurs most commonly in adults, usually those older than the age of 45 years (277). Children and infants can be affected, however (284). The incidence of zoster in childhood ranges from 20 to 63 cases per 100,000 person-years (284). Zoster usually presents as a vesicular rash involving thoracic dermatomes. Approximately 50% of children with zoster have fever; whereas, lymphadenopathy or pain, a common feature of zoster in adults, is infrequent. In the majority of healthy children, zoster remits within 3 weeks (285). Postherpetic neuralgia, a complication that affects 9% to 14% of all patients with zoster, rarely affects children (286).

Potential neurologic complications of zoster include neuropathies, encephalitis, aseptic meningitis, and myelitis (275,287–290). Neuropathies, motor or sensory, usually involve the dermatome affected by the rash (290). Patients with Ramsay Hunt syndrome, for example, have seventh cranial nerve paralysis in association with facial pain and zoster of the ear canal, external ear, and tympanic membrane (291,292).

Encephalitis, a rare complication of zoster, usually occurs within 2 weeks of the onset of the rash (287–289). This disorder resembles the encephalitis that complicates primary VZV infections. Another rare complication of zoster, herpes zoster ophthalmicus and contralateral hemiparesis, has been attributed to VZV-induced angiitis (293).

VZV can also severely damage the developing nervous system when infection is acquired congenitally (294,295).

Infection early in gestation has been associated with low birth weight, limb hypoplasia, chorioretinitis, cutaneous scars, and cataracts. CNS defects include cortical atrophy and severe hydrocephalus.

The CSF findings in these disorders usually consist of a lymphocytic pleocytosis, mild elevation in protein content, and a normal glucose concentration (276,281). In some patients, such as those with cerebellar ataxia, the CSF may be entirely normal. Approximately 25% of patients with varicella have an abnormal EEG (296), although the specific features of the EEG vary with the clinical syndrome. CT head scans are usually normal. In a 5-year-old child with VZV encephalopathy, MRI revealed abnormal signals in the midbrain and middle cerebellar peduncle (242).

In the vast majority of patients, the diagnosis of VZV infection can be established on clinical grounds. VZV can be isolated from the oropharynx or skin vesicles. In patients with VZV encephalitis, VZV-specific antibodies can be detected in CSF (297).

The pathogenesis of VZV-induced neurologic disorders has not been established with certainty (274). Encephalitis presumably represents direct virus invasion, but VZV has rarely been recovered from CNS tissues. The pathologic findings in this disorder consist of perivascular cuffing, edema, leptomeningeal inflammation, and occasionally, necrosis. In some cases, perivascular demyelination has been observed, a feature of immunologically mediated disorders. Because few, if any, patients with VZV-induced cerebellar ataxia die during their illness, little pathologic data about such patients exist.

The therapy of VZV-induced neurologic disorders must be individualized to the clinical syndrome and the patient's underlying immune state. Patients with immunodeficiency disorders must be treated aggressively and antiviral therapy initiated early (298–300). Acyclovir, 500 mg/m^2 every 8 hours, has been shown to prevent dissemination and reduce the duration of virus persistence in skin vesicles.

The role for acyclovir in the therapy of VZV-induced neurologic disorders has not extensively investigated. The drug should be considered in cases of encephalitis, however, using dose regimens analogous to those used for HSV infections. In the pre-antiviral era, mortality in VZV encephalitis ranged from 5% to 35%, and neurologic sequelae were reported in 10% to 20% of survivors (276,281). The majority of children with neuropathies or cerebellar ataxia recover without disability.

OTHER VIRUSES

Lymphocytic Choriomeningitis Virus

Lymphocytic choriomeningitis (LCM) virus, a member of the arenavirus family, occasionally causes influenza-like illness, meningitis, or meningoencephalitis in humans. The virus naturally infects the common mouse, *Mus musculus,* and other rodents, like hamsters (301), which develop chronic LCM virus infection and excrete the virus in their urine, nasal secretions, and feces. Human infections result from contact with infected rodents or inhalation of dust contaminated with the virus and often occur in winter, when infected mice enter human dwellings. Outbreaks of LCM virus infections have been linked to exposure with pet hamsters (302–304).

After an incubation period of 1 to 3 weeks, humans infected with LCM virus develop fever, headache, malaise, myalgias, and vomiting. Neurologic features, present in approximately 20% of infected individuals, consist of headache, photophobia, meningeal signs, altered mental status, and occasionally, focal deficits (302,303). In most patients, the disorder lasts less than 2 weeks. Occasional patients, however, experience a chronic or relapsing illness lasting several weeks (302).

The CSF usually shows a lymphocytic pleocytosis with counts ranging as high as several thousand, mildly increased protein content, and a normal or slightly decreased glucose concentration (302,303,305). The diagnosis of LCM virus infection can be made by isolating LCM virus from the CSF or detecting serologic responses using complement fixation or immunofluorescence methods.

Treatment consists of supportive care. The majority of patients have a self-limited illness and recover without sequelae. Rarely, patients have communicating hydrocephalus, a complication attributed to the striking CSF inflammatory response or protein elevation (302).

LCM virus can also infect infants prenatally. Between 1974 and 1981 approximately 20 cases were reported worldwide (306). Almost all of these infants had hydrocephalus and chorioretinitis, and most had adverse outcomes with death or spastic quadriparesis. The diagnosis of congenital LCM virus infection was established by isolating LCM virus from CSF or detecting virus-specific antibodies in the infant's serum.

Papovaviruses

The JC polyomavirus, a member of the papovavirus family, causes progressive multifocal leukoencephalopathy (PML), an uncommon neurodegenerative disorder that typically occurs in immunosuppressed patients (307–309). The vast majority of patients are adults, usually between the ages of 30 and 60 years. However, PML has been reported in children as young as 5 years (310,311).

Conditions associated with PML consist primarily of those with abnormal cell-mediated immunity (308). These include AIDS (309), congenital immunodeficiency syndromes, and disorders requiring immunosuppressive therapy, such as leukemia, lymphoma, systemic lupus erythematosus, or renal transplantation.

Although PML rarely occurs, seroepidemiologic studies suggest that the majority of adults in the United States have been infected with the JC virus. Padgett and Walker, surveying more than 400 persons in Wisconsin, detected antibodies to the virus in nearly 60% (312). Seropositivity rates were low in children younger than 4 years of age, but rose progressively in childhood such that 65% of 14-year olds had serologic evidence of prior infection.

Patients with PML insidiously develop mental deterioration, visual loss, sensory deficits, paralysis, speech disturbances, and ataxia (308–310). Seizures, headaches, or fever are unusual. The CSF may occasionally show a mild lymphocytic pleocytosis, but the glucose and protein content are typically normal. The EEG usually demonstrates diffuse or focal slowing, and CT or MRI head scans reveal white-matter lesions and cortical atrophy (313).

The diagnosis of PML can currently be established only by examining brain tissue (308,314). The neuropathologic features, which consist of intranuclear inclusions in oligodendrocytes and multifocal demyelination, are diagnostic. JC virus infection can be confirmed by immunohistochemistry, electron microscopy, or detection of JC virus DNA by in situ hybridization (315).

Although the clinical course varies from patient to patient, most deteriorate relatively rapidly and die within 6 months (308,309,314–317). Antiviral therapy with such agents as cytosine arabinoside or adenine arabinoside has been ineffective (316,317).

Unconventional Agents

Certain rare neurodegenerative disorders of humans and animals, termed *slow virus infections,* have been linked to infection with unconventional viral agents (318–320). Unlike conventional viruses, these agents do not incite an inflammatory response in neural tissues, do not cause CSF pleocytosis or protein elevation, and do not stimulate identifiable immunologic responses.

Creutzfeldt-Jakob disease (CJD), the most important human disorder linked to an unconventional agent, accounts for approximately one in 10,000 deaths in the United States and other countries annually (321–323). Although CJD usually occurs in mid to late adulthood, CJD has been reported in adolescents and young adults (322–327). CJD in young adults can occur spontaneously but has been linked in several instances to iatrogenic exposure to the CJD agent, either by therapy with human growth hormone extracted from human pituitary glands (322,323) or inoculation during electrocorticography (325).

CJD begins insidiously with behavioral change and intellectual deterioration (322,323). Other common features include myoclonus, cerebellar signs, and visual disturbances. The majority of patients with CJD deteriorate rapidly, becoming vegetative within a few months. Occasional patients, comprising approximately 10% of all CJD cases, have a protracted course that can last several years (328). The condition is uniformly fatal.

The CSF in patients with CJD is normal. EEG typically reveals diffuse slowing, often with periodic triphasic waves, whereas neuroimaging studies show progressive cortical atrophy. Brain biopsy, the only confirmatory test, discloses neuronal loss, gliosis, and status spongiosis, a change consisting of vacuolation of axons and neurons.

REFERENCES

1. Johnson RT. Viral Infections of the Nervous System. New York: Raven Press, 1982.
2. Bell WE, McCormick WF. Neurologic Infections in Children; 2nd ed. Philadelphia: W.B. Saunders, 1981.
3. Koskiniemi M, Rautonen J, Lehtokoski-Lehtiniemi E, et al. Epidemiology of encephalitis in children: a 20 year study. Ann Neurol 1991;29:492–497.
4. Johnson RT. Selective vulnerability of neural cells to viral infections. Brain 1980;103:447–472.
5. Roizman B. Multiplication of viruses. In: Fields BN, Knipe DM, Chanock RM, et. al, eds. Virology Chap. 5. New York: Raven Press. 1990;87–94.
6. Johnson RT, Mims CA. Pathogenesis of viral infections of the nervous system. N Engl J Med 1968;278:23–30, 54–92.
7. Murphy FA. Rabies pathogenesis: A brief review. Arch Virol 1977;54:279–297.
8. Baringer JR. Recovery of herpes simplex virus from human sacral ganglions. N Engl J Med 1974;291:828–830.
9. Baringer JR, Swoveland P. Recovery of herpes simplex from human trigeminal ganglions. N Engl J Med 1973;288:648–650.
10. Cook ML, Bastone VB, Stevens JG. Evidence that neurons harbor latent herpes simplex virus. Infect Immun 1974;9:946–951.
11. Davis LE, Johnson RT. An explanation for the localization of herpes simplex encephalitis. Ann Neurol 1979;5:2–5.
12. Ennis FA, ed. Human immunity to viruses. New York: Academic Press, 1983.
13. Johnson KP, Wolinsky JS, Ginsberg AH. Immune mediated syndromes of the nervous system related to virus infections. In: Vinken PJ, Bruyn GW, eds. Handbook of Clinical Neurology; Vol. 34. Amsterdam: Elsevier, 1978;391–434.
14. Gendelman HE, Wolinsky JS, Johnson RT, et al. Measles encephalomyelitis: Lack of evidence of viral invasion of the central nervous system and quantitative study of the nature of demyelination. Ann Neurol 1984;15:353–360.
15. Prineas JW. Pathology of the Guillain-Barré syndrome. Ann Neurol 1980;9 Suppl:6–19.
16. Paterson PY. Neuroimmunologic diseases of animals and humans. Rev Infect Dis 1979;1:468–482.
17. Chernesky MA, Ray RC, Smith TF. Laboratory diagnosis of viral infections. Cumitech 15. Am Soc Microbiol, Washington, D.C., 1982.
18. Grandien M, Olding-Stenkvist E. Rapid diagnosis of viral infections in the central nervous system. Scand J Infect Dis 1984;16:1–8.
19. Haase A, Brahic M, Stowring L, et al. Detection of viral nucleic acids by in situ hybridization. Methods Virol 1984;7:189–226.
20. Spector SA, Rua JA, Spector DH. Detection of human cytomegalovirus in clinical specimens by DNA-DNA hybridization. J Infect Dis 1984;150:121–126.
21. Jeffries DJ. Viruses and intensive care. Intensive Care Med 1983;9:105–107.
22. Whitley RJ, Alford CA, Hirsch MS, et al. Vidarabine versus acyclovir therapy in herpes simplex encephalitis. N Engl J Med 1986;314:144–149.
23. Barza M, Pauker SG. The decision to biopsy, treat, or wait in suspected herpes encephalitis. Ann Intern Med 1980;92:641–649.
24. Hanley DF, Johnson RT, Whitley RJ. Yes, brain biopsy should be a prerequisite for herpes simplex encephalitis treatment. Arch Neurol 1987;44:1289–1290.
25. Fishman RA. No, brain biopsy need not be done in every patient suspected of having herpes simplex encephalitis. Arch Neurol 1987;44:1291–1292.
26. Pasternak JF, Devivo DC, Prensky AL. Steroid-responsive encephalomyelitis in childhood. Neurology 1980;30:481–486.
27. Dunn V, Bale JF, Zimmerman RA, et al. MRI in children with postinfectious disseminated encephalomyelitis. MRI 1986;4:25–32.
28. The Guillain-Barré study group. Plasmapheresis and acute Guillain-Barré syndrome. Neurology 1985;35:1096–1104.
29. Centers for Disease Control. Arboviral infections of the central nervous system. MMWR 1986;35:341–350.
30. Potter ME, Currier RW, Pearson JE, et al. Western equine encephalomyelitis in horses in the northern red river valley, 1975. JAMA 1977;170:1396–1399.
31. Leech RW, Harris JC, Johnson RM. 1975 encephalitis epidemic in North Dakota and Western Minnesota. Minn Med 1981;545–548.
32. Medovy H. Western equine encephalomyelitis in infants. J Pediatr 1943;22:308–318.
33. Shinefield HR, Townsend TE. Transplacental transmission of western equine encephalomyelitis. J Pediatr 1953;43:21–25.
34. Sekla LH, Stackiw W. Laboratory diagnosis of western encephalitis. Can J Public Health 1976;67 Suppl:33–39.
35. Calisher CH, Berardi VP, Muth DJ, et al. Specificity of immunoglobulin M and G antibody responses in humans infected with eastern and western equine encephalitis viruses: Application to rapid serodiagnosis. J Clin Microbiol 1986;23:369–372.
36. Medovy H. The history of western encephalitis in Manitoba. Can J Public Health 1976;67 Suppl:13–14.
37. Earnest MP, Goolishian HA, Calverley JR, et al. Neurologic, intellectual, and psychologic sequelae following western encephalitis. Neurology 1971;21:969–974.
38. Hayes RO, Hess AD. Climatological conditions associated with outbreaks of eastern encephalitis. Am J Trop Med Aug 1964;13:851–959.
39. Levi HL, Lovejoy F, Daniels J. Eastern equine encephalitis in Massachusetts: First human case in 14 years. N Engl J Med 1971;284:540.

40. Farber S, Hill A, Connerly ML, et al. Encephalitis in infants and children caused by the virus of the eastern variety of equine encephalitis. JAMA 1940;114:1725–1731.

41. Ayres JC, Feemster RF. The sequelae of eastern equine encephalomyelitis. N Engl J Med 1949;240:960–962.

42. Przelomski MM, O'Rourke E, Grady GF, et al. Eastern equine encephalitis in Massachusetts: A report of 16 cases, 1970–1984. Neurology 1988;38:736–739.

43. Center for Disease Control. St. Louis encephalitis in the United States, 1975. J Infect Dis 1977;135:1014–1016.

44. Luby JP. St. Louis encephalitis. Epidemiol Rev 1979;1: 55–73.

45. Brinker R, Paulson G, Monath T, et al. St. Louis encephalitis in Ohio, September, 1975. Clinical and EEG studies in 16 cases. Arch Intern Med 1979;139:561–566.

46. Southern PM, Smith JW, Luby JP, et al. Clinical and laboratory features of epidemic St. Louis encephalitis. Ann Intern Med 1969;71:681–689.

47. Monath TP, Nystrom RR, Bailey RE, et al. Immunoglobulin M antibody capture enzyme-linked immunosorbent assay for diagnosis of St. Louis encephalitis. J Clin Microbiol 1984;20:784–790.

48. Cooperative study group. Epidemic St. Louis encephalitis in Houston, 1964. JAMA 1965;193:139–146.

49. Calisher CH. Taxonomy, classification and geographic distribution of California serogroup bunyaviruses. Prog Clin Biol Res 1983;123:1–16.

50. Thompson WH, Kalfayan B, Anslow R. Isolation of California encephalitis group virus from a fatal human illness. Am J Epidemiol 1964;81:245–253.

51. Center for Disease Control. LaCrosse encephalitis in West Virginia. MMWR 1988;37:79–82.

52. Watts DM, Thompson WH, Yuill TM, et al. Overwintering of LaCrosse virus in Aedes triseriatus. Am J Trop Med Hyg 973;23:694–700.

53. Balfour HH, Edelman CK, Bauer H, et al. California arbovirus (LaCrosse) infections. III. Epidemiology of California encephalitis in Minnesota. J Infect Dis 1976;133: 293–301.

54. Balfour HH, Siem RA, Bauer H, et al. California arbovirus (LaCrosse) infections I. Clinical and laboratory findings in 66 children with meningoencephalitis. Pediatrics 1973;52: 680–691.

55. Hilty MD, Haynes RE, Azimi PH, et al. California encephalitis in children. Am J Dis Child 1972;124:530–533.

56. Johnson KP, Lepow ML, Johnson RT. California encephalitis I. Clinical and epidemiological studies. Neurology 1968; 18:250–254.

57. Dykers TI, Brown KL, Gundersen CB, et al. Rapid diagnosis of LaCrosse encephalitis: Detection of specific immunoglobulin M in cerebrospinal fluid. J Clin Microbiol 1985;22: 740–744.

58. Grabow JD, Matthews CG, Chun RW, et al. The electroencephalogram and clinical sequelae of California arbovirus encephalitis. Neurology 1969;19:394–404.

59. World Health Organization. Japanese encephalitis. MMWR 1984;119–125.

60. Spruance S, Bailey A. Colorado tick fever. Arch Intern Med 1973;131:288–293.

61. Smith R, Woodall JP, Whitney MS, et al. Powassan virus infection. Am J Dis Child 1974;127:691–693.

62. Zehmer RB, Dean PB, Sudia WD, et al. Venezuelan equine encephalitis epidemic in Texas, 1971. Health Serv Rep 1974;89:278–282.

63. Wenger F. Venezuelan equine encephalitis. Teratology 1977;16:359–362.

64. Johnson RT, Burke DS, Elwell M, et al. Japanese encephalitis: immunocytochemical studies of viral antigen and inflammatory cells in fatal cases. Ann Neurol 1985;18:567–573.

65. Burke DS, Lorsomrudee W, Leake CJ, et. al. Fatal outcome in Japanese encephalitis. Am J Trop Med Hyg 1985;34: 1203–1210.

66. Melnick J. Portraits of viruses: The picornaviruses. Intervirol 1983;20:61–100.

67. Kim-Farley RJ, Schonberger LB, Nkowane BM, et al. Poliomyelitis in the USA. Lancet 1984;II:1315–1318.

68. Nathanson N. Epidemiologic aspects of poliomyelitis eradication. Rev Infect Dis 1984;6:308–312.

69. Schonberger LB, McGowan JE, Gregg MB. Vaccine-associated poliomyelitis in the United States 1961–1972. Am J Epidemiol 1976;104:202–211.

70. Horstmann DM. Poliovirus (poliomyelitis). In: Feigin R, Cherry JD, eds. Textbook of Pediatric Infectious Diseases. Philadelphia: W.B. Saunders, 1981;1186–1192.

71. Assaad F, Ljungars-Esteves K. World overview of poliomyelitis: Regional patterns and trends. Rev Infect Dis 1984; 6:302–307.

72. Weinstein L, Shellokov A, Seltser R, et al. A comparison of the clinical features of poliomyelitis in adults and in children. N Engl J Med 1952;246:296–302.

73. Baker AB. Bulbar poliomyelitis: Its mechanism and treatment. Am J Med 1949;6:614–619.

74. Plum F. Sensory loss with poliomyelitis. Neurology 1956; 6:166–172.

75. Mendex-Cashion D, Sanchez-Longo LP, Valcore M, et al. Acute cerebellar ataxia in children associated with infection with poliovirus 1. Pediatrics 1962;29:808–815.

76. Smith E, Harris IL, Rosenblatt P. Acute poliomyelitis. J Pediatr 1953;43:9–20.

77. Lopez C, Biggar WD, Park BH, et al. Nonparalytic poliovirus infections in patients with severe combined immunodeficiency disease. J Pediatr 1974;84: 497–502.

78. Wright PF, Hatch MH, Kasselberg AG, et al. Vaccine-associated poliomyelitis in a child with sex-linked agammaglobulinemia. J Pediatr 1977;91:408–412.

79. Cherry JD, Nelson DB. Enterovirus infections: Their epidemiology and pathogenesis with particular reference to coxsackie A16 virus. Clin Pediatr 1966;5:659–664.

80. Kibrick S, Benirschke K. Acute aseptic myocarditis and meningoencephalitis in the newborn child infected with coxsackie virus group B, type 3. N Engl J Med 1956;255: 883–889.

81. Adler JL, Mostow SR, Mellin H, et al. Epidemiologic investigation of hand, foot and mouth disease. Infection caused by coxsackievirus A16 in Baltimore, June through September 1968. Am J Dis Child 1970;120:309–313.

82. Dery P, Marks MJ, Shapera R. Clinical manifestations of coxsackievirus infections in children. Am J Dis Child 1974;128:464–468.

83. Grist NR, Bell EJ, Assaad F. Enteroviruses in human disease. Prog Med Virol 1978;24:114–157.

84. Roden VJ, Cantor HE, O'Connor DM, et al. Acute hemiplegia of childhood associated with coxsackie A9 viral infection. J Pediatr 1975;86:56–58.

85. Kuban KC, Ephros MA, Freeman RL, et al. Syndrome of opsoclonus-myoclonus caused by coxsackie B3 infection. Ann Neurol 1982;13:69–71.

86. Grist NR, Bell EJ. Enteroviral etiology of the paralytic poliomyelitis syndrome. Studies before and after vaccination. Arch Environ Health 1970;21:382–387.

87. Cramblett HG, Moffet HL, Black JP, et al. Coxsackie virus infections. Clinical and Laboratory Studies. J Pediatr 1964; 64:406–414.

88. Chemtob S, Reece ER, Mills EL. Syndrome of inappropriate secretion of antidiuretic hormone in enteroviral meningitis. Am J Dis Child 1985;139:292–294.

89. Berg R, Jelke H. Acute cerebellar ataxia in children associated with coxsackie viruses group B. Acta Pediatr Scand 1965;54:497–502.

90. Cooper JB, Pratt WR, English BK, et al. Coxsackievirus B3 producing fatal meningoencephalitis in a patient with X-linked agammaglobulinemia. Am J Dis Child 1983;137:82.

91. Sells CJ, Carpenter RL, Ray CG. Sequelae of central-nervous system enterovirus infections. N Engl J Med 1975;293:1–4.

92. Bergman I, Painter MJ, Wald ER, et al. Outcome in children with enteroviral meningitis during the first year of life. J Pediatr 1987;110:705–709.

93. Linnemann CC, Steichen J, Sherman WG, et al. Febrile illness in early infancy associated with ECHO virus infection. J Pediatr 1974;84:49–54.

94. Lake AM, Lauer BA, Clark JC, et al. Enterovirus infections in neonates. J Pediatr 1976;89:787–791.

95. McAllister R, Hummeler K, Coriell L. Acute cerebellar ataxia. Report of a case with isolation of type 9 ECHO virus from the cerebrospinal fluid. N Engl J Med 1959;261: 1159–1162.

96. Vrano T, Kawase T, Kodaira K, et al. Guillain-Barré syndrome associated with ECHO virus type 7 infections. Pediatrics 1970;45:294–295.

97. Johnson DA, Eger AW. Myelitis associated with an echovirus. JAMA 1967;301:637–638.

98. Singer JI, Mauer PR, Riley JP, et al. Management of central nervous system infections during an epidemic of enteroviral aseptic meningitis. J Pediatr 1980;96:559–563.

99. Sabin AB, Krumbiegel ER, Wigand R. ECHO type 9 virus disease. Am J Dis Child 1958;96:197–219.

100. Haynes RE, Cramblett HG, Kronfol HJ. Echovirus 9 meningoencephalitis in infants and children. JAMA 1969;208:1657–1660.

101. Wilfert CM, Thompson RJ, Sunder TR, et al. Longitudinal assessment of children with enteroviral meningitis during the first three months of life. Pediatrics, 1981;67:811–815.

102. Bardelas JA, Winkelstein JA, Seto DS, et al. Fatal ECHO 24 infection in a patient with hypogammaglobulinemia: Relationship to dermatomyositis-like syndrome. J Pediatr 1977;90:396–399.

103. Wilfert CM, Buckley RH, Mohanakumar T, et al. Persistent and fatal central nervous system echovirus infections in patients with agammaglobulinemia. N Engl J Med. 1977;296:1485–1489.

104. Bodensteiner JB, Morris HH, Howell JT, et al. Chronic ECHO type 5 virus meningoencephalitis in X-linked hypogammaglobulinemia: Treatment with immune plasma. Neurology 1979;29:815–819.

105. Wadia NH, Katrak SM, Misra VP, et al. Polio-like motor paralysis associated with acute hemorrhagic conjunctivitis in an outbreak in 1981 in Bombay, India: Clinical and serologic studies. J Infect Dis 1983;147:660–667.

106. Center for Disease Control. Case of paralytic illness associated with enterovirus 71 infection. MMWR 1988;37: 104–114.

107. Melnick JL. Enterovirus 71 infections: A varied clinical pattern sometimes mimicking paralytic poliomyelitis. Rev Infect Dis 1984;6 Suppl 2:387–390.

108. Weller TH, Neva FA. Propagation in tissue culture of cytopathic agents against patients with rubella-like illnesses. Proc Soc Exp Biol Med 1962;111:215–225.

109. Krugman S. Present status of measles and rubella immunization in the United States: A medical progress report. J Pediatr 1977;90:1–12.

110. Clarke M, Schild GC, Miller C, et al. Surveys of rubella antibodies in young adults and children. Lancet 1983;1:7–669.

111. Forbes JA. Rubella: Historical aspects. Am J Dis Child 1969;118:5–11.

112. Steen E, Torp KH. Encephalitis and thrombocytopenic purpura after rubella. Arch Dis Child 1956;31:470–473.

113. Simpson REH. Rubella and polyarthritis. Br Med J 1940; 1:830–831.

114. Center for Disease Control. Rubella and congenital rubella, 1984–1986. MMWR. 1987;36:664–675.

115. Sherman FE, Michaels RH, Kenny FM. Acute encephalopathy (encephalitis) complicating rubella. JAMA 1965;192: 675–681.

116. Walker JM, Nahmias AJ. Neurologic sequelae of rubella infection. Clin Pediatr 1966;5:699–702.

117. Connolly JH, Hutchinson WM, Allen IV, et al. Carotid artery thrombosis, encephalitis, myelitis, and optic neuritis associated with rubella virus infections. Brain 1975;95:583–594.

118. Saeed AA, Lange LS. Guillain-Barré syndrome after rubella. Postgrad Med J 1978;54:333–334.

119. Gregg N McA. Congenital cataract following German measles in the mother. Trans Ophthalmol Soc Aust 1941; 3:35–46.

120. Ueda K, Nishida Y, Oshima K, et al. Congenital rubella syndrome: Correlation of gestational age at time of maternal rubella with type of defect. J Pediatr 1979;94:763–766.

121. Dudgeon JA. Congenital rubella. J Pediatr 1975;87: 1078–1086.

122. Desmond MM, Fisher ES, Vorderman AL, et al. The longitudinal course of congenital rubella encephalitis in nonretarded children. J Pediatr 1978;93:584–591.

123. Chess S, Fernandez P, Korn S. Behavioral consequences of congenital rubella. J Pediatr 1978;93:699–703.

124. Menser MA, Forrest JM. Rubella: High incidence of defects in children considered normal at birth. Med J Austral 1974;1:123–126.

125. Townsend JJ, Baringer JR, Wolinsky JS, et al. Progressive rubella panencephalitis: Late onset after congenital rubella. N Engl J Med 1975;292:990–993.

126. Weil ML, Itabashi HH, Cremer NE, et al. Chronic progressive panencephalitis due to rubella virus simulating subacute sclerosing panencephalitis. N Engl J Med 1975;292: 994–998.

127. Wolinsky J, Berg BO, Maitland CJ. Progressive rubella panencephalitis. Arch Neurol 1976;33:722–723.

128. Kilbourne ED. Epidemiology of influenza. In: Kilbourne ED, ed. Influenza Viruses and Influenza. New York: Academic Press, 1975;483.

129. Wright PF, Ross KB, Thompson J, et al. Influenza A infections in young children. N Engl J Med 1977;296:829–834.

130. Webster RG, Laver WG. Studies on the origin of pandemic influenza: I antigenic analysis of A2 influenza viruses isolated before and after the appearance of Hong Kong influenza using antisera to the isolated hemagglutinin subunit. Virology 1972;48:433–444.

131. Kilborne ED. Recombination of influenza A viruses of human and animal origin. Science 1968;160:74–76.

132. Bennett AE, Turk RE. Acute encephalitis and death following Asian influenza. Calif Med 1957;87:411–412.

133. Wells CEC. Neurological complications of so-called "influenza": A winter study in southeast Wales. Br Med J 1971;1:369–373.

134. Price DA, Postlethwaite RJ, Longson M. Influenza virus A2 infections presenting with febrile convulsions and gastrointestinal symptoms in young children. Clin Pediatr 1976;15:361–367.

135. Wells CEC, James WRL, Evans AD. Guillain-Barré syndrome and virus of influenza A (Asian strain). AMA Arch Neurol Psychiatr 1959;81:699–705.

136. Partin JC, Partin JS, Schubert WK, et al. Isolation of influenza virus from liver and muscle biopsy specimens from a surviving case of Reyes syndrome. Lancet 1976;2: 599–602.

137. Center for Disease Control. Implementation of recommendations for influenza control. MMWR 1985;34: 639–642.

138. Bryson YJ. The use of amantadine in children for prophylaxis and treatment of influenza A infections. Pediatr Infect Dis 1982;1:44–46.

139. Morgan EM, Rapp F. Measles virus and its associated diseases. Bacteriol Rev 1977;41:636–666.

140. Cherry JD, Feigin RD, Lobes LA Jr, et al. Urban measles in the vaccine era: A clinical, epidemiologic and serologic study. J Pediatr 1972;81:217–230.

141. Center for Disease Control. Measles—United States, 1986. MMWR 1987;36:301–305.

142. Enders JF, McCarthy K, Mitus A, et al. Isolation of measles virus at autopsy in cases of giant-cell pneumonia without rash. N Engl J Med 1959;261:875–896.

143. Siegel MM, Walter TK, Ablin AR. Measles pneumonia in childhood leukemia. Pediatrics 1977;60:38–40.

144. LaBoccetta AC, Tornay AS. Measles encephalitis: Report of 61 cases. Am J Dis Child 1964;107:247–255.

145. Miller HG, Stanton JB, Gibbons JL. Parainfectious encephalomyelitis and related syndromes. Q J Med 1956; 25:427–505.

146. Tyler HR. Neurologic complications of rubeola (measles). Medicine 1957;36:147–167.

147. Aarli JA. Nervous complications of measles: Clinical manifestations and prognosis. Eur Neurol 1974;12:79–93.

148. Johnson RT, Griffin DE, Hirsch RL, et al. Measles encephalomyelitis: Clinical and immunologic studies. N Engl J Med 1984;310:137–141.

149. Douglas JWB. Ability and adjustment of children who have had measles. Br Med J 1964;2:1301–1303.

150. Payne FE, Baublis JV. Measles virus and subacute slerosing panencephalitis. Perspect Virol 1971;7:179–195.

151. Jabbour JT, Duenas DA, Serv JL, et al. Epidemiology of subacute sclerosing panencephalitis (SSPE). A report of the SSPE Registry. JAMA 1972;220:959–962.

152. Modlin JF, Jabbour JT, Witte JJ, et al. Epidemiologic studies of measles, measles vaccine, and subacute sclerosing panencephalitis. Pediatrics 1977;59:505–512.

153. Zilber N, Rannon L, Alter M, et al. Measles, measles vaccination and risk of subacute sclerosis panencephalitis (SSPE). Neurology 1983;33:1558–1564.

154. Zeman W, Kolar O. Reflections on the etiology and pathogenesis of subacute sclerosing panencephalitis. Neurology 1968;18:1–7.

155. La Piana FG, Tso MO, Jenis EH. The retinal lesions of subacute sclerosing panencephalitis. Ann Ophthalmol 1974;6: 603–610.

156. Silva CA, Paula-Barbosa MM, Pereira S, et al. Two cases of rapidly progressive subacute slerosing panencephalitis. Arch Neurol 1981;38:109–113.

157. Gilden DH, Ronke LB, Tanaka R. Acute SSPE. Arch Neurol 1981;32:644–646.

158. Krawiecki NS, Dyken PR, Gammal TE. Computed tomography of the brain in subacute sclerosing panencephalitis. Ann Neurol 1984;15:489–492.

159. Jones CE, Huttenlocher PR, Dyken PR, et al. Inosiplex therapy in subacute sclerosing panencephalitis. Lancet 1982;1: 1034–1037.

160. DuRant RH, Dyken PR. The effect of inosiplex on the survival of subacute sclerosing panencephalitis. Neurology 1983;33:1053–1055.

161. Cobb WA, Morgan-Hughes JA. Nonfatal subacute sclerosing leukoencephalitis. J Neurol Neurosurg Psychiatr 1968;31:115–123.

162. Lorand B, Nagy T, Tariska S. Subacute progressive panencephalitis. World Neurol 1982;3:376.

163. Haddad FS, Risk WS, Jabbour JT. Subacute sclerosing panencephalitis in the Middle East: Report of 99 cases. Ann Neurol 1977;3:211–217.

164. Murphy JV, Yunis EJ. Encephalopathy following measles infection in children with chronic illness. J Pediatr 1976; 88:937–942.

165. Aicardi J, Govtieres F, Arsenio-Nunes ML, et al. Acute measles encephalitis in children with immunosuppression. Pediatrics 1977;59:232–239.

166. Roos RP, Graves MC, Wollman RL, et al. Immunologic and virologic studies of measles inclusion body encephalitis in an immunosuppressed host: The relationship to subacute sclerosing panencephalitis. Neurology 1981;31:1263–1270.

167. Center for Disease Control. Mumps. United States, 1984–1985. MMWR 1986;35:216–219.

168. Brunell PA, Brickman A, O'Hare D, et al. Ineffectiveness of isolation of patients as a method of preventing the spread of mumps. N Engl J Med 1968;279:1357–1361.

169. Brunell PA. Mumps. In: Feigin RD, Cherry JD, eds. Textbook of Pediatric Infectious Diseases. Philadelphia: W.B. Saunders, 1981;1231–1235.

170. Beard CM, Benson RC, Kelalis PP, et al. The incidence and outcome of mumps orchitis in Rochester, Minnesota, 1935 to 1974. Mayo Clin Proc 1977;52:3–7.

171. McLean DM, Larke RPB, Cobb C, et al. Mumps and enteroviral meningitis in Toronto, 1966. Can Med Assoc J 1967;96:1355–1361.

172. Koskiniemi M, Donner M, Pettay O. Clinical Appearance and outcome in mumps encephalitis in children. Acta Paediatr Scand 1983;72:603–609.

173. Thomas FB, Perkins RL, Saslaw S. Paralytic mumps infection in two sisters. Arch Intern Med 1968;121:45–49.

174. Azimi P, Crablett MG, Haynes RE. Mumps meningoencephalitis in children. JAMA 1969;207:509–512.

175. Bang HO, Bang J. Involvement of the central nervous system in mumps. Acta Med Scand 1943;113:487–505.

176. Vuori M, Lahikainen EA, Peltonen T. Perceptive deafness in connection with mumps. A study of 298 servicemen suffering from mumps. Acta Otolaryngol 1962;55:231–236.

177. Davis LE, Harms AC, Chin TDY. Transient cortical blindness and cerebellar ataxia associated with mumps. Arch Ophthalmol 1971;85:366–368.

178. Ghosh S. Guillain-Barré syndrome complicating mumps. Lancet 1967;1:895.

179. Lennette EH, Caplan GE, Magoffin RL. Mumps virus infection simulating paralytic poliomyelitis. Pediatrics 1960;25:788–797.

180. Bray PF. Mumps: A cause of hydrocephalus? Pediatrics 1972;49:446–449.

181. Johnson RT, Johnson KP, Edmonds CJ. Virus-induced hydrocephalus: Development of aqueductal stenosis in hamsters after mumps infection. Science 1967;157:1066–1067.

182. Herndon RM, Johnson RT, Davis LE, et al. Ependymitis in mumps virus meningitis. Arch Neurol 1974;30:475–479.

183. Turner GS. A review of the world epidemiology of rabies. Trans R Soc Trop Med Hyg 1976;70:175–178.

184. Baer GM, ed. The Natural History of Rabies. New York: Academic Press, 1975.

185. Winkler WG, Fashinell TR, Leffinwell L, et al. Airborne rabies transmission in a laboratory worker. JAMA 1973;226:1219–1221.

186. Baer GM, Shaddock JH, Houff SA, et al. Human rabies transmitted by corneal transplantation. Arch Neurol 1982;39:103–107.

187. Anderson LJ, Nicholson KG, Tauxe RV, et al. Human rabies in the United States 1960 to 1979: Epidemiology, diagnosis and prevention. Ann Intern Med 1984;100:728–735.

188. Center for Disease Control. Human rabies—California, 1987. MMWR 1988;37:305–308.

189. Dupont JR, Earle KM. Human rabies encephalitis. Neurology 1965;15:1023–1034.

190. Chopra JS, Banejee AK, Murthy JMK, et al. Paralytic rabies: A clinicopathological study. Brain 1980;103:789–802.

191. Porras C, Barboza JJ, Fuenzalida E, et al. Recovery from rabies in man. Ann Intern Med 1976;85:44–48.

192. Bernard KW, Roberts MA, Sumner J, et al. Human diploid cell rabies vaccine: Effectiveness of immunization with small intradermal or subcutaneous doses. JAMA 1982;247:1138–1142.

193. Wiktor TJ, Plotkin SA, Koprowski H. Development and clinical trials of the new human rabies vaccine of tissue culture (human diploid cell) origin. Dev Biol Stand 1978;40:3–9.

194. Bernard KW, Smith PW, Kader FJ, et al. Neuroparalytic illness and human diploid cell rabies vaccine. JAMA 1982;248:3136–3168.

195. Spencer MJ, Cherry JD. Adenoviral Infections. In: Feigen RD, Cherry JD, eds. Textbook of Pediatric Infectious Diseases. Philadelphia: W.B. Saunders, 1981;1279–1298.

196. Sohier R, Chardonnet Y, Prunieras M. Adenoviruses: Status of current knowledge. Prog Med Virol 1965;7:253–325.

197. Foy HM, Cooney MK, Maletzky AJ, et al. Incidence and etiology of pneumonia, croup, and bronchiolitis in preschool children belonging to a prepaid medical care group over a four-year period. Am J Epidemiol 1973;97:80–92.

198. Lelong M, Lepine P, Alison F. La pneumoniae virus du groupe A, B, C, chez de hourrison isolement du virus: Les lesions antomohistoliques. Arch Fr Pediatr 1956;13:1092–1094.

199. Kelsey DS. Adenovirus meningoencephalitis. Pediatrics 1978;61:291–293.

200. Kim KS, Gohd RS. Acute encephalopathy in twins due to adenovirus type 7 infection. Arch Neurol 1983;40:58–59.

201. Similia S, Jouppila R, Salmi A, et al. Encephalomeningitis in children associated with adenovirus type 7 epidemic. Acta Pediatr Scand 1970;59:310–316.

202. Faulkner R, Van Rooyen CE. Adenovirus types 3 and 5 isolated from the cerebrospinal fluid of children. Can Med Assoc J 1962;87:1123–1125.

203. Pereira MS, MacCallum FO. Infection with adenovirus type 12. Lancet 1964;1:198–199.

204. Roos R, Chou SM, Basnight M, et al. Isolation of an adenovirus 32 strain from human brain in a case of subacute encephalitis. Proc Soc Exp Biol Med 1972;139:636–640.

205. Ho M. Cytomegalovirus: Biology and Infection. New York: Plenum, 1982.

206. Krech V, Jung M, Jung F. Cytomegalovirus Infections of Man. Basel: Karger, 1971.

207. Weller TM. The cytomegaloviruses: Ubiquitous agents with protean clinical manifestations. N Engl J Med 1971;285:203–214, 267–274.

208. Bale JF, Jr, Jordan MC. Cytomegalovirus. In: Vinken PJ, Bruyn GW, eds. Handbook of Clinical Neurology; Vol. 56. Amsterdam: Elsevier, 1989;263–279.

209. Pass RF, August Am, Divorsky M, et al. Cytomegalovirus infection in a day care center. N Engl J Med 1982;307:477–479.

210. Adler SP. The molecular epidemiology of cytomegalovirus transmission among children attending a day care center. J Infect Dis 1985;152:760–768.

211. Murph JR, Bale JF, Jr., Murray JC, et al. Cytomegalovirus transmission in a midwest day care center: Relationship to child care practices. J Pediatr 1986;109:35–39.

212. Bale JF, Jr. Human cytomegalovirus infection and disorders of the nervous system. Arch Neurol 1984;41:310–320.

213. Pass RF, Stagnos S, Myers GJ, et al. Outcome of cytomegalovirus infection: Results of long-term longitudinal follow-up. Pediatrics 1980;66:758–762.

214. Bale JF, Jr., Bray PF, Bell WE. Neuroradiographic abnormalities in congenital cytomegalovirus infection. Pediatr Neurol 1985;1:42–47.

215. Conboy TJ, Pass RF, Stagnos S, et al. Early clinical manifestations and intellectual outcome in children with symptomatic congenital cytomegalovirus infection. J Pediatr 1987;111:343–348.

216. Conboy TJ, Pass RF, Stagnos S, et al. Intellectual development in school-aged children with asymptomatic congenital cytomegalovirus infection. Pediatrics 1986;77:801–806.

217. Saigal S, Luny KO, Larke RPB, et al. The outcome of children with congential cytomegalovirus infections. Am J Dis Child 1982;132:896–901.

218. Riikonen R. Cytomegalovirus infection and infantile spasms. Dev Med Child Neurol 1978;20:570–579.

219. Dowling PC, Cook SD. Role of infection in Guillain-Barré syndrome: Laboratory confirmation of herpes virus in 41 cases. Ann Neurol 1981;9 Suppl:44–55.

220. Post MJD, Curless RG, Gregorios JB, et al. Reactivation of congenital cytomegalic inclusion disease in an infant with HTLV-III associated immunodeficiency. A CT-pathologic correlation. J Comput Assist Tomogr 1986;10:533–536.

221. Jamison RM, Hathorn AW. Isolation of cytomegalovirus from cerebrospinal fluid of a congenitally infected infant. Am J Dis Child 1978;132:63–64.

222. Bale JF, Jr, O'Neil ME, Hart MN, et al. Human cytomegalovirus nucleic acids in tissues from congenitally infected infants. Pediatr Neurol 1989;5:216–220.

223. Collaborative DHPG Treatment Study Group. Treatment of serious cytomegalovirus infections with 9-(1,3-dihydroxy-2-propoxymethyl) guanine in patients with AIDS and other immunodeficiencies. N Engl J Med 1986;314:801–805.

224. Andiman WA. The Epstein-Barr virus and EB virus infections in childhood. J Pediatr 1979;95:171–182.
225. Grose C. The many faces of infectious mononucleosis: The spectrum of Epstein-Barr virus infection in children. PIR 1985;7:35–44.
226. Sumaya CV, Ench Y. Epstein-Barr virus infectious mononucleosis in children; I. Clinical and general laboratory findings. Pediatrics 1985;75:1003–1010.
227. Heath CW Jr, Brodsky AL, Potolsky A. Infectious mononucleosis in a general population. Am J Epidemiol 1972;95:46–52.
228. Miller G, Niederman JC, Andrews LL. Prolonged oropharyngeal excretion of Epstein-Barr virus after infectious mononucleosis. N Engl J Med 1973;228:229–232.
229. Grose C, Henle W, Henle G. Primary Epstein-Barr virus infections in acute neurologic diseases. N Engl J Med 1975;292:392–395.
230. Leavell R, Ray G, Ferry PC. Unusual acute neurologic presentations with Epstein-Barr virus infection. Arch Neurol 1986;43:186–188.
231. Silverstein A, Steinberg G, Nathanson N. Nervous system involvement in infectious mononucleosis. Arch Neurol 1972;26:353–358.
232. Baker FJ, Kotchmer GS Jr, Fushee WS, et al. Acute hemiplegia of childhood associated with Epstein-Barr virus infection. Pediatr Infect Dis 1983;2:136–138.
233. Bergen D, Grossman H. Acute cerebellar ataxia of childhood associated with infectious mononucleosis. J Pediatr 1975;87:832–833.
234. Cleary TG, Henle W, Pickering LK. Acute cerebellar ataxia associated with Epstein-Barr virus infection. JAMA 1980;243:148–149.
235. Erzurum S, Kalavsky SM, Watanakunakorn C. Acute cerebellar ataxia and hearing loss as initial symptoms of infectious mononucleosis. Arch Neurol 1983;40:760–762.
236. Diaz-Mitoma F, Vanast WJ, Tyrrell DJ. Increased frequency of Epstein-Barr virus excretion in patients with new daily persistent headaches. Lancet 1987;1:411–415.
237. DeSimone PA, Snyder D. Hypoglossal nerve palsy in infectious mononucleosis. Neurology 1978;28:842–848.
238. Frey T. Optic neuritis in children with infectious mononucleosis as an etiology. Doc Ophthalmol 1973;34:183–188.
239. Russell J, Fisher M, Zivin JA, et al. Status epilepticus and Epstein-Barr virus encephalopathy. Arch Neurol 1985;42:789–792.
240. Bonforte RJ. Convulsion as a presenting sign of infectious mononucleosis. Am J Dis Child 1967;114:429–432.
241. Whitley RJ, Soong SJ, Hirsch MS, et al. Herpes simplex encephalitis. Vidarabine therapy and diagnostic problems. N Engl J Med 1981;304:313–318.
242. Bale JF Jr, Andersen RD, Grose C. Magnetic resonance imaging of the brain in childhood herpesvirus infections. Pediatr Infect Dis J 1987;6:644–647.
243. Halsted CC, Chang RS. Infectious mononucleosis and encephalitis: Recovery of EB virus from spinal fluid. Pediatrics 1979;64:257–258.
244. Sumaya CV, Ench Y. Epstein-Barr virus infectious mononucleosis in children, II. Heterophil antibody and viral-specific responses. Pediatrics 1985;75:1011–1019.
245. Nahmias AJ, Roizman B. Infection with herpes simplex viruses 1 and 2. N Engl J Med 1973;289:667–674, 719–725, 781–790.
246. Straus SE, Rooney JF, Sever JL, et al. Herpes simplex virus infection. Biology, treatment, and prevention. Ann Intern Med 1985;103:404–419.
247. Juretic M. Natural history of herpetic infection. Helv Paediatr Acta 1966;21:356–368.
248. Corey L, Adams HG, Brown ZA, et al. Genital herpes simplex virus infections: Clinical manifestations, course, and complications. Ann Intern Med 1983;98:958–977.
249. Whitley R. Diagnosis and treatment of herpes simplex encephalitis. Ann Rev Med 1981;32:335–340.
250. Baringer JR. Herpes simplex virus infections of the nervous system. In: Vinken PJ, Bruyn GW, eds. Handbook of Clinical Neurology; Vol. 34. Amsterdam: North-Holland Publishing, 1978;145–159.
251. Whitley RJ, Soong SJ, Linneman C, et al. Herpes simplex encephalitis: Clinical assessment. JAMA 1982;247:317–320.
252. Griffith JF, Chien CT. Herpes simplex encephalitis: Diagnostic and treatment considerations. Med Clin N Am 1983;67:991–1008.
253. Chien LT, Boehm RM, Robinson H, et al. Characteristic early electroencephalographic changes in herpes simplex encephalitis. Arch Neurol 1977;34:361–364.
254. Zimmerman RA, Russell EJ, Leeds NE, et al. CT in the early diagnosis of herpes simplex encephalitis. AJR 1980 134:61–66.
255. Schroth G, Gawehn J, Thron A. Early diagnosis of herpes simplex encephalitis by MRI. Neurology 1987;37:179–183.
256. Koskiniemi M, Vaheri A, Taskinen E. Cerebrospinal fluid alterations in herpes simplex virus encephalitis. Rev Infect Dis 1984;6:608–618.
257. Nahmias AJ, Whitley RJ, Visintine AN, et al. Herpes simplex virus encephalitis: Laboratory evaluations and their diagnostic significance. J Infect Dis 1982;145:829–836.
258. Morawetz RB, Whitley RJ, Murphy DM. Experience with brain biopsy for suspected herpes encephalitis: A review of forty consecutive cases. Neurosurgery 1983;12:654–657.
259. Frank AL, Tucker G. Isolation of herpes simplex type 1 from ventricular fluid of an infant with encephalitis. J Pediatr 1978;92:601–602.
260. Kohl S, James AR. Herpes simplex virus encephalitis during childhood: Importance of brain biopsy diagnosis. J Pediatr 1985;107:212–215.
261. Whitley RJ, Nahmias AJ, Visintine AM. The natural history of herpes simplex virus infection of mother and newborn. Pediatrics 1980;66:489–494.
262. Whitley RJ, Nahmias AJ, Soong SJ, et al. Vidarabine therapy of neonatal herpes simplex virus infection. Pediatrics 1980;66:495–501.
263. Arvin AM, Yeager AS, Bruhn FW. Neonatal herpes simplex infection in the absence of mucocutaneous lesions. J Pediatr 1982;100:715–721.
264. Montgomery JR, Flanders RW, Yow MD. Congenital anomalies and herpes virus infection. Am J Dis Child 1973;126:364–366.
265. Hutto C, Arvin A, Jacobs R, et al. Intrauterine herpes simplex virus infection. J Pediatr 1987;110:97–101.
266. Mizrahi EM, Tharp BR. A characteristic EEG pattern in neonatal herpes simplex encephalitis. Neurology 1982;32:1215–1220.
267. Whitley RJ, Arvin A, Corey L, et al. Vidarabine versus acyclovir therapy of neonatal herpes simplex virus infection. Pediatr Res 1986;20:323A.
268. Smith JB, Groover RV, Klass DW. Multicystic cerebral degeneration in neonatal herpes simplex virus encephalitis. Am J Dis Child 1977;131:568–572.

269. Shturman-Ellstein R, Borkowsky W, Fish I, et al. Myelitis associated with genital herpes in a child. J Pediatr 1976;88:523.

270. Craig CP, Nahmias AJ. Different patterns of neurologic involvement with herpes simplex virus types 1 and 2. Isolation of herpes simplex virus type 2 from the buffy coat of two adults with meningitis. J Infect Dis 1973;127:365–372.

271. McCormick DP. Herpes simplex virus as a cause of Bell's palsy. Lancet 1972;1:937–939.

272. Faden HS, Bybee BL, Overall JC, et al. Disseminated herpesvirus hominis infection in a child with acute leukemia. J Pediatr 1977;90:951–953.

273. Charette RP, Bale JF Jr, Overall JC, et al. Fatal disseminated herpes simplex virus type 1 infection in a child receiving ACTH: Failure of vidarabine therapy. Pediatr Infect Dis 1983;2:245–247.

274. Griffith JF, Salam MV, Adams RD. The nervous system diseases associated with varicella. Acta Neurol Scand 1970;46:279–300.

275. McKendall RR, Klawans HL. Nervous system complications of varicella-zoster virus. In: Vinken PJ, Bruyn G, eds. Handbook of clinical neurology; Vol. 34. Amsterdam: North-Holland Publishing, 1978, 161–183.

276. Johnson R, Milbourn PE. Central nervous system manifestation of chickenpox. Can Med Assoc J 1970;102:831–834.

277. Weller TH. Varicella and herpes zoster: Changing concepts of the natural history, control and importance of a not-so-benign virus. N Engl J Med 1983;309:1362–1368.

278. Dolin R, Reichman RC, Mazur MH, et al. Herpes zoster-varicella infections in immunosuppressed patients. Ann Intern Med 1978;89:375–378.

279. Morgan ER, Smalley LA. Varicella in immunocompromised children. Am J Dis Child 1983;137:883–885.

280. Fleisher G, Henry W, McSorley M, et al. Life-threatening complications of varicella. Am J Dis Child 1981;135:896–899.

281. Appelbaum E, Rachelson MH, Dolgopol VB. Varicella encephalitis. Am J Med 1953;15:223–230.

282. Goldston AS, Millichap JG, Miller RH. Cerebellar ataxia with preeruptive varicella. Am J Dis of Child 1963;106:197–200.

283. Kamholz J, Tremblay G. Chickenpox with delayed contralateral hemiparesis caused by cerebral angiitis. Ann Neurol 1985;18:358–360.

284. Guess HA, Broughton DD, Melton LJ, et al. Epidemiology of herpes zoster in children and adolescents: A population-based study. Pediatrics 1985;76:512–517.

285. Latif R, Shope TC. Herpes zoster in normal and immunocompromised children. Am J Dis Child 1983;137:801–802.

286. Watson PN, Evans RJ. Postherpetic neuralgia, a review. Arch Neurol 1986;43:836–840.

287. McCormick WF, Rodnitzky RL, Schochet SS, et al. Varicella-zoster encephalomyelitis. Arch Neurol 1969;21:559–570.

288. Appelbaum E, Kreps SI, Sunshine A. Herpes zoster encephalitis. Am J Med 1962;32:25–31.

289. Rose FC, Brett EM, Binston J. Zoster encephalomyelitis. Arch Neurol 1964;11:155–172.

290. Thomas JE, Howard FM. Segmental zoster paresis: A disease profile. Neurology 1972;22:459–466.

291. Ohaki M, Chiba S, Nakao T. Bell palsy in infants associated with varicella-zoster virus infection. J Pediatr 1974;84:103–104.

292. Hunt JR. On herpetic inflammation of the geniculate ganglion: A new syndrome and its complications. J Nerv Ment Dis 1907;34:73–96.

293. Hilt DC, Buchholz D, Krumholz A, et al. Herpes zoster ophthalmicus and delayed contralateral hemiparesis caused by cerebral angiitis: Diagnosis and management approaches. Ann Neurol 1983;14:543–553.

294. Alkalay AL, Pomerance JJ, Rimoin DL. Fetal varicella syndrome. J Pediatr 1987;111:320–323.

295. Cuthbertson G., Weiner CP, Giller RH, et al. Prenatal diagnosis of second-trimester congenital varicella syndrome by virus specific immunoglobulin M. J Pediatr 1987;111:592–595.

296. Gibbs FA, Gibbs EL, Carpenter PR. Electroencephalographic abnormality in "uncomplicated" childhood diseases. JAMA 1959;171:1050–1059.

297. Gershon A, Steinberg S, Greenberg S, et al. Varicella-zoster-associated encephalitis: Detection of specific antibody in cerebrospinal fluid. J Clin Microbiol 1980;12:764–767.

298. Prober CG, Kirk LE, Keeney RE. Acyclovir therapy of chickenpox in immunosuppressed children—a collaborative study. J Pediatr 1982;101:622–625.

299. Balfour HH. Intravenous acyclovir therapy for varicella in immunocompromised children. J Pediatr 1984;104:134–136.

300. Shepp DH, Dandliker PS, Meyers JD. Treatment of varicella-zoster virus infection in severely immunocompromised patients. N Engl J Med 1986;314:208–212.

301. Lehmann-Grube F. Lymphocytic choriomeningitis virus. Virol Monogr 171;10:1–173.

302. Hirsch MS, Moellering RC, Pope HG. Lymphocytic choriomeningitis virus infection traced to a pet hamster. N Engl J Med 1974;291:610–612.

303. Bigger RJ, Woodall JP, Walter PD, et al. Lymphocytic choriomeningitis outbreak associated with pet hamsters. JAMA 1975;232:494–500.

304. Deibel R, Woodall JP, Decher WJ, et al. Lymphocytic choriomeningitis virus in man. Serologic evidence of association with pet hamsters. JAMA 1975;232:501–504.

305. Chesney PJ, Katcher ML, Nelson DB, et al. CSF eosinophilia and chronic lymphocytic choriomeningitis virus meningitis. J Pediatr 1979;94:750–752.

306. Sheinbargas MM, Lewis VJ, Thacker WL. Serological diagnosis in children infected prenatally with lymphocytic choriomeningitis virus. Infect Immun 1981;31:837–838.

307. Padgett BL, Walker DL, Zurhein GM, et al. Cultivation of papova-like virus from human brain with progressive multifocal leukoencephalopathy. Lancet 1971;1:1257–1260.

308. Walker DL. Progressive multifocal leukoencephalopathy: An opportunistic viral infection of the central nervous system. In: Vinken PJ, Bruyn GW, eds. Handbook of Clinical Neurology; Vol. 34. Amsterdam: North-Holland Publishing, 1978;307–329.

309. Berger JR, Kaszovitz B, Dickinison G. Progressive multifocal leukoencephalopathy associated with human immunodeficiency virus infection. Ann Intern Med 1987;106:73–87.

310. Rhein GM, Padgett BL, Walker DL, et al. Progressive multifocal leukoencephalopathy in a child with severe combined immunodeficiency. N Engl J Med 1978;229:256–257.

311. Grinnell BW, Padgett BL, Walker DL. Distribution of nonintegrated DNA from JC papovavirus in organs of patients with progressive multifocal leukoencephalopathy. J Infect Dis 1983;147:669–675.

312. Padgett BL, Walker DL. Prevalence of antibodies in human sera against JC virus, an isolate from a case of progressive multifocal leukoencephalopathy. J Infect Dis 1973;127:467–470.

313. Krupp LB, Lipton RB, Swerdlow ML, et al. Progressive multifocal leukoencephalopathy: Clinical and radiographic features. Ann Neurol 1985;17:344–349.

314. Schlitt M, Morawetz RB, Bonnin J, et al. Progressive multifocal leukoencephalopathy: Three patients diagnosed by brain biopsy, with prolonged survival in two. Neurosurgery 1986;18:407–414.

315. Aksamit AJ, Mourrain P, Sever JC, et al. Progressive multifocal leukoencephalopathy: Investigation of three cases using in situ hybridization with JC virus biotinylated DNA probe. Ann Neurol 1985;18:490–496.

316. Bauer WR, Turel AP, Johnson KP. Progressive multifocal leukoencephalopathy and cytarabine. JAMA 1973;266:174–176.

317. Rand KH, Johnson KP, Rubenstein L, et al. Adenine arabinoside in the treatment of progressive multifocal leukoencephalopathy. Ann Neurol 1977;1:458–462.

318. Brooks BR, Jubelt B, Swarz JR, et al. Slow viral infections. Ann Rev Neurosci 1979;2:309–340.

319. Gajdusek DC. Unconventional viruses and the origin and disappearance of Kuru. Science 1977;197:943–960.

320. Prusiner SB. Prions and neurodegenerative diseases. N Engl J Med 1987;317:1571–1581.

321. Bobowick AR, Brody JA, Mathews MR, et al. Creutzfeldt-Jakob disease: A case control study. Am J Epidemiol 1973;98:381–394.

322. Koch TK, Berg BO, DeArmand SJ, et al. Creutzfeldt-Jakob disease in a young adult with idiopathic hypopituitarism: Possible relationship to administration of cadaveric human growth hormone. N Engl J Med 1985;313:731–733.

323. Brown P. Human growth hormone therapy and Creutzfeldt-Jakob disease: A drama in three acts. Pediatrics 1988;81:85–92.

324. Masters CL, Harris JO, Gajdusek C, et al. Creutzfeldt-Jakob disease: Patterns of worldwide occurrence and significance of familial and sporadic clustering. Ann Neurol 1979;5:177–188.

325. Bernoulli C, Siegfried J, Baumgartner G, et al. Danger of accidental person-to-person transmission of Creutzfeldt-Jakob disease by surgery. Lancet 1977;1:478–479.

326. Monreal J, Collins GH, Masters CL, et al. Creutzfeldt-Jakob disease in an adolescent. J Neurol Sci 1981;52:341–350.

327. Packer RJ, Cornblath DR, Gonatas NK, et al. Creutzfeldt-Jakob disease in a 20 year old woman. Neurology 1980;30:492–496.

328. Brown P, Rodgers-Johnson P, Cathala F. Creutzfeldt-Jakob disease of long duration: Clinicopathological characteristics, transmissibility, and differential diagnosis. Ann Neurol 1984;16:295–304.

Chapter 11
Mycotic and Parasitic Infections

Elizabeth Martina Bebin and Manuel R. Gomez

MYCOTIC INFECTIONS

Although fungi are widely distributed in nature, only a few species are pathogenic to the healthy human. Development of fungal infections are dependent, as other infections, on cellular and humoral factors that play an important role in the host defense system. The fungus virulence, host resistance, and the dose of infecting organism are also important in these defense mechanisms. Debilitating diseases and immunosuppressed states of the host facilitate invasion of the central nervous system (CNS) by fungi. There is an increased incidence of some mycoses, particularly candidiasis, phycomycosis, and cryptococcosis, in patients with debilitating diseases (leukemias, lymphomas, aplastic anemia). Patients with deficiency of cellular immunity may become victims of reactivated latent infections.

The incidence of mycotic infections increases with the use of antibiotics, corticosteroids, cytotoxic drugs, and immunosuppressor agents, but the mechanisms underlying these predisposing factors are not well understood. Diminished resistance to fungal infections has been attributed to superinfection of the reticuloendothelial system, the reduction of antibody production, and neutrophil migration.

The classification of fungi is variable and depends on the author's perspective. Fungi are considered as yeasts or molds. Yeasts are unicellular organisms that reproduce by budding. The yeasts most commonly causing CNS infection in humans are *Cryptococcus neoformans, Histoplasma capsulatum, Candida albicans,* and *Blastomyces dermati-tidis.* Molds are multicellular organisms, have a mycelium, but often have a yeast phase in tissue.

Most fungi are ubiquitous in nature and are usually found in soil and decaying vegetation. Man is infected by inhalation of dust or by puncture wounds contaminated by fungi; the invasion of the CNS is usually secondary to pulmonary infection via hematogenous dissemination. Only in rare instances, CNS fungal infections result from direct extension into cranial or vertebral epidural spaces or from intravenous injections.

Lyons and Andriole have suggested that fungal infections were of two clinical types: infections that occur in healthy hosts, and those infections of the immunosuppressed host (1). In the United States (US), fungal infections of healthy subjects are caused by *C. neoformans, Coccidioides immitis, B. dermatitidis,* and *H. capsulatum.* Fungal infections of immunosuppressed hosts include *C. albicans,* an organism commonly found in normal flora of human mucous membranes and phycomycosis (mucormycosis).

Fungal infections should be suspected in all cases of meningitis or brain abscess. *Cryptococcus, Histoplasma, Coccidioides,* and Candida infections may be initially manifested as meningitis; whereas, Nocardia infections usually cause an intracranial abscess. Phycomycosis should be considered in patients with diabetes, lactic acidosis, uremia or other debilitating diseases. Brain abscesses are rare complications of chronic skin fungal infections, but may result from maduromycosis caused by *Petriellidium boydii (Allescheria boydii)* infections (2).

Examination of the cerebrospinal fluid (CSF) is necessary in all cases of CNS fungal infections. The opening pressure is usually increased, there is increased protein and low or normal glucose concentrations. Fungi may be cultured from the CSF in some systemic mycotic infections, but failure to identify the fungus by direct examination or varied culture techniques does not rule out the presence of CNS mycosis. It is prudent to examine several samples of CSF when fungal infection is considered. The precise identification of fungal infections, however, can be established only by isolation of the fungus in pure culture. Pathogenic fungi may be cultured from lesions, exudates, blood, in addition to CSF.

Immunologic studies of the CSF may be helpful in establishing the diagnosis. The complement fixation test is considered diagnostic for coccidioidal meningitis (3). Determination of cryptococcal polysaccharide antigen in blood or CSF by the complement fixation test is widely utilized in the diagnosis of cryptococcosis.

The CNS response to fungal infection may include meningeal inflammatory reaction, formation of miliary microabscesses, formation of large single or multiple abscesses, granulomatous reactions, and infarcts. A characteristic feature of mucormycosis is vascular invasion, leading to thrombotic occlusions and resulting in infarcts. *Cryptococcus, Histoplasma,* and *Coccidioides* species can produce subacute or chronic meningitis, and abscesses may be observed in candidiasis, nocardiosis, actinomycosis, and aspergillosis.

The treatment of CNS fungal infections usually requires long-term administration of potentially toxic antifungal agents. Medications used may adversely affect the hematopoietic system and kidneys. The CSF should be frequently examined to monitor the progress of the illness. At present, the most widely-used antifungal agents include Amphotericin B, flucytosine (5-fluorocytosine), ketoconazole, and miconazole. Amphotericin B, the principal drug for treatment of systemic mycosis, binds to the fungal cytoplasmic membrane, increasing its permeability. It also binds to serum proteins and body tissues. The drug is excreted over weeks (4); it can be detected in the urine up to seven weeks after discontinuing treatment.

Flucytosine has a narrow therapeutic spectrum but when administered in combination with Amphotericin B, there is a synergistic effect in treatment of *Cryptococcus* and *Candida* infections. Ketoconazole is effective in treating blastomycosis and histoplasmosis infections. It can be given orally and is less toxic than Amphotericin B, but it is less effective in treating severe acute systemic mycotic infections. Miconazole, a synthetic imidazole derivative, is active against yeasts and filamentous fungi and is usually reserved for fungal infections that have not responded to treatment with Amphotericin B. Sulfonamides, administered singly or in combination with cycloserine or trimethoprin/sulfamethoxazole, are used for Nocardia infections.

Penicillin is the drug of choice for treating actinomyces infections.

Cryptococcosis

Cryptococcosis is caused by *C. neoformans,* a budding encapsulated saprophytic yeast found in domestic and wild animals, pigeon droppings, and soil. It is a naturally acquired disease of animals and man, but its transmission from either man or animal to man has not been documented (5). Males and Caucasians are primarily affected and there is an increased incidence of the disease in patients receiving corticosteroids or suffering from lymphoreticular malignancies, especially leukemia, Hodgkin disease, diabetes, collagen vascular diseases and acquired immunodeficiency syndrome (AIDS). *C. neoformans* enters the respiratory tract with inhaled dust, and by way of hematogenous spread reaches the CNS, liver, spleen, bone marrow, and skeleton. Though uncommon in children, the CNS can be involved at any age (6). Eighty-five percent of cryptococcal infections occur in adults 20 to 60 years of age (7), the majority of which are males (8,9). In one autopsy series, 90% of all cases had involvement of the CNS (10).

CNS cryptococcosis usually results in diffuse subacute or chronic meningoencephalitis. Soluble anticryptococcal factors that are present in normal serum are absent in the CSF, which is a good culture medium for growth of *C. neoformans* (11). An inflammatory response to cryptococci is usually absent in the human brain (12). There is no significant activation of the complement pathway detectable in the CSF of either patients with the cryptococcal infection or in normal controls, although cryptococci can activate the alternative complement pathway in serum. Thus, it leads to a deficiency of chemotactic and opsonic factors in the CSF, allowing the lesions to progress in the brain while inflammatory reactions clear the foci outside the CNS (13).

The onset of the disease is usually insidious. Symptoms including headache, nausea, dizziness, irritability, somnolence, and behavioral changes may be present for weeks or months prior to diagnosis. Seizures usually occur late in the course of the illness. Ocular symptoms and signs include diplopia, photophobia, and internuclear ophthalmoplegia. Cranial nerve palsies and communicating hydrocephalus can develop as a result of chronic basilar meningitis (5). Papilledema is sometimes present, and many patients have intermittent hyperthermia. As the CNS disease progresses, patients may develop hemiparesis, seizures, lethargy, and coma.

The opening CSF pressure at lumbar puncture (LP) is often elevated; the glucose concentration is decreased; whereas, the concentration of protein is elevated, 60 to 400 mg/dL in most cases The white blood cell count is increased, ranging from 40 to 400 leukocytes/mm^3 with predominance of lymphocytes. Cryptococci will grow in

CSF or urine culture and may be visualized when the CSF smear is stained with India ink. A positive smear should be confirmed by CSF culture. Several serologic tests have been developed for detection of cryptococcal polysaccharide capsular antigen (CPCA) in blood and CSF. The latex agglutination test detects antigen in CSF or serum or both in over 90% of patients with cryptococcal meningitis and has replaced the less sensitive complement fixation test. False positive reactions, however, can occur and appear to be related to the presence of rheumatoid factor (14). Anticryptococcal antibodies are detectable in one-third of patients with cryptococcal meningitis, but they are sometimes present in normal subjects. A latex agglutination titer in CSF of 1:8 or greater is considered significant (15,16).

The pathologic findings observed in cryptococcal meningoencephalitis are varied. The meninges are sometimes cloudy, and in some cases the subarachnoid space is filled with white exudate, that is usually more prominent at the base of the brain and dorsal aspect of the cerebellum. The cerebral blood vessels are often congested and minute nodules may be observed along their course. Hydrocephalus is sometimes present, and is associated with chronic meningitis (Figure 11.1). Small cystic spaces, 1 mm to 2 mm in diameter, are evident in the cerebral cortex (Figure 11.2), often involving superficial areas of the cerebral and cerebellar cortex, and can sometimes be observed in the basal ganglia. These cysts result from destruction and enlargement of the perivascular spaces.

In contrast to other fungi, *C. neoformans* elicits limited cellular reaction to the organism. The inflammatory reaction is minimal in some cases; however, granulomatous reactions are present in others. This reaction consists of lymphocytes, plasma cells, and large macrophages containing organisms. The ventricular ependymal lining appears granular and the choroid plexuses may be infiltrated by *C. neoformans*. Loculation of the infection within the

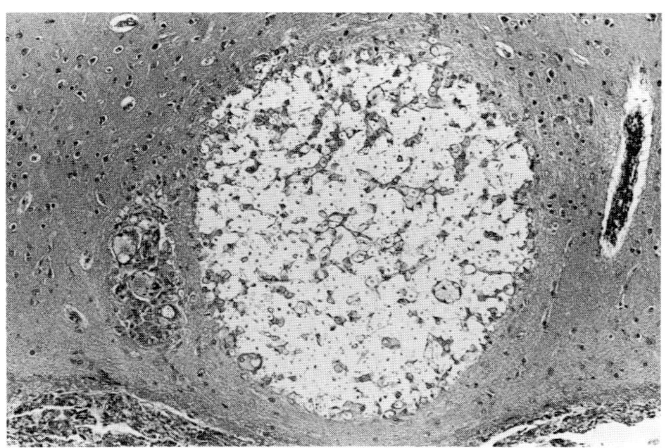

FIGURE 11.2   Cryptococcosis: cerebral cortex with a cyst filled with *C. neoforman*. H&E ×200 before a 49% reduction.

ventricular system may resemble a large brain abscess. *C. neoformans* can be identified histologically by using PAS or silver methenamine stains that outline yeast-like ovoid budding bodies, 2 mm to 15 mm in diameter. The mucoid capsule of cryptococcus is best demonstrated by mucicarmine staining method that stains the capsule rose-red, but does not stain other fungi with similar morphologic characteristics.

CNS cryptococcosis can resemble other mycotic infections, as well as tuberculous meningitis, viral encephalitis, and meningeal carcinomatosis. The absence of localizing neurologic signs reduces the suspicion of intracranial neoplasm. Computed tomographic (CT) head scans with contrast have facilitated the detection of clinically asymptomatic cryptococcal infections by demonstrating enhancing areas that must be differentiated from pyogenic abscesses, tuberculous infections, and neoplasms.

Untreated cryptococcal meningoencephalitis is a fatal disease, with the majority of patients dying within one year after symptom onset. Recent studies suggest the combination of Amphotericin B and 5-fluorocytosine is the treatment of choice for cryptococcal meningitis. This drug combination permits administration of lower doses of Amphotericin B, thereby, decreasing the incidence of nephrotoxicity. The recommended dosage of Amphotericin B is 0.3 mg/kg/day administered intravenously (IV), and 5-fluorocytosine 37.5 mg/kg/day given orally every 6 hours for 6 weeks. Children may tolerate doses of 1.0 mg/kg/day (17). Intrathecal administration of Amphotericin B is recommended for severe infections with rapid clinical deterioration, as well as for patients who developed nephrotoxicity with intravenous (IV) drug administration.

Miconazole has been administered to patients who had inadequate response to combined treatment. The drug is well tolerated and has few adverse effects. Miconazole penetrates the CSF poorly, requiring intrathecal drug administration to treat meningitis (18). The recommended dose is 30 mg/kg/day given intravenously in divided doses every 8

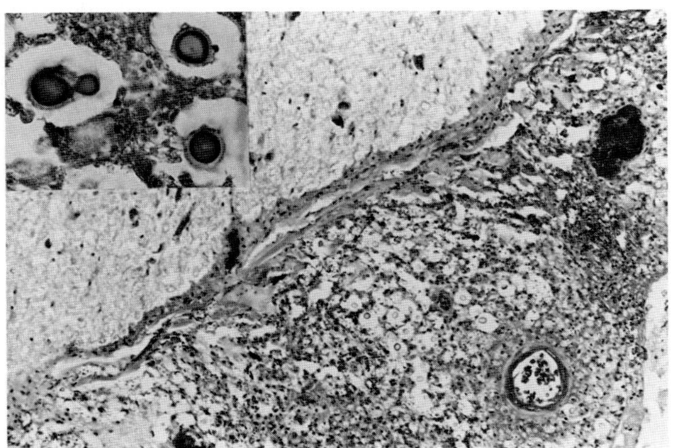

FIGURE 11.1   Crytococcosis: spinal cord with changes of *C. neoformans* granulomatous meningitis. H&E X200. Inset: budding forms of organism with a narrow attachment. Mucicarmine —×400 before a 49% reduction.

hours over a 30-minute period. Large lesions, greater than 3 cm in diameter, may not respond to antibiotic treatment and require surgical resection (19).

Coccidioidomycosis

Coccidioidomycosis, caused by the fungus *C. immitis,* has two morphologic forms; namely, a spherule with endospores, and a hypha with arthrospores. *C. immitis* exists in the soil in the mycelial phase and as it matures, the hypha fragments and liberates spores (arthrospores) that become air-borne and can be inhaled by an animal host. In the host, the spores swell, become spherical, and develop a thick wall thus forming a new structure called the spherule which produce endospores. When the endospores are released, they can develop into a new spherule (parasitic cycle). If the endospore returns to the soil it forms an elongated bud and then hyphae, and the saprophytic phase begins again. If infected material is cultured, the fungus reverts to the mycelial phase.

Coccidioides is endemic in certain regions of North, Central, and South America, usually characterized by arid climate, hot summers, low altitude, mild winters, and sparse flora. Endemic regions in the US include parts of California, especially the San Joaquin Valley, central and western Arizona, southwestern Texas, southern New Mexico, and southwest Utah.

There have been reports of a few patients who contracted *C. immitis* outside the endemic areas; however, they either were exposed to the disease while traveling through those areas, or they had reactivation of an infection acquired earlier while living there. Occupations associated with exposure to dust facilitate infections, especially for immigrant workers who may have no immunity to the organism.

Coccidioides is not contagious from person-to-person. *C. immitis* enters the body by way of the respiratory tract or in a small number of cases, through cutaneous inoculation (20). Many patients have asymptomatic infections only manifested by positive skin tests. Forty percent of patients develop symptoms of primary infection 1 to 3 weeks after the exposure. Symptoms include productive cough, chest pain, malaise, fever, chills, anorexia, and weakness. Erythema nodosum or erythema multiforme involving the upper trunk and extremities may also occur. Chest radiographs may be normal or show evidence of infiltrates, pleural effusions, or hilar nodes. Five percent of patients have residual pulmonary findings consisting of a pulmonary nodule that may calcify or cavitate. If pulmonary symptoms do not resolve, the patient may develop progressive pneumonia leading to potentially fatal chronic pulmonary disease.

Disseminated coccidioidomycosis occurs in only about 0.5% of patients, but this disease form has a significant mortality rate. Any anatomical structure can be involved, including lung, bone, skin, and meninges; lung dissemination resembles miliary tuberculosis. Coccidioides osteomyelitis usually involves long bones (radius, ulna, tibia) and occasionally the skull or vertebrae. Vertebral involvement is often associated with a paraspinal abscess. Dissemination of the organism and fatal disease are more common in men, pregnant women, immunocompromised hosts, and dark-skinned races (American Indians) (21).

Congenital infection is rare even if the placenta is involved. The risk of dissemination before puberty seems not to occur (21,22). The mortality rate of disseminated coccidioides in infancy is higher than that recorded in older children or adults (23). CNS dissemination is most frequently manifested as meningitis, but granulomas of variable size may occur within the brain or spinal cord. Meningitis usually develops within 6 months after primary infection (24). The most common symptoms are headache, fever, weakness, confusion, seizures, abnormal behavior, nuchal rigidity, and vomiting. Focal neurologic symptoms and signs may occur. The CSF is consistently abnormal, with a pleocytosis of 50 to 500 primarily mononuclear cells, decreased glucose and elevated protein concentrations. Eosinophilia is present in some cases.

Coccidioidal meningitis is characterized by a granuloma chiefly affecting the basilar meninges (Figure 11.3). Small granulomas may be present on the cortical surface and in the subarachnoid space; abscesses occasionally occur. Hydrocephalus may be a late complication of chronic basilar meningitis. The organism, *C. immitis,* can be identified in tissue sections stained with hematoxylin and eosin (H&E). The round or oval endospores are demonstrable with silver methenamine stains. The characteristic form is the spherule, up to 60 μ in diameter, filled with endospores (Figure 11.4).

The diagnosis of coccidioides meningitis should be suspected in patients with abnormal CSF who develop persistent headaches, meningeal signs, and who live or have traveled through endemic areas. Supportive evidence for the diagnosis includes the presence of serum antibodies to

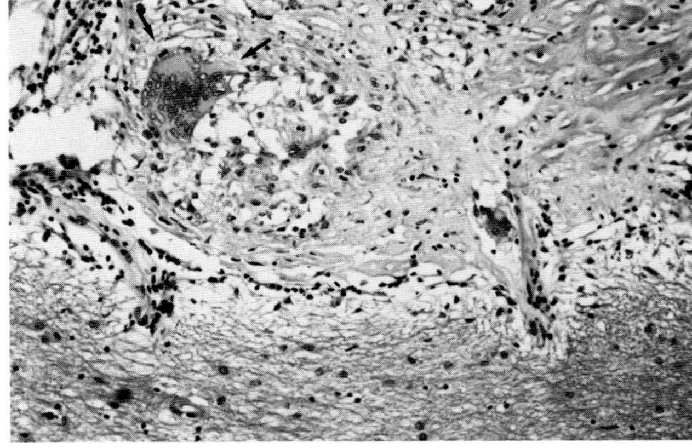

FIGURE 11.3 Coccidioidomycosis: section of cerebral cortex and meninges in graulomatous meningitis. (see arrows) H&E ×200 before a 49% reduction.

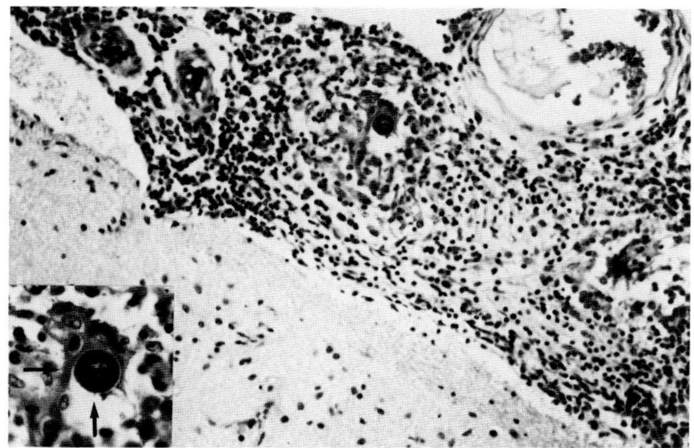

FIGURE 11.4 Coccidioidomycosis: section of cortex and meninges in chronic granulomatous meningitis. Inset shows typical spherules (arrows) filled with endospores. H&E ×200 before a 49% reduction.

C. immitis, a positive coccidioidin skin test, and exclusion of other causes of chronic meningitis. The diagnosis is confirmed by culture or positive complement fixation test. Prompt diagnosis is important since early treatment correlates with successful outcome. The differential diagnosis includes tuberculosis, cryptococcosis, as well as other fungal infections. Sarcoidoses and carcinomatous meningitis should not be overlooked.

The mycelial phase antigen, coccidioidin, is most useful in detecting humoral antibodies. In 75% of cases, serum IgM precipitins appear 1 to 3 weeks after onset of symptoms of primary infection and disappear within 4 months (20). Serum IgG antibodies occur later and may last 6 months. Within 3 months after onset of the disease, 50% to 90% of the patients with symptomatic primary infection have positive antibody titers. Ninety percent of affected patients show precipitins or complement fixing antibodies (CFA). The hallmark of disseminated disease is elevated titers of CFA; 61% of patients have a titer of at least 1:32, and 41% have titers at least 1:64. The CFA titers parallel the course of the disease (20). The latex agglutination test is the most sensitive test for precipitin antibodies; however, there is a false-positive rate of 6% to 10%. In meningeal coccidioidomycosis, CFA are present in the CSF in 70% of the patients on initial examination and in almost all patients as the disease progresses (20).

Skin hypersensitivity tests to *C. immitis* in symptomatic patients with a primary infection are positive within 1 month of symptom onset. Skin testing is important only as an epidemiologic tool or in assessing the status of cellular immunity in patients with documented coccidioidal disease. Confirmation of the diagnosis of coccidioidomycosis depends on isolation of the organism, its identification in tissue by microscopic examination, or both. The characteristic spherules are best demonstrated by the silver methenamine method.

Most patients with symptomatic primary infection recover without therapy; however, it is generally agreed that patients with severe primary infection should receive antifungal therapy. Amphotericin B given intravenously or intrathecally is the treatment of choice for coccidioidal meningitis. The initial intrathecal dose is 0.1 mg for the first 2 or 3 injections, followed by gradually increasing doses of 0.25 mg to 0.5 mg 2 to 4 times per week. Because of the nature of the disease, the treatment of coccidioidal meningitis must be prolonged. Periodic CT head scans will commonly show development of hydrocephalus that may require shunting. In disseminated coccidioidomycosis, Amphotericin B is administered IV in courses of 1 g to 2.5 g, with an extended course if the patient does not respond. Ketoconazole, an alternative antifungal drug, is administered orally in doses of 200 mg to 400 mg/day (25). Treatment results are favorable in all forms of coccidioidomycosis except in the case of meningitis. Relapse rates can be as high as 25% (26). Miconazole has a relapse rate as high as 56% to 78% in patients who had initially responded to treatment.

Candidiasis

Candida species are regarded as a constituent of normal flora of the oral cavity, pharynx, intestinal tract, vagina, and skin of healthy individuals. The organisms seldom produce lesions in the absence of predisposing factors such as diabetes, leukemia, or immunosuppressive therapy.

Candida is a common cause of dermatitis and oral lesions in newborn infants, and of vulvovaginitis in adults. The lesions, in general, are benign and respond to local treatment. Bronchial and pulmonary candidiasis as well as esophagitis are often diagnosed at autopsy. A rare disorder of autosomal-recessive inheritance known as mucocutaneous candidiasis is an association of endocrinopathies, anemia, diabetes (27,28), and immunodeficiency.

Disseminated candidiasis occurs in patients with lymphoma, leukemia, sepsis, immunodeficiency syndromes, other debilitating diseases, prolonged administration of broad-spectrum antibiotics or cytotoxic agents. In these conditions, *C. albicans* can produce systemic infection with multiple organ involvement. In disseminated candidiasis, the kidneys are consistently involved, followed by the heart, lungs, gastrointestinal tract, and brain (29).

There are no characteristic clinical findings in disseminated candidiasis. The disease is often identified fortuitously in blood cultures or unexpectedly at autopsy. Fever is a consistent symptom in children with disseminated candidiasis along with irritability, lethargy, and vomiting. These patients often have hepatosplenomegaly, petechiae, cardiorespiratory symptoms and signs, and a variety of neurologic signs when the CNS is involved. Endophthalmitis has been detected with increasing frequency in recent years (30) and is characterized by focal, glistening, white retinal lesions that may be solitary or multiple, and often associated with vitreous inflammation (31).

In disseminated candidiasis, involvement of the CNS may be present in immunosuppressed patients or those with chronic debilitating illness. *C. albicans* is the most common species of *Candida* that produces lesions in the CNS (7). In a review of 42 patients with cerebral candidiasis, 7 had no predisposing factors while 35 had some underlying disease which increased susceptibility to fungal infection; 27 had meningitis and 15 had cerebral abscesses, microabscesses, or granulomatous lesions. Twelve of the 42 patients were neonates (32).

The symptoms and signs of CNS involvement depend to some degree on whether the process is meningeal, cerebromeningeal, or intraparenchymal (abscess). The initial symptoms and signs are fever, vomiting, seizures, and lethargy that may rapidly progress to coma. Common signs and symptoms of meningitis include fever, headache, nuchal rigidity and focal neurologic signs. The CSF is usually clear, often with increased pressure and pleocytosis, predominantly neutrophils and mononuclear cells; the concentration of protein is elevated and the glucose may be normal or decreased. Most patients will have a positive culture for Candida, and a positive Gram stain. In patients with intraparenchymal lesions, the CSF shows little change and cultures are usually negative.

The neuropathologic changes observed in candidiasis include meningitis that is predominantly basilar, and miliary nodules closely related to blood vessels. *Candida* may invade the wall of cerebral vessels, causing thrombosis and resulting in brain infarction. The meningeal inflammatory infiltrate consists primarily of lymphocytes, plasma cells, and polymorphonuclear leukocytes (33). Parenchymal lesions consist of necrotic foci surrounded by polymorphonuclear leukocytes and macrophages. Abscesses and granulomata are common in disseminated candidiasis (Figure 11.5) and are usually small and often observed only

at microscopic examination. Meningeal and cerebral blood vessels may be thrombosed resulting in infarction of the surrounding brain. Candida is demonstrated by Grocott methenamine silver or periodic acid-Schiff stains and appears as pseudohyphae, which should be distinguished from *Aspergillus* with its septate hyphae (Figure 11.6).

One should suspect an opportunistic infection such as candidiasis when an unexplained fever, neurologic symptoms or signs, or pulmonary infiltrates present in an immunodeficient or leukopenic patient who has received prolonged antibiotic or corticosteroid therapy, or who has an indwelling intravascular catheter. The diagnosis is usually established by isolation and culture of the fungus from blood, CSF, or other body fluids. Serologic methods are not widely available; agglutinating antibody titers are reputed to be reliable (34).

Disseminated candidiasis associated with meningoencephalitis is a life-threatening disease; however, successful therapeutic efforts have been obtained with administration of Amphotericin B. The prognosis of CNS candidiasis is better in patients with meningitis rather than in those with encephalitis. Amphotericin B is the drug of choice for the treatment of disseminated candidiasis, and there is a synergistic effect when combined with 5-fluorocytosine, allowing the dosage of Amphotericin to be reduced. The antifungal agent 5-fluorocytosine has excellent penetration into the CSF (35). Treatment is continued for 6 to 12 weeks with the duration of therapy determined by clinical and laboratory response, and as influenced by the drug's toxic effects. Miconazole is an alternative drug but its value in treatment of candida meningitis has not been well established (36).

Aspergillosis

Aspergillosis, a disease produced by species of the fungus Aspergillus, is attributed to antigenic stimulation, coloniza-

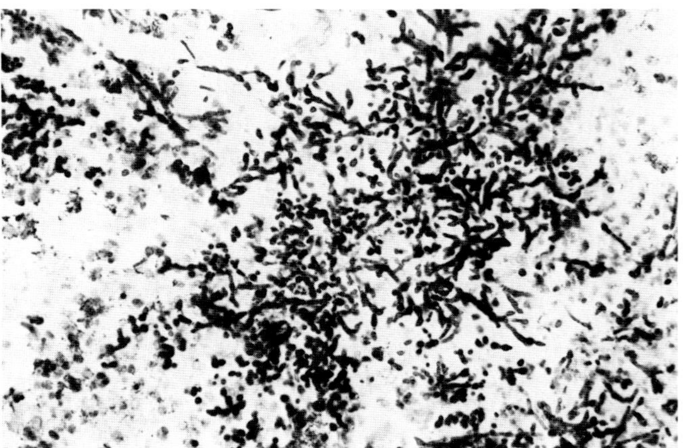

FIGURE 11.5 Candidiasis: cerebrum with inflammatory foci containing abundant forms of *Candida albicans*. H&E ×200 before a 49% reduction.

FIGURE 11.6 In higher magnification (×400) with a 49% reduction, *Candida* appear in tissue as round or elongated forms. Silver methenamine.

tion, or tissue invasion by the fungus. Although over 300 species of genus *Aspergillus* are recognized, few are pathogenic to man. *Aspergillus fumigatus* is the usual cause of aspergillosis and *Aspergillus flavus* is the second most important pathogenic species. The *Aspergillus* species is identified by the appearance of colony and spore-bearing structures; they produce a variety of toxins in vitro, none of which are known to be produced in the infected host (37). *Aspergillus* species are ubiquitous in the environment throughout the world and grow well in hay, grain, or decaying vegetation. They have also been found in hospital air (38) and, according to Bennett, are present in the air of oncology wards year round (39).

Aspergillosis is acquired by inhalation of airborne spores (2.5 μ to 3.0 μ) that reach the pulmonary alveoli or paranasal sinuses. Although exposure to *Aspergillus* is universal, aspergillosis is an uncommon disease. Occupation may be an important factor in acquiring the disease by facilitating exposure to contaminated dust or birds. Infection occurs more frequently in individuals with debilitating diseases such as tuberculosis, leukemia, lymphoma, or cancer. Prolonged therapy with antibiotics, corticosteroids, cytotoxic drugs, or antimetabolites predispose to infection with *Aspergillus*, especially in severely immunosuppressed patients. The disease may be localized or diffuse.

Aspergillus can grow in bronchi, cysts or cavities of the lungs, or paranasal sinuses for months or years without invading the lung tissue. Primary pulmonary aspergillosis results in granuloma or abscess formation, which has a characteristic radiographic appearance of round densities within a cavitary lesion. Severely immunosuppressed patients show infarction, necrosis, and vessel invasion by the fungus without granulation tissue. When a fungus ball is visible radiographically, IgG antibody to *Aspergillus* can be readily demonstrated in patients. Massive inhalation of *Aspergillus* by normal children may be followed by fever, dyspnea, and a miliary infiltrate on chest radiograph within 24 hours. Improvement begins spontaneously in 2 to 4 weeks, leading to recovery. In patients with progressive disease, a chronic granulomatous disease develops (40). Immunosuppressed patients are prone to an acute and usually fatal pneumonia. The disease begins with high fever followed by pulmonary extension and hematogenous dissemination to the CNS, heart, liver, and other organs. Death usually occurs in 1 to 3 weeks (41–43).

Aspergillosis of the CNS is relatively rare but may affect patients with severe immunosuppression or chronic debilitating diseases. Most patients with CNS involvement have multiple affected organs, and 60% of disseminated cases of aspergillosis have CNS lesions (44). The fungus reaches the brain by hematogenous dissemination secondary to pulmonary colonization, self-administration of street drugs, or extension of adjacent lesions in the paranasal sinuses or orbits. In some patients the neurologic manifestations of the disease are minimal, and the disease is only recognized at autopsy. Invasion of the CNS by *Aspergillus* results in either formation of granulomas or abscesses and in many cases both are present (45), sometimes simulating expanding intracranial lesions such as neoplasms. Meningeal involvement produces a subacute or chronic meningitis.

The CSF is usually clear and under normal pressure; a pleocytosis of less than 600 cells with neutrophil and mononuclear cell predominance is common. Concentrations of protein and glucose are elevated and normal, respectively. Attempts to isolate *Aspergillus* from the CSF are usually unsuccessful. *Aspergillus* in the CNS provokes an acute inflammatory reaction, often associated with vascular thrombosis and infarction resulting from fungal invasion of the vascular wall. The vascular lumen is thrombosed by masses of hyphae leading to hemorrhage and necrosis of variable sizes. Vascular involvement is not limited to small arteries and arterioles, but may include large arteries like the internal carotid artery (46). The chronic lesions are granulomatous in nature, composed of inflammatory cells, including plasma cells, occasional giant cells, abundant fibrous connective tissue, and areas of hemorrhage and necrosis.

The diagnosis of CNS aspergillosis is confirmed by demonstration of *Aspergillus* at culture and microscopic examination. The appearance of the *Aspergillus* hyphae in a smear or biopsy can be very suggestive, but is not diagnostic (Figure 11.7). Blood and CSF serologic tests for aspergillosis are rarely positive.

Amphotericin B is the drug of choice for treatment of invasive aspergillosis. Treatment efficacy is best when the diagnosis is made early, there is little or no immunosuppression, and the dose of Amphotericin B rapidly attains therapeutic levels (47). In CNS aspergillosis, Amphotericin should be administered systemically and intrathecally. The combined use of Amphotericin B and 5-fluorocytosine or rifampin has an additive effect (48); however, the clinical

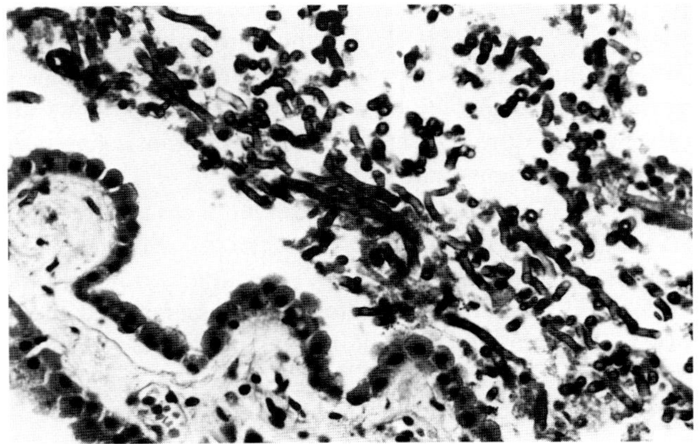

FIGURE 11.7 Aspergillosis: choroid plexus invaded by organisms, appearing as branching septate hyphae. Silver methenamine. H&E ×400 before a 49% reduction.

evidence of their effectiveness when combined in treatment, is not sufficiently established.

Histoplasmosis

Infection caused by Histoplasma capsulatum is largely asymptomatic and is most commonly manifested as a benign pulmonary infection. Histoplasma capsulatum infections are virtually universal in highly endemic areas. In the US, endemic areas include Ohio, the central Mississippi valleys, Appalachian mountains, and parts of North Carolina. The infective agent is the airborne spore of *Histoplasma capsulatum,* usually arising from the soil in endemic areas, although pulmonary histoplasmosis may result from exposure to chicken, bird, or bat excrement. In an outbreak of the disease in Ohio, 384 students developed clinical symptoms and signs of pulmonary histoplasmosis after clearing a school courtyard contaminated with starling and black bird excrement (49). There is, in general, no apparent sex predisposition to histoplasmosis in children. In the majority of cases the primary disease is asymptomatic or so mild that its etiology is unrecognized. The diagnosis may be suspected in calcified pulmonary foci on radiographs, and is usually made by a positive histoplasmin skin test. Occasionally it is a complication of debilitating disease such as diabetes, tuberculosis, leukemia, or lymphoma. Common symptoms of acute pulmonary histoplasmosis include fever, chills, headaches, myalgias, fatigue, chest pain, and cough. Pulmonary infiltrates are usually bilateral as observed on chest radiographs during the acute phase. With resolution of the infection, lymph nodes become more apparent and tend to calcify. Rarely, chronic cavitary pulmonary lesions are produced.

Progressive disseminated histoplasmosis is infrequent but is reported to occur in infancy (50), or in patients with predisposing or debilitating conditions. The prevalence of disseminated histoplasmosis has been estimated as 2 to 10 per 1 million infected persons per year, but may be as high as 46 per 100,000 (51,52). During outbreaks of infection, 50% of patients suffer from a serious underlying illness or are immunocompromised; the remainder of patients are otherwise healthy. Disseminated histoplasmosis has been reported in patients with AIDS.

The clinical manifestations of disseminated histoplasmosis include fever, malaise, cough, weight loss, diarrhea, nausea and vomiting, anorexia, weakness, chills, and abdominal pain. Fulminant forms of disseminated histoplasmosis occur mainly in infants, but adults may develop a subacute or chronic form characterized by focal organ involvement including intestinal ulceration and perforations (37%), Addison disease (16%), endocarditis (16%), meningitis and cerebritis (5%), and spinal cord compression (5%). The chest radiograph is abnormal in less than 33% (51). Hematologic abnormalities such as low hematocrit (less than 30) or leukopenia may be present.

CNS involvement in histoplasmosis is relatively rare. Schultz found lesions in the brain or meninges in 12 cases of 120 autopsies of histoplasmosis. Three cases were in children less than 2 years of age and 9 were adults (53). The majority of neurologic manifestations occurred in patients with underlying diseases including leukemia, lymphoma, renal transplants, hypoimmunoglobulinemia (54). Histoplasma meningitis occurs in 10% of cases of disseminated histoplasmosis and is indistinguishable from other meningitides when it develops in an acute and rapidly progressive manner (55). It may also present as a subacute granulomatous process.

Goodwin et al. (51) consider disseminated histoplasmosis as an infection of the macrophage system, for *Histoplasma capsulatum* is often found in macrophages in which they multiply. Macrophages are often distended by massive numbers of organisms appearing histologically intact but there is a lack of organism destruction.

The following three patterns of tissue reaction may be observed: diffuse histiocytosis, often with massive accumulations of infected macrophages throughout the reticuloendothelial system with little evidence of response by other cells; focal histiocytosis with development of central, often perivascular necrosis especially in the CNS and adrenal gland; and granuloma formation resembling tuberculosis.

Three types of CNS histoplasmosis have been described, the first type of which is meningitis of varying severity with predilection for the basal cisterns. When the meningeal reaction is pronounced, there is a thick yellow exudate, and in chronic cases, a meningeal fibrosis (Figure 11.8). This reaction is comprised of phagocytes containing yeast and, on occasion, single or multiple caseating granulomas. A second type is a focal cerebritis, consisting of multiple granulomas scattered throughout the brain parenchyma (Figure 11.9); and a third type includes large granulomas, similar to tuberculomas, sometimes reaching several centimeters in diameter (55). In tissue section the fungi appear as small

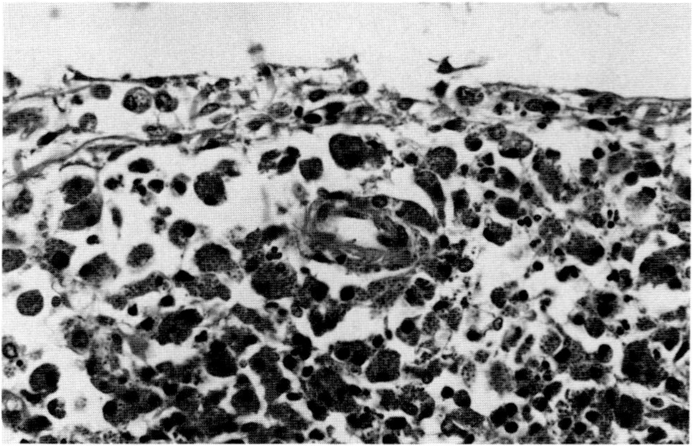

FIGURE 11.8   Histoplasmosis: The subarachnoid space is diffusely infiltrated by lymphocytes and plasma cells. *H. capsulatum* are within cytoplasm of macrophages. H&E ×600 before a 49% reduction.

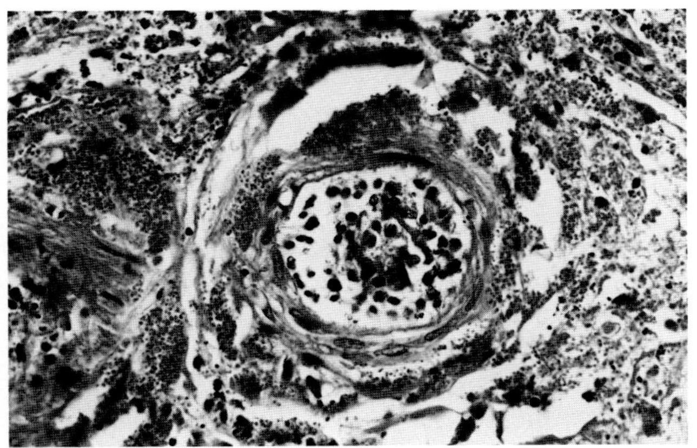

FIGURE 11.9 Histoplasmosis: small meningeal artery surrounded by a cellular infiltrate consisting of lymphocytes and plasma cells. Note numerous organisms within macrophages. H&E ×600 before a 49% reduction.

ovoid bodies, 1 μ to 5 μ, that stain well with PAS and Grocott silver methenamine stains. In H & E preparations, the ovoid bodies appear smaller because only the central portion of the fungus is well demonstrated. *H. capsulatum* should be distinguished from other fungi and from *Toxoplasma gondi* which develop pseudocysts in other cells than the reticuloendothelial system (RES).

CNS involvement in disseminated histoplasmosis is suggested by development of neurologic symptoms and signs associated with abnormal CSF. The clinical diagnosis should be confirmed, if possible, by organism identification in cultures of blood, bone marrow, CSF, or sputum, recognizing that only about 50% of CSF cultures are positive. Early diagnosis depends on biopsy from oropharyngeal mucosa, bone marrow, or lymph nodes. The histoplasmin skin test is of limited value in the diagnosis; the test is almost uniformly positive in people living in endemic areas. Serologic tests such as complement fixation and immunodiffusion are important adjuncts to diagnosis.

Recommended treatment for initial infection is Amphotericin B (18). Ketoconazole has also been effective in the treatment of disseminated histoplasmosis, but not in *H. capsulatum* meningitis because of poor penetration of the blood-brain barrier (18).

Pulmonary histoplasmosis is usually managed conservatively. The progressive disseminated form of histoplasmosis is treated with Amphotericin B administered intravenously. Intrathecal administration of Amphotericin B should be considered in chronic infection.

Blastomycosis

Blastomycosis, caused by *Blastomyces dermatitidis,* is found predominantly in the US, Canada, and Mexico, and is endemic in the Ohio and Mississippi valleys as well as the southern and southeastern states (56). It is a sporadic disease primarily affecting adult males. Immunocompromised patients are not predisposed to this infection. The infective organism is a dimorphic fungus depending on the temperature and site of growth. At room temperature, it produces filamentous colonies that can be converted to a yeast form by transfer to brain-heart-glucose-agar at 37 C°. In the human host, blastomyces appear almost invariably as a spherical, thick walled budding yeast. The fungus gains access to the body via the respiratory tract disseminating further via lymphatic and hematogenous systems to involve skin, oral or nasal mucosa, bone, genitourinary tract, and rarely the CNS (57).

Although the source of blastomyces is obscure, it is accepted that the majority of cases are acquired from contaminated soil (58). There is no transmission from man to man nor from animal to man.

In 63 cases reported by Duttera and Osterhout (59), cutaneous lesions were present in 57%, pulmonary infection in 52%, bone involvement in 19%, and CNS lesions in 6%. CNS blastomycosis is estimated to occur in 6% to 30% of patients with blastomycosis (59).

Primary pulmonary lesions are usually benign and are associated with influenza-like symptoms. They may be complicated by pleural effusions or in chronic states resembling pulmonary tuberculosis with other organ involvement. Primary cutaneous blastomycosis is rare and usually follows a primary pulmonary infection with metastases to skin and subcutaneous tissues. Cutaneous blastomycosis begins as a papule that progressively enlarges and becomes an indurated, elevated, irregular, crusted lesion with a violaceous color. Regional lymphangitis and lymphadenitis may develop. Osteolytic lesions can be present in disseminated blastomycosis and cranial and vertebral lesions may become suppurative, extending into the epidural space and resulting in spinal cord or brain compression.

Blastomycosis of the CNS is usually secondary to hematogenous dissemination from the lungs; the majority of these patients have evidence of disease elsewhere (Figure 11.10). Cutaneous and subcutaneous lesions are common

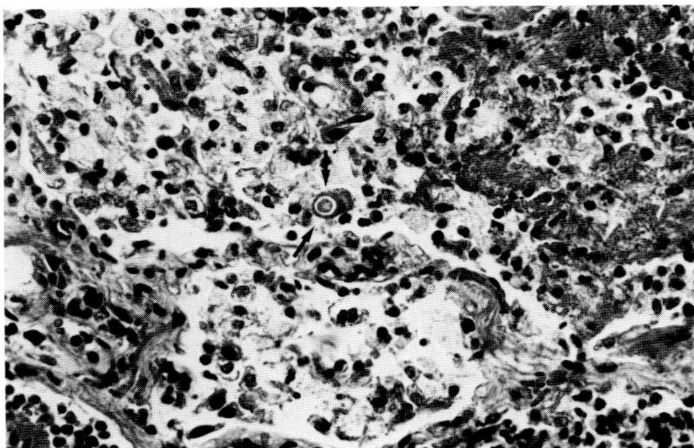

FIGURE 11.10 Blastomycosis: severe pneumonitis showing the fungus in center field (arrows). It is spherical and has a thick clear wall. H&E ×400 before a 49% reduction.

and frequently precede the neurologic manifestations. Meningeal involvement is clinically manifested by headaches, vomiting, confusion, and nuchal rigidity. The process may be acute or chronic with great variation in severity of the symptoms. CSF examination is characterized by increased opening pressure, pleocytosis, increased protein and decreased glucose concentrations. The fungus can be cultured from the CSF, and the organism is sometimes observed on dried smears. Cerebral lesions may be single or multiple, and patients with intracranial abscess or granulomas have symptoms and signs of increased intracranial pressure. Intracranial and extradural spinal abscesses may occur in association with cranial and vertebral osteomyelitis. Paraplegia may be secondary to spinal cord compression by vertebral blastomycotic osteomyelitis.

Leptomeningitis is common and fibropurulent or frank purulent exudate is observed in the subarachnoid space primarily in the basilar regions of the brain. In chronic meningitis, the leptomeninges are adherent to the dura mater. The characteristic microscopic lesions are microabscesses with a central core of necrosis and neutrophils, surrounded by lymphocytes, epithelial cells, and multinucleated giant cells. The lesions resemble those of tuberculosis. The diagnosis of CNS blastomycosis can be established with certainty by culture and identification of *B. dermatitides* in secretions, exudate, CSF, or tissue sections. *B. dermatitides* are seen free or within multinucleated giant cells as round or oval, thick walled organisms 6μ to 15μ in diameter. The fungus characteristically multiplies by a single bud that is released from the parent cell by a wide septum.

Untreated CNS blastomycosis is fatal. The treatment of disseminated blastomycosis requires not only long-term therapy but, when necessary, surgical removal of large granulomatous lesions and drainage of abscessses. The most effective treatment includes Amphotericin B and 2-hydroxystilbamidine. Success in removal of brain granulomas in conjunction with administration of Amphotericin B has been reported (60). Meningitis due to *B. dermatitides* has been successfully treated with Amphotericin B (61).

Mucormycosis

The phycomycoses are diseases caused by any fungi of the class Phycomycetes. The term mucormycosis indicates infections caused by species of the genus *Mucor,* class Phycomycetes. The organisms are present in soil and often in decaying vegetation. Mucormycosis has a predilection for patients with uncontrolled diabetes or ketoacidosis, leukemia, lymphoma, cancer, or other patients receiving immunosuppressive therapy.

Mucormycosis is a rare disease but has been reported in all races and age groups. In infancy, mucormycosis complicates severe debilitating diseases associated with dehydration, acidosis, or uremia (62). In older children and adults,

the most significant related factor is acute diabetic ketoacidosis, which is present in over 50% of reported cases beyond infancy (63).

The disease often begins in the nose or nasopharynx, and in susceptible patients extends to the paranasal sinuses and through the ethmoidal cribriform plate into the intracranial cavity, meninges, and brain. Pulmonary involvement occurs frequently, even in the absence of other organ involvement; the gastrointestinal tract is less commonly involved. Cutaneous and subcutaneous mucormycosis has also been reported as nosocomial contamination. Hematogenous dissemination of the disease may originate from any of these foci.

Patients may have unilateral orbital or facial pain with erythema and periorbital edema which rapidly becomes indurated. Proptosis, external ophthalmoplegia, mydriasis, and visual loss are present, and ophthalmoscopy may show retinal vein engorgement or ischemia. Facial paralysis may develop. Neurologic signs and symptoms include alteration of consciousness, headache, papilledema, hemiparesis, obtundation, seizures, coma, and unless successful and early treatment has been given, death.

The opening CSF pressure at lumbar puncture is initially normal and only later becomes elevated. The CSF is generally clear but can be xanthochromic if hemorrhagic infarction has occurred. Pleocytosis may be minimal or as high as 1,000/mm³, with neutrophilic predominance. Protein concentration is usually elevated, while glucose is normal or increased. CT head scans demonstrate enlarged ventricles and lesion localization. When CNS infection is an extension from the paranasal sinuses or orbit, lesions may be found in the inferior aspect of the frontal lobes; whereas, in hematogenous dissemination, lesions may be scattered throughout the cerebral hemisphere(s). Infarcts are common in mucormycosis and are usually hemorrhagic with focal areas of subarachnoid hemorrhage. Thrombosed blood vessels, both large and small, with necrotic walls are present in and around the infarcted area (Figure 11.11).

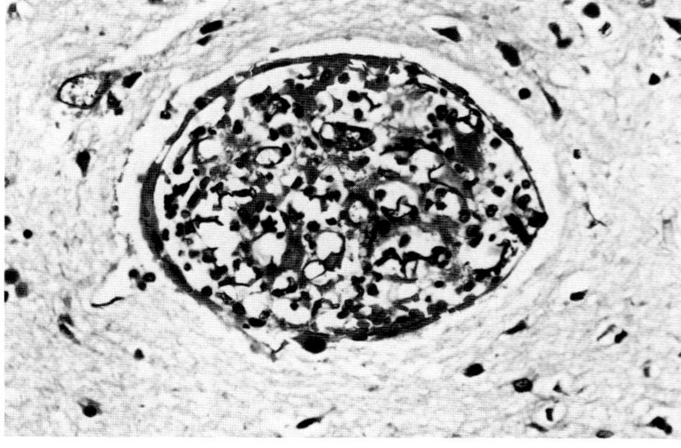

FIGURE 11.11   Cerebral mucormycosis: small cerebral vessel thrombosed by hyphae. H&E × 400 before a 49% reduction.

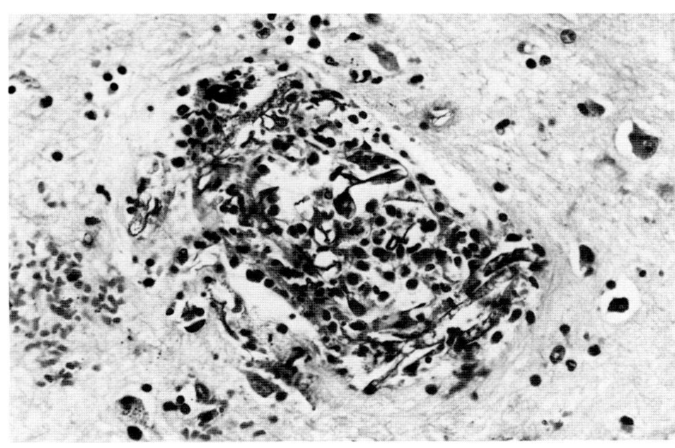

FIGURE 11.12 Cerebral mucormycosis: small cerebral blood vessels with numerous nonseptate hyphae within and extending through the vessel wall into adjacent tissue. H&E × 400 before a 49% reduction.

Numerous branching hyphae are found within the thrombi as well as penetrating the brain parenchyma (62) (Figure 11.12). The reaction of brain tissue to the fungus is variable. At the periphery of the infarct, moderate neutrophilic infiltration is common; suppuration is rare and granulomatous reaction may be seen. Meningeal inflammation and infiltration of the meninges with hyphae is usually moderate.

The diagnosis of mucormycosis is made on the basis of clinical presentation and the demonstration of nonseptate, branching hyphae 15μ to 25μ in width in tissues. The organisms in tissue sections stain well with H&E, PAS, and Grocott silver methenamine.

Mucormycosis affecting the CNS should be considered a life threatening condition that demands immediate therapy. Hale described 36 cases of mucormycosis in children of which 34 died (64).

PARASITIC INFECTIONS

Parasites are more commonly found in tropical and subtropical regions of the world, but are not confined to these regions and some have worldwide distribution. Their prevalence in tropical regions is related to warm climate and poor sanitary conditions. Malaria, toxoplasmosis, and amebiasis are more widely disseminated throughout the world, while American and African trypanosomiasis are found in subtropical South America and Equatorial Africa, respectively. Schistosomiasis and Paragonimiasis are common infections of the Orient and Southeast Asia; whereas, cestode and nematode infections are usually found in Central and South America, Eastern Europe, India, and Australia. Parasites of medical significance belong to the Helminth (worm) or Protozoa (unicellular organisms) classes. They may infect man or animals and serve as an intermediary source of human infection.

Helminthic Infections

Helminths, or worms, are probably the most prevalent of human parasites; and it is estimated that 54 million persons in the US may be infected by these organisms (65). They are classified into three groups including: Nematodes (round worms), Trematodes (flukes), and Cestodes (tapeworms). These parasites infect man by ingestion, direct skin penetration, or by inoculation of an insect vector.

The life cycle of helminths may be simple. For example, in enterobiasis and trichuriasis, eggs pass from the gut, embryonate, and when ingested, develop into egg-producing adult worms. In similar manner ingested larvae in meat or vegetables enter the intestine where they develop into tapeworms or flukes. Sometimes, the life cycle includes ingestion of egg, hatching, and penetration of the intestinal wall by larvae. Embryos of cestodes penetrate the intestinal wall and lymphatics and portal venules carry them to the liver and to the lungs; the systemic circulation transports them to their final destination, the brain or spinal cord. Massive CNS involvement suggests larval multiplication of the parasite. The larvae of the nematodes *Trichinella spiralis* and *Toxocara canis* also gain access to CNS through the systemic circulation.

Parasites within the CNS may affect nervous tissue mechanically, by liberating toxic metabolites inducing immunologic responses, and competing for essential nutrients. The frequently observed eosinophilia in helminthiasis is believed to be related to the immunologic reaction of the host. These mechanisms suggest the following four clinical pathologic syndromes: symptoms and signs of space occupying lesions as in cysticercosis and hydatidosis; inflammatory response of meningitis or meningoencephalitis as in trichinosis and many cases of schistosomiasis; competition for a vital factor producing a deficiency syndrome as in diphyllobothriasis; and the association of two or all three syndromes (66).

The diseases produced by helminthic CNS invasion, while not homogeneous, have certain common features. Infections caused by each species of helminth have characteristic clinical features within a particular geographic region primarily determined by socioeconomic, sanitary, and cultural conditions. CNS cysticerosis and hydatidosis are two conditions with high prevalence and morbidity that could be elminated with effective sanitary measures. Less common CNS parasitosis in the US are schistosomiasis, paragonimiasis, trichinosis, coenurosis, and toxocariasis.

Toxocariasis (Visceral larva migrans)

Toxocariasis is a parasitic infection caused by larvae of *Toxocara canis*. Human infection with *T. canis* was recognized by Wilder (67), who discovered the larvae within a child's retinal granuloma. Beaver et al. (68) described 3 children with eosinophilia and multisystem disease caused by *T. canis* and suggested the name of visceral larva migrans (VLM).

The adult parasite *T. canis* is 7 cm to 12 cm in length, smaller than the Ascaris. It enters the dog's intestines where eggs are produced and excreted in the dog's feces. The life cycle of *T. canis* in humans begins with ingestion of embryonated eggs. The larvae hatch within the intestine penetrate the gut wall, migrate via the portal system to the liver and lungs and sometimes other organs including kidney; eye, one of the most severely affected; and brain. They become encysted in these organs, evoking the host's granulomatous response. The larvae of *T. canis* secrete proteolytic enzymes that facilitate movement through the lesions. The host response to the infection is an intense eosinophilic inflammation, and when the larva dies, its concentrated protein stimulates the granulomatous reaction.

VLM is more common, though not limited to children between the ages of 1 and 4 years. The higher prevalence of VLM in children is attributed to increased exposure to infective eggs and poor habits of hygiene. The primary source of infective eggs are puppies and nursing bitches, both of which are capable of excreting eggs in their feces. After 2 to 3 weeks the eggs become infective and may remain viable and infective for years.

The clinical manifestations range from an asymptomatic state associated with eosinophilia to severe infection with multiple organ involvement. Asymptomatic and minimally symptomatic forms are the most common and are usually unreported. In the symptomatic cases, fever, lower respiratory symptoms (bronchospasm resembling asthma), and abdominal discomfort are the most frequent symptoms. Myocarditis, nephritis, and involvement of the CNS have also been described. A serious consequence of VLM is involvement of the retina that may result in blindness. Usually one eye is affected. The infection can cause diffuse endophthalmitis and retinal detachment. Focal lesions may form macular and paramacular granulomas (69); optic neuritis has been reported (70).

There are few reports of symptomatic CNS involvement by *T. canis* (71–73). Anderson et al. (1975) published a case of an 18-month-old child with serologic evidence of *T. canis* infection who developed a spastic hemiparesis associated with eosinophilia in the blood and CSF (74). Schochett (1967) described a child with Toxocara encephalitis manifested by recurrent seizures, rapid coma, and death. At autopsy multiple granulomas were found in the brain, one of which contained *T. canis* larvae (73). The diagnosis of VLM in a child is usually made clinically on the basis of fever, hepatomegaly, and eosinophilia. Because the adult worm rarely develops in humans, the diagnosis cannot be made by searching for eggs in the stools.

In many cases, the diagnosis of *T. canis* infections is made primarily on an immunologic basis. The enzyme-linked immunoabsorbent assay (ELISA), which employs antigens secreted by the second stage larvae, has sufficient specificity for this infection. Eighty percent of those infected are positive in this test (75). Other helpful laboratory findings to support the diagnosis of VLM include the following: leukocytosis with marked blood eosinophilia, elevation of gamma globulin (especially IgG, IgM, and IgE), serum aspartic succinic transaminase (AST or SGOT), and CSF eosinophilia.

VLM is, in general, a self-limiting disease. The migratory larvae evoke an inflammatory response from the host and eventually become encapsulated and quiescent. In most cases, the symptomatic period correlates with the larval migration and resolves spontaneously, but blood eosinophilia persists for months.

Antilarval therapy is ineffective. Diethylcarbamazine has been used with inconclusive results to treat human VLM. Thiabendazole, a broad-spectrum antihelminthic, has been used with some success (76). Prophylaxis should be directed to prevent close contact with dogs (puppies and nursing bitches).

Trichinosis (Trichinellosis)

Trichinosis, an infection caused by the small nematode *Trichinella spiralis,* prevails in regions where pork is consumed. It is common in Poland, Russia, Bulgaria, Chile, Argentina, Central and North America, including the Arctic region. Recent surveys in the US show 10 to 12 million persons are infected with *T. spiralis* (77). Only 100 to 200 cases are reported to the Centers for Disease Control each year, but more than 200,000 new infections are calculated to occur each year (78).

T. spiralis always has a parasitic existence. The 1.4 mm to 1.6 mm long male worms and the 3 mm to 4 mm long female worms live in the small intestine of man, pigs, bears, and other carnivores. These animals serve as definitive hosts, bearing both adult and larval parasites. Man is usually infected by eating uncooked pork containing *T. spiralis* larvae encysted in its muscles. Once the larvae are liberated by action of digestive enzymes, they reach the proximal small intestine, penetrate the intestinal mucosa, and within 30 hours are adult worms. Five to 7 days after mating, females within the intestinal mucosa begin to deposit larvae which enter the mesenteric lymphatics and thoracic duct to reach the systemic circulation. The larvae emerge from the capillaries into the parenchyma and except for the skeletal muscle fibers, most cells will die as a result of this invasion. The muscle and, to a lesser extent the brain, support growth of the larvae, and after 20 days they become encysted. They eventually die and become calcified.

During their intestinal transit, *T. spiralis* causes inflammation with hyperemia, swelling of the intestinal villi and Peyer patches, and eosinophilic infiltration of the lamina propria. The muscles of the limbs, external ocular muscules, the masseters, and diaphragm are most frequently affected. Larvae penetrate the muscle fibers causing their degeneration and an inflammatory reaction (Figure 11.13). Within several weeks encystment begins, a collagen layer develops around the cyst and is completed in three months. Within a few months the lesion is calcified. Larvae in heart muscle produce a transient and inconsequential myocarditis, but do not encyst. When *T. spiralis* invades the CNS, it causes cerebral edema, perivascular lymphocytic infiltration, petechial hemorrhages, and granulomatous lesions that may contain larvae. The meninges may also be inflamed.

Trichinosis can mimic many clinical syndromes and as a consequence is often misdiagnosed. The onset of symptoms begins one to three weeks after eating infected pork meat. In subclinical forms of the disease only blood eosinophilia may be fortuitously discovered. In mild infections the eosinophilia may be associated with facial and periorbital edema, myalgia of the neck and low back, and transient diarrhea. In severe infections the intestinal phase is characterized by anorexia, abdominal pain, and diarrhea; and during the muscle invasion phase there is fever, headache, periorbital and facial edema, myalgia, muscle tenderness, and weakness (79). Encephalitis, meningitis, myocarditis, bronchopneumonia, and nephritis may occur in severe infections and these complications may be fatal although recovery may occur after several weeks. Eosinophilia is present in most patients, but does not parallel the severity of the infection. Hypoalbuminemia is frequent in severe infections and the serum enzymes including creatine kinase (CK) are usually elevated in cases with muscle involvement.

Involvement of the CNS in the 1st week resembles any acute meningoencephalitis with headache, lethargy, and confusion. Two to 3 weeks later partial seizures, hemiparesis, dysphasia, and ataxia appear alone or in combination. Examination of the CSF may be normal or demonstrate increased pressure, pleocytosis and increased protein concentration.

Patients with myositis and eosinophilia with the recent history of eating raw or improperly cooked pork meat

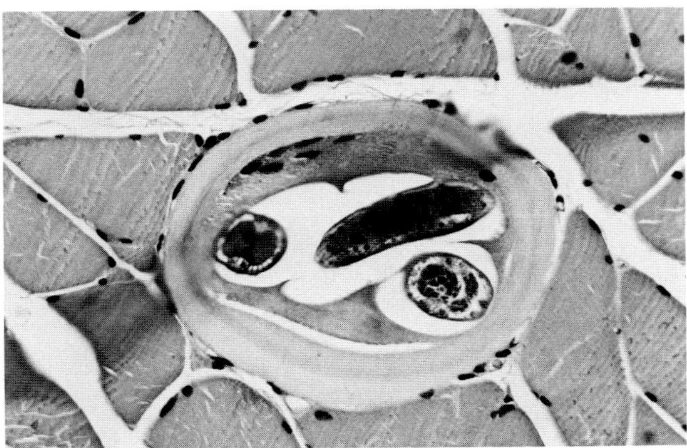

FIGURE 11.13 Trichinosis of skeletal muscle showing a single coiled T spiralis larva. H&E × 200 before a 49% reduction.

should suggest trichinosis as first diagnosis. Homemade sausage and similar pork products may have escaped proper inspection. The definitive diagnosis is made by identification of the larvae in the patient's muscle biopsy, but this valuable diagnostic test should not be performed before the 3rd week after onset of symptoms. The preferred muscles for biopsy are deltoid and gastrocnemius.

Intradermal skin and precipitin tests are available but their specificity is in doubt. The most reliable and specific laboratory aid is the complement fixation test.

There is no specific treatment for trichinosis. Symptomatic treatment consists of antipyretics and analgesics, and severely ill patients may require corticosteroids. Thiabendazole has been shown experimentally to kill larvae and is recommended for severe infections. Prevention of trichinosis may be accomplished by thoroughly cooking or freezing pork.

Tenia solium

Tenia solium belongs to the class Cestodea which includes the most common helminths parasitic to man: *Tenia saginata, T. solium, Dyphyllobothrium latum,* and *Echinococcus granulosus.* Humans acquire teniasis by ingesting inadequately cooked infested pork. The worms develop in the intestine of the host and may reach a length of 10 to 20 feet. *T. solium* consists of a head or scolex, a thin unsegmented neck, and a segmented portion or strobila composed of individual proglottids. Some species of tapeworms have one animal as a final host and another as an intermediary host. In the case of *T. solium,* man is the final host and the intermediary host is the pig. However, if man ingests the eggs of *T. solium,* the life cycle of the *T. solium* changes and cysticercosis, an infestation of tissues by larvae, develops.

The helminthiasis (teniasis) produced by *T. solium* is most common in Eastern Europe, Central and South America, parts of Africa, China, and India, and is rare in the US. The infection results from ingestion of *T. solium* eggs in contaminated food. It is possible that eggs released from proglottids and regurgitated to the stomach re-enter the intestine and initiate the life cycle. The shell or cuticle covering the egg dissolves in the host's stomach or proximal small intestine. An oncosphere, or infectious embryo, emerges and penetrates the intestinal wall and enters the blood stream to be passively carried to the tissue of other organs such as muscle, lung, heart, eyes, and brain, where they encyst and grow causing cysticerosis. The *Cysticercus* consists of a liquid filled vesicle of variable size with an invaginated scolex (Figure 11.14).

The clinical manifestations of the teniasis may be inapparent or mild. Some infected persons complain of abdominal discomfort. Eosinophilia may be present in response to this infection. The diagnosis is made by examining the feces for eggs and proglottids of *T. solium.*

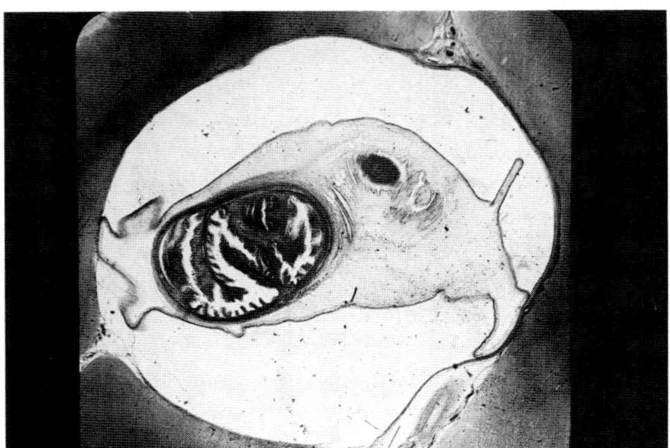

FIGURE 11.14 Cerebral cysticercosis: the scolex of cysticercus is invaginated and surrounded by fluid. H&E ×50 before a 49% reduction.

The treatment of *T. solium* is the same as for T. saginata. The drug Niclosamide is administered orally (2 g) and chewed thoroughly (80). The drug has a direct toxic effect on the worm causing its release from the intestinal mucosa and degeneration. Precautions taken to avoid the disease include cooking pork thoroughly and controlling fecal contamination of pig feeding areas.

Cysticercosis is caused by the larval forms of *T. solium*. Humans become the intermediate host in the parasite's life by ingesting food or water contaminated with human feces (most common source), autoinfection from anus to mouth by persons with adult *T. solium,* and least likely reverse peristalsis and intestinal infection.

The oncospore develops rapidly after penetrating the host's intestinal wall. Within three weeks the scolex is visible in the cyst and by 10 weeks is a fully infective larva. The cyst is initially 0.5 cm to 1 cm in diameter, and contains the invaginated scolex and a yellowish fluid; it remains viable for 3 to 5 years and then degenerates (81). At this time the cyst evokes an inflammatory reaction. Cysticercus show a strong affinity for muscles, liver, lung, heart, subcutaneous tissue, and brain.

Cysticercosis is most common in Mexico, Central and South America, and certain parts of Africa and India. It is occasionally reported in the border states of the Southwestern US. McCormick et al. reported 127 cases of CNS involvement during a 10-year period in Los Angeles (82). Reports of cysticercosis in infants and children are less common than in adults. The majority of patients had seizures and all symptomatic children had increased intracranial pressure. No sex or race predominance has been reported. The incubation period is difficult to establish but may average 4 to 8 years. In the early stages of the disease when the larvae may be passively disseminated, there are usually no symptoms or only myalgia due to focal myositis. Occasionally the presence of cysts is revealed by the presence of multiple subcutaneous nodules or radiographic calcifications.

Cerebral cysticercosis produces a variety of symptoms and signs that develop when the death of the parasite elicits an inflammatory reaction. The cysts may be located anywhere within the brain but there is preference for the cerebral gray matter, followed by the brain stem, cerebellum, and the spinal cord in that order. An unusual racemose form of cysticercosis may be seen when the parasite develops in the basal cisterns, the ventricles, or the spinal subarachnoid space. The cysts grow to form large vesicles with projections and loculations. The racemose cyst is sterile; it has no scolex and is formed by an abnormal growth of the cysticercus wall (Figure 11.15). Racemose cysts may block CSF circulation, producing obstructive hydrocephalus.

The typical cysticercus cellulosae has a life span of from 2 to 5 years after which calcification occurs. The cysts within the brain may be single or multiple, and are found in cavities produced by displacement atrophy of the surrounding brain tissue. Recently developed cysts have a capsule of variable thickness and brain tissue around them shows minimal astrocytic reaction. As cysts enlarge and age, and tissue response is more apparent and when the parasite dies, there is an inflammatory and foreign body reaction with mononuclear and giant cells. Cysticercus arteritis is a characteristic reaction of the small cerebral arteries. When the cysticercus affects the meninges, a severe granulomatous inflammation develops with obliteration of the subarachnoid spaces and development of hydrocephalus.

One of three clinical presentations may predominate in CNS cysticercosis: seizures, increased intracranial pressure, or psychiatric symptoms. Additional clinical features may include headache, visual disturbances, nausea, vomiting, ataxia, and most commonly, papilledema. Seizures may occur and are partial or generalized, sometimes presenting initially as status epilepticus. Increased intracranial pressure is commonly present and may begin abruptly. The psychiatric symptoms are frequent and vary from minor memory loss to delusional states and sometimes dementia. Spinal cysticercosis is a rare form of the disease accounting for only 5% of all cases of CNS cysticercosis. In one review

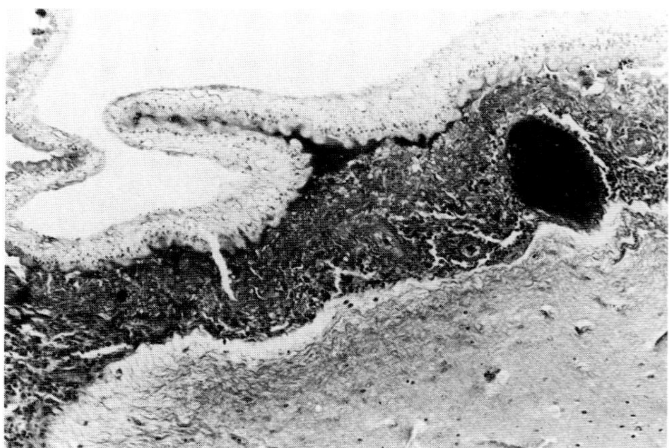

FIGURE 11.15 Cysticercus racemosa membrane and severe meningeal reaction.

of cases, there were only 15 patients with intramedullary and 40 with extramedullary cysticercosis (83). The disease may progress or exhibit long periods of exacerbation and remission, and may sometimes quickly resolve.

The CSF is usually clear and under normal or increased pressure; there is a lymphocytic pleocytosis when active meningitis is present. In an analysis of 89 cases of cysticercosis in children, 50% had abnormal CSF (84). The glucose concentration tends to be low and the protein elevated in active meningitis. Slight to moderate eosinophilia in the peripheral blood is frequent but inconsistent.

Confirmation of the clinical diagnosis of cysticercosis is aided by serologic tests. The indirect hemagglutination appears to be the most reliable; however, false-positives occur in 2% to 15% of cases. An ELISA has been developed to measure specific antibodies to cysticercus antigens. High immunoglobulin levels are present in the CSF and serum when meningitis or ependymitis are present. The elevated immunologic response in the CSF appears to be related to the death of the parasite. Serologic examination of both serum and CSF should be performed (85).

Completion of MRI and CT head scans without enhancement usually demonstrate the radiolucent cysts, cerebral edema, and calcification in dead cysticerci (Figure 11.16). CT with enhancement may show the hyperemic ring around a young cyst (Figure 11.16). Plain skull radiographs may show findings consistent with increased intracranial pressure or the punctate calcification of a dead cysticercus or both.

The treatment of cerebral cysticercosis may require surgical intervention to remove the individual cysts responsible for focal neurologic deficits or to relieve obstruction in the CSF circulation by ventriculostomy or shunt placement. Symptomatic treatment includes the control of seizures, and reduction of cerebral edema with steroids when necessary.

Mebendazole and Praziquantel have been reported to be effective in killing the larval stage of cysticercus (86). However, the value of drug therapy may be limited because the parasite may already be degenerating at the time symptoms appear. Prevention of infection by control of human excrement deposits is important. Inspection of meat products, especially pork, will also reduce the disease.

Schistosomiasis (Bilharziasis)

Schistosomiasis is caused by any of three species of *Schistosoma* worms of the class Trematoda (flukes): *S. mansoni, S. japonicum,* and *S. haematobium.* These parasites affect millions of persons worldwide and their prevalence is increasing. In the US the number of individuals with schistosomiasis has been estimated to exceed 400,000 persons (87), most of whom are immigrants from endemic areas. Infections with *S. mansoni,* a parasite transmitted to man by the snail, prevail in Africa, South America, and the

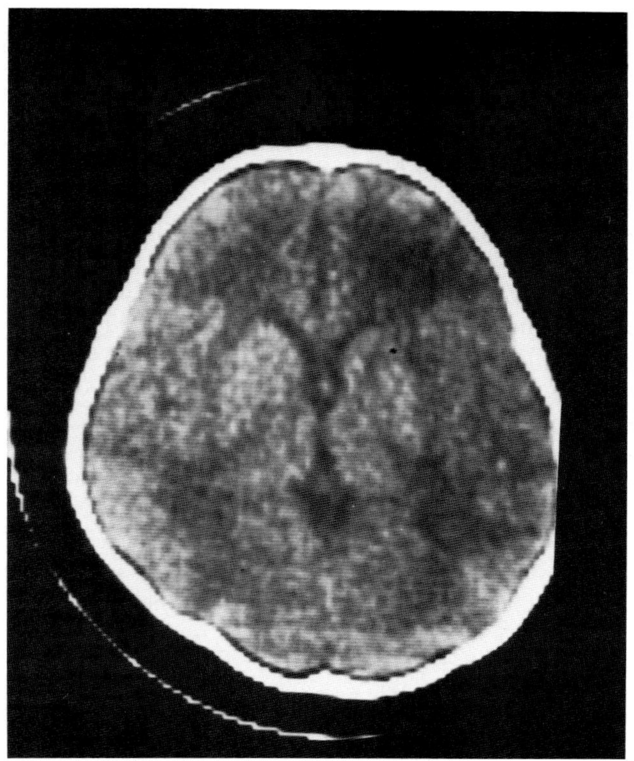

FIGURE 11.16   **A:** CT head scan without contrast of a patient with cerebral cysticerosis showing edema of the white matter. **B:** CT head scan with contrast of the same patient showing multiple enhancing lesions in both cerebral hemispheres.

West Indies. *S. japonicum* is found only in Asia—China, Malaysia, the Philippines, and Japan. The intermediate host is the snail while dogs, monkeys, rats, pigs, and cattle serve as reservoirs. *S. haematobium* also has a snail as the intermediate host and the human disease is prevalent in Africa, the Middle East, and Southeastern India.

S. japonicum lives in the superior mesenteric veins and some organisms find their way to the brain, choroid plexus, and veins around the spinal cord. *S. haematobium* is found in the visceral plexus. The female organisms lay eggs throughout their lives. The eggs of *S. mansoni* are oval and possess a lateral spine; those of *S. japonicum* are globular and lack a spine, while those of *S. haematobium* are oval with a terminal spine.

The human is the definitive host for the three *Schistosoma* species. Adult worms living in the intestinal venous system or the urinary bladder start the sexual life cycle by passing their eggs into urine or stool. In fresh water the eggs hatch, releasing ciliated motile miracidia that soon penetrate into the body of the specific snail intermediate host. It is the absence of a specific snail species in the US that prevents the transmission of the infection in this country.

The miracidia multiply asexually in the snail and within 4 to 5 weeks, hundreds of mobile cercaria emerge. The cercaria are the infective form and penetrate the skin of the human host where they change into adult forms that migrate to the lungs and liver. Within 6 weeks the adult worm moves through the venous system reaching its final habitat.

The clinical manifestations of schistosomiasis are only present in heavily infected persons and are rarely seen in occasional travelers through endemic areas. Three major syndromes have been described: dermatitis, Katayama fever, and the chronic fibro-obstructive sequelae. The penetrating cercaria have been associated with a pruritic rash called swimmer's itch resulting from a sensitization phenomenon since it occurs in previously exposed persons. When the worms have matured and the deposition of eggs begins, Katayama fever or acute schistosomiasis may be observed with fever, generalized lymphadenopathy, hepatomegaly, and splenomegaly. It is suggested to result from immunocomplex formation by massive antigen challenge from the eggs. Neither swimmer's itch nor Katayama fever consititute a serious clinical problem, but the chronic stage is directly related to the intensity of the infection. The host reaction to eggs retained in the tissues results in a granulomatous response. Hepatomegaly is secondary to portal vein fibrosis and splenomegaly follows. Portal vein obstruction may lead to hematemesis from bleeding of esophageal varices. The terminal stage of hepatosplenomegaly is liver failure, secondary infections, and uremia. Pulmonary schistosomiasis may be manifested by signs and symptoms of cor pulmonale, obstruction of pulmonary blood flow secondary to arteritis, and granuloma formation (88).

Involvement of the CNS is rare, accounting for 3% of complications of *S. japonicum* (89). Although the majority

of reported cases of CNS schistosomiasis results from *S. japonicum* infections (89), there are occasional cases secondary to *S. mansoni*, and *S. haematobium*. In one report of 95 cases of schistosomiasis affecting the CNS, organisms involved included: *S. japonicum*, identified in 60 cases with 2 involving a spinal cord; *S. mansoni* in 26 cases with 1 case involving the spinal cord; and *S. haematobium* was found in 11 cases, 8 of which involved the spinal cord involvement (90).

The clinical manifestations of CNS schistosomiasis may be in the form of an acute encephalopathy with altered sensorium, confusion, seizures, and coma; meningeal signs may be present. The tissue response is a granulomatous reaction resembling tuberculosis, with the center of the lesion necrotic, containing the eggs, eosinophils, and spindle shaped cells. There is a middle zone of epithelioid cells and lymphocytes, and a granulation tissue zone with lymphocytes, plasma cells, fibroblasts, and macrophages, surrounded by a peripheral zone of gliosis (Figure 11.17).

Spinal cord involvement in the disease may be manifested as: a myelitic form with destruction, vacuolation, and atrophy of the cord; intrathecal granuloma production; or radicular form with microscopic granulomas and fibrosis over the cauda equina and conus medullaris (91,92).

Schistosomiasis more commonly affects the brain than spinal cord but the manner by which the schistosoma eggs reach the brain or the cord is not determined. The onset of cerebral disease may occur from 2 to 3 months after exposure, as an acute encephalopathy (93). In some cases the CNS symptoms appear later, up to 6 months after symptoms of systemic disease. Patients may have focal neurologic signs resulting in long-term sequelae. Spinal cord symptoms are generally low back pain with leg cramps, followed by paraplegia and sphincter disturbances. Functional recovery is rare, and death from widespread spinal cord necrosis has been reported (94). The CSF generally shows a lymphocytic pleocytosis with increased concentration of protein.

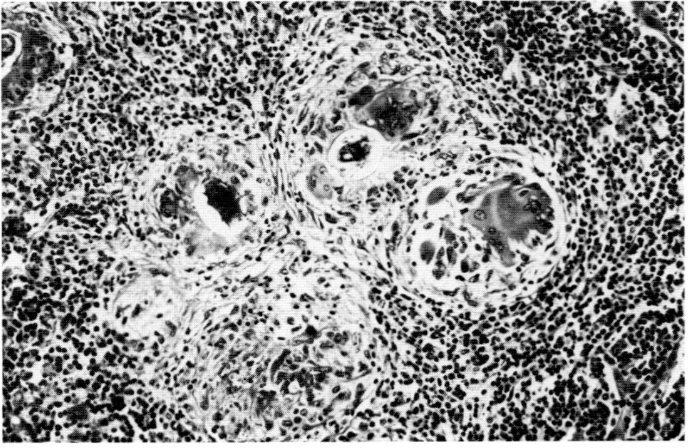

FIGURE 11.17 Cerebral schistosomiasis showing the parasite and granulomatous reaction with lymphocytes, epithelioid and giant cells. H&E ×200 before a 49% reduction.

The diagnosis of CNS schistosomiasis is difficult to establish in nonendemic areas. The definitive diagnosis can be made by finding eggs in feces, urine, or biopsy specimens. In CNS infections without evidence of eggs in feces, urine, or rectal mucosa, a positive serologic test will support the diagnosis (95).

Human schistosomiasis is treated with Praziquantel, a broad-spectrum antihelminthic agent, which is effective against all *Schistosoma* species (96); side effects are minimal. Other oral preparations are also effective but with limited range of parasite specificity. Mitrifonale is effective in treating *S. haematobium* infection and oxamniquine has been effective in treating *S. mansoni*. In cases where intracerebral granulomas progressively enlarge and result in increased intracranial pressure, surgical removal of the lesions may be required.

Paragonimiasis

Paragonimiasis is essentially a pulmonary parasitic disease caused by the trematode *Paragonimus westermani* (lung fluke). The disease is prevalent in the Far East and Southeast Asia, but also occurs in parts of Africa and South America.

Humans, the final hosts, acquire the infection from eating raw or undercooked crab or crayfish (97). Occasionally, the disease is acquired by handling crab when preparing food, and by giving crawfish juice as a medicine to infants and young children with measles (Korea), or drinking crab juice as an antifebrile medication (Japan).

The parasite *P. westermani* is a reddish-brown fluke measuring 5 mm × 10 mm; the ova measure 85 μ × 55 μ. The eggs coughed up in the sputum are expectorated, develop in fresh water and hatch. The miracidia penetrate the appropriate snails and undergo asexual multiplication. Cercaria emerging from the snails then enter the fresh water crabs or crayfish and transform to encysted metacercariae. When ingested by man the cysts are digested and the parasites penetrate the intestinal wall, pass to the peritoneal cavity, penetrate the diaphragm and pleura, and reach the lung where they develop into adult worms. Symptoms do not occur until the stage of inflammatory reaction around the worm and eggs. Onset of signs and symptoms is usually insidious with fever, sporadic cough, and production of blood-tinged sputum. Gross hemoptysis and severe pleuritic chest pain may occur. The disease may spontaneously arrest at any stage. Worms in the abdominal cavity can cause hepatitis, enteritis, lymphadenitis, or draining fistulae.

CNS paragonimiasis is serious and sometimes fatal. The parasite may reach the brain via the blood stream or by migrating from the primary lesion in the lung along the wall of the jugular veins, entering the skull through the jugular foramen (98). Within the cranial cavity, the parasite continues along the dural sinus and veins to the parietotemporal and occipital regions where the larvae mature into adult worms. The CNS lesions are varied but are generally of three histopathologic types, including: (stage I) meningoencephalitic, (stage II) granulomatous, and (stage III) the form of organization and calcification (99,100).

The meningoencephalitic form is characterized by nonencapsulated, early necrotizing granuloma formation. The meninges are diffusely infiltrated by purulent inflammatory exudate containing lymphocytes. The encephalitic features include perivascular infiltrates, glial nodules, and occasional vasculitis. The granulomatous form (stage II) consists of an encapsulated granuloma, sometimes multiloculated and cystic with a necrotic center containing the eggs of *P. westermani*. In Stage III the granuloma becomes organized and the cystic necrotic center calcifies; eggs are not easily seen. Charcot-Leyden crystals are surrounded by thick collagenous tissue. In spinal cord disease, the common lesion is an extradural granuloma in the thoracic region manifested by spastic paraplegia, radicular pain, paresthesias, and spincter disturbances.

The CSF may be under increased pressure with a primarily lymphocytic pleocytosis and occasional eosinophils. The CSF protein may be elevated. Skull radiographs and CT head scans may demonstrate intracranial calcification, and in one report, calcification was observed in one-half of all patients with CNS disease (101).

Demonstration of *P. westermani* in the sputum, stools, or pleural fluid would confirm the diagnosis. The complement fixation test in the CSF is positive in 42% of cases (102).

The treatment of choice is administration of bithionol which halts egg production and kills the parasites (103). The drug is also effective in the acute and subacute phases of cerebral paragonimiasis, but is ineffective in the chronic stages of the disease. Surgical removal or drainage of an abscess or granuloma may be necessary.

Echinococcosis (Hydatid Cyst)

Hydatid disease is caused by the larvae of the tapeworm *Echinococcus granulosus*, a parasite of dogs, the definitive natural host to the adult form of *E. granulosus*. The larvae may develop in humans resulting in hydatid cysts.

Echinococcosis is widely distributed throughout the world and consitutes a serious problem in sheep and cattle raising countries, particularly Australia, New Zealand, and Iceland. Other endemic areas include Greece, Rumania, Spain, Italy, Argentina, Uruguay, South Africa, Russia, Turkey, Lebanon, Syria, and Egypt. Indigenous infections are also seen in California, Utah, and Arizona.

The adult *E. granulosus* is a small tapeworm, 3 mm to 6 mm in length, and is composed of 4 or 5 segments. The hydatid cysts are white, spherical, and filled with fluid, varying in size from a few mm to several cm in diameter.

Children and adults acquire the disease by direct contact with dog excreta or by consumption of uncooked contaminated food. Following their ingestion, eggs hatch in the duodenum, releasing larvae that penetrate the intestinal wall, and are carried to the liver, lungs, and other organs by hematogenous dissemination where they develop into hydatid cysts. For the parasite to complete its life cycle, the hydatid cyst with its contents must be ingested by a canine host as in the case of slaughtered infected sheep whose organs containing hydatid cysts are fed to sheep dogs.

The hydatid cyst increases in size by about 1 cm yearly, compressing adjacent host structures as it enlarges. When a cyst ruptures it may produce an anaphylactic reaction, and the cyst contents may seed the area, producing a second generation of hydatid cysts. The most common location for their occurrence include the liver (63%), lungs (25%), muscles (5%), and bones (3%). Involvement of brain has been estimated to occur in 1% to 2% of cases. About one-half of patients with hydatid disease are children (104).

Intracranial hydatid cysts are usually subcortical, single, and spherical, commonly involving the temporal and temporoparietal regions. They may become quite large. Multiple cerebral cysts are rare and result from dissemination of scolices or rupture of a cyst during attempts at surgical removal. The brain tends to accommodate to the slowly enlarging mass without causing notable neurologic signs (105).

Children may initially have signs and symptoms of increased intracranial pressure. Focal signs occur, and seizures may be present. Intraspinal cysts are uncommon but may cause spinal cord compression. CT and MRI head scans are most important in demonstrating structural abnormalities. Serologic tests including complement fixation and indirect hemagglutination tests are available, but not of uniform reliability.

The treatment of cerebral hydatid cysts is complete surgical removal of the cyst, avoiding its puncture to prevent seeding and recurrence of symptoms. Although there is no specific drug therapy for hydatid disease, Mebendazole administered over a period of at least several months has been attempted with some success (106).

Coenurosis

Coenurosis is a parasitic disease of humans when they become the intermediary host of the tapeworm larvae of *Multiceps multiceps*, a cestode. The adult tapeworm *M. multiceps* inhabits the intestinal tract of dogs, foxes, coyotes, and wolves. The eggs ingested by sheep, cattle, horses, and mammals develop into coenurus. The life cycle of this tapeworm is similar to that of *E. granulosus*.

Humans are accidentally infected by ingesting the eggs, usually from dog excreta. The oncospheres hatch in the intestine, penetrate the intestinal wall, and enter the circulation and may reach the CNS where larvae develop into coenurus, a cyst with multiple scolices, but without capsules or daughter cysts (107). Human CNS coenurosis is rare: there are only occasional reports in sheep raising countries, especially South Africa (108).

The parasitic larvae of *M. multiceps* have a predilection for the CSF pathways and are found scattered in the basal cisterns, and the third and fourth ventricles. They produce signs and symptoms of increased intracranial pressure and can be clinically manifested as acute or chronic intermittent hydrocephalus. Examination of the CSF shows pleocytosis and elevated concentration of protein. The majority of cases of coenurosis has been reported in adults, and only occasionally will the disease affect children. A fatal instance of multilocular coenurosis in the posterior fossa has been reported in a child (109), and 14-year-old patient had paraplegia secondary to intramedullary coenurosis (110). Ocular involvement has been described (111). The diagnosis is generally established at surgery, with the identification of the parasitic cyst that differs from a hydatid cyst because of its smaller size and having several scolices.

Protozoal Diseases

Protozoa, found throughout nature as free living organisms, are a complex group of unicellular organisms. They are eukaryotic, uni- or multinucleated, and reproduce sexually and asexually. Sexual reproduction takes place within the definitive host and results in the formation of a zygote. As parasites they can infest all species of vertebrates and many invertebrates.

Protozoa are classified morphologically as flagellates, amebas, sporozoa, and ciliates. The flagellates may be parasitic in humans as in the case of trypanosomes, and like trichomonades may occupy only the intestine or genital tract. Amebas are primarily inhabitants of humans; some species are free living and may become parasitic to invade the CNS. The sporozoae include organisms that have asexual and sexual reproductive cycles. Plasmodia have an asexual cycle in mammals and a sexual cycle in mosquitoes, and *Toxoplasma* have an asexual cycle in the epithelial cells of feline intestinal walls and a sexual cycle in the mouse. This discussion is limited to protozoal diseases that affect the human central nervous system.

Toxoplasma Infections

Toxoplasma gondi, an obligate intracellular protozoan ubiquitous in nature, is the cause of toxoplasma infections (toxoplasmosis). Toxoplasma infections, widespread in a large portion of the world human population, may be acute or chronic, and symptomatic or asymptomatic. The acute infection is usually asymptomatic, but when symptoms occur they are usually of short duration and self limited. In most cases, tissue cysts of organisms persist but the patient has no manifestation of clinical disease. Toxoplasmosis, however, can cause persistent or recrudescent clinical symptoms. Toxoplasmosis occurring in immunocompromised patients can be life threatening, causing encephalitis, myocarditis, or pneumonia. Fetal toxoplasma infections can result in congenital cerebral and ocular anomalies (112).

T. gondi can infect birds and all mammals including man. It is usually acquired by humans who ingest undercooked or raw meat. All human toxoplasma infections are derived from cats, the only definitive host known to harbor the parasite in its asexual stage. The only exception is transmission by organ transplantation (113). Frenkel recognized two patterns of transmission, one in children and the other in adults (114). Childhood infections begin about the age of one year from contact with sand or soil contaminated with cat feces. Fifty percent to 70% of children have developed antibodies by the time of adolescence. Adult infections start late in adolescence and continue throughout adult years.

T. gondi exists in the following three forms: tachyzoites (trophozoites), tissue cysts, and oocysts. Tachyzoites are oval or crescentic in shape and are $4 \mu \times 8 \mu$ in size. They invade all human cells except non-nucleated erythrocytes. Proliferation of tachyzoites produce foci of necrosis with intense mononuclear reaction and development of humoral and cellular immunity.

Tissue cysts vary in size from 100μ to 200μ and may contain as many as 3,000 organisms. Toxoplasma infection is transmitted to humans and other carnivores by ingestion of tissue cysts in raw or uncooked meat. The digestive enzymes disrupt the cyst wall and release the organisms which then invade the intestinal mucosa, and by hematogenous dissemination are spread throughout the body. Tissue cysts can be found in any organ, especially brain, heart, and muscle; they remain viable for the remainder of the host's life and are responsible for the chronic phase of the disease. This constitutes the asymptomatic or chronic toxoplasma infection (115). The oocysts are ovoid, 10μ to 12μ in diameter and are produced only in the intestine of the cat.

The CNS can be severely affected in patients with congenital infection, patients treated with immunosuppressant drugs, and those patients with HIV (AIDS). In these cases, acute focal or diffuse meningoencephalitis and extensive areas of brain necrosis with vasular involvement may be observed (Figure 11.18). Periventricular and periaqueduc-

tal necrosis are characteristic of toxoplasmosis. The lesions may become calcified and are readily apparent on skull radiographs. Hydrocephalus may develop and is usually secondary to aqueductal obstruction. In immunodeficient adult patients, the major finding is necrotizing encephalitis with small, diffusely distributed lesions (Figure 11.19). Large abscesses may also occur. Typical ocular lesions (116) include acute chorioretinitis with severe inflammation and necrosis, necrotizing retinitis and granulomatous chorioretinitis (116). The myocardium and skeletal muscle may contain tissue cysts without inflammation or there may be widespread myositis.

Congenital toxoplasmosis is the result of acute, usually asymptomatic infection, acquired by the mother during the pregnancy. If the pregnant woman is infected before conception, there is no risk of transmission of the organism to the fetus (115). Maternal antibodies acquired from infection prior to pregnancy prevents fetal infection. Fetal infection occurs via the placenta but does not occur during the 1st 2 months of pregnancy; it is found in 2 to 3 per 1,000 births (115). During the 2nd trimester the risk of infection increases and continues to increase during the 6th and 7th month of gestation. There is a high incidence of premature births.

Toxoplasma proliferates in the ependymal lining and subependymal regions and spreads widely because of the lack of antibodies. Morphologic changes include lymphocytic infiltration of meninges, destructive lesions of both grey and white matter, and focal periventricular and periaqueductal calcifications. Microcephaly and chorioretinitis are common sequelae of the congenital infection.

Clinical signs of toxoplasma infection are evident during the neonatal period (115). Premature infants may have severe CNS and ocular disease during the first few months of life. Term infants develop a milder disease with hepatomegaly usually appearing in the first two months of life. Symptoms of CNS involvement generally appear later. Eichenwald reported 152 infants with toxoplasmosis:

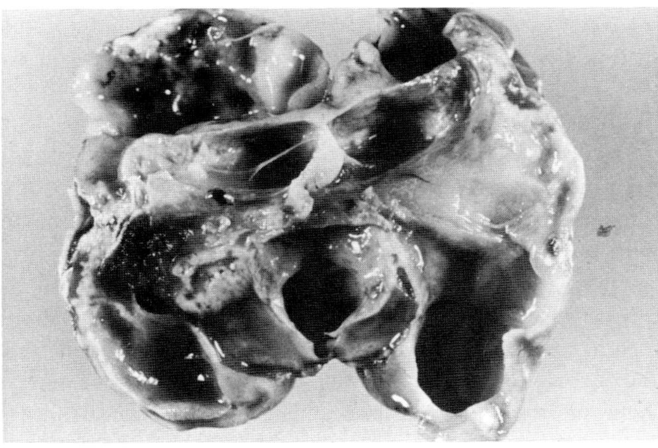

FIGURE 11.18   Neonatal cerebral toxoplasmosis showing extensive necrosis and cavitation of the white matter with hydrocephalus.

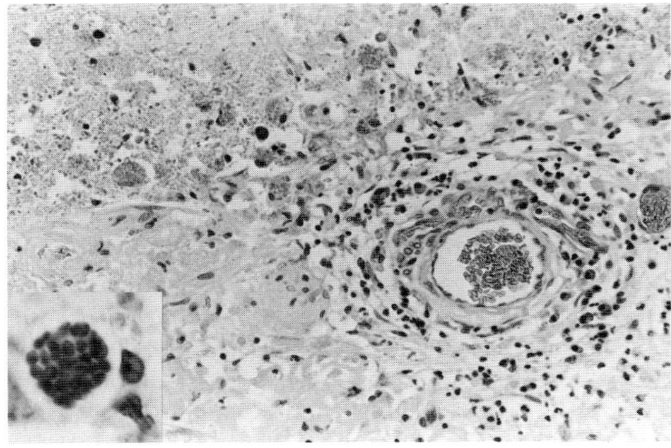

FIGURE 11.19   Cerebral toxoplasmosis showing small arteriole with inflammatory reaction. Inset shows a toxoplasma cyst. H&E ×400 before a 49% reduction.

neurologic manifestations were prominent in 108, chorioretinitis in 95%, abnormal CSF findings in 55%, convulsions in 50%, intracranial calcification in 50%, obstructive hydrocephalus in 28%, and microcephaly in 30%. A four year follow-up evaluation of 100 patients showed: 80% of patients were mentally retarded; 81% had seizures; 70% have some motor deficit; hydrocephalus or microcephaly or both were present in 42% and deafness in 16%. Only 11% were considered normal (117). Silent infection was found to be most common in retrospective studies (118–120). Congenital toxoplasmosis must be distinguished from other congenital infections of the TORCH group, including rubella, herpes simplex, and cytomegalovirus.

The diagnosis of toxoplasmosis in older children depends on serologic tests and the isolation of *T. gondi.* Isolation of toxoplasma from blood or other body fluids establishes that the infection is acute. In neonates isolation of the organism from any tissue including the placenta is diagnostic of congenital toxoplasmosis (115). If antibodies are present, a definite diagnosis of toxoplasmosis requires demonstration of the organism, usually in cyst form in stained preparations of brain, liver or spleen. The presence of tachyzoites in tissue sections or smears of body fluids will also establish the diagnosis (115).

Cerebrospinal fluid findings include mononuclear pleocytosis, elevation of protein concentration and normal glucose. Serologic tests, which indicate specific antibodies to toxoplasma, are useful in establishing the diagnosis in many cases. The most commonly used serologic test is the Indirect Fluorescent Antibody test and IgG ELISA that has replaced the Sabin-Feldman dye test.

IgG antibodies may be transferred passively from the mother to the fetus across the placenta. IgG antibody titer is present in a newborn by the third month of life. For detection of IgM antibody, the ELISA method is preferred because of its greater sensitivity. The demonstration of IgM antibodies in the neonate is diagnostic of congenital toxoplasmos.

Treatment consists of the administration of pyrithamine, a folic acid antagonist that may cause bone marrow suppression. It is necessary to carefully monitor the patient for leukopenia and thrombocytopenia. Sulfadiazine can be used in combination as treatment for tachyzoites. The treatment period is 4 to 6 weeks. The cystic form of toxoplasma is resistant to presently available drugs.

Acute acquired toxoplasmosis in pregnant women should be treated to lessen the incidence of fetal infection. Therapeutic regimens vary from country to country. If the infection is confirmed, the patient should be treated with pyrimethamine and sulfadiazine until there is evidence that the patient has adequate immunity. The duration of optimal treatment varies from several months to 1 year, depending on the clinical status of the patient (115). Spiramycin is less toxic and though not available in the US, it has been useful in treating pregnant women and infants with congenital toxoplasmosis. Only controlling the spread of oocysts of cats will prevent the transmission of the infection to humans.

Cerebral Malaria

Malaria, an infection caused by a protozoan of the genus *Plasmodium,* is transmitted to humans by infected Anopheles mosquitoes. It is one of the most prevalent diseases in the world (121), with more than 200 million people affected and 1 million consequent deaths estimated to occur annually. The disease, previously found throughout the world is, for the most part, restricted to tropical and subtropical regions. It was eradicated from the US in the late 1940s, but the increase in travel to and from endemic areas in recent years has resulted in a greater number of sporadic cases in this country.

Only four species of the genus *Plasmodium* infect humans, as follows: *Plasmodium falciparum, Plasmodium vivax, Plasmodium malariae,* and *Plasmodium ovale.* Each species has morphologic and biologic characteristics that permit their identification. *P. falciparum,* the most pathogenic of human malarias, causes cerebral malaria and accounts for the majority of fatal cases. The organism is identified by the presence of small ring-stage trophozoite in erythrocytes. As trophozoites mature, they become sequestered in the capillaries of the heart, brain, spleen, and muscle. In the life cycle of Plasmodia, asexual reproduction occurs in humans and sexual reproduction occurs in the mosquito. When the infected Anopheles mosquito penetrates the skin to suck blood, it inoculates its salivary fluids containing sporozoites which initiate the infection. After passing into the peripheral blood, the sporozoites reach the liver, invade the hepatocytes, and undergo asexual reproduction (Schizogonia). A single sporozoite produces between 2,000 and 40,000 merozoites, and 1 to 6 weeks later they are released into the circulation initiating the clinical phase of the disease. Merozoites attach themselves to erythrocytes in which they enlarge and divide. Not all merozoites divide asexually, but differentiate into sexual forms (gametogenesis) called macrogametocyte (female) and microgrametocyte (male), which complete their development within the gastrointestinal tract of the appropriate mosquito. The zygotes penetrate the gut and form oocytes within 24 hours of ingestion of blood meal. Sporozoites then develop and mature in 10 to 14 days forming oocytes which reach the salivary glands. When the mosquito bites the human host, the cycle begins again.

The clinical and pathologic manifestations of malaria result from invasion of erythrocytes by merozoites. The rupture of erythrocytes, and eventually phagocytosis of hemoglobin, and malarial pigment are the consequences of their parasitism. The clinical manifestations are apparent during the erythrocyte phase of the infection. The invasion, growth, maturation, rupture, and re-invasion of the erythrocytes by the asexual parasites cause chills, fever, sweating, and other symptoms associated with malaria. In malaria due to *P. falciparum*, anemia is caused by severe hemolysis and bone marrow depression. Complications can result from capillary blockage by parasitized erythrocytes leading to shock, lung, liver, and renal failure, and mesenteric ischemia (122)(Figure 11.20).

Cerebral malaria is the most severe complication and is caused by blockage of cerebral capillaries with infected erythrocytes which adhere to the vascular endothelium. In fatal cases of cerebral malaria, the brain is edematous with vascular congestion and petechiae in the white matter (123) (Figure 11.21). On occasion, there is selective congestion of the white matter that helps to distinguish cerebral malaria from viral encephalitis in which congestion predominates in the gray matter. Microscopically, examination of the brain shows diffuse edema, congestion with diapedesis of erythrocytes, thrombosis of blood vessels, and perivascular areas of demyelination. Ring hemorrhages, Durck's granulomas (cerebral capillaries surrounded by glial proliferation), and focal areas of demyelination are not specific of cerebral malaria; these lesions are also found in cases of fat emboli. The pathophysiology of cerebral malaria is more complex. Maegraith supported the view that the thromboses of capillaries are terminal events, not essential to the pathogenesis of cerebral malaria (122). The early change is an alteration of the vascular endothelium with disruption of the blood-brain barrier (124). This damage may be initiated by the presence of specific antigen-antibody complexes in the blood (125).

The neurologic manifestations of cerebral malaria include: disturbances of consciousness ranging from somnolence to coma; acute organic brain syndrome with behavioral changes, delirium, hallucinations; partial or generalized seizures; focal signs including extensor plantar response, tremor, myoclonus, hemiparesis, and choreiform movements. Lumbar puncture may show increased CSF pressure, pleocytosis, and increased concentration of protein.

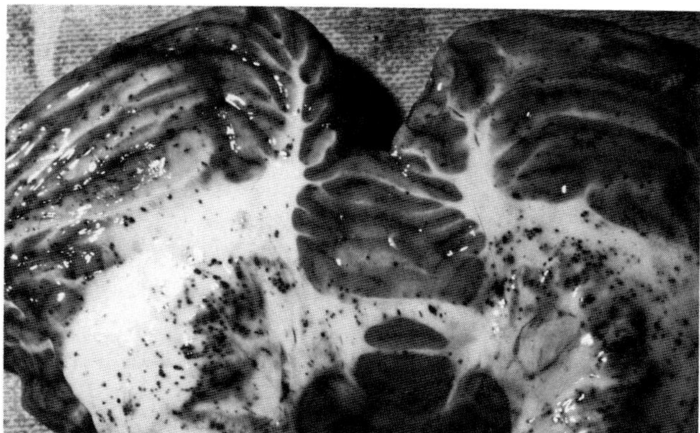

FIGURE 11.21   Cerebral malaria showing petechial hemorrhages in the cerebellar cortex, white matter, and basal ganglia.

Cerebral malaria in children has a dramatic onset during the acute illness. After the onset of fever and headache, the child becomes unresponsive or develops generalized convulsions. These symptoms are often preceded by confusion, obtundation, and tremulousness. Meningeal signs and focal neurologic deficits are rare presenting symptoms in children. Death may occur secondary to status epilepticus associated with hyperthermia, but with appropriate treatment, recovery without sequelae is not infrequent.

The treatment of cerebral malaria is considered to be a medical emergency (126) and includes intravenous administration of chloroquine. Efforts should be made to determine if the patient has traveled in an area of chloroquine resistant *P. falciparum* or has taken chloroquine prophylaxis. In these cases, the patient should be treated with combination chemotherapy including quinine, sulfanilamide, and pyrimethamine. When *P. falciparum* is resistant to all chemotherapeutic agents, intravenous quinine has been suggested for treatment (127). Fluoroquinoline methanol is effective against chloroquine-resistant *P. falciparum* infection. Dexamethasone is no longer recommended and may be deleterious in cerebral malaria (128). Dehydration, hyponatremia, renal failure, and pulmonary edema may develop in these patients.

Amebiasis

Two serious CNS diseases can be produced by protozoa of the group *Entamoeba,* including brain abscess caused by the *Entamoeba histolytica,* and primary meningoencephalitis caused by free living amebas *(Naegleria* and *Acanthamoeba).* Amebic brain abscesses are caused by *E. histolytica,* which is found throughout the world. It inhabits the lumen and mucosa of the large intestine and is the causative agent of amebic dysentery and less frequently extraintestinal infections.

Amebiasis is a common disease in tropical and subtropical climates, affecting up to 50% of the population in underdeveloped areas. *E. histolytica* exists in two forms,

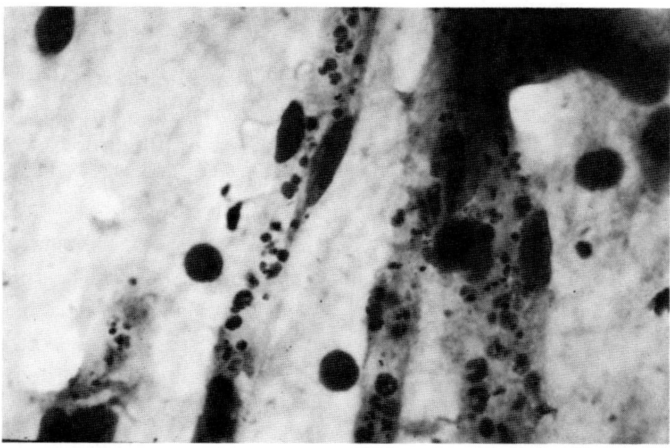

FIGURE 11.20   Malaria: parasitized red cells in cerebral capillaries.

trophozoites and cysts. Trophozoites invade the tissues of the large intestine, may erode the wall to gain entrance into the blood stream, and reach all parts of the body. It most commonly establishes an infection in the liver, and may reach the brain. In extraintestinal amebiasis no cysts are produced. The trophozoites continue to divide by binary fission. Involvement of the CNS in amebiasis is rare, and is usually a late complication of hematogenous dissemination from a primary intestinal infection or, more rarely, from pulmonary or hepatic foci.

Meningoencephalitis caused by *E. histolytica* is very rare and occurs in 0.9% to 8.1% of fatal cases (129). The lesions are found in the well vascularized gray matter, cortex, and basal ganglia. Odunjo found a frequency of 4% in 135 autopsy cases in Nigeria (130).

The earlier lesions consist of a softened area surrounded by petechial hemorrhages, which may cavitate. The abscess wall consists of an inner zone of necrotic tissue, and an outer zone of neovascularization and congestion. The surrounding brain tissue undergoes degeneration, with an inflammatory reaction of primarily lymphocytes, plasma cells, few polymorphonuclear cells, and reactive astrocytosis. The trophozoites are identified in the necrotic abscess wall. The prognosis of patients with brain abscess is very poor and only few surviving cases have been reported (131).

Diseases caused by free living amebas that ordinarily live a nonparasitic existence in soil and fresh water are uncommon. Two genera of ameba are pathogenic for animals and humans, including the better known *Naegleria,* which causes primary ameba meningoencephalitis in man, and the less common *Acanthamoeba,* which is associated with cerebral necrosis in laboratory animals and may cause granulomatous lesions in humans.

Primary Amebic Meningoencephalitis (PAM)

The free living ameba of the genus *Naegleria,* a fresh water ameba-flagellate, causes PAM. *Naegleria flowleri* is responsible for most reported human cases. *Naegleria* has been found in almost every continent (132) and many cases of Naegleria infection have been reported in the US, England, Belgium, Brazil, Australia, Zambia. Healthy children and young adults are primarily affected in summer and fall. The infection is acquired by swimming in fresh water ponds or swimming pools contaminated with ameba.

N. fowleri is 10 μ in diameter with large pseudopodia and a large nucleus with a prominent karyosome. Its life cycle includes trophozoite replication. *N. fowleri* is found in large numbers in fresh water with heavy growth of algae or bacteria (133). The organism gains access to CNS through the nasal mucosa covering the cribriform plate, reaching the nervous tissue which is an appropriate environment for multiplication. Postmortem findings and experimental work by Martinez et al. support this hypothesis. *N. fowleri* produces extensive damage to the

meninges, the olfactory bulbs, and penetrates the brain following the perivascular spaces (134). Clinical manifestations of the disease include severe frontal headaches, lethargy, fever, progressing to nausea, vomiting, and nuchal rigidity, followed by convulsions and coma. The disease is usually fatal within 2 to 7 days.

Lesions produced by *N. fowleri* may be found anywhere in the CNS, including the spinal cord. The involved areas are swollen, soft and congested with the appearance of an acute necrotizing and hemorrhagic meningoencephalitis. The purulent meningeal exudate consists of mononuclear cells and lymphocytes. Hemorrhages present in affected areas are associated with brain tissue destruction and vascular thrombosis. Diffuse meningeal involvement is evident in the CSF with elevated concentrations of protein and low glucose. The ameba *N. fowleri* can be seen in the subarachnoid exudate but may be difficult to distinguish from macrophages. Diagnosis can be confirmed by identification of the parasite in the CSF, biopsy specimen, or culture. Numerous treatment methods have been unsuccessful and most cases of Naegleria meningoencephalitis have been fatal. A few patients have responded to Amphotericin B given intravenously or intrathecally (135–137).

Granulomatous Amebic Encephalitis

Amebas of the *Hartmannella-Acanthamoeba* group cause an acute meningoencephalitis similar to that caused by the Naegleria infection; however, they produce multifocal chronic disease in debilitated patients or in immunosuppressed individuals. Affected persons range from 5 to 58 years of age with equal sex distribution; a history of swimming in pools has not been reported. In one series of 15 patients reviewed by Martinez, 13 suffered from other diseases including liver disease, diabetus mellitus, Hodgkin disease; and all patients were receiving antibiotic therapy, radiotherapy, or steroid therapy. Two patients were pregnant and three were alcoholics (138); few cases with no pre-existing illness have been recorded (139). The clinical course is longer than in encephalitis due to *N. fowleri* and varies from 12 to 120 days.

The clinical symptoms include mental abnormalities, seizures, headaches, hemiparesis, and less frequently, ataxia, aphasia, and visual disturbances. In human cases of granulomatous amebic encephalitis, intracranial arteritis has been reported (140).

The microscopic findings of the affected CNS consist of diffuse meningitis with areas of hemorrhage and necrosis in the cerebrum, cerebellum, or brain stem. Vasculitis of arteries and veins, with associated thrombi occur. Trophozoites can be found in vessel walls and in areas free of inflammation. Some human cases have shown granulomas, arteritis, and mycotic aneurysms (140).

Diagnosis is confirmed by demonstrating CSF pleocytosis, increased concentration of protein, and the presence of amebas in CSF. Meningoencephalitis due to *Hartmannella-Acanthameba* is a fatal disease and no effective treatment has been found. Sulfadiazine and clotrimazole appear effective against some strains of *Acanthomoeba* (139). Other drugs that have been used include 5-fluorocytosine and hydroxystilbamidine isethionate (135).

Trypanosomiasis

The diseases caused by flagellate protozoa of the genus *Trypanosoma* include approximately 20 species, two of which are pathogenic for humans. *Trypanosoma gambiense* and *Trypanosoma rhodesiense* cause sleeping sickness in Africa, and *Trypanosoma cruzi* is responsible for Chagas disease in South and Central America. Endemic areas of African sleeping sickness and Chagas disease do not overlap; there are significant differences in the mode of transmission, pathogenesis, and clinical course.

African Trypanosomiasis (Sleeping Sickness)

There are two variants of sleeping sickness; Eastern (acute) and Western (chronic). Eastern African trypanosomiasis is caused by *T. rhodesiense,* and Western African trypanosomiasis by *T. gambiense.*

Sleeping sickness is endemic through equatorial Africa. The infecting trypanosomes tend to remain extracellular in the host's connective tissue. Immune reaction to trypanosomes and antibody production lead to appearance of circulating immune complexes in blood and CSF (141). A few days after the insect bite, the inoculated parasites invade the blood stream and reach various organs. The parasites live extracellularly in the blood, CSF, and interstitial spaces. Invasion of the blood stream is accompanied by fever, erythema, edema, and tachycardia. In the fly's gut the trypanosomas multiply and transform into metatrypanosomes, which are infective to humans. The minimum infective dose for most hosts is 300 to 500 organisms. The two African trypanosomes cause similar clinical symptoms but the course is different.

The disease caused by *T. rhodesiense* usually follows an acute course, with an incubation period of 3 to 4 weeks and a clinical course of several weeks. The brain is invaded after 3 to 4 weeks causing severe meningoencephalitis and involvement of the lymphoid system. There are numerous foci of perivascular lymphocyte or plasma cell infiltrates in the brain parenchyma. The presence of plasma cells with pyknotic nuclei and vacuolated cytoplasm filled with Russell bodies are distinctive features. Neuronal injury and demyelination are rare. Trypanosomes, rarely demonstrable in tissue sections, are found in the the blood or CSF.

T. gambiense disease has an incubation period of several weeks to months and the brain invasion occurs much later. CNS involvement is heralded by headache, an indifference to the environment, neck stiffness, and somnolence, alternating with insomnia at night. There are also disorders of thermoregulation, progressive mental deterioration, focal neurologic signs, seizures, tremors, and palsies. Patients may progress to coma and die, usually from associated complications such as bronchopneumonia. Trypanosomiasis is more likely to be missed in its early stages in children (142,143). The disease progresses rapidly, often not discovered until there are psychiatric symptoms. The patient may develop seizures and progress to coma.

The diagnosis of trypanosomiasis is suggested in persons with a history of travel in endemic regions, and especially if bitten by the tsetse fly. Definite diagnosis depends on finding the trypanosome in blood, CSF, or lymph node aspirate. Serologic tests are not reliable for the clinical diagnosis of the disease.

Treatment should begin before the manifestations of CNS involvement because the most effective drugs do not cross the blood-brain barrier. The intravenous adminstration of suramin is the treatment of choice. Pentamidine isethionate, an alternative drug, has many side effects. Melarsoprol is the recommended drug for patients with advanced disease and CNS involvement, but it may cause myocarditis, renal failure, and peripheral neuropathy (80).

South American Trypanosomiasis (Chagas Disease)

Chagas disease, caused by *Trypanosoma cruzi,* is predominant in South American countries and Panama. It is transmitted by a Triatomid (reduviid) bug which characteristically feeds at night. When the infected bug has a blood meal, it defecates immediately near the puncture wound and parasites in these feces are deposited around the skin wound. Patients infected by conjunctival entry of the organism have unilateral edema and violaceous discoloration of the eye lids (Romaña sign) with conjuctivitis, and there may be an erythematous nodule that develops in the skin (chagoma) at the site of the bite. The trypomastigotes enter a wide variety of cells where they multiply, become amastigotes and fill the host cell. When released from the infected cells, they enter the blood stream and disseminate throughout the body.

The disease is usually acquired during childhood and may be acute in children, and either acute or chronic in children and adults. The infection may remain dormant for 10 to 20 years (144). The acute state of Chagas disease is characterized by hematogenous dissemination of the parasite with invasion of various tissues and organ systems. In addition, patients may have fever, enlargement of lymph nodes, liver, and spleen. Skeletal muscle, myocardium, adrenal gland, and the CNS are the most heavily invaded. The chronic stage of the disease is the result of gradual tissue destruction. Some patients have the cardiac conduction system replaced by a fibrous tissue, and in the gut, destruction of the myenteric plexus is responsible for development of megaesophagus. Encephalitis is more common during the acute than in chronic stage of the disease. Other neurologic abnormalities include changes of mental function, aphasia, hemiplegia, and movement disorders.

The brain of patients who die during the acute illness show edema, congestion, and petechial hemorrhages in the white matter; parasites may be found in glial cells. It is believed that organisms invade the vascular endothelium before passing into the astrocytes (145). The cortical neurons are relatively preserved. Demyelination has been observed when cellular aggregates are present. The autonomic ganglion cells degenerate during the acute stage of the disease before an inflammatory infiltrate appears. Ten percent of acute cases of Chagas disease evolve into a chronic illness in which the heart, hollow viscera, and autonomic ganglia are affected (146).

Congenital cases of Chagas disease are well recognized. The infection can occur during any maternal phase (147) and may lead to abortion or premature birth. Most infants born with *T. cruzi* die within a few days from meningoencephalitis. The acute stage of Chagas disease can be missed because it may be clinically asymptomatic. The infection that occurs in childhood usually persists for life. There is an incubation period of 4 to 12 days after invasion by the parasite. The acute phase lasts approximately 2 months and patients who recover from acute phase enter the chronic phase. The two most common clinical forms of the disease are cardiac and gastrointestinal.

The diagnosis of acute Chagas disease is made by finding trypomastigotes in the blood or at biopsy of tender muscles. It can also be diagnosed by xenodiagnosis. The indirect immunofluorescence test can detect the infection 2 weeks after the infection. The complement fixation test becomes positive 6 weeks after the infection.

T. cruzi is not susceptible to most drugs thus far investigated. The efficacy of Nifurtimox in patients with acute and chronic Chagas disease is controversial; it appears to eradicate parasites during the acute infection but there is no evidence it will reverse chronic Chagas disease. Nifurtimox has serious side effects including anorexia, vomiting, polyneuritis, seizures, and sleep disorders. Bendazole has undergone limited trials in patients with Chagas disease and has similar efficacy to Nifurtimox. The duration of therapy is limited by development of a peripheral neuropathy or bone marrow suppression.

The authors are grateful to Dr. Jose Bebin of the University of Mississippi School of Medicine, Department of Pathology for providing all illustrations except Figures 16, 18, and 19.

REFERENCES

1. Lyons RW, Andriole VT. Fungal infections of the CNS. In: Booss JM, Thornton GF, eds. Infectious Diseases of the Central Nervous System. Neurol Clin 1986;4(1):159–170.
2. Anderson RL, Carroll TF, Harvey JT, et al. Petriellidium (Allescheria) boydii orbital and brain abscess treated with intravenous miconazole. Am J Ophthalmol 1984;97:771–775.
3. Smith CE, Saito MT. Serologic reactions in coccidioidomycosis cases. J Chronic Dis 1957;5(4):571–579.
4. Christianson KJ, Bernard EM, Gold JWM, et al. Distribution and activity of amphotericin B in humans. J Infect Dis 1985;152(5):1037–1043.
5. Littman ML, Walter JE. Cryptococcosis: Current status. Am J Med 1968;45:922–932.
6. Emanuel B, Ching E, Lieberman AD, et al. Cryptococcus meningitis in a child successfully treated with amphotericin B, with a review of the pediatric literature. J Pediatr 1961;59:577–591.
7. Bell WE, McCormick WF. Neurological Infections in Children, 2nd edition. Philadelphia: W.B. Saunders, 1981;503–513.
8. Butler WT, Alling DW, Spickard A, et al. Diagnostic and prognostic value of clinical and laboratory findings in cryptococcal meningitis. A follow-up study of forty patients. N Engl J Med 1964;270:59–67.
9. Edwards VE, Sutherland JM, Tyrer JH. Cryptococcosis of the central nervous system. Epidemiological, clinical and therapeutic features. J Neurol Neurosurg Psychiatry 1970;33:415–425.
10. Fetter BF, Klintworth GK, Wilson SH. Cryptococcosis. Mycosis of the central nervous system. Baltimore: Williams and Wilkins, 1967;89–123.
11. Igel HJ, Bolande RP. Humoral defense mechanisms in cryptococcosis: substances in normal human serum saliva and cerebrospinal fluid affecting the growth of *cryptococcus neoformans*. J Infect Dis 1966;116:75–83.
12. Grosse G, Misrha SK, Staib F. Selective involvement of the brain in experimental murine cryptococcosis: II. Histopathological observations. Zentralbl Bakteriol Hyg 1975;233:106.
13. Macher AM, Bennett JE, Gadek JE, et al. Complement depletion in cryptococcal sepsis. J Immunol 1978;120:1686–1690.
14. Bennett JE, Bailey JW. Control for rheumatoid factor in the latex test for cryptococcosis. Am J Clin Pathol 1971;56:360–365.
15. Bindschadler DD, Bennett JE. Serology of human cryptococcosis. Ann Intern Med 1968;69:45–62.
16. Snow RM, Dismukes WE. Cryptococcal meningitis. Diagnostic value of cryptococcal antigen in cerebrospinal fluid. Arch Intern Med 1975;135:1155–1157.
17. Wilson R, Feldman S. Toxicity of amphotericin B in children with cancer. Am J Dis Child 1979;133:731–734.
18. Terrell CL, Hermans PE. Antifungal infections used for deep seated mycotic infections. Mayo Clin Proc 1987;62:1116–1128.
19. Penar PL, Kim J, Chyatte D, et al. Intraventricular cryptococcal granuloma. J Neurosurg 1988;68:145–148.
20. Stevens DA. Coccidioides immitis. In: Mandell GL, Douglas RG, Bennett JE, eds. Principles and Practice of Infectious Diseases, 2nd ed. New York: John Wiley & Sons, 1985;1485–1492.
21. Pappagianis D. Epidemiology of coccidioidomycosis. In: Stevens DA, ed. Coccidioidomycosis: A Text. New York: Plenum Medical, 1980;63.

22. Smith CE, Beard RR, Whiting EG, et al. Varieties of coccidiodal infection in relation to the epidemiology and control of the diseases. Am J Public Health 1946;36: 1394–1402.

23. Smith CE. Coccidioidomycosis. Pediatr Clin North Am 1955;2:109–125.

24. Bouza E, Dreyer JS, Hewitt WL, et al. Coccidioidal meningitis. An analysis of thirty-one cases and review of the literature. Medicine 1981;60:139–172.

25. Galgiani JN. Ketoconazole treatment of coccidioidomycosis. Drugs 1983;26:347–354.

26. Stevens DA, Stiller RL, Williams PL, et al. Experience with ketoconazole in three major manifestations of progressive coccidioidomycosis. Am J Med 1983;74(1B):58–63.

27. Blizzard RM, Gibbs JH. Candidiasis: Studies pertaining to its association with endocrinopathies and pernicious anemia. Pediatrics 1968;42:231–237.

28. Kroll JJ, Einbinder JM, Merz WG. Mucocutaneous candidiasis in a mother and son. Arch Dermatol 1973;108: 259–262.

29. Louria DB, Stiff DP, Bennett B. Disseminated moniliasis in the adult. Medicine 1962;41:307–337.

30. Haning HAL, Johnston R, Touloukian R, et al. Successfully treated candida endophthalmitis in a child. Pediatrics 1973; 51:1027–1031.

31. Edwards JE, Montgomerie JZ, Foos RY, et al. Experimental hematogenous endophthalmitis caused by *Candida albicans.* J Infect Dis 1975;131:649–657.

32. Black JT. Cerebral candidiasis: case report of brain abscess secondary to *Candida albicans,* and review of the literature. J Neurol Neurosurg Psychiatry 1970;33:864–870.

33. Roessmann, U, Friede RL. Candidal infection of the brain. Arch Pathol 1967;84:495–498.

34. Preisler HD, Hasenclever HF, Levitan AA, et al. Serologic diagnosis of disseminated candidiasis in patients with acute leukemia. Ann Intern Med 1969;70:19–30.

35. Montgomerie JZ, Edwards JE, Guze LB. Synergism of amphotericin B and 5-fluorocytosine for *Candida* species. J Infect Dis 1975;132:82–86.

36. Balk MW, Crumrine MH, Fischer GW. Evaluation of miconazole therapy in experimental disseminated candidiasis in laboratory rats. Antimicrob Agents Chemother 1978; 13:321–325.

37. Ciegler A, Burmeister HR, Vesonder RF. Poisonous fungi: Mycotoxins and mycotoxicosis. In: Howard DH, ed. Fungi Pathogenic for Humans and Animals. New York: Marcel Deker, 1983;3 part, 413–469.

38. Mullins J. Harvey R, Seaton A. Sources and incidence of airborne *Aspergillus fumigatus.* Clin Allergy 1976;6:209–217.

39. Bennett JE. *Aspergillus* species. In: Mandell GL, Douglas RG, Bennett JE, eds. Principles and practice of infectious diseases, 2nd edition. New York: John Wiley & Sons, 1985; 1447–1451.

40. Altman AR. Thoracic wall invasion secondary to pulmonary aspergillosis. AJR 1977;129:140–142.

41. Young RC, Bennett JE, Vogel CL, et al. Aspergillosis. The spectrum of the disease in 98 patients. Medicine 1970;49: 147–173.

42. Mangurten HH, Fernandez B. Neonatal aspergillosis accompanying fulminant necrotising entercolitis. Arch Dis Child 1979;54:559–562.

43. Gonzalez-Crussi F, Mirkin LD, Wyllie RM, et al. Acute disseminated aspergillosis during the neonatal period. Clin Pediatr 1979;18:137–143.

44. Grevic N, Matthews WF. Pathological changes in acute disseminated aspergilllosis. Am J Clin Pathol 1959;32: 536–551.

45. Amromin GD, Gildenhorn VB. Massive cerebral aspergillus abscess in a leukemic child. Case report. J Neurosurg 1971; 35:491–494.

46. McCormick WF, Schochet SS, Weaver PR, et al. Disseminated aspergillosis. Aspergillus endophthalmitis, optic nerve infarctions and carotid artery thrombosis. Arch Pathol 1975;99:353–359.

47. Henze G, Aldenhoff P, Stephani U, et al. Successful treatment of pulmonary and cerebral aspergillosis in an immunosuppressed child. Eur J Pediatr 1982;138:263–265.

48. Arroyo J, Medoff G, Kobayashi G. Therapy of murine aspergillosis with amphotericin B in combination with Rifampin or 5-fluorocytosine. Antimicrob Agents Chemother 1977; 11:21–25.

49. Brodsky AL, Gregg MB, Loewenstein MS, et al. Outbreak of histoplasmosis associated with 1970 Earth Day activities. Am J Med 1973;54:333–342.

50. Holland P, Holland NH. Histoplasmosis in early infancy. Hematologic, histochemical and immunological observations. Am J Dis Child 1966;112:412–421.

50. Goodwin RA, Shapiro JL, Thurman SS, et al. Disseminated histoplasmosis: clinical and pathological correlations. Medicine 1980;59:1–33.

52. Sathapatayavongs B, Batteiger BE, Wheat J, et al. Clinical and laboratory features of disseminated histoplasmosis during two large urban outbreaks. Medicine 1983;62: 263–270.

53. Schulz DM. Histoplasmosis of the central nervous system. JAMA 1953;151:549–551.

54. Couch JR, Abdou NI, Sagawa A. Histoplasma meningitis with hyperactive suppressor T cells in cerebrospinal fluid. Neurology 1978;28:119–123.

55. Nelson JD, Bates R, Pitchford A. Histoplasma meningitis: Recovery following amphotericin B therapy. Am J Dis Child 1961;102:218–223.

56. Harrell ER, Curtis AC. North American blastomycosis. Am J Med 1959;27:750–766.

57. Schwarz J, Baum GL. Blastomycosis. Am J Clin Pathol 1951;21:999–1029.

58. Sarosi GA, Davies SF. Blastomycosis. Am Rev Respir Dis 1979;120:918–938.

59. Duttera MJ, Osterhout S. North American blastomycosis: A survey of 63 cases. South Med J 1969;62:295–301.

60. Waisbren BA, Ullrich D. An isolated blastomycetoma of the posterior cranial fossa treated successfully with surgery and amphotericin B. Am J Med 1962;32:621–624.

61. Carmody EJ, Tappen W. Blastomycosis meningitis: Report of a case successfully treated with amphotericin B. Ann Intern Med 1959;51:780–791.

62. Borland DS. Mucormycosis of the central nervous system. Am J Dis Child 1959;97:852–856.

63. Abramson E, Wilson D, Arky RA. Rhinocerebral phycomycosis in association with diabetic ketoacidosis: Report of two cases and a review of clinical and experimental experience with amphotericin B therapy. Ann Intern Med 1967; 66:735–742.

64. Hale LM. Orbital-cerebral phycomycosis. Report of a case and a review of the disease in infants. Arch Ophthalmol 1971;86:39–43.

65. Warren KS. Helminthic diseases endemic in the United States. Am J Trop Med Hyg 1974;23:723–730.

66. Garcia-Maldonado E, Gonzáles J, Céspedes G. Helminthiasis of the nervous system. In: Vinken PJ, Bruyn GW, eds. Handbook of Clinical Neurology: Infections of the Nervous System. Amsterdam: North Holland, 1978;35(Part 3), 209–229.

67. Wilder HC. Nematodes endoophthalmitis. Trans Am Acad Ophthalmol Ortolaryngol 1950;55:99–104.

68. Beaver PC, Snyder CH, Carrera GM, et al. Chronic eosinophilia due to visceral larva migrans: Report of three cases. Pediatrics 1952;9:7–19.

69. Wilkinson CP, Welch RB. Intraocular toxocara. Am J Ophthalmol 1971;71:921–930.

70. Bird AC, Smith JL, Curtin VT. Nematode optic neuritis. Am J Ophthalmol 1970;69:74–77.

71. Beautyman W, Woolf A. An ascaris larva in the brain in association with acute anterior polyomyelitis. J Pathol Bacteriol 1951;63:635–647.

72. Moore MT. Human toxocara canis encephalitis with lead encephalopathy. J Neuropathol Exp Neurol 1962;21:201–217.

73. Schochett SS. Human toxocara canis encephalopathy in a case of visceral larva migrans. Neurology 1967;17:227–229.

74. Anderson DC, Greenwood R, Fishman M, et al. Acute infantile hemiplegia with cerebrospinal fluid eosinophilic pleocytosis: An unusual case of visceral larva migrans. J Pediatr 1975;84:247–249.

75. Katz M, Dickson DD, Gwadz RW. Nematodes. Toxocara canis. In: Parasitic diseases. New York: Springer-Verlag, 1982;54–58.

76. Ohesen EA. Visceral larva migrans and other unusual helminth infections. In: Mandell GL, Douglas RG, Bennet JE, eds. Principles and Practice of Infectious Diseases, 2nd ed. New York: John Wiley & Sons, 1985;1584–1588.

77. Zimmerman WJ, Steel JH, Kagan IG. Trichinosis in the US population (1966–1970). Prevalence, epidemiologic factors. Health Serv Rep 1973;88:606–623.

78. Love JR, Ogilvie BM, McLaren DJ. The immune mechanism which expells the intestinal stage of Trichinella spirales from rats. Immunology 1976;30:7–16.

79. Davis MS, Cilo M, Plactakis A, et al. Trichinosis: Severe myopathic involvement with recovery. Neurology 1976;26:37–40.

80. Medical Letter Editors: Drugs for parasitic infections. Med Lett Drugs Ther 1986;28:9–17.

81. Marquez-Monta H. In: Marcial-Rojas RA, ed. Pathology of Protozoal and Helminthic Diseases and Clinical Correlation. Baltimore: Williams and Wilkins, 1971;592–626.

82. McCormick GF, Zee CS, Heidey J. Cysticercosis cerebri: Review of one hundred twenty-seven cases. Arch Neurol 1982;39:534–539.

83. Trelles JG, Trelles L. Cysticercosis. In: Vinken PJ, Bruyn GW, eds. Handbook of Clinical Neurology: Infections of the Nervous System. Amsterdam: North Holland, 1978;35 (Part 3), 291–320.

84. Hernandez AL, Garaizer C. Analysis of eighty-nine cases of infantile cerebral cysticercosis. In: Flisser A, ed. Cysticercosis: Present State of Knowledge and Perspectives. New York: Academic Press, 1982.

85. Meller BL, Heimer D, Goldberg MP. The immunology of cerebral cysticercosis. Bull Clin Neurosci 1983;48:18–23.

86. Gemmell MA, Johnstone PD. Cestoides. Antibiot Chemother 1981;30:54–114.

87. Warren KS, Mahmoud AAF, Cummings P, et al. Schistosomiasis mansoni in Yemeni in California. Duration of infection, presence of disease, therapeutic management. Am J Trop Med Hyg 1974;23:902–909.

88. Mahmoud AAF. Schistosomiasis. In: Warren KS, Mahmoud AAF, eds. Tropical and Geographical Medicine. New York: McGraw-Hill, 1984;443.

89. Kane CA, Most H. Schistosomiasis of the central nervous system. Experiences in World War II and a review of the literature. Arch Neurol Psychol 1948;59:141–181.

90. Marcial-Rojas RA, Fiol RE. Neurological complications of schistosomiasis. Review of the literature and report of two cases of transverse myelitis due to *S. mansoni*. Ann Intern Med 1963;59:215–230.

91. Bird AV. Acute spinal schistosomiasis. Neurology 1964;14:647–656.

92. Bird AV. Spinal cord complications of bilharziasis. S Afr Med J 1965;39:158–162.

93. Blankfein RJ, Chiroco RM. Cerebral schistosomiasis. Neurology 1965;15:957–967.

94. Queiroz L de S, Nucci A, Facure NO, et al. Massive spinal cord necrosis in schistosomiasis. Arch Neurol 1979;36:517–519.

95. Peters PA, Mahmoud AAF, Warren KS, et al. Field studies of a rapid accurate means of quantifying Schistosoma haematobium eggs in urine samples. Bull WHO 1976;54:159–162.

96. Pearson RD, Guerrant RL. Praziquantel: A major advance in antihelminthic therapy. Ann Intern Med 1983;99:195–198.

97. Yokogawa M. Paragonimus and paragonimiasis. Advanc Parasitol 1965;3:99–158.

98. Yokogawa S, Suyemori S. An experimental study of the intracranial parasitism of the human lung fluke (Paragonimus westermani). Am J Hyg 1921;1:63–78.

99. Oh SJ. Cerebral and spinal paragonimiasis — A histopathological study. J Neurol Sci 1969;9:205–236.

100. Oh SJ. Paragonimiasis in the central nervous system. In: Vinken PJ, Bruyn GW, eds. Handbook of Clinical Neurology: Infections of the Nervous System. Amsterdam: North Holland, 1978;(part 3), 243–266.

101. Oh SJ. Roentgen findings in cerebral paragonimiasis. Radiology 1968;90:292–299.

102. Oh SJ. Cerebral paragonimiasis. J Neurol Sci 1968;8:27–48.

103. Yokogawa M, Yoshimura H, Okura T, et al. Chemotherapy of paragonimiasis with bithionol-II. Clinical observations on the treatment of bithionol. Jap J Parasitol 1961;10:317–327.

104. Pearl M, Kotsilimbos DG, Lehrer HZ, et al. Cerebral echinococcosis a parasitic disease: Report of two cases with one successful five-year follow-up. Pediatrics 1978;61:915–920.

105. Arana-Iniquez R, San Julian J. Hydatid cysts of the brain. J Neurosurg 1955;12:323–335.

106. Cheris RAF. Mebendazole in surgical and non-operative management of hydatid disease. Med J Aust 1976;2:580.

107. Becker BJP, Jacobson S. Infestation of the human brain with coenurus cerebralis. Report of 3 cases. Lancet 1961;2:198–202.

108. Johnstone HG, Jones OW. Cerebral coenurosis in an infant. Am J Trop Med 1950;30:431–441.

109. Hermos JA, Healy GR, Schultz MG, et al. Fetal human cerebral coenurosis. JAMA 1970; 213:1461–1464.

110. Landolls JW. Intramedullary cyst of spinal cord due to the cestode multiceps in coenurus stage: A report of a case. J Clin Pathol 1949;2:61–63.

111. Epstein E, Proctor NSF, Heinz HJ. Intraocular coenurus infestation. S Afr Med J 1959;33:602–604.

112. Wolf A, Cowen D, Paige BH. Human toxoplasmosis: Occurrence in infants as encephalomyelitis. Verification by transmission to animals. Science 1939;89:807–814.

113. Britt RH, Enzmann DR, Remington JS. Intracranial infection in cardiac transplant and recipients. Ann Neurol 1981;9:107–119.

114. Frenkel JK. Toxoplasmosis. Pediatr Clin North Am 1985; 32:917–931.

115. Remington JS, Desmonts G. Toxoplasmosis. In: Remington JS, Klein JO, eds. Infectious Diseases of the Fetus and Newborn Infant. Philadelphia: W. B. Saunders, 1983; 143–263.

116. O'Connor GR. Manifestations and management of ocular toxoplasmosis. Bull N Y Acad Med 1974;50:192–210.

117. Eichenwald HF. A study of congenital toxoplasmosis. In: Siim J Chr. ed. Human Toxoplasmosis. Copenhagen: Munksgaard, 1960;41–49.

118. Alford CA, Foft JW, Blankenship WJ, et al. Subclinical central nervous system disease of neonates: A prospective study of infants born with increased levels of IgM. J Pediatr 1969;75(6 Pt 2):1167–1178.

119. Alford CA, Stagnos S, Reynolds DW. Congenital toxoplasmosis. Clinical, laboratory and therapeutic considerations with special reference to subclinical disease. Bull N Y Acad Med 1974;50(2):160–181.

120. Desmonts G, Couvreur J. Congenital toxoplasmosis. A prospective study of 378 pregnancies. N Engl J Med 1974;290:1110–1116.

121. Wernsdorfer WH. The importance of malaria in the world. In: Krier JP, ed. Malaria. New York: Academic Press, 1980;V:1–95.

122. Maegraith BG. Other pathological process in malaria. Bull WHO 1974;50:187–193.

123. Toro G, Roman G. Cerebral malaria. A disseminated vasculomyelinopathy. Arch Neurol 1978;35:271–275.

124. Migasena P, Maegraith BG. Pharmacological action of antimalarial drugs. Action of chloroquin and hydrocortisone on blood-brain barrier in *Plasmodium kowlesi* malaria. Trans R Soc Trop Med Hyg 1967;61:6.

125. Rest JR, Wright DH. Electron microscopy of cerebral malaria in golden hamsters infected with *Plasmodium berghei*. J Pathol 1979;127:115–120.

126. Jeliffe DB. The therapy of cerebral malaria in children. Editorial comment. J Pediatr 1966;69:483.

127. Phillips RE, Warrell DA, White NS, et al. Intravenous quinidine for the treatment of severe falciparum malaria. N Engl J Med 1985;312:1273–1278.

128. Warrell DA, Looareesuwan S, Warrell MJ, et al. Dexamethasone proves deleterious in cerebral malaria. N Engl J Med 1982;306:313–319.

129. Lombardo L, Alonso P, Amoyo LS, et al. Cerebral amebiasis. Report of 17 cases. J Neurosurg 1964;21:704–709.

130. Odunjo EO. Pathological manifestations of amebiasis in Nigerians. W Afr Med J 1969;18:117–120.

131. Becker GL, Knep S, Lance KP, et al. Amebic abscess of the brain. Neurosurgery 1980;6:192–194.

132. Culbertson CG. Amebic meningoencephalitis. In: Binford CH, Connor DH, eds. Pathology of Tropical and Extraordinary Disease, Vol. I. Washington, DC, Armed Forces Institute of Pathology 1976:317–324.

133. Neva FA. Amebic meningoencephalitis, a new disease. N Engl J Med 1970;282:450–452.

134. Martinez AJ, Duma RJ, Nelson E, et al. Experimental Naegleria meningoencephalitis in mice. Penetration of the olfactory mucosal epithelium by Naegleria and pathologic changes produced: A light and electron microscopic study. Lab Invest 1973;29:121–133.

135. Seidel J. Primary amebic meningoencephalitis. Pediatr Clin North Am 1985;32:881–892.

136. Seidel JS, Harmatz P, Visvesvara GS, et al. Successful treatment of primary meningoencephalitis. N Engl J Med 1982;306:346–348.

137. Appley J, Clarke SKR, Roome APCH, et al. Primary amoebic meningoencephalitis in Britain. Br Med J 1970; 1:596–599.

138. Martinez AJ, Garcia CA, Halko-Miller M, et al. Granulomatous amebic encephalitis presenting as a cerebral mass lesion. Acta neuropathol 1980;51:85–91.

139. Martinez AJ. Acanthoamoebiasis and immunosuppression. J Neuropathol Exp Neurol 1982;41:548–557.

140. Martinez AJ, Sotelo-Avila C, Alcalá H, et al. Granulomatous encephalitis, intracranial arteritis and mycotic aneurysms due to free living ameba. Acta Neuropathol 1980;49:7–12.

141. Lambert PH, Berney M, Kazyumba G. Immune complexes in serum and in cerebrospinal fluid in African trypanosomiasis. J Clin Invest 1981;67:77–85.

142. Buyst H. Sleeping sickness in Zambia. East Afr Med J 1976;53:452–458.

143. Cramet R. La maladie due sommeil chez l'infant et ses sequelles á distance. A propos de 110 observations personelles á l'hôpital de Fontem (Cameroun). Med Trop (Mars) 1982;42(1):27–31.

144. Laranja FS, Dias E, Nobrega G, et al. Chagas' disease. A clinical, epidemiologic, and pathologic study. Circulation 1956;14:1035–1060.

145. Alencar A. Chagas' disease. In: Minkler J, ed. Pathology of the Nervous System. New York: McGraw-Hill, 1972; 3:2559–2569.

146. Brown WJ, Voge M. Neuropathology of Parasite Infections. Oxford, England: Oxford Univ Press, 1982;70–81.

147. Bittencourt AL. Congenital Chagas' disease. Am J Dis Child 1976;130:97–103.

Chapter 12
Rickettsial and Spirochetal Infections

Mary L. Zupanc and Raymond W. M. Chun

SPIROCHETAL INFECTIONS

The spirochetal infections that cause human diseases are found in the Treponemataceae family of Spirochetales order. The three genera in this family include *Treponema*, *Leptospira*, and *Borrelia*. All three genera contain organisms that can cause disease in humans. *Treponema pallidum* causes syphilis; *Leptospira icterohemorragiae* causes leptospirosis; *Borrelia recurrentis* results in relapsing fever; and *Borrelia burgdorferi*, a newly described spirochete, is the etiologic agent of Lyme disease.

Spirochetes are small, coiled, helix-shaped bacteria that are motile. Their motility is the result of axial fibrils; whereas, other bacteria rely on flagella or cilia for motion. They are heterotropic organisms that survive poorly outside their host. Of all bacteria that infect the human body, spirochetal infections are among the most tenacious and can affect virtually every organ system of the body. Two of the most common spirochetal infections are Lyme disease and syphilis, the new and the old. Syphilis and its neurologic manifestations have been described for centuries; Lyme disease and its neurologic manifestations are only beginning to be described.

Lyme Disease

Lyme disease was first described in the European literature. In 1900, there was a description of the rash, erythema chronicum migrans (ECM), which is now associated with the disease. ECM is initially characterized by a red macule or papule, followed by an expanding ring with central clearing (Figure 12.1). There can be one or multiple lesions. In 1922, Garin and Bujadoux (1) described some neurologic manifestations of the disease including isolated muscle paralysis, meningitis, and sensory radiculitis that occurred several months after ECM. Reports of similar patients followed, but the etiology remained unknown.

Bannwarth (2) first recognized the association of tick bites, radicular pain, and chronic meningitis. The arthropod vector theory was confirmed by subsequent reports, but the causative organisms remained elusive. In 1966, Schaltenbrand (3) described 50 patients with tick bites who later developed chronic meningitis and peripheral neuritis; 2/3 had a skin rash typical of erythema chronicum migrans (ECM). In 1973, Horstrup and Ackermann (4) gave a similar account of 47 patients and named the disease tick-borne meningopolyneuritis.

Lyme disease was first recognized in the United States when a cluster of cases occurred in 1975 near Lyme, Connecticut. Most patients had an oligoarticular arthritis (5); moreover, the fact that the ECM was a common feature of the disease suggested that it might be arthropod borne.

In 1983 Steere et al. (6,7), isolated the spirochete from the *Ixodes Dammini* tick as well as from the blood and cerebrospinal fluid (CSF) of several patients who had typical signs and symptoms associated with the disease (Figure 12.2). The spirochete, *Borrelia burgdorferi*, has since been isolated in many patients with Lyme disease. In Europe, the arthropod carrier is the *Ixodes ricinus*. Endemic areas have been identified in Europe, Australia, and the northeastern and midwestern regions of the United States, as well as California and Oregon.

Ixodes dammini ticks require a blood meal during each of their three stages (larval, nymphal, and adult) of their life cycle. Larval and nymphal ticks prefer white-footed mice (Peromyscus leucopus) and adult ticks prefer deer, but the ticks will attach to any mammal, including humans. Mice and deer are the natural reservoirs for the *B. burgdorferi* organisms. The ticks become infected by feeding on an infected mammal. Transovarial transmission of *B. burgdorferi* rarely occurs. Nymphal ticks feed during May through early August. They are very small and difficult to detect, which probably explains why the peak onset of early stage Lyme disease in humans corresponds to this time period. Adult ticks have a greater chance of being

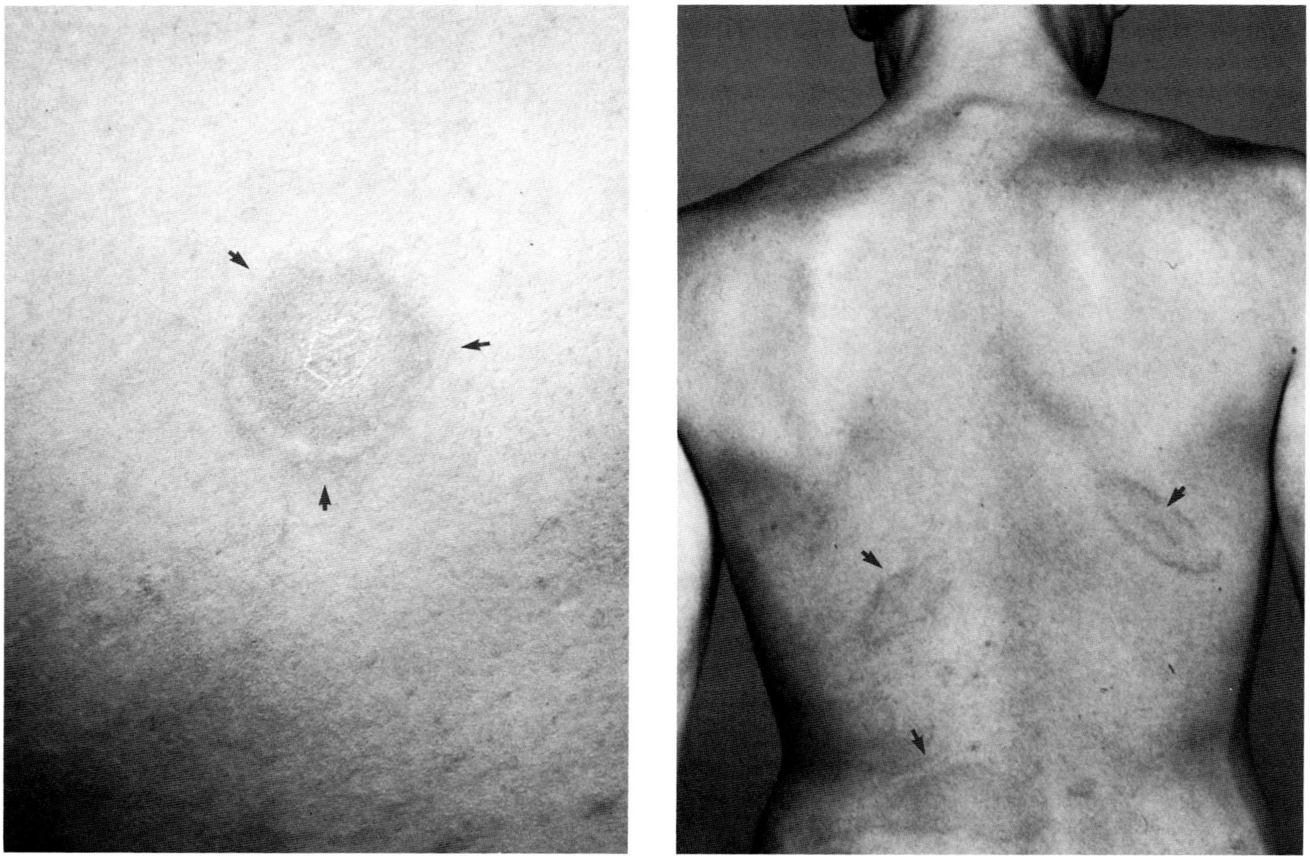

FIGURE 12.1 (A) An erythematous macular lesion, typical of early Lyme disease. (B) There may be one or multiple lesions that become an expanding erythematous ring with central clearing. Courtesy of Gunderson Medical Foundation, LaCrosse, WI.

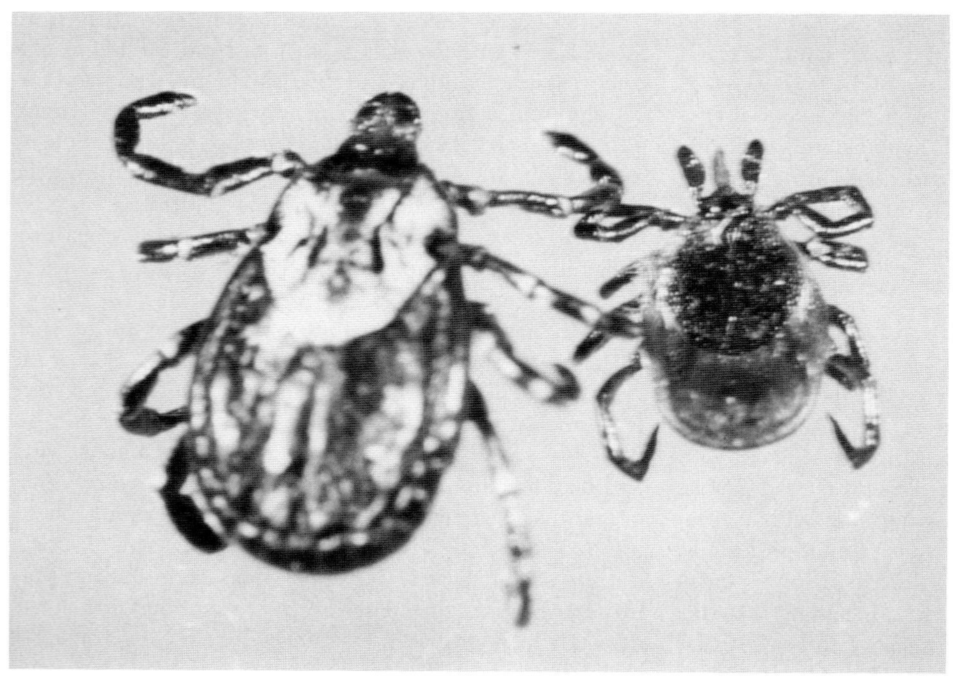

FIGURE 12.2 The Lyme disease spirochete is transmitted by certain ixodes ticks including *I. dammini* (right), which is about 5 mm in length. The common wood tick is noted on the left.

infected with *B. burgdorferi,* but they are larger and more easily seen by the naked eye, prompting removal from the skin. The ticks probably need to attach for 24 hours or longer before transmitting the *B. burgdorferi* spirochete to humans. While person to person transmission of *B. burgdorferi* is theoretically possible through direct contact with human blood, it has never been reported.

Clinical Features

Lyme disease affects multiple organ systems including the skin, heart, joints, and nervous system. Males are affected more often than females, a fact that may be related to lifestyle rather than to inherent sexual differences in susceptibility. Three typical stages are currently described but as knowledge of this disorder increases, the clinical descriptions may change.

The 1st stage is the development of ECM (8), which generally begins 1 to 4 weeks after the tick bite and is usually accompanied by systemic symptoms such as fever, malaise, stiff neck, myalgia, arthralgia, and headache. The rash typically lasts about 3 weeks and consists of several lesions.

The 2nd stage develops weeks to months later and involves the nervous system and heart (9,10). It is currently believed that approximately 11% of patients develop abnormalities of the nervous system (9). The neurologic abnormalities are protean, and because of many presentations, are only beginning to be appreciated. The most frequent cardiac abnormality is heart block.

The 3rd stage is an asymmetric mono- or oligoarticular inflammatory arthritis in the large joints (11) that usually develops 1 to 24 months after the neurologic symptoms. However, it is now appreciated that chronic neurologic or skin involvement can occur years after the onset of *Borrelia* infection. Stage 3 central nervous system infection is incompletely defined but includes chronic fatigue, neuropsychiatric manifestations, and focal CNS lesions.

Some investigators claim that the European disease is different from the manifestations of the disease observed in the United States (12). Encephalitis, arthritis, and carditis are uncommonly described by Europeans, and their reports have not emphasized the recurrent nature of the disease. Additionally, radicular pain found in the dermatomal segment of the arthropod bite has been well described in Europe but not in the United States. The differences in the disease spectrum have been hypothesized to be on the basis of different antigens on the surface of the European and American *Borrelia* isolates. Altered host susceptibility may also affect the expression of the disease. Other investigators dispute the different disease theory, however, and claim that perceived differences can be explained on a clinical basis (13). For example, Europeans have been treating Lyme disease for years with antibiotics. This early therapeutic intervention probably plays a role in the decreased incidence of arthritis in European patients.

Neurologic Manifestation

The current descriptions of neurologic abnormalities are multifocal and protean in adult patients. Among patients with signs and symptoms of nervous system involvement, 40% recall the initial tick bite, although virtually all have lived in or visited endemic areas (14). Sixty-eight percent to 80% describe a skin rash reminiscent of ECM (14,15). The first neurologic complications may occur approximately 1 to 6 months after the onset of ECM, but there are patients who develop ECM and neurologic manifestations concomitantly. Approximately 40% of patients with Lyme disease subsequently develop arthritis (11). These statistics may change as the illness is better recognized and treated earlier.

Most often, a lymphocytic meningitis develops during stage 2 of the infection. The vast majority of patients complain of meningeal symptoms such as headache, stiff neck, nausea, and vomiting. Examination of the CSF usually shows a lymphocytic pleocytosis with normal concentrations of glucose and protein. Oligoclonal banding has been reported in these patients (14–16).

Many patients with meningitis also have findings suggestive of a mild meningoencephalitis. The symptoms described include somnolence, emotional lability, depression, poor memory and concentration, and behavioral changes (14,17). Only sparse neuropsychologic testing of patients with Lyme disease has been performed, however, and subtle symptoms of encephalitis may have been missed. Electroencephalograms (EEGs) of patients with symptoms of encephalitis have been abnormal with mild generalized slowing as the most frequently observed abnormality.

Cranial neuritis is also common during stage 2 of Lyme disease and most often occurs in patients who also have meningeal symptoms. The incidence of cranial neuritis in patients with Lyme disease and neurologic symptoms and signs is about 55% (9,18). Peripheral, often bilateral, facial-nerve palsy is most frequently reported; however, optic atrophy and involvement of cranial nerves V, VIII, IX, and X may occur (9,19).

Polyradiculitis, reported in a less than half of patients with neurologic complaints (20), is the other neurologic manifestation of stage 2 Lyme disease. It may be under reported because although many patients have prominent limb paresthesias, most have normal neurologic examinations. Electrophysiologic testing, however, reveals significantly abnormal results (20).

Stage 3 central nervous system Lyme disease, known as tertiary neuroborreliosis, is incompletely defined. The majority of patients complain of neuropsychiatric symptoms, such as memory loss, personality change, and cognitive impairments. It is felt to be uncommon. Transverse myelitis has also been reported as well as encephalomyelitis (16,17,21). Movement disorders, particularly chorea, and cerebellar ataxia have been observed (16). A Guillain-

Barré-like syndrome (16,20), cerebral arteritis, myopathy, and a multiple sclerosis-like illness have also been reported (22–26), in addition to chronic fatigue syndrome.

The neurologic manifestations of Lyme disease in children are thus far not prominently recorded in the medical literature, and virtually all that is known in this regard comes from recent European literature (16–21). Fifty-five percent of patients initially had ECM, and all had early symptoms of headache, fatigue, nausea, and arthralgia. In those patients who remembered a tick bite, neurologic symptoms developed after a latent period of 3 to 5 weeks. Nearly all patients (89%) presented with meningitis, manifesting nuchal rigidity, headache, nausea, and vomiting. Examination of the CSF showed lymphocytic pleocytosis in all cases. Twenty-two percent of patients had concomitant encephalitis or peripheral facial palsy, or both. When compared to the adult population, few had complaints or evidence of polyradiculitis. The prevalence of tertiary neuroborreliosis in children is unknown.

Diagnosis

The diagnosis of Lyme disease can be elusive, but a carefully obtained history may reveal several key points including a tick bite, ECM, and travel or residence in an endemic area of Lyme disease. The onset of first neurologic symptoms commonly occurs between June and December, and those symptoms are usually recurrent, chronic, and affecting various parts of the central and peripheral nervous system.

The diagnosis, in the setting of an appropriate clinical picture, depends on the presence of significant antibody titers. Because the growth of the bacteria is relatively slow, isolation of the organism, *Borrelia Burgdorferi,* is usually not helpful in establishing an early diagnosis. Antibody titers provide quick, sensitive evidence for the *Borrelia burgdorferi* organism and can be obtained from serum, CSF, or joint fluid by means of indirect immunofluorescent antibody assay (IFA), enzyme linked immunosorbent assay (ELISA), and Western blot analysis. IgM antibody titers peak between 3 to 6 weeks after onset of ECM. Early and appropriate antibiotic therapy may blunt measurable antibody responses. The serologic assays have also been found to give false negatives in as many as 50% of *early* cases, making repeat testing after 2 to 6 weeks essential. An additional problem has been intra- and interlaboratory variability of test results (26a). The IgG titers rise more slowly and generally peak between 8 to 12 months when arthritis is present. The serum IgG antibody response in patients with meningitis may be slow, with significant levels attained 5 to 10 weeks after symptom onset; the CSF titers rise faster. Ninety percent of reported patients with involvement of the central nervous system (CNS), heart, and joints, have significantly elevated IgG titers (6). All reported patients with arthritis have had significantly elevated IgG titers. Specific IgG response persists throughout the infection and may be

detectable for years irrespective of the patient's clinical status. The erythrocyte sedimentation rate is frequently elevated, and cryoglobulins are reported in 83% of patients with Lyme disease (14).

The diagnostic criteria for tertiary CNS Lyme disease is not well defined. Because it can present months after the initial infection, CSF studies and other tests may be negative. The diagnosis is currently made if (1) the patient has a history suggestive of Lyme disease, (2) the IgG serum titers to *B. borgdorferi* are high, (3) there is an absence of another reasonable diagnosis, and (4) a reasonable response to appropriate antibiotic therapy is achieved (26b).

Computed tomographic (CT) brain scans in patients with meningitis or encephalitis have been normal; however, magnetic resonance imaging (MRI) brain scans of several patients with probable encephalitis have revealed high-density signals in the white matter of both cerebral hemispheres, in both T1 and T2 weighted images. No mass effect has been observed. These findings suggest an inflammatory response, consistent with observations usually present in mild encephalomyelitis (17). Electrophysiologic studies of patients with polyradiculitis are abnormal, often demonstrating delayed nerve conduction velocities. Nerve biopsy specimens have usually shown a mild axonal process with secondary demyelination (20).

EEGs of patients with Lyme disease, except in those patients with symptoms and signs of encephalitis, are usually normal. Serial neuropsychologic testing of some patients with mild encephalopathy have demonstrated initial deficiencies and significant improvement following treatment. The recorded deficiencies include immediate and delayed memory—auditory, visual, and verbal; diminished ability to learn new information; poor attention and concentration; difficulty in perceptual motor tasks; decreased ability of problem solving; and diminished conceptual flexibility (17).

The treatment of Lyme disease depends on the stage at which the diagnosis is made. During the ECM stage, the treatment of choice is the administration of oral erythromycin, penicillin, or amoxicillin. The oral administration of tetracycline to adults and children older than the age of 8 years is also used. It is believed that this treatment will decrease the incidence of subsequent manifestations of the disease.

The treatment of choice in patients with neurologic abnormalities is the intravenous (IV) administration of high dose penicillin (adults: 20 to 24 million units per day for 14 days; children: 250,000 U/kg/day [maximum 20 million units]) (27), which has a 50% response rate. Patients with intractable symptoms are given ceftriaxone (adults: 2 g twice a day for 14 days; children: 100 mg/kg/day [maximum 2 g]) resulting in fair-to-good results (28). Retreatment may be necessary (26b).

Early appropriate antibiotic treatment can prevent progression of disease. Unfortunately, 1/3 of patients do not develop ECM prior to the onset of neurologic symptoms.

The relatively poor success of antibiotic treatment after onset of ECM may reflect a change in the pathophysiology of the disease, with ECM being the direct result of organism invasion, and the neurologic, cardiac, and joint manifestations a result of immune complex formation. This would explain, for example, why the use of steroids during these stages may result in improvement of the patient's clinical status.

The major preventive measures include avoiding contact with ticks by wearing trousers tucked into boots, long sleeved shirts, and hats while in tick infested areas; limiting exposure of skin, using tick repellent, frequent inspection of skin, and "deticking." Ticks probably need to attach for 24 hours or longer to transmit *B. borgdorferi.*

Syphilis

Syphilis is the result of spirochetal infection that is capable of involving almost every organ system of the body. The causative organism, *Treponema pallidum,* is a slender spirochete that constitutes a great threat to all humans, particularly children. In the past, syphilis was one of the most common venereal diseases, but the introduction of penicillin and readily available serologic screening tests has made it a controllable and preventable disease. Unfortunately, syphilis is still prevalent, and the disease incidence is more recently increasing (29).

Clinical Features

Congenital syphilis is the result of fetal infection that occurs by transplacental transmission of spirochetes from an infected mother to the fetus. It is both preventable and curable in utero. The incidence of fetal infection is greatest if the pregnant woman has primary, secondary, or early latent syphilis, when the spirochetes are present in the blood. It was once thought that the *T. pallidum* could not cross the placenta until the placenta was fully formed, but it is now believed that the organism can cross the placenta at an early stage. The clinical signs and symptoms of syphilis do not develop, however, until the fetus has the capability of producing delayed immune cellular responses that are needed to produce the lesions of syphilis (30). Because cellular immunity occurs after 16 weeks of gestation, fetal infection takes place after organogenesis and is, therefore, not associated with major congenital malformations. Stillbirths occur in approximately 30% of fetuses infected with syphilis (29). Those infants born in the presence of maternal syphilis may be asymptomatic for weeks or months after birth, but more commonly, exhibit signs and symptoms of congenital syphilis at or shortly after birth. Neurosyphilis may develop years later if congenital syphilis goes untreated, and the *T. pallidum* spirochetes invade the blood-brain barrier (usually asymptomatically) during the congenital stage. Approximately 10% to 20% of infants with untreated congenital syphilis will develop neu-

rosyphilis. The severity of the disease depends on the time of fetal infection, the severity of the infection in the mother, the dose of *T. pallidum* spirochetes, maternal treatment, and the state of maternal immunity.

Early Congenital Syphilis

Early congenital syphilis is comparable to the secondary stage of acquired syphilis. The infant may exhibit early nonspecific signs and symptoms such as fever, anemia, failure to thrive, restlessness, or listlessness. Skin lesions may appear before other nonspecific constitutional findings. The characteristic skin lesions of early congenital syphilis include a macular, maculopapular, annular, nodular, or pustular rash, which may be diffuse or circumscribed. In addition, "snuffles" (rhinitis), mucous patches, periostitis, osteochondritis, hepatosplenomegaly, jaundice, and lymphadenopathy, are usually observed; and in the majority of cases anemia is present. Excoriations about the nose and lip, resulting from the copious rhinitis and ulceration of the nasal mucosa, can result in a saddle nose deformity. Mucous patches may be present about the mouth, genitalia, or perianal regions. The scars left from these moist, irritating lesions are called *rhagades.* Periostitis, osteochondritis, and their bony deformities often result in pseudoparalysis of one or more limbs. This pseudoparalysis is not the result of a specific neurologic deficit. The CSF and leptomeninges can become infected if organisms cross the blood-brain barrier via the meningeal or choroidal vessels and enter the CSF or are trapped in the leptomeninges.

During the first 6 months to 2 years after contracting congenital syphilis, 30% to 50% of infants develop meningovascular meningitis (31,32), which, though usually asymptomatic, may be symptomatic. Symptomatic basilar meningitis is present because of the abundant blood supply at the base of the brain and the accumulation of CSF in the pontine and chiasmatic cisterns. Inflammation of the leptomeninges blends peripherally with the perineurium of the cranial nerves of which II, III, VII, and VIII are most vulnerable (33).

The eighth cranial nerve is especially vulnerable to infection because the arachnoidal space lines the nerve for some distance before it merges with the perineural connective tissue. Treponemes in the CSF bathe the nerve, readily resulting in inflammation of the perineurium. Infiltration of inflammatory cells, hemorrhage, and deposits of fibrin lead to severe degeneration of the spiral ganglion, the organ of Corti, and the eighth nerve fibers (34). Hearing loss is usually bilateral. This form of syphilitic deafness is reversible if treatment is prompt and appropriate (35). Inflammation of the optic nerve may result in optic atrophy and blindness (36–38), which can also be reversed by the prompt administration of appropriate antibiotics. In addition to cranial-nerve involvement, communicating hydrocephalus, seizures, cerebrovascular accidents, and mental retardation are often sequelae of early symptomatic meningitis.

Late Congenital Syphilis

Late congenital syphilis occurs when there is progression of the disease. The most common stigmata of late congenital syphilis are gummata, which are deep, palpable infiltrations with or without ulceration. Nasopalatine, nasopharyngeal, mucocutaneous, subperiosteal, and hepatic gummata occur. Other somatic stigmata of late congenital syphilis include saddle nasal bridge deformity secondary to bony destruction from excoriating syphilitic rhinitis; frontal bossing resulting from periostis; rhagades (linear or reticular scarring) caused by atrophy of elastic tissue of the lips, chin, cheeks, or perianal skin; enlargement of the medial third of the clavicle (Higoumenakis sign); epiphyseal enlargement; saber shin, secondary to bowing of the tibia and enlargement of the middle third of the tibia from periostitis and osteitis; Clutton joints that result from chronic symmetric synovitis of the knee joints; and dental malformations (Hutchinson incisors) (30,33).

Ophthalmologic complications are commonly noted during late congenital syphilis. The most frequent manifestation is interstitial keratitis, a result of corneal clouding from lymphocytic infiltration. Photophobia, lacrimation, and blindness are also common symptoms of interstitial keratitis. The corneal opacity may lead to blindness within a period of weeks to months. Optic atrophy, chorioretinitis, retinitis, or vascular occlusions may also occur (37).

Neurosyphilis

If early or late congenital syphilis is unrecognized and untreated, approximately 10% to 20% of patients develop neurosyphilis, which usually appears in adolescence. The manifestations of neurosyphilis are protean. An acute meningovascular meningitis, usually affecting the basilar meninges can occur. An abrupt cerebrovascular accident can be the initial presentation or may occur sometime later during the course of the illness. Other sequelae of meningitis include seizures, hydrocephalus, optic atrophy, or deafness (or both). Deafness that occurs during acute inflammation of the perineural sheath is reversible with therapy.

Neurosyphilis more commonly presents as a chronic meningitis/encephalitis. The typical patient will have below-average intelligence or mental retardation, similar to the dementia observed in adult patients with neurosyphilis. This dementia (juvenile paresis) is progressive and reflects the vulnerability of the brain parenchyma to syphilis. Behavioral problems including irritability, temper tantrums, antisocial behavior, emotional instability, depression, delusions, poor concentration, and memory deficits are commonly associated conditions. Eighth-nerve deafness can occur in isolation or associated with these symptoms. The sensorineural hearing loss following chronic inflammation is not readily reversible.

Tabes dorsalis, though unusual in children, has been reported. The signs and symptoms include lightning-like pains in the legs, gait unsteadiness, sensory changes, and the loss of stretch reflexes. The gait ataxia is more prominent in the dark. The hyperesthesias and parethesias increase with time. There is loss of bladder sensation leading to retention of urine, eventual urinary incontinence, and recurrent urinary-tract infections.

In addition to deafness that may result from acute or chronic inflammation of the leptomeninges and perineural sheath, approximately 10% of patients with late congenital syphilis have a chronic, gummatous osteomyelitis and periostitis of the temporal bones that erode and slowly destroy the cochlear and vestibular receptors. The enchondral bone is nearly avascular. Additionally, the gummata are associated with arteritis. Even with appropriate antibiotic therapy, the *treponemes* can survive, subsequently reactivate, and cause rapid progressive deafness. Eventually the spirochetes invade the inner ear, resulting in labyrinthitis (39,40). Disturbance of vestibular function, tinnitus, and hearing loss are the prominent symptoms (41,42). Usually, the symptoms are bilateral, but they may be unilateral and mimic Menière disease. Periods of quiescence and exacerbations of symptoms reflect the different stages of activity of the various gummata (43–45). This form of deafness has been reported to improve with administration of penicillin in combination with prednisone.

Diagnosis

The diagnosis of neurosyphilis is often not considered because the varied neurologic manifestations mimic other diseases. Serologic studies are the standard tests for diagnosis. The isolation and culture of the organism can be difficult, especially in the later stages of the disease. Early syphilis can be diagnosed, however, by demonstrating under darkfield microscopy the motile *T. pallidum* spirochetes from scrapings of a cutaneous lesion or a lymphnode aspirate (46).

There are two categories of serologic tests used to diagnose syphilis including the nonspecific reagin antibody, either complement fixation or flocculation tests, and specific antibody tests. The first category of serologic studies includes the Kolmer test (complement fixation test) and the Venereal Disease Research Laboratory (VDRL), a flocculation test (47), which measures antibodies against lipoidal antigens derived from the *treponeme* organism itself or from its interaction with the host tissue. Although these tests are sensitive, they are not as specific as the 2nd category of tests; moreover, there may be false-positive reactions to non-treponemal antigens.

False-positive reactions to non-treponemal antigens are of two types, the first group of which includes acute infectious diseases, such as infectious mononucleosis, infectious hepatitis, viral pneumonia, malaria, varicella, rubeola, as well as with immunizations against yellow fever, typhoid, and small pox. The second group of false-positive reactions occurs with chronic autoimmune diseases such as lupus erythematosis, rheumatoid arthritis, and periarteritis nodosa, as well as drug addiction (heroin), leprosy, hepatitis, and brucellosis (48–50).

The 2nd major category of tests are antibody tests that are more sensitive and specifically directed against the treponemal organism; they are, therefore, not likely to produce false-positives. Commonly used tests of this group are the fluorescent treponemal antibody absorption test (FTA-ABS) or the treponemal hemagglutination test.

Reagin antibody tests can be negative in late congenital syphilis or neurosyphilis; however, these studies are very helpful in documenting successful antibiotic treatment of early syphilis because the titers will fall and the test will become nonreactive. The treponemal specific serologic tests are most helpful in the diagnosis of late syphilis in which the reagin test will be negative. The treponemal specific antibody tests will remain positive for years, even after adequate treatment. They are, therefore, not reliable indicators of cure.

The diagnosis of syphilis in the newborn is complicated by the fact that there is passive transfer of both reagin and treponemal antibodies across the placenta. The infant's titer of reagin antibodies, such as the VDRL, should not be greater than that of the mother's titer and should decrease over a few months. Until recently, however, there was no specific serologic test that separated infected infants from those with passively transferred maternal antibodies. Active neonatal infection can now be detected by the IgM-FTA-ABS test. This test uses labelled antihuman IgM to detect antitreponemal IgM antibodies. It is based on the fact that the primary antibodies that cross the placenta are maternal IgG antibodies; whereas, infants respond to infection by producing specific IgM antibodies. The IgM-FTA-ABS test is standardized and highly sensitive (51).

Treatment and Prevention

The treatment of choice for syphilis is the administration of penicillin, the dosage of which will vary, depending on the extent of involvement. Examination of the CSF prior to initiation of therapy is imperative. If the CSF is normal, benzathine penicillin G, 50,000 U/kg, administered intramuscularly (IM) in a single dose, is curative. If the CSF is abnormal, there are two treatment recommendations: either aqueous crystalline penicillin G, 50,000 U/kg, administered IM or IV daily in two divided doses for 14 to 21 days; or aqueous procaine penicillin G, 50,000 U/kg, administered IM daily for 14 to 21 days. In older children with clinical neurosyphilis, procaine penicillin G, 6 to 12 million units administered for 2 to 3 weeks, is recommended treatment. In patients with juvenile paresis, 12 to 24 million units of procaine penicillin G given for 2 or 3 weeks is recommended. Unfortunately, the results of treatment of juvenile paresis are poor (30, 52). In the case of

auditory nerve involvement secondary to gummata osteomyelitis, administration of penicillin in combination with prednisone has been shown to be superior to penicillin alone (35,53,54).

Patients with neurosyphilis must be followed carefully for at least 3 years. Clinical and CSF examinations should be conducted every 6 months. There is evidence that the *treponeme* organism remains in the perilymph and ocular tissue for years, even after treatment.

Given the severity of untreated congenital syphilis, the best therapy is prevention. Resources for accessible early prenatal care with adequate screening for syphilis in pregnant women are essential. Even in populations with a low prevalence of syphilis, screening in the prenatal clinics is cost effective (55).

Relapsing Fever

A spirochetal infection less common than syphilis that may produce neurologic manifestations in children, is relapsing fever, caused by *Borrelia recurrentis*. This loosely coiled spirochete is microaerophilic, vector-borne, and is transmitted by either lice or ticks. The louse-borne variety of relapsing fever occurs in patients who are living under conditions of crowding, poor hygiene, or cold weather (or both). The tick-borne variant is found in patients who are likely to be campers, hikers, or be frequently out of doors.

The incubation period of relapsing fever is 5 to 11 days, and the initial symptoms are systemic manifestations of high fever, chills, headache, and myalgias. These initial symptoms last 3 to 6 days, and the patient becomes asymptomatic, only to have a "relapse," days to weeks later.

Southern and Sanford (56) conducted an extensive review of relapsing fever and found neurologic manifestations in approximately 10% of tick-borne and 30% of louse-borne cases of relapsing fever. Neurologic complications include meningeal irritation, cranial nerve palsies, hemiplegia, seizures, neuralgias, myelitis, iridocyclitis, and psychiatric disturbances (57). One case of vocal-cord paralysis associated with a multifocal neuropathy has also been reported (58).

The diagnosis of relapsing fever depends on taking a careful, complete clinical history. Confirmation of the disease is established by observing *Borrelia* organisms on smears examined with Wright stain, as well as by serologic tests. The treatment of choice is oral or parenteral tetracycline 30 mg/kg/day in four divided doses for 10 days. Erythromycin and chloramphenicol have also been used (59).

Leptospirosis

Leptospirosis was first described by Alfred Weil in 1886, but the causal agent, *spirocheta icterohemorrhagiae* was not identified until 1915 by Inada and colleagues (60). It is a multisystem disease transmitted from an animal carrier to a human host. It is now recognized that there is a family of Leptospirae, with multiple serogroups and serotypes. The three most important serogroups include: *Leptospire icterohemorrhagiae*, in which rats and mice serve as the animal reservoir; *Leptospire canicola*, in which the dog serves as the animal reservoir; and *Leptospire pomona*, with swine as the animal reservoir. The Leptospirae cause disease worldwide and have a predilection for the kidneys of the animal carrier, shedding the organisms in the urine. The infection in humans is spread by contact with leptospirae containing urine or its contaminants, such as soil and water; as such the disease tends to follow occupational lines, affecting, for example, young men who work on farms. Though not common, the disease can affect children, in whom the usual animal carrier is the dog.

Clinical Features

Leptospirosis is most prevalent between July and October, coinciding with exposure to lakes, ponds, and soil, which can harbor the *Leptospire* organism. Leptospirae enter the human body by penetration through conjunctivae, mucous membranes, and abraded skin. The incubation time is approximately 7 to 10 days, and the signs and symptoms vary considerably. The mild infection may present with only headache, fever, malaise, and myalgias; whereas, severe infection can be fatal, with symptoms of high fever, hepatitis, and hypotension (60).

Leptospirosis is usually manifested as a biphasic disease. During the first stage, there is septicemia associated with an abrupt onset of fever and chills, headache, myalgias, and malaise. Conjunctivitis is commonly observed. Leptospirae are recoverable from the blood and CSF. There is usually a leukocytosis and an elevated sedimentation rate; examination of the CSF shows normal cell count and normal concentrations of protein and glucose. This phase lasts about 1 week, and then the signs and symptoms diminish. If the infection is severe and affects the liver, however, the signs and symptoms of hepatitis persist. The second stage of leptospirosis begins in the 2nd and 3rd week after symptom onset. Generally, there is recurrence of fever, and signs and symptoms of neurologic involvement appear during this phase; aseptic meningitis is the most commonly observed neurologic abnormality.

Neurologic Manifestations

During the first stage of leptospirosis, headache and malaise are uniformly seen. In addition, confusion, delirium, hallucinations, and mood disturbances have been reported (61,62).

During the second stage of the disease, a CSF pleocytosis indicative of meningeal inflammation occurs in 80% of patients; whereas, only 50% develop symptoms of aseptic meningitis (60), such as headache, vomiting, and stiff neck.

The CSF initially has a polymorphonuclear leukocytosis, with a mononuclear leukocytosis developing after a few days. The protein concentration can be normal or elevated, and the glucose is either normal or low. The *Leptospire* organism cannot be isolated or cultured from the CSF at this stage, which is the basis for the theory that this phase of the disease represents as immune reaction (63,64). Encephalitis, myelitis, peripheral neuritis (commonly the brachial plexus), cranial-nerve involvement, upper motor neuron disturbance, seizures, and findings consistent with Guillain-Barré syndrome have all been reported in the second stage of leptospirosis (60–62,65–68). Neuropathologic studies show perivascular infiltration of blood vessels in affected areas including the spinal cord, basal ganglia, hippocampus, and white matter (69).

Despite the intensity of the immune response during this second stage, complete recovery is the general rule. Aseptic meningitis usually lasts only 1 to 2 days, but other neurologic manifestations can be more prolonged. The more severe form of leptospirosis, with impaired hepatic and renal function, can produce an alteration of consciousness, confusion, and hallucinations. This is thought to be secondary to the accompanying metabolic perturbations. This type of leptospirosis has a 5% to 10% mortality rate, with vascular collapse and hemorrhage occurring frequently.

Diagnosis

Leptospirosis can be diagnosed by isolation of the organism or by serologic testing. The organism can be isolated from blood and CSF only during the 1st week; however, leptospiruria can persist for weeks. Serologic testing, the more common method of diagnosis, can be carried out by using different serologic techniques, including microscopic agglutination, complement fixation, indirect immunofluorescence, and hemagglutination. The antibody titer rises 7 to 10 days after exposure to the *Leptospire* organisms (60).

Prevention and Treatment

Preventive measures are the best way to control the disease. Good hygiene, protective clothing, rodent control, and avoidance of contaminated areas like ponds, are simple, effective ways to prevent infection. For those individuals who have high risk occupations, immunizations have been used with fairly good success (70).

Leptospirosis is usually a self-limiting disease. Aqueous penicillin G in doses of 6 to 8 million units/M^2, given over a 24-hour period in 6 divided doses, has been shown to minimize the symptoms, if given early in the disease course (60,71). Alternatively, tetracycline can be given to children older than the age of 10 years or adults, in doses of 10 to 20 mg/kg/day, divided 4 times a day for a period of 1 week. If the medication is administered later than 7 days after onset, treatment is less effective. Attention to fluid and electrolyte balance and other supportive measures are essential.

Leptospirosis is a disease not commonly found in children but may have a diversity of neurologic manifestations in its 2nd or immune stage. Unlike the other spirochetal infections, however, leptospirosis is distinctive in that the neurologic manifestations tend to be self-limiting.

RICKETTSIAL DISEASE

Rickettsiae have characteristics that are common to bacteria and viruses. They resemble viruses because they are obligate intracellular parasites and require the environment of living cells for growth and reproduction. They are similar to bacteria because of similar properties: multiplication is by binary fission; they contain both RNA and DNA; at least one species contains muramic acid; they possess enzymes of the Kreb cycle of electron transport and of protein synthesis; and growth is inhibited by antibacterial agents (72). Rickettsiae are, therefore, considered to occupy a taxonomic position between bacteria and viruses.

The organism is named after Dr. H.T. Ricketts who, at the turn of the century, discovered the agent causing Rocky Mountain Spotted Fever (RMSF). These microorganisms are small, pleomorphic coccobacilli appearing as spherical forms, as short rods, or as thin rods under the light microscope. Rickettsiae stain poorly with Gram stain but with Gimenez stain have a characteristic red color. Infections caused by rickettsiae produce agglutinins to the OX19, OX2, or OXK strains of the bacillus Proteus vulgaris (Weil-Felix reaction), complement-fixing, and immunofluorescent antibodies (73).

The rickettsial microorganisms have a wide range of natural hosts including insects, ticks and mites, birds, and mammals. In mammals, rickettsiae are primarily transmitted through the bite of insects (lice and fleas) and arachnids (ticks and mites). Arthropod vectors frequently serve as carrier and host in which rickettsiae are transovarially transmitted to its progeny from generation to generation (74).

In humans, rickettsial infections often result in characteristic clinical features manifested by an infectious disease with fever, headache, and skin rash. Early in the course of the illness, the infections are susceptible to certain broad-spectrum antibiotics (tetracycline and chloramphenicol). The severity of illness of a rickettsial infection varies from a benign self-limiting condition (rickettsialpox) to one that may have a fulminating course (RMSF). On the basis of clinical characteristics, etiologic agents, vectors, serologic reactions, and epidemiologic characteristics, the rickettsial diseases can be classified into five groups (75). The groups include spotted fever, typhus, scrub typhus, Q fever, and trench fever. Partial or complete immunity is conferred against an infection by any of the rickettsiae of the same group. Little or no cross immunity is conferred against infections caused by agents of different groups. Because infections by some of these groups of microorganisms

rarely cause neurologic symptoms in children, only RMSF and louse-borne typhus fever will be discussed.

Rocky Mountain Spotted Fever

RMSF is classified with the spotted fever group of diseases. These diseases are transmitted by ticks and are also called tick typhuses. The occurrence of RMSF is not limited to the foothills of the Rocky Mountains of the United States, for identical diseases occur in other parts of this country and other countries of the Western Hemisphere (Sao Paulo fever). Tick-borne typhus fever occurring in other parts of the world, for example those occurring in Europe, Australia, Africa and elsewhere, are considered as variants of the same disease. The clinical manifestations of the spotted fever diseases occurring in other parts of the world are, however, usually less severe than those noted in individuals with RMSF.

Pathology

The primary pathologic lesion of RMSF and of virtually every rickettsial disease, is found in the vascular system. Rickettsiae have a predilection for endothelial cells and the media of capillaries and arterioles. Organisms multiply within the cells lining blood vessels, and platelets then adhere to the surface of the rickettsial infected endothelial cells (76). In the brain, as in other organs, the primary histologic lesion is a destructive or destructive-proliferative thrombovasculitis (77), and if severe, the diffuse vasculitis causes vessel thrombosis, necrosis, and other tissue damage. Microinfarctions of brain parenchyma are common. The effects of the vasculitis appear to account for some but not all of the prominent clinical manifestations of RMSF.

Etiology and Transmission

RMSF is caused by *Rickettsia rickettsii*. This *rickettsia* is an obligate parasite and multiplies not only in the cytoplasm, but primarily in the nuclei of cells of susceptible animals. The principal carriers and vectors transmitting the organism are the Western wood tick, *Dermacentor andersoni*, the Eastern dog tick, *Dermacentor verabilis*, and *Amblyomma Americanum*, in the southwestern United States. Rickettsiae are passed from one generation of ticks to another by transovarian transmission and survive the winter months (overwinters) in cells of the arthropod vector. Adult female ticks require a blood meal from animals to initiate the ovarian cycle, lay eggs, and increase the virulence and transmissibility of the microorganism (78). Rickettsiae are also transmitted from an infected male to a previously uninfected female through venereal transmission during the mating process (79). The disease is transmitted to humans, an incidental host, usually by the bite of an adult tick.

The incidence of RMSF in this country increased markedly after 1960 at which time there was a shift of distribution of cases to the eastern United States. The disease occurs from May to September during the period of the greatest tick activity. Because children often play with dogs and engage in outdoor activity during the warm weather months they have increased opportunities for exposure to the vector. Approximately 2/3 of patients with RMSF are younger than 15 years of age.

Clinical Features

The onset of symptoms occurs 2 to 8 days after the bite of an infected tick. The principal clinical features include fever, headache, rash, tick bite, confusion, and myalgia. The temperature rapidly rises to 40° C and may remain persistently elevated or have a spiking course. The child often appears acutely ill. The headache is intense and not readily amenable to therapy. The rash of RMSF is an important diagnostic feature of the disease and usually appears on the 2nd or 3rd day after onset of symptoms, although it may appear later. The initial lesions are erythematous macules, which blanch on pressure, but they rapidly become maculopapular, petechial, and even hemorrhagic. The rash initially appears on the wrist or ankles and within hours spreads up the extremities to the trunk. The rash characteristically appears on the palms and soles of affected patients (Figure 12.3).

Neurologic Manifestations

CNS involvement in RMSF is manifested by changes in the level of consciousness, mental confusion, hallucinations, seizures, and coma. Retinal venous engorgement, retinal edema, papilledema, and corticospinal tract signs have been reported (77). The early clinical features of RMSF including fever, nuchal rigidity, headache, and skin rash may mislead the physician into making a diagnosis of bacterial meningitis or meningococcemia. When it is not possible to carefully and clearly differentiate RMSF, bacterial meningitis, or meningococcemia, specific antibiotic therapy against these diseases must be initiated immediately and should not be delayed until a specific diagnosis can be made. Delay in administering specific antibiotics for rickettsial infections is the most important reason for the continuing mortality rate of 5% to 10% in RMSF.

Diagnosis

Unfortunately during the early stages of the disease, no laboratory test is available that can readily establish the diagnosis of RMSF. Routine laboratory studies may show normal white-blood-cell count or leukocytosis with shift to the left, or thrombocytopenia without significant clotting abnormalities, and hyponatremia. The major clinical manifestations associated with low serum sodium concentration

and thrombocytopenia are helpful in recognition of this infection (80). Serologic tests that are used to confirm the diagnosis usually become positive in the 2nd week of the illness. Immunoflourescent staining of a punch biopsy of the skin rash with specific antibody (81) and specific immunofluorescent assays become positive during the 1st week of the illness. These techniques, however, may not be readily available in many laboratories. The Weil-Felix Reaction is a useful test because it is readily available, it can be performed quickly, and is positive in a high proportion of untreated patients with RMSF. The test relies on the fact that these rickettsiae share common antigens with two strains of Proteus, the OX19 and OX2. Rising titers, or titers of 1 : 160 or greater, in a patient with clinical signs of RMSF are significant. The standard complement-fixation antibody test, when positive, is highly specific. A rise in titer may not be present until 10 to 12 days after the onset of the illness. Acute and convalescent titers should be determined.

Therapy and Prevention

Tetracycline and chloramphenicol are highly effective antibiotics when administered early in the course of the disease. In seriously ill patients, chloramphenicol can be administered IV in a dose range of 30 to 50 mg/kg/24 hours. It can be changed to oral administration of 50 mg/kg/24 hours when conditions warrant. Tetracycline may be given IV at a dose of 20 mg/kg/24 hours, but can be given orally at a dose of 30 to 40 mg/kg/24 hours. Because of possible adverse effects of tetracycline on the permanent teeth when administered to patients younger than 8 years of age, the administration of chloramphenicol is preferred. Treatment can be terminated when the temperature remains normal for several days. Doxycycline has also been used to treat some patients with the rickettsial infections of the spotted fever group, but it has not been recommended for the treatment of patients with RMSF (82). The careful management of fluids and electrolytes and of symptomatic thrombocytopenia with fresh platelet concentrates are major considerations in the care of a child with RMSF.

The major preventive measures include avoiding contact with ticks and the use of vaccines. Avoiding tick contact can be reduced by tucking trousers into boots, limiting exposure of skin, using tick repellent, frequent inspection of the skin, and "deticking." Vaccines have been given to high-risk patients, and annual booster immunization is recommended.

Louse-Borne (Epidemic) Typhus Fever

The typhus fevers are comprised of louse-borne (epidemic) typhus, flea-borne (murine/endemic) typhus, and recrudescent (Brill-Zinsser) typhus. Because flea-borne typhus is a relatively mild infection characterized by headache, fever,

FIGURE 12.3 (A) Typical maculopapular erythematous rash of Rocky Mountain Spotted Fever that initially appears on the wrists or ankles of infected patients but within hours spreads to the extremities and trunk. (B) Close-up view of a maculopapular and petechial rash of Rocky Mountain Spotted Fever. Courtesy of Gunderson Medical Foundation, LaCrosse, WI.

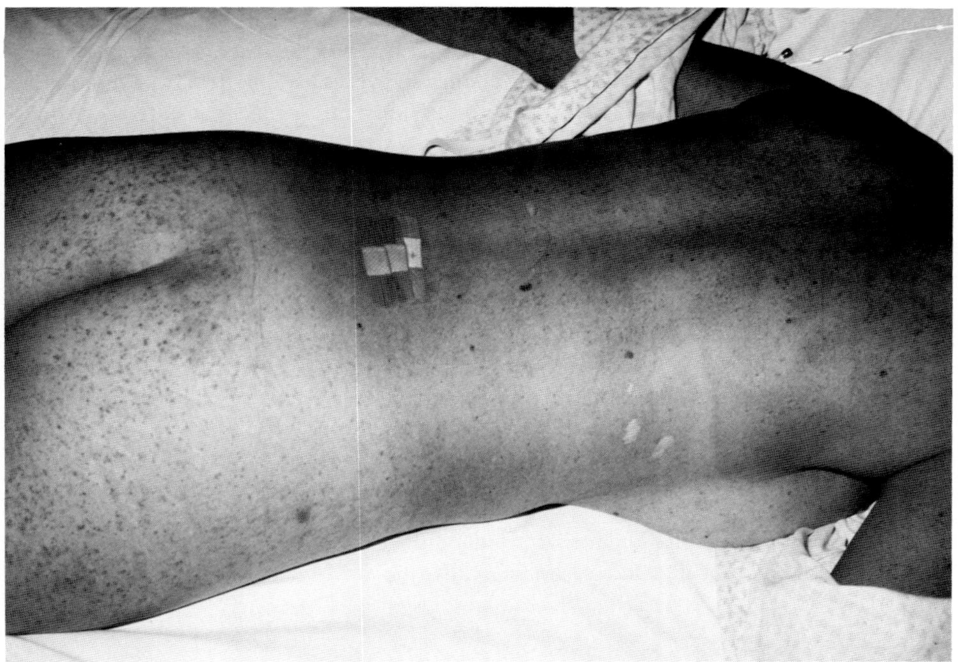

A

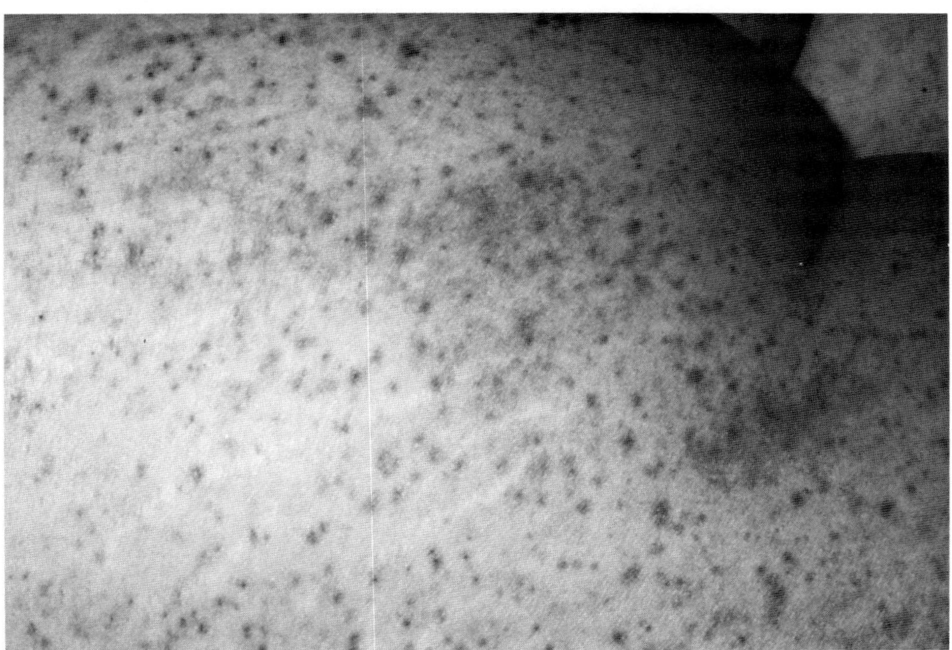

B

malaise, and a maculopapular rash, and the Brill-Zinsser typhus is a recrudescence of epidemic typhus with similarly mild symptoms, this section describes only the louse-borne typhus.

Etiology and Transmission

During periods of social upheaval as in the time of war, severe poverty, and famine, the body louse multiples in great numbers. Although epidemic typhus has not been reported recently in the United States, epidemics have occurred in other parts of the world, including Europe, Africa, and Asia. The etiologic agent is *Rickettsia prowazekii,* and humans and lice *(Pediculus Humanus humanus)* are the only significant hosts. The louse becomes infected during a blood meal from febrile patients with rickettsemia. After an incubation period, rickettsiae appear in the louse feces. Infected feces are transmitted when the material is scratched into the bite wound or can be transmitted when infectious matter is rubbed into the mucous membranes of the eye or inhaled into the respiratory tract. The pathologic findings in cases of louse-borne typhus are similar to those reported in RMSF.

Clinical Features

Symptoms occur 1 to 2 weeks after the bite and include headache, fever, and rash. The rash appears on the trunk by the 4th to the 7th day and spreads peripherally to the extremities, sparing the palms of the hands and soles of the feet. The rash is initially maculopapular but then becomes petechial and purpuric in the second week of the illness. In untreated patients with a severe attack, the illness may be accompanied by paranoia, delirium, hallucinations, mental excitability, and deafness.

During an epidemic, the diagnosis is made with relative ease and often on clinical grounds. Serologically, the Weil-Felix reaction is almost always positive for the Proteus OX19 and often with OX2. Complement-fixation serologic tests and immunofluorescent staining of skin biopsy specimens are confirmatory studies.

Therapy and Prevention

Patients with epidemic typhus should be deloused by bathing with soap and water and dusting with delousing powder. Tetracycline or chloramphenicol should be administered early in the disease with recommended doses similar to those used in treating RMSF. Doxycycline, a derivative of tetracycline, in a single oral dose of 100 mg for adult patients and 50 mg for children younger than 10 years of age, has been effective in treating epidemic typhus (83). The dose of doxycycline may need to be increased or administered for a longer period of time when it is used in the treatment of other types of typhus fever infections.

REFERENCES

1. Garin C, Bujadoux C. Paralysie par les Tiques. J Med Lyon 1922;71:765–767.
2. Bannwarth A. Chronische lymphocytare meningitis, entzundliche polyneuritis und "Rheumatismus." Arch Psychiatr Nervenkr 1941;113:284–376.
3. Schaltenbrand G. Durch Arthropoden ubertragene infektionen der Haut and des Nervensystems. Münch Med Wochenschr 1966;108:1557–1562.
4. Horstrup P, Ackermann R. Durch zecken ubertragene meningopolyneuritis (Garin-Bujadoux, Bannwarth). Fortsch Neurol Psychiatr 1973;41:583–606.
5. Steere AC, Malawista SE, Snydman DR, et al. Lyme Arthritis: An epidemic of oligoarticular arthritis in children and adults in three Connecticut communities. Arthritis Rheum 1977;20:7–17.
6. Steere AC, Grodzick RL, Kornblatt AN, et al. The spirochetal etiology of Lyme disease. N Engl J Med 1983;308:733–740.
7. Benach JL, Bosler EM, Hanrahan JP, et al. Spirochetes isolated in the blood of two patients with Lyme disease. N Engl J Med 1983;308:740–742.
8. Steere AC, Bartenhagen NH, Craft JE, et al. The early clinical manifestations of Lyme disease. Ann Intern Med 1983;99:76–82.
9. Pachner AR, Steere AC. The triad of neurologic manifestations of Lyme disease: Meningitis, cranial neuritis, and radiculoneuritis. Neurology 1985;35:47–53.
10. Steere AC, Batsford WP, Weinberg M, et al. Lyme carditis: Cardiac abnormalities of Lyme disease. Ann Intern Med 1980;93(Part I):8–16.
11. Steere AC, Malawista SE, Hardin JA, et al. Erythema chronicum migrans and Lyme arthritis: The enlarging clinical spectrum. Ann Intern Med 1977;86:685–698.
12. Muhlemann MF, Wright DJM. Emerging patterns of Lyme disease in the United Kingdom and Irish Republic. Lancet 1987;1:260–262.
13. Dattwyler RJ, Volkman DJ, Luft BJ, et al. Lyme disease in Europe and North America. Lancet 1987;1:681.
14. Reik L, Steere AC, Bartenharge NH, et al. Neurologic abnormalities of Lyme disease. Medicine 1979;58:281–294.
15. Steere AC, Broderick TF, Malawista SE. Erythema chronicum migrans and Lyme arthritis: Epidemiologic evidence of a tick vector. Am J Epidemiol 1978;108:312–321.
16. Christen H, Hanefeld F. Neurologic complications of erythema migrans disease in childhood clinical aspects. Zentralbl Bakteriol Mikrobiol Hyg. 1986;263:337–342.
17. Halperin JJ, Pass HL, Anand AK, et al. Nervous system abnormalities in Lyme disease. Unpublished. Presented at the International Symposium on Lyme Disease, 1987.
18. Clark JR, Carlson RD, Pachner AR, et al. Facial paralysis in Lyme disease. Laryngoscope 1985; 95:1341–1345.
19. Reik L, Burgdorfer W, Donaldson JO. Neurologic abnormalities in Lyme disease without erythema chronicum migrans. Am J Med 1986;81:73–78.
20. Halperin JJ, Little BW, Coyle PK, et al. Lyme disease—cause of a treatable peripheral neuropathy. Neurology 1987;37:1700–1706.
21. Christen H, Hanefeld F. Lyme Borreliosis in children—A prospective clinical epidemiological study. Annals of the New York Academy of Sciences, In press.
22. Midgard R, Hofstad H. Unusual manifestations of nervous system *Borrelia burgdorferi* infection. Arch Neurol 1987;44:781–783.
23. Schmutzhard E, Willeit J, Gerstenbrand F. Meningopolyneuritis Bannwarth with focal nodular myositis. Klin Wochenschr 1986;64:1204–1208.
24. Pachner AR, Steere AC. Neurologic involvement in the third stage of Lyme disease: CNS manifestations can mimic multiple sclerosis and psychiatric illness. Neurology 1986;36 Suppl 1:286.
25. Hansen K, Rechnitzer C, Pederson NS, et al. *Borrelia meningitis* and demyelinating CNS disease. Second International Symposium on Lyme Disease and related disorders. Vienna, Austria, Sept 17–19, 1985:45.

26. Reik L, Smith L, Khan A, et al. Demyelinating encephalopathy in Lyme disease. Neurology 1985;35:267–269.

26a. *Lyme Borreliosis in Wisconsin.* Marshfield, WI: Marshfield Medical Press, 1991.

26b. Davis J, Schell W. *Lyme Disease: A Clinician's Guide,* Maddison, WI, Wisconsin Department of Health and Social Services, January 1989.

27. Steere AC, Pachner AR, Malawista SE. Neurologic abnormalities of Lyme disease: Successful treatment with high dose intravenous Penicillin. Ann Intern Med, 1983;99:767–772.

28. Dattwyler RJ, Halperin JJ, Pass HL, et al. Ceftriaxone as effective therapy in refractory Lyme disease. J Infect Dis 1987;155:1322–1325.

29. Congenital syphilis—US, 1983–1985. JAMA, 1986;256:3206–3208.

30. Speck WT, Toltzis P. Syphilis. In: Behrman RE, Vaughan VC, eds. Nelson Textbook of Pediatrics. 12th ed. Philadelphia: W.B. Saunders, 1983, 728–733.

31. Curtis AC, Philpott OS. Prenatal syphilis. Med Clin North Am 1964;48:707.

32. Peterson JC. Congenital syphilis: A review of its present status and significance in pediatrics. South Med J 1973;66:257.

33. Tavs LE. Syphilis. In: Solomon LM, Esterly NB, Loeffel D, eds. Major problems in clinical pediatrics, Vol. 19. Philadelphia: W.B. Saunders, 1978;19:222–256.

34. Vercoe GS. The effect of early syphilis on the inner ear and auditory nerves. J Laryngol Otol 1976;86:853–861.

35. Saltiel P, Melmed C, Portnoy D. Sensorineural deafness in early acquired syphilis. Can J Neurol Sci 1983;10:114–116.

36. Bush JA, Ryan EJ. Syphilitic optic perineuritis. Am J Ophthalmol 1981;9:404–406.

37. Spoor TC. Ocular syphilis—acute and chronic. J Clin Neurol-ophthalmol, 1983;3:197–203.

38. Sacks JG, Osher RH, Elconin H. Progressive visual loss in syphilitic optic atrophy. Clin Neuro-ophthalmol 1983;3:5–8.

39. Mayer O, Fraser JS. Pathological changes in the ear in late congenital syphilis. J Laryngol Otol 1936;51:683–755.

40. Harmondy CS, Schuknecht HF. Deafness in congenital syphilis. Arch Otolaryngol 1966;83:18–27.

41. Hendershot EL. Luetic deafness. Laryngoscope 1983;83:865–870.

42. Hendershot EL. Luetic deafness. Otolaryngol Clin North Am 1978;11:43–47.

43. Karmody C, Schuknecht H. Deafness in congenital syphilis. Arch Otolaryngol 1966;83:44.

44. Perlman HB. Late congenital syphilis. Proceedings of the symposium on sensorineural hearing processes and disorders. Detroit, Henry Ford Hospital, 1967.

45. Perlman HB, Leek J. Late congenital syphilis of ear. Laryngoscope 1952;62:1175.

46. Alpert G, Plotkin SA. A practical guide to the diagnosis of congenital infections in the newborn infant. Pediatr Clin North Am 1986;33:465–479.

47. Harris A, Rosenberg AA, Riedel IM. A microflocculation test for syphilis using cardiolipin antigen. J Vener Dis Inform 1946;27:169.

48. Catterall RD. Systemic disease and the biological false positive reaction for syphilis. Br J Vener Dis 1972;48:1.

49. Harvey AM, Schulman LE. Connective tissue disease and the chronic biologic false positive test for syphilis. Med Clin North Am 1966;50:1271.

50. Tuffanelli DL. False positive reactions for syphilis. Arch Dermatol 1968;98:606.

51. Muller F. Specific immunoglobulin M and G antibodies in the rapid diagnosis of human treponemal infections. Diagn Immunol 1986;4:1–9.

52. Wilfert C, Gutman L. Syphilis. In: Feigin RD, Cherry CD, eds. Textbook of Pediatric Infectious Disease: Vol. 1. Philadelphia: WB Saunders, 1981, 388–400.

53. Becker GD. Late syphilitic hearing loss: A diagnostic and therapeutic dilemma. Laryngoscope 1979;89:1273–1288.

54. Steckelberg JM, McDonald TJ. Otologic involvement in late syphilis. Laryngoscope 1984;94:753–757.

55. Stray-Pederson B. Economic evaluation of maternal screening to prevent congenital syphilis. Sex Transm Dis 1983;10:167–172.

56. Southern PM, Sanford JP. Relapsing fever. Medicine 1969;48:129–149.

57. Scott RB. Neurological complications of relapsing fever. Lancet 1944;1:436–438.

58. Olchovsky D, Pines A, Sodeh M, et al. Multifocal neuropathy and vocal cord paralysis in relapsing fever. Eur Neurol 1982;21:340–342.

59. Boyer KM. *Borrelia:* Relapsing fever. In: Feigin RD, Cherry CD, eds. Textbook of Pediatric Infectious Diseases, Vol. 1. Philadelphia: WB Saunders, 1981, 825–828.

60. Feigin RD, Anderson DC. Leptospirosis. In: Feigin RD, Cherry CD, eds. Textbook of Pediatric Diseases, Vol. 1. Philadelphia: WB Saunders, 1981, 895–911.

61. Edwards GA, Domm BM. Human leptospirosis. Medicine (Balt) 1960;39:117–156.

62. Heath CW, Jr, Alexander AD, Galton MM. Leptospirosis in the US. N Engl J Med. 1965;273:857–922.

63. Babudieri B. Animal reservoirs of leptospires. Ann NY Acad Sci 1958;70:393–413.

64. Gsell O. Leptospirosis. Bern: Hans Huber Verlag, 1952.

65. Elian M, Tamir M, Bornstein B. Unusual case of brachial plexitis in relation to leptospires and Coxsackie virus. Confin Neurol 1965;26:1–6.

66. McCulloch WF, Braun JL, Robinson RG. Leptospiral meningitis. J Iowa Med Soc 1962;52:728–731.

67. Middleton JE. Canicola fever with neurological complications. Br Med J 1955;2:25–26.

68. Van Thiele PH. The leptospiroses. Leiden: Universitaire Pers Leiden, 1948.

69. Koppisch E, Bond WM. The morbid anatomy of human leptospirosis: A report on thirteen fatal cases. In: Symposium on the Leptospiroses, December 11–12, 1952. Medical Science Publication No. 1. Washington, DC: U.S. Government Printing Office, 1953, 83–105.

70. Turner LH. Leptospirosis. Trans R Soc Trop Med Hyg 1967;61:842–855.

71. Kocen RS. Leptospirosis, a comparison of symptomatic and penicillin therapy. Br Med J 1962;1:1181–1183.

72. Murray ES. Rickettsial disease. In: Feigin RD, Cherry CD, eds. Textbook of Pediatric Infectious Diseases, Vol. 2. Philadelphia: WB Saunders, 1981, 1437–1449.

73. Tayler JP, Tanner WB, Rawlings JA, et al. Serological evidence of subclinical Rocky Mountain Spotted Fever infections in Texas. J Infect Dis 1985;151:367–369.

74. Farhang-Azad A, Traub R, Bagar S. Transovarial transmission of murine typhus rickettsiae in xenopsylla cheopis fleas. Science 1985;227:543–544.

75. Riley HD Jr. Rickettsial disease. In: Wedgwood RJ, Davis SD, Ray CG, et al., eds. Infections in Children, Vol. 1. Philadelphia: Harper and Row, 1982, 1027–1031.

76. Silverman DJ. Adherence of platelets to human endothelial cells infected by rickettsia rickettsii. J Infect Dis 1986; 153:694–700.

77. Bell WE, Lascari AD. Rocky mountain spotted fever. Neurology 1970;20:841–847.

78. Riley HD Jr. Rocky Mountain Spotted Fever. In: Wedgwood RJ, Davis SD, Ray CG, et al., eds. Infections in Children, Vol. 1. Philadelphia: Harper and Row, 1981, 1045–1076.

79. Phillip CB. Some epidemiologic considerations in Rocky Mountain Spotted Fever. Public Health Rep 1959; 74:595.

80. Bradford WD, Hawkins HK. Rocky Mountain Spotted Fever in childhood. Am J Dis Child 1977;131:1228–1232.

81. Woodward TE, Peterson CE, Oster CN, et al. Prompt confirmation of Rocky Mountain Spotted Fever: Identification of rickettsiae in skin tissue. J Infect Dis 1976;134:297–305.

82. Yagupsky P, Gross EM, Alkan M, et al. Comparison of two dosage schedules of doxycycline in children with rickettsial spotted fever. J Infect Dis 1987;155:1215–1219.

83. Wisserman CL. Typhus fever. In: Hoeprich PD, ed. Infectious Disease; Vol. 3. Philadelphia: Harper and Row, 1983, 908–914.

Chapter 13
Neurosarcoidosis

Paul R. Dyken

Besnier-Boeck-Schaumann disease, also called benign lymphogranuloma, or simply sarcoidosis is a systemic disorder of unknown cause that is characterized by the development of small, noncaseating epithelioid granulomas in almost any organ. The term sarcoidosis is a noun that represents a disease and should be distinguished from the adjective, sarcoid. A sarcoid lesion may be secondary to a wide variety of diseases. The term comes from Boeck who named the lesion for a fancied resemblance to sarcoma. Sarcoidosis is a systemic disease in which there are sarcoid lesions. The diagnosis of sarcoidosis rests with the clinician and not the pathologist (1).

The history of sarcoidosis illustrates some confusing aspects of the disease (1–3). Jonathan Hutchinson in 1869 was the first to describe a patient with presumed sarcoidosis. He actually described 2 patients, naming the condition Mortimer malady, after a woman who was afflicted with disfiguring facial skin lesions. In 1889, Besnier described lupus pernio, which is characterized by a large bulbous, violaceous nose, ubiquitously pictured in texts of physical diagnosis. Lupus pernio is also characterized by disfiguring lesions in the interphalangeal joints, and it has since been recognized as a form of sarcoidosis.

In 1899, Ceasar Boeck described the histologic appearance of skin and lymph-gland lesions. In his doctorate thesis, Schaumann (1914) grouped all of these various disorders under one name, benign lymphogranuloma, to distinguish them from malignant lymphogranuloma or Hodgkin disease. Neurologic aspects of sarcoidosis were recognized earlier by Licharew in 1908, who described a peculiar form of muscular wasting in a patient with lupus pernio; and in 1909 Heerfordt coined the term uveoparotid fever. Even with the enlightened work of Schaumann, the subject seemed in later years to devolve into clinical and pathologic chaos. A helpful step was taken by the National Research Council Conference on Sarcoidosis in 1948, when the disease was given definition (4). The 1980s have shown an expansion and refinement in definition (5).

The many clinical syndromes of this condition are dependent upon the organ or tissue involved. The lungs, reticuloendothelial system, eyes, skin, and parotid glands are most commonly affected, but all organ systems have been implicated at one time or another (6–9).

The condition of sarcoidosis with neurologic symptoms has been referred to as neurosarcoidosis (10,11). This condition alone represents a significant clinical problem. Although data suggesting the incidence of neurosarcoidosis is variable and dependent upon the time, location, and selective bias of the reporter (12–18), it has been estimated that symptomatic neurologic manifestations associated with sarcoid vary from 5% to 16% of reported cases (15,16). It is generally accepted that many of the patients with neurosarcoidosis, perhaps as many as 50%, present with neurologic involvement only (11). Frequent neurologic manifestations before histologic confirmation of the diagnosis, include isolated cranial and peripheral neuropathy, aseptic meningitis, hydrocephalus, symptoms of hypothalamic and pituitary parenchymatous involvement, mass lesions in the brain, symptoms resulting from multifocal meningeal and parenchymatous involvement, and myopathy.

Several reviews of sarcoidosis in childhood have emphasized the relative infrequency of the disease in this age group (19,20). In 1983, fewer than 350 cases of sarcoidosis in children had been reported, mostly as isolated case reports or as a small series of patients (21–25). This general figure might be compared to an estimated 6000 cases reported in the world, suggesting that about 6% of all instances of sarcoidosis occurs in children. Weinberg and associates (21) surveyed 261 pediatric cases of sarcoidosis and found that 23 (9%) had neurologic involvement. Three of those patients with neurologic involvement were less than 4 years old. Thus, it appears that neurologic syndromes of sarcoidosis in children represent a similar percentage of the total pediatric cases as in adult patients. James and Williams (6) surveyed the clinical features of 818

Table 13.1 Comparison of adults and children with sarcoidosis*

	*Adults** (17 yrs or greater)*	*Children*** (3 mos to 18 yrs)*
Total No.	818	261
% Neurologic Manifestations	9%	9%
% Females	61%	52%
Symptoms/Signs Before 4 years	74%	—
Symptoms/Signs After 4 years	—	87%

*Used with permission from Wyngaarden JB, Smith LH. In: Cecil Textbook of Medicine, 17th ed. Philadelphia: WB Saunders, 1985.

**Used with permission from Clinical Pediatrics 1983;22: 447–481.

patients with sarcoidosis and discovered that only 9% had nervous system findings (Table 13.1).

Even though sarcoidosis, in general, represents a disease of young adults, neurosarcoidosis is an important diagnostic entity and one of which pediatric neurologists should be well aware. Neurosarcoidosis should be considered in the differential diagnosis of otherwise unexplained neurologic symptoms in children.

PATHOPHYSIOLOGY

The pathologic reactions of sarcoidosis are dependent upon two somewhat independent mechanisms. One is the simple compressive or space occupying phenomenon that depends upon symptoms produced by local involvement of granulomas, whether diffuse, single, multiple nodules, small or as large solitary collections represented classically as the giant granuloma of the central nervous system (CNS). The second pathologic mechanism emphasized by Zeman (8), consists of the noncompressive effect possibly due to angiitis or involvement of small vessels, resulting from toxic or immune factors. Complete facial nerve palsy usually results from direct granulomatous involvement of the facial nerve and its compression. The diffuse symptomatology associated with another common manifestation of neurosarcoidosis syndrome, polyneuropathy, cannot be explained by compressive phenomena alone, nor can the symptoms usually seen in the uncommon syndrome of sarcoidotic muscular dystrophy (26–28).

The cause of sarcoidosis remains unclear though infectious, toxic, immunologic, allergic, and genetic mechanisms have all been implicated in the production of granulomas and angiitis. Although a specific etiology has not been proven, all of the above noxious agents may be responsible in causing the pathophysiologic mechanisms of neurosarcoidosis. Even though the cause of sarcoidosis is unknown, the basic infectious nature of the disease seems supported by the clinical similarity of the disease to known infections such as tuberculosis. The presence of identified fungi and viruses or bacterial agents in patients with proven sarcoidosis probably reflects coincidental rather than causal events. Immunopathic etiologic factors also stand out. Sarcoidosis represents a proven lymphoproliferative disorder (6). In sarcoidosis, there is evidence of depression of delayed-type hypersensitivity, activated thymus mediated T4-helper cells, hyperreactive B cells, and frequent circulating immune complexes. Again, there is some question whether these factors are the cause or are rather a secondary result of the disorder. There is little evidence that patients are immunocompromised as in Acquired Immunodeficiency Syndrome (AIDS), although these disorders show some vague similarities. There have been claims that a hypersensitivity reaction to certain antigens is important in producing sarcoid lesions, and ultimately sarcoidosis. Implicated noxious antigens in sarcoidosis include pine pollen, peanut dust, clay, pine pitch, zirconium, and beryllium. These noxious antigens are not related to all patients with the disease. It would seem, however, that there may be some genetic predisposition to the disease. Women seem more susceptible to the disease, especially if they are of child-bearing age. American blacks are more susceptible to sarcoid than Orientals with similar geographic distribution, and Japanese sarcoidosis is a well-known entity. Sarcoidotic erythema nodusum commonly occurs in early pregnancy and in women taking oral contraceptives. Arthritis and skin lesions of sarcoidosis occur more often in persons who are HLA-B8, AI, CW7, and DR3 types. These HLA (human leukocyte antigen) typings are associated with short-course illness and good prognosis; whereas, HLA-B13 is more likely associated with chronicity (6) and poorer prognosis.

Sarcoid granulomas are believed to be formed by an antigen-antibody reaction after a noxious antigen stimulates the host's cellular and humoral immune responses. T-lymphocytes liberate monocyte attracting substances (7); these attracted monocytes, in turn, are precursors of specific macrophages, which are further stimulated by the local antigen. The stimulated macrophages coalesce and ultimately form the well-recognized epithelioid cells that later coalesce to form larger, more mature, usually multinucleated, giant cells. The typical granuloma formation has then occurred. Granulomas are not associated with the extensive caseation or cheese-like necrosis so typical of granulomas seen in other granulomatous diseases such as tuberculosis.

T-helper cells are mobilized and stimulate B-cell overactivity. The activated T4-helper cells are known to secrete interleukin-2, which leads to a clonal proliferation of similar T4-cells. Anergy develops away from the site of the lesion. The T-cells also produce various lymphokines, whereas the B-cells produce immunoglobulins. Enzymes secreted by the granuloma include angiotensin-converting enzyme (ACE), lysozyme, glucuronidase, collagenase, and elastase. Calcitriol, the active form of vitamin D, may also be formed in the granuloma and causes increased intestinal calcium absorption, which leads to hypercalcemia and hypercalciuria. The aging granuloma is infiltrated by fibroblasts that deposit intracellular reticulin. Reticulin is ultimately replaced by collagen and then structureless, eosinophilic-hyaline material.

The center of the granuloma is usually found to have more epithelioid and giant cells than at the periphery. The periphery contains more monocytes, macrophages, interdigitating cells, and simple histiocytes. Interaction continues to occur between the macrophages and suppressor-cytotoxic T-cells in the periphery of the granuloma and between the epithelioid and helper T-cells in the center. The antigen stimulated macrophages produce interleukin-1, which activates T4-helper-inducer cells to produce interleukin-2, signalling clonal proliferation. Interleukin-1, acting on T-cells, does so by a prostaglandin-induced feedback mechanism that, in turn, can be inhibited by prostaglandin inhibitors such as indomethacin (6).

The pathophysiologic mechanisms that produce neurologic manifestations are similar to those that produce other systemic manifestations of sarcoidosis. The reticuloendothelial system is less well-developed in the nervous system than in other organ systems, and granulomas possibly tend to be smaller. This relative hypotrophy in granuloma formation suggests that a more diffuse angiitic basis for symptomatology is important in the production of many neurologic symptoms. The relative hypotrophy of CNS granulomas could explain lesser neurologic involvement in sarcoidosis as compared to other more active organ systems that have a more generous reticuloendothelium, such as the respiratory system, skin, liver-spleen-lymph nodes, and the eye. Involvement of these tissues is estimated to occur in 94%, 52%, 49%, and 27% respectively, in a large series of patients with sarcoidosis (6). These figures are comparable to the 9% occurrence of nervous system involvement in children and adults.

NEUROPATHOLOGY

Sarcoid granulomas can form in the extradural and subdural spaces, the leptomeninges, and in the parenchyma of the brain, spinal cord, and optic nerves (Figures 13.1 and 13.2). In addition, involvement of cranial and peripheral nerves is well-known, as is the frequent involvement of skeletal and cardiac muscle (6). Distant angiitic lesions in polyneuritis, aseptic meningitis, retinitis, and even stroke have been reported and emphasized by neuropathologists (8). Granulomatous angiopathy occurs after infiltration of small blood vessels of the meninges, brain, and spinal cord, and may result in small-to-moderately large infarctions or frank hemorrhage (8,16). Opportunistic infections rarely occur in sarcoidosis related to associated immunopathy.

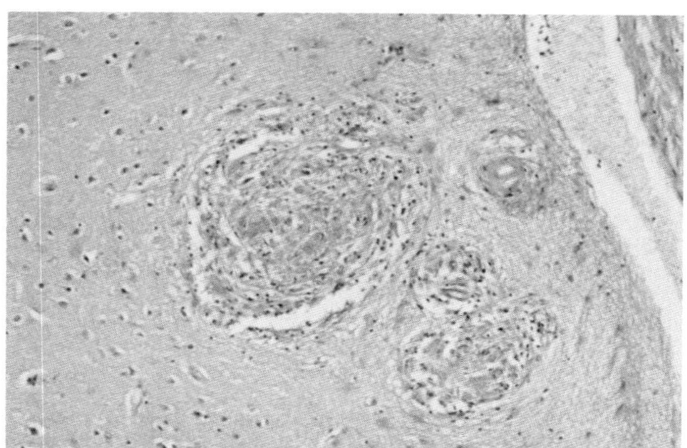

FIGURE 13.1 Multiple sarcoid granulomas just below the cortical surface at the base of the brain; the leptomeninges were involved by the granulomatous process. (Courtesy of Dr. R. L. Davis, University of California Medical Center, San Francisco).

Progressive multifocal leukoencephalopathy, herpes simplex encephalitis, nocardia, and cryptococcal meningitis have all been described in neurosarcoidosis (6).

Intracranial lesions take the form of either single-giant granulomas or multiple-smaller granulomas, which are found in many sites. Solitary mass lesions can occur in almost any location of the brain and cerebellum. The multiple-small granulomas have no specific localization, but deposits in the white matter or at the gray-white junction, especially in the hypothalamus, seem preferred.

Meningoencephalitis characteristically takes the form of chronic granulomatous leptomeningitis with basal distribution. These lesions frequently involve the neighboring parenchyma and are especially prone to affect the neuropituitary, pituitary stalk, and hypothalamic areas. Mass lesions in these areas, even though usually small, tend to obstruct the cerebrospinal fluid (CSF) pathways.

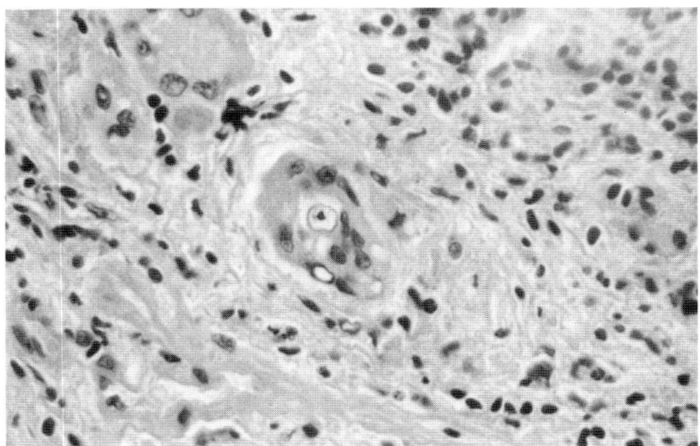

FIGURE 13.2 Typical epithelioid and giant cells found in the sarcoid granuloma. The periphery of the granuloma was composed of monocytes, macrophages, interdigitating cells, and simple histiocytes. (Courtesy of Dr. R. L. Davis, University of California Medical Center, San Francisco, California).

Obstruction to normal CSF flow is prone to occur and if severe, results in obstructive hydrocephalus. Extraventricular hydrocephalus usually results from obstruction of CSF flow at the exit foramina of the fourth ventricle; whereas, intraventricular obstruction seems to occur at the Aqueduct of Sylvius, the fourth ventricle, and less commonly at the Foramen of Monro. Since basal meningitis also involves the optic nerves and chiasm, optic atrophy may occur as a manifestation of neurosarcoidosis, as well as diabetes insipidus, which is secondary to hypothalamic and neuropituitary involvement. Involvement of the rostral brain and hemispheric convexities occurs less often and is associated with randomly-scattered, small granulomas and solitary-confined mass lesions (giant granulomas). As expected, the diffuse granulomas produce symptoms of more diverse nature. If small lesions occur in the brain stem or spinal cord, they may produce rapidly developing and usually dramatic symptoms. Scattered lesions in the cerebral cortex and subcortical white matter may lead to dementia and refractory seizures, with or without associated hydrocephalus. The clinical distinction between the compressive effects of multiple-scattered, small granulomas and angiitic phenomena is difficult to establish even though the pathologic differences may be dramatic.

Optic nerve involvement is common and takes the form of granulomas localized on the papilla or in the retina. They are easily visible at funduscopy. Frank papilledema, obvious optic atrophy, and retrobulbar neuritis may all be encountered in sarcoidosis and also have characteristic funduscopic features. An angiitic mechanism that produces eye involvement also seems likely. Such angiitic phenomena may account for patches of retinal atrophy, diffuse retinitis, retrobulbar neuritis, and retinal infarction. Mass lesions in the retina, though usually small, are similar to lesions in the brain, spinal cord, and peripheral nervous system and may be demonstrated in each of these areas by current neuroimaging techniques (10,11,29,30). Retinal perivenous sheathing, which is often sausage-shaped and nearly transparent, may be observed in neurosarcoidosis (31).

Solitary spinal cord granulomas can occur in both extra- or intramedullary locations, and cause diffuse subacute or chronic myelopathy without prominent granuloma formation (32,33).

The neuropathologic aspects of the peripheral nervous system and muscle are similar to other tissues showing multiple, noncaseating epithelioid granulomas and angiitic features (1,23,26,34,35).

CLINICAL MANIFESTATIONS

Because of the variability of anatomic distribution of granulomas and the pathophysiologic mechanisms involved, the clinical manifestations of sarcoidosis are many. There can be variability in the same sample tissue. For example, in the case of peripheral neuropathy, compressive factors may produce mononeuritis or if multiple, a mononeuritis multiplex; whereas, angiitic factors cause a more symmetrical polyneuritis. Although developmental factors are usually important in manifestations of clinical disease of children, it is surprising that this does not appear to be of great importance in sarcoidosis, for the neurologic manifestations of sarcoid are generally similar in adults and children.

In spite of the wide clinical variability on neurosarcoidosis, several well-recognized clinical syndromes are produced in children and adults including cranial neuropathy, meningoencephalopathy, hypothalamic-pituitary involvement, hydrocephalus, spinal cord involvement, peripheral neuropathy, and involvement of muscle. Only five of these six well-recognized syndromes of neurosarcoidosis have been reported in children (Table 13.2) (21).

Cranial Neuropathy

Cranial nerve involvement is the most common neurologic manifestation of sarcoidosis in children. In the study of Weinberg and associates (21), 12 of the 23 patients (52%) with neurosarcoidosis were found to have cranial neuropathies either alone or associated with other neurologic symptoms. In their review, 6 patients had facial nerve palsies, 4 patients had optic nerve involvement, 2 patients had acoustic nerve involvement, 2 had anosmia or pathologically confirmed infiltration of the olfactory nerve with granulomas, and 1 had dysphagia believed to be due to glossopharyngeal/vagus nerve lesions. Obviously, 3 patients had multiple-cranial nerve palsies. It is believed that the multiple-cranial nerve palsy syndrome is secondary to an associated basal granulomatous meningitis and resulting either from direct nerve compression by granulomatous lesions or distant nerve infarction. It is more difficult to

Table 13.2 Comparison of adults and children with neurosarcoidosis

Site	Adults* (18 to 66 yrs)	Children † (3 mos to 18 yrs)	Total
Meningoencephalopathy	15/23 (65%)	8/23 (35%)	50%
Cranial neuropathy	10/23 (43%)	12/23 (52%)	48%
Hypothalamic/pituitary	5/23 (22%)	7/23 (30%)	26%
Hydrocephalus	6/23 (26%)	4/23 (17%)	22%
Spinal cord	2/23 (09%)	1/23 (04%)	07%
Peripheral nerve/muscle	4/23 (17%)	0/23 (0%)	09%

Note: Patients may have had multiple sites of involvement that are more commonly observed in adults.

*Used with permission from Delaney P. Neurological manifestations of sarcoidiosis. Ann Intern Med 1977;87:336–345.
†Used with permission from Weinberg S, Benne HH, Weinstock I. CNS manifestations of sarcoidosis in children. Clin Pediatr 1983;22:447–448.

explain isolated cranial nerve palsies on a meningitic basis. Optic nerve involvement may be manifested as optic neuritis or papillitis, resembling papilledema. In these cases, the granulomatous lesions of sarcoid are found in the optic nerves, chiasm, or tracts (31). Review of the more extensive medical literature of adult patients suggests similar distribution of cranial nerve involvement.

According to Delaney (16), the facial nerve, either unilateral or bilateral, is the most commonly involved cranial nerve in neurosarcoidosis, followed in order of decreasing frequency by the optic, glossopharyngeal/vagus, acoustic, olfactory, trigeminal, oculomotor/trochlear/abducens, spinal accessory, and hypoglossal nerves. This general order of frequency of cranial nerve involvement seems to be present in children as well. The facial nerve palsy represents an interesting phenomenon because it may or may not be associated with parotid swelling. When facial palsy and parotitis occur with associated uveitis, the condition has been called uveoparotid fever. Facial palsy may precede or follow parotitis, or may not be associated with parotid abnormality. In many cases, dysgeusia is associated with complete facial palsy suggesting the site of involvement is proximal to the parotid gland, as one might expect with lesions associated with basal meningitis. Auditory nerve involvement ranked high in frequency in Colover's earlier adult study in 1948 (12). In the study of Weinberg and associates (21), only 2 of 23 patients had confirmed neurosensory involvement of the auditory nerve.

Meningoencephalopathy

Cerebral involvement in pediatric neurosarcoidosis may be manifested by a number of syndromes including symptomatology associated with chronic granulomatous basal meningitis, isolated seizure activity, and a solitary mass lesion. To the author's knowledge, although not yet reported in children, two other unique syndromes of neurosarcoidosis observed in adult patients have implications for pediatricians. They are isolated extrapyramidal syndrome manifested by chorea, ballism, or Parkinson-like symptoms or both and associated with granulomatous infiltration of the basal ganglia, and progressive multifocal leukoencephalopathy, an uncommon, subacute-demyelinating disease of the CNS that develops in adults with malignancies or chronic immunopathies (36). In the review of Weinberg et al. (21), three postmortem examinations of granulomatous meningitis were performed in which the children had fibrous thickening of the basal meninges and multiple noncaseating epithelioid granulomas. As in adult patients, the granulomatous meningitis in these cases preferentially involved the basal leptomeninges. The granulomatous invasion generally seems to follow the CSF into perivascular spaces, often involving the optic tract and chiasm, hypothalamus, cerebral cortex, and the cerebellum. In the three cases reviewed, symptoms of encephalopathy and

seizures predominated. It is of note that the clinical symptoms suggesting encephalopathy and parenchymal involvement in other patients were manifested by memory impairment, headache, and deterioration of higher cortical function. Patients with these symptoms had extensive pathologic involvement of the CNS on postmortem examinations. The basal meningitis of childhood neurosarcoidosis, as in adults, follows a chronic course, and is characterized by acute or subacute exacerbations. When lumbar puncture is performed during an exacerbation of symptoms, there is often a pleocytosis, primarily lymphocytic, and increased CSF protein concentration. Less often is there significant hypoglycorrachia.

The often cited youngest case of neurosarcoidosis, described by Naumann (1938), was a 3-month-old who had signs of meningitis, seizures, and abnormal CSF. After a 5 week course, the patient died and at autopsy revealed subdural and basal granulomatous meningoencephalopathy. If Naumann's case was an example of Letterer-Siwe disease (8), as has been suggested, a 9-month-old reported by Berger (37), but not reviewed by Weinberg and associates (21), may be the youngest case of neurosarcoidosis reported in the literature (1).

Seizure activity is believed by some to be unusual in sarcoidosis; however, Delaney (16) reported 6 of 23 (26%) adult neurosarcoidosis patients had seizures. Of the 23 children reported by Weinberg et al. (21), 4 (17%) had seizures, but the authors note in their discussion that 6 of the reported patients in their study had seizures, 2 of which were partial seizures and 4 were generalized in type. Although Weinberg and associates claim that seizures occur more frequently in children with neurosarcoidosis than adults, this does not seem to be the case. There have been no reports of children with acute or chronic cerebrovascular accidents; however, transient ischemic attacks, though rare, have been reported in adults (16,29,38).

In the review of Weinberg et al. (21), only 2 patients were found to have definite cerebellar involvement. One of these patients showed intention tremor, nystagmus, and scanning speech; a spastic quadriparesis eventually developed, with infiltration of the brainstem (12). Another patient with an unusual gait and ataxia (39) had granulomatous infiltration of the tegmentum of the brain stem, cerebellar cortex, and anterior portion of the vermis on postmortem examination. In Delaney's series of adult patients (16), 6 of 23 patients had either brain stem or cerebellar dysfunction that correlated well with pathologic findings. Cerebellar involvement, like all other forms of neurosarcoidosis, may remain clinically asymptomatic and only be detected at postmortem examination.

Hypothalamic and Pituitary Involvement

Involvement of the hypothalamus and pituitary gland occurs frequently in sarcoidosis patients of all age groups (40). In the large pediatric series, 7 patients had hypothalamic-pituitary abnormalities; 5 were reported as having isolated diabetes insipidus, 1 had hypopituitarism and 1 patient, without clinical evidence of hypothalamic-pituitary dysfunction, had small focal collections of epithelioid cells in the hypothalmus at autopsy. In one series of adult patients with sarcoidosis (14), it was reported that 35% had diabetes insipidus. In an earlier study of adult patients, Colover (12) found 20% to 25% of the patients had hypothalamic-pituitary dysfunction.

Hydrocephalus

Hydrocephalus without signs of other clinical abnormality is uncommon in neurosarcoidosis in adults and children. In the two comparative series of Delaney (16) and Weinberg and associates (21), a total of 10 patients of 46 studied, showed signs of hydrocephalus. Neither in adults (6/23 affected) nor in children (4/23 affected) was hydrocephalus the only clinical neurologic manifestation of the disease. All 6 adult patients with hydrocephalus had associated meningoencephalopathy. In 3 of 4 children with hydrocephalus, there was an associated meningoencephalopathy; whereas, in 1 case reported by Reed (25), papilledema alone existed, possibly representing a papillitis from inflammation of the optic nerve. The pathogenesis of hydrocephalus in sarcoidosis is multifactorial: resulting from granulomatous infiltration of the ependyma and choroid plexuses and altering CSF dynamics; chronic meningitis causing obliteration of the subarachnoid spaces; and from aqueductal stenosis or outlet obstruction of the fourth ventricle by intraventricular granulomas.

Spinal Cord

Spinal cord abnormalities resulting from thickened meninges and collections of granulomatous tissue both intra- and extramedullary were reported in one child patient (39). Delaney (16) reported two patients with spinal sarcoidosis, one of which had spinal cord dysfunction as the only neurologic manifestation; whereas, the other patient had cranial nerve dysfunction and encephalopathy. Spinal cord involvement is generally considered uncommon even in adults but with improved neuroimaging techniques, better visualization of spinal cord pathology is expected (11).

Peripheral Nerve and Muscle

Although no report of peripheral nerve or muscle involvement was observed by Weinberg et al. (21), it is anticipated that many examples of minimal or asymptomatic involvement exist even in children. Colover (12) estimated that 15% of neurosarcoidosis patients have peripheral neuropathy and 3 of Delaney's (16) 23 patients had peripheral neuropathy. Peripheral nerve involvement in sarcoidosis includes practically all types of nerve involvement including isolated mononeuritis, mononeuritis multiplex, and polyneuropathy. Usually vague symptoms and signs, such as paresthesias or decreased myotatic reflexes are not considered evidence of peripheral neuropathy when perhaps they should be. Although a wide variety of different causes of peripheral neuropathy exists, Oh (33) pointed out that axonal degeneration seen in his patient was the secondary result of panangiitis and periangiitis, as well as compression by perineural sarcoid granuloma. He did not believe the neuropathy was due to segmental demyelination alone as suggested by Delaney (16).

No children with symptomatic muscle disease were reported by Weinberg et al. (21); however, 2 adult patients were reported by Delaney (16) and 1 other patient was noted to have muscle involvement but without symptoms. Muscle involvement in neurosarcoidosis is varied and includes: asymptomatic infiltration of skeletal muscle with granulomas, painful nodules in muscle, acute myopathy with myalgia, and chronic myopathy resembling muscular dystrophy. The most common clinical manifestation of muscle involvement in sarcoid, though rare, is chronic progressive myopathy (26). It has never been reported in children.

DIAGNOSIS

The diagnosis of sarcoidosis during life requires a compatible clinical course and histologic findings of noncaseating epithelioid granulomas observed at biopsy. One must be careful to exclude other diseases capable of producing similar clinical findings. It is important to recognize that neurosarcoidosis is often a diagnosis of exclusion; yet, it should always be kept in mind when attempting to answer unexplained clinical questions.

It has been suggested that the majority of patients with sarcoidosis showed distinctive bilateral hilar lymphadenopathy with or without peritracheal adenopathy on chest radiographs and may be asymptomatic. Clinical manifestations of respiratory sarcoidosis are not essential for the diagnosis of neurosarcoidosis; however, the presence of bilateral hilar lymphadenopathy in a patient with symptoms consistent with neurosarcoidosis is very important. The histologic confirmation of the disease is made by biopsy, usually of a palpable lymph node or cutaneous lesion. It has been reported that random biopsy of minor salivary glands is positive for granuloma in about 60% of the cases; whereas, percutaneous liver biopsy demonstrates noncaseating granuloma in 65% to 75% of cases (6,7). Other sites of biopsy include transbronchial biopsy of the lungs and biopsy of random or selected skeletal muscles. It is of note that CNS involvement tends to occur in earlier stages of the disease and prior to involvement of other organ systems. Peripheral nerve involvement in sarcoidosis characteristically occurs in the chronic stages of the disease and with multisystem manifestations.

Hypercalcemia is found in 2% to 10% of patients with sarcoidosis. Calcium absorption is altered by hypersensitivity of Vitamin D, which enhances intestinal absorption of calcium; hypercalcinuria is actually more common than hypercalcemia. Serum ACE is elevated in 50% to 80% of the patients with sarcoidosis. In general, serum ACE is highest in untreated patients with active disease and then falls toward normal during spontaneous remission, or with advent of corticosteroid therapy. Elevated ACE has been shown to come from epithelioid cells in the granuloma, as well as other sites including lymph nodes, liver, skin, and the lung. In addition, ACE can be excreted by activated macrophages within the CSF. It has been estimated (7) that the T-lymphocytes stimulate epithelioid cell ACE production. The incidence of false-positive elevated ACE levels in patients with diseases mimicking sarcoidosis is about 15%. In patients with neurosarcoidosis, spinal fluid ACE is often elevated (41,42).

Sarcoid granulomas, if active, take up gallium, enabling gallium scanning to act as marker of involved lymph nodes, lung parenchyma, and extrapulmonary granuloma sites, such as the parotid and lacrimal glands. Gallium scanning combined with serum ACE screening have a diagnosis confirmation rate of about 99% for sarcoidosis (7). There is, however, no specificity of gallium studies for neurosarcoidosis. Lysozyme is a weakly proteolytic enzyme found in cells of the monocyte-macrophage system. Serum elevation of lysozyme is a nonspecific finding in extrapulmonary sarcoidosis, and may also be found in other granulomatous diseases including tuberculosis, fungal infections, and Wegener granulomatosis. Elevated serum lysozyme correlates best with extrapyramidal sarcoidosis and especially with involvement of the spleen.

With few exceptions, the clinical features of neurosarcoidosis are not distinctive and, therefore, histologic confirmation by biopsy of even extraneural tissues is desirable. Any accessible lesions, such as enlarged lymph nodes or the characteristically inflamed nodularly conjuctiva, should be biopsied. Muscle biopsy often shows granulomas even in asymptomatic patients, and is more likely positive in acute or subacute, initial or exacerbating sarcoidosis, than in the chronic forms. Sural nerve biopsy has been useful to support the diagnosis of peripheral neuropathy.

The Kveim test is of little use in establishing a diagnosis of sarcoid. In this test a saline suspension of sarcoid tissue is injected subcutaneously and if the test is positive, a nodule with the distinctive histology of sarcoid develops in about 6 weeks. The nature of the antigen in sarcoidosis or the induced reactions are not understood and expert interpretation is required, for testing often produces mixed results. Even under ideal circumstances, the Kveim test is positive in only 43% of cases of sarcoidosis without thoracic involvement (18); a positive Kveim test may be inhibited by steroid treatment. It is of note that a tuberculin skin test is negative in over 60% of the cases of sarcoidosis because of anergy.

In all forms of sarcoidosis of the CNS, the CSF total protein concentration is almost always increased, sometimes to levels beyond those observed in other similar disease (43). Oligoclonal bands in the IgG have been reported (44). There is little evidence of intrathecal synthesis of IgG in neurosarcoidosis (18). The white cell count is often increased, showing lymphocytes, reticulomonocytes, neutrophilic granulocytes, and occasionally eosinophils in excessive numbers. Bizarre multinucleated cells in the CSF are occasionally seen (45). The CSF glucose concentration is rarely decreased. Recent studies suggest that the cerebrospinal fluid ACE may prove to be of diagnostic value in indicating activity of neurosarcoidosis (41,42). Neuroimaging studies with computed tomography (CT) and magnetic resonance imaging (MRI) may show distinctive features (10,11,29,30), but mass lesions are not distinctive. Sarcoid meningoencephalitis often shows enhancing lesions scattered in the basal or convexity meninges. These lesions, of course, may involve adjacent parenchymal structures, notably in the cerebral cortex and hypothalamus. Without contrast enhancement, the small-multiple lesions may not be seen. Lesions in the ventricular wall are somewhat characteristic of sarcoid (10).

TREATMENT

In accordance with authoritative views (6,7), the common indications for treatment of sarcoidosis with corticosteroids include progressive pulmonary involvement and respiratory symptoms, ocular involvement, myocardial and muscular involvement, CNS symptoms and lesions, disfiguring cutaneous lesions, and persistent hypercalcemia or hypercalcuria with renal insufficiency. It is not known precisely how corticosteroid therapy works in sarcoidosis. Prednisone is the most commonly used drug with the recommended initial dose of approximately 30 mg per day, a dose which is at least adequate for pulmonary sarcoidosis. Corticosteroid therapy usually produces clinical improvement in 1 to 2 weeks, but maximum improvement usually occurs in 1 to 2 months. Corticosteroids should be continued from 6 to 12 months. Prolonged treatment is necessary since more than half of the patients will relapse when therapy is discontinued, particularly if medication is abruptly discontinued. Alternate day therapy is effective in maintaining improvement and helps minimize the long-term effects of corticosteroids (6,7). The effects of corticosteroids should be closely monitored, especially in patients with respiratory disease, when serial chest radiographs and pulmonary function tests should be performed.

According to Delaney (16), patients with cranial nerve involvement, encephalopathy, hypothalamic-pituitary involvement, peripheral neuropathy, and acute myopathy, all have a favorable response to steroids. The response to steroids, however, is only fair in patients with meningitis, seizures treated with anticonvulsants, space occupying lesions—whether or not surgery has been performed—cerebellar lesions, and muscular nodular disease. Patients with involvement of the brain stem and spinal cord, and those with chronic myopathy, have unpredictable or variable responses.

The natural history and prognosis of cranial mononeuropathy is thought to be excellent, but the prognosis of peripheral neuropathy is less predictable. It is important to remember that spontaneous recovery can occur in neurosarcoidosis. Retrobulbar optic nerve lesions also have a good prognosis for spontaneous regression.

According to Matthew (18), the natural prognosis in proved sarcoid meningoencephalitis is poor and the response to steroid therapy disappointing. Substantial remissions from cerebral hypothalamic symptoms have been occasionally reported (46), or the disease may appear to be arrested. Even in these cases, however, the CSF protein concentration may remain greatly elevated in clinical remission, suggesting continued activity. Cerebrospinal ACE levels continue to be elevated.

Cytotoxic agents have been sporadically administered in the treatment of neurosarcoidosis, but without reported success. Some response to radiotherapy has been claimed in a single case (47). Neurosurgical procedures have been of some benefit in the treatment of neurosarcoidosis, depending on the particular syndrome. Ventriculo-peritoneal shunting has temporarily relieved the symptoms of increased intracranial pressure of hydrocephalus when associated with a giant cell granuloma in the cerebrum (18,48). In a review of spinal cord sarcoidosis, one patient derived benefit from surgery (32).

REFERENCES

1. Dyken PR. Neurological aspects of sarcoidosis. J Indiana Med Assoc 1963;56:1511–1515.
2. Longcope W, Freiman D. A study of sarcoidosis. Medicine 1952;31:1–14.
3. Harvey JC. A myopathy of Boeck's sarcoid. Am J Med 1959;26:356–363.
4. Conference on Sarcoidosis. National Research Council, Division of Medical Sciences, Army Institute of Pathology, Washington, Feb. 11, 1948.
5. Tenth International Conference on Sarcoidosis. Ann N Y Acad Sci 1986; 465.
6. James DG, Williams WJ. Sarcoidosis. In: Wyngaarden JB, Smith LH, eds. Cecil Textbook of Medicine. 18th ed. Philadelphia: W.B. Saunders, 1988;69:451–457.
7. Winterbauer RH. Sarcoidosis. In: Petersdorf RG, Adams RD, Braunwald E, et al., eds. Harrison's Principles of Internal Medicine. 10th ed. New York: McGraw-Hill, 1983; 235:1248–1253.
8. Zeman W. Morbus Besnier-Boeck-Schaumann. In: Handbuch der Speziellen Pathologischen Anatomie and Histologie. Berlin: Springer-Verlag, 1958;13/2:1100–1112.
9. James DG, Jones Williones W. Sarcoidosis and other granulomatous disorders. Philadelphia: W.B. Saunders, 1984.
10. Brooks BS, El Gammal T, Hungerford GD, et al. Radiological evaluation of neurosarcoidosis: World of computed tomography. Am J Neuroradiol 1982;3:513–521.
11. Cooper SD, Brady MB, Williams JP, et al. Neurosarcoidosis: Evaluation using CT and MRI. J Comput Assist Tomogr 1988;12:96–99.
12. Colover J. Sarcoidosis with involvement of the nervous system. Brain 1948;71:451–475.
13. Ricker W, Clark M. Sarcoidosis. Am J Clin Pathol 1949;19:725–732.
14. Pennell WH. Boeck's sarcoid involvement of the central nervous system. Arch Neurol Psychiatry 1951;66:728–737.
15. Silverstein A, Feuer MM, Silzbach LE. Neurologic sarcoid: Study of 18 cases. Arch Neurol 1965;43:595–597.
16. Delaney P. Neurological manifestations of sarcoidosis. Ann Intern Med 1977;87:336–345.
17. Adams RD, Victor M. Sarcoidosis (Besnier-Boeck-Schaumann Disease). In: Adams RD, Victor M, eds. Principles of Neurology. 3rd ed. New York: McGraw-Hill, 1985; 31:528–529.
18. Matthew WB. Neurologic manifestations of sarcoidosis. In: Asbury AK, McKhann GM, McDonald WI, eds. Diseases of the Nervous System: Clinical Neurobiology. 1st ed. Philadelphia: W.B. Saunders, 1986;129:1563–1570.
19. Denny FW. Sarcoidosis. In: Behrman RE, Vaughn VC, eds. Nelson Textbook of Pediatrics, 13th ed. Philadelphia: W.B. Saunders, 1987;26.3:1484–1485.
20. Bell WE. Sarcoidosis. In: Swaiman KF, Wright FS, eds. The Practice of Pediatric Neurology, 2nd ed. St. Louis: C.V. Mosby, 1982;27:688–689.
21. Weinberg S, Bennett H, Weinstock I. CNS manifestations of sarcoidosis in children. Clin Pediatr 1983;22:447–481.
22. Cone RB: A review of Boeck's sarcoid with analysis of 12 cases occurring in children. J Pediatr 1948;32:629–635.
23. McGovern JP, Merrit DM. Sarcoidosis in children. Pediatrics 1956;8:97–101.
24. Naumann O. Kasuistischer Bertrag zur Kenntnis der Schaumannschen benignen granulomatose (Moebus Besnier-Boeck-Schaumann). Kinordterheilkd 1938;60:1–8.
25. Reed WG. Sarcoidosis: A review and report of 8 cases in children. J Tenn Med Assoc 1969;62:27–33.
26. Dyken PR. Sarcoidosis of skeletal muscle: A case report and review of the literature. Neurology 1962;12:643–651.
27. Hinterbruchner CN, Hinterbruchner LP. Myopathic syndrome in muscular sarcoidosis. Brain 1964;87:355–366.
28. Silverstein A, Silzbach LE. Muscle involvement in Sarcoidosis. Asymptomatic myositis and myopathy. Arch Neurol 1969; 21:235–241.
29. Sethi KD, El Gammal T, Patel BP, et al. Dural sarcoidosis presenting with transient neurologic symptoms. Arch Neurol 1986;43:595–597.
30. Ketonen L, Oksanen V, Kuuliala I, et al. Hypodense white matter lesions in computed tomography of neurosarcoidosis. J Comput Assist Tomogr 1983;10:181–183.
31. Caplan L, Corbett J, Goodwin J, et al. Neuro-ophthalmologic signs in the angiitic form of neurosarcoidosis. Neurology 1983;33:1130–1135.

32. Day AL, Sypert GW. Spinal cord sarcoidosis. Ann Neurol 1976;1:79–85.
33. Oh SJ. Sarcoid polyneuropathy: A histologically proven case. Ann Neurol 1980;7:178–181.
34. Wallace SL, Lattes R, Malia JP, et al. Muscle involvement in Boeck's sarcoid. Ann Intern Med 1958;48:497–501.
35. Myers GB, Gottlieb AM, Matman PE, et al. Joint and skeletal muscle manifestations in sarcoidosis. Am J Med 1952; 12:161–165.
36. Christensen E, Fog M. A case of Schilder's disease in an adult with remarks to the etiology and pathogenesis. Acta Psychiatr Scand 1955;30:141–154.
37. Berger H. Morbus Boeck Der Gehirns und Meningitis Tuberculosa. Ann Paediatr 1952;154:346–350.
38. Case records of the Massachusetts General Hospital (No. 46–1975). N Engl J Med 1975;293:1138–1145.
39. Camp WA, Frierson JG. Sarcoidosis of central nervous system. Arch Neurol 1962;7:432–441.
40. Schealy CN, Kahana L, Engel FL. Hypothalamic-pituitary sarcoidosis. A report on 4 patients, one with prolonged remission of diabetes insipidus following steroid therapy. Am J Med 1961;30:46–55.
41. Chan Seem CP, Norfolk G, Spokes EG. CSF angiotensin-converting enzymes in neurosarcoidosis. Lancet 1985; 1:456–457.
42. Oksanen V, Fyhrquist F, Grohagen-Riska C, et al. CSF angiotensin-converting enzyme in neurosarcoidosis. Lancet 1985;1:1050–1051.
43. Gaines JD, Eckman PB, Remington JS. Low CSF glucose in sarcoidosis involving the central nervous system. Arch Neurol 1973;23:981–989.
44. Kinnman J, Link H. Intrathecal production of oligoclonal IgM and IgG in CNS sarcoidosis. Acta Neurol Scand 1984; 69:97–106.
45. Dyken P. Cerebrospinal fluid cytology: Practical clinical usefulness. Neurology 1975;25:210–217.
46. Griggs RC, Markesberg WR, Condemi JJ. Cerebral mass due to sarcoidosis. Neurology 1973;23:981–989.
47. Grizzanti JN, Knapp AB, Schecter AJ, et al. Treatment of sarcoid meningitis with radiotherapy. Am J Med 1982; 73:605–608.
48. Ross JA. Uveal parotid sarcoidosis with cerebral involvement. Br Med J 1955;2:593–596.

Chapter 14
Reye Syndrome

Doris A. Trauner

In the 25 years since the initial description of metabolic encephalopathy with fatty degeneration of the viscera by Reye (1) in Australia and Johnson (2) in the United States (US), a great deal has been learned about the clinical, metabolic, and pathologic features of this often fatal disease. Although the disorder is rare, it is one of the most common causes of death from virus-related diseases.

EPIDEMIOLOGY

Reye syndrome (RS) has been reported in many parts of the world and in all races. Both sexes are affected equally. Although primarily recognized in children, the disease can affect adults as well (3). The annual incidence of RS reported to the Centers for Disease Control (CDC) varies from 0.15 to 0.88 cases per 100,000 children under the age of 18 years in the US (4). However, many of the milder cases may remain undiagnosed, and it is possible that the true incidence of the disorder is closer to 3.5 cases per 100,000 children per year (5). The relative frequency of RS in adults has not been established, most likely because the disorder goes largely unrecognized in that age group. The highest frequency of the disease in children is found in the age ranges 0 to 4 years and 10 to 14 years (4).

In children over 1 year of age, RS is most prevalent among white, middle-class children in suburban and rural areas. Recent data indicate that 85% to 90% of all RS cases occur in white children (4,6). In infants, however, the opposite is true (7,8). The majority of infants with RS are from minority groups, and are more likely to be inner city dwellers from lower socioeconomic classes. The reason for these differences is not clear. One possibility is that poor children in urban settings with crowded living conditions receive their initial exposure to a particular virus at an earlier age than do children in middle-class settings. Another potential explanation is the different levels of awareness of the parents or caretakers regarding the use of various medications for their children during times of acute febrile illness. Whether these or other factors are the cause for the observed differences remains to be clarified.

An antecedent, usually viral illness, precedes the onset of RS in at least 85% of cases. The most frequently associated agent, particularly in case clusters, is *Influenza* B. The peak incidence of RS occurs in late winter and early spring, consistent with temporal associations with influenza. Varicella accounts for the antecedent illness in up to 29% of sporadic cases occurring throughout the year. Numerous other viruses have been associated with the prodromal illness in infrequent instances.

The epidemiologic aspects of RS in the US appear to have changed in recent years (9). Previously, epidemics of *Influenza* B have been associated with an increased incidence of RS. However, from December 1985 through November 1986, a period of high influenza activity, the number of cases of RS was far lower than in previous influenza epidemic years (5). Also, the incidence of RS in the 0 to 10 year age range appears to be decreasing, while the number of cases in children older than 10 years is remaining stable or increasing.

Explanations for the apparent change in frequency and distribution of RS cases revolve primarily around the issue of salicylate use. Between 1980 and 1982, independent reports from three regions of the US suggested a possible association between salicylate use during the prodromal illness, and subsequent development of RS (10–12). Although there were methodologic problems associated with these studies, public awareness of a potential concern with salicylate use during viral illnesses increased. These studies also resulted in the placement of warning labels on aspirin bottles to inform users of the potential link. In 1985, a pilot study of RS and medication use conducted by the Public Health Service reported a strong epidemiologic association between the use of salicylates and the occurrence of RS (13). This was followed by a larger study of 27 patients with stage II or greater RS, and 140 case controls

(14). Again, a strong statistical association between salicylate use and RS was observed.

Although a causal relationship between salicylates and RS has not been demonstrated, one explanation for the declining incidence of RS is a reported decrease in use of aspirin for symptoms of varicella and respiratory illnesses (9,15). The decline in usage appears to be greatest in the age range of 0 to 9 years, although older children and adolescents are using less aspirin for these conditions as well. However, information from both Australia (16) and Japan (17) suggest that the incidence of RS is decreasing in those countries as well, but that there appears to be no association between RS and aspirin use. In fact, salicylate use among children in Australia has been extremely low for over 25 years, well before any changes in the frequency of RS occurred. Thus, it is possible that the reported association between aspirin use and RS in the US is coincidental. This possibility will be difficult to test for several more years, until more data have been accumulated on the RS incidence trends following long-term reduction in aspirin use.

Another possible explanation for the decreasing frequency of RS is the recognition of a number of inborn errors of metabolism that may mimic the symptoms of RS. One disorder of fatty acid oxidation in particular, medium-chain acyl-Coenzyme-A (acyl-CoA) dehydrogenase deficiency, has only been described in the past few years, and is being identified with increasing frequency. It is likely that some of the cases reported as RS in the early 1980s were, in reality, metabolic disorders, and that the proper identification of these disorders has been responsible for some of the apparent decline in the incidence of RS.

PATHOPHYSIOLOGY

Despite extensive investigation, the underlying mechanisms involved in producing RS remain unknown. Theories relating to the pathogenesis of RS primarily involve the role of viruses, exogenous and endogenous toxins, and viral-toxin interactions.

The mitochondria are the primary organelles involved pathologically. Assessment of various metabolic abnormalities indicates that cytosolic enzyme activities are normal; whereas, activities of mitochondrial enzymes such as those of the urea cycle are diminished (18). Thus, any hypothesis relating to the pathogenesis of RS must take into account the ability to cause severe mitochondrial dysfunction.

Since RS is almost always preceded by a viral infection, could it be the result of direct viral involvement of liver and brain? There has been no pathologic evidence of inflammatory changes in these organs that would support such a hypothesis. An experimental model of RS developed by Davis et al. (19) utilized influenza B injection into mice to produce a syndrome similar to RS. No evidence of infection in liver or brain was found, but active virus was necessary for the production of symptoms. Several viral antigens were found within hepatocytes, suggesting incomplete viral replication in that organ. Such partial replication could induce a toxic host factor that causes secondary damage to the liver and brain. Pursuing that hypothesis, Trauner and Davis (20) used the mouse model to study its effects on fatty acid oxidation, and found an inhibition of palmitate oxidation in mouse liver mitochondria following influenza injection. Previous studies by Trauner et al. (21) had demonstrated accumulation of serum short-chain fatty acids in children with RS, and experimental studies suggested that infusion of a short-chain fatty acid into laboratory animals could produce clinical, biochemical, and pathologic changes similar to those found in children with RS (22,23). One hypothetical mechanism based on these studies is that viral infection may inhibit the ability of mitochondria to oxidize fatty acids, leading to accumulation of excessive amounts of these compounds, which then may produce the clinical, biochemical, and pathologic changes associated with RS.

The other endogenous toxin that has been most frequently implicated as a cause for the encephalopathy is ammonia (24). Activities of the two mitochondrial enzymes of the urea cycle, ornithine transcarbamylase and carbamyl phosphate synthetase, are reduced during the acute stages of RS (25), perhaps as a result of virus-initiated diffuse mitochondrial dysfunction. This, in addition to the increased nitrogen load precipitated by illness and poor food intake, may explain the hyperammonemia found uniformly in this disorder. In experimental animals, very high blood ammonia concentrations are capable of producing coma and hyperventilation (26), although an effective model of RS has not been produced using hyperammonemia alone. There appears to be a synergistic effect between ammonia and short-chain fatty acids in producing encephalopathy (26), and it is more likely that the diffuse mitochondrial dysfunction allows accumulation of multiple toxins which, in combination, act to cause the clinical manifestations of RS.

One of the earliest implications of an environmental toxin was based on information from Thailand (27), where a disease resembling RS, called Udorn encephalopathy, was found to be caused by ingestion of aflatoxin B1, a metabolite of the fungus *Aspergillus flavus* which is found in corn and peanut products. Experimental studies utilizing aflatoxin B1 produced a Reye-like syndrome in macaques (28). Subsequently, aflatoxin was identified in blood or liver specimens from a few patients in the US (29), but no evidence of widespread aflatoxin exposure in children with RS has been found (30). Other environmental toxins that have been considered as possible causative agents include pesticides, herbicides, other plant toxins, anti-emetic medications, camphor, and salicylates.

Salicylates have been of particular interest, because in toxic doses they produce symptoms, such as hyperventilation and coma (31), that are similar to those of RS. Salicylate intoxication also causes metabolic acidosis, liver dysfunction, uncoupling of oxidative phosphorylation in mitochondria, and fatty changes in liver (32). There is controversy, however, regarding the extent of the pathologic similarities in these two disorders (33,34). Although intriguing, the hypothesis that RS and salicylism are the same, or that salicylates cause RS, fails to explain the occurrence of RS in children who have had no exposure to salicylates (16,17).

PATHOLOGY

The primary pathologic changes in RS are found in the liver (35,36). Light microscopic studies demonstrate swelling of hepatocytes, with preservation of the normal hepatic lobular architecture. Hematoxylin and eosin stains show a uniform foaminess of the hepatocyte cytoplasm. Fat stains, such as Oil Red O, of frozen liver sections demonstrate diffuse, intracellular, microvesicular lipid vacuoles in a panlobular distribution. There is depletion of glycogen stores. There is notable absence of inflammatory changes or hepatocellular necrosis. Histochemical stains show depletion of succinic dehydrogenase enzyme activity.

Ultrastructural changes include large amounts of fat in small droplets; a swelling and pleiomorphism of mitochondria, with a distortion or fragmentation of cristae and an absence of matrix dense bodies; an increase in the number of peroxisomes and a clustering of these organelles; and the proliferation of the smooth endoplasmic reticulum.

Pathologic changes of the brain are inconsistent (37). Light microscopic findings are often nonspecific, demonstrating neuronal necrosis secondary to anoxia, or diffuse cerebral edema. Inflammatory changes are absent in brain tissue as well. Evidence of cerebral edema is also found at ultrastructural examination, with swelling of astrocytic foot processes. Changes in brain mitochondria similar to those found in the liver have been reported in some patients.

CLINICAL MANIFESTATIONS

Reye syndrome is a biphasic illness. The clinical presentation is fairly consistent in children over the age of 1 year. The initial symptoms are of a viral illness, usually with gastrointestinal or upper respiratory symptoms, or varicella. The child is recovering from the initial phase when he or she develops recurring vomiting, which progresses rapidly to include alterations in consciousness. In the mildest case, the child only appears sleepy, and this is often considered normal for an ill child. However, even at this point an electroencephalogram (EEG) will reveal generalized slowing, indicating that the child is encephalopathic.

As the encephalopathy progresses, the child goes through a phase of disorientation, and during this time may be extremely combative. Because of this, a diagnosis of drug ingestion or toxic reaction is sometimes suspected. The combativeness lasts only a few hours, and is followed by further depression of the sensorium, with delirium, obtundation, and finally coma.

Infants under the age of 1 year may have a more subtle presentation (38). Vomiting may be less pronounced or even absent. The initial manifestations of the illness may be respiratory in nature, with hyperventilation or apnea. Seizures are more likely to occur during the early stages of the disease in this age group.

The neurologic examination of the infant or child with Reye syndrome includes depressed sensorium with preservation of brain stem reflexes (until late in the course), diffuse hyperreflexia, and no consistent focal abnormalities. Funduscopic examination may demonstrate papilledema, but this finding may be absent even when intracranial pressure (ICP) is greatly elevated. Thus, a normal fundus examination is not useful in determining diagnosis, severity of illness, or magnitude of ICP elevation in this disease.

Generalized, usually motor seizures, can occur at any time during the course of the illness, particularly in the more advanced stages, in up to 50% of children (39). The incidence is higher in infants. Rarely, partial as well as myoclonic seizures have been observed.

Hyperventilation is present in most children, particularly after stage I. This appears to be centrally mediated and is often sufficient to produce a marked respiratory alkalosis. Hyperthermia is another common occurrence, even without evidence to suggest active infection. This manifestation is most likely the result of central neurogenic dysfunction as well.

Laboratory evaluation of children with Reye syndrome reveals evidence of liver dysfunction with elevation of serum transaminases and prolonged prothrombin time. Hyperammonemia is present in virtually all cases, particularly when the blood ammonia concentration is measured within the first 24 hours of the onset of encephalopathy. Initial or peak ammonia concentrations appear to have a correlation with outcome, in that levels greater than 450 μg/dL correspond with greater mortality and morbidity (40). However, ammonia concentrations begin to decline rather rapidly in many cases, and may return to normal levels, regardless of eventual outcome.

The concentration of serum bilirubin is normal and serum glucose concentrations are normal or low. The latter finding is particularly true in children under 4 years of age and, in fact, is quite rare in older children. Lactic acidosis and elevated levels of creatine kinase are common.

The cerebrospinal fluid (CSF) is acellular with normal protein concentration. CSF glucose concentration may be low, reflecting systemic hypoglycemia. CSF pressure may be increased.

The electroencephalographic abnormalities associated with RS are nonspecific, but are consistent with any metabolic or toxic encephalopathy. Generalized slowing of background activity in the theta or delta range is typically found without any focal changes. The occurrence of 14 and 6 cycle/second positive bursts has been reported in children between the ages of 7 and 14 years (41); however, the significance of this is unclear. Occasionally, generalized spikes or sharp waves can be seen and, rarely, electrographic seizure activity is present. In the most advanced cases, there may be a burst-suppression pattern or isoelectric EEG. Aoki and Lombroso (39) proposed an EEG classification for patients with RS, and suggested that the EEG might have prognostic value. Trauner and Stockard (40) found a correlation between the severity of the EEG and the degree of elevation in serum short-chain organic acid levels. More recent studies have failed to replicate the prognostic value of EEG during the acute illness (42).

Somatosensory evoked potentials (SEP) are abnormal in children with RS, demonstrating the absence or marked depression of all components of the SEP early in the course of the illness (43). Progressive recovery of the primary cortical components of the SEP appears to correlate with survival, whereas lack of recovery is associated with a fatal outcome. Recovery of later components (beyond 100 msec) is associated with good clinical outcome; whereas, failure of these late components to return appears to signify the presence of residual neuropsychologic deficits.

Neuroimaging procedures such as computed tomographic (CT) head scans do not demonstrate a specific lesion. Slit-like ventricles associated with diffuse cerebral edema may be found.

DIAGNOSIS

There is no single test that will document the presence or absence of Reye syndrome. Rather, the diagnosis is based on the constellation of history, clinical symptoms, laboratory abnormalities, and the absence of other illnesses that might mimic Reye syndrome. The Centers for Disease Control have established guidelines for the diagnosis of this disorder (4) (Table 14.1).

Approximately 85% of cases have had an antecedent viral illness. This information, in addition to a history of

Table 14.1 CDC guidelines for the diagnosis of Reye syndrome

1. Acute noninflammatory encephalopathy with alteration in level of consciousness; CSF leukocyte count of 8/mm³ or less, or histological sections of brain demonstrating lack of inflammation.

2. Evidence of hepatic dysfunction including a threefold or greater elevation in serum glutamic-oxaloacetic transaminase, serum glutamic-pyruvic transaminase, or serum ammonia concentration; or biopsy or autopsy tissue considered to be diagnostic of Reye syndrome.

3. No more reasonable explanation for the cerebral or hepatic abnormalities.

Adapted from CCD. Reye Syndrome surveillance—United States, 1986. MMWR 1987;36:689–691.

repeated vomiting and altered sensorium, with laboratory evidence of hepatic dysfunction, should raise the suspicion of Reye syndrome. However, there are numerous conditions that can produce similar clinical pictures, and thus it is important to rule out these other disorders.

The differential diagnosis of Reye syndrome (44) includes severe systemic infections (especially when they are associated with disseminated intravascular coagulation), infections of the nervous system such as bacterial meningitis, viral (in particular herpes) encephalitis, varicella hepatitis and encephalitis, anoxia, salicylism, other toxin ingestions (such as aflatoxin, hypoglycin A, methanol, *Amanita falloides*), valproic acid hepatotoxicity, acute hepatic encephalopathy from liver failure, and various inborn errors of metabolism.

Severe systemic infections may be difficult to distinguish from Reye syndrome. The child is typically febrile, and may be encephalopathic; the presence of disseminated intravascular coagulation (DIC) will result in prolonged prothrombin time. However, other features of DIC (prolongation of partial thromboplastin time, presence of fibrin split products, and evidence of hemolysis) are not typical of RS and serve to differentiate the two conditions. Also, marked hyperammonemia is unusual with systemic infections.

Infections of the central nervous system (CNS) can usually be readily identified by the presence of an increased number of white blood cells in the CSF. Rarely, viral encephalitis will not produce a cellular response, but the liver is unlikely to be involved unless there is a concurrent hepatitis. This can occur with varicella infection, and may be clinically indistinguishable from RS. In that instance, the presence of cells in the CSF or evidence of inflammation on liver biopsy will help to differentiate the two conditions.

Anoxia can result in multi-system injury, including the liver and brain. With the exception of nonaccidental injuries, the history is usually obvious. In the latter instance, evidence of trauma can aid in making the correct diagnosis.

Toxin ingestion or drug overdose should be considered in any child with acute alteration in consciousness. A detailed history of possible toxin exposure, and a toxicology screen should be a routine part of the diagnostic evaluation, even if RS is considered the most likely possibility. In areas of the world where Ackee fruit is grown, such as Jamaica, the possibility of ingestion of hypoglycin A from the unripe Ackee fruit is high. Hypoglycin A produces a clinical picture identical to RS (45).

Acute liver failure, for example as a result of a hepatotoxin such as *Amanita* or carbon tetrachloride, or secondary to acute hepatitis, is often accompanied by encephalopathy. However, the liver dysfunction usually differs sufficiently from that of RS that the two disorders are not confused. In liver failure, the serum bilirubin concentration is typically markedly elevated (until the very advanced stages); whereas, in RS the bilirubin levels are normal or only minimally increased. Bilirubin concentrations greater than 5 mg% are not typically found in RS. In questionable cases, a liver biopsy will differentiate the two conditions.

Some presentations of inborn errors of metabolism are not easily distinguished from RS (46), nor is there an immediate laboratory test that can separate the two in many cases. They most likely comprise some of the Reye syndrome cases reported in the early literature, in particular the recurrent and familial cases. It is important to pursue the possibility of an inborn metabolic disorder, since such children often require specific treatment for the metabolic dificiency; also, the symptoms are likely to recur at a later date if the appropriate diagnosis is not made. Since these disorders are inherited, accurate diagnosis is necessary to identify other siblings with the same problem before they exhibit clinical symptomatology. Infectious diseases can precipitate acute symptoms of underlying metabolic disorders; thus, the fact that the child had an antecedent viral illness does not preclude the diagnosis of an inborn error of metabolism.

Disorders of urea cycle metabolism can present with acute encephalopathy, hyperammonemia, elevated serum transaminase levels, and respiratory alkalosis (See Chapter 2). Diagnosis rests on the finding of abnormal metabolites in the urine in some instances, or on measurement of specific enzyme activity in liver biopsy tissue in others.

Several organic acidurias, including methylmalonic acidemia and propionic aciduria, can mimic RS in their acute presentations. A helpful differentiating factor is the presence of a marked metabolic acidosis in the organic acid disorders.

In systemic carnitine deficiency (47), there is defective production of carnitine from its precursors. Carnitine is necessary for the transport of long-chain fatty acids across the mitochondrial membrane to undergo beta-oxidation. Symptoms and signs are identical to those of RS. Diagnosis is aided by measurements of plasma and liver carnitine levels, which are reduced in this disorder.

Medium-chain acyl-CoA dehydrogenase deficiency (48) is the most recently defined disorder which bears a striking resemblance to RS. This is an inborn error of fatty acid beta oxidation which results in deficient acyl-CoA production. Fasting or illness precipitates acute symptoms of persistent vomiting and lethargy, with hypoglycemia and hyperammonemia. These children typically have little or no ketonuria despite prolonged fasting and hypoglycemia. Abnormal elevations of dicarboxylic acids are present in the urine during the acute stages. Definitive diagnosis can be made by measuring enzyme activity in cultured fibroblasts or liver biopsy tissue.

MANAGEMENT

Since the pathogenesis of RS is unknown, there is no specific treatment. Management of the acute illness consists primarily of comprehensive and intensive supportive care, and treatment of the metabolic and neurologic complications of the disorder (49). The degree of intervention used depends on the severity of the encephalopathy. Several staging systems have been proposed to assess the disease severity. The National Institutes of Health Consensus Development Conference on the Diagnosis and Treatment of Reye syndrome (50) urged that a uniform staging system be used by all centers treating RS patients, in order to achieve better correlations between treatment and outcome across institutions (Table 14.2). Stage III and above signify severe illness, and qualify for aggressive management techniques. Duncan et al. (42) believe that the Glasgow Coma Scale (GCS), a 15-point classification for evaluation of level of consciousness that is widely used for head trauma patients, provides a more accurate indicator of progressive nervous system dysfunction than other methods, and may correlate better with the presence of increased intracranial pressure (ICP). A GCS of 8 or below indicates markedly depressed levels of consciousness (severe RS), and correlates with a high probability of raised ICP. Since most treatment regimens rely on a 5-point staging system, this will be employed for the remainder of the discussion.

GENERAL CONSIDERATIONS

Any child with suspected RS, even in the very mild stages, should be hospitalized in a pediatric intensive care unit, so that there is continuous visual observation of the child. These patients can deteriorate quite rapidly (within a few hours) to more severe levels. Vital signs should be monitored frequently. Oral feedings should be withheld, and a 10% dextrose solution with appropriate electrolyte concentrations for age should be administered intravenously at maintenance rates. There is evidence that prompt treatment with hypertonic glucose in the early stages prevents progression of the disease (5).

Laboratory investigations should initially include a complete blood count, serum pH, hepatic and renal function tests, determination of serum ammonia concentration, toxicology screen, and lumbar puncture. A liver biopsy should

Table 14.2 NIH consensus development conference guidelines for the staging of Reye syndrome

Stage 1.   Vomiting and lethargy. Responses to verbal stimuli are appropriate.

Stage 2.   Disorientation, combativeness, delirium. Responses to painful stimuli are appropriate.

Stage 3.   Obtundation or coma. Response to painful stimuli is decorticate posturing. Pupillary and oculocephalic reflexes are preserved.

Stage 4.   Coma. Response to painful stimuli is decerebrate posturing. Pupillary and oculocephalic reflexes may be incomplete.

Stage 5.   Coma and flaccid paralysis. No response to painful stimuli. Pupillary and oculocephalic reflexes may be absent.

Adapted from Diagnosis and treatment of Reye's syndrome, Consensus Conference. JAMA 1981;246:2441–2444.

be considered, particularly in infant patients, if other family members have had a similar disorder, or if it is a recurrent or atypical case. Plans should be made to evaluate the child for other metabolic disorders that may mimic Reye syndrome.

TREATMENT OF ADVANCED REYE SYNDROME

If the child's condition deteriorates to stage III or worse, an aggressive approach to therapy is warranted. Nasotracheal intubation should be performed, and the child placed on a mechanical ventilator. Central venous and arterial catheters should be inserted so that continuous measurements of these parameters are possible. Sedation, for example, with a short acting barbiturate may be required, or paralysis with a neuromuscular blocking agent such as pancuronium bromide, if the child is fighting the respirator. A nasogastric tube and indwelling urinary catheter should be inserted, and strict intake and output monitored. Intravenous solutions containing 15% dextrose with appropriate electrolyte concentrations should be administered at a rate that will maintain serum osmolality below 320 mOsm.

Hyperthermia is frequently present in these children. Reduction or maintenance of body temperature within the normal range may be accomplished with the use of a cooling blanket. Careful chest physiotherapy and suctioning of secretions from the endotracheal tube and mouth can reduce the problem of mucus plug accumulation, which may result in increased intrathoracic pressure and, secondarily, increased intracranial pressure.

Reversal of metabolic and clotting abnormalities is an important component of treatment for this disorder. Use of neomycin, by nasogastric tube or enema, alone or in combination with lactulose, is effective in reducing serum ammonia levels. Administration of fresh, frozen plasma will aid in correcting prolonged prothrombin time. Some centers continue to use exchange transfusion to correct metabolic derangements, clear potential toxins from the circulation, and correct clotting disorders.

Recent evidence suggests that children with RS may develop a secondary carnitine deficiency. Based on this information, some centers are administering intravenous L-carnitine as an adjunct to therapy during the acute stages.

Since increased intracranial pressure is a significant complication of this disorder, it is important to monitor ICP directly, using either surface or intraventricular monitoring devices, so that treatment can be carried out before there are clinical signs of deterioration. Brain function is compromised if cerebral perfusion pressure (CPP) is inadequate. CPP represents the difference between mean arterial blood pressure (MABP) and ICP. If CPP falls below 50mm Hg,

cerebral ischemia can occur, potentially leading to permanent damage. Thus, rather than attempting to maintain a specific ICP in any individual patient, the goal of therapy should be to maintain a CPP of at least 50mm Hg.

Intravenous mannitol, 0.25 g/kg/dose, lowers ICP within 5 to 10 minutes (51). Mannitol may be administered as often as necessary to control ICP, and the individual dose may be increased if needed. Mannitol is most effective if the serum osmolality is low; thus, it is useful to keep the serum osmolality below 320 mOsm in order to achieve maximal response to mannitol, and also to prevent complications of hyperosmolar states, such as renal damage.

Additional methods to control ICP include controlled hyperventilation to a pCO_2 of 25 to 40mm Hg, elevation of the head to 30 degrees, and hypothermia. If all of these measures fail to adequately reduce ICP to a level sufficient to allow adequate CPP, barbiturate therapy may be utilized (52,53). This may take the form of small doses of short-acting barbiturates as needed when ICP is unacceptably high, or of large, frequently repeated doses to induce an iatrogenic burst-suppression pattern on the EEG (barbiturate coma). The latter approach is often complicated by systemic hypotension, which may require the addition of pressor agents to the therapeutic regimen.

RESULTS

Mortality rates for RS have remained fairly constant over recent years at approximately 30%. Most survivors over the age of 1 year return to normal levels of function (54); however, transient neurologic, speech, and cognitive deficits may be found for many months after the acute illness (55). In some children, learning disabilities, motor speech problems, and subtle cognitive deficits may persist indefinitely (56–58). Rarely, seizure disorders, mental retardation, and fixed motor deficits follow recovery from the acute illness. In general, the presence of long-term impairments correlates with the severity of the initial illness.

Infants under 1 year of age are at particular risk to develop significant neurologic and intellectual sequelae. This may reflect, in part, the difficulty of diagnosing RS in infants, since the clinical presentation is often subtle and not as consistent as in older children. The rapidly developing brain in the 1st year of life may also be highly susceptible to the effects of metabolic derangements.

Early identification of potential RS cases, and rapid treatment with hypertonic glucose, may prevent worsening of the disease and, in turn, possibly reduce the potential sequelae of this disorder.

REFERENCES

1. Reye RDK, Morgan G, Baral J. Encephalopathy and fatty degeneration of the viscera: A disease entity in childhood. Lancet 1963;2:749–752.

2. Johnson GM, Scurletis TD, Carroll NB. A study of sixteen fatal cases of encephalitis-like disease in North Carolina children. N C Med J 1963;24:464–469.

3. Meythaler JM, Varma RR. Reye's Syndrome in adults: Diagnostic considerations. Arch Int Med 1987;147:61–64.

4. CDC. Reye Syndrome surveillance—United States, 1986. MMWR 1987;36:689–691.

5. Lichtenstein PK, Heubi JE, Daugherty CC, et al. Grade I Reye's Syndrome: A frequent cause of vomiting and liver dysfunction after varicella and upper-respiratory-tract infection. N Engl J Med 1983;309:133–139.

6. CDC. Reye Syndrome—United States, 1984. MMWR 1985;34:13–16.

7. Huttenlocher PR, Trauner DA. Reye's Syndrome in infancy. Pediatrics 1978;62:84–90.

8. Sullivan-Bolyai JZ, Nelson DB, Morens DM, et al. Reye Syndrome in children less than 1 year old: Some epidemiologic observations. Pediatrics 1980;65:627–629.

9. Barrett MJ, Hurwitz ES, Schonberger LB, et al. Changing epidemiology of Reye Syndrome in the United States. Pediatrics 1986;77:598–602.

10. Starko KM, Ray CG, Dominguez LB, et al. Reye's Syndrome and salicylate use. Pediatrics 1980;66:859–864.

11. Waldman RJ, Hall WN, McGee H, et al. Aspirin as a risk factor in Reye's Syndrome. JAMA 1982;247:3089–3094.

12. Halpin TJ, Holtzhauer FJ, Campbell RJ, et al. Reye's Syndrome and medication use. JAMA 1982;248:687–691.

13. Hurwitz ES, Barrett MJ, Bregman D, et al. Public Health Service study on Reye's Syndrome and medications: Report of the pilot phase. N Engl J Med 1985;313:849–857.

14. Hurwitz ES, Barrett MJ, Bregman D, et al. Public Health Service study of Reye's Syndrome and medications: Report of the main study. JAMA 1987;257:1905–1911.

15. Arrowsmith JB, Kennedy DL, Kuritsky JN, et al. National patterns of aspirin use and Reye Syndrome reporting, United States, 1980 to 1985. Pediatrics 1987;79:858–863.

16. Orlowski JP, Gillis J, Kilham HA. A catch in the Reye. Pediatrics 1987;80:638–642.

17. Yamashita F, Ono E, Kimura A, et al. Reye's Syndrome in Asian countries. In: Pollack JD, ed. Reye's Syndrome IV. Bryan, Ohio: National Reye's Syndrome Foundation, 1985:47–60.

18. Mitchell RA, Ram ML, Arcinue EL, et al. Comparison of cytosolic and mitochondrial hepatic enzyme alterations in Reye's syndrome. Pediatr Res 1980;14:1216–1221.

19. Davis LE, Cole LL, Lockwood SJ, et al. Experimental influenza B virus toxicity in mice: A possible model for Reye's Syndrome. Lab Invest 1983;48:140–147.

20. Trauner DA, Davis LE. Effect of influenza virus on β-oxidation in mouse liver mitochondria: Importance for Reye's Syndrome. Neurology 1988;38:239–241.

21. Trauner DA, Nyhan WL, Sweetman L. Short-chain organic acidemia and Reye's Syndrome. Neurology 1975;25:296–298.

22. Trauner DA, Huttenlocher PR. Short-chain fatty acid-induced central hyperventilation in rabbits. Neurology 1978;28:940–944.

23. Trauner DA. Pathologic changes in a rabbit model of Reye's syndrome. Pediatr Res 1982;16:950–953.

24. Shannon DC, De Long R, Bercu B, et al. Studies on the pathophysiology of encephalopathy in Reye's syndrome: Hyperammonemia in Reye's syndrome. Pediatrics 1975;56:999–1004.

25. Brown T, Hug G, Lansky L, et al. Transiently reduced activity of carbamyl phosphate synthetase and ornithine transcarbamylase in liver of children with Reye's syndrome. N Engl J Med 1976;294:861–867.

26. Zieve RJ, Zieve L, Doizaki WM, et al. Synergism between ammonia and fatty acids in the production of coma: Implication for hepatic coma. J Pharmacol Exp Ther 1974;191:10–21.

27. Olson LC, Bourgeois CH, Cotton RB, et al. Encephalopathy and fatty degeneration of the viscera in Northeastern Thailand: Clinical syndrome and epidemiology. Pediatrics 1971;47:707–712.

28. Bourgeois CH, Shank RC, Grossman RA, et al. Acute aflatoxin B1 toxicity in the macaque and its similarities to Reye's syndrome. Lab Invest 1971;24:206–213.

29. Ryan NJ, Hogan GR, Hayes AW, et al. Aflatoxin B1: Its role in the etiology of Reye's syndrome. Pediatrics 1979;64:71–75.

30. Nelson DB, Kimbrough R, Landrigan PS, et al. Aflatoxin and Reye's syndrome: A case control study. Pediatrics 1980;66:865–869.

31. Dove DJ, Jones T. Delayed coma associated with salicylate intoxication. J Pediatr 1982;100:493–496.

32. Temple AR. Pathophysiology of aspirin overdosage toxicity with implications for management. Pediatrics 1978;62 (suppl):873–876.

33. Starko KM, Mullick FG. Hepatic and cerebral pathology findings in children with fatal salicylate intoxication: Further evidence for a causal relation between salicylate and Reye's syndrome. Lancet 1983;1:326–329.

34. Partin JS, Daugherty CC, McAdams J, et al. A comparison of liver ultrastructure in salicylate intoxication and Reye's syndrome. Hepatology 1984;4:687–690.

35. Bove KE, McAdams AJ, Partin JC, et al. The hepatic lesion in Reye's syndrome. Gastroenterology 1975;69:685–697.

36. Partin JC, Schubert WK, Partin JS. Mitochondrial ultrastructure in Reye syndrome (encephalopathy and fatty degeneration of the viscera). N Engl J Med 1971;285:1339–1343.

37. Partin JC, Partin JS, Schubert WK, et al. Brain ultrastructure in Reye's syndrome (encephalopathy and fatty alteration of the viscera). J Neuropathol Exp Neurol 1975;34:425–444.

38. Huttenlocher PR, Trauner DA. Reye's syndrome in infancy. Pediatrics 1978;62:84–90.

39. Aoki Y, Lombroso CT. Prognostic value of electroencephalography in Reye's syndrome. Neurology 1973;23:333–343.

40. Trauner DA, Stockard JS. Electrophysiological studies in Reye's syndrome: A case report. Arch Neurol 1977;34:116–118.

41. Yamada T, Tucker RP, Kooi KA. Fourteen and six c/sec positive bursts in comatose patients. Electroencephalogr Clin Neurophysiol 1976;40:645–653.

42. Duncan CC, Ment LR, Shaywitz BA. Evaluation of level of consciousness by the Glasgow coma scale in children with Reye's syndrome. Neurosurgery 1983;13:650–653.

43. Goff WR, Shaywitz BA, Goff GD, et al. Somatic evoked potential evaluation of cerebral status in Reye syndrome. Electroencephalogr Clin Neurophysiol 1983;55:388–398.

44. Robinson RO. Differential diagnosis of Reye's syndrome. Dev Med Child Neurol 1987;29:110–120.

45. Hassall CH, Reyle K. The toxicity of the akee (Blighia sapida) and its relationship to the vomiting sickness of Jamaica. West Indian Med J 1955;4:91–98.

46. Greene CL, Blitzer MG, Shapira E. Inborn errors of metabolism and Reye syndrome: Differential diagnosis. J Pediatr 1988;113:156–159.

47. Stumpf DA, Parker WDJ, Angelini C. Carnitine deficiency, organic acidemia, and Reye's syndrome. Neurology 1985;35:1041–1045.

48. Taubman B, Hale DE, Kelley RJ. Familial Reye-like syndrome: A presentation of medium-chain acyl-coenzyme A dehydrogenase deficiency. Pediatrics 1987;79:382–385.

49. Trauner DA. Treatment of Reye's syndrome. Ann Neurol 1980;7:2–5.

50. Diagnosis and treatment of Reye's syndrome, Consensus Conference. JAMA 1981;246:2441–2444.

51. Trauner DA, Brown F, Ganz E, et al. Treatment of elevated intracranial pressure in Reye syndrome. Ann Neurol 1978;4:275–278.

52. Marshall LF, Shapiro HM, Rauscher A, et al. Pentobarbital therapy for intracranial hypertension in metabolic coma—Reye's syndrome. Crit Care Med 1978;6:1–5.

53. Shaywitz BA, Rothstein P, Venes JL. Monitoring and management of increased intracranial pressure in Reye syndrome: Results in 29 children. Pediatrics 1980;66:198–204.

54. Shaywitz SE, Cohen PM, Cohen DJ, et al. Long-term consequences of Reye syndrome: A sibling-matched, controlled study of neurologic, cognitive, academic, and psychiatric function. J Pediatr 1982;100:41–46.

55. Brunner RL, O'Grady DJ, Partin JC, et al. Neuropsychologic consequences of Reye syndrome. J Pediatr 1979;95:706–711.

56. Reitman MA, Casper J, Coplan J, et al. Motor disorders of voice and speech in Reye's syndrome survivors. Am J Dis Child 1984;138:1129–1131.

57. Quart EJ, Cruickshank WM, Sarnaik A. Prior history of learning disabilities in Reye's syndrome survivors. J Learn Disab 1985;18:345–349.

58. Quart EJ, Buchtel HA, Sarnaik AP. Long-lasting memory deficits in children recovered from Reye's syndrome. J Clin Exp Neuropsychol 1987;10:409–420.

Part III

Neurologic Manifestations of Organ System Disorders

Chapter 15
Neurologic Aspects of Cardiovascular Disease

Richard S. K. Young

Stroke is the most dramatic manner in which the heart affects the brain. The cardiovascular system may also alter neurologic function in more subtle ways by producing syncope, amaurosis, or amnesia. Cardiac disease produces nueurologic symptoms when there is curtailment of delivery of oxygen and fuel to the brain. Disorders of the blood vessels create neurologic deficits through embolization, thrombosis, or hemorrhage. The incidence of ischemic and hemorrhagic stroke in children is estimated to be 2.52 cases per 100,000 per year (1–5). In recent reviews of childhood stroke, a cardiac etiology was present in 35% of subjects (Table 15.1); however, when all disorders of the heart and blood vessels are included, the percentage is twofold greater.

The functioning of the cardiovascular and nervous systems are inextricably intertwined. The heart is responsible for providing a continuous supply of blood and substrate to the brain. The brain, through the autonomic nervous system, regulates arterial blood pressure and heart rate. The dependency of the brain on the heart has been recognized for centuries. Only recently have we appreciated that the functioning of the heart requires an intact brainstem.

Table 15.1 Etiology of cerebrovascular disease in childhood

	Cornell(2)	St. Louis(3)	Mayo(4)	Iowa(5)
I. Ischemic Stroke				
Thrombosis/ atherosclerotic	16	25		39
Trauma	11			
Infection	11			
Cardiac disease	10		18	35
Hematologic/ sickle cell	5		5	22
Venous thrombosis		11		
Vasculopathy				39
Moyamoya disease			3	
Miscellaneous	4		17	10
II. Hemorrhagic Stroke				
Subarachnoid or intraventricular hemorrhage		45		
Intracerebral hemorrhage		11		
Arteriovenous malformation	4	14	13	
Aneurysm		4	6	
Unknown	25		12	
TOTALS:	86	110	74	145

DEVELOPMENTAL PHYSIOLOGY OF THE CEREBRAL CIRCULATION

Developmental Changes

Recent research has clarified the volume, rate, and responsiveness of cerebral blood flow (CBF) in the human infant and child. There is an early adjustment of cerebral perfusion in the term newborn infant resulting from closure of the ductus arteriosus and the foramen ovale, and from opening of pulmonary capillary beds. Following this, the neonate maintains a constant cerebral blood flow (6).

The xenon technique has been employed to measure CBF in both the premature and the full term infant. CBF in the preterm infant (30 weeks gestation) is estimated to be 48.4 ± 14.9 mL/100g/min (7). In the full term infant, CBF has been determined to be 87 mL/100g/min in grey matter and 17.2 mL/100g/min in white matter (8). Measurements of CBF with positron emission tomography (PET) have ranged from 9.0 to 73 mL/100g/min in term infants and 4.9 to 23 mL/100g/min in preterm infants (9). Cerebral blood flow reaches a peak in the growing child and then decreases to adult values by the late teenage years (10).

Doppler analysis of cerebral blood flow velocity provides an indirect estimate of CBF in the human neonate. These studies disclose that intracranial vascular resistance increases during the first one-half hour of life. Thereafter, the pulsatility index (v systolic–v diastolic) decreases during the first several days of life, due to a fall in diastolic flow velocity (11).

Measurements of CBF with the radioactive xenon technique are comprised by the inability to discriminate flow in the extracranial vessels. Recent studies employing PET (9) have the advantage of spatial resolution, but the disadvantages associated with radioactive isotopes. In the future, nuclear magnetic resonance (NMR) may provide a noninvasive method of measuring CBF using nonradioactive tracers such as D_2O.

Autoregulation of the Cerebral Circulation

The flow of blood from heart to brain is not pressure passive, but is closely monitored by the autonomic nervous system (12,13). The ability of such organs as the brain and kidney to self-govern the flow of blood received over a wide range of blood pressures is termed *autoregulation* (Figure 15.1). Through dilation or constriction of the small and medium-sized arteries of the brain, cerebral blood flow to the various regions increases or decreases to accommodate to changes in posture, blood pressure, hematocrit, oxygen tension, carbon dioxide tension, or acid–base status.

The autoregulatory plateau of the human newborn

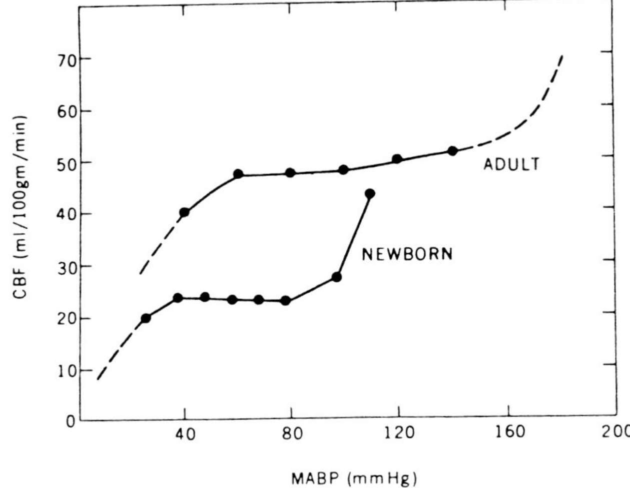

FIGURE 15.1 Pressure-blood flow curves show that the plateau of autoregulation is lower and shifted to the left in the neonatal compared to the adult dog. (Reprinted with permission from Drs. R.C. Vannucci and M.J. Hernandez.)

infant is substantially lower than that in the adult human (Figure 15.1). Younkin et al. (8) established autoregulatory limits of 60 to 84 mm Hg of blood pressure in healthy newborn human infants, although it is likely that a substantially wider range exists. A lower rate of CBF and metabolism is teleologically advantageous during parturition when hypoxia or hypotension may supervene.

Several studies have shown that factors which affect CBF during development in animals such as the dog also affect CBF in the human neonate (14,15,16). Data show that the autoregulatory plateau of newborn dogs is 27 to 97 mm Hg. The limit of autoregulation at which blood flow begins to fail may be lower for white matter than for grey matter (15).

Responsiveness of the Cerebral Circulation

CBF is responsive to a variety of stimuli including hypoxemia, hypo- and hypercarbia, acidosis, and alterations in hematocrit. Hypoxemia produces marked compensatory increase in cerebral blood flow. Hypercarbia causes vasodilation and increase in cerebral blood flow; whereas, hypocarbia reduces CBF. Acidosis induced by infusion of lactic acid increases hindbrain blood flow. The hematocrit is the major determinant of blood viscosity. Lowering the hematocrit is associated with an increase in CBF and, depending on the degree, an increase in oxygen delivery. The increase in CBF is maximal during periods of increased metabolic demand such as that which occurs during seizures (16) or hypoglycemia (17). An increase in CBF during physiologic activation (speech, reading, singing) is typically heterogeneous.

TRANSIENT CEREBRAL ISCHEMIA

Syncope

Syncope is the most common cause of transient neurologic dysfunction in childhood and occurs in approximately 15% of children (18). Syncopal episodes can be caused by either neurologic or cardiac disorders (Table 15.2). The mechanism of reflex syncope involves increased vagal tone, triggered by unpleasant physical and psychologic experiences. Prodromal symptoms of hunger, heat, and pain often precede the faint, while cough and micturition may initiate the syncopal episode. During syncope, there is a sudden drop in blood pressure and bradycardia. Consciousness is rapidly restored when the individual assumes a recumbent posture and cerebral blood flow is restored. Camfield and Camfield suggest that there is a familial tendency toward syncope (19).

Patients with orthostatic hypotension are frequently syncopal. Causes of orthostatic hypotension include dysautonomic syndromes (Riley-Day syndrome), diabetes mellitus, excessive diuretic therapy, or prolonged bed rest. Syncope can also result from contraction of the intravascular volume secondary to anorexia or dehydration. Measurement of the pulse and blood pressure in supine and erect positions is an essential part of the examination. More definitive testing involves a graded tilt test, exercise test, and determination of plasma catecholamines. Thilenius and associates cite the tilt test as a cost-effective means for the evaluation of unexplained, recurrent syncope in childhood (20).

Table 15.2   Differential diagnosis of syncope

Type	Age	Duration	Features
Vascular reflex			
Vasovagal	Any	< 1 min	Rapid return of consciousness, no bodily injury
Breath holding spell	Infants	< 1 min	Associated with crying
Cardiac			
Arrhythmia	Any	Brief	No precipitating event
Obstructive	Any	Brief	No precipitating event
Neurologic			
Myoclonic seizure	Any	Seconds	EEG abnormal; bodily injury
Cataplexy	Older children	Seconds	Associated with narcolepsy
3rd Ventricular tumor	Any	Short	Headache, vomiting
Metabolic			
Hypoglycemia, hypocalcemia, hyponatremia, hypokalemia, anemia	Any		Rare, as a cause of syncope

The majority of syncopal episodes are benign, and a careful history and physical examination may be all that is necessary to establish the diagnosis. However, the presence of an arrhythmia, a family history of cardiomyopathy or sudden death, warrants detailed cardiologic investigation. Bodily injury (e.g. tongue biting), incontinence, or postictal confusion may be evidence for a seizure disorder. Children with anoxic seizures due to vagal stimulation may be identified by digital ocular compression during an electrocardiographic (EKG) recording which reveals a brief period of asystole (21). The treatment of syncopal episodes is predicated upon the etiology. Vasovagal syncope may be aborted by teaching the child to recognize the premonitory symptoms and to assume a prone position. Education and treatment with β-adrenergic blockers can be helpful in patients (often young girls) who develop palpitations from sinus tachycardia consequent to slight physiologic stress (hyperbeta adrenergic syndrome) (22). Patients with hypovolemia and exaggerated venous pooling may require treatment with mineralocorticoids or anti-gravity stockings.

Cardiac Arrhythmias and Stokes-Adams Attacks

In the mid 1800s, Stokes and Adams described the phenomenon of cardiovascular syncope. It is now recognized that a variety of cardiac disorders may induce syncope. These include aortic stenosis, idiopathic hypertrophic subaortic stenosis, heart block, and Wolf-Parkinson-White syndrome. Tachy- or bradyarrhythmias producing prolonged periods of asystole may be a cause of episodic unconsciousness. The long QT interval syndrome, inherited as an autosomal dominant trait, causes syncopal episodes in children between the ages of 2 and 6 years. Exertion or fright can precipitate sudden death in children with inherited QT interval prolongation (23). Right ventricular cardiomyopathy may present first as palpitations, syncopal episodes, or sudden death (24). Paroxysmal familial ventricular fibrillation may similarly be a cause of syncope or sudden death (25). A characteristic EKG pattern (short P-R interval and U wave) is present, but Holter monitoring, exercise testing, and electrophysiologic studies of the cardiac conduction system may be required for thorough evaluation.

Hypoglycemia

Hemiparesis due to hypoglycemia may be mistaken for a primary cerebral ischemic event. The mechanism of focal neurologic deficits occurring during a presumed global substrate deficiency is not understood but may represent a selective metabolic vulnerability (26).

1. Brain Oxygen Requirement $=$ Cerebral metabolic rate$_{O_2}$ ($ml_{O_2}/g_{brain}/min$) $\times$ brain weight (g)

$= 0.05 \times 1{,}000$

$= \boxed{50\ ml_{O_2}/min.}$

2. Arterial Oxygen Content $=$ Oxygen$_{Hgb\text{-}bound}$ $+$ Oxygen$_{dissolved}$

$= [Hgb\ (g/ml_{blood}) \times O_2\ \text{carrying capacity of Hgb}\ (ml_{O_2}/g_{Hgb}) \times O_2\ Sat.] + [ml_{O_2}/ml_{blood} \times mm\ Hg]$

$= [0.04 \times 1.39 \times 0.975] + [0.00003 \times 100]$

$= 0.0542 + 0.003$

$= \boxed{0.0572\ ml_{O_2}/ml_{blood}}$

3. Total Oxygen Delivered to Brain $=$ Cerebral Blood Flow ($ml_{blood}/g_{brain}/min$) $\times$ Brain Weight (g) $\times$ Arterial Oxygen Content (ml_{O_2}/ml_{blood})

$= 0.75 \times 1000 \times 0.0572$

$= \boxed{42.9\ ml_{O_2}/min}$

FIGURE 15.2 Severe anemia led to reduction of cerebral oxygen delivery to marginal levels. (Reprinted with permission from Stroke, 1983.)

Anemic Hypoxia

Profound anemias in childhood may reduce oxygen delivery to the brain to the extent that syncope, hemiparesis, or infarction result. The anemia usually develops slowly so that the intravascular volume remains normal. When the hemoglobin is less than 3 g/dL, oxygen delivery to the brain reaches precarious levels (27) (Figure 15.2).

Migraine

The development of transient neurologic deficits such as aphasia, hemiparesis, and hemianopsia during attacks of migraine are referred to as complicated migraine. It is critical to note that migraine is a diagnosis of exclusion and that infectious, metabolic, and physiologic causes must be excluded. Measurements of CBF during attacks of complicated migraine disclose an initial hypoperfusion followed by hyperperfusion in the hemisphere contralateral to the deficit (28). In some patients, CBF studies show global oligemia. Normal cerebral physiologic function may be altered during migraine and the increase in regional CBF typically seen during cortical activity may be impaired.

The incidence of migrainous strokes is 3.4 per 100,000 (29). The association between migraine and ischemic stroke is significantly increased in patients with classic migraine,

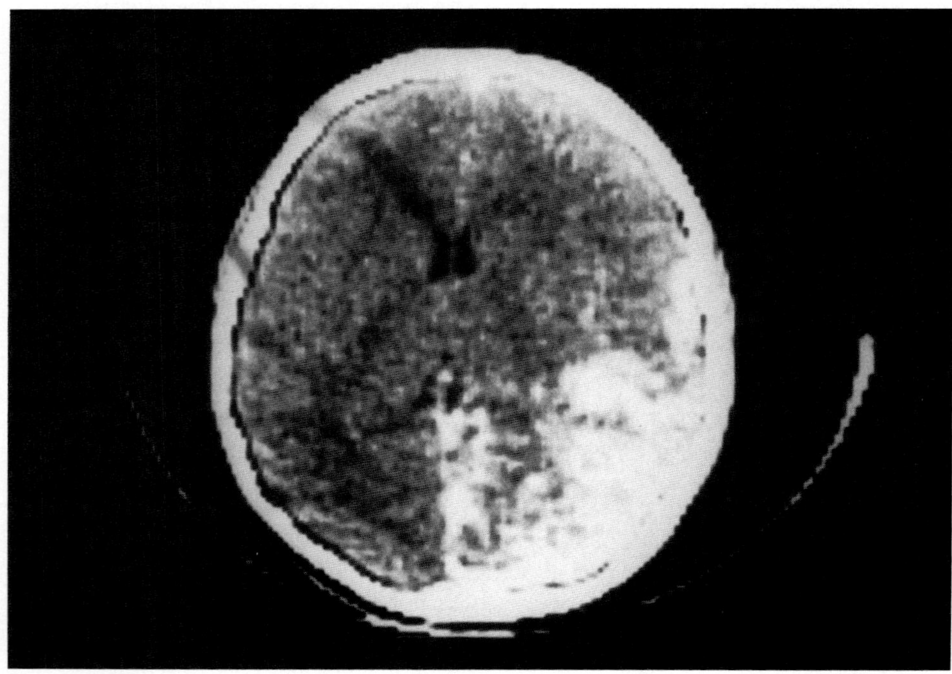

FIGURE 15.3 The initial complaint in this teenager was unilateral headache. A large arteriovenous malformation is supplied by both middle and posterior cerebral arteries. Hemispheric asymmetry is present.

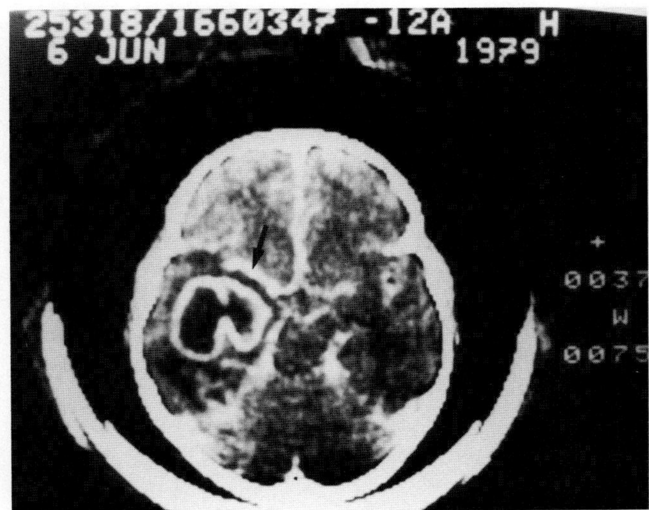

FIGURE 15.4 This child with unrepaired ventricular septal defect was diagnosed by a neurologist as having migraine. A CT brain scan shows a temporal lobe brain abscess with formation of a daughter cyst. There is anterior displacement of the middle cerebral artery (arrow).

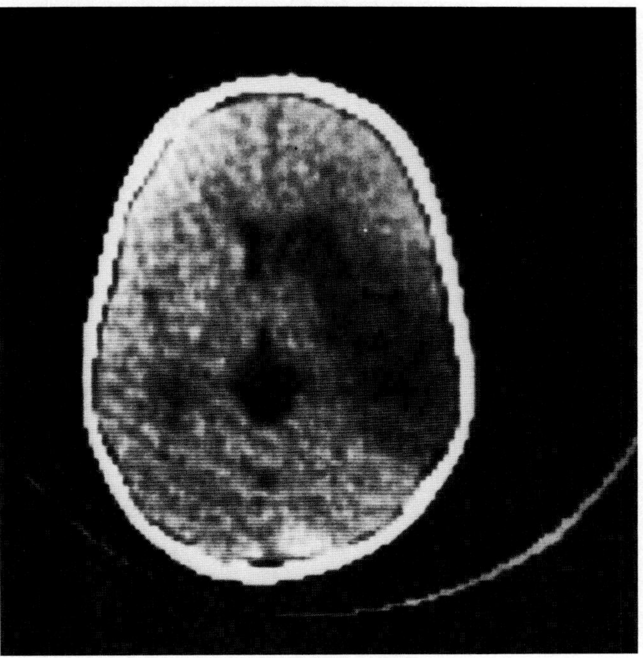

FIGURE 15.5 An infarction in the distribution of the middle cerebral artery occurred in this neonate with ventricular septal defect.

but not common migraine (29). Stroke can occur in the absence of migraine attack (30,31). In Adams's study, 14% of 144 young adults with nonhemorrhagic stroke had vascular headache, but only 3% had migraine as the cause of cerebral infarction (5). The cause of cerebral infarction in migraine is presumed to result from ischemia due to vasospasm. No cardiac or arterial anomaly was found in 91% of patients (31).

Migraine-related infarcts may occur in the anterior circulation or subcortically. Hemicranial pain due to arteriovenous malformation (Figure 15.3), brain abscess (Figure 15.4), or tumor can masquerade as migraine. There is disagreement about whether "basilar artery migraine" can result in stroke (1,29).

CARDIAC SOURCES OF CEREBROVASCULAR DISEASE

Hypotensive Injury

A major cause of cerebral infarction is hypotension due to low cardiac output ("pump failure"). When the lower range of autoregulation is exceeded, blood flow fails. Ischemic injury to the brain leads to a variety of patterns of neuropathologic damage reflecting arterial irrigation beds as well as the selective vulnerability of neurons. These patterns include: infarction in the distribution of a major vessel (Figure 15.5); border zone infarction (Figure 15.6); selective neuronal necrosis (Figure 15.7); and cystic encephalomalacia (Figure 15.8).

Ischemic injury is frequently multisystemic with collateral damage to the heart, kidneys, and gut. The metabolic

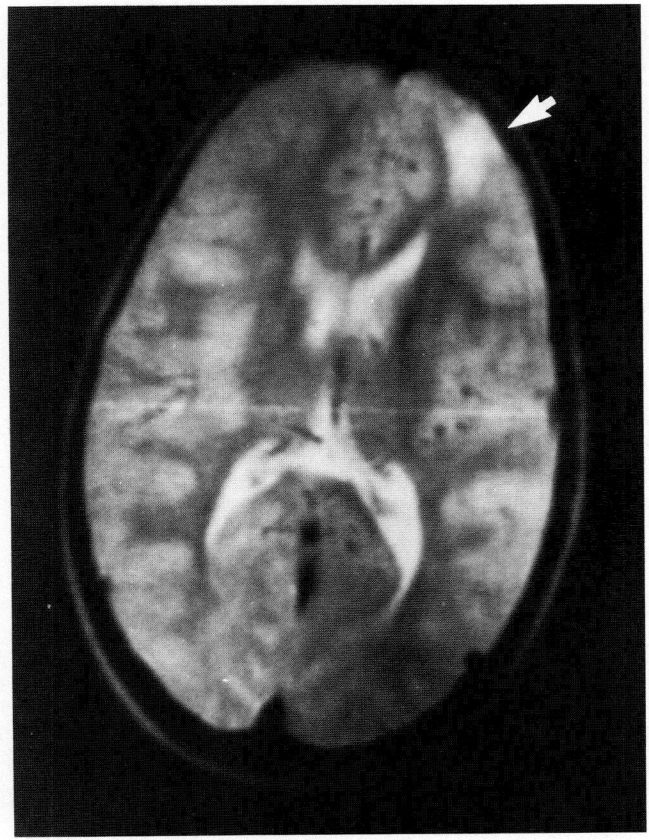

FIGURE 15.6 Magnetic resonance image demonstrating a border zone (watershed) infarct (arrow) in the cerebral cortex between the anterior and middle cerebral artery distributions in a patient with sickle cell disease. (Reprinted with permission of Dr. S.J. Pavlakis and Annals of Neurology.)

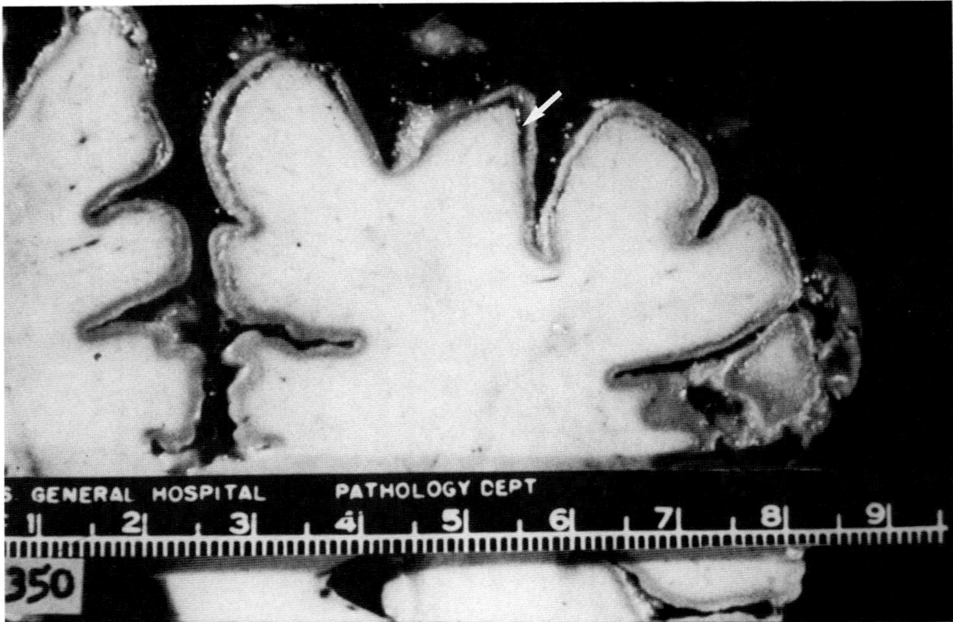

FIGURE 15.7 Necrosis of the cortical grey matter (arrow) with sparing of the subcortical white matter has resulted from the relative vulnerability of neurons.

profile of impaired oxidative metabolism includes a decrease in phosphocreatine levels and an increase in inorganic phosphate as documented by ^{31}P neuromagnetic resonance (NMR) spectroscopy in the asphyxiated human infant (32). All infants with phosphocreatine/inorganic phosphate ratios less than 1.0 died or developed cerebral atrophy. Cardiac arrest during hypothermia is a singular exception to the rule that brain injury follows global ischemia (33). Intelligence scores in children who have undergone cardiac arrest during hypothermia are not significantly different from those of their siblings (34).

Cardiogenic Emboli

Cardiac emboli account for approximately one-fourth of childhood strokes (5) (Figure 15.9; Table 15.3). Embolic stroke is typically preceded by headache, maximal at onset, and is associated with alteration of consciousness. Approximately 12% of patients with embolic stroke have a seizure at the onset of symptoms. In contrast, seizures during cerebral thrombosis are only one-fourth as likely to occur (35). Neurologic deficits due to cerebral embolism include hemiparesis, hemisensory symptoms, aphasia, and visual loss.

Cardiac emboli typically lodge in the middle cerebral artery. They are infrequently found in the posterior cerebral or basilar arteries and are seldom in the anterior cerebral artery. A history of prior cerebral (Figure 15.10) or systemic embolization suggests cardiogenic emboli. Symptoms of cardiac disease, such as chest pain, palpitations, tachy- or bradyarrthyhmia, also implicate a cardiac source of emboli.

Infective Endocarditis

Fever, cardiac murmur, and focal neurologic deficit are the clinical bellwethers of infective endocarditis (36,37). Approximately one-half of patients with infective endocarditis present with neurologic deficits such as seizures, hemiplegia, or toxic encephalopathy. Patients may have protean complaints of fever, arthralgia, myalgia, and weakness. Patients with a history of intravenous drug abuse are

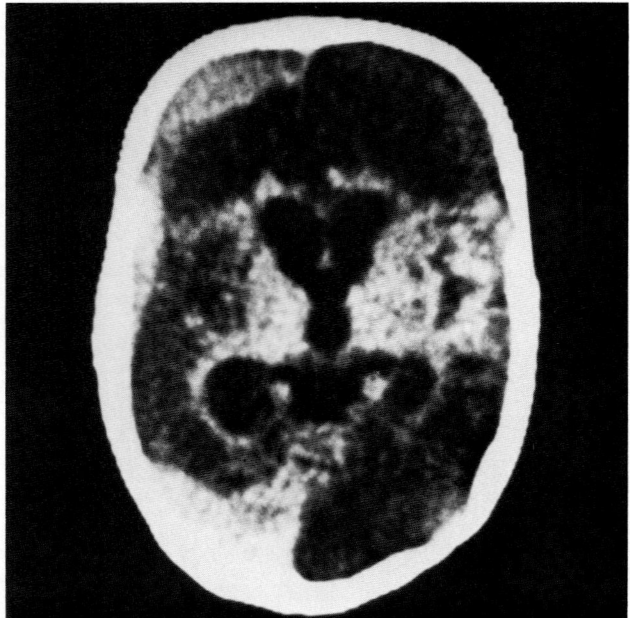

FIGURE 15.8 This neonate underwent a surgical procedure and had considerable blood loss. Cystic encephalomalacia developed as a consequence of a prolonged period of hypotension.

FIGURE 15.9 A clot is present in the apex of the left ventricle (LV and RV, left and right ventricles; LA and RA, left and right atria.) (Courtesy of Dr. C. Jaffe.)

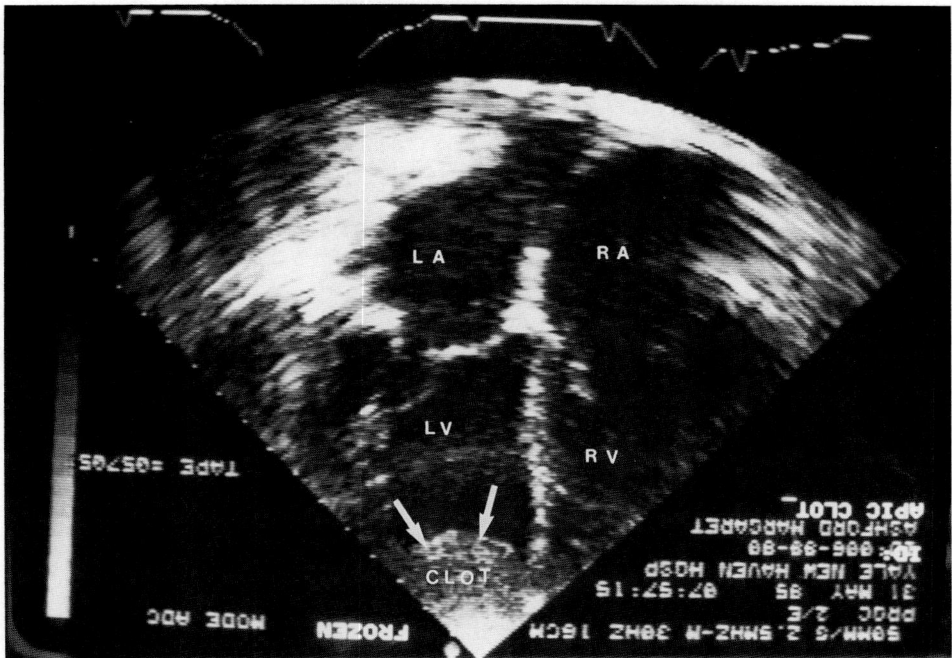

at particular risk for the development of infective endocarditis. Systemic as well as cerebral embolization can occur. Secondary neurologic complications of infective endocarditis include meningoencephalitis, arteritis, intracerebral hemorrhage, mycotic aneurysm formation, and brain abscess. Brain embolism may be fatal in 80% of patients (38). Children with bacterial endocarditis and cyanotic congenital heart disease are predisposed to development of brain abscess (Figure 15.4). The pathophysiology involves paradoxical septic embolism, right to left shunting of bacteria, or secondary bacterial colonization of an infarct.

Table 15.3 Laboratory evaluation for cerebrovascular disease Yale stroke program

Standard Evaluation	Collagen Vascular Screen
Complete blood count	Protein C and Protein S
Platelet count	Antithrombin III
Electrolytes	Rheumatoid factor
Glucose	Antinuclear antibody
BUN and creatinine	Lupus anticoagulant
Alkaline phosphatase	Serum protein electrophoresis
Total bilirubin	C3, C4, CH50
SGOT, LDH, SGPT, CK	
Total protein	
Uric acid	
Calcium, phosphate	
Cholesterol and triglycerides	
PT, PTT	
Erythrocyte sedimentation rate and serum viscosity	
Hemoglobin electrophoresis (if appropriate)	
EKG and Holter monitor	
Urinalysis	
Imaging Studies	**Optional—(pending initial assessment)**
Magnetic resonance imaging	CK isoenzymes
Chest X-ray	Fibrinogen
Carotid ultrasound	VDRL
Angiography	Platelet function test
Cardiac ultrasound	HDL cholesterol
Exercise tolerance test	Magnesium
EEG	Lumbar puncture
Tilt test	Thyroid function tests
	Blood cultures

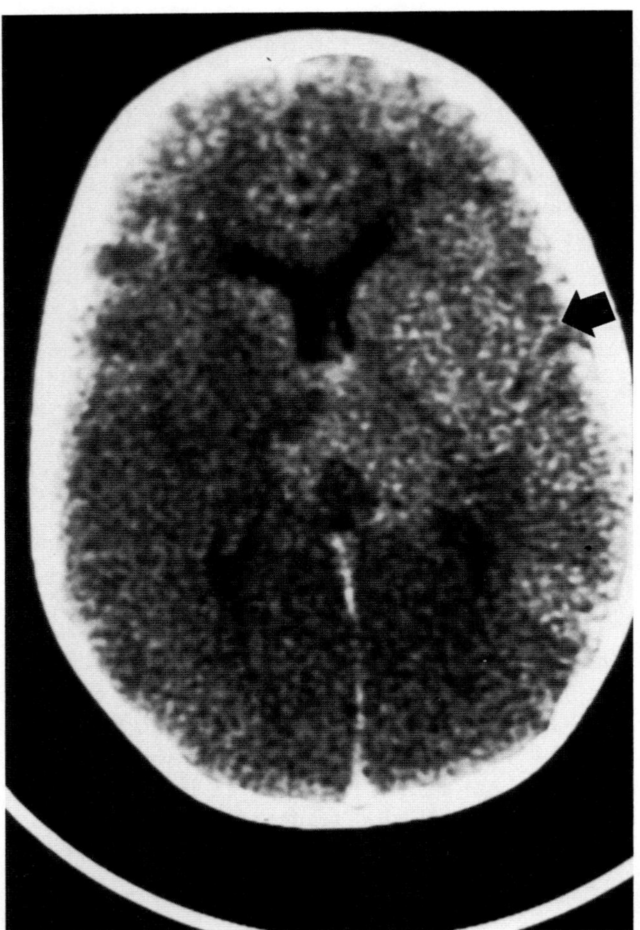

FIGURE 15.10 This child with Down syndrome initially presented with sudden left hemiplegia. Subsequently, he developed sudden right hemiplegia, accompanied by seizure and coma. There is infarction of the territory supplied by the left posterior cerebral artery and right middle and posterior cerebral arteries. There is sparing of the left middle cerebral artery territory (arrow.) No source of emboli was identified.

A high degree of suspicion is needed for prompt diagnosis of brain abscess. Serial blood cultures are essential. Patients at increased risk include those with congenital heart disease, rheumatic heart disease, dental caries, drug abuse, parenteral hyperalimentation, and immunosuppression (HIV infections). Two dimensional echocardiography is more sensitive than M-mode echocardiography in detecting cardiac valvular vegetations. Appropriate cultures should be obtained and antibiotics administered to any child with cyanotic congenital heart disease who presents with stroke. In Kanter and Hart's series (36), neurologic complications occurred more often when the offending pathogen was *Staphylococcus aureus* than when it was *Streptococcus viridans* (e.g., frequency of stroke, 39% versus 9%). Group D *streptococcus* is the organism typically found in intravenous drug abusers, while non-Group D *streptococcus* is a common pathogen in nonaddicted patients (37).

Fungal Emboli

Fungal emboli can develop in patients who are immunosuppressed or have altered immune function. Fungal cultures should be obtained in patients who have had embolic stroke and in whom bacterial cultures are negative. Neonates whose surface cultures for fungi are positive may be at particular risk for cerebral fungal embolization (Figure 15.11).

Rheumatic Heart Disease

In rheumatic heart disease, hypersensitization of the cardiac tissue by a streptococcal infection leads to an initial pancarditis, followed by the development of a valvulitis. Calcifications and verrucae along cusp borders are sources of thromboemboli. About 10% to 20% of patients with rheumatic heart disease will experience systemic embolization; one-half of them will have a recurrence. Both mitral stenosis and mitral regurgitation are associated with embolization. When atrial fibrillation is present, the risk of stroke may increase tenfold or more. Anticoagulation reduces the risk of systemic embolism to 10% to 20% of the natural incidence (39). The prevalence of rheumatic heart disease has declined sharply because of improved health and the widespread use of antimicrobial agents.

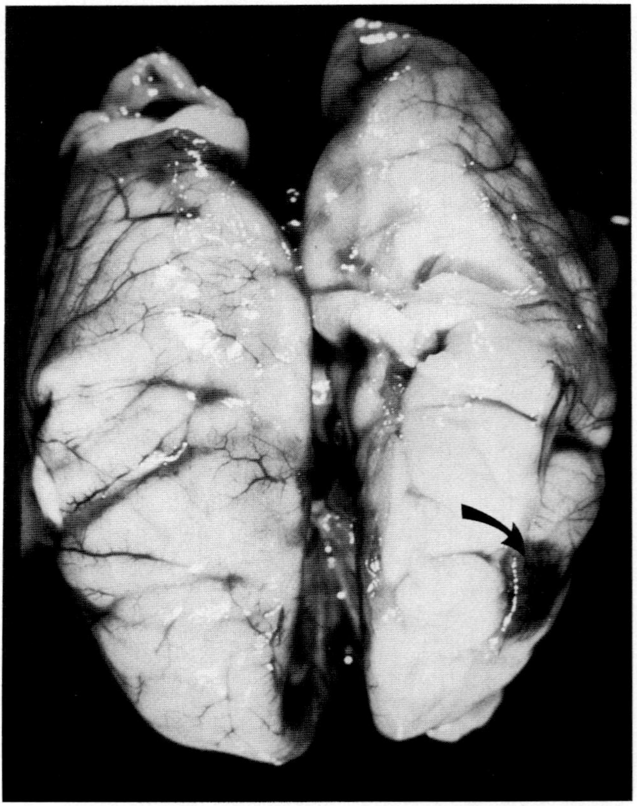

FIGURE 15.11 A neonate with a fungal embolus that produced an infarct (arrow) in the right parieto-occipital area.

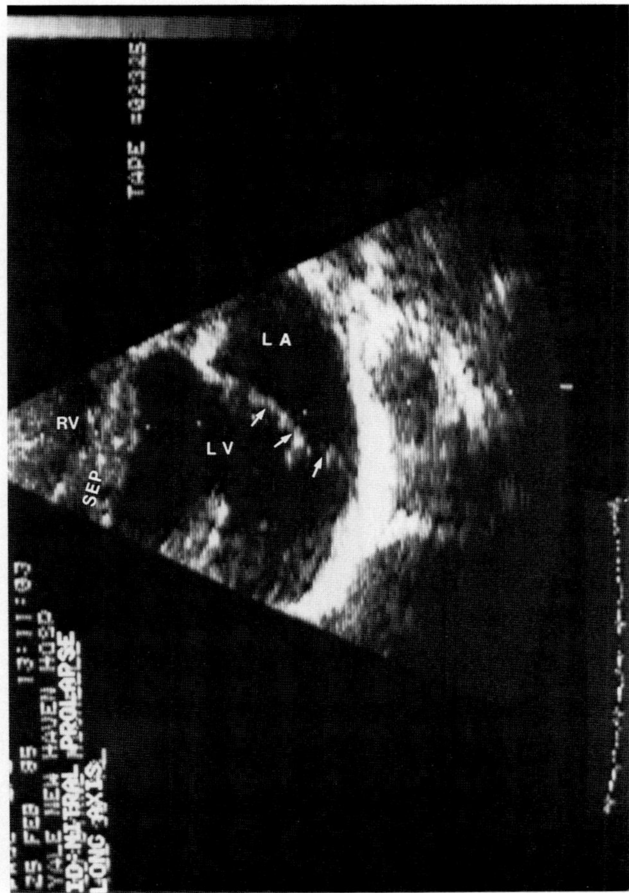

FIGURE 15.12   Mitral valve prolapse (arrows) occurs when the mitral valve extends beyond the plane of the cusps during systole (RV, right ventricle; SEP, septum; LV, left ventricle; LA, left atrium.) (Courtesy of Dr. C. Jaffe.)

Prosthetic Heart Valves

The degeneration of prosthetic heart valves or the accumulation of fibrin on the surface of the valve may be a source of cerebral emboli. Mechanical valves are more likely to deteriorate than tissue valves, although rates of thromboembolism depend upon the valve type and anticoagulation regimen. It is uncertain whether children require less intensive anticoagulation therapy than adults with similar valve models (40).

Mitral Valve Prolapse

Mitral valve prolapse (MVP) is defined as the protrusion of one or both mitral leaflets beyond the plane of the mitral annulus into the left atrium during systole (Figure 15.12). The prevalence of MVP is estimated at 5% to 10% of the population (41) with an overall risk of MVP-associated stroke estimated to be 1 in 6,000 patients in one study, although some of the patients had other risk factors (5). It

has also been associated with noninfective thromboembolism, an increased incidence of arrhythmias, mitral regurgitation, bacterial endocarditis, and sudden death (41). Although MVP may occur as an isolated defect, it may also be a component of heritable connective tissue disorders such as osteogenesis imperfecta, Ehlers Danlos syndrome, or Marfan syndrome (42).

Arrhythmia

Atrial fibrillation predisposes to stroke, because stasis of blood within the left atrium encourages the formation of thrombi. Embolism most commonly occurs shortly after onset of atrial fibrillation and may be recurrent. Sinoatrial dysfunction ("sick sinus syndrome") may be a source of both tachy- and bradyarrhythmias and is seen in children with rheumatic heart disease, myotonic dystrophy, and Friedreich ataxia. The development of intraventricular thrombi with subsequent embolization (Figure 15.13) can also occur in the setting of abnormal myocardial contractility or disorders of the septum (idiopathic hypertrophic subaortic stenosis or asymmetrical septal hypertrophy). Stressful emotional stimuli are thought to occasionally trigger paroxysmal familial ventricular fibrillation (25).

Paradoxical Cerebral Emboli

A paradoxical cerebral embolus crosses from the right to the left side of the heart through a patent foramen ovale or

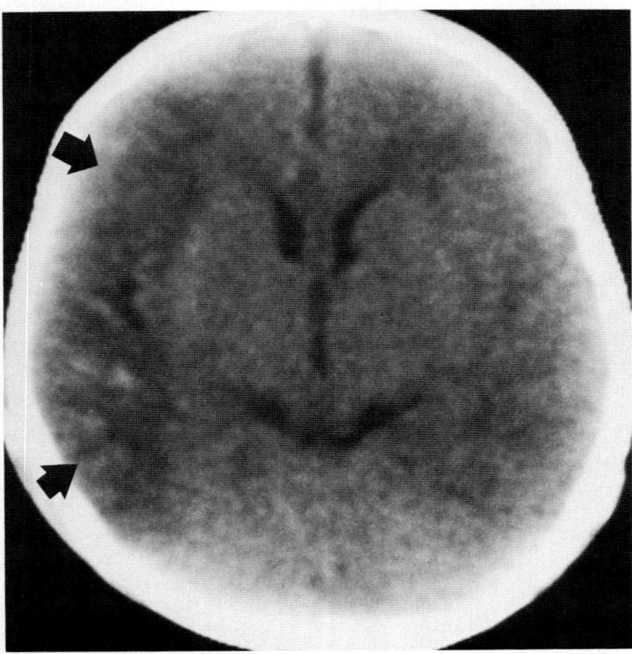

FIGURE 15.13   An infarct (arrow) in the territory of the right middle cerebral artery occurred in this child two hours following extracorporeal membrane oxygenation (ECMO) and was heralded by contralateral focal arm and leg seizures. (Courtesy of Dr. T.M. Voorhies.)

an occult atrial septal defect. Criteria for the diagnosis of paradoxical cerebral emboli include evidence for source of venous thrombosis; a pulmonary lesion causing acute increased right atrial pressure, such as pulmonary embolus; and an intracardiac defect permitting right to left shunt or pulmonary arteriovenous fistula (43).

The concomitant rise in right atrial pressure due to Valsalva maneuver can contribute to paradoxical cerebral emboli. The incidence of cerebral infarction due to paradoxical emboli is estimated at 4% (44). If routine M-mode and two-dimensional echocardiography are normal, contrast echocardiographic studies may be needed to rule out the potential for paradoxical cerebral embolism.

Cardiac Myxoma

Symptoms of myxomas are constitutional, obstructive, and embolic (45,46,47). Cerebral embolization is often the presenting problem in individuals with atrial myxoma. Emboli are found in the systemic circulation in 60% of children with atrial myxoma and in the cerebral circulation of 30% (Figure 15.14, 15.15). When situated in the left atrium, myxomas can obstruct cardiac outflow and cause

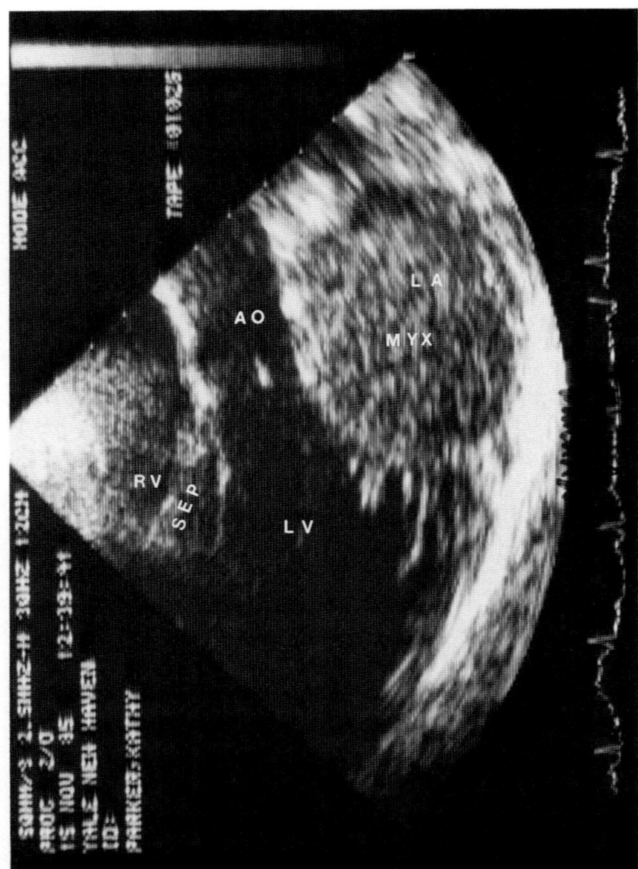

FIGURE 15.14 A myxoma occupies the left atrium (MYX, myxoma; LA, left atrium; LV, left ventricle; RV, right ventricle; S, septum.) (Courtesy of Dr. C. Jaffe.)

symptoms of heart failure, weakness, fatigue, weight loss, and syncope.

Approximately 20% of patients with familial cardiac myxomas have a genetic disorder inherited as an autosomal dominant trait (42). Myxomatous degeneration of the heart valves is particularly common in tuberous sclerosis. Magnetic resonance imaging (MRI) is a new diagnostic tool that may ultimately prove superior to echocardiography for establishing the diagnosis of atrial myxoma. Continued follow-up is essential in atrial myxoma because the lesions may reappear in 5% of patients. Myxomas that form intracerebral aneurysms can later cause subarachnoid hemorrhage. Myxomas can be surgically removed with low mortality rate and a low risk of delayed neurologic events (47).

Marantic Endocarditis

Patients with serious underlying diseases such as cancer or other systemic illnesses (48) can develop marantic endocarditis (nonbacterial thrombotic endocarditis). The malignancies which are most commonly associated with marantic endocarditis are mucin producing adenocarcinomas, although hematologic malignancies may also be involved. Trauma to the cardiac valves may be etiologically important. These verrucous growths (Figure 15.16) often embolize systemically and result in hematuria, skin necrosis, or peritonitis.

Fat Emboli

Fat embolism typically occurs after a fracture of a long bone or, less commonly, as a sequel of cardiopulmonary bypass or surgical lengthening of the femora (49). Following a 12 to 48 hour period free of symptoms, patients develop respiratory distress, fever, tachycardia, and neurologic dysfunction. Fat emboli lodge primarily in lungs or brain. Severe cases may progress to hypoxemia or hypotension (50).

Neonatal Cerebral Infarction

Barmada et al. (51) noted that 5.4% of 592 unselected infants had cerebral infarction at postmortem examination. The diagnosis is most readily confirmed by MRI; whereas, ultrasonography detected only 79% of lesions, and computed cerebral tomography (CT) less than one-half (52). The etiology of neonatal cerebral infarction may be multifactorial (53), and some neonatal cerebral infarctions occur in utero or are asymptomatic. For instance, contributory causes of cerebral infarction in neonates with meconium aspiration include hypoxemia, acidosis, or hyperviscosity.

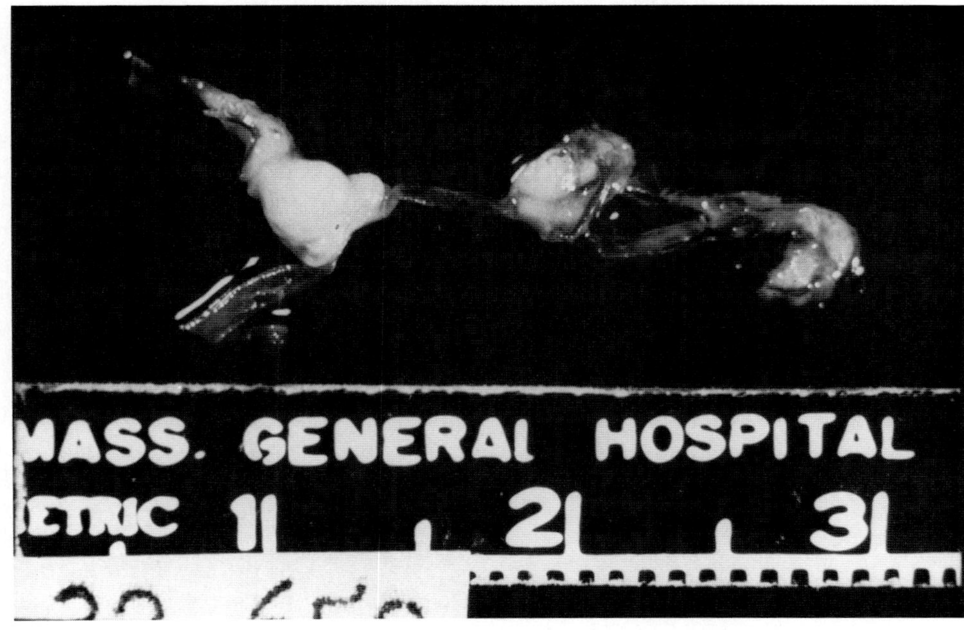

FIGURE 15.15 Myxomatous material which has embolized to the cerebral vessels.

Catheterization

Catheterization of either the umbilical artery or vein may result in cerebral embolization. Thrombotic complications in umbilical venous catheterization range from 3% to 33%. Emboli from thrombosed hepatic veins can migrate through the foramen ovale to the left middle cerebral artery (54). Temporal artery catheterization, a procedure now abandoned, may cause infarction in the middle cerebral artery territory, presumably from retrograde flow.

Polycythemia

Polycythemia occurs in 2% to 5% of all newborn infants and may produce cardiorespiratory, gastrointestinal, renal, and central nervous system signs. The mechanisms of thrombosis include decreased laminar flow and increased viscosity. With elevation of the hematocrit, viscosity increases substantially. Neurologic disorders associated with polycythemia include stroke, movement disorders, and developmental delay.

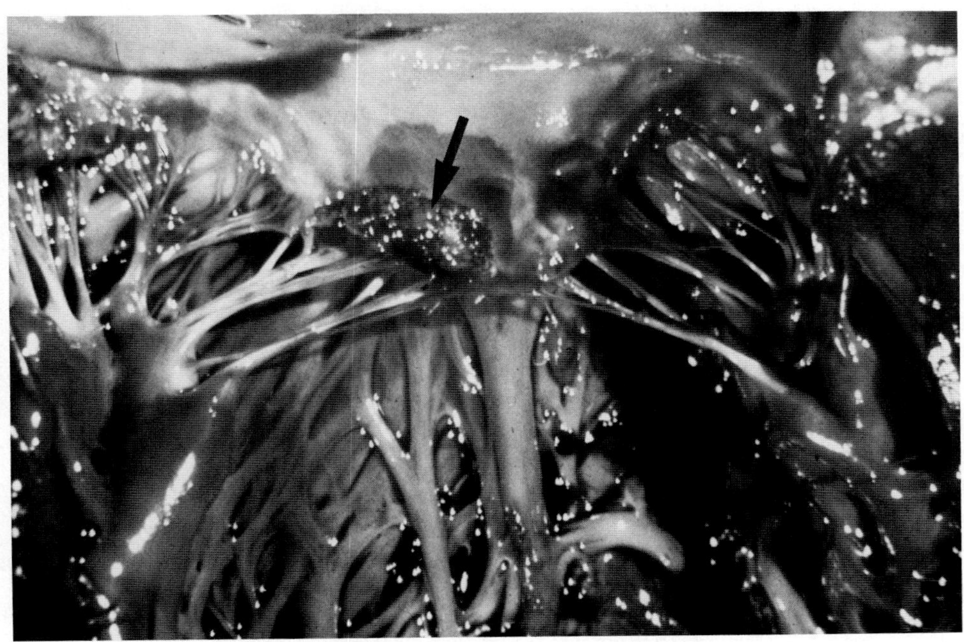

FIGURE 15.16 Verrucous material (arrow) is present on the heart valve of this child with marantic endocarditis (nonbacterial thrombotic endocarditis).

Extracorporeal Membrane Oxygenation

Extracorporeal Membrane Oxygenation (ECMO) has been used in some centers to oxygenate infants in whom conventional methods have failed. ECMO necessitates ligation of a major vessel, typically the carotid artery. Distal field cerebral infarction may result from hypotension or embolization (Figure 15.13). Cerebral infarction secondary to hypoxic-ischemic injury may antedate initiation of ECMO. Cerebral hemorrhage may result from increased CBF due to ligation of the contralateral carotid. Schumacher et al. noted that 8 of 59 survivors of neonatal ECMO suffered ipsilateral hemispheric injury (55).

DISORDERS OF THE BLOOD VESSELS

Arteriopathies

Arteriopathies which damage the luminal surface can predispose to cerebral infarction in a variety of ways including (Table 15.4): damage to the endothelium may form a surface for thrombus formation; nonlaminar blood flow may predispose to formation of thrombi; and abnormal proteins may predispose to thrombosis. Abnormalities of the vascular tree which was demonstrable by angiography include occlusions, luminal irregularities, beading, tortuosity, and evidence of collateralization.

Sickle Cell Disease

Sickle cell disease is a cause of both ischemic and hemorrhagic stroke (56–60) (Figures 15.17, 15.18). Symptomatic cerebral infarction occurs in 10% of children homozygous for the sickle gene (56), and asymptomatic cerebral infarction may be present in 25% of patients. Ischemic injuries most commonly occur in the distal branches of the internal carotid artery (57), and the area between the anterior and middle cerebral arteries constitutes a boundary or border

Table 15.4   Arteriopathies

Atherosclerosis
Hemoglobinopathies (Sickle cell disease)
Drug abuse
Collagen vascular disease (vasculitis)
Isolated angiitis of the central nervous system
Inflammatory bowel disease
Fibromuscular dysplasia
Homocystinuria
MELAS (mitochondrial encephalopathy, lactic acidosis, stroke)
Infections
Localized (mastoiditis, meningitis)
Generalized (meningitis, herpes zoster arteritis)
Trauma (oral, cervical)
Cancer (local malignancy), chemotherapy, radiation vasculopathy
Neurocutaneous disorders

zone ("watershed" infarction). Ischemic cerebrovascular disease occurs three times more frequently than cerebral hemorrhage. The mechanism of brain infarction in sickle cell disease may be due to log jamming of sickled cells. Alternatively, the rigid cells may injure the endothelium causing subintimal reactive fibrous proliferation (58); both large and small vessels may be injured by sickled cells.

Patients with sickle cell disease who are at risk for cerebral infarction should be hypertransfused to suppress erythropoiesis because strokes may recur in more than one-half of patients without a hypertransfusion regimen. It is recommended that the hemoglobin S level be maintained below 30%. Hypertransfusion is not risk free and over a prolonged period of time, poses the risk of iron overload. Angiography is not a reliable method of following arteriolar damage due to sickle cell disease. CBF may increase with transfusion therapy and then decrease as the hematocrit falls following cessation of transfusion therapy. In the nontransfused patient, CBF may be elevated in response to vasodilatation and chronic hypoxemia (59)(See Chapter 19).

Transient neurologic deficits have been reported in 5% of patients heterozygous for the sickle cell gene (60), although the incidence of cerebral arterial occlusion in

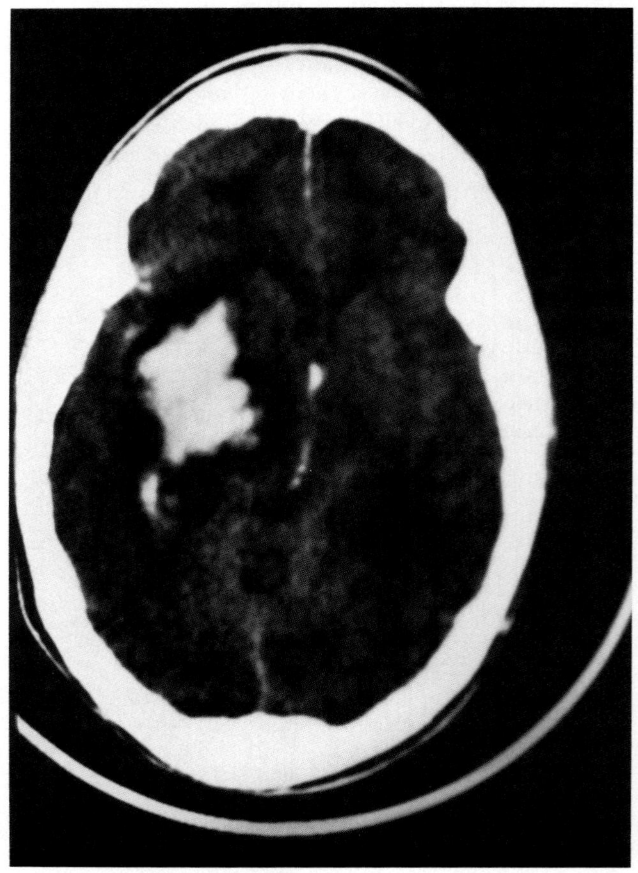

FIGURE 15.17   Fatal basal ganglial hemorrhage with ventricular extension occurred in this adolescent with sickle cell disease.

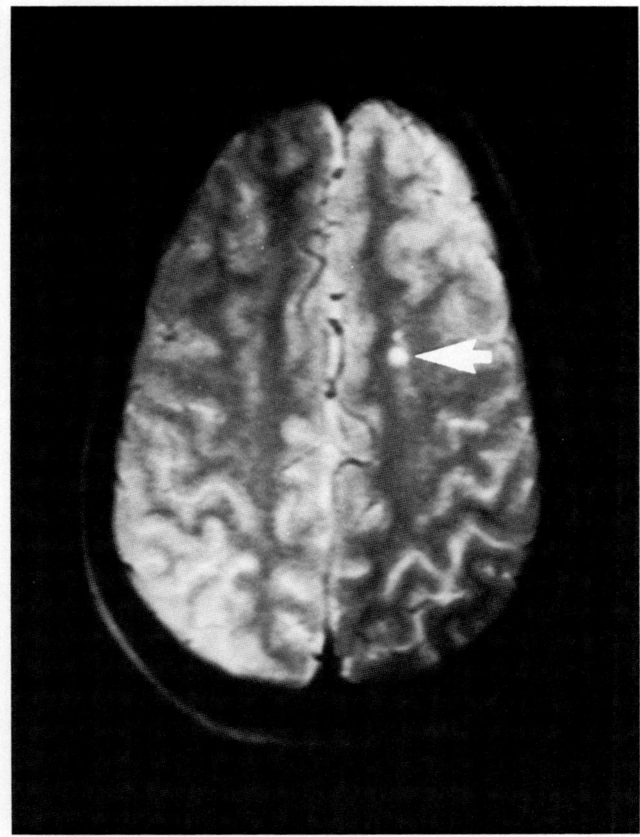

FIGURE 15.18 Magnetic resonance image showing an infarct (arrow) in the centrum semiovale of this patient with sickle cell disease. Small infarcts in the cerebral white matter may be asymptomatic. (Reprinted with permission of Dr. S.J. Pavlakis and Annals of Neurology.)

individuals with sickle cell trait is not increased compared to controls (sickle cell trait, 1.7%; African-American controls, 1.8%). Cerebral venous thromboses have been reported in patients with sickle cell trait (50). Sudden death due to hypoxemia and acidosis at high altitude is a rare event. Hemoglobin SC disease seldom produces stroke (42).

Homocystinuria and Fabry Disease

Several inborn errors of metabolism are associated with cerebrovascular disease. Homocystinuria, a disorder inherited as an autosomal recessive trait, is characterized by the inability to convert homocysteine to cystathione or to methionine (see Chapter 1). Patients with this disorder characteristically have a marfanoid habitus, cataracts, osteoporosis, mental retardation, and premature atherosclerosis (42). Although homocystinuria is an unusual cause of stroke in young patients, the frequency of heterozygosity is 1 in 70. Recent evidence suggests that heterozygosity may predispose to the development of premature occlusive arterial disease including peripheral vas-

cular disease, renovascular hypertension, and ischemic stroke (61).

Fabry disease (angiokeratoma corporis diffusum) is a sex-linked recessive disorder that may produce cerebrovascular disease, including stroke. Males with this disorder typically have pain in the extremities, corneal opacities, angiokeratomas of the skin, and chronic renal failure. Cerebrovascular complications of Fabry disease include multifocal small and large vessel involvement, aneurysm formation, and hypertensive hemorrhage (42).

Inflammatory Bowel Disease

Patients with inflammatory bowel disease may develop cerebral thromboembolic disease, but systemic thromboembolism is more common (62). The etiology of stroke in patients with inflammatory bowel disease has been ascribed to coagulation defects, increased levels of fibrinogen and factor V, and elevated platelet counts.

Systemic Lupus Erythematosus

Antiphospholipid autoantibodies in patients with systemic lupus erythematosus (SLE) are associated with focal cerebral and ocular ischemia (Figure 15.19) (63). The lupus anticoagulant, a circulating immunoglobulin in the IgG or IgM class, has been associated with thromboembolism in one fourth to one-half of patients who are anticoagulant positive. One-third of patients with lupus anticoagulants have SLE (64), while the remainder acquire the anticoagulant spontaneously or have some other systemic illness. Lupus anticoagulants seldom produce cerebral hemorrhage, except in the setting of thrombocytopenia or disseminated intravascular coagulopathy (DIC). Levine and Welch (63) reviewed 70 cases of focal cerebral ischemia associated with lupus anticoagulant. The majority were young women (mean age, 39 years), some of whom had symptoms remniscent of migraine.

Isolated angiitis of the central nervous system, a designation preferable to "granulomatous angiitis", is a fatal inflammatory disease that is characterized clinically by headaches and multifocal neurologic deficits. There is a predilection for small blood vessels (65). Unlike SLE, systemic symptoms and serologic evidence of inflammation (elevated ESR, ANA, rheumatoid factor, immune complexes) are absent. Treatment with prednisone and cyclophosphamide may induce prolonged remissions.

Mitochondrial Myopathy, Encephalopathy, Lactic Acidosis and Stroke

Mitochondrial myopathy, encephalopathy, lactic acidosis, and stroke (MELAS) is a syndrome that may be either familial or sporadic (66). The elevation of plasma lactate is indicative of a disorder of oxidative phosphorylation, but the biochemical abnormality can be variable. Infarcts cross

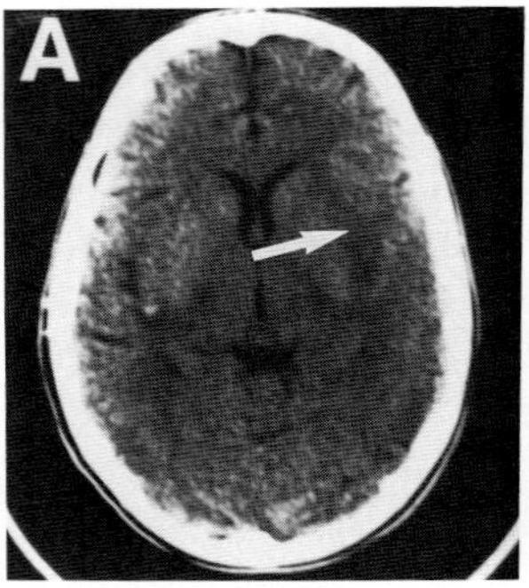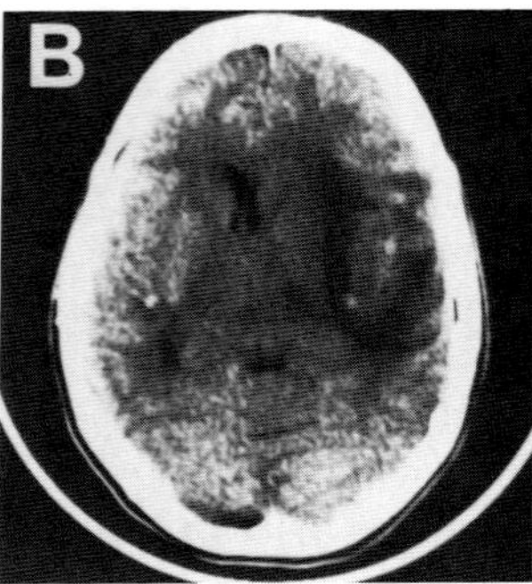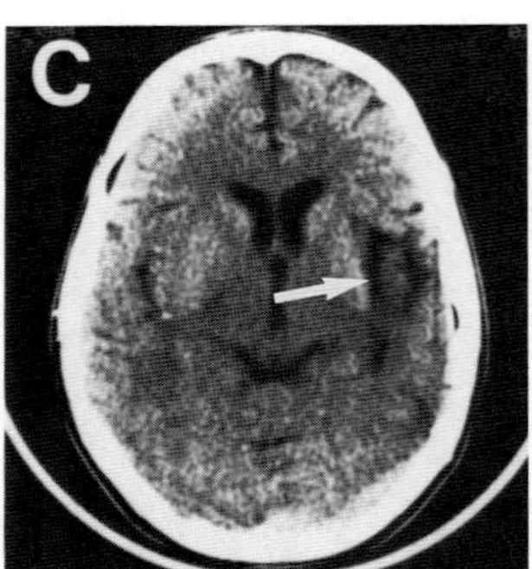

FIGURE 15.19   A: This adolescent with systemic lupus erythematosus had subacute onset of aphasia and right hemiplegia. The initial CT brain scan showed an area of low attenuation (arrow); **B:** There was subsequent development of cerebral edema and midline shift resulting in coma; **C:** CT scan during the recovery phase shows tissue loss (arrow) and mild ventricular asymmetry. After a prolonged period of rehabilitation, the patient's speech and gait returned to normal.

vascular territories and are more common in the parieto-occipital region. Matthews and associates recently reported a specific MRI finding on T2-weighted images consisting of multifocal areas of hyperintense signal confined to the cerebral and cerebellar cortex and subjacent white matter (67). The cause of cerebral infarction is uncertain. Pathologic examination discloses swollen capillary cells in the systemic circulation.

Fibromuscular Dysplasia

Fibromuscular dysplasia is a rare angiopathy of unknown cause. Small saccular dilatations due to destruction of the media develop in the small to medium sized cerebral arteries. The characteristic angiographic features are of multiple small arterial dilations ("string of beads") (68). Fibromuscular dysplasia occurs most commonly in children and young women and consists of episodes of transient ischemic attacks, intracranial hemorrhage, and cerebral infarction.

Arterial Dissections

Arterial dissections typically occur between the internal elastic lamina and media (subintimal dissection) producing the characteristic angiographic finding of a double lumen. Intracranial dissection aneurysms are unusual in childhood. The typical patient is male with a history of trauma, prodromal headache, and seizures. The treatment for arterial dissection has been disappointing, and anticoagulation, corticosteroids, or surgical decompression have not been of proven benefit. The majority of patients develop massive brain edema and herniation (69).

Traumatic Arterial Occlusions

Injuries to the neck are recognized as a known cause of cerebral arterial occlusions (Figure 15.20). Chiropractic manipulation of the spine, gymnastic exercises, yoga posi-

tions, and athletic injuries can damage the vertebral arteries which course through restrictive bony canals from C2 through the atlas to the foramen magnum. Possible mechanisms include stretching of the vessel, endothelial damage, and platelet aggregation. Traction injuries result in more damage than hyperextension and rotation injuries (70). Individuals with Klippel-Feil syndrome, odontoid aplasia (71), or other disorders of the vertebrae in the cervical region may also be predisposed toward infarction in the posterior circulation (Figure 15.21). Perforating trauma in the region of the soft palate may lead to thrombosis of the internal carotid artery (72).

Atherosclerosis

Atherosclerosis is an important cause of nonhemorrhagic stroke in as many as one fourth of children with stroke (5). Glueck and associates (73) noted that 10 of 11 children with unexplained ischemic cerebrovascular disease had abnormal levels of high density lipoproteins, cholesterol or triglycerides.

Children may develop stroke due to one of the inherited lipoprotein abnormalities (74). Nine of 11 patients with lipoprotein abnormalities developed premature coronary artery disease or suffered stroke. Decreased levels of high density lipoproteins may be associated with familial hypoalphalipoproteinemia and familial hypercholesterolemia, both of which are inherited as autosomal dominant traits. Patients with type IV hyperabetalipoproteinemia are also at risk for developing premature atherosclerosis and stroke.

Moyamoya Disease

Moyamoya disease is a condition in which the internal carotid artery becomes stenotic at its terminal bifurcation (74). The mechanism may involve a dysplastic process of the vessel wall; a true arteritis has not been documented. Collateral channels arise from the external carotid, the

Cerebral Venous Thrombosis

Thrombosis of the sagittal sinus or other cerebral veins occurs in a variety of disorders (Table 15.5) and is present in one percent of all routine autopsies (76). Possible mechanisms include hypercoagulability in the nephrotic syndrome (77), inflammation due to L-asparaginase, and mechanical occlusion from neuroblastoma (78). Neonates with congenital heart disease or polycythemia are at increased risk for developing sagittal sinus thrombosis.

Thrombosis of the sagittal sinus is often heralded by the presence of seizures, lethargy or coma, and increased intracranial pressure (Figure 15.22). The definitive diagnosis can be made by cerebral angiography, making certain that sufficient time is allowed to compensate for filling delay. Magnetic resonance imaging or digital subtraction angiography may aid in confirming the diagnosis. Treatment remains controversial. A definite beneficial effect of anticoagulation has not yet been demonstrated. Should raised intracranial pressure supervene, it may be necessary to initiate hyperventilation and osmotherapy.

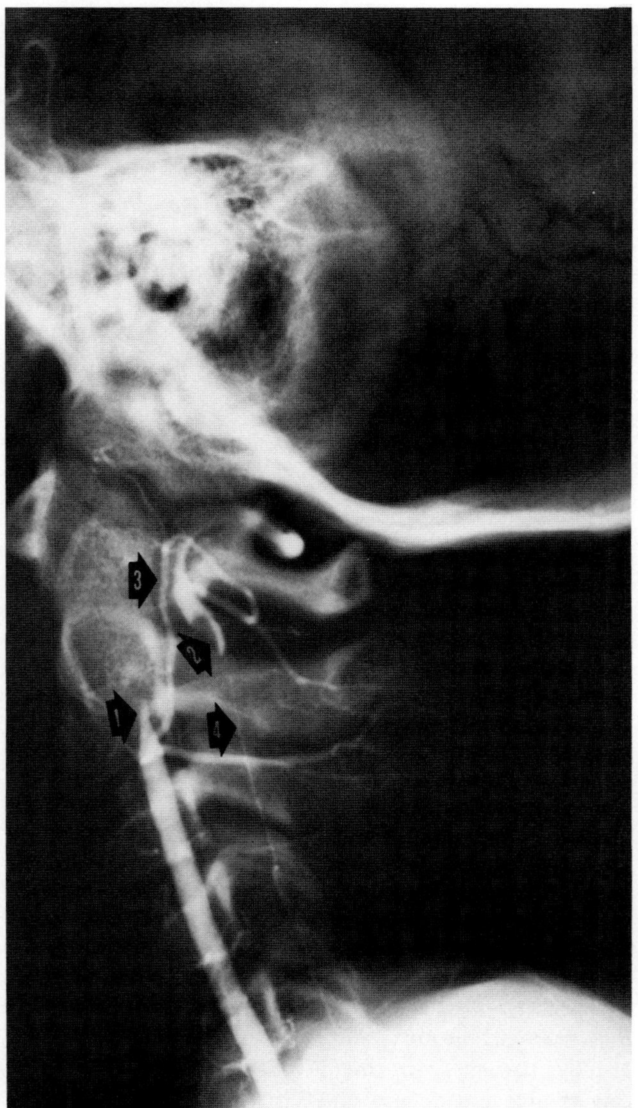

FIGURE 15.20 Following chiropractic manipulation, this child developed severe headache and left facial weakness, vomiting, diplopia, ataxia, and right hemiparesis. Selective left vertebral angiogram demonstrates: **1:** occlusion of left vertebral artery at level of C-2; **2:** distal vertebral artery with intraluminal thrombus; **3:** collateral vascular channel filling the distal vertebral artery; and **4:** anterior spinal artery. (Reprinted with permission of Dr. A. Zimmerman and Neurology.)

vertebral arteries, and from transdural anastamoses of the middle meningeal and superficial temporal arteries. The disease is frequently bilateral and typically affects children less than 15 years of age (75). The clinical manifestations of moyamoya disease include sudden hemiplegia and movement disorder; dementia and cerebral hemorrhage are less common. Treatment of stroke in individuals with moyamoya disease is supportive; however, a variety of vascular anastomatic procedures are being performed with some degree of success (75a).

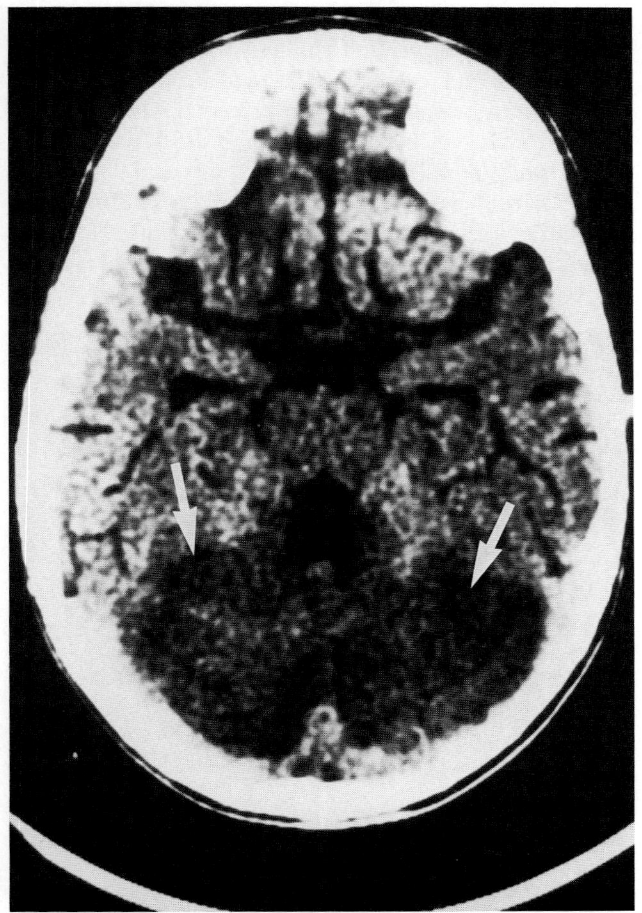

FIGURE 15.21 Bilateral cerebellar infarction (arrows) occurred in this child with abnormalities of the cervical spine.

Table 15.5   Causes of cerebral venous thrombosis

Cachexia
Coagulopathy
Oral contraceptives
Pregnancy
Puerperium
Dehydration
Congestive heart failure
Hemolytic anemia
Sickle cell disease
Cerebral arterial occlusions
Trauma
Neoplasm
Nephrotic syndrome with coagulopathy
Sepsis
Mastoiditis or other localized infection

Coagulopathies, Sepsis, and Meningitis

Sepsis and disseminated intravascular coagulopathy (DIC) may produce multiple acute or chronic lesions of the vessel walls, with formation of fibrin-platelet thrombi. In one study, 9 of 11 patients with sepsis had multiple small areas of necrosis surrounded by blocked small arteries and arterioles in multiple organs. A focal arteritis due to leptomeningitis may also lead to cerebral arterial thrombosis.

Patients with sepsis and children with cancer (78) may also have a high incidence of DIC and stroke. A procoagulant factor is postulated to be present in promyelocytic leukemic cells which is released upon cell lysis. Neonates may be predisposed to hypercoagulability and depletion of fibrinolysins due to the respiratory distress syndrome.

A variety of proteins and cofactors regulate the activity of the coagulation cascade by inhibiting activated factors V

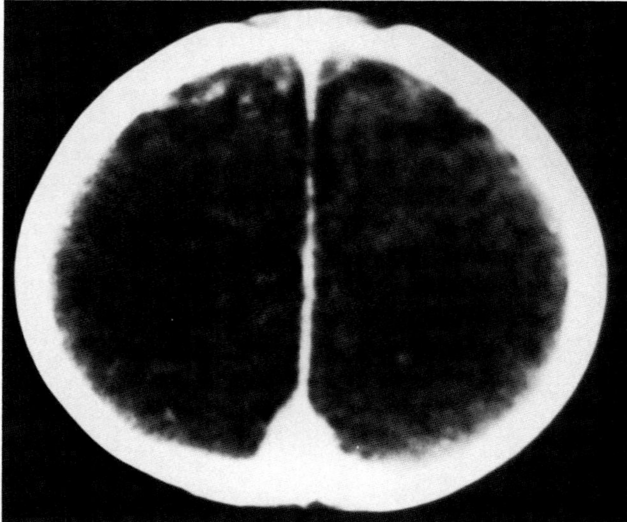

FIGURE 15.22 The radiographic features of sagittal sinus thrombosis are opacification of the sinus and the torcula on a non-contrast CT brain scan.

and VIII. Partial deficiency of protein C and protein S may cause recurrent thromboses in the cerebral or systemic circulations of neonates and young adults (79).

HEMORRHAGIC DISORDERS

Cerebral hemorrhage can occur as a result of coagulopathy (Factor VIII and IX deficiencies) or platelet abnormalities (idiopathic and isoimmune thrombocytopenic purpura) (80), as well as from aneurysms and arteriovenous malformations.

Cerebral Arteritis

Arteritis may develop in patients with a history of collagen vascular disease, intravenous drug abuse (81), or intracranial infections (82). Ulcerative colitis, systemic lupus erythematosis, polyarteritis, and rheumatoid arthritis are collagen vascular disorders that may cause arteritis and subsequent subarachnoid hemorrhage. One-third of patients with systemic lupus erythmatosus studied by Gonzalez-Scarano and associates had either intracerebral hemorrhage or cerebral infarction. Sulcal or generalized atrophy is present in the majority of patients with SLE and has been attributed to microinfarction (83).

Coarctation of the Aorta

Cerebral hemorrhage is a recognized complication of coarctation of the aorta and may occur in as many as 10% of older patients with this disorder (84). The mechanism may involve aneurysms of the Circle of Willis and the presence of systemic hypertension. The causal role of systemic hypertension in the production of cerebral hemorrhage is uncertain, but it is possible that during sudden hypertension, the upper limit of the autoregulatory plateau is exceeded.

Hypertension and Renal Disease

Sudden increase in arterial blood pressure due to sympathomimetic agents may cause CBF to break through the upper end of the autoregulatory plateau resulting in cerebral hemorrhage. Cocaine, methamphetamine, and amphetamine abuse have all been associated with intracerebral hemorrhage, and, less commonly, ischemic stroke (81). The etiology of stroke due to drug abuse may be related to injury of the vascular wall. Cerebral angiography may demonstrate occlusion of intracranial arteries or arterial beading.

Renal hypertension may also elevate arterial blood pressure, leading to cerebral hemorrhage. Subarachnoid hemorrhage may develop during an episode of acute poststreptococcal glomerulonephritis (85) because of hypertension or hemodynamic injury to the blood vessels. Other types of renal parenchymal disease may also predispose to subarachnoid hemorrhage, including polyarteritis nodosa, Henoch-Schönlein purpura, systemic lupus erythematosus, and Goodpasture syndrome.

Congenital Aneurysms

Aneurysms are deemed congenital if an acquired cause is ruled out and if developmental abnormalities of the vessel wall can be demonstrated. Ten percent of children with congenital aneurysms may have other malformations, such as coarctation of aorta and polycystic kidneys.

Aneurysms in children may be focal defects in vessel walls developing at sites where embryonic vessels or vascular buds developed but had failed to disappear normally (86). Aneurysms may also represent part of a more generalized disorder of the connective tissue such as Marfan disease or Ehlers-Danlos syndrome. The most common sites for the formation of aneurysms in children are the internal carotid (38%), anterior communicating, and middle cerebral arteries. Multiple aneurysms are present in 15% of patients. Congenital berry aneurysms may lack the media or internal elastic lamina.

The clinical course of aneurysms is often explosive with subarachnoid hemorrhage producing intense headache, vomiting, lethargy, or coma (Figure 15.3). Surgical clipping

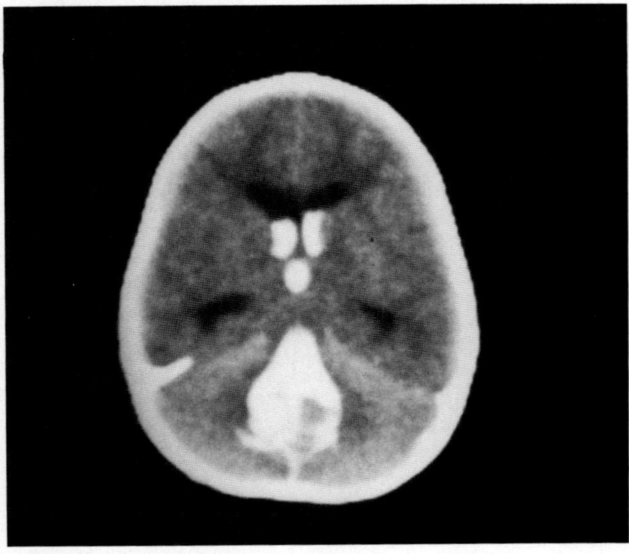

FIGURE 15.23 Fatal subarachnoid and intraventricular hemorrhage in this infant was due to rupture of a basilar artery aneurysm.

of aneurysms is associated with a mortality rate of approximately 5% and a morbidity of 10% (87). Surgery was not performed in some patients because they were moribund or because the aneurysm had disappeared at a second angiographic study. The prognosis is considerably better for patients with arteriovenous malformations.

Basilar artery aneurysms are rare in children. These aneurysms are typically saccular (Figure 15.23), but may be fusiform when due to arteriopathies (88). Examination of the basilar artery aneurysm in a child with alpha-glucosidase deficiency disclosed fibrous thickening and calcification of the intima, fragmentation and segmental loss of the internal elastic lamina, and marked vacuolation of the medial smooth muscle (89). Rarely, large aneurysms may exert mass effect and present as a progressive brain stem syndrome.

CARDIOVASCULAR MANIFESTATIONS OF SYSTEMIC DISORDERS

Tuberous Sclerosis

Cardiac rhabdomyomas may develop in patients with Tuberous Sclerosis (see Chapter 23); and subsequently, some of these myxomatous tumors embolize. Cerebrovascular segmental ectasia and distal branch occlusion may also occur (35).

Friedreich Syndrome

Cardiomyopathy develops in approximately one-half of patients with Friedreich ataxia, some of whom die from cardiac arrhythmia or congestive failure. A degeneration of the cardiac muscle fibers or of the conduction system is present.

Kearns-Sayre Syndrome

The triad of progressive external ophthalmoplegia, pigmentary degeneration of the retina, and juvenile onset constitute Kearns-Sayre syndrome. Heart block, cerebellar syndrome, and increased cerebrospinal protein concentration are frequently present. The disorder is sporadic. Blood lactate is elevated in this mitochondrial myopathy and a defect of coenzyme Q10 was reported in one patient (90).

THERAPY OF CEREBROVASCULAR DISEASE

Throughout this chapter, an emphasis is placed on the appropriate diagnostic and therapeutic measures to be taken for patients with cerebrovascular disease. Some therapies are of known benefit, such as anticoagulation for patients with cardiac valve replacement and hemodilution for neonates with hyperviscosity. In other disorders such as carotid artery dissection, sickle cell disease, and isolated angiitis, treatment is either unproven or associated with serious side effects.

Although there is no known treatment for acute cerebral infarction at the present time, a wave of research breaks upon the shoals of stroke. Tissue plasminogen activator (tPA) is currently being tested for its thrombolytic action on stroke (91). Antagonists to the n-methyl-d-aspartate subclass of glutamate receptors (92) ameliorate cerebral infarction in experimental animals (39).

Cerebrovascular disease is the third leading cause of death, and cardiovascular disease is the principal cause of death in adults in the United States. One of the most important preventive measures that can be taken to reduce the mortality from cerebro- and cardiovascular disease is to encourage the development of health-promoting habits in our young patients: abstinence from tobacco, limitation of dietary fat, and frequent, vigorous exercise.

REFERENCES

1. Rothner AD, Cruse RP. Cerebrovascular disease in children and adolescents. Int Pediatr 1987;2:124–128.
2. Solomon GE, Hilal SK, Gold AP, et al. Natural history of hemiplegia in children. Brain 1970;93:107–120.
3. DeVivo D, Holmes SJ, Dodge PR. Cerebrovascular diseases in the pediatric population. Ann Neurol 1977;2:261–262.
4. Schoenberg BS, Mellinger JF, Schoenberg DG. Cerebrovascular disease in infants and children: A study of incidence, clinical features, and survival. Neurology 1978;28:763–768.
5. Adams HJ, Butler MJ, Biller J, et al. Nonhemorrhagic cerebral infarction in young adults. Arch Neurol 1986; 43:793–796.
6. Sonesson S, Winberg P, Lundell B. Early postnatal changes in intracranial arterial blood flow velocities in term infants. Pediatr Res 1987;22:461–464.
7. Ment LR, Duncan CC, Ehrenkranz RA. Perinatal cerebral infarction. Semin Perinatol 1987;11:142–154.
8. Younkin DP, Reivich M, Jaggi JL, et al. The effect of hematocrit and systolic blood pressure on cerebral blood flow in newborn infants. J Cereb Blood Flow Metab 1987;7:295–299.
9. Altman DI, Powers WJ, Perlman JM, et al. Cerebral blood flow requirement for brain viability in newborn infants is lower than in adults. Ann Neurol 1988;24:218–226.
10. Kennedy C, Sokoloff L. An adaptation of the nitrous oxide method to the study of the cerebral circulation in children; normal values for cerebral blood flow and cerebral metabolic rate in childhood. J Clin Invest 1957;36:1130–1137.
11. Daven JR, Milstein JM, Guthrie RD. Cerebral vascular resistance in premature infants. Am J Dis Child 1983;137:328–331.
12. Volpe JJ. Neurology of the Newborn. Philadelphia: WB Saunders, 1987;119–123.
13. Lou HC, Lassen NA, Friis-Hansen B. Impaired autoregulation of cerebral blood flow in the distressed human newborn infant. J Pediatr 1979;94:118–121.
14. Hernandez MJ, Brennan RW, Bowman GS. Autoregulation of CBF in the newborn dog. Brain Res 1980;184:199–202.
15. Young RSK, Hernandez MJ, Yagel SK. The selective reduction of cerebral blood flow of white matter during severe hypotension in newborn dogs: A possible mechanism of periventricular leukomalacia. Ann Neurol 1982;12:445–458.
16. Young RSK, Cowan BE, Petroff OAC, et al. In vivo ^{31}P and in vitro ^{1}H nuclear magnetic resonance study of hypoglycemia during neonatal seizure. Ann Neurol 1987;22:357–361.
17. Anwar M, Vesta F, Koons A, et al. Changes in regional cerebral blood flow in response to hypoglycemia in newborn dogs. Pediatr Res 1987;21:460A.
18. Ruckman RN. Cardiac causes of syncope. Pediatr Rev 1987;9:101–108.
19. Camfield PR, Camfield CS. Syncope in childhood: A controlled study of the familial tendency to faint. Ann Neurol 1987;22:419.
20. Thilenius OG, Quinones JA, Husayni TS, et al. Tilt test for diagnosis of unexplained syncope in pediatric patients. Pediatrics 1991;87:334–338.
21. Stephenson JBP. Reflex anoxic seizures ("white breath-holding"): Nonepileptic vagal attacks. Arch Dis Child 1978;53:193–200.
22. Fouad FM, Maloney JD. Orthostatic hypotension: Circulatory dynamics and clinical spectrum. In: Furlan AJ, ed. The Heart and Stroke. New York: Springer-Verlag, 1987;235–248.
23. Levine SR, Patel VM, Welch KMA, et al. Are heart attacks really brain attacks? In: Furlan AJ, ed. The Heart and Stroke. New York: Springer-Verlag, 1987;185–216.
24. Thiene G, Nava A, Corrado D, et al. Right ventricular cardiomyopathy and sudden death in young people. New Engl J Med 1988;318:129–133.
25. McRae JR, Wagner GS, Rogers MC, et al. Paroxysmal familial ventricular fibrillation. J Pediatr 1974;84:515–518.
26. MacDonald JT, Brown DR. Acute hemiparesis in juvenile insulin-dependent diabetes mellitus. Neurology 1979;29:893–896.
27. Young RSK, Rannels DE, Hilmo A, et al. Severe anemia in childhood presenting as transient ischemic attacks. Stroke 1983;13:491–494.
28. Andersen AR, Friberg L, Olsen T, et al. Delayed hyperemia following hypoperfusion in classic migraine. Arch Neurol 1988;45:154–159.
29. Henrich JB, Horwitz RI. A controlled study of ischemic stroke risk in migraine patients. J Clin Epidemiol 1989;42:773–780.
30. Broderick JP, Swanson JW. Migraine-related strokes. Arch Neurol 1987;44:868–871.
31. Bogousslavsky J, Regli F, Van Melle G, et al. Migraine stroke. Neurology 1988;38:223–227.
32. Hamilton PA, Hope PL, Cady EB, et al. Impaired energy metabolism in brains of newborn infants with increased cerebral echodensities. Lancet 1986;1:1242–1246.
33. Young RSK, Zalneraitis EL, Dooling EC: Neurologic outcome in cold water near drowning. JAMA 1980;244(I):1233–1235.

34. Stevenson JG, Stone EF, Dillard DH, et al. Intellectual development of children subjected to prolonged circulatory arrest during hypothermic open heart surgery in infancy. Circulation 1974;50:54–59.

35. Easton JD, Sherman DG. Management of cerebral embolism of cardiac origin. Stroke 1980;11:433–441.

36. Kanter MC, Hart RG. Neurologic complications of infective endocarditis. Neurology 1991;41:1015–1020.

37. Nelson RJ, Harley DP, French WJ, et al. Favorable ten-year experience with valve procedures for active infective endocarditis. J Thorac Cardiovasc Surg 1984;87:493–502.

38. Kurlan R, Griggs RC. Cyanotic congenital heart disease with suspected stroke. Arch Neurol 1983;40:209–212.

39. Salgado ED, Furlan AJ, Conomy JP. Cardioembolic sources of stroke. In: Furlan AJ, ed. The Heart and Stroke. New York: Springer-Verlag, 1987;47–62.

40. Hart RG. Prevention and treatment of cardioembolic stroke. In: Furlan AJ, ed. The Heart and Stroke. New York: Springer-Verlag, 1987;117–138.

41. Barnett HJM, Boughner DR, Taylor DW, et al. Further evidence relating mitral valve prolapse to cerebral ischemic events. N Engl J Med 1980;302:139–144.

42. Natowicz M, Kelley RI. Mendelian etiologies of stroke. Ann Neurol 1987;22:175–192.

43. Jones HR, Caplan LR, Come PC, et al. Cerebral emboli of paradoxical origin. Ann Neurol 1983;13:314–319.

44. Biller J, Johnson MR, Adams HP, et al. Echocardiographic evaluation of young adults with nonhemorrhagic cerebral infarction. Stroke 1986;17:608–612.

45. Bobo H, Evans OB. Intracranial aneurysms in a child with recurrent atrial myxoma. Pediatr Neurol 1987;3:230–232.

46. St. John Sutton MG, Mercier L, Giuliani ER, et al. Atrial myxomas. Mayo Clin Proc 1980;55:371–376.

47. Knepper LE. Biller J, Adams HP, et al. Neurologic manifestations of atrial myxoma. Stroke 1988;19:1435–1440.

48. Young RSK, Zalneraitis EL. Marantic endocarditis in children and young adults. Stroke 1981;12:635–639.

49. Ganel A, Israeli A, Horoszowski H. Fatal complications of femoral elongation in an achondroplastic dwarf. Clin Orthop 1984;185:69–71.

50. Kamenar E, Burger PC. Cerebral fat embolism: A neuropathological study of a microembolic state. Stroke 1980;11:477–485.

51. Barmada MA, Moossy J, Shuman RM. Cerebral infarcts with arterial occlusion in neonates. Ann Neurol 1979;6:495–502.

52. Keeney SE, Adcock EW, McArdle CB. Prospective observations of 100 high-risk neonates by high-field (1.5 Tesla) magnetic resonance imaging of the central nervous system. II. Lesions associated with hypoxic-ischemic encephalopathy. Pediatrics 1991;87:431–438.

53. Clancy R, Malin S, Laraque D, et al. Focal motor seizures hearlding stroke in full-term neonates. Am J Dis Child. 1985;139:601–606.

54. Ruff RL, Shaw CM, Beckwith JB, et al. Cerebral infarction complicating umbilical vein catheterization. Ann Neurol 1979;6:85.

55. Schumacher RE, Barks JDE, Johnston MV, et al. Right sided brain lesions in infants following extracorporeal membrane oxygenation: Neurodevelopmental outcome at 1 year of age. Pediatrics 1989;83:72–78.

56. Scott RB. Advances in the treatment of sickle cell disease in children. Am J Dis Child 1985;1219–1222.

57. Rothman SM, Fulling KH, Nelson JS. Sickle cell anemia and central nervous system infarction: A neuropathological study. Ann Neurol 1986;20:683–690.

58. Rao C, Kozlowski PB, Brown A, et al. Neuropathological findings in sickle cell anemia. Ann Neurol 1986;20:432.

59. Prohovnik I, Pavlakis S, DeVivo D, et al. Sickle cell disease, cerebral hyperemia, and stroke. Ann neurol 1986;20:432.

60. Feldenzer JA, Bueche MJ, Venes JL, et al. Superior sagittal sinus thrombosis with infarction in sickle cell trait. Stroke 1987;18:656–660.

61. Boers GH, Smals AG, Trijbels FJ, et al. Heterozygosity for homocystinuria in premature peripheral and cerebral occlusive arterial disease. N Engl J Med 1985;313:709–715.

62. Mayeux R, Fahn S. Strokes and ulcerative colitis. Neurology 1978;28:571–574.

63. Levine SR, Welch KMA. The spectrum of neurologic disease associated with antiphospholipid antibodies. Arch Neurol 1987;44:876–883.

64. Grotta JC, Current medical and surgical therapy for cerebrovascular disease. N Engl J Med 1987;317:1505–1516.

65. Moore PM. Diagnosis and management of isolated angiitis of the central nervous system. Neurology 1989;39:167–173.

66. DiMauro S, Bonilla E, Zeviani M, et al. Mitochondrial myopathies. Ann Neurol 1985;17:521–538.

67. Matthews PM, Tampieri D, Berkovic SF, et al. Magnetic resonance imaging shows specific abnormalities in the MELAS syndrome. Neurology 1991;41:1043–1046.

68. Pappada G, Panzarasa G, Sani R, et al. Intracranial fibromuscular dysplasia. J Neurosurg Sci 1987;31:13–18.

69. Nass R, Hays A, Chutorian A. Intracranial dissecting aneurysms of childhood. Stroke 1983;13:204–207.

70. Zimmerman AW, Kumar AJ, Gadoth N, et al. Traumatic vertebobasilar occlusive disease in childhood. Neurology 1978;28:185–188.

71. Phillips PC, Lorentsen KJ, Shropshire LC, et al. Congenital odontoid aplasia and posterior circulation stroke in childhood. Ann Neurol 1988;23:410–413.

72. Fritsch G. Acute infantile hemiplegia caused by cerebral ischemic infarction. Padiatr Padol 1984;19:287–301.

73. Gleuck CJ, Daniels SR, Bates S, et al. Pediatric victims of unexplained stroke and their families: familial lipid and lipoprotein abnormalities. Pediatrics 1982;69:308–316.

74. Bruno A, Yuh WTC, Biller J, et al. Magnetic resonance imaging in young adults with cerebral infarction due to Moyamoya. Arch Neurol 1988;45:303–306.

75. Suzuki J, Kodama N. Moyamoya disease—A review. Stroke 1983;14:104–109.

75a. Hoffman HJ, Griebel RW. Moyamoya syndrome in children. In: Edwards MSB, Hoffman HJ, eds. Cerebral vascular disease in children and adolescents. Baltimore: Williams and Wilkins, 1989;229–237.

76. Averback P. Primary cerebral venous thrombosis in young adults: The diverse manifestations of an underrecognized disease. Ann Neurol 1978;3:81–86.

77. Lau SO, Bock GH, Edson JR, et al. Sagittal sinus thrombosis in the nephrotic syndrome. J Pediatr 1980;97:948–950.

78. Packer RJ, Rorke LB, Lange BJ, et al. Cerebrovascular accidents in children with cancer. Pediatrics 1985;76:194–201.

79. Israels SJ, Seshia SS. Childhood stroke associated with protein C or S deficiency. J Pediatr 1987;111:562–564.

80. Zalneraitis EL, Young RSK, Krishnamoorthy KS: Intracranial hemorrhage in utero as a complication of isoimmune thrombocytopenia. J Pediatr 1979;90:611–613.

81. Rothrock JF, Rubenstein R, Lyden PD. Ischemic stroke associated with methamphetamine inhalation. Neurology 1988; 38:589–592.

82. Edwards KR. Hemorrhagic complications of cerebral arteritis. Arch Neurol 1977;34:549–552.

83. Kaell AT, Shetty M, Lee BCP, et al. The diversity of neurologic events in systemic lupus erythematosus. Arch Neurol 1986;43:273–276.

84. Young RSK, Liberthson RR, Zalneraitis EL: Cerebral hemorrhage in neonates with coarctation of the aorta. Stroke 1983; 13:491–494.

85. DeBeukelaer MM, Young GF. Subarachnoid hemorrhage complicating acute poststreptococcal glomerulonephritis. Arch Neurol 1978;35:473–474.

86. Keren G, Barzilay Z, Cohen BE. Ruptured intracranial arterial aneurysm in the first year of life. Arch Neurol 1980; 37:392–393.

87. Pasqualin A, Mazza C, Cavazzani P, et al. Intracranial aneurysms and subarachnoid hemorrhage in children and adolescents. Childs Nerv Syst 1986;2:185–190.

88. Read D, Esiri MM. Fusiform basilar artery aneurysm in a child. Neurology 1979;29:1045–1049.

89. Makos MM, McComb RD, Hart MN, et al. Alpha-glucosidase deficiency and basilar artery aneurysm. Ann Neurol 1987;22:629–633.

90. Pavlakis SG, Rowland LP, DeVivo DC, et al. Mitochondrial myopathies and encephalomyopathies. In: Plum F, ed. Advances in Contemporary Neurology. Philadelphia: FA Davis Co., 1988;95–133.

91. Grotta JC. Current medical and surgical therapy for cerebrovascular disease. N Engl J Med 1987;17:1505–1516.

92. Young RSK, Petroff OAC, Aquila WJ, et al. Effects of glutamate, quisqualate, and n-methyl-d-aspartate in neonatal brain. Exper Neurol 1991;111:362–368.

93. Zivin JA, Choi DW. Stroke Therapy. Sci Am 1991;265: 56–63.

Chapter 16
Disorders of the Respiratory System

Francis J. DiMario, Jr. and Donald Younkin

NEUROLOGIC CONTROL OF RESPIRATION

Respiration facilitates the supply of oxygen (O_2) and the elimination of carbon dioxide (CO_2). To accomplish this, there is a gas reservoir (lung), a passive gas exchanger (alveolus), a pump (rib cage, respiratory muscles), and a control mechanism (peripheral receptors, central respiratory centers). The control mechanism is capable of sensing the need for O_2 and CO_2 and adjusting the reservoir and pump to maintain arterial O_2 (P_aO_2) and CO_2 (P_aCO_2) in the most efficient manner (1,2).

The peripheral receptor system is comprised of arterial chemoreceptors in the carotid and aortic bodies, mechanoreceptors in the upper airways, and intrapulmonary receptors (3–6). The carotid bodies are located at the carotid bifurcation; the aortic bodies in the anterior and posterior portion of the ascending aorta. The peripheral chemoreceptors mediate increasing respiratory drive in response to decreasing P_aO_2, increasing P_aCO_2 or increasing arterial pH (pH_a). Peripheral receptors have a variable response to decreasing P_aO_2. There is a progressive increase in chemoreceptor activity as P_aO_2 falls below 500 mm Hg; a rapid increase from 100 mm Hg to 30 mm Hg; and an inability to sustain firing when P_aO_2 falls below 30 mm Hg. In contrast, peripheral chemoreceptors have a linear res-

ponse to increases in P_aO_2 from 20 to 60 mm Hg, and in pH_a from 7.2 to 7.7. Increased chemoreceptor activity due to changes in P_aO_2 is potentiated by simultaneous changes in P_aCO_2 or pH_a. Chemoreceptor activity also increases when blood flow in the aortic and carotid bodies decreases during hypotension or sympathetic activity (vasoconstriction).

The carotid chemoreceptor afferents travel in the carotid sinus nerve to join the glossopharyngeal nerve and terminate in the region of the nucleus tractus solitarius. Activation of the chemoreceptors causes activation in numerous structures in the lower brainstem, including the nucleus tractus solitarius, dorsal and lateral reticular formation, paramedian nucleus, and the dorsal and ventral respiratory groups (6–8). It is likely that the afferent fibers terminate on small interneurons that control respiration via a central pattern generator. These interneurons are probably located in the medial portion of the nucleus tractus solitarius.

The activity in the peripheral chemoreceptors is controlled by neurotransmitters. The afferent nerve terminals act directly as chemoreceptors and when stimulated, the afferent nerve terminals release excitatory neurotransmitters. In turn, the excitatory neurotransmitters stimulate the globus cells, causing the release of dopamine, which inhibits impulse generation in the afferent nerve terminals (9,10).

In addition to the peripheral chemoreceptors, there are central chemoreceptors located near the surface of the ventrolateral medulla. The central receptors respond to changes in extracellular fluid PCO_2 and pH, but are not affected by changes in PO_2.

Mechanoreceptors are located throughout the upper airways (5,11–14). The afferent fibers from these receptors travel to the medulla via the trigeminal nerve (nasal mucosa), pharyngeal branch of the glossopharyngeal nerve (pharynx), superior laryngeal nerve (larynx) and the vagus (trachea). Stimulation of these mechanoreceptors causes sneezing, coughing, or apnea; moreover, there are secondary cardiovascular effects including hypertension and bradycardia.

There are three types of intrapulmonary receptors that project to the caudal medulla via the vagus nerve (5). These receptors monitor the resistance of the airways and compliance of the lung and chest wall. Pulmonary stretch receptors are located in airway smooth muscle, and lung distention causes activation of the stretch receptors, resulting in prolonged expiration time and slowed respiratory rate (Hering-Breuer reflex) (14). "J" receptors located in the pulmonary capillary wall monitor interstitial fluid volume and pulmonary congestion. Irritant receptors in airway epithelial cells are excited by chemical and particulate irritants. In some individuals with asthma, stimulation of irritant receptors by histamine may activate respiratory centers in the medulla and, in turn, cause bronchospasm; therefore, the central nervous system (CNS) may be causally involved in some asthmatic patients.

The peripheral receptors relay information to the central controller, located in the lower brain stem and upper cervical spinal cord. Within the pons and medulla there are several distinct respiratory centers (7,14–16); in this context, however, the term *center* does not refer to a circumscribed collection of neurons, but rather to a region associated with a specific function (7,15,16).

The pneumotaxic center (PNC) is located in the dorsolateral portion of the rostral pons. Transection of the brainstem rostral to the PNC does not alter the breathing pattern. Isolation of the PNC from the brainstem results in slow deep breathing with prolonged inspiration (apneusis) (17–19). Electrophysiologic recordings have identified 3 different units in the PNC: one discharges slowly during inspiration, another during expiration, and a 3rd in a phase spanning manner. Although the PNC was originally believed to be the primary respiratory rhythm generator, it is more likely that the PNC sets threshold levels for inputs to the CNS from peripheral receptor systems; once these threshold levels are reached, inspiration is terminated or expiration prolonged.

Destruction of the PNC results in apneustic breathing (2 to 3 second pause at the end of inspiration, often associated with end-expiratory pauses and other irregularities of the respiratory rhythm). In humans, apneustic breathing is usually associated with extensive brainstem injury, most commonly pontine infarction secondary to basilar artery occlusion (17–19). Apneustic breathing is rarely associated with transtentorial herniation, which tends to involve medial structures, thus sparing the PNC.

The apneustic center (APC) has not been associated with any specific group of neurons. It lies in the region of the striae acousticae at the pontomedullary border and must remain in continuity with more caudal structures for apneusis to be observed. Although it is clear that apneusis occurs in humans and animals, the exact role of the APC in normal respiration has not been defined. One possibility is that the APC is the site of the normal inspiratory cut-off switch.

Within the medulla there are 2 compact groups of respiratory neurons. In the dorsal medulla, close to the obex and associated with the ventrolateral nucleus of the tractus solitarius is the dorsal respiratory group (DRG). In the ventral medulla, in the rostral nucleus ambiguus and the caudal aspect of the nucleus retroambigualis, is the ventral respiratory group (VRG).

The DRG is predominantly composed of inspiratory neurons and subserves several vital functions. DRG neurons project to the contralateral spinal cord and probably serve as the principal input to the phrenic motor neurons. DRG neurons are also second-order neurons in several respiratory reflexes, including the Hering-Breuer reflex, and as such, the DRG has a primary role in viscerosensory respiratory motor acts. DRG neurons project to the VRG, but they do not receive input from the VRG. Respiratory phase switching and possibly the primary respiratory pattern generation may reside in the DRG.

The 2 nuclei that make up the VRG contain inspiratory and expiratory neurons. The respiratory cells in the nucleus ambiguous are primarily cranial motor neurons. They receive input from the DRG and innervate the laryngeal muscles and accessory muscles of respiration. Cells in the nucleus retroambigualis drive expiratory intercostal and abdominal motor neurons and may inhibit inspiratory intercostal motor neurons (20–27).

The medulla probably contains the neurons responsible for yawning, but they have not been identified or definitely localized. Yawning may help to maintain lung compliance, but its primary function is not known.

Pathologic lesions in the medulla characteristically produce ataxic breathing—an irregular pattern with deep and shallow breaths, irregular pauses, and slow respiratory rate (17,18). In ataxic breathing, there is usually progressive slowing of the respiratory rate, leading to apnea. In compressive lesions of the medulla, respiration fails before circulation.

Although breathing does not require input from structures above the pons, these structures obviously influence respiration, and such fundamental acts as speaking or voluntary breath holding require higher cortical input. The forebrain, especially the limbic system, appears to inhibit respiration, and apnea has been recorded as an ictal event

(28). Pathologic lesions involving the hemispheres can cause posthyperventilation apnea. Lesions that are deep in both hemispheres or involving the diencephalon cause Cheyne-Stokes respirations (hypernea alternating with apnea) (17,18). In cats, electrical stimulation of the mesencephalon causes hyperventilation, and increasing the temperature of the anterior hypothalamus results in panting. Lesions of the rostral brainstem tegmentum can cause central neurogenic hyperventilation (increased P_aO_2, increased pH_a, decreased P_aCO_2), but this is rarely seen in humans. Instead, most cases of primary hyperventilation are caused by pulmonary congestion with secondary stimulation of lung receptors and are not related to destructive CNS lesions (24,29,30). The cerebellum can also exert an inhibitory influence on respiration, but it is not known whether this is caused by projections to the pontomedullary complex or to segmental levels.

Efferent fibers from the cortex and pontomedullary complex descend in separate pathways to the phrenic, intercostal, and abdominal motor neurons of respiration. Descending cortical fibers travel in the lateral corticospinal or corticorubrospinal tracts; involuntary or rhythmic respiration fibers are located in the ventrolateral cord. Diminished rhythmic ventilation can occur following high cervical anterolateral cordotomies, and selective loss of voluntary respiration has been reported following partial cervical transverse myelitis (17–19).

The integration of descending input and local spinal reflexes occurs at a segmental level, and as expected, inspiratory neurons are inhibited during expiration, and expiratory neurons inhibited during inspiration. This inhibition is not via a typical spinal reflex mechanism, however. Instead, there is active supraspinal inhibition of antagonist muscles during agonist contraction.

The phrenic nerve is formed by rootlets that arise in motor neurons in the ventral horn of C_3, C_4, and C_5. Intercostal motor neurons extend throughout the thoracic cord and innervate external (inspiratory) and internal (expiratory) intercostal muscles. Abdominal respiratory muscles are expiratory muscles, and their innervation is similar to that of the internal intercostal muscles.

DEVELOPMENT OF RESPIRATORY CONTROL IN THE FETUS AND NEWBORN

The development of respiratory control in the fetus and newborn has been extensively investigated in the past few years (29–38). The obvious difference between respiration in the fetus and newborn or adult is that fetal respiration is not required for gas exchange. Fetal respiration begins during early gestation, is intermittent, and correlates best with the behavioral state. During wakefulness and active sleep, there is sustained respiratory effort; during quiet sleep, there is apnea. It is likely that fetal respiration facilitates neuronal integration and strengthens respiratory muscles for continuous function after birth.

Although there is minimal correlation between fetal respiration and P_aO_2 or P_aCO_2, the fetal peripheral and central chemoreceptors are readily excited by physiologic changes in P_aO_2 or P_aCO_2 (7,33–39). It is not known why changes in fetal arterial blood gases do not have a greater effect on fetal respiratory patterns, but most investigators postulate that there is a central inhibitory mechanism that blocks brainstem respiratory centers, preventing fetal respirations from increasing during fetal hypoxemia or hypercapnia.

In addition to diminished respiratory responses to changes in fetal blood gases, the fetus and newborn have a different pattern of response, especially to hypoxemia (40,41). Acute reduction of fetal P_aO_2 causes a biphasic change in fetal respiration. Initially, there is increased peripheral chemoreceptor activity and increased minute ventilation; within 1 to 2 minutes, however, minute ventilation decreases despite continued chemoreceptor activity. There may be a central inhibitory mechanism that causes the decreased ventilation and ultimately leads to apnea. The central inhibitory mechanism may persist into early postnatal life, causing apnea during postnatal hypoxic events.

Regular respiration begins within a few seconds of birth and is controlled by the feedback mechanisms discussed earlier; however, the feedback mechanisms are not fully developed at birth (33,34–36,41). Fetal arterial blood gases ($P_aO_2 \sim 25$ mm Hg, $P_aCO_2 \sim 50$ mm Hg) are much different from newborn blood gases ($P_aO_2 \sim 70$ mm Hg, $P_aCO_2 \sim 40$ mm Hg), and it takes several days for chemoreceptors to "reset" to new threshold values. The ventilatory response of the newborn to changes in P_aCO_2 is more mature than the response to hypoxia, and it takes a few days for the oxygen chemoreceptors to become the major controller of breathing. During this time, the newborn may be at greater risk of sustaining hypoxic injury.

Sleep influences newborn respiratory patterns via central and peripheral mechanisms (39,42–44). During sleep, periodic breathing is accentuated and respiratory pauses prolonged. In quiet sleep, periodic breathing is "regular," with the length of breathing intervals and apneas being constant, and during active sleep, periodic breathing is irregular, with breathing intervals and apneas that are variable in duration. Periods of apnea are more common, longer, and more frequently associated with bradycardia during active sleep (44,45). Active sleep also affects the respiratory muscles, with decreased intercostal muscle tone and activity and decreased functional residual capacity. Under normal conditions, sleep modulates rather than determines breathing patterns; however, when central respiratory centers are injured, sleep may be a critical element in triggering life-threatening apnea (29,46).

There are numerous mechanical differences in the pulmonary pump of infants and adults (12), but most of the differences are not relevant to a discussion of neural mechanisms of respiration. One area of interest is the composition of diaphragmatic muscle fibers (47,48). Relative to adults, the newborn diaphragm has a lower proportion of type I fibers (slow oxidative, fatigue-resistant) and a higher proportion of type IIa fibers (fast oxidative, fatigue-sensitive). In theory this should predispose the newborn to diaphragmatic fatigue and may contribute to respiratory failure in preterm babies.

BREATHING

The process of respiration can be separated into 4 general categories including: the exchange of air between atmosphere and alveoli; diffusion of oxygen (O_2) and carbon dioxide (CO_2) between alveoli and blood; transport of O_2 and CO_2 to and from the cells; and the regulation of ventilation (49,50). Disturbances that affect the process of respiration most commonly produce varying degrees of hypoxia or hypercapnia (or both) with secondary alterations in acid–base balance. The CNS effects of hypoxia and hypercapnia vary with the acuity of the changes. In response to hypoxemia, cerebral blood flow (CBF) increases to maintain cerebral oxygen delivery. This response is adequate until PaO_2 falls below 25 mm Hg. Hypoxia and hypercapnia can cause alterations of consciousness.

Airway obstruction or pulmonary arrest can cause acute hypoxemia and hypercarbia. Mild acute hypoxia (PaO_2 50 mm H_2O) can induce inattentiveness, poor judgement, and motor incoordination. Severe acute hypoxia (PaO_2 25 mm H_2O) or anoxia cause loss of consciousness within seconds (51); seizures, pupillary dilation, and bilateral extensor plantar responses can follow within hours. The severity of the CNS injury and the degree of recovery depend on several factors including: the time required to reestablish normal cerebral oxygenation; the amount of cerebral lactate produced; the degree of alteration of cerebral calcium homeostasis; and the extent of excitotoxin and possible oxygen free radical exposure (52,53). At present, one cannot correlate hypoxemia directly with the CNS injury. Some patients may fully recover from an acute hypoxic event; whereas, others may be left with a permanent disability.

A relatively uncommon phenomenon after an hypoxic event is delayed post-anoxic encephalopathy (54), in which there is an initial complete recovery from the hypoxic episode severe enough to cause coma. Several weeks later, however, a sudden relapse characterized by confusion, irritability, or agitation occurs. Many patients continue to deteriorate, eventually progressing to coma and death (54).

Acute hypercarbia will cause dilation of the cerebral vessels, increased cerebrospinal fluid (CSF) production, and increased cerebral blood volume; it may lead to vascular headache. There are few causes of pure hypercarbia, but it can be seen in mechanically ventilated patients or when there is excess respiratory dead space.

Chronic hypoxia, as observed in bronchopulmonary dysplasia or widespread bronchiectasis, may produce a non-specific constellation of symptoms and signs. As the degree of hypoxia increases, errors in judgement, disorientation, and lethargy occur, followed by periodic breathing and hyperreflexia. Ultimately, multifocal myoclonus, rigidity, and focal neurologic signs occur as arterial PaO_2 falls below 25 mm Hg (55).

Pulmonary diseases in which there is chronic inadequacy of respiratory effort or ventilation can result in hypercapnia as sometimes noted in cystic fibrosis. This is generally accompanied by reduction in arterial oxygenation, and as a consequence, secondary polycythemia, cor pulmonale, and heart failure are often present. The patient can experience headaches, mental dullness, drowsiness, confusion, asterixis, tremor, fasciculations, and coma. Papilledema with elevated CSF pressure can also occur in this context (56). The severity of the neurologic signs and symptoms tends to correlate with the degree of CO_2 induced acidosis as measured in the CSF (57). The CSF pH in respiratory acidosis may deviate from normal as much as, or more than, that of the pH_a. The homeostatic mechanisms involved in maintaining normal CSF pH in other acid–base disturbances appear nonfunctional during this specific disturbance (56). Brain metabolism during respiratory acidosis is affected by both hypoxia and the acidosis itself. Assuming normal oxygenation, a lower CSF pH occurs primarily because the CSF bicarbonate is reduced; thus, the relatively higher CSF PCO_2 may affect brain function by way of its passage across brain cell membranes, causing both an intracellular and extracellular acidosis (57).

Disorders of acid–base balance can also affect the nervous system indirectly by causing neuromuscular dysfunction. Acute respiratory acidosis particularly in the framework of chronic renal insufficiency can precipitate hyperkalemia and lead to hyperkalemic paralysis (58). Respiratory alkalosis, on the other hand, especially when it accompanies acute hyperventilation, can produce paresthesias and precipitate tetany (58).

COMMON RESPIRATORY-TRACT ABNORMALITIES

The common congenital and acquired abnormalities of the respiratory tract and their direct or indirect neurologic associations or consequences are presented within the framework of the anatomy of the respiratory tract (Table 16.1).

Upper Tract

Ear

Conditions affecting the ears in children are commonly encountered in pediatric practice. Normally, the ear serves as a complex unit subserving hearing as well as equi-

Table 16.1 Respiratory-tract abnormalities and related nervous system considerations

Respiratory Tract Abnormality	Nervous System Considerations
Upper Tract	
Ear	
Malformed/malpositioned auricle	Hearing loss, syndromes, CHARGE
Middle ear anomalies	Hearing loss
Cholesteatoma	Facial-nerve palsy
Otitis media	Contiguous CNS infection
Nose/Sinuses/Oropharynx	
Malformed/malpostioned nares	CNS malformation
Choanal atresia/nasal septal defects	CHARGE
Chronic rhinitis/sinusitis	Neoplasia, neurodegenerative disorders, ataxia–telangiectasia, vasculitis, Pott puffy tumor, ADEM, AHLE, GBS
Yellow-Orange tonsils	Tangier disease
Lower Tract	
Larynx/Trachea	
Persistent hoarse voice/stridor	Recurrent laryngeal nerve paresis; Moebius sequence, CNS malformation, familial
Tracheo-esophageal fistula	VATER
Bronchi/Lung	
Agenesis/hypoplastic lung	Anencephaly, Down syndrome
Pneumothorax	Tuberous sclerosis
Bronchitis/Pneumonia	ADEM, AHLE, GBS

VATER   = Vertebral anomalies, anal atresia, T-E fistula, radial and renal dysplasia
CHARGE = Coloboma, heart defects, choanal atresia, retarded growth and development, genital hypoplasia, ear anomalies
ADEM   = Acute disseminated encephalomyelitis
AHLE   = Acute hemorrhagic leukoencephalitis
GBS   = Guillain-Barré syndrome

librium. It is composed of three distinct parts; viz., the external ear, which serves as a sound collector, the middle ear, which functions as a sound conductor, and the inner ear, which converts sound waves to nerve impulses, as well as signaling changes in equilibrium.

Malformations of the external ear are frequently associated with conductive hearing loss and malformations of the middle ear (59,60); whereas, they are rarely associated with inner-ear anomalies. The most common external malformations noted are the occurrences of pits, tags, anomalies of the pinna, protruding ears, low set, and small ears. The majority of children with these minor malformations do not have accompanying CNS abnormalities; however, they can signal the occurrence of a chromosomal aberration such as trisomy 18, a recognizable genetic condition like Treacher-Collins syndrome, or be part of a constellation of malformations such as the CHARGE syndrome (coloboma of the iris or retina, heart defects, choanal atresia, retarded growth and development, genital hypoplasia, and ear anomalies (60, 61). The size of the external ear can also suggest neurologic abnormality. For example, exceptionally small ears are generally seen in children with Down syndrome (62), and unusually large ears are found in children with the fragile-X syndrome (63). Another abnormality of the external ear occasionally observed is a cholesteatoma, an acquired or congenital rest of epithelial tissue seen as a white cyst within the external auditory canal. If not identified and removed, cholesteatomas can enlarge, causing bony destruction and the eventual spread

to the intracranial cavity (64), sometimes resulting in facial palsy.

Middle-ear malformations in the absence of external-ear malformations generally manifest as congenital or progressive hearing loss (65). These anomalies can be associated with a variety of recognizable syndromes and associated internal malformations (65).

Acquired disorders of the ear are numerous. Otitis media is the most common of these disorders in childhood, and neurologic complications can include hearing loss, facial-nerve palsy, and the contiguous spread of infection, resulting in mastoiditis, venous sinus thrombosis, meningitis, subdural empyema, cerebritis and cerebral abscess (64).

Nose/Sinuses/Oropharynx

The normal anterior migration of the forebrain is responsible in part for anterior midline facial development (66). The face, particularly the nose, sinuses, and oropharynx, can serve as external markers of underlying CNS malformations (66). Holoprosencephaly, for example, causes median facial underdevelopment of varying degrees. These facial anomalies can be as simple as the absence of the philtrum or nasal septum to the complex, as a single tube-like proboscis and cyclopsia (66). An underlying encephalocele can also be encountered. As noted, choanal atresia may be encountered as one component of several underlying defects comprising the CHARGE association (61).

Of all acquired disorders of the naso-pharynx and sinuses, rhinitis and sinusitis are the most common. Clear nasal discharge, particularly in the setting of nasal trauma, can signal an underlying fracture of the cribriform plate with CSF rhinorrhea and result in meningitis and possibly brain abscess. A variety of other causes of nasal discharge exists, including infection, allergy, nasal-spray overuse, substance abuse, and neoplasia. Chronic nasal and sinus discharge may also be a sign of an underlying neurodegenerative process. Awareness of coarse or dysmorphic features, visceral enlargement, and developmental delay should heighten suspicion of these disorders (vide infra). Chronic or persistent sinusitis, particularly if recurrent pulmonary infections are also encountered, may be the first indication of ataxia–telangiectasia (AT) (chapter 24)(67). In early childhood the typical conjunctival and facial telangiectatic vessels are not always evident, and the ataxia can be insidious in development. Recurrent respiratory disease can, therefore, be manifest as the most prominent early symptoms and signs of AT. Systemic vasculitides, especially Wegener granulomatosis, can be manifested as chronic sinusitis (68), and in this context, both cranial and peripheral neuropathy can be associated features. An uncommon complication of sinus infection is osteomyelitis, particularly of the frontal sinus in the adolescent age group. This can develop into a focal periosteal inflammation of the inner bony table of the skull producing a "Pott puffy tumor," which can cause CNS signs and symptoms secondary to mass effect, inflammatory responses, or direct extension of infection into the CNS (69,70).

Among the varied signs and symptoms of oropharyngeal disease are enlarged yellow-orange tonsils or plaques overlying the tonsils, the hallmark of Tangier disease (71). This rare disorder, inherited as an autosomal recessive trait, is characterized by a deficiency of plasma high-density lipoproteins with deposition of cholesterol esters in tonsils, spleen, liver, bone marrow, and corneas. Older patients have an associated relapsing polyneuropathy manifested by analgesia or the reduction of pain and temperature sensation with decreased stretch reflexes (72).

Lower Tract

Larynx/Trachea

Webs, clefts, atretic segments, and other deformities can occur in the larynx and trachea, but they are generally not associated with CNS abnormalities. Persistent hoarseness of the voice or stridor (or both) can be a sign of neurologic dysfunction; moreover, unsuspected trauma to the neck of newborns may injure the recurrent laryngeal nerve, causing a temporary paralysis of the vocal cords (73,74). Other cranial nerve deficits, usually the VIth, VIIth, and Xth, are affected as part of the Moebius sequence (75,76). Hoarseness and stridor, especially with an altered respiratory pattern or apnea, difficulties with suck or swallow, and hydrocephalus suggest the occurrence of an Arnold-Chiari malformation (77,78). This and other structural lesions of the posterior fossa, lower brainstem, and high cervical spinal cord can present with apnea (79). A rare familial vocal-cord dysfunction has been reported in 3 siblings who presented in the neonatal period with stridor. It was suggested that defective chemical regulation of breathing via ventilatory reflex neural pathways led to stridor in these children (80).

Tracheo-esophageal (T–E) fistulas are generally not associated with nervous system abnormalities. However, when they are a component of the VATER association (vertebral anomalies, anal atresia, T–E fistula, radial limb and renal dysplasia), middle-ear defects and conductive hearing loss can be present (64,81,82). This syndrome can be associated with other CNS abnormalities such as hypotonia, facial paralysis, pachygyria, polymicrogyria, foramen magnum defects, as well as the lack of ventricular ependymal lining (83).

Bronchi/Lung

Congenital agenesis or severe hypoplasia of the lung, or both, is rare and generally incompatible with life. Bilateral lung hypoplasia of lesser degree is commonly seen in Down syndrome and has been associated with anencephaly (84,85). There is decreased proximal branching of the distal airways during lung development and a smaller alveolar surface area, with a decreased total number of alveoli accompanied by a loss of capillary surface area (84). This can play a role in the pathogenesis of pulmonary hypertension found in patients with Down syndrome (85). Abnormal fetal respiration has been considered a possible common etiology (84).

Spontaneous pneumothorax can occur in a variety of primary respiratory disorders. Insofar as its association with nervous system disorders is concerned, it is an often fatal, albeit rare, manifestation of tuberous sclerosis found almost entirely in young women (chapter 23)(86).

Infections, aspiration, toxic substances and drugs, hypersensitivity reactions, and radiotherapy can all produce significant bronchial and pulmonary disease. Many of these clinical states can produce CNS effects either indirectly by disrupting the normal ventilatory process or directly by their systemic effects on the nervous system. A more subtle and sometimes delayed effect of infections of the respiratory tracts are postinfectious/postvaccinal demyelinating syndromes, which are thought to be a consequence of an indirect immune-mediated mechanism in which small-vessel injury and perivascular demyelination occur (87). The process can involve the CNS, the peripheral nervous system, or both simultaneously. Among the postinfectious demyelinating syndromes are acute disseminated encephalomyelitis (ADEM), acute hemorrhagic leukoencephalitis (AHLE), Guillain-Barré syndrome (GBS), transverse myelitis, optic neuritis, and acute cerebellar ataxia (88–90).

ADEM typically manifests during the recovery phase of a relatively minor respiratory-tract infection. Its development is accompanied by low-grade fever and resurgence of systemic symptoms like malaise and headache. A diminished level of consciousness or seizures (or both) accompanied by the development of long-tract signs (spasticity, hyperreflexia, and extensor plantar responses) gradually evolve over 7 to 10 days. These signs reflect the anatomic localization of the immune-mediated white-matter injury. Signs and symptoms of ADEM tend to resolve over several weeks or months as remyelination takes place.

AHLE, a rare entity that develops several days after the patient has recovered from a respiratory-tract illness, manifests with the sudden onset of headache and progressive deterioration of mental status. Seizures, long-tract signs, and increased intracranial pressure, usually accompany the process. Perivascular hemorrhages occur within the brain parenchyma during the early phases of its evolution, and most patients die within the first few days to a week of its development. The few survivors are generally left with significant neurologic sequelae.

GBS, a multifocal peripheral demyelinating polyneuropathy, usually develops more insidiously than do either ADEM or AHLE (see chapter 24). Several days to weeks after recovery from a minor respiratory-tract illness, patients typically develop paresthesias or dysasthesias of the feet, followed by gradually ascending symmetric weakness of the lower limbs. Weakness may eventually involve all muscle groups. Autonomic dysfunction can be a prominent feature. Progressive ascending weakness, decreased to absent stretch reflexes, variable alterations of sensation, respiratory insufficiency occasionally associated with cranial-nerve deficits and ataxia, in the absence of meningitis, suggest the diagnosis of GBS. There is usually spontaneous recovery within 2 to 4 weeks after the disease has reached its nadir. Plasmapheresis has been of benefit in altering the clinical course of the disease (91).

DISORDERS ASSOCIATED WITH CESSATION OF BREATHING

Apnea is a particularly problematic issue in neonates and infants and can be symptomatic of a wide variety of underlying disorders not limited to the nervous and respiratory systems (Table 16.2). It is convenient to think of apnea as resulting from a central or diaphragmatic cause that implies the absence of air flow and respiratory effort, an obstructive phenomenon implying the absence of air flow but with preserved respiratory effort, and a mixed variety of abnormalities in which there is an initial cessation of air flow and effort followed by a resumption of effort without air flow (92). There are multiple causes of apnea including abnormalities of ventilatory control, decreased chemoreceptor

Table 16.2   Diseases with intermittent cessation of breathing

Apnea
Sudden infant death syndrome
Broncho-pulmonary dysplasia
Breath-holding spells
Sleep apnea
Central alveolar hypoventilation (Ondine Curse)

sensitivity, autonomic nervous dysfunction; neurologic disorders, such as seizures, intracranial hemorrhage, structural anomalies; systemic processes including sepsis, metabolic abnormalities, and toxins; cardiac abnormalities such as electrocardiographic aberrations, congestive heart failure; gastrointestinal processes such as gastroesophageal reflux, T–E fistula; mechanical problems causing air obstruction; the stimulation of various reflexes within the respiratory tract; and elevated endogenous opioid peptides (79,92–101). Whether or not apnea has any role in the etiology of sudden infant death syndrome (SIDS) is yet to be determined (95,96,98,101).

Multiple theories have been presented to explain the occurrence of apnea and its relationship to SIDS. Insofar as these hypotheses relate to the CNS, however, they are at least partly based on the following mechanisms: a primary failure of the central inspiratory generator in the brainstem; an abnormal chemoreceptor function to carbon dioxide and oxygen; an abnormal pulmonary reflex inhibition of the central inspiratory generator function; and an abnormal suprapontine inhibition of the central inspiratory generator. Data concerning these mechanisms have been reviewed (100,101).

Bronchopulmonary dysplasia, a chronic progressive lung disease occurring in infants following mechanical ventilation for severe respiratory-distress syndrome, has been associated with neurologic sequelae that appear to occur more commonly in infants with bronchopulmonary dysplasia than in the general low-birth-weight infant population (102–104). Neurologic deficits are usually considered in two categories: a nonprogressive disease characterized by motor deficits and/or developmental delay with or without blindness; and a progressive disease characterized by abnormal motor signs, developmental delay with deterioration, visual impairment, intractable seizures, and eventual death secondary to continued and progressive respiratory compromise (105). There are, however, infants with bronchopulmonary dysplasia who have a normal outcome. It is of interest that at least some survivors with bronchopulmonary dysplasia have been noted to have had decreased incidence of bronchospasm during the course of illness (105). Infants with the nonprogressive neurologic disease have a higher incidence of intraventricular and intracerebral hemorrhage (105).

Breath-holding spells are a well recognized self-limited clinical entity (106) that typically appear during the 1st 2 years of life but rarely before 6 months of age; they spontaneously remit by age of 6 to 8 years (107,108). The child may be frightened, hurt, or angered, begin to cry for one or two breaths, and then "holds his breath," which is actually a prolonged expiratory apnea. There are two clinical forms of breath-holding spells; viz., the cyanotic and the pallid types, which refer to the color of the child during the spell (106). Once the "breath-holding" begins, the child becomes cyanotic within several seconds, then becomes limp, and falls to the ground. Alternatively, after a brief period of crying, the onset of a pallid-type spell is followed by the sudden loss of consciousness. Cyanotic spells have been associated with clonic activity, and it is important to determine whether the cyanosis precedes or follows the onset of clonic movements (108,109). This is helpful to distinguish seizure phenomena in which cyanosis can follow the tonic–clonic activity. The pallid type of breath-holding spell is associated with a sudden asystole mediated by the vagus nerve; atropine has been used as a preventative treatment (110). In both forms of breath-holding spells, the child can assume an opisthotonic posture, but in neither form are there neurologic sequelae (108). It is most important to distinguish breath-holding spells from convulsive disorders and syncope. The laboratory evaluation of patients may include an electroencephalogram accompanied by ocular compression, because in patients with the pallid breath-holding spells, ocular compression can induce an exaggerated bradycardia or asystole leading to a clinical spell. The normal response involves a reflex via the trigeminal nerve afferent fibers and the vagal nerve efferent fibers, causing a slowing of the heart rate (111). The typical course of breath-holding spells is one of a decreasing frequency and duration of episodes after 2 years of age. An increased frequency or duration with age should prompt suspicion of an alternative diagnosis. An unsuspected tumor of the medulla has been observed in this setting (112).

DISEASES WITH PULMONARY INFILTRATES (Table 16.3)

Asthma

Asthma is a complex syndrome of recurrent, reversible airways obstruction caused by airways hyperreactivity and characterized by wheezing, coryza, breathlessness, and increased sputum production (113). There are many causative factors of asthma, including allergy, infection, environmental exposures, chemicals and drugs, exercise, vasculitis, and an idiopathic variety (114). The CNS is rarely implicated but there is evidence suggesting a causal relationship between asthma and an imbalance of components of the autonomic nervous system (115). This imbalance is demonstrated by a blunted β-adrenergic response, and hyperreactive α-adrenergic and cholinergic responses. Each of these contribute to the production of bronchial constriction (115).

Table 16.3 Lung infiltration and associated nervous system dysfunction

Asthma
Cystic fibrosis
Sickle cell anemia
Amyloidosis
Chediak-Higashi syndrome
Sarcoidosis
Histiocytosis-X
Hereditary hemorrhagic telangiectasia
Pulmonary neoplasms
Connective tissue diseases/vasculitides

Asthma and asthma therapy can also influence the CNS. Altered respiratory function may cause hypoxia, hypercapnea, acid–base disturbances, and secondary changes of mental status. Neurologic toxicity and complications of therapy, such as seizures following the administration of theophylline and terbutaline are well recognized (48,116). Cerebellar and brainstem infarction secondary to vertebral artery dissection during status asthmaticus has been observed (117). The etiology of the vertebral artery dissection is unknown, however, but it can occur as the result of mechanical trauma to the vessel during coughing or through possible changes in intravascular pressures during tussive events.

A related issue involves the sudden unexplained death of ambulatory asthmatic patients. In a study of 13 patients from the Children's Hospital of Philadelphia, the authors concluded that three possible causes of death existed: medication related as exemplified by patient abuse of inhaled adrenergic drugs, poor compliance of prescribed drugs, and physician failure to prescribe corticosteroids; an unsuspected pulmonary pathology; and sudden intense airways narrowing (118). A primary CNS pathogenesis has not been implicated.

An unusual combination of flaccid paralysis of one or more extremities following asthmatic attacks (Hopkins syndrome) has been described (119). In a review of this poliomyelitis-like syndrome, all patients had been immunized against polio. Seventeen developed monoplegia, 2 hemiplegia, and 1 diplegia (120). The paralysis was permanent. The most likely pathogenetic mechanism is that the paralysis was caused by a neurotropic virus that coincidentally triggered an asthmatic attack. Enteroviruses were isolated in 4 of the cases. It has been suggested that the concurrent use of corticosteroids could render asthmatic patients more susceptible to viral invasion of the anterior horn cells (120).

The Churg-Strauss syndrome, an unusual vasculitic process that causes asthma, is characterized by necrotizing vasculitis, eosinophilic tissue infiltration, and peripheral eosinophilia with intracranial extravascular granulomatosis (121,122). This type of vasculitis is unique among the vasculitides in that there is a high incidence of pulmonary vascular involvement as well as severe asthma.

Chest radiographs show a spectrum of abnormalities ranging from a diffuse interstitial process to patchy or nodular parenchymal infiltration (122). In addition to the respiratory tract, other organ systems are involved including the gastrointestinal tract, kidneys, bone, skin, and the nervous system (122). Peripheral neuropathy has been present in as many as 65% of patients, manifested as a mononeuritis multiplex (121,122). Although not a prominent feature, asthma has been reported in patients with adrenoleukodystrophy and homocystinuria (123).

Cystic Fibrosis

Cystic fibrosis (CF), inherited as an autosomal recessive trait, is a multisystem disorder that affects all exocrine glands to some degree, with the eccrine sweat glands producing increased levels of sodium and chloride (124). Dysfunction of mucous secreting glands and other exocrine glands leads to obstructive pulmonary disease, pancreatic insufficiency, intestinal obstruction, gallstones, biliary cirrhosis, and electrolyte imbalance (124–126).

Abnormalities of the autonomic nervous system have been demonstrated in patients with CF, and include an increased sensitivity to α-adrenergically stimulated pupillary constriction, parotid saliva secretion, and eccrine sweat secretion (127). There is also a decreased responsiveness to β-adrenergic stimulation of the cardiovascular system, circulating lymphocytes, and granulocytes (127). Aside from the pupillary abnormalities noted, other ocular findings include capillary engorgement, microaneurysms, retinal hemorrhages, papilledema, preganglionic oculosympathetic paresis, and decreased light contrast sensitivity (128). It has been suggested that the autonomic nervous system plays a role in the pathophysiology of the disease in affected patients and obligate heterozyotes for CF (129).

As a result of pancreatic insufficiency, gastrointestinal malabsorption, particularly of vitamins E and D, can have profound effects on peripheral nerve and muscle function. A slowly progressive impairment of vibratory and position sense perception can produce a disabling sensory ataxia. This proprioceptive impairment associated with nystagmus and areflexia has been reported secondary to vitamin E deficiency in CF (130). Proximal myopathy in the presence of rickets, and neurologic deficits similar to those seen with vitamin E deficiency, have been encountered in a patient with CF and vitamin D deficiency (131). The rickets and myopathy resolved after vitamin replacement; however, the other neurologic signs persisted (131).

A rare complication of CF in children is the development of secondary amyloidosis (85), which has typically manifested as proteinuria; thyroid enlargement and hepatosplenomegaly have also been encountered (132). Although typical amyloidosis affects peripheral nerves, no evidence of nervous system involvement has been reported in children with CF and secondary amyloidosis (130).

Sickle Cell Anemia

Sickle cell anemia is a severe chronic hemolytic anemia occurring in patients homozygous for the sickle cell gene (133). The manifestations of sickle cell anemia vary with the age of the patient. In the child, acute painful crises are usually associated with intercurrent infection (133). Pulmonary dysfunction is usually caused by atelectasis, pulmonary infarction, and pulmonary infections (133–135). Pulmonary infarction can be the result of thromboses of the pulmonary micro-circulation by sickled red cells and/or thrombo-emboli from fat and bone marrow elements. The frequency of thrombo-embolic events increases with age (134), and cor pulmonale may result from chronic and recurrent pulmonary infarctions (136)(see chapter 19).

The major neurologic complication of sickle cell anemia is cerebral infarction (137), which primarily results from thromboses of large and small arteries, dural sinuses, and cortical veins, secondary to the sickling phenomenon and rarely from fat emboli (137). Both ischemic and hemorrhagic infarctions throughout the entire neuroaxis can occur (137–140). Children at greatest risk for cerebral infarction have a mean age at symptom onset of 7.7 years, with a recurrence rate of 67% (137). There tends to be a temporal clustering of recurrences within 36 months of the initial infarction (138). Subarachnoid or intracerebral hemorrhages are generally observed in adolescents and young adults (141,142) and are frequently associated with such vascular defects as aneurysms (138,141–142). Other neurologic complications of sickle cell anemia include a reversible recurrent organic mental syndrome and headaches that are thought to be secondary to transient ischemia of multifocal small vessels (143). Partial or generalized seizures may herald a stroke or recur as a chronic seizure disorder (137,140). A retinopathy as well as transient visual and hearing loss may also occur (137,144).

Amyloidosis

Amyloidosis is uncommon in childhood. It is caused by the deposition of amyloid, an insoluble amorphous material composed of fine fibrils of protein that can be deposited in a focal or diffuse manner, resulting in tissue enlargement and dysfunction. Amyloidosis, considered as a primary or secondary disorder, can involve the lungs as well as the peripheral nervous system, but rarely at the same time (145,146). Primary amyloidosis occurs as a heredofamilial disease in association with plasma cell dyscrasias or as an idiopathic form. The secondary form is usually associated with an underlying chronic illness such as collagen vascular disease, neoplasms, or chronic suppurative infections (147,148). Familial Mediterranean fever is the most common heredofamilial form of amyloidosis in childhood and has prominent pulmonary involvement (145,148). This disease, inherited as an autosomal recessive trait, is found primarily in patients of Mediterranean, and Middle Eastern Jewish extraction. Agammaglobulinemia, a plasma cell dyscrasia, has also been reported to cause amyloidosis in a child (149). Secondary systemic amyloidosis has been observed most often in association with juvenile rheumatoid arthritis, chronic suppurative infections, and in cystic fibrosis (132,145). Primary focal tracheobronchial amyloidosis has also been reported in a child (150). Pulmonary involvement may be diffuse with deposition of amyloid in the alveolar septae, pulmonary vessels and capillary membranes, or focal with nodular lesions in the lung and tracheobronchial tree (145–150). Despite deposition throughout the respiratory tract, the process generally causes no signs or symptoms of pulmonary disease and only rarely causes dyspnea and impaired gas exchange (147).

Neurologic involvement has not been reported in children with amyloidosis; adult patients, however, can have involvement of the peripheral nervous system with symmetric sensorimotor polyneuropathy or carpal tunnel syndrome (151). The disease has a predilection for small autonomic and sensory nerves; therefore, autonomic signs and symptoms such as orthostatic hypotension, bowel dysfunction, and diminished sweating, may be the manifesting features. Painful paraesthesias and numbness are more prominent than are other sensory abnormalities and typically appear before motor weakness. Muscle involvement manifested by weakness, stiffness, and muscle enlargement is rarely seen as amyloid becomes deposited between muscle fibers (152). It is unclear why children have not been observed to have involvement of the peripheral nervous system.

Chediak-Higashi Syndrome

The Chediak-Higashi syndrome, inherited as an autosomal recessive trait, is characterized by partial oculocutaneous albinism with photophobia, nystagmus, decreased lacrimation, peripheral neuropathy, and a propensity to pyogenic infections, episodic fevers, and lymphoreticular malignancy (153). The hallmark of the disorder is the presence of giant peroxidase positive cytoplasmic granules found in leukocytes. Disseminated and focal collections of mononuclear cells can be found in multiple organs including the lungs and the central and peripheral nervous systems (153). Pyogenic infections occur throughout the respiratory tract causing otitis media, sinusitis, pharyngitis, bronchitis, bronchopneumonia, and lobar pneumonia. The most common neurologic problem is a chronic polyneuropathy with features of axonal degeneration and demyelination, manifested as weakness, absence of deep-tendon reflexes, and a sensory deficit in a stocking-glove distribution (154). CNS manifestations of the disorder include mental retardation, seizures, a form of spinocerebellar degeneration, and movement disorder (153,155). Patients have nystagmus, cerebel-

lar ataxia, and overall clumsiness; a parkinsonian-like syndrome has also been described with a resting tremor, mask-like facies, bradykinesia, and mild cogwheel rigidity (155).

Sarcoidosis

Sarcoidosis is a multisystem granulomatous disease of unknown etiology seldom affecting children younger than the age of 15 years (156,157). It most often manifests with diffuse interstitial reticular-nodular pulmonary infiltrates, hilar adenopathy, and eye or skin manifestation (156–162). The nervous system can be affected (see chapter 13).

Histiocytosis-X

Histiocytosis-X is a disorder of the reticuloendothelial system in which there is hyperplasia of histiocytes in the absence of lipid inclusions (163). There are 3 variants of the disorder; viz., Letterer-Siwe disease, Schüller-Christian disease, and eosinophilic granuloma of the lung or bone. Thus, histiocytosis-X can be manifested as a localized or generalized process. Frequent clinical findings include painful bone lesions, seborrheic skin rash, hepatosplenomegaly and lymphadenopathy, chronic otitis media, dyspnea, and hypothalamic dysfunction with growth retardation, hypothyroidism, and diabetes insipidus (164). Pulmonary involvement, when manifested as dyspnea, tachypnea, or pneumothorax, can be an ominous sign; however, when pulmonary disease is evident on chest radiographs in the absence of clinical signs or symptoms, it tends to occur in patients with a more favorable outcome (164,165). Radiographic evidence of bilateral reticular or reticular-nodular interstitial infiltration can be present and progress to interstitial fibrosis, developing a cystic honeycomb appearance with emphysematous blebs (163,164). The blebs may, in turn, rupture and produce recurrent pneumothoraces.

Neurologic involvement can include cerebellar infiltration, demyelination, and calcification of the dentate nuclei (164). Enlargement of the fourth ventricle and subarachnoid cisterns of the posterior fossa have been described (166). An unusual manifestation of the disease is the deposition of histocytes along the cauda equina, resulting in a cauda equina syndrome (167).

Hereditary Hemorrhagic Telangiectasia (Osler-Weber-Rendu Disease)

Hereditary hemorrhagic telangiectasia, inherited as an autosomal dominant trait with variable expression, is manifested by dermal, mucosal, and visceral telangiectasias and a tendency to form arteriovenous fistulas (168). Patients have multiple pinpoint spider and/or nodular telangiectasias over the tongue, skin, lips, mucous membranes, nailbeds, and other sites that have a tendency to bleed. Recurrent episodes of epistaxis and hemorrhage of the lung, intestinal tract, kidney, brain, and other organs have been reported (168–172).

The signs and symptoms of pulmonary disease include hemoptysis and those secondary to left to right vascular shunting through pulmonary arteriovenous fistulas (168,173), which can result in polycythemia, clubbing of the nails, dyspnea, cyanosis on exertion, and pulmonary hypertension. Chest radiographs frequently show nodular densities with vascular connections extending into the hilus (173).

About 36% of patients with CNS complications have neurologic manifestations as a direct consequence of CNS vascular malformations or indirectly from vascular malformations in other organs (171,172). Cerebral vascular abnormalities include telangiectasias and angiomas, arteriovenous malformations, aneurysms, carotid-cavernous sinus fistula formation, and spinal cord arteriovenous malformations. These lesions can produce focal static, progressive, or transient deficits, including infarction, transient ischemic attacks, hydrocephalus, ataxia, visual disturbances, seizures, and recurrent headache (172). Spontaneous bleeding has resulted in subarachnoid, intracerebral, intraventricular, and intramedullary spinal cord hemorrhages (171,172). Indirect neurologic complications can arise as a consequence of vascular shunting through pul-

Table 16.4   Primary pulmonary neoplasms of childhood*

Benign
Hamartoma
Inflammatory pseudotumor
Leiomyoma
Mucous gland adenoma
Myoblastoma
Neurogenic tumors
Malignant
Adeno-carcinoma
Bronchial adenoma
Bronchogenic carcinoma
Bronchiolo-alveolar carcinoma
Bronchial carcinoid
Hemangiopericytoma
Leiomyosarcoma
Lymphoma
Mesothelioma
Mucoepidermoid carcinoma
Myxosarcoma
Plasmacytoma
Pulmonaryblastoma
Rhabdomyosarcoma
Teratoma

*Modified from Hartman GE, Shochat ST. Primary pulmonary neoplasms of childhood: A review. Ann Thorac Surg 1983; 36:108–119.

Table 16.5   Pediatric neoplasms with cerebral and pulmonary metastases

Leukemia
Lymphoma
Wilms tumor
Neuroblastoma
Osteogenic sarcoma
Ewing tumor
Rhabdomyosarcoma
Melanoma
Histiocytosis-X
Hepatoblastoma/Hepatocarcinoma

monary arteriovenous fistulas (172), which can produce symptoms secondary to decreased arterial oxygen saturation and a propensity to cerebral vascular thromboses from increased blood viscosity, associated with polycythemia and paradoxical emboli (172,174). Embolization can result in cerebral infarction or, if septic, brain abscess. Hepatic encephalopathy can develop if significant portal-systemic shunting occurs (172).

Pulmonary Neoplasms

Primary pulmonary neoplasms in childhood are rare. Hartman and Shochat reported a variety of histologic types, of which approximately 2/3 were malignant (175). The most common benign tumors are hamartomas; whereas, bronchial adenomas are the most common malignant lesions. Other malignant tumors include primary adenocarcinoma, bronchiolo-alveolar carcinoma, and malignant mesothelioma (Table 16.4)(176–178). Recurrent pneumonitis with cough and hemoptysis are most often associated with malignant tumors. Cerebral metastatic lesions are reported in patients with primary pulmonary rhabdomyosarcoma, leiomyosarcoma, and adenocarcinoma (175,176,179). It is clear, however, that any malignant process, particularly when involving the lung, has the potential to metastasize to the brain via hematogenous spread (Table 16.5). Primary neurogenic tumors of the lungs have been reported and are generally limited to neurofibromas and neurilemmomas (175).

CONNECTIVE TISSUE DISEASES/VASCULITIDES (See chapter 24)

The connective tissue diseases and vasculitides include a broad spectrum of clinical disorders in which pulmonary pathologic changes include serosal inflammation, pleural thickening, interstitial fibrosis and pneumonitis, alveolar hemorrhage, cystic changes, and bronchopneumonia. An overview of disorders that have both pulmonary and nervous system involvement is presented (Tables 16.6,16.7).

Table 16.6   Connective tissue diseases/vasculitides

Connective-Tissue Diseases
  Juvenile rheumatoid arthritis
  Juvenile ankylosing spondylitis
  Systemic lupus erythematosus
  Dermatomyositis/polymyositis
  Scleroderma
  Mixed connective tissue disease

Vasculitides
  Mucocutaneous lymph node syndrome
  Anaphylactoid purpura
  Polyarteritis nodosa
  Churg-Strauss syndrome
  Wegener granulomatosis
  Behçet syndrome

Juvenile Rheumatoid Arthritis

Juvenile rheumatoid arthritis (JRA) is the most common disease of connective tissue in children. There are 3 distinct types of onset including polyarthritis, oligoarthritis, and a systemic form of the disease (180–184). Associated pulmonary disease, though uncommon, can occur with the systemic and polyarticular types (185). Extensive interstitial pulmonary fibrosis and pulmonary arteriolar intimal hypertrophy with arterial occlusion can lead to the development of pulmonary hypertension, cor pulmonale, and sudden death (186). In a review of 16 unselected pediatric patients with JRA, pulmonary function was studied, demonstrating that carbon monoxide diffusing capacity was abnormal in 34% after correcting for volume and was compatible with diffuse vascular or parenchymal lung disease (187). Rheumatoid lung nodules are more often seen in adult patients.

CNS complications of JRA are more common than those observed in the respiratory tract (178). Mental status changes can occur secondary to metabolic abnormalities, fever, aspirin toxicity, and associated systemic disease. Fifteen to 20% of the patients will manifest an encephalopathy with irritability and lethargy accompanied by transient electroencephalographic abnormalities (185,187); menin-gismus and seizures have also been observed (185,188). Ocular complications, particularly iridocyclitis found in 17% of patients, occur most often as an accompaniment of an oligoarticular disease in females (189). Amyloidosis complicating JRA may also occur (145).

Juvenile Ankylosing Spondylitis

Juvenile ankylosing spondylitis, a chronic inflammatory arthritis of the appendicular and axial skeleton, is frequently associated with HLA–B27 antigen and unaccompanied by serum rheumatoid factor or antinuclear antibody (190). Although decreased chest expansion is common, associated pleuropulmonary disease is rare in children. In a series of adult patients, 1.3% of 2,080 patients with ankylosing spondylitis had apical fibrobullous lesions that appeared on chest radiographs as interstitial markings and cystic spaces in the apical lung fields (191). An important neurologic complication of juvenile ankylosing spondylitis is atlantoaxial subluxation (192), which can produce cervical pain radiating into the occiput and has the potential to cause cervical cord compression. Cervical spine radiographs are needed to confirm the diagnosis.

Systemic Lupus Erythematosus

Systemic lupus erythematosus (SLE) is a multisystem disease primarily seen in females and characterized by episodic, diffuse autoimmune inflammatory changes of blood vessels and connective tissues (191). Pulmonary involvement is often overshadowed by other organ system disease. Pleural effusions and migratory interstitial infiltrates suggestive of pneumonitis are the most common findings, with signs and symptoms ranging from cough and dyspnea to chest pain and hemoptysis. Pulmonary hemorrhage rarely occurs (193,194).

The nervous system is often involved in SLE and may have protean manifestations (193,195). Headache, changes of mental status, pseudotumor cerebri, seizures, and stroke are among the more common problems (193,195). Of chil-

Table 16.7   Clinical spectrum of connective tissue diseases*

	Chest Radiograph	*CNS*	*Ocular*	*PNS*	*Muscle*
JRA	Interstitial fibrosis/nodules	+ +	+ +	+	−
JAS	Apical fibrobullae	+	−	−	−
SLE	Interstitial fibrosis/hemorrhage	+ +	−	+	+
D/P	Interstitial fibrosis/pneumonitis	+	+	+	+ +
S	Interstitial fibrosis/bullae	+	−	−	−
MCTD	Increased vascular markings/interstitial fibrosis/pneumonitis	+ +	−	+	+

−	not identified	JRA	= Juvenile rheumatoid arthritis	S	= Scleroderma
+	rare or occasional	JAS	= Juvenile ankylosing spondylitis	D/P	= Dermatomyositis/Polymyositis
+ +	frequent	SLE	= Systemic lupus erythematosis	MCTS	= Mixed connective-tissue disease

*See text for details

dren with CNS manifestations of lupus, up to 81% had signs and symptoms of CNS disease at the onset of SLE (195). Mild myositis, manifested by muscle pain and tenderness with elevations in serum aldolase but generally normal serum creatine phosphokinase levels (196), has been reported in about 8% of young adults with SLE. Infrequently, a distal sensory or sensorimotor polyneuropathy can be present.

Dermatomyositis/Polymyositis

Dermatomyositis is characterized by nonsuppurative inflammation of skin and striated muscle (197). Polymyositis is uncommon in childhood, but is characterized by the same muscle pathology without the skin rash. Vasculitis, a feature observed in both processes, is manifested by perivascular inflammatory cells in affected striated muscles (181,182). Pulmonary manifestations can result from weakness of affected intercostal and abdominal muscles, leading to dyspnea, cough, and a predisposition to recurrent aspiration pneumonitis. Even in pediatric patients without pulmonary complaints, about 78% have significant restrictive decrease of ventilatory capacity (195). Fatal lung involvement secondary to a diffuse progressive pulmonary fibrosis has occurred in some children (198). Chest radiographs can show diffuse lower lung field interstitial infiltrates and, infrequently, pneumothoraces (181,199,200).

The predominant manifestations of dermatomyositis/polymyositis are muscle pain and insidious weakness; however, as many as 40% of children will have no muscle discomfort (200). Limb weakness is symmetric, affecting initially the proximal muscles with gradual involvement of distal muscles. There is a proclivity for involvement of anterior neck flexor muscles in polymyositis. CNS abnormalities such as neuropsychiatric disorders and seizures have been noted during long-term follow-up of patients (201); iridocyclitis has also been reported (201).

Scleroderma

Scleroderma is a multisystem disease characterized by vascular inflammatory and fibrotic changes in the skin and internal organs (202). The disease can be manifested as a localized or a diffuse systemic disease. Pulmonary manifestations include dyspnea on exertion , with linear and nodular fibrosis on chest radiographs (203). Severe reduction of the alveolar spaces and rupture of septae into emphysematous blebs are salient pathologic features (203). Neurologic complications are unusual; however, an associated progressive CNS vasculitis can lead to seizures, visual disturbances, and hemiparesis (204).

Mixed Connective Tissue Disease

Mixed connective tissue disease is a rheumatic disease primarily seen in females (80%) that has elements of SLE, JRA, scleroderma, and dermatomyositis/polymyositis and is associated with antibody titers to extractable nuclear antigen (ENA) (205–207). The ENA has been resolved into a soluble ribonucleoprotein and a glycoprotein designated as Sm antigen. Pulmonary manifestations of the disease consist of restrictive lung changes on pulmonary function studies and pulmonary hypertension. Recurrent aspiration pneumonitis can occur secondary to esophageal dysmotility. Chest radiographs have shown basal pulmonary cysts, increased vascular markings, and pleural effusions. Shortness of breath with an associated abnormal diffusing capacity for carbon monoxide has been reported with development of interstitial fibrosis (205).

Neurologic abnormalities occur in 10% to 30% of children with mixed connective tissue disease, usually manifested as headaches and depression. Less commonly reported problems include seizures, encephalopathy, aseptic meningitis with elevated CSF protein, cerebral hemorrhage, myositis, and peripheral neuropathies (205,206).

Mucocutaneous Lymph Node Syndrome

Mucocutaneous lymph node syndrome (Kawasaki disease, MLNS) is an acute febrile illness primarily affecting infants and children and is associated with a systemic vasculitis (208). Establishing the diagnosis is dependent on the identification of five of six cardinal features including fever of more than 5 days, bilateral conjunctivitis, lip and oral cavity lesions, changes of peripheral extremities, skin rash, acute nonpurulent swelling of cervical lymph nodes, and the exclusion of other similar diseases (Table 16.8)(209).

Abnormalities of the respiratory tract are not prominent, but can include mild transient cough, coryza, or hoarseness. Chest radiographic findings include pneumonitis and pleural effusions (208). Tonsilar exudates and otitis media can be present.

The nervous system is commonly involved in MLNS. Aseptic meningitis accompanied by irritability, lethargy, and nuchal rigidity is frequent; other abnormalities can include encephalopathy, facial nerve palsy, and seizures (210). Because aneurysmal dilations tend to silently evolve over the 1st 3 weeks and may persist into the convalescent and chronic stages of illness, surveillance for the development of arterial aneurysms, as well as thrombosis and stenosis of medium-sized arteries particularly of the coronary vessels is of paramount importance (211). There are rare reports of death secondary to aneurysmal rupture as well as cerebral infarction from occlusion of branches from the right middle cerebral artery (212,213).

Table 16.8   Clinical spectrum of vasculitides*

	Chest Radiograph	CNS	Ocular	PNS	Muscle
MLNS	Increased interstitial markings, pneumonitis, pleural effusion	+ +	+ +	−	−
HSP	Hemorrhage	+	+	+	−
PAN	Increased interstitial markings	+ +	+	+ +	−
CSS	Increased interstitial markings	−	−	+ +	−
WG	Increased interstitial markings/cavitary nodules	+	+ +	+	−
BS	Reticular–nodular densities	+ +	+	−	−

−	not indentified	MLNS	= Mucocutaneous lymph node syndrome	CSS	= Churg-Strauss syndrome
+	rare or occasional	HSP	= Henoch-Schönlein purpura	BS	= Behçet syndrome
+ +	frequent	PAN	= Polyarteritis nodosa	WG	= Wegener granulomatosis

*See text for details

Anaphylactoid Purpura

Anaphylactoid purpura (Henoch-Schönlein Purpura), a vasculitic syndrome of the capillary vessels, is characterized by nonthrombocytopenic purpura, arthritis and arthralgia, abdominal pain, and nephritis (214,215). There is usually a preceding upper-respiratory tract infection (90%), but the specific etiology and pathogenesis of anaphylactoid purpura are unknown (214).

Rarely pulmonary hemorrhage can occur during the course of illness (215). Neurologic complications of anaphylactoid purpura are probably more common than recognized, and in a review of the world literature, 48% of 79 reported children manifested a depressed state of consciousness; seizures occurred in 44%, and 23% manifested other behavioral changes (216). Headaches commonly occurred. Focal deficits, including aphasia, hemiparesis, cortical blindness, ataxia, and other neurologic signs and symptoms, were reported in up to 14% of the patients (214). Hemorrhage into brain parenchyma and the subarachnoid space has also been observed (215). Peripheral nervous system abnormalities have been reported in 2% to 3% of patients, including mononeuropathies affecting the sciatic, femoral, peroneal, and ulnar nerves, as well as the IInd and VIIth cranial nerves (214,216). Polyneuropathy has been infrequently observed (2l6). Neurologic complications associated with hypertension and renal failure can occur (214).

Polyarteritis Nodosa

Polyarteritis nodosa is a rare vasculitic syndrome of childhood, manifested as a necrotizing process of small- and medium-sized arteries (121). The regions of vascular branching are particularly involved. The skin, kidneys, heart, and liver are most often affected (60% to 90%), with the respiratory tract, the CNS, and other systems involved less frequently (217,218). The diagnosis is established by demonstrating the characteristic vascular pathology on tissue biopsy.

Pulmonary complications are more often found in children than in adults. Upper-respiratory-tract infection, pulmonary infiltrates, and perforation of the nasal septum have been commonly associated with childhood polyarteritis nodosa. Neurologic complications are common and varied and are manifested as the presenting complaint in about 10% of adults; about 15% of patients will have involvement referable to the CNS at some time during the course of illness (121). The predominant CNS manifestations are changes of mental status and seizures; however, stroke, visual abnormalities, papilledema, and cranial neuropathies have also been observed (121,217,218). Involvement of the peripheral nervous system occurs in up to 60% of patients as mononeuritis multiplex, mononeuritis, distal sensorimotor polyneuropathy, or cutaneous neuropathy (121,218).

The Churg-Strauss syndrome or allergic granulomatosis is a clinical variant of the polyarteritis nodosa group of disorders and is distinguished by its predominant pulmonary symptomology (asthma), and an accompanying peripheral eosinophilia (121,122). Mononeuritis multiplex occurs in up to 65% of patients with this syndrome (vida supra). Wegener granulomatosis, an immune necrotizing granulomatous angiitis of unknown etiology, chiefly affects the respiratory tract and kidneys (68,219,220). It is generally observed in older persons, but has been reported in children younger than the age of 10 years (221). The disease tends to be progressive with destructive granulomatous lesions of the upper- and lower-respiratory tracts associated with a systemic necrotizing vasculitis. Respiratory-tract disease (sinuses, nasopharynx, lung) is present in up to 81% of pediatric patients at disease onset (221). Upper-respiratory-tract lesions include otitis media, sinusitis, necrotizing mucosal ulceration, and saddle nose deformity (219). Common complaints are those of purulent rhinorrhea, sinus pressure, and ear infection. Lower-respiratory-tract disease manifests as cough, hemoptysis, dyspnea, and pleuritis (68). The characteristic pulmonary findings are multiple nodular infiltrates, that tend to cavitate, pleural effusions, and atelectasis (68).

The ocular manifestations of the disease include conjunctivitis, episcleritis, uveitis, optic neuritis, and corneoscleral ulceration and are present in up to 39% of pediatric patients; whereas, nervous system involvement is noted in 16% of patients (222).

The most prominent neurologic problem associated with Wegener granulomatosis is mononeuritis multiplex. Multiple cranial nerve dysfunction (II, V, VII, VIII, IX, XII) is a manifestation of CNS involvement (173,174,220). Intracranial granuloma causing parenchymal compression may lead to focal deficits.

Behçet Syndrome

Behçet syndrome, a multisystem disorder, is characterized by ocular, mucocutaneous, articular, and neurologic abnormalities (121,222,223). It is rarely reported in childhood. In older patients and particularly in females, genital ulcers are a frequent site of mucosal lesions; whereas, recurrent oral aphthous ulcers are the most common mucous membrane lesions in children. Pulmonary artery aneurysms and thrombophlebitis have been observed and can manifest as massive hemoptysis secondary to bronchial erosion from an aneurysm. Pleural effusions, transient infiltrates, and reticular-nodular densities are more commonly seen (223).

Neurologic signs and symptoms occur in about 30% of adults and children. Manifestations of CNS involvement include recurrent meningoencephalitis, pseudotumor cerebri, seizures, headache, mental status changes, focal brainstem syndromes, hemiparesis, and quadriparesis. Ocular findings including uveitis, keratoconjunctivitis, and iritis are more frequently seen in adult patients.

NEUROLOGIC DISORDERS AND ASSOCIATED RESPIRATORY DYSFUNCTION

Neurologic disorders that involve respiratory function can be considered in several categories including neuromuscular and metabolic diseases, selected neurocutaneous disorders (see chapter 23), and CNS tumors (Table 16.9). Respiratory dysfunction as a manifestation of neuromuscular disease is generally secondary to muscle weakness, resulting in respiratory insufficiency. Metabolic diseases, on the other hand, are secondary to specific involvement of the CNS (Table 16.10). Some tumors of the CNS can metastasize to the lung or pleura (Table 16.11).

Table 16.9 Neurologic disorders and associated abnormalities of respiration

Neurocutaneous disorders*
Syndrome of palatal myoclonus
Rett syndrome
Metabolic encephalopathies
CNS neoplasms
Neurogenic pulmonary edema

*See chapter 23

Table 16.10 Metabolic disease and associated respiratory signs*

Recurrent upper-respiratory infections, respiratory insufficiency, and persistent coryza
Mucopolysaccharidosis I
Mucopolysaccharidosis II
Mucopolysaccharidosis III
Mannosidosis
Fucosidosis
Aspartylglucosaminuria
Mucolipidosis II
Respiratory Insufficiency from Pulmonary Infiltration
Infantile Niemann-Pick disease
Infantile Gaucher disease
Farber disease
Hyperventilation
Leigh disease
Congenital lactic acidosis
Aminoacidopathies with metabolic acidosis
Recurrent Upper-Respiratory Infection and Dyspnea
GM_1-gangliosidosis I
Dyspnea Due to Laryngeal Infiltration
Farber disease
Asthma
Homocystinuria
Adrenoleukodystrophy
Chronic Pulmonary Insufficiency
Fabry disease

*Modified with permission from Adams RD, Lyon G. Neurology of Hereditary Metabolic Diseases of Children. Bristol, PA: Hemisphere, 1982.

Rhythmic Palatal Myoclonus

Rhythmic palatal myoclonus is a rare entity, characterized by rapid (up to 200 per minute), rhythmic oscillations of the soft palate. It is generally associated with lesions interrupting the dentato–rubro–thalamic tract in the brainstem (224). The myoclonus can be accompanied by respiratory muscle incoordination as well as rhythmic vocal-cord closure, which may cause an extrathoracic airways obstruction. The causes of the brainstem injury include vascular lesions, an inflammatory process, traumatic injuries, demyelination, and others. If intubation results in the relief of symptoms, tracheostomy is suggested.

Table 16.11 Pediatric CNS tumors with metastases to lung or pleura*

Malignant glioma
Ependymoma
Pinealoma
Papillary meningioma
Meningeal fibrosarcoma
Choroid plexus papilloma
Medulloblastoma
Chordoma

*References 233–239

Rett Syndrome

Rett syndrome is a poorly understood progressive encephalopathy currently recognized only in females and manifested by autism, ataxia, and dementia (225–228). Patients present with a gradual arrest of developmental progress, followed by deterioration of higher cortical function after the first 6 to 18 months of life, with a simultaneous loss of motor abilities. Affected patients typically exhibit mental retardation, autistic behavior, and a peculiar writhing movement of fingers and hands, which gradually deteriorates to the loss of any purposeful movement. Associated findings include truncal ataxia, an acquired microcephaly, occasionally seizures, spasticity, intermittent hyperventilation, apnea, and breath holding (216–218). The etiology of Rett syndrome is unknown. Levels of both homovanillic acid and metabolites of norepinphrine in the CSF have been identified in some patients with Rett syndrome. Recent evidence to suggest the possibility of an underlying disorder in biogenic amines has since been questioned (229). Seizures are present in up to 80% of patients (228), and electroencephalograms have shown poor maturation of background and multifocal epileptiform discharges. Other electrophysiologic and neuroimaging studies have been normal (226).

Central Nervous System Neoplasms

Extracranial metastases of primary CNS tumors in children, though extremely rare, are known to occur (Table 16.11)(230–236). There is always a question of whether an operative procedure to remove the intracranial neoplasm may have produced hematogenous metastases extracranially.

Neurogenic Pulmonary Edema

Pulmonary edema is generally considered to be caused by increased pulmonary vascular pressure or increased pulmonary vascular permeability. Neurogenic pulmonary edema (NPE) occurs after some neurologic insult and cannot be considered in either category (237–249).

NPE can be manifested as an acute form, occurring within minutes to hours of an insult to the nervous system or as a delayed form that evolves over several days (250). Patients experience dyspnea, mild chest pain, and hemoptysis in the face of hyoxemia. Chest radiographs show bilateral central alveolar filling which can resolve over 24 to 48 hours. Tachycardia, tachypnea, fever, and leucocytosis can accompany the process. The acute form is most often seen after generalized tonic–clonic seizures; whereas, the delayed type of NPE usually follows head trauma (Table 16.12)(251–254).

There is a complex interaction of the CNS autonomic nervous system, mediated by neurotransmitters. The hypo-

Table 16.12   Nervous system insults and neurogenic pulmonary edema*

Seizures
Intracerebral hemorrhage
Subarachnoid hemorrhage
Cervical spinal cord injury
Head trauma
Cerebral air embolism
Vertebral artery ligation
Brain tumor
Guillain-Barré syndrome
Reye encephalopathy
Lesions of the medulla oblongata
Bulbar poliomyelitis

*References 244–258

thalamus and several loci within the medulla, particularly areas Al, A5, nuclei of tractus solitarius, and the area postrema have been implicated in the pathogenesis. There appears to be a pulmonary endothelial defect, resulting in high protein transvascular fluid flux and an increased pulmonary venoconstriction, all of which result in development of pulmonary edema (238–240).

A variety of nervous system lesions result in NPE, and increased intracranial pressure has been suggested as a common denominator. Correlations of intracranial and intravascular pressures and the clinical outcome have pointed to increased pulmonary vascular resistance as the most important predictor of outcome (255).

Neuromuscular Disorders

The hallmarks of neuromuscular disease include weakness, muscle cramps, fasciculations, and sensory abnormalities (256–258). The muscles of respiration are commonly involved, and weakness can occur as an acute and reversible process as in botulism and GBS or as a chronic irreversible process such as Duchenne muscular dystrophy or amyotrophic lateral sclerosis (259). The most prominent associated symptoms of neuromuscular diseases affecting respiration are dyspnea and respiratory distress.

Respiratory compromise can be worsened by development of skeletal abnormalities like scoliosis and rib deformity, resulting in reduced lung volume and proclivity for developing atelectasis. Moreover, recurrent aspiration can result in lung infiltrates and pneumonia. Somnolence, plethora, and impaired consciousness, as observed in CO_2 retention, is typically a late manifestation of respiratory fatigue (260,261).

Treatment is individualized and may include administration of antibiotics, immunosuppressive therapy, plasmapheresis, and surgery (thymectomy) as in the case of myasthenia gravis (262). Mechanical ventilation is often required, but its use is sometimes controversial in progressive neuromuscular diseases (250).

REFERENCES

1. Berger AJ, Mitchell RA, Severinghaus JW. Regulation of respiration. N Engl J Med 1977; 297:92–97,138–143, 194–201.
2. Bianki AL, Denavit-Saubiem. Neurogenesis of Central Respiratory Rhythms. Lancaster, England: MTP Press, 1985;25–471.
3. Dejours P. Chemoreflexes in breathing. Physiol Rev 1967; 42:335–358.
4. Fisher JT, Sant'Ambrogio G. Airway and lung receptors and their reflex effects in the newborn. Pediatr Pulmonol 1985; 1:112–126.
5. Widdicombe JG. Nervous receptors in the respiratory tract and lungs. In: Hornbein TF, ed. Regulation of Breathing; Vol. 1. New York: Marcel Dekker, 1987;429–472.
6. St. John WM. Central nervous system regulation of ventilation. In: Davies DG, Barnes CD, eds. Regulation of Ventilation and Gas Exchange. New York: Academic Press, 1978;1–30.
7. Rigatto H. A critical analysis of the development of peripheral and central respiratory chemosensitivity during the neonatal period. In: von Euler C, Lagercrantz H, eds. Central Nervous Control Mechanisms in Breathing. Oxford: Pergamon, 1979;137–148.
8. Mitchell RA, Berger A. Neural regulation of respiration. Am Rev Resp Dis 1975;111:206–224.
9. Chernick V. Endorphins and ventilatory control. N Engl J Med 1981;304:1227–1228.
10. Brandt NJ, Terenius L, Jacobsen BB, et al. Hyperendorphin syndrome in a child with necrotizing encephalomyelopathy. N Engl J Med 1980;303:914–916.
11. Davis GM, Bureau MA. Pulmonary and chest wall mechanics in the control of respiration in the newborn. Clin Perinatol 1987;14:551–579.
12. Kalia MP. Anatomical organization of central respiratory neurons. Am Rev Physiol 1981;43:105–20.
13. Karczewski WA. Organization of the brain stem respiratory complex. In: Widdicombe JG, ed. MTP International Review of Science: Ser I. Physiology; Vol. 2. Baltimore: University Park Press, 1974;197–219.
14. Remmers J, Bartlett D. Reflex control of expiratory airflow and duration. J Appl Physiol 1977;42:80–87.
15. Mitchell RA, Berger AJ. Neural regulation of respiration. In: Hornbein TF, ed. Regulation of Breathing; Vol. 2. New York: Marcel Dekker, 1981;541–620.
16. Mueller RA, Landberg D, Breese G, et al. The neuropharmacology of respiratory control. Pharmacol Rev 1982; 34: 255–78.
17. Plum F. Neurological integration of behavioral and metabolic control of breathing. In: Porter R, ed. Breathing: Hering Breuer Centenary Symposium. London: Churchill-Livingstone, 1970;159–175.
18. Plum F, Leigh RJ. Abnormalities of central mechanisms. In: Hornbein TF, ed. Regulation of Breathing; Vol. 2. New York: Marcel Dekker, 1981;989-1067.
19. North JB, Jennett S. Abnormal breathing patterns associated with acute brain damage. Arch Neurol 1974;31: 338–344.
20. Cohen MI. Neurogenesis of respiratory rhythm in the mammal. Physiol Rev 1979;59:1105–1173.
21. Dawes GS, Gardner WM, Johnston BM, et al. Breathing in fetal lambs: The effect of brainstem section. J Physiol (Lond) 1983;355:535–553.
22. Polgar G, Weng TR. The functional development of the respiratory system. Am Rev Respir Dis 1979;120:625–637.
23. Purves D, Lichtman JW. Principles of Neural Development. Sunderland, MA: Sinauer Association, 1985;435.
24. Simon RP. Respiration. In: Asbury AK, McKhann GM, McDonald WI, eds. Diseases of the Nervous System; Vol. 1. Philadelphia: WB Saunders, 1986;651–664.
25. Von Euler C, Lagercrantz H, eds. Neurobiology of the Control of Breathing. New York: Raven Press, 1986.
26. Wyman RJ. Neural generation of the breathing rhythm. Ann Rev Physiol 1977;39:417–448.
27. Von Euler C. Brain stem mechanisms for generation and control of breathing pattern. In: Cherniach N, Widdicombe J, eds. Handbook of Physiology. Bethesda: American Society of Physiology, 1986;1–68.
28. Nelson DA, Ray CD. Respiratory arrest from seizure discharges in limbic system. Arch Neurol 1968;19:199–207.
29. Oren J, Kelly DH, Shannon DC. Long-term follow-up of children with congenital central hypoventilation syndrome. Pediatrics 1987;80:375–380.
30. Simon RP. Neurogenic pulmonary edema. Semin Neurol 1984;4:490–496.
31. Strang LB. Neonatal respiration. Physiological and Clinical Studies. London: Mosby, 1978.
32. Walker DW. Peripheral and central chemoreceptors in the fetus and newborn. Ann Rev Physiol 1984;46:687–703.
33. Blanco CE, Hanson MA, McCooke HB. Studies in utero of the mechanisms of chemoreceptor resetting. In: The Physiologic Development of the Fetus and the Newborn. London: Academic Press, 1985;639–641.
34. Bureau MA, Begin R. Postnatal maturation of the respiratory response to O_2 in awake newborn lambs. J Appl Physiol 1982;52:428–433.
35. Davis GM, Hobbs S, Bureau MA. Limitation of the ventilatory response to CO_2 in newborn lambs. Am Rev Respir Dis 1986;133Suppl:A136.
36. Guthrie RD, Sandaert TA, Hodson WA, et al. Development of CO_2 sensitivity: Effects of gestational age, postnatal age, and sleep state. J Appl Physiol 1981;50:956–961.
37. Lagercrantz H. Neuromodulators and respiratory control in the infant. Clin Perinatol 1987;14:683–695.
38. Long Se, Duffin J. The medullary respiratory neurons: A review. Can J Physiol Pharmacol 1984;62:161–182.
39. Rigatto H: Control of ventilation in the newborn. Ann Rev Physiol 1984;45:661–674.
40. Haddad GG, Mellins RB. Hypoxia and respiratory control in early life. Ann Rev Physiol 1984;46:629–643.
41. Rigatto H, Brady JP, Verduzco RT: Chemoreceptor reflexes in premature infants. I. The effect of gestational and postnatal age on the ventilatory response to inhalation of 100% and 15% oxygen. Pediatrics 1975;55:604–613.
42. Read DJC, Henderson-Smart DJ. Regulation of breathing in the newborn during different behavioral states. Ann Rev Physiol 1984;46:675–685.
43. Bryan AC, Bowes G, Maloney JE. Control of breathing in the fetus and neonate. In: Cherniack NS, Widdicombe JD, eds. Handbook of Physiology, Respiration, Control of Breathing. Baltimore: Williams & Wilkins, 1986;621–649.

44. Moss IR, Condorelli S, Scarpelli EM. Progressive onset of spontaneous and induced fetal breathing. Respir Physiol 1981;45:299–308.

45. Brazy JE, Kinney HC, Oakes WJ. Central nervous system structural lesions causing apnea at birth. J Pediatr 1987;111:163–175.

46. Broddy K, Dawes GS, Fisher R, et al. Fetal respiratory movements, electrocortical and cardiovascular response to hypoxia and hypercapnia in sheep. J Physiol (Lond) 1974;243:599–618.

47. Keens TG, Bryan AC, Levison H, et al. Developmental pattern of muscle fibre types in human ventilatory muscle. J Appl Physiol 1978;909–913.

48. Keens TG, Ianuzzo CD. Development of fatigue-resistant muscle fibres in human ventilatory musculature. Ann Rev Respir Dis 1979;119Suppl:139–141.

49. Silverstein A. ed. Neurological Complications of Therapy. Mount Kisco, NY: Futura, 1982.

50. Guyton AC. Textbook of medical physiology. Philadelphia: W. B. Saunders, 1976;516–529.

51. Rossen R, Kabat H, Anderson JP. Acute arrest of cerebral circulation in man. Arch Neurol Psychiatr 1943; 50: 510–528.

52. Weinberger LM, Gibbon MH, Gibbon JH, Jr. Temporary arrest of the circulation to the central nervous system. I. Physiologic effects. Arch Neurol Psychiatr 1940; 43:615–634.

53. Weinberger LM, Gibbon MH, Gibbon JH, Jr. Temporary arrest of the circulation to the central nervous system. II. Pathologic effects. Arch Neurol Psychiatr 1940;43:961–986.

54. Plum F, Posner JB, Hain RF. Delayed neurologic deterioration after anoxia. Arch Intern Med 1962;110:18–25.

55. Plum F, Posner JB. The diagnosis of stupor and coma. Philadelphia: F. A. Davis, 1980;177–304.

56. Austen FK, Carmichael MW, Adams RD. Neurologic manifestations of chronic pulmonary insufficiency. N Engl J Med 1957;257:579–590.

57. Posner JB, Swanson AG, Plum F. Acid base balance in cerebrospinal fluid. Arch Neurol 1965;12: 479–496.

58. Layzer RB: Neuromuscular manifestations of systemic disease, Philadelphia: F.A. Davis, 1985;47–78.

59. Konigsmark BW. Hereditary deafness in man (Part One). N Engl J Med 1969;281:713–719.

60. Melnick M. The etiology of external ear malformations and its relation to abnormalities of the middle ear, inner ear and other organ systems. Birth Defects 1980;26:303–331.

61. Pagon RA, Graham JM, Jr, Zonana J, et al. Coloboma, congenital heart disease and choanal atresia with multiple anomalies; CHARGE association. J Pediatr 1981; 99:223–227.

62. Rex AP, Preu SM. A diagnostic index for Down syndrome. J Pediatr 1982;100:903–906.

63. Hagerman RJ. The Fragile X syndrome. Curr Probl Pediatr 1987;17:625–674.

64. Bluestone CD. Recent advances in the pathogenesis, diagnosis and management of otitis media. Pediatr Clin North Am 1981;28:727–753.

65. Bergstrom L. Assessment and consequence of malformations of the middle ear. Birth Defects 1981;26:217–241.

66. DeMeyer W, Zeman W, Palmer CG. The face predicts the brain: Diagnostic significance of median facial anomalies for holoprosencephaly. Pediatrics 1964;34:256–263.

67. McFarlin DE, Strober W, Waldman TA. Ataxia-telangiectasia. Medicine 1972;51:281–314.

68. Wolf SM, Fauci AS, Horn RG, et al. Wegner's granulomatosis. Ann Intern Med 1974;81:513–525.

69. Wells RG, Sty JR, Landers D. Radiological evaluation of Pott Puffy tumor. JAMA 1986;255:1331–1333.

70. Wald ER, Pang D, Milmor GJ, et al. Sinusitis and its complications in the pediatric patient. Pediatr Clin North Am 1981;28:777–795.

71. Kocen RS, Lloyd JK, Lascelles PT, et al. Familial alphalipoprotein deficiency (Tangier disease) with neurological abnormalities. Lancet 1967;1:1341–1345.

72. Engel WK, Dorman JD, Levy RJ, et al. Neuropathy in Tangier disease: Alpha-lipoprotein deficiency manifesting as familial recurrent neuropathy and intestinal lipid storage. Arch Neurol 1967;17:1–9.

73. Hollinger D. Etiology of stridor in the neonate, infant and child. Ann Otorhinolaryngol 1980;89:397–400.

74. Quin-Bogard AL, Potsic WP. Stridor in the first year of life. The clinical evaluation of the persistant or intermittent noisy breather. Clin pediatr 1977;16:913–919.

75. Myerson MD, Toushee DR. Speech language and hearing in Moebius syndrome. Devel Med Child Neurol 1978; 20:357–365.

76. Henderson JL. The congenital facial diplegia syndrome. Clinical features, pathology and etiology. A review of sixty-one cases. Brain 1939;62:381–403.

77. Papasozomenos S, Roessmann U. Respiratory distress and Arnold-Chiari malformation. Neurology 1981;31: 97–100.

78. Hollinger PC, Hollinger LD, Reichert TJ, et al. Respiratory obstruction and apnea with bilateral abductor vocal cord paralysis with meningocele, hydrocephalus, and Arnold-Chiari malformation. J Pediatr 1978;92:368–373.

79. Brazy JE, Kinney HC, Oakes WJ. Central nervous system structural lesions causing apnea at birth. J Pediatr 1987; 111:163–175.

80. Cunningham MJ, Eavey RD, Shannon DC. Familial vocal cord dysfunction. Pediatrics 1985;76:750–753.

81. Rapin I, Ruben RJ. Patterns of anomalies in children with malformed ears. Laryngoscope 1976;86:1469–1502.

82. Quan L, Smith DW. The VATER association; vertebral defects, anal atresia, TE fistula with esophageal atresia, radial and renal dysplasia: A spectrum of associated defects. J Pediatr 1973;82:104–102.

83. Weaver DD, Mapstore CL, Yu P. The VATER association: Analysis of 46 patients. Am J Dis Child 1986;140:225–229.

84. Reale FR, Esterly JR. Pulmonary hypoplasia: A morphometric study of the lungs of infants with diaphragmatic hernia, anencephaly, and renal malformations. Pediatrics 1973;51:91–96.

85. Conney TP, Thurlbeck WM. Pulmonary hypoplasia in Down's syndrome. N Engl J Med 1982;307:1170–1173.

86. Rudolph RI. Pulmonary manifestations of tuberous sclerosis. Cutis 1981;27:82–84.

87. Hart MN, Earle KM. Hemorrhagic and perivenous encephalitis: A clinical-pathological review of 38 cases. J Neurosurg Psychiatry 1975;38:585–591.

88. Sriram S, Steinman L. Post-infectious and post vaccinal encephalomyelitis. Neurol Clin North Am 1984;2:341–353.

89. Reik L, Jr. Disorders that mimic CNS infections. Neurol Clin North Am 1986;4:223–248.

90. Asbury AK. Diagnostic considerations in Guillain-Barré syndrome. Ann Neurol 1981;9 Suppl:1–5.

91. The Guillain-Barré Study Group: Plasmapharesis and acute Guillain-Barré syndrome. Neurology 1985;35:1096–1104.

92. Kelly DH, Shannon DC. Neonatal and infantile apnea. In: Mulinsky A, Friedman E, Gluck L, eds. Advances in Perinatal Medicine; Vol. 1. New York: Plenum 1981;1–44.

93. Shannon DC, Kelly DH, O'Connell K. Abnormal regulation of ventilation in infants at high risk for sudden infant death syndrome. N Engl J Med 1977;297:747–750.

94. Clancy RR, Spitzer AR. Cerebral cortical function in infants at high risk for sudden infant death syndrome. Ann Neurol 1985;18:41–47.

95. Valdes-Dapena MA. Sudden infant death syndrome: A review of the medical literature 1974–1979. Pediatrics 1980;66:597–614.

96. Sadek D, Shannon DC, Abboud S, et al. Altered cardiac repolarization in some victims of sudden infant death syndrome. N Engl J Med 1987;317:1501–1505.

97. Shannon DC, Kelly DH. SIDS and near-SIDS. N Engl J Med 1982;306:959–965.

98. Myer EC, Morris DL, Adams ML, et al. Increased cerebrospinal fluid B-endorphin immunoreactivity in infants with apnea and in siblings of victims of sudden infant death syndrome. J Pediatr 1987;111:660–666.

99. Martin RJ, Miller MJ, Carlo WA. Pathogenesis of apnea in preterm infants. J Pediatr 1981;109:733–741.

100. Hunt CD, Brouillette RT. Sudden infant death syndrome: 1987 perspective. J Pediatr 1987;110:669–678.

101. Southall DP. Role of apnea in the sudden infant death syndrome: A personal view. Pediatrics 1988;80:73–84.

102. Northway WH, Rosan RC, Porter DO. Pulmonary disease following respiratory therapy of hyaline-membrane disease: Bronchopulmonary dysplasia. N Engl J Med 1967;276:357–368.

103. Northway WH. Observations on bronchopulmonary dysplasia. J Pediatr 1979;95:815–818.

104. Vohr BR, Bell EF, Oh W. Infants with bronchopulmonary dysplasia. Growth pattern and neurologic and developmental outcome. Am J Dis Child 1982;136:443–447.

105. Campbell LR, McAlister W, Volpe JJ. Neurologic aspects of bronchopulmonary dysplasia. Clin Pediatr 1988;27:7–13.

106. Meigs JR. A Practical Treatise on the Disease of Children. Philadelphia: Lindsay and Blakiston, 1848;417–418.

107. Livingston S. Breath-holding spells in children. Differentiation from epileptic attacks. JAMA 1970;212:2231–2235.

108. Lombroso CT, Lerman P. Breath-holding spells (cyanotic and pallid infantile syncope). Pediatrics 1967;39:563–581.

109. Gauk EW, Kidd L, Prichard JS. Mechanism of seizures associated with breath-holding spells. N Engl J Med 1963;268:1436–1441.

110. McWilliam RC, Stephenson JBP. Atropine treatment of reflex anoxic seizures. Arch Dis Child 1984;59:473–485.

111. Stephenson JBP. Reflex anoxic seizures and ocular compression. Devel Med Child Neurol 1980;22:380–383.

112. Southall DP, Lewis GM, Buchanan R, et al. Prolonged expiratory apnoea (cyanotic breath-holding) in association with a medullary tumor. Devel Med Child Neurol 1987;29:784–804.

113. American Academy of Pediatrics Section on Allergy and Immunology. Management of Asthma. Pediatrics 1981;68:874–879.

114. Kaliner M, Eggleston PA, Mathews KP. Rhinitis and asthma. JAMA 1987;258:2851–2873.

115. Kaliner M, Shelhamer JH, Davis PB, et al. Autonomic nervous system abnormalities in allergy. Ann Intern Med 1982;96:349–357.

116. Friedman R, Zitelli B, Jardine D, et al. Seizures in a patient receiving terbutaline. Am J Dis Child 1982;136:1091–1092.

117. DiMario FJ, Jr. Personal observation, unpublished data, 1987.

118. Kravis LP, Kolsig B. Unexplained death in childhood asthma. Am J Dis Child 1985;139:558–563.

119. Hopkins IJ, Shield LK. Poliomyelitis-like illness associated with asthma in childhood. Lancet 1974;1:76.

120. Nihei K, Naitoh H, Ikeda K. Poliomyelitis-like syndrome following asthmatic attack (Hopkins syndrome). Pediatr Neurol 1987;3:166–168.

121. Fauci AS. Vasculitis. J Allergy Clin Immunol 1983;72:211–223.

122. Chumbley LC, Harrison EG, Jr., DeRemee RA. Allergic granulomatosis and angiitis (Churg-Strauss syndrome) report and analysis of 30 cases. Mayo Clin Proc 1977;52:477–484.

123. Adams RD, Lyon G. Neurology of Hereditary Metabolic Diseases of Children, Bristol, PA: Hemisphere, 1982.

124. Wood RE, Boat TF, Doershuk CF. State of the art: Cystic fibrosis. Am Rev Respir Dis 1976;113:833–876.

125. DiSant'Aghese PA, Davis PB. Cystic fibrosis in adults: 75 cases and a review of 232 cases in the literature. Am J Med 1979;66:121–132.

126. Schwachman H, Kowalski M, Khaw KT. Cystic fibrosis: A new outlook. Medicine 1979;56:129–149.

127. Davis PB, Kaliner M. Autonomic nervous system abnormalities in cystic fibrosis. J Chron Dis 1983;36:269–279.

128. Spaide RF, Diamond G, D'Amico RA, et al. Ocular findings in cystic fibrosis. Am J Ophthalmol 1987;103:204–210.

129. Davis PG. Physiologic implications of the autonomic aberrations in cystic fibrosis. Horm Metab Res 1986;18:271–220.

130. Bye AME, Muller DPR, Wilson J, et al. Symptomatic vitamin E deficiency in cystic fibrosis. Arch Dis Child 1985;60:162–164.

131. Scott J, Elias E, Moult PJA, et al. Pancreatic rickets in adult cystic fibrosis with myopathy and proximal renal tubular dysfunction. Am J Med 1977;63:488–492.

132. Castile R, Shwachman H, Travis W, et al. Amyloidosis as a complication of cystic fibrosis. Am J Dis Child 1985;139:728–732.

133. Powars DR. Natural history of sickle cell disease—the first ten years. Semin Hematol 1975;12:267–285.

134. Oppenheimer EH, Esterly JR. Pulmonary changes in sickle cell disease. Am Rev Resp Dis 1971;3:858–859.

135. Ponez M, Kane E, Gill FM. Acute chest syndrome in sickle cell disease: Etiology and clinical correlation. J Pediatr 1985;107:861–866.

136. Moser KM, Shea JG. The relationship between pulmonary infarction, cor pulmonale and the sickle states. Am J Med 1957;22:561–579.

137. Sarnaik SA, Lusher JM. Neurologic complications of sickle cell anemia. Am J Pediatr Hematol Oncol 1982;4:386–394.

138. Powars D, Wilson B, Imbus C, et al. The natural history of stroke in sickle cell disease. Am J Med 1978;65:461–471.

139. Rothman SM, Nelson JS. Spinal cord infarction in a patient with sickle cell anemia. Neurology 1980;30:1072–1070.

140. Stockman JA, Nigro MA, Mishkin MM, et al. Occlusion of large cerebral vessels in sickle cell anemia. N Engl J Med 1972;287:846–849.

141. Overby MC, Rothman AS. Multiple intracranial aneurysms in sickle cell anemia. J Neurosurg 1985;62:430–484.

142. Van Hoff J, Ritchey AK, Shaywitz BA. Intracranial hemorrhage in children with sickle cell disease. Am J Dis Child 1985;139:1120–1123.

143. Haruda F, Friedman JH, Ganti SR, et al. Rapid resolution of organic mental syndrome in sickle cell anemia in response to exchange transfusion. Neurology 1981;31:1015–1016.

144. Condon PI, Whitelocke RAF, Bird AR, et al. Recurrent visual loss in homozygous sickle cell disease. Br J Ophthalmol 1985;69:700–706.

145. Strauss RG, Schubert WK, McAdams AJ. Amyloidosis in children. J Pediatr 1969;74:272–282.

146. Glenner GG, Terry WD, Isersky C. Amyloidosis: It's nature and pathogenesis. Semin Hematol 1973;10:65–86.

147. Kyle RA, Bayrd ED. Amyloidosis: Review of 236 cases. Medicine 1975;54:271–299.

148. Sohar E, Gafni J, Pras M, et al. Familial mediterranean fever. A survey of 470 cases and review of the literature. Am J Med 1967;43:227–253.

149. Pick AI, Versano I, Schreibman S, et al. Agammaglobulinemia, plasma cell dyscrasia and amyloidosis in a 12 year old child. Am J Dis Child 1977;131:682–686.

150. Gottlieb LS, Gold WM. Primary tracheobronchial amyloidosis: Am Rev Resp Dis 1972;105:425–429.

151. Kelly JJ, Kyle RA, O'Brien PC, et al. The natural history of peripheral neuropathy in primary systemic amyloidosis. Ann Neurol 1979;6:1–7.

152. Ringel SP, Claman HN. Amyloid associated muscle hypertrophy. Arch Neurol 1982;39:413–417.

153. Bheme RS, Wolff SM. The Chediak-Higashi syndrome: Studies in four patients and a review of the literature. Medicine 1972; 51:247–280.

154. Lockman LA, Kennedy WE, White JG. The Chediak-Higashi syndrome: Electrophysiological and electron microscopic observations on the peripheral neuropathy. J Pediatr 1967;70:942–951.

155. Pettit PE, Berdal KR. Chediak-Higashi syndrome: Neurologic appearance. Arch Neurol 1984;41:1001–1002.

156. McGovern JP, Merritt DH. Sarcoidosis in childhood. Adv Pediatr 1956;8:97–135.

157. Jasper PL, Denny FW. Sarcoidosis in children with special emphasis on natural history and treatment. J Pediatr 1968;73:499–512.

158. Kendel FA, Moschella SL. Sarcoidosis: An updated review. J Am Acad Dermatol 1984;11:1–19.

159. Weinberg S, Bennett H, Weinstock I. Central nervous system manifestations of sarcoid in children. Clin Pediatr 1983;22:477–481.

160. Camp WA. Sarcoid of the central nervous system. Arch Neurol 1962;7:432–441.

161. Kataria S, Trevathan GE, Holland JE, et al. Ocular presentation of sarcoid in children. Clin Pediatr 1983;22:793–797.

162. Gardner-Thorpe C. Muscle weakness due to sarcoid myopathy. Neurology 1972;22:917–928.

163. Nesbit ME Jr, Krivit W. Histiocytosis. In: Bloom HJG, Lemerle J, Neidhardt MR, et al. Cancer in Children: Clinical Management. Berlin: Springer-Verlag, 1975;193–199.

164. Nezelof C, Frileux-Herbet F, Cronier-Sachot J. Disseminated histiocytosis-X. Analysis of prognostic factors based on a retrospective study of 50 cases. Cancer 1979;44:1824–1838.

165. Lahey MW. Histiocytosis-X, an analysis of prognostic factors. J Pediatr 1975;87:184–189.

166. Adornato BT, Eil C, Head GL, et al. Cerebellar involvement in multifocal eosinophilic granuloma: Demonstrated by computerized tomographic scanning. Ann Neurol 1980;7:125–129.

167. Hewlett RH, Ganz JC. Histiocytosis-X of the cauda equina. Neurology 1976;26:472–476.

168. Hodgson CH, Kaye RE. Pulmonary arteriovenous fistula and hereditary hemorrhagic telangiectasia: A review and report of 35 cases of fistula. Dis Chest 1963;43:449–455.

169. Jacobson G, Krause U. Hereditary hemorrhagic telangiectasia localized to the gastrointestinal tract. Scand J Gastroenterol 1970;5:283–288.

170. DeCenzo JM, Morrisseau PM, Marrocco G. Osler-Weber-Rendu syndrome. Urologists View. Urology 1975;5:549–552.

171. Sobel D, Norman D. CNS manifestations of hereditary hemorrhagic telangiectasia. AJNR 1984;5:569–573.

172. Roman G, Fisher M, Perl DP, et al. Neurological manifestations of hereditary hemorrhagic telangiectasia (Rendu-Osler-Weber disease): Report of 2 cases and review of the literature. Ann Neurol 1978;4:130–144.

173. Lande A, Bedford A, Schechter LS. The spectrum of arteriographic findings in Osler-Weber-Rendu disease. Angiology 1976;27:223–240.

174. Hewes RC, Auster M, White RI Jr. Cerebral embolism—first manifestation of pulmonary arteriovenous malformation in patients with hereditary hemorrhagic telangiectasia. Cardiovasc Intervent Radiol 1985;8:151–155.

175. Hartman GE, Shochat SJ. Primary pulmonary neoplasms of childhood: A review. Ann Thorac Surg 1983;36:108–119.

176. Sawyer KC, Sawyer RB, Lubchenco AE, et al. Fatal primary cancer of the lung in a teenage smoker. Cancer 1967;20:451–457.

177. Brody JS: Clinicopathological case: 4–1976. N Engl J Med 1976;294:210–217.

178. Grundy GW, Miller RW. Malignant mesothelioma in childhood. Cancer 1972;30:1216–1218.

179. Ownby D, Lyon G, Spock A. Primary leiomyosarcoma of the lung in childhood. Am J Dis Child 1976;130:1132–1133.

180. Cassidy JT. Textbook of Pediatric Rheumatology. New York: John Wiley, 1982.

181. Eisenberg H. The interstitial lung disease associated with the collagen-vascular disorders. In: Fulmer JD, ed. Clin Chest Med. Philadelphia: W.B. Saunders, 1982;3:565–578.

182. Dreisim RB. Pulmonary vasculitis. In: Fulmer JD, ed. Clin chest med. Philadelphia: W.B. Saunders, 1982;3:602–618.

183. Schaller JG. Juvenile rheumatoid arthritis; Series 1. Arthritis Rheum 1977;20:165–170.

184. Stillman JS, Barry PE. Juvenile rheumatoid arthritis; Series 2. Arthritis Rheum 1977;20:171–175.

185. Calabro JJ. Other extra-articular manifestations of juvenile rheumatoid arthritis. Arthritis Rheum 1977;20:237–240.

186. Jordan JD, Snyder CH. Rheumatoid disease of the lung and cor pulmonale. Observations in a child. Am J Dis Child 1964;108:174–180.

187. Wagener JS, Taussig LM, DeBenedetti C, et al. Pulmonary function in juvenile rheumatoid arthritis. J Pediatr 1981;99:108–110.

188. Jan JE, Hill RH, Low MD. Cerebral complications in juvenile rheumatoid arthritis. Can Med Assoc J 1972;107:623–625.

189. Chylack LT Jr. The ocular manifestations of juvenile rheumatoid arthritis. Arthritis Rheum 1977;20:271–273.

190. Schaller JG. Ankylosing spondylitis of childhood onset. Arthritis Rheum 1977;20:398–401.

191. Rosen EL, Strimlan CV, Mukm JR, et al. Pleuropulmonary manifestations of ankylosing spondylitis. Mayo Clin Proc 1977;52:641–649.

192. Reid GD. Atlantoaxial subluxation in juvenile ankylosing spondylitis. J Pediatr 1978;93:531–532.

193. King KK, Kornreich HK, Bernstein BH, et al. The clinical spectrum of systemic lupus erythematosus in childhood. Arthritis Rheum 1977;20:287–294.

194. Alarcon-Segovia D, Alarcon DG. Pleuropulmonary manifestations of systemic lupus erythematosus. Dis of Chest 1961;39:7–17.

195. Yancey CL, Doughty RA, Athreya BH. Central nervous system involvement in childhood systemic lupus erythematosus. Arthritis Rheum 1981;24:1389–1395.

196. Tsokos CC, Noutsopoulos HM, Steinberg AD. Muscle involvement in systemic lupus erythematosus. JAMA 1981;246:766–768.

197. Pachman LM, Cooke N. Juvenile dermatomyositis: A clinical and immunologic study. J Pediatr 1980;96:226–234.

198. Park S, Nyhan WL. Fatal pulmonary involvement in dermatomyositis. Am J Dis Child 1975;129:723–726.

199. Olsen GN, Swanson EW. Polymyositis and interstitial lung disease. Am Rev Resp Dis 1972;105:611–617.

200. Sullivan DB, Cassidy JT, Petty RE. Dermatomyositis in the pediatric patient. Arthritis Rheum 1977;20:327–331.

201. Miller JJ. Late progression in dermatomyositis. J Pediatr 1973;83:543–548.

202. Cassidy JT, Sullivan DB, Dabich L, et al. Scleroderma in children. Arthritis Rheum 1977;20:351–354.

203. Weaver AL, Divertie MB, Titus JL. Pulmonary scleroderma. Dis Chest 1968;54:4–12.

204. Kornreich HK, King KK, Berstein GH, et al. Scleroderma in childhood. Arthritis Rheum 1977;20:343–350.

205. Singsen BH, Bernstein BH, Kornreich HK, et al. Mixed connective tissue disease in childhood. J Pediatr 1977;90:893–900.

206. Singsen BH. Mixed connective tissue disease in childhood. Ped Rev 1986;17:309–314.

207. Mattioli M, Reichlin M. Physical association of two nuclear antigens and the mutual occurence of their antibodies: The relationship of the SM and the RNP protein (Mo) systems in SLE sera. J Immunol 1973;110:1318–1324.

208. Kawasaki T, Kosaki F, Okawa S, et al. A new infantile acute febrile mucocutaneous lymph node syndrome (MLNS) prevailing in Japan. Pediatrics 1974;54:273–276.

209. Melish ME, Hicks RV, Reddy V. Kawasaki syndrome: An update. Hosp Pract 1982;3:99–106.

210. Amano S, Hazama F. Neural involvement in Kawasaki disease. Acta Pathol Jpn 1980;30:365–373.

211. Hicks RV, Melish ME. Kawasaki syndrome. Pediatr Clin North Am 1986;33:1151–1175.

212. Tamaka N, Seikimoto K, Naoe S. Kawasaki disease relationship to infantile periarteritis nodosa. Arch Pathol Lab Med 1976;100:81–86.

213. Lapointe JS, Nugent RA, Graeb DA, et al. Cerebral infection and regression of widespread aneurysms in Kawasaki syndrome: Case report. Pediatr Radiol 1984;14:1–5.

214. Emery H, Larter W, Schaller JG. Henoch-Schönlein vasculitis. Arthritis Rheum 1977;20:385–388.

215. Silber DL. Henoch-Schönlein syndrome. Pediatr Clin North Am 1972;19:1061–1070.

216. Belman AL, Leicher CR, Moshe' SL, et al. Neurologic manifestations of Schöenlein-Henoch purpura: Report of three cases and review of the literature. Pediatrics 1985;75:687–692.

217. Reimold EW, Weinberg AG, Fink CW, et al. Polyarteritis in children. Am J Dis Child 1976;130:534–541.

218. Magilary DB, Petty RE, Cassidy JT, et al. A syndrome of childhood polyarteritis. J Pediatr 1977;91:25–30.

219. Wolff Sm, Fauci AS, Horm RG, et al. Wegener's granulomatosis. Ann Intern Med 1974;81:513–525.

220. Fauci AS, Haynes DB, Katz P, et al. Wegener's granulomatosis: Prospective clinical and therapeutic experience with 85 patients for 21 years. Ann Intern Med 1983;98:76–85.

221. Hall SI, Miller LC, Duggan E, et al. Wegener's granulomatosis in pediatric patients. J Pediatr 1985;106:739–744.

222. Mundy TM, Miller JJ III. Behçet's disease presenting as chronic aphthous stomatitis in a child. Pediatrics 1978;62:205–207.

223. Ammann AJ, Johnson A, Gyfe GA, et al. Behçet's syndrome. J Pediatr 1985;107:41–43.

224. Bollinger MS, Menkes HA, Benjamin JJ, et al. The syndrome of rhythmic palatal myoclonus: A cause of significant extrathoracic airway obstruction. Am Rev Resp Dis 1974;110:803–806.

225. Hagberg B, Aicardi J, Dias K, et al. A progressive syndrome of autism, dementia, ataxia, and loss of purposeful hand use in girls: Rett's syndrome: Report of 35 cases. Ann Neurol 1983;14:471–479.

226. Suzuki H, Natsuzaka T, Hirayama T, et al. Rett's syndrome: Progression of symptoms from infancy to childhood. J Child Neurol 1986;1:137–141.

227. The Rett Syndrome Diagnostic Criteria Work Group: Diagnostic criteria for Rett syndrome. Ann Neurol 1988;23:425–428.

228. Zoghbi HY, Perez AK, Glaze DG, et al. Reduction of biogenic amine levels in the Rett syndrome. N Engl J Med 1985;313:921–924.

229. Perry TL, Dunn HG, Ho HH, et al. Cerebrospinal fluid values for monoamine metabolites, γ-aminobutyric acid, and other amino compounds in Rett syndrome. J Pediatr 1988;112:234–238.

230. Cohen ME, Duffner PK. Brain tumors in children. Principles of Diagnosis and Treatment. New York: Raven press, 1984.

231. Klein M, Festa R. Central nervous system malignancies. In: Langkowsky P, ed. Pediatric Oncology: New York: McGraw-Hill, 1984.

232. Glasauer FE, Yuan RHP. Intracranial tumors with extracranial metastases. Case report and review of the literature. J Neurosurg 1963;20:474–493.

233. Brander WL, Turner DR. Extracranial metastases from a glioma in the absence of surgical intervention. J Neurol Neurosurg Psychiatry 1975;38:1133–1135.

234. Vannucci RC, Baten M. Cerebral Metastatic disease in childhood. Neurology 1974;24:981–985.

235. Ludwin SK, Rubinstein LJ, Russel DS. Papillary meningioma: A malignant variant of meningioma. Cancer 1975;36:1363–1373.

236. Brooks LJ, Afshani E, Hidalgo C, et al. Clivus chordoma with pulmonary metastases appearing as failure to thrive. Am J Dis Child 1981;135:713–715.

237. Shanies HM. Noncardiogenic pulmonary edema. Med Clin North Am 1977;61:1319–1337.

238. Colice GL. Neurogenic pulmonary edema. In: Mattaq MA, ed. Clin Chest Med. Philadelphia: W.B. Saunders, 1985;6:473–489.

239. Colice GL, Matthay MA, Bass E, Matthay RA. Neurogenic pulmonary edema. Am Rev Respir Dis 1984;130:941–948.

240. Simon RP. Neurogenic pulmonary edema. Semin Neurol 1984;4:490–496.

241. Mulroy JJ, Mickell JJ, Tong TK, et al. Postictal pulmonary edema in children. Neurology 1988;35:403–405.

242. Terrence CF, Rao GR, Perper JA. Neurogenic pulmonary edema in unexpected, unexplained death of epileptic patients. Ann Neurol 1981;9:458–464.

243. Carlson RW, Schaeffer RC, Michaels SG, et al. Pulmonary edema following intracranial hemorrhage. Chest 1979;75:731–734.

244. Fein IA, Rackow EC. Neurogenic pulmonary edema. Chest 1982;81:318–320.

245. Poe RH, Reisman JL, Rodenhouse RG. Pulmonary edema in cervical spinal cord injury. J Trauma 1978;18:71–73.

246. Baigelman W, O'Brien JC. Pulmonary effects of head trauma. Neurosurgery 1981;9:729–740.

247. Rittenhouse EA, Merendino KA. Acute pulmonary edema in the absence of left ventricular failure. Circulation 1969;40:823–827.

248. Waters HR, Gooding MR. Pulmonary edema following vertebral artery ligation. Anaesthesia 1972;27:450–453.

249. Felman AH. Neurogenic pulmonary edema. AJR 1971;112:393–396.

250. Bredin DP. Guillain-Barré syndrome: The unresolved cardiovascular problems. Ir J Med Sci 1977;146:273–279.

251. Lansky LL, Linn CR, Mathewson HS, et al. Neurogenic pulmonary edema and intracranial pressure monitoring in severe Reye syndrome. Ann Neurol 1978;9:191, 1978.

252. Schlesinger B. Neurogenic pulmonary edema due to puncture wound of the medulla oblongata. J Nerv Ment Dis 1945;102:247–255.

253. Brown RH Jr, Beyerl BD, Iseke R, et al. Medulla oblongata edema associated with neurogenic pulmonary edema. J Neurosurg 1986;64:494–500.

254. Baker AB. Poliomyelitis: A study of pulmonary edema. Neurology 1957;7:743–751.

255. Popp JA, Gottlieb ME, Paloski WH, et al. Cardiopulmonary hemodynamics in patients with serious head injury. J Surg Res 1982;32:416–421.

256. Brooke MH. A clinician's view of neuromuscular disease. Baltimore: Williams & Wilkins, 1986.

257. Fenichel G, Swaiman KF, Wright FS. Neuromuscular disease. In: Swaiman KF, Wright FS, eds. The Practice of Pediatric Neurology. St. Louis: C.V. Mosby, 1982;1139–1294.

258. Lewis DW, Berman PH. Progressive weakness in infancy and childhood. Pediatr Rev 1987;43:189–197.

259. Serisier DE, Mastaglia FL, Gibson GJ. Respiratory muscle function and ventilatory control. I. In patients with motor neuron disease. II. In patients with myotonic dystrophy. Q J Med 1982;202:205–226.

260. Roussos CS, Macklem PT. Diaphragmatic fatigue in man. J Appl Physiol 1977;43:189–197.

261. Rochester DF, Findley LJ. The lungs and neuromuscular and chest wall diseases. In: Murray JF, Nadel JA, eds. Textbook of respiratory medicine. Philadelphia: W.B. Saunders, 1988;1942–1971.

262. Braum SR, Sufit RL, Giovannoni BA, et al. Intermittent negative pressure ventilation in the treatment of respiratory failure in progressive neuromuscular disease. Neurology 1987;37:1874–1875.

Chapter 17
Neurologic Manifestations of Renal Disease

Martin S. Polinsky

Central and peripheral nervous system dysfunction is responsible for substantial morbidity in patients with severe chronic renal failure (1–3), and it becomes increasingly prevalent as the glomerular filtration rate (GFR) decreases below 5 mL/min/1.73 m^2, the level of function which defines end stage renal disease (ESRD). It is at this degree of renal insufficiency that the need generally arises to initiate maintenance dialysis or perform renal transplantation, in lieu of continuing conservative management with dietary and drug therapy. Adequate dialysis and successful renal transplantation usually result in stabilization or improvement of ESRD-related neurologic dysfunction; yet, both treatment modalities can interfere with nervous system function in unique and clinically significant ways. While the prevalence and severity of the disturbances tend to vary with patient age and the premorbid state of the nervous system (4), their clinical features and management are similar in adults and children. This chapter will review the neurologic manifestations attributable to acute and chronic renal failure (ARF, CRF) in children, adolescents, and in adults, where relevant, including those resulting from complications of ESRD therapy with drugs, dialysis, and transplantation. These manifestations comprise the syndromes of uremic, hypertensive, and drug- and aluminum-induced encephalopathy, and peripheral and cranial neuropathies.

NEUROLOGIC COMPLICATIONS OF ACUTE AND CHRONIC RENAL FAILURE

Uremic Encephalopathy

Uremia (Gr. ouron, urine; haima, blood—'urine in the blood') can be defined as a state of systemic intoxication "caused by severe glomerular insufficiency associated with disturbances in tubular and endocrine functions of the kidney. It is characterized by retention of toxic metabolites derived mainly from protein metabolism associated with changes in volume and electrolyte composition of the body fluids and excess or deficiency of various hormones" (5).

Pathogenesis

The pathogenesis of uremic encephalopathy is incompletely understood, although a variety of biochemical, metabolic, and physiologic disturbances have been observed in the brains of humans studied both ante- and postmortem and in experimental animal models of ARF and CRF. Cerebral energy metabolism is abnormal, as evidenced by the decreased oxygen and glucose consumption measured in adults with ESRD (6) and in crude homogenates of uremic rat brain (7). The utilization of high energy phosphate is also decreased in rats and dogs with acute and chronic uremia, whose cerebral adenosine triphosphate (ATP), creatine kinase, and glucose stores were found to be normal to increased, while the levels of their respective metabolites, adenosine diphosphate (ADP), adenosine monophosphate (AMP), and creatine, were normal or low (7,8). Total brain energy stores, energy charge, and redox state were normal, however, indicating that lower energy consumption resulted from decreased demand instead of limited supply (8).

The permeability of the blood-brain barrier to various electrolytes, organic acids, and sugars, is also abnormal in uremia so that the rates of entry of ^{42}K, ^{35}SO$_4$, ^{14}C inulin, and ^{14}C sucrose are all increased, while those of ^{24}Na and ^{14}C penicillin are diminished (9–11). Brain and cerebrospinal fluid (CSF) urea nitrogen and osmolality are increased in ARF and CRF (12,13), but in proportion to the corresponding changes in their plasma levels, so that water content is normal and cerebral edema does not occur (10,12,13). This is consistent with observations made by computed tomography (CT) that cerebral density measurements are normal in adults with ESRD prior to initiation of maintenance dialysis (14). Early studies in rats (7,10) indicated that the activity of whole brain Na, K activated ATPase was normal in uremia. A decrease in the activity of this enzyme in uremia, however, was subsequently reported by Minkoff et al.(15). This has recently been confirmed by Fraser et al.(16), who demonstrated that veratridine-stimulated sodium transport is increased in cerebral synaptosomes from uremic rats.

The electrolyte content and pH of uremic brain and CSF are normal except for an increase in the calcium content of the cerebral cortex and hypothalamus, as shown in dogs with ARF and CRF (12,13,17,18); the latter was also identified in the brains of four adults who died with CRF and secondary hyperparathyroidism (HPTH) (19). Cerebral subcortical and basal ganglia calcifications were also identified by CT in a 5-year-old boy with Down syndrome and severe secondary HPTH (20). The observed elevations of brain calcium content in the animals were at least partly dependent upon the presence of concomitant secondary HPTH, as was the excessive slowing of their electroencephalogram (EEG) background rhythms (18); moreover, when parathyroidectomy was performed prior to induction of uremia, the EEG remained normal (18). Finally, in adults with ARF and CRF, comparable slowing of the EEG background rhythm resolved following either recovery or subtotal parathyroidectomy (21). Thus, parathyroid hormone (PTH) can be responsible for some disturbances of brain function and composition that are seen in humans and in experimental models of uremia, although arguments to the contrary have also been proposed (22).

Finally, disturbances in cerebral amino acid metabolism and associated neurotransmitter levels have been reported (23,24). Concentrations of gamma-amino butyric acid (GABA) are low (23,24) while those of dopamine and serotonin are elevated (25). Cerebral uptake of glutamine, a GABA precursor, is diminished, along with that of valine and isoleucine, while glycine and 1/2 cystine extraction is increased (23). It has been suggested that the disordered balance between these stimulatory and inhibitory neurotransmitters and their amino acid precursors may contribute to the development of cognitive and motor dysfunction in uremia (25). Nonetheless, the true significance of these observations regarding the pathogenesis of uremic encephalopathy is not known.

Pathologic Changes

No pathologic lesions have been identified as being uniquely characteristic of uremic encephalopathy. The histologic changes present in the brains of 104 patients dying of terminal uremia were described by Olsen (26) and included: focal neuronal degeneration, most prominent in the cerebral cortex, brain stem sensory nuclei, and reticular formation in all patients; acute necrosis of the granular layer of the cerebellar cortex in 62 of 104 (59.6%); necrotic foci scattered through the pons and corpus striatum in 23 of 104 (22.1%); and focal glial proliferation in 6 of 104 (5.8%). Changes were nonspecific and frequently could be attributed to superimposed insults; for example, peripheral vascular collapse, severe hypertension, atherosclerosis, infection, diabetes mellitus, or anoxia. No clinicopathologic correlations could be established. Olsen's failure to identify a specific anatomic lesion, however, is nonetheless consistent with the fact that most or all of the cognitive, motor, and electrophysiologic disturbances seen in patients with uremic encephalopathy are reversible with adequate dialysis or renal transplantation.

Cerebral atrophy has been identified in adults and children with ESRD by CT (27–30) and appears to be most pronounced in children and young adults (27,28) in whom an inverse linear relationship between degree of atrophy and patient age has been shown (27). The majority of patients were asymptomatic, and significant relationships could not be established between the degree of atrophy and either the duration of CRF or dialysis or a history of prior steroid therapy. Patients with cerebral atrophy, however, tended to have received maintenance dialysis for a longer time; those patients without cerebral atrophy tended to have had a previously functioning allograft for a greater period of time (29,30). Moreover, cerebral atrophy in some children has been identified during evaluation for symptomatic aluminum intoxication or other causes of progressive encephalopathy associated with severe CRF in early life (29,31–37)(vide infra). Cerebral atrophy, therefore, appears to be a relatively common finding in patients with ESRD, the etiology of which is probably multifactorial (29). As an isolated finding, its significance regarding the pathogenesis of uremic encephalopathy remains unclear.

Clinical Manifestations

The clinical manifestations of uremic encephalopathy include disturbances of cognitive and motor function and are usually accompanied by characteristic electrophysiologic abnormalities. The precise nature and severity of the clinical features, however, can vary, depending on the rate at which renal insufficiency progresses (2,38) and the patient's premorbid personality (39). Thus, while typical cognitive disturbances are common at GFR's below 10 mL/min and in association with blood urea nitrogen (BUN) concentrations to greater than 250 to 300 mg/dL (40,41), they have also developed in a patient whose BUN was only 48 mg/dL (42). In this regard, it is important to note that clinical manifestations of ARF and CRF do not differ qualitatively, but tend to be more severe, and to develop more rapidly, and at relatively lower levels of BUN in the former condition (2,38).

Disturbances of Cognition. As encephalopathy develops, cognitive dysfunction is initially manifested as clouding of consciousness (sensorial clouding)(43), characterized by a "reduced clarity of awareness of the environment with reduced capacity to shift, focus, and sustain attention to environmental stimuli" (44). Patients typically exhibit episodes of apathy, preoccupation, and fatigue, which alternate with periods of relatively normal reactivity, making early diagnosis more difficult. As the disease progresses, however, concentration and attention span become more consistently affected (2,3,43,45) and can be identified by the patient's inability to perform repetitive mental arithmetic, (for example, subtracting serial 7's), (2,43) and by a reduced speed of decision making (46). The latter may be quantitatively assessed with the Choice Reaction Time test (CRT) and Continuous Performance Task (CPT), which are measures of sustained and selective attention (vigilance). Performance on these tests has been shown to correlate significantly with the level of renal insufficiency in adults (46) but not in children (47).

The appearance of deficits in recent memory indicates a more advanced stage of encephalopathy, as does the presence of more severe personality changes such as petulance and a refusal to cooperate (2,43). Much later, remote memory fails. With further progression, episodes of lucid behavior become less frequent; confusion and disorientation become more persistent and are followed by progression to lethargy, stupor, and ultimately, coma (2). If dialysis is not instituted, respiratory depression supervenes; Kussmaul breathing appears, followed by Cheyne-Stokes respiration and then apnea (39).

Patients with uremic encephalopathy can also present with the clinical features of delirium or toxic psychosis (2,43), particularly when renal functional deterioration has occurred rapidly, as in developing ARF. In such situations, visual hallucinations, agitation, and slurred speech can predominate; the latter can also be caused by drug intoxication that must be ruled out.

Cognitive performance has been assessed in clinically stable, conservatively managed children and adolescents with severe CRF and ESRD (47–53). Of 34 children with moderate-to-severe CRF who were managed conservatively with dietary restriction and medication for 5 to 19 (mean 7.3) years, psychomotor development was found to be normal by school performance in 31 (91.2%)(47). More objective assessments of visuoanalytic and general intellectual functioning, using the Wechsler Intelligence Scale for Children (WISC-R) and the Raven's Progressive Coloured Matrices, have yielded results in the average range, and not significantly different from controls matched for age, sex, and level of parental education (47,52). Children and adolescents with ESRD, however, tended to perform more poorly than controls on tests of vigilance (CPT), memory, and distractibility (Auditory Consonant Trigrams Tasks)(52,53). Furthermore, performance on the latter two sets of studies were significantly correlated, suggesting that memory disturbances seen in the children with ESRD were related in part to a deficit in attention span (52).

In these studies, quantitative correlations between levels of residual renal function and cognitive performance could not be established, as had been done previously in adults (46). Nonetheless, linear regression analysis showed a tendency for lesser degrees of impairment to be present in children who were older at the time of onset of renal insufficiency and who had had the disease for fewer years (50). This has been substantiated by Crittenden et al. (51), who noted that median IQ scores of children who experienced onset of CRF prior to 1 year of age were lower than those of patients whose diagnoses were made after the age of 3 years. In this regard, a recent literature survey (54) summarized results of 95 neurodevelopmental assessments performed in 85 children with severe CRF from infancy and showed that: microcephaly was present in 33 of 51 patients (64.7%); mild delay in one or more areas of development was present in 60 of 95 (63.2%); of 20 patients evaluated prior to 1 year of age, 17 (85%) were at least mildly delayed; gross motor and language development were most consistently affected. Patients at greatest risk for occurrence of developmental delay appear to be those in whom severe reductions in GFR occur (less than 10% to 15% of normal) within the first 2 months of life (34,35,55,56). The precise level of GFR at which specific cognitive functions first become impaired in infants and children remains to be determined.

A number of factors known to complicate the course of severe CRF may contribute to temporary or permanent cognitive dysfunction in affected children. Undernutrition is a major problem in pediatric renal patients (57,58) and may interfere with brain growth during the critical period of glial proliferation in early infancy (59–62). The problems noted above with severe secondary HPTH, as well as aluminum intoxication (vide infra), chronic anemia, the depressant effects of anticonvulsant medications (63) and the psychosocial consequences of severe CRF for patients and parents, (54) may also interfere with normal infant and early childhood development.

Motor Disturbances. Disturbances of motor function are invariably present as uremic encephalopathy progresses including: muscle cramps, increased neuromuscular excitability, myopathy, weakness, and seizures (Table 17.1). Early manifestations include muscle cramps, tremor, and asterixis. Tremor, the earliest of these findings, is a sensitive indicator of developing encephalopathy (43) and is an action and postural tremor, usually exacerbated by attempts to elicit asterixis. First described in 1949, asterixis is a sudden and dramatic lapse of position that is accompanied by electrical silence on the electromyogram (EMG) and as such, is not a movement disorder (43,64). It must be elicited (that is, it does not generally appear during routine activity) and can be demonstrated at the wrist or ankle (45). The development of asterixis usually coincides with

Table 17.1 Motor disturbances in ESRD*

Disturbance	Clinical Setting	Etiology
1. Muscle cramps	"Early" Uremic Encephalopathy	Decreased muscle intracellular pH.(2) Fluid shift into muscle cells.(62) Effects of uremic toxins.(62)
2. Muscle tremor	"Early" Uremic Encephalopathy	"Increased CNS irritability."(62)
3. Asterixis	"Early" Uremic Encephalopathy	"Diffuse CNS dysfunction of a metabolic nature."(62)
4. Myoclonus	"Advanced" Uremic Encephalopathy	"Diffuse neuronal dysfunction." (2) Elevated blood, neuronal urea concentrations.(3)
5. Fasciculations	"Advanced" Uremic Encephalopathy	Elevated CSF K^+:Ca^{++} ratio.(2) Elevated CSF P_4^{-3} concentration.(2)
6. Distal muscle weakness, wasting	Advanced Peripheral Neuropathy (GFR $\leq$ 5–13 mL/min/1.73m(2))	Multiple uremic toxins implicated.(176)
7. Proximal muscle weakness, wasting	(a) Severe Secondary Hyperparathyroidism	Skeletal muscle ischemia due to circumferential medial arteriolar calcinosis and intimal fibrosis.(66,67)

	(b) Primary Polymyopathy
	  (i) Mild (weakness only)
	  (ii) Severe
		Nonspecific, minor changes on muscle biopsy.(2)
		Skeletal muscle ischemia due to luminal arteriolar phospholipid deposition.

	(c) Hemodialysis patients with osteomalacia and multiple bone fractures	Aluminum accumulation in bone.(69)

*Modified with permission from Fine RN., Gruskin AB. ESRD in Children. Philadelphia: W.B. Saunders, 1984.

the appearance of sensorial clouding in uremic encephalopathy; however, it can be seen with other metabolic disorders as well (64). Muscle cramps typically affect the distal extremities (65) and initially occur at night but subsequently extend into waking hours. They ultimately tend to disappear as uremia progresses (2) but can be worsened by marked volume overload.

Myoclonus and muscle fasciculations are present in advanced encephalopathy. Uremic myoclonus is typically multifocal and stimulus-sensitive and is believed to originate in the brain stem reticular formation (reticular reflex myoclonus) (42,66,67). Other clinical manifestations of increased neuromuscular excitability include heightened muscle tone, stretch reflex asymmetry, the appearance of frontal-release signs (paratonia, snouting, rooting, and grasp reflexes), tetany unresponsive to calcium, meningismus, opisthotonus, and decorticate posturing (2,42,43, 44,68). Muscle weakness is usually prominent in both acute (68) and chronic renal failure (43)(Table 17.1). Distal muscle weakness usually occurs secondary to severe peripheral neuropathy and, as such, tends to more commonly involve the lower extremities. Proximal muscle weakness can occur due to vascular metastatic calcification resulting from severe secondary HPTH (69,70); with aluminum-induced osteomalacia in adults (71,72) and children (73); and in patients who have developed a primary myopathy characterized by weakness, wasting, and tenderness involving proximal musculature (2,74). The last of these diagnoses must be made by excluding the first two, as well as polymyositis (2). Proximal muscle weakness with severe pelvic girdle involvement was the presenting manifestation of CRF in a 13-year-old boy with a 3 year history of slowly progressive debility; it was attributed primarily to severe secondary HPTH (75).

Vitamin deficiencies can occur in association with the poor nutrition characteristic of severe CRF, as in the case of a 12-year-old girl who had ataxia and oculomotor palsy, consistent with the Wernicke encephalopathy (76); clinical improvement followed treatment with thiamine.

Seizures are not uncommon in uremic encephalopathy and have been reported to occur in 17% to 39% of patients with acute (41,68) and 33% to 46% of those with CRF (39,40). They occur more often in patients with severe azotemia (41), can be partial or generalized, and are usually seen late in the clinical course when stupor or coma has supervened (43). Other superimposed causes of seizures that must be considered in patients with uremia, include hypertension, electrolyte imbalance, aluminum and drug toxicity, and infection (Table 17.2).

Lumbar puncture can show mildly elevated opening pressures and CSF protein concentrations; less commonly, pleocytosis is present (2,42,43). Nonetheless, elevated CSF protein concentration or pleocytosis should be considered evidence of infection until proven otherwise.

In the differential diagnosis of uremic encephalopathy (Table 17.2), uremia is unique in causing signs of cerebral excitation (for example, multifocal myoclonus and tetany) and depression (2,42,43). Papilledema or isolated focal neurologic signs suggest the presence of hypertensive encephalopathy and/or intracranial hemorrhage, since uremia per se is not associated with cerebral edema, and more characteristically causes multifocal abnormalities (43,45).

The development of uremic encephalopathy is an indication for prompt initiation of dialysis. Once the diagnosis

Table 17.2   Differential diagnosis of uremic encephalopathy*†

1. Hypertensive encephalopathy
2. Drug-induced encephalopathy
3. Electrolyte imbalance
   a) Water intoxication (dilutional hyponatremia)
   b) Hypocalcemia
   c) Severe acidemia
4. Aluminum encephalopathy
5. CNS infection
6. Pre-existing neuropsychiatric conditions
   a) Functional psychiatric disorders
   b) CNS vasculitis associated with multisystem disease
      (e.g., systemic lupus erythematosus)
   c) Idiopathic seizure disorder

*All conditions can be associated with seizures
†Modified with permission from Fine RN., Gruskin AB. ESRD in
  Children. Philadelphia: W.B. Saunders, 1984.

is suspected, consultation with a pediatric nephrologist
should be requested for this purpose and to obtain recommendations regarding appropriate dietary protein, phosphorus, and potassium restrictions. The use of phosphate
binders (vide infra), vitamin D metabolites, alkali therapy,
and antihypertensive medications, can also be indicated.
Clonazepam has been very effective in controlling
myoclonus (66,67).

Electrophysiologic Manifestations.   In acute and chronic
renal failure, changes in the electroencephalogram (EEG)
can be seen at BUN concentrations as low as 60 mg/dL (2);
however, in early uremic encephalopathy, the EEG can be
normal, or show a predominance of low voltage activity
(2). With progression, there is a decrease in clearly defined
alpha rhythm expected for age. Thereafter, in both ARF
and CRF, increasingly poor regulation of the background
rhythm is seen, followed by the appearance of paroxysmal
bursts of bilaterally synchronous, irregular slow waves,
with the largest amplitudes seen over the anterior
parasagittal regions (2,3,77). These alterations are not
specific for uremia and can be present in other metabolic
disorders, such as hepatic encephalopathy (2). This is also
true of the tendency for some patients with ARF to exhibit
photic driving (2), a phenomenon also observed in alcohol
withdrawal and after discontinuation of sedatives. Other
electrophysiologic disturbances seen predominantly in uremic encephalopathy include a paradoxical response to eye
opening, abnormal arousal responses, and photomyo-
clonus (77). Normalization of the EEG in acute uremia has
been noted during the diuretic phase of recovery from renal
failure (21) and following initiation of maintenance dialysis
for ESRD (vide infra).

Early attempts to relate these disturbances to cognitive
dysfunction in adults suggested that an EEG record containing any epochs with activity less than 6 Hz was a sensitive indicator of early uremic encephalopathy; it was also
noted that cognitive dysfunction was likely when excessive
slowing was present in at least 40% of the record (78). Ini-

tial efforts to relate abnormal brain electrical activity to
attendant clinical and metabolic disturbances, however,
were hampered by the need to derive data from visual analysis of EEG recordings. Thus, manual and automated
methods were developed to overcome these problems
(20,79–82). Several useful indices were derived to quantitate the excessive slow-wave activity observed in patients
with ARF and CRF by determining the percent of all
frequencies below 5 and 7 Hz (80,81); the percent of all
EEG power below 5 Hz (80); and the amount of slow
wave-associated EEG power as a function of total energy
(calculated as: % Power [(3 − 7)/(3 − 13) Hz × 100])(46).
A significant inverse linear correlation was demonstrated
between the latter index and level of renal function in
patients with serum creatinine concentrations between 2
and 29 mg/dL (46). Progressively slower background
rhythms can be expected in adults with renal insufficiency
of increasing degrees of severity.

The quantitation of brain electrical activity in children is
more difficult because the frequency distribution of the
EEG background rhythm is age-dependent (83). This problem was addressed by Balzar et al. (84) by comparing absolute and relative EEG power (microvolts) in the delta, theta,
and beta frequency bands in 9 children with ESRD to the
same measures in 9 age- and sex-matched controls. Both
absolute and relative power in the delta and theta bands
were shown to be significantly greater in the patients with
ESRD versus controls. A more comprehensive approach
was used in the development of neurometrics (85). Using
computer analysis of brain electrical activity recorded at
rest, an age-specific normative data base for the EEG frequency distribution was developed from studies performed
in several hundred children and adolescents 5 to 21 years of
age (83). Neurometrics has been used to study patterns of
brain electrical activity in 26 children with CRF and ESRD
and their relationship to attendant clinical and biochemical
derangements (86). Data collected from scalp electrodes
were quantitated by computer and referenced to age-
related normative values by z-transformation. From these,
a multivariate statistic, the EEG Severity Index (SI), was
derived to represent the probability that each patient's
overall pattern of brain electrical activity was likely to be
seen in a normal child of the same age. Using this method,
significant linear relationships were identified between the
SI and: GFR (estimated from the calculated creatinine
clearance) (87); and the duration of CRF (4). These results
are similar to those obtained in adults using the percent of
slow wave-associated EEG power (46) and show that quantitative indices can be derived from brain electrical activity
in children with CRF, which can then be used to study the
effects of various uremia-related clinical, biochemical, and
metabolic disturbances on their cerebral function.

Event-related Potentials in Chronic Renal Failure.   The
latencies of various components of visual and auditory
event-related potentials (ERPs) have been studied in several

small groups of adolescents and adults with CRF (46,88,90). The mean latency of the first characteristic major negative component (N_{75}) of the visual evoked potential (VEP) elicited in response to strobe light, was significantly prolonged in a group of 56 patients with CRF, when compared to normals (46); a weakly significant correlation (r = 0.26, $P<0.05$) between latency and BUN was identified in 48 patients. VEP P_{100} component latencies were prolonged in 3 of 6 asymptomatic patients with normal visual acuity, when studied by Cohen et al. (88). Peak V, and I–V and III–V interpeak latencies of brain stem auditory evoked responses (BAERs) were significantly prolonged in 6 of 17 adolescents and adults with CRF (90) (Figure 17.1). The wave I–III interpeak latency was significantly correlated with BUN, but not with serum creatinine or PTH concentrations (90). Likewise, neither BUN nor serum creatinine concentrations were significantly related to the degree of prolongation of VEP N_{75} or P_{100} component latencies in 12 adolescents and adults with CRF receiving either conservative management or maintenance hemodialysis (89). In patients studied to date, therefore, no consistent relationships have been documented between the degree of prolongation of various ERP component latencies and the presence and severity of CRF or its associated metabolic complications, so that their clinical usefulness in the management of children with ESRD remains to be established.

Hypertensive Encephalopathy

Hypertensive encephalopathy is a potentially life-threatening but reversible disorder characterized by the subacute onset of cerebral dysfunction resulting from sudden and marked increase in blood pressure over pre-existing levels (91–93). Previously normotensive patients in whom de novo severe hypertension develops are more likely to experience symptoms at lower blood pressures than are patients with established hypertension in whom a secondary abrupt

increase occurs. Hypertensive encephalopathy in children most commonly results from kidney disease (94) and thus represents an important potential cause of cerebral dysfunction complicating the course of CRF in pediatrics.

Both generalized and focal cerebral dysfunction occur in hypertensive encephalopathy. The pathogenesis of generalized dysfunction that is seen more commonly involves the development of cerebral edema, a prominent finding noted in the brains of patients dying with this disorder (91,93,95). It is not clear whether edema results from a primary failure of cerebral vascular autoregulation (breakthrough) or from excessive arteriolar vasospasm (96). According to the breakthrough theory, systemic hypertension causes increased hydraulic pressure in, and excessive fluid leakage from capillaries in the brain. The latter theory holds that severe cerebral arteriolar vasospasm is the primary insult and results in tissue ischemia. Either theory can explain the development of cerebral edema in these patients. Focal neurologic signs can be present and have been attributed to the development of fibrinoid necrosis in cerebral arterioles and petechial hemorrhages and microinfarcts in brain parenchyma (91,97).

The clinical manifestations of hypertensive encephalopathy typically appear from 12 to 48 hours following an abrupt rise in blood pressure. Initially, severe generalized headache develops and can be present for hours to 1 to 2 days as an isolated finding; restlessness is common (91). Alterations of the level and content of consciousness appear and progress from sensorial clouding and drowsiness to coma, if the condition remains untreated. Meningismus, vomiting, visual disturbances including blurring and blindness, transient and migratory focal neurologic signs including VIth and VIIth cranial nerve palsies, muscle twitching and myoclonus, and seizures, either generalized or focal, can be present (91,93,96). Of these findings, convulsions are the most common complication in children, occurring in up to 92% of cases (98). Severe retinal-arteriolar vasospasm is almost always present, but papilledema can be

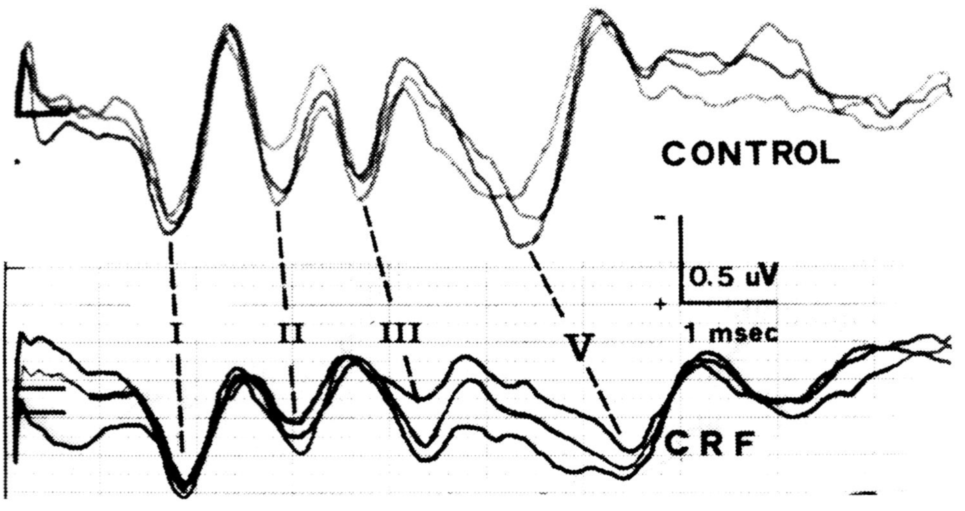

FIGURE 17.1 BAERs in an adult female control subject (A) and a patient with chronic renal failure (B). Significant delays are present for peak III, IV, and V, and interpeak I–III and I–V latencies. Reprinted with permission from Electroencephalography and Clinical Neurophysiology 1984;57:507–514.

observed in as few as 35% of children and, in general, its presence should no longer be considered essential to the diagnosis (98,99).

Lumbar puncture is indicated if the diagnosis is in question, particularly if infection or subarachnoid hemorrhage is suspected. The presence of increased intracranial pressure as identified by CT head scans, however, should first be ruled out. CSF pressure can be normal or increased and is of little diagnostic significance because of its lability (100). Protein concentrations are normal or elevated; pleocytosis is suggestive of subarachnoid hemorrhage. The EEG shows bilateral slowing, particularly in the presence of underlying uremia; focal slowing can be more prominent over areas corresponding to clinically apparent, transient focal neurologic deficits (93,96). The brain scan is normal (96). CT brain scans typically show supratentorial edema, particularly involving cerebral white matter (101,102). In more severe cases, infratentorial edema of the cerebellar white matter and the brain stem can be visualized.

In children and adolescents with CRF, hypertensive encephalopathy should strongly be suspected when cerebral dysfunction develops in the presence of severe hypertension or an abrupt rise in blood pressure from pre-existing levels and in association with retinal-arteriolar vasospasm. Uremia can also alter mental status and cause seizures, and can be present with hypertensive encephalopathy; however, headache, visual disturbances, and funduscopic findings as noted above are usually not as prominent. Moreover, since the hallmark of hypertensive encephalopathy is severe hypertension, the prompt resolution of clinical findings following blood pressure reduction remains the most important clue to this diagnosis (91,92,97). Nonetheless, full resolution of clinical findings can take up to 1 to 7 days. Other conditions to be considered including subdural hematoma, subarachnoid hemorrhage, brain abscess, cerebral infarction, or thromboembolism (91,96) should be suspected when symptoms fail to respond promptly to adequate blood pressure control, particularly when focal neurologic signs persist or progress thereafter. The latter indicates the need for additional diagnostic studies to rule out an intracranial mass lesion. CT is invaluable in this regard but should be performed without administration of radiographic contrast.

The management of hypertensive encephalopathy consists of prompt reduction of blood pressure using rapidly acting parenteral agents, which do not appreciably alter mental status. The drugs of choice for this purpose are nitroprusside, diazoxide, and labetalol. Nitroprusside, a direct arteriolar and venodilator, is the drug of choice in patients with concomitant congestive heart failure (CHF) or suspected intracranial hemorrhage, since it does not cause reflex tachycardia or increase in left ventricular work (103). Its antihypertensive effect is dose dependent, peaking within 1 to 2 minutes, and disappearing promptly upon discontinuation; this allows accurate titration of the blood pressure to a predetermined level, thus minimizing potential complications associated with relative hypotension (vide infra). Nitroprusside is given by continuous intravenous (IV) infusion in doses of 0.5 to 8 to 10 μg/kg/min; an infusion rate of 3 μg/kg/min should reduce diastolic blood pressure by 30% to 40% (104,105). Doses in excess of 10 μg/kg/min, however, have been required for brief periods of time (103). The solution must be protected from light and should be administered in an intensive care setting with continuous blood pressure monitoring, ideally via an intraarterial cannula. The major cause of toxicity associated with the use of nitroprusside is accumulation of thiocyanate, which is eliminated via the kidneys. Thus, blood levels of this metabolite should be monitored regularly in patients with ESRD and the drug discontinued if plasma levels exceed 10 μg/mL (92). Thiocyanate is removed by hemo- and peritoneal dialysis (103,105).

Diazoxide is a direct arteriolar vasodilator; it increases venous return and cardiac output and, therefore, is a less desirable agent for use in patients with CHF or suspected intracranial hemorrhage (106). It is given intravenously in an initial dose of 0.5 to 1.0 mg/kg over 5 to 10 seconds, with constant blood pressure monitoring. The peak antihypertensive effect is seen at 2 minutes, with some rebound occurring, usually 15 minutes after administration; residual antihypertensive activity may be noted for up to 12 to 24 hours (104,106). Although the above-noted dose is substantially lower than that previously recommended (96), smaller initial boluses are now used to avoid causing excessive hypotension (105); if ineffective, our practice has been to repeat the bolus at twice the initial dose within 5 to 10 minutes. This can be continued to a maximum dose of 10 mg/kg or 300 mg. Infusions of 5 mg/kg to 10 mg/kg over 15 to 30 minutes have also been administered with success (105).

Labetalol is an antihypertensive agent with both selective alpha$_1$- and nonselective beta adrenergic blocking properties and, therefore, is contraindicated in patients with CHF, greater than first-degree heart block, or a history of asthma. It is given in an initial IV dose of 0.1 mg/kg to 0.2 mg/kg, which should lower blood pressure within 5 minutes; thus, pressures should be monitored frequently after administration. Repeat doses can be administered every 10 minutes in amounts of up to 0.5 mg/kg each (maximum 300 mg/24 hours in adults) to achieve the desired degree of antihypertensive effect. Adverse central nervous system (CNS) effects include headache, tremor, depression, and nightmares (107).

The lowering of blood pressure in patients with hypertensive encephalopathy has been associated with development of temporary or permanent blindness and hemi- or paraplegia, which has been attributed to ischemic injury to the optic nerves, occipital cortex, and spinal cord (100,108–114). In at least two affected children (108) and one adult (109), vision was diminished even before initiation of therapy so that a clear cause-and-effect relationship could not be established in these cases between the degree of relative hypotension recorded and the development of neurologic sequelae. In 2 other cases (111,112), however, the blood pressure had been lowered gradually over 12 to 24 hours, in one instance by using only oral antihypertensive medication. Since the lower limit of cerebral autoregulation is known to be abnormally increased in at least some patients with severe hypertension (115), it is wise to avoid excessive lowering of the blood pressure during the initial course of therapy, particularly in ESRD patients, in whom peripheral vascular resistance is often chronically elevated. It has been suggested (93,116) that a reduction of mean arterial pressure of 40% or more is likely to exceed cerebral autoregulatory capacity, whereas a 25% to 30% decrease should be safer. Since prompt reduction in blood pressure is indicated to avoid permanent neurologic injury or death due to cerebral edema, the aforementioned data at least provide guidelines for blood pressure lowering that can be followed until more definitive information becomes available.

Drug-Induced Encephalopathy

Cerebral dysfunction attributable to drug toxicity commonly occurs in patients with CRF, with antibiotics, sedative-hypnotics, and antipsychotic tranquilizers heading the list of responsible agents (117,118). These medications were held responsible for 1/3 of 178 episodes of neurologic derangement reported in adults with CRF (118). Patients with severely diminished or absent kidney function may be at increased risk for the development of drug-induced CNS toxicity for several reasons including: the plasma concentration of many drugs and their active metabolites are increased due to diminished urinary elimination (119); the free plasma concentrations of many acidic drugs such as phenytoin, barbiturates, salicylates, the penicillins, and diazepam, a basic compound, are increased due to diminished protein binding (120). The effect of both of the above phenomena is to increase the availability of these drugs and their active metabolites for entry into the CNS via the choroid plexus organic acid transport system (117); and accumulation of organic acid waste products may result in competitive inhibition of outward transport across the blood-brain barrier via the choroid plexus (117).

The clinical manifestations of drug toxicity seen most commonly in patients with CRF are those of delirium (toxic psychosis) or decreased consciousness. Seizures, myoclonus, and asterixis can also be seen. A toxic psychosis, characterized by agitation, confusion, disorientation, and visual hallucinations, has been observed following treatment with therapeutic doses of chlorpromazine, diphenhydramine, and cyproheptadine, when administered alone or in various combinations for 2 to 8 days (124,127). The clinical picture resembled that of the central anticholinergic syndrome caused by drugs with atropine-like side effects, except for the absence of systemic signs of toxicity; for example,

mydriasis, cycloplegia, hyperthermia, constipation, xerostomia, cutaneous flushing, and tachycardia, which are usually present (126,128). In 5 patients, therapy with diazepam or flurazepam was temporally related to the development of a reversible syndrome of confusion, disorientation, and short-term memory loss accompanied by asterixis (129). Confusion, hallucinations, and inappropriate behavior developed after 2 to 4 weeks of antihypertensive therapy with prazosin in 3 adults with CRF (123). The penicillins are known neurotoxins and are likely to cause CNS dysfunction when CSF levels exceed 10 μg/mL (130). This is more likely to occur in the presence of renal insufficiency; doses of penicillin G in excess of 25 million units/day, when administered to affected adults and children, has resulted in an encephalopathy characterized by coma, myoclonus, and seizures, generally within 8 to 24 hours of the initial dose (131). Myoclonus, asterixis, hyperreflexia, hallucinations and subsequently, decreased consciousness, followed 3 weeks of therapy with ticarcillin in an adult with ESRD (132). Reversible psychic disturbances, seizures, and decreased consciousness have also developed in patients with ESRD receiving other antibiotics (aminoglycosides, colistin), barbiturates, and haloperidol (118).

Drug intoxication should be suspected in any child or adolescent with ARF or CRF who has experienced the abrupt and unexpected onset of seizures, myoclonus, asterixis, or alterations in the level or content of consciousness. If withdrawal of the suspected drug results in clinical improvement, the diagnosis is most likely correct and further therapy may be unnecessary. Reported recovery times, however, are variable and depend upon the agent responsible: 1 to 4 weeks for the phenothiazines; (124) 4 to 5 days for the benzodiazepines; (129) 2 months for prazosin; (123) 12 to 72 hours for the penicillin G; (131) and 7 to 14 days for ticarcillin (132). In the presence of respiratory depression, cardiac arrhythmias, or other potentially life-threatening manifestations of the central anticholinergic syndrome, physostigmine salicylate may be administered and should alleviate symptoms within 30 minutes (128). Physostigmine should not, however, be used to treat less serious degrees of toxicity in patients with renovascular hypertension, since its use is generally contraindicated in such patients (126). Finally, for those drugs for which metabolism is altered in renal failure, toxicity is best avoided by following recommendations for modifying dosage or interval of administration or both, and by monitoring blood levels where appropriate (119).

Aluminum Encephalopathy in Pediatric Patients with Chronic Renal Failure

During the past 15 years, it has become increasingly apparent that aluminum accumulates in the CNS and other tissues of patients with CRF and has been responsible for the development of a syndrome of progressive neurologic deterioration initially associated with mortality rates in excess of 85% in adults (133–136) and children (31–36,137–140). Pathologic examination of brains from adults and children dying of this disorder has revealed cortical gray-matter aluminum concentrations of 4 to 25 times those of control brains (33,135–137); no other histopathologic findings are characteristic (134). The pathophysiology of the cerebral dysfunction attributed to excessive brain aluminum accumulation is not well understood although interruption of cerebral perfusion and altered blood-brain barrier permeability have been suggested as possible mechanisms (141). Interference with brain function at the cellular level may occur: aluminum binds to nuclear chromatin and, thus, may interfere with DNA replication or RNA transcription or both (142). It also interferes with the function of enzymes such as dihydropteridine reductase, ferroxidase, and hexokinase, the last of which is important in cerebral glucose utilization (141,142). Interference with the activity of dihydropteridine reductase, an enzyme essential for the synthesis of tyrosine, could reduce the availability of the cerebral neurotransmitter, dopamine (141,142).

The pathogenesis of enhanced cerebral aluminum accumulation in patients with CRF is attributable to one or more of the following: increased exposure to aluminum-containing solutions and compounds; increased bioavailability; and decreased urinary excretion. For children with CRF, the major source of environmental exposure has been the aluminum-containing phosphate binding gels taken to control hyperphosphatemia. Substantial amounts of ingested aluminum are absorbed from the gastrointestinal (GI) tract in normal individuals and those with chronic renal disease (143,144). Serum aluminum levels are significantly correlated with phosphate binder dose in children and adults (73,145–150); and in fact, for most children with aluminum intoxication reported to date, these compounds were the only available source of this trace metal from which excessive exposure could possibly have occurred (31,35,36,73,137,138,146,147). Aluminum-containing phosphate binders are a particular problem for infants with severe CRF, since their major source of nutrition is milk-based formulas that generally contain large amounts of phosphorus. Consequently, infants frequently require higher mg per kg doses of these compounds than do older children. Moreover, an inverse linear correlation between plasma levels and age has been identified in infants and children with documented aluminum intoxication (84). These observations explain why the majority of pediatric cases of progressive encephalopathy have occurred in patients younger than 2 years of age (54).

Recently, aluminum was found in high concentrations in a wide variety of commercially available milk formulas marketed in North America, Europe, and Australia (140,152–154). Concentrations in these formulas ranged from 85 to greater than 5,000 µg/L and were highest in soy-based preparations and lowest in human breast milk (152,153). Two infants with severe CRF who died at 1 and

3 months of age were receiving formulas subsequently found to contain elevated aluminum concentrations (126 to 391 µg/L)(140); neither had been receiving phosphate binders. At autopsy, brain gray matter aluminum concentrations were 6.4 and 47.4 µg/g (normal below 0.1) dry weight (wt). Very high aluminum concentrations have also been found in a variety of solutions available for IV use, including 25% human serum albumin, sodium and potassium phosphate, 5% and 10% calcium gluconate, and heparin (152,154–156). Bone aluminum loading has been documented in premature infants receiving IV therapy for at least 3 weeks (152) and in adults with normal renal function receiving long-term parenteral nutrition (157). Thus, in patients with severe CRF who have been receiving these formulas or parenteral solutions for more than 2 to 3 weeks, routine periodic monitoring of serum aluminum levels is mandatory.

The bioavailability of aluminum is influenced by several factors. PTH has been shown to enhance GI aluminum uptake and deposition in brain gray matter (158–160). Thus, secondary HPTH, which is common in children with severe CRF, may be a risk factor for development of cerebral aluminum intoxication. This problem may be self limiting (73), however, since aluminum also accumulates in the parathyroid glands (161) and appears to suppress PTH release after an as-yet undetermined period of time (162,163). The bioavailability of ingested aluminum may also be increased during the routine administration of vitamin D metabolites (calcitriol and 1-alpha hydroxyvitamin D) to treat renal osteodystrophy (164,165) and as a consequence of iron deficiency anemia (166).

Clinical Manifestations

As initially described, the clinical manifestations of CNS aluminum intoxication in children are those of progressive encephalopathy associated with microcephaly, disturbances in motor function, seizures, and characteristic electroencephalographic changes (131,167). Nearly all affected patients have had congenital nephropathies that were diagnosed during infancy. All had severe renal insufficiency, usually by 1 to 2 years of age, with GFR's below 30 mL/min/1.73 m², where reported (31–37,139,140,146). The results of a multicenter international questionnaire survey (167a) conducted to determine the scope of this problem worldwide, indicated that all affected patients had been receiving aluminum-containing phosphate binding gels, and that over 90% had had secondary HPTH prior to the development of neurologic deterioration. The duration of phosphate binder therapy prior to onset ranged from 9 to 62 months in reported cases (31,35,36,137–139). In all patients a similar pattern of progressive deterioration occurred in three stages. Initially, there occurred an arrest in the acquisition of new motor skills. Declining school performance was also one of the earliest, although nonspecific, indications of developing encephalopathy (36). Dysmetria was apparent in the infants and very young children; ambulatory patients developed ataxia, and tremor, hyperreflexia, and extensor plantar reflexes were present. With disease progression, regression of developmental milestones occurred, and hypotonia, myoclonus, and seizures developed. Speech disturbances were present, as characterized by dysarthria and lingual apraxia. Ultimately, a chronic vegetative state developed with unresponsiveness to visual and auditory stimuli, generalized myoclonus, marked hypotonia, and absence of voluntary movement. CT in affected patients showed evidence of cortical atrophy in 83% of 31 cases in which it had been performed (31,37). Serial EEGs revealed progressive slowing of the background rhythm with superimposed bursts of sharp waves and 2 to 4 Hz polyspike-wave discharges (Figure 17.2), a pattern similar to that seen in Dialysis Dementia, or Dialysis Encephalopathy Syndrome, the syndrome of aluminum-related progressive encephalopathy initially described in hemodialyzed adults with ESRD (vide infra).

The clinical and EEG deterioration characteristic of aluminum intoxication typically have proceeded in parallel, and have followed a subacute or chronic course, evolving over periods of 1 to 12 months in most reported cases (31–33,36,137–139). In some children and adults at risk due to long-term oral aluminum loading, however, encephalopathy has developed acutely, over periods of days to weeks (35,138,169–170). In these patients, acute deterioration has followed intercurrent infection (138), immobilization (168,169) and surgery, including that for renal transplantation with the concomitant administration of corticosteroids (35,138,168–171). In all of these cases, intercurrent stresses occurred that were capable of inducing a catabolic state in which tissue breakdown could lead to the acute mobilization of bone and, thus, of its aluminum content. Since bone aluminum levels are typically elevated in patients with CRF who have been ingesting phosphate binding gels for prolonged periods of time, it is possible that substantial quantities of the metal could be released to acutely redistribute in cerebral cortex. The resulting symptoms might then develop in a manner analogous to that in which acute encephalopathy may be precipitated in a previously asymptomatic child with chronic lead poisoning (172). Thus, children receiving long-term therapy with aluminum-containing phosphate binders should be considered at-risk for development of encephalopathy during severe intercurrent illnesses, even if they have not previously been symptomatic.

Blood and tissue aluminum levels do not always correlate well; however, plasma concentrations in excess of 133 to 200 (normal <10 to 30 µg/L) (73,146) have predicted the presence of aluminum-related bone disease with a sensitivity of 60% to 93% (173,174). Moreover, plasma

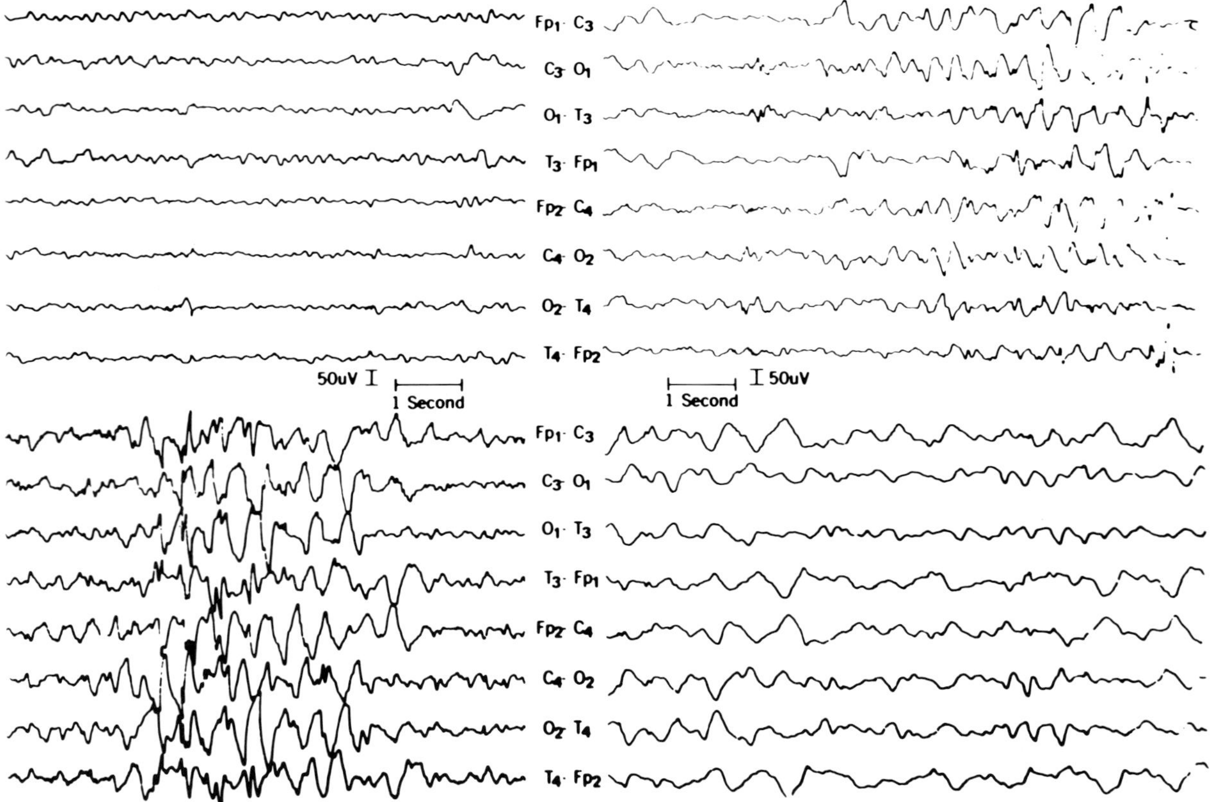

FIGURE 17.2 Serial tracings from EEG recordings obtained at 6-month intervals beginning at 3 1/2 years of age, in a boy with progressive encephalopathy. See text for interpretation. (Earliest tracing is in upper left; latest, lower right.) Reprinted with permission from Fine RN, Gruskin AB. ESRD in Children. Philadelphia: W.B. Saunders, 1984.

concentrations in excess of 100 μg/L were found in children with oral intakes of elemental aluminum in excess of 75 mg/kg/day, all of whom showed clinical evidence of aluminum toxicity (146). Plasma aluminum levels may, therefore, be of value in assessing the risk of developing encephalopathy.

In children with severe CRF, the differential diagnosis of aluminum intoxication should include uremic encephalopathy and severe hypercalcemia and hypophosphatemia. As already discussed, uremic encephalopathy may cause delirium or dementia, and myoclonus. Since most cases of aluminum intoxication in children appear prior to the initiation of maintenance dialysis, differentiating the two conditions may prove difficult on clinical grounds. The fully developed EEG changes seen with aluminum intoxication are not characteristic of uremia and are helpful in this regard. Demonstration of markedly elevated plasma or bone aluminum concentrations may also prove useful. Most importantly, uremic encephalopathy should respond promptly to initiation of maintenance dialysis, whereas aluminum intoxication will not. Acute hypercalcemia and severe phosphate depletion may also cause clinical syndromes similar to those of aluminum intoxication. To date, these have only been reported in patients receiving maintenance dialysis as discussed below.

Peripheral Neuropathy

Etiology and Pathogenesis

Clinically apparent peripheral neuropathy is a major manifestation of the uremic syndrome, occurring in 11% to 75% of patients evaluated prior to the initiation of maintenance dialysis (175)(Table 17.3). It is, fortunately, much less common in younger patients, having been reported in only eight children and adolescents, all of whom were over 11 years of age (175–180). The etiology of uremic peripheral neuropathy remains controversial. Histologic examination of biopsy specimens from sural nerves has revealed variable degrees of paranodal segmental demyelination and remyelination and degeneration of axis cylinders (181–184). Axonal degeneration is more marked distally than proximally and may be present in the absence of demyelination (182). While considerable controversy has existed regarding its pathogenesis, recent reviews of available clinical and experimental data (185,186) indicate that uremic neuropathy most likely represents a form of axonopathy or dying back neuropathy (187). Consistent with this view are the observations that in uremia, neuropathy is slow to develop and clinically insidious in onset (13,175); it affects the most distal portions of large, long axons in the lower extremities earliest, producing a stocking-glove sensory deficit and diminished deep-tendon reflexes (DTRs) at the ankles (185,186); and unlike a myelinopathy, it produces less severe depression of motor nerve conduction velocities (MNCVs), from which recovery occurs slowly following successful transplantation, and with the potential for residual deficits (187–189). Uremic peripheral neuropathy does not develop during ARF, either in humans (21) or laboratory animals (13).

The manner in which uremia leads to neuronal changes is not known. Various abnormal metabolites isolated from the blood of affected patients have been advanced as so-called uremic toxins (186), the concentrations of which were shown to correlate with observed degrees of depression of MNCVs in animal studies. In most cases, however,

Table 17.3   Drugs associated with peripheral neuropathy*

Clinical Presentation	Antimicrobial Drugs	Antineoplastic Drugs	Cardiovascular Drugs	Hypnotics and Psychotropics	Antirheumatic Drugs	Other Drugs
Sensory neuropathy	Ethionamide Chloramphenicol Thiamphenicol Diamines	Procarbazine Nitrofurazone				Calcium Carbimide Sulfoxone Ergotamine Propylthiouracil
Paresthesiae only	Colistin Streptomycin Nalidixic Acid	Cytarabine	Propranolol	Phenelzine		Sulthiame Chlorpropamide Methysergide
Sensorimotor neuropathy	Isoniazid† Ethambutol Streptomycin Nitrofurantoin Clioquinol Metronidazole	Vincristine Podophyllum Chlorambucil	Perhexiline Hydralazine† Amiodarone Disopyramide Clofibrate	Thalidomide Methaqualone Glutethimide Amitriptyline	Gold Indomethacin Colchicine Chloroquine Phenylbutazone	Phenytoin Disulfiram Carbutamide Tolbutamide Chlorpropamide Methimazole
Predominantly motor	Sulfonamides Amphotericin			Imipramine		Dapsone
Localized neuropathies	Amphotericin Penicillin	Mustine Ethoglucid				Anticoagulants

*British Medical Journal 1979;1:663 with permission.
†Pyridoxine-responsive

these results have not been reproducible in humans, and the degree of correlation between blood levels of the putative toxin in question and the degree of depression of nerve conduction velocity (NCV), has been weak. In this regard, it has been suggested by Nielsen (190) that for a compound to be considered a uremic neurotoxin, the degree of correlation between its blood levels and slowing of NCVs must be more highly significant than that observed between the latter and GFR per se (r = −0.68, P < 0.001); this criterion has not yet been fulfilled by any compound (186). For example, PTH was proposed as a peripheral neurotoxin, the serum levels of which were found to correlate significantly with the degree of depression of MNCVs in 42 uremic patients (195); however, the degree of correlation observed (r = −0.45, P < 0.01) clearly failed to meet Nielsen's criterion. Moreover, attempts to duplicate these findings have been unsuccessful (186,192,193).

The likelihood of developing clinically apparent peripheral neuropathy is determined by a patient's age, sex, and the severity and duration of their renal insufficiency (194). In adults, clinical evidence of peripheral neuropathy is generally absent until the GFR fall below 5 to 13 mL/min/1.73 m², or the serum creatinine concentration exceeds 5 mg/dL (195–198). Males are uniformly affected more frequently than females who generally have more severe reductions in GFR when symptomatic neuropathy develops (194,199). It is likely that reductions in GFR even more dramatic than those noted above are necessary for neuropathy to become symptomatic in children. Using stepwise discriminant analysis, a significant positive linear correlation was identified between GFR (creatinine clearance) and age of male patients with and without moderate-to-severe clinical neuropathy (194). The data indicated that in children under 15 years of age, GFR would have to decrease below 2 mL/min/1.73 m² before clinical evidence of neuropathy could be expected. Since most children and adolescents begin receiving maintenance dialysis well before this level of decompensation is reached, the above data may explain why clinically significant peripheral neuropathy is, in fact, uncommon in pediatric patients. Moreover, it has been shown that peripheral nerve anatomy and function tend to deteriorate with increasing age (184,200,201), so that the lower prevalence of clinical neuropathy in young patients may also be due to the healthier premorbid state of their peripheral nerves.

The clinical manifestations are those of a mixed, bilaterally symmetric sensorimotor polyneuropathy in which the distal portions of the lower extremities are affected earliest and, ultimately, most severely (2,65,175,180). Clinical involvement of the upper extremities is less common, particularly proximally, although evidence of neuropathy in one 13-year-old female was limited to paresis and atrophy involving the muscles of the hypothenar eminence (175). The earliest sensory and motor symptoms are those of paresthesias and dysesthesias, and muscle cramps and restless legs, respectively (2,175,176,195). Paresthesias are generally experienced in the fingers and toes, but the soles of the feet were involved exclusively in two adolescents evaluated prior to beginning maintenance dialysis (176). They are the symptoms of peripheral neuropathy that correlate best with the presence of objective signs (180). Muscle cramps and later, restless legs, tend to involve the lower extremities. Cramps are usually painful, initially nocturnal and episodic; they gradually become more persistent and occur during the day as well (2). The restless legs syndrome was described by Callaghan (179) as "peculiar creeping, crawling, prickling and itchy sensations experienced in the lower limbs," most commonly in the calves. They have also been described in the arms and hands of a 17-year-old female (179). Typically, the sensations appear later in the course of progressive renal failure than do muscle cramps. They are worst during periods of inactivity, for example, at night, and are relieved by movement. Other symptoms, less common and also generally seen at a more advanced stage of renal insufficiency, include pain, burning feet, and muscle weakness. The burning foot syndrome is characterized by painful paresthesias of the dorsal and plantar surfaces of the feet (2). It has been associated with severe nutritional deficiency and may actually be a manifestation of thiamine deficiency (202). The earliest sign of muscle weakness is an inability to dorsiflex the big toe due to selective involvement of the extensor digitorum brevis (203).

The earliest signs of peripheral neuropathy are diminished vibratory sensation over the pulp of the big toe and medial malleolus and diminished stretch reflexes, most commonly at the ankles and knees (180,195,197). The former may be quantitatively assessed by determining the vibratory perception threshold (VPT)(180,204); in this way, vibratory sensation may be shown to deteriorate abruptly over a period of weeks (205). Screening for both hyporeflexia and an increased VPT should permit accurate diagnosis in over 90% of patients with clinically significant peripheral neuropathy (180). If the diagnosis of uremia is not made and dialysis initiated, however, neuropathy will continue to progress with the development of stocking-glove anesthesia and more generalized lower and, eventually, upper extremity muscle weakness and atrophy.

Electrophysiologic Studies in Uremic Neuropathy

Sensory and motor NCVs are commonly used to evaluate peripheral nerve function in patients with CRF because they may provide a more sensitive index of functional integrity than does the physical examination, since abnormal NCVs have been reported with serum creatinine concentrations as low as 2.1 mg/dL in adults (196) and 1.5 mg/dL in children (206). Both sensory and motor NCVs correlate significantly with levels of residual renal function in adults (190,196,198), although comparable studies have not been performed in children. Nonetheless, abnormally low NCVs, particularly those involving the motor components of the common peroneal nerve, are present in most adults and children with ESRD when studied just prior to initiation of maintenance dialysis (177–179,190,195,196, 198,199,201,206,207).

Differential Diagnosis and Management

Given the relative infrequency with which peripheral neuropathy produces clinical symptoms in children, its appearance should prompt a search for nonuremia-related causes. Poor nutrition can be associated with thiamine or pyridoxine deficiency, which can cause peripheral neuropathy. This is unusual, however, except when B vitamin supplements have not been prescribed or taken by patients receiving maintenance dialysis which removes them from the blood. If thiamine or pyridoxine deficiency is suspected in a child with peripheral neuropathy, blood levels of both vitamins should be obtained to confirm the diagnosis. Peripheral neuropathy can also be a complication of drug therapy (Table 17.3)(208). The use of medications known to cause this problem should be avoided in children with chronic renal disease. When necessary, doses should be adjusted to compensate for altered urinary excretion (119).

Uremic peripheral neuropathy is treated by initiation of maintenance dialysis. The restless legs syndrome in adults has been successfully treated with clonazepam, at a starting dose of 0.5 mg given at 6 P.M. and bedtime (209).

Cranial Neuropathy

Visual disturbances occur infrequently in patients with CRF. Transient episodes of blindness (uremic amaurosis) have been reported to develop over several hours and to resolve within several days (2); their occurrence has not been associated with funduscopic or pupillary reflex abnormalities and has been attributed to focal cerebral edema involving the white matter of the occipital cortex. Transient blindness can occur during or as a sequela of cerebral edema due to hypertensive encephalopathy (vide supra). Other, subtler changes in visual function have also been described. Contrast sensitivity thresholds were found to be reduced in 10 asymptomatic patients with ESRD and to improve following acute dialysis (210). Snellen visual acuities were normal in all patients in this study, so that the clinical significance of these findings is unclear. Spontaneously occurring, asymptomatic retinal hemorrhages were noted in 21 of 115 maintenance dialysis patients aged 11 to 64 years, and salt-and-pepper degenerative changes involving the retinal pigment epithelium were seen in 13 (211); the latter findings were felt to represent the sequelae of old hypertensive disease. Optic atrophy was seen in 3 patients in the same study.

Electroretinographic evaluations in adults receiving maintenance dialysis have revealed progressively smaller evoked response amplitudes to a given stimulus intensity and decreasing slope of the intensity-response curve with increasing time on dialysis (212), funduscopic findings in these patients were remarkable only for hypertensive changes. Electrical activity of the retina normalized following successful transplantation.

Sensorineural hearing loss has been reported in 61% to 70% of adult and 47% of pediatric patients with ESRD (213,215). In children and adolescents this was most frequently attributed to congenital diseases other than Alport syndrome (31%) and to acquired causes (31%); that is, recurrent otitis and drug toxicity (215). Antibiotics commonly associated with hearing loss in patients with CRF include the aminoglycosides and furosemide (2); it has been irreversible in some cases (216). Despite the hepatic route of metabolism of erythromycin, its pharmacokinetics are altered in CRF, presumably because of increased bioavailability (217), and it, too, has been associated with ototoxicity in adolescents and adults so affected (218). Regardless of etiology, the hearing loss observed in most patients with CRF tends to involve higher frequencies, to remain relatively stable over long periods of time (215) and to be unaffected by maintenance dialysis (214).

Taste acuity is frequently diminished in children with CRF, as characterized by abnormally increased detection and discrimination thresholds that are, respectively, the lowest concentrations at which tastes are distinguishable from water and from each other (219–221). However, taste sensitivity, that is the ability to distinguish between different suprathreshold concentrations of the same taste, and preference for different tastes, is normal (222). Diminished taste acuity has uniformly been associated with inadequate caloric intake and, where red blood cell (RBC) or hair zinc levels have been determined, with hypozincemia (220,221).

These findings indicate the need to perform routine periodic audiologic and ophthalmologic evaluations in all children and adolescents with severe CRF.

NEUROLOGIC COMPLICATIONS ASSOCIATED WITH DIALYSIS

Beneficial Effects

The clinical manifestations of uremic encephalopathy are promptly reversed following institution of maintenance dialysis (39,68). When compared to studies obtained prior to initiation, individual performances on tests of cognitive function (CPT and CRT) improve significantly, in some cases within weeks, in adults receiving adequate hemodialysis (46,223). Similarly, in an early report (224), the behavior of 5 of 18 children who were considered emotionally disturbed or intellectually retarded normalized within weeks to months following initiation of dialysis. More recently, however, formal IQ testing using either the Stanford-Binet or WISC-R failed to show significant improvement in the performances of children studied prior to and following initiation (51); nor have tests of vigilance, visuospatial perception and reasoning, or memory yielded significantly different results when dialyzed children with ESRD are compared to those still being conservatively managed (52,53). This is possibly because dialysis was initiated well before uremic encephalopathy had developed.

No appreciable deterioration in cognitive function has been detected in adults dialyzed for more than five years, as long as environmental aluminum exposure is minimized (225). Maintaining effective metabolic control of uremia appears to be important in this regard, however, as evidenced by the results of the National Cooperative Dialysis Study (226); patients receiving relatively inefficient dialysis reported increased difficulty concentrating significantly more often than those in whom azotemia was better controlled. Moreover, hemodialysis appears to be more effective when performed 3 times instead of twice weekly (223). Evaluations performed in adults (227) and children (228) before and after isolated treatments have failed to demonstrate any acutely beneficial or detrimental effects of dialysis on cognitive function.

Neurobehavioral testing has failed to show significant differences in cognitive function between adults receiving maintenance hemo- versus peritoneal dialysis (229). There is some evidence, however, that children receiving maintenance hemodialysis may be more distractible than those being treated with continuous ambulatory peritoneal dialysis and, therefore, perform more poorly on tests of selective memory function such as the Auditory Consonant Trigrams Test (52). Further study is clearly indicated to evaluate the differential effects of various dialysis modalities on neurobehavioral function, particularly in infants and young children.

Electrophysiologic Studies

EEG Changes: Following initiation of maintenance dialysis, a trend toward normalization of the EEG background rhythm becomes apparent in most adults, as characterized by a progressive decrease in the percent of slow wave-associated EEG power with successive treatments (46,83). Although comparable data are not available for children, in those studied prior to and following a single treatment, computer analysis of absolute and relative EEG power has also shown a reduction in slow wave activity and a shift toward higher frequencies (84). Adequate dialysis, therefore, has a beneficial effect upon brain electrical activity in children as well as adults; early reports of deterioration of the EEG, or of de novo development of electroencephalographic abnormalities during dialysis, were probably a consequence of dialysis disequilibrium due to overly aggressive therapy (230)(vide infra).

Paroxysmal EEG abnormalities are commonly seen in children receiving maintenance dialysis (231); of 54 EEG recordings from 37 patients with ESRD aged 2.3 to 18 years, epileptiform discharges unassociated with clinical seizure activity occurred in 16 (43.2%). These were characterized by generalized bursts of spike-wave complexes and occipital intermittent rhythmic delta activity. Their clinical significance, regarding the presence of associated deficits in attention and memory, has not yet been investigated.

Event-related Potentials.   Pattern shift VEPs performed in patients receiving maintenance hemodialysis demonstrate abnormal prolongation of P100 group mean latencies, but to an extent not significantly different from those seen in individuals with CRF (89). When determined prior to and following initiation of dialysis, however, patient comparisons have shown a significant decrease in VEP component latencies toward normal (46). Nonetheless, these latencies have been abnormal in as many as 50% to 67% of dialysis patients reported (88,232). Abnormal prolongation of BAER component latencies have been seen in 25% to 28% of maintenance dialysis patients and 36% of adults with CRF still receiving conservative management, an insignificant difference (90,232). Therefore, maintenance dialysis does not appear to have a consistently beneficial effect on the functional integrity of those neural pathways involved in the generation of the ERP components studied to date.

Peripheral Neuropathy

In adults, peripheral neuropathy usually stabilizes or improves clinically after 3 to 12 months of adequate dialysis (197,198,205); continued deterioration during the first months of therapy is an indication that treatment time may be inadequate (197,198,226). Serial physical examinations should document whether or not progressive improvement is occurring. In this regard, determination of the VPT can provide a more quantitative indicator of progress; by this method objective improvement has been shown to occur after 3 months of maintenance dialysis (205). As noted, most children and adolescents do not develop clinically significant peripheral neuropathy with ESRD, and they remain asymptomatic following initiation of dialysis (207,233).

The response of NCVs to maintenance dialysis is less predictable. With adequate therapy, sensory and motor NCVs have stabilized in some patients for periods of 1 to 10 years (185,199,205). In others, deterioration continued during the first year of maintenance dialysis, with gradual improvement occurring thereafter (197,198,234). Prior to initiation of dialysis, NCVs may be normal or depressed in children and adolescents (206,207,233). Thereafter, abnormally decreased peroneal or posterior tibial MNCVs have been noted in 18% to 57% of patients, and have remained stable for periods of 12 to 24 months (206,233). Median sensory latencies have remained normal in 73% to 91% of those studied (206,233).

NCVs and Adequacy of Dialysis.   Once the clinical signs and symptoms of peripheral neuropathy were found to respond to adequate dialysis, quantitative indices were sought that could be used as a numerical guide to assess adequacy of therapy and the use of NCVs for this purpose seemed reasonable initially (235); however, the clinical and electrophysiologic features of uremic neuropathy do not correlate well. For example, 20 of 59 patients of Jennekens et al. (195) had abnormally decreased NCVs, but so did 19 of 27 individuals without associated signs or symptoms; and none of the patients of Mentser et al. (207) had clinical findings despite the fact that most of them had abnormally low MNCVs. Unlike the clinical findings, NCVs show gradual and progressive slowing that proceeds in parallel in both upper and lower extremities, so that the ratio between the two remains constant (201,236,237). Moreover, the intrapatient variation in NCVs may be as high as 25% when daily testing is performed (237). In general, NCVs are not a useful measure of the efficacy of treatment in either children or adults receiving maintenance dialysis. However, the unexpected development of symptoms or signs of peripheral neuropathy in a patient with ESRD remains an indication to perform NCVs and to search for a cause (4). In patients receiving maintenance hemodialysis, acute changes in NCVs may result from rapid ultrafiltration of fluid (238), the repeated use of dialyzers with inappropriately large surface areas (239,240) or, conversely, from

inadequate dialysis (226). Rapid shifts in the serum potassium concentration (185) or the use of high magnesium-containing dialysate (241) can also alter NCVs, as can intercurrent Hepatitis B infection (242), or interruption of the blood supply to peripheral nerves due to vasa nervorum ischemia associated with severe hyperreninemic hypertension (177,242).

Neurologic Complications Attributable to Dialysis

The Dialysis Disequilibrium Syndrome

The Dialysis Disequilibrium Syndrome (DDS) is an acute, reversible neurologic syndrome observed primarily in patients receiving maintenance dialysis and is most common early in the clinical course; that is, during the first few treatments (2,38,244). Its incidence in early reports was 8% in adults and 33% in children (1,224) although it has probably become less common in recent years due to the avoidance of overly rapid dialysis.

The pathogenesis of the DDS (Figure 17.3) has been attributed to the development of a blood-brain osmotic gradient during rapid hemodialysis, resulting in cerebral

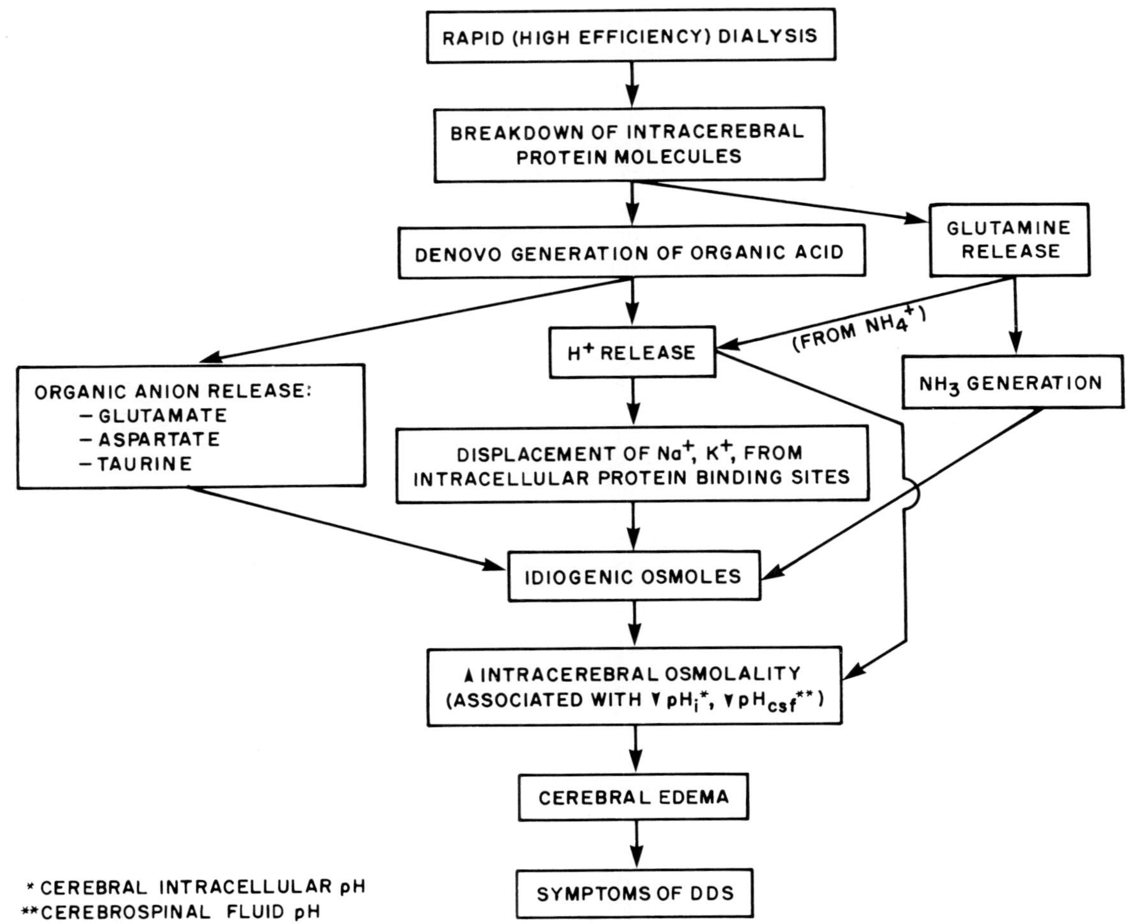

FIGURE 17.3 Suggested pathogenesis of the dialysis disequilibrium syndrome (DDS). Reprinted with permission from Fine RN, Gruskin AB. ESRD in Children. Philadelphia: W.B. Saunders, 1984.

edema (1,230,244–247). In adults, even in the absence of the DDS, brain water content is known to increase to some extent during hemodialysis as evidenced by changes in cerebral density measurements performed by CT (14,248). Moreover, intraocular pressure was shown to rise, an average of 8.1 mm Hg during prolonged (10 to 12 hr) hemodialysis treatments (249). It was also demonstrated that the symptoms and EEG changes characteristic of the DDS could be lessened by infusions of osmotically active solutes, such as fructose (230) or 3% sodium chloride (250), or by dialyzing patients against hypertonic glucose-containing dialysate (251). This intercompartmental osmotic dysequilibrium was initially attributed to hyponatremia (252) and to the reverse urea effect (230); the latter relates to the fact that urea is cleared more rapidly from the extracellular than intracellular compartment, thus creating a transcellular osmotic gradient for several hours. Rapid dialysis of dogs against dialysate containing high concentrations of sodium or urea, however, failed to prevent cerebral edema (246). In this experimental model, it was also shown that the development of a blood-brain osmotic gradient and cerebral edema during rapid hemodialysis was associated with a decrease in intracerebral and CSF pH, and with the formation of idiogenic osmoles; none of these changes were seen during routine dialysis (246,253). Addition of mannitol to the dialysate during rapid hemodialysis prevented these changes; glycerol did the same, and also prevented appearance of the EEG abnormalities seen in the DDS (vide infra)(253). Thus, the cerebral edema that develops during rapid hemodialysis appears to result from generation of idiogenic osmoles in association with a decrease in intracerebral pH and can be partially or completely corrected by treatment with mannitol or glycerol. The source of the idiogenic osmoles may be intracerebral organic acids (Figure 17.3).

The characteristic clinical picture of DDS develops at or toward the end of a dialysis treatment with the appearance of irritability and restlessness, accompanied by complaints of headache, nausea, muscle cramps, weakness, and fatigue (1,38,65). Vomiting is occasionally seen. If not recognized and treated, hypertension, muscle twitching, fasciculations, asterixis, (1) and confusion develop. Seizures and decreasing consciousness can occur, the latter occasionally progressing to coma. Transient blindness and death due to brainstem herniation have occurred in children and an adolescent (254–256). In recent years only the milder symptoms are commonly seen, since earlier recognition and treatment are the rule (257). The characteristic EEG changes in DDS consist of bursts of bilaterally symmetric, high-voltage rhythmic delta waves. At times this has occurred superimposed on a high-voltage bisynchronous polyrhythmic background (230,251,255).

The differential diagnosis of the DDS includes other causes of altered mental status, neuromuscular hyperirritability, hypertension, and seizures in maintenance dialysis patients (Table 17.4). When hypertension, seizures, or decreased consciousness are present, hypertensive encephalopathy or intracranial hemorrhage should be considered, particularly in the presence of focal neurologic signs.

Management of the DDS involves prophylactic as well as therapeutic intervention. In children and adolescents, mannitol can be used to reduce the likelihood that DDS will develop during the first few treatments, or when the predialysis BUN exceeds 100 mg/dL (257). For this purpose, mannitol (0.5 g/kg) can be given intravenously at onset, followed by an additional 0.25 g/kg at the end of the first and second hours; the cumulative dose should not exceed 1 g/kg, or a total of 50 g per treatment. In patients with mild DDS, mannitol (0.5 g/kg) can be given and repeated once; it should not be given during the final hour of dialysis so that residual drug will not remain in the blood post-treatment. If symptoms persist or progress, the blood flow should be reduced promptly. Should these measures fail or seizures develop, dialysis should be discontinued immediately.

The use of excessive mannitol should be avoided in oligoanuric patients, since it can cause dilutional hyponatremia and symptomatic water intoxication (258), or intravascular volume overload, congestive heart failure, and pulmonary edema (259). Hyponatremia due to mannitol overdose is accompanied by a difference between the measured and calculated serum osmolalities.

Headaches and Muscle Cramps

Isolated headaches are a common complaint during maintenance hemodialysis and have been noted in as many as 72% of patients (260). They most commonly occur during periods of hypotension and become increasingly prevalent as the percent reduction in body weight due to fluid removal (ultrafiltration) increases (261). They occur less frequently during peritoneal than hemodialysis (261). Isolated headaches are also more common in patients with hyporeninemia and have been attributed to mild cerebral hypoperfusion with resultant ischemia (260). However, intradialytic headaches may also occur due to hypertension or intracranial hemorrhage (vide infra).

Muscle cramps occur almost as frequently as headaches and are also more common during hemodialysis than peritoneal dialysis treatments, particularly those resulting in the ultrafiltration of large fluid volumes (261). The use of low, instead of high sodium-containing dialysate (132 versus 145 mEq/L) more frequently results in the development of painful muscle cramps (262). Thus, cramps, as headaches, appear to be precipitated by rapid intravascular volume contraction, presumably due to decreased muscle blood flow and tissue ischemia.

Electrolyte Imbalance

Acute changes in fluid, electrolyte, and acid base balance occur in patients with ESRD. Depending upon the severity of these changes and the rapidity with which they develop, they can profoundly affect the level and content of consciousness, motor activity, and cognition. In general, slow changes are better tolerated than rapid ones. These disturbances include hypo- and hypernatremia, acidemia, hypo- and hypercalcemia, hypophosphatemia, and severe hyperosmolality.

Sodium Imbalance.   In most patients with ESRD, hyponatremia is dilutional; that is, it almost always results from excessive free water intake (264). However, either hypo- or hypernatremia can develop acutely during a hemodialysis session. With the newer central proportioning systems currently in use, hyponatremia is likely to develop only if the concentrate container is not properly connected or appropriate conductivity limits have not been set (265). Because the peritoneum is more permeable to water than sodium, the ultrafiltrate produced during peritoneal dialysis tends to be hypotonic (266); hypernatremia can develop, particularly when rapid fluid ultrafiltration is attempted by using high dextrose concentrations and frequent, short exchanges (267,268). Symptomatic hypo- or hypernatremia usually appears at sodium concentrations below 120 or above 160 mEq/L, respectively (264,269); however, even smaller deviations from the normal range (130 to 150 mEq/L) can produce symptoms if they occur rapidly. The neurologic manifestations of hyponatremia associated with water intoxication include anxiety, headache, irritability, restlessness, abdominal pain, and decreasing consciousness, which can progress to coma if treatment is not initiated. Decreased muscle tone and hyporeflexia are characteristic, and seizures can occur (265,270). Hypothermia, pseudobulbar palsy, and Cheyne-Stokes respiration can also be present (271). If hyponatremia develops acutely during dialysis, the resulting decrease in serum osmolality will also cause pain in the extremity to which blood is returning as an early sign (265). Severe hypernatremia manifests with intense thirst, headache, nausea, and vomiting; if untreated, drowsiness develops, and can progress to coma. Seizures are more common than with hyponatremia (265). Muscle tone is characteristically increased.

In children and adolescents with ESRD, symptomatic dilutional hyponatremia should be treated with fluid restriction. In addition, 3% NaCl should be given judiciously to raise the serum sodium concentration at an appropriate rate to 125 mEq/L, a level at which neurologic disturbances should resolve (269). Thereafter, ongoing fluid restriction should allow further correction to continue. Hypernatremia is managed by administration of hypotonic saline solutions at a rate calculated to allow the serum sodium concentration to fall by approximately 0.5 to 0.6 mEq/L/hr. If the patient experiences seizures during dialysis, the treatment should be promptly discontinued and not resumed until control has been achieved and vital signs have stabilized.

Acidosis.   In patients with ESRD, mild-to-moderate degrees of metabolic acidosis are common and do not generally interfere with CNS function. Rapid changes in pH,

however, may precipitate seizures, particularly in the presence of pre-existing moderate-to-severe acidosis (245). Moreover, abrupt increases in blood pH can lower the serum ionized calcium concentration, further increasing the risk that seizures may develop. Correction of metabolic acidemia can be initiated with small doses of oral alkali as $NaHCO_3$ or Na citrate, 1 to 2 mEq/kg/day in 2 to 4 divided doses; however, full correction is best achieved during dialysis, since the dialysate used contains calcium (3.5 mEq/L).

Calcium Imbalance.   Hypocalcemia is not a complication of maintenance dialysis per se, but is common in newly diagnosed and as-yet untreated patients with ESRD in whom it usually manifests as tetany or seizures. Calcium-responsive seizures also have been reported in a 10-year-old hypocalcemic female following her first peritoneal dialysis treatment (272); these were attributed to delayed metabolism of the lactate, contained in peritoneal dialysate, to bicarbonate, with a subsequent acute rise in blood pH and fall in the ionized calcium fraction. Hypocalcemic seizures can initially be treated with 10% Ca gluconate, 0.5 to 1.0 mL/kg given by *slow* intravenous infusion over 3 to 5 minutes with continuous cardiac monitoring (273). The infusion is stopped if the heart rate falls below 60/min. Once control has been achieved additional calcium can be given by oral supplementation, or by an IV infusion of 4 mg elemental Ca/kg/hr; for every hour the latter is continued, the serum calcium concentration can be expected to rise by no more than 1 mg/dL. The serum calcium x phosphorus product must be monitored and maintained below 70, the level above which metastatic calcification can occur (274); thus, hyperphosphatemia should be treated simultaneously, using a combination of phosphate binding gels, dietary restriction, and dialysis.

In patients receiving treatment for ESRD, hypercalcemia can develop due to severe secondary HPTH, therapy with calcium supplements and vitamin D metabolites, or enhancement of the calcemic effects of PTH on bone (274). The latter has been attributed to removal of circulating inhibitors of bone resorption by dialysis (274). Iatrogenic hypercalcemia has also occurred due to addition of excessive amounts of calcium salts to the dialysate bath (276). The clinical manifestations of hypercalcemia include headache, irritability, and decreased consciousness, accompanied by muscle weakness, hypotonia, and hyporeflexia (265,270). Management includes temporary withdrawal of calcium supplements and vitamin D metabolites; subtotal parathyroidectomy can be indicated in patients with severe secondary HPTH unresponsive to conservative therapy, and in whom renal transplantation is not a possibility in the near future.

Hypophosphatemia.   The combination of dietary restriction, dialysis, and therapy with phosphate binders has resulted in symptomatic hypophosphatemia, particularly in ESRD patients whose food intake is poor due to severe anorexia (277,278). Symptoms usually appear at serum concentrations below 1 mg/dL and are variable; except for the absence of hallucinations, they can resemble those of delirium, a functional psychosis, or the dialysis encephalopathy syndrome (279,280)(vide infra). Treatment should consist of the temporary discontinuation of phosphate binders and administration of parenteral phosphate, followed by oral supplementation (278,281).

Hyperosmolality. The repeated use of peritoneal dialysate relatively high in glucose concentration (4.25% or 7%) has resulted in the development of nonketotic hyperosmolar coma in nondiabetic patients (282,283). In these patients, confusion, facial twitching, focal and generalized seizures, and coma developed at blood glucose concentrations of 900 to 2,400 mg/dL, and were more common following dialysis against the 7% solutions, which are no longer used in pediatric patients. Adequate ultrafiltration can usually be achieved by using combinations of 1.5% and 4.25% glucose-containing dialysate. When the frequent use of 4.25% dialysate is necessary, however, blood glucose concentrations should be monitored, and the addition of insulin directly to dialysate containers considered as a means of controlling hyperglycemia (284).

Cerebrovascular Accidents During Maintenance Dialysis

Subdural hematoma is a serious and often life-threatening complication of maintenance hemodialysis seen in 0.6% to 9.8% of patients (1,285–287). The major factors predisposing to intracranial hemorrhage have been hypertension and long-term oral anticoagulation therapy, the latter prescribed to maintain vascular access patency (286,288). The inadvertent use of excessive amounts of heparin during dialysis (289,290) and the coagulation disturbances associated with intercurrent hepatitis (288) have also been contributory factors. Minor head trauma or the inadvertent use of hypertonic hemodialysate has precipitated intracranial bleeding in hypertensive patients or those receiving supplemental oral anticoagulation (286,288). Finally, a nontraumatic subdural hematoma has been reported in a young adult with ESRD and osteogenesis imperfecta (291). The hematoma was attributed to platelet dysfunction and abnormal capillary fragility.

The clinical manifestations of subdural hematoma include protracted headache, nausea and vomiting, confusion, and decreased consciousness. As such, it can be mistaken for the DDS or even hypertensive encephalopathy, since elevated blood pressures are often present (286). The presence of fluctuating focal or multifocal neurologic signs in as many as 77% of patients, however, and the tendency for these signs, and altered consciousness, to progressively worsen during successive treatments independent of changes in blood pressure, should favor the diagnosis of an expanding intracranial mass lesion (286,288,291). CT or magnetic resonance imaging (MRI) should be performed in patients with any of the above-noted findings; cerebral angiography is also a useful neuroimaging study (286). The appropriate treatment is usually surgical evacuation of the hematoma. Mortality rates as high as 85% have been reported (286); fortunately, this complication is uncommon in pediatric patients (224,288,292).

Dialysis Encephalopathy Syndrome

The Dialysis Encephalopathy Syndrome (DES) is a syndrome of progressive neurologic deterioration initially described in adults receiving maintenance hemodialysis (133). It has occurred in both epidemic and sporadic forms with a worldwide distribution of reported cases (134,293,294). As noted earlier, it is generally accepted that DES is caused by aluminum intoxication (135,136) and that a major source of this metal in adults has been the water used to prepare dialysate (295–297). Although initially described in hemodialysis patients, intoxication in adults, as in children, can follow oral aluminum loading (151,298–300), which can precede initiation of maintenance hemodialysis (301,302). Symptomatic intoxication has also occurred in patients receiving peritoneal dialysis (303,304).

The clinical syndrome typically begins with speech disturbances that have been characterized by progressive mixed dysarthria, apraxia of speech, and aphasia (134, 254). Within months, motor disturbances develop, including tremulousness, myoclonus, asterixis, movement dyspraxia, and memory loss associated with an inability to concentrate. Seizures, personality changes, and frank psychosis can occur (133,134). Initially, the aforementioned cognitive and motor disturbances worsen during dialysis and improve between treatments. Ultimately, however, they persist and patients have become unable to walk or feed themselves. Apneic spells have occurred in advanced disease (306), and death has ensued within months due to sepsis, pneumonitis, or suicide (134).

Characteristic EEG changes occur that are indistinguishable from those seen in children with aluminum intoxication and can antedate the onset of clinical manifestations by months (134). The EEG has, therefore, served as a screening test to identify patients at risk for development of clinically apparent DES.

In the differential diagnosis of DES, acute hypercalcemia (276) and phosphate depletion (279) should be considered. In the former, a syndrome characterized by delirium, dysarthria, myoclonus, and seizures followed an acute rise in serum calcium concentration to 11.8 to 13.7 mg/dL in four maintenance hemodialysis patients and resolved following successful treatment of the hypercalcemia. The neurologic complications of severe hypophosphatemia were described earlier. Finally, intracranial hemorrhage must be considered as a cause of neurologic disturbances that appear to worsen during successive dialysis treatments.

Until 1980, no definitive therapy for aluminum intoxication had been available, although the associated myoclonus was shown to respond well to clonazepam (307,308). As in children (31), successful renal transplantation did not uniformly result in improvement (309,310), possibly because of increased movement of aluminum from bone associated with surgical stress, immobilization, and steroid therapy (169,171). Subsequently, Ackrill et al. (311) and others (312–314) reported dramatic improvement in the speech and motor disturbances in patients with advanced DES following the repeated IV administration of deferoxamine during or following hemodialysis or hemoperfusion. Deferoxamine is most effective in promoting aluminum removal when used in conjunction with charcoal-activated hemoperfusion (315). It has also been effective, however, when added to peritoneal dialysate (316). Recently, Andreoli et al. (317) reported the successful treatment of both CNS and bone manifestations of aluminum intoxication in a 7-year-old boy receiving continuous ambulatory peritoneal dialysis, by the intraperitoneal instillation of deferoxamine, 7.5 mg/kg to each of three daily 750 mL exchanges. Within 3 months school performance, muscle strength, and seizure control improved, and his EEG began to normalize. Thus, the efficacy of this form of therapy has now been established in children.

The presence of clinical and EEG evidence of DES is an indication for discontinuation of aluminum-containing phosphate binders and initiating chelation therapy with deferoxamine, particularly in the presence of: serum aluminum concentrations consistently greater than 100 µg/L, a level that has been associated with increased risk for the development of toxic sequelae (36,73,146,318); an increase in plasma aluminum concentration of greater than 200 µg/L following infusion of deferoxamine, 40 mg/kg IV over 2 hours (174) (This test is particularly helpful in patients with evidence of persistent, unexplained encephalopathy, in whom serum aluminum levels are normal or only mildly elevated)(314); and bone histopathology consistent with aluminum accumulation (73). In conjunction with hemodialysis or hemoperfusion, deferoxamine may be given intravenously at doses of up to 15 mg/kg/hr for the first 2 hours of each treatment (319); serum aluminum concentrations can be expected to rise within 5 hours as tissue stores are mobilized. Therapy should be continued until predialysis serum aluminum concentrations have decreased and stabilized and maximum clinical improvement has been achieved or until evidence of drug toxicity appears (317,319).

The use of deferoxamine in doses of 34 to 175 mg/kg/day for periods of two months to four years, has been associated with ocular and ototoxicity, and fungal infections (320–325). Auditory toxicity has manifested as high frequency sensorineural hearing loss, identified by audiometry in 24.7% of 89 patients, 13 of whom were symptomatic (320,324). Ocular complications have included decreased visual acuity associated with optic atrophy, and asymptomatic changes in the retinal pigment epithelium (320). These complications were reversible to a variable extent upon discontinuation of deferoxamine therapy and occurred infrequently at doses of less than 40 to 50 mg/kg/day (320). Fatal rhinocerebral mucormycosis has occurred in adults receiving maintenance hemodialysis and therapy with deferoxamine (325); it has been suggested that the drug may serve as a growth factor for *Rhizopus* species. Because of these potential complications, the prevention of aluminum encephalopathy is obviously more desirable than the need for chelation therapy. Progressive aluminum loading and intoxication may be minimized by adhering to the following recommendations:

1. Hyperphosphatemia should be controlled with dietary restriction and calcium carbonate as the initial phosphate binder of choice (326,327). Only if adequate control cannot be achieved with calcium carbonate should the addition of an aluminum-containing binder be considered, in which case the total daily dose should not exceed 30 mg elemental aluminum/kg/day (145,146). Nonetheless, even at this dose progressive body aluminum accumulation can occur (327a), indicating that therapy with aluminum-containing phosphate binders may be hazardous at any level of administration. In dialysis patients, magnesium-containing salts have also been successfully used to control hyperphosphatemia (328,329). They must, however, be used with magnesium-free dialysate to avoid development of hypermagnesemia;

2. Infant formulas containing high concentrations of aluminum, particularly soy-base preparations (152,153), should be avoided in patients with severe CRF. Likewise, when formulating total parenteral nutrition orders for such patients, the long-term use of additives high in aluminum content should be avoided if possible. When necessary, patients receiving them should have serum aluminum concentrations monitored at regular intervals;

3. Measures should be instituted to control secondary HPTH, in order to minimize the potential for this hormone to stimulate GI aluminum absorption (158–160);

4. Although uncommon in CRF patients, iron deficiency anemia should be identified and treated to avoid any possible stimulatory effect which it may have on GI aluminum absorption (166);

5. In patients receiving maintenance dialysis, the aluminum concentration of the dialysate should be monitored periodically and ideally maintained below 6 µg/L, a value corresponding to the ultrafilterable fraction of the aluminum concentration in normal serum (20%) (141,330).

Other Dialysis-Related Neurologic Complications

The B vitamins are water soluble and are removed from blood during hemo- and peritoneal dialysis. Failure to replace them with daily supplements has led to the development of neurologic complications, including Wernicke encephalopathy (76) and pyridoxine-responsive seizures in a 1-year-old patient receiving maintenance peritoneal dialysis (331). Vitamin deficiency syndromes should always be considered in the differential diagnosis of neurologic dysfunction in pediatric dialysis patients who have not been receiving oral supplements. The daily oral intake of thiamine (1.5 mg) and pyridoxine (1 mg) is sufficient to compensate for dialysis-related losses (332).

NEUROLOGIC COMPLICATIONS OF RENAL TRANSPLANTATION

Beneficial Effects On Cognitive Function and Neuropathy

Following successful renal transplantation, cognitive function improves in many adults and children when assessed by performance on tests of speed of decision making, vigilance, verbal memory, and susceptibility to distraction (46,47,52,53). When compared to performance prior to transplantation, the results of tests of IQ and overall intellectual function are improved in some reports (47,51), but not in others (50,52), suggesting that these measures of global intelligence may not be sufficiently selective to identify the specific areas of cognitive dysfunction present in patients with severe CRF. Although catch up growth in head circumference and, therefore, in brain size, and improvement in neurodevelopmental status has been observed posttransplantation even among infants with ESRD (56,333), permanent neurologic sequelae can also occur in these patients (37). Moreover, in a study of one set of identical twins (48), one with and one without congenital nephropathy, significant differences in cognitive function were still present at 1 year posttransplantation, suggesting that realization of full intellectual potential may not occur even after normalization of renal function when severe disease has been present from early infancy.

Within weeks of successful transplantation, clinical signs of peripheral neuropathy begin to improve (188). Recovery begins proximally and proceeds distally and tends to follow a biphasic course, with rapid improvement occurring initially and further, more gradual resolution occurring over several months. Generally, any residual deficit which has not begun to resolve within 6 months of transplantation tends to persist (188). NCVs begin improving by 1 to 2 months posttransplantation, in a pattern consistent with both segmental remyelination and axonal regeneration (189,334). In most children, ulnar MNCVs are normal by 12 to 36 months posttransplantation; whereas, those in the peroneal nerve have remained low in 82% of patients for up to 25 to 36 months (206). A further trend toward normalization of brain electrical activity is seen, as evidenced by a significant decrease in the percent of slow-wave associated EEG power (46). Normalization of VEP component latencies has also been demonstrated (46,89).

Adverse Effects of Transplantation

Peripheral Nervous System

Femoral and ulnar neuropathies have developed in children and adults in the immediate post transplant period and appear to result from nerve compression by surgical retractors, hematomas, or direct pressure (335–339); they cause muscle weakness, hyporeflexia, paresthesia, hypesthesia, numbness and hypalgesia, which have tended to resolve over days to weeks. Extradural fat accumulation resulting from corticosteroid therapy has caused spinal cord compression with paraparesis in an adolescent male (340). Cytomegalovirus-associated transverse myelitis (341) and parainfectious polyradiculopathy (342) have also occurred.

Central Nervous System

CNS infections.   Infection remains a major cause of death in pediatric renal transplant recipients (343,344). In nondiabetic patients the risk of developing serious CNS infections and the types of agents responsible for them depend on the amount and duration of immunosuppression administered (345,346); thus, they are uncommon during the first posttransplant month, when cumulative immunosuppressive doses are still relatively low. Thereafter, bacterial infections due primarily to *Listeria monocytogenes* but also to *Streptococcus pneumoniae* have occurred at any time from 2 months to 4 years following graft placement (346–348). *Listeria* most commonly causes acute meningitis or meningoencephalitis, and has been reported in patients as young as 11 years of age (349); fever, headache, meningismus, and an elevated CSF cell count and protein concentration are prominent findings. Altered consciousness and focal neurologic signs can be present (347). *Listeria* can also cause brain abscess (347), cerebritis (350), and pontomedullary infection (351). Viral encephalitis, including fatal CNS infection with Varicella-Zoster virus, has occurred in children and adults between 1 and 30 months after transplantation (348,352). CMV is commonly acquired when seronegative patients receive renal allografts from seropositive donors and is an important cause of systemic infection in transplant recipients (353). Typical manifestations include hepatitis, glomerulitis, leukopenia, arthralgias, and pneumonitis (354). CMV retinitis occurs in patients with chronic viremia and was responsible for the development of acute, reversible blindness in a 13-year-old female, 6 months following transplantation (M. Polinsky, unpublished observation, 1984). Encephalitis due to CMV also occurs (355).

Fungal infections are most commonly due to *Cryptococcus* and *Aspergillus* species, which together with *Listeria* account for 75% to 90% of all CNS infections in renal transplant recipients (345,346). Candidiasis, nocardiosis, histoplasmosis, coccidiosis, sporotrichosis, and (rhinocerebral) mucormycosis have also occurred in adolescents and adults (346,356–360). *Cryptococcus* usually presents more than 4 months posttransplantation with a clinical picture of subacute or chronic meningitis, while *Aspergillus* and other fungi more commonly produce brain abscess or other focal infections that often develop earlier, at 1 to 4 months (345). Clinical presentation is usually manifested by fever, delirium, and seizures, while headache, meningismus, and focal neurologic signs are less common. Evidence of pulmonary involvement with cough and a positive chest radiograph is seen in over 87% of patients and, along with fever, is important in differentiating CNS infection from neoplasia (65,356).

Focal cerebral involvement due to toxoplasmosis (361) and cystercercosis (362) has been reported in two patients, 19 and 17 years old, at 10 and 14 days posttransplantation, respectively. Neither case occurred in the United States.

The initial diagnostic evaluation of all patients with suspected CNS infection should include nonenhanced CT followed by lumbar puncture, unless intracranial pressure is increased. Aseptic meningitis has developed within 72 hours of beginning therapy with OKT$_3$ for acute transplant rejection and should be considered in the differential diagnosis of suspected CNS infection in patients receiving this drug (363). Institution of definitive therapy for CNS infection is contingent upon identification of the responsible organism.

Hypertensive Encephalopathy. Some degree of hypertension has complicated the immediate posttransplant course in 19% to 100% of pediatric patients in various series (348,364–367). It is usually attributable to sodium and water retention associated with initial allograft nonfunction due to vasomotor nephropathy, corticosteroid therapy, and to acute rejection (344,348,364). Subsequently, renal artery stenosis can cause hypertension in as many as 15% of patients (344,364). Late hypertension more commonly results from acute or chronic rejection (348,365). Hypertensive encephalopathy has been reported to occur in 4.7% to 15.6% of pediatric transplant recipients (348,368), and appears to be more common in children than adults (369); the typical presentation is with seizures (368–370). The management of hypertensive encephalopathy was described earlier.

Rejection encephalopathy is a recently described neurologic syndrome seen primarily in children and adolescents, and characterized by headache, altered mental status, seizures, focal neurologic signs, and papilledema (371). Its occurrence has coincided with and, presumably, was related to the severity of episodes of acute rejection. Elevated blood pressures, however, occurred in 14 of 15 episodes and the clinical features of the syndrome were indistinguishable from those of hypertensive encephalopathy. In another report (372), seizures and transient blindness developed in a 12-year-old patient 48 to 72 hours following administration of a dose of IV methylprednisolone, and 24 hours after parenteral diazoxide was given to control blood pressure

elevations to 180/120 mm Hg. Again, it was not possible to exclude hypertension as having contributed to the development of encephalopathy in this patient. The data available to date do not permit characterization of rejection encephalopathy as a new and unique posttransplant neurologic syndrome in children and adolescents.

Drug-Related Neurologic Complications

Corticosteroids can affect cerebral function independent of their tendency to promote sodium and water retention. Acute psychotic reactions or isolated euphoria have occurred in 2.9% of 718 patients receiving oral prednisone and resolved following dosage reduction (373). High dose corticosteroids can cause hyperglycemia and glycosuria, and were responsible for development of nonketotic hyperosmolar coma in a nondiabetic adult transplant recipient (374). Finally, corticosteroids can interfere with glial proliferation and cortical myelination when administered to newborn rats, and have been associated with EEG disturbances and developmental delay in premature infants (54). Whether renal transplantation in young infants would lead to transient or permanent neurodevelopmental sequelae attributable to corticosteroid administration is not clear at present; further investigation of this issue is necessary before transplantation can be accepted as a routine treatment for ESRD during infancy.

Cyclosporin A (CyA), now used for routine immunosuppression following bone marrow and solid organ transplantation, can cause seizures (375,376); CyA blood levels in patients so affected were markedly elevated to 533 to 1,583 ng/mL (normal therapeutic range <400 ng/mL). Tremor, ataxia, muscle weakness, paresthesias, and altered mental status (drowsiness, confusion, and amnesia) have also been described, and usually resolve following dosage reduction (376,377). The use of valproic acid has been recommended when an anticonvulsant is required, since it does not affect corticosteroid or CyA metabolism (378).

Cerebrovascular Complications

Stroke due to thromboembolic phenomena has occurred in 4% to 9.4% of renal transplant recipients and is more common in patients over 40 years old; virtually all reported cases have occurred in individuals 18 years of age or older (343,379–383). No definite period of greatest risk has been identified since strokes have developed at 1 week to 5 years posttransplantation (380,381,384). Predisposing factors include blood hypercoagulability associated with surgery, corticosteroid and CyA therapy, hypertriglyceridemia, malignant hypertension, systemic infection, fat embolization, and preexisting cerebral atherosclerosis (380–388). Stroke has been responsible for 3% to 4% of reported deaths in renal transplant recipients (384); that due to malignant hypertension was the cause of death in 2 pediatric patients (383). By comparison, subarachnoid hemorhage and subdural hematoma were responsible for the deaths of only 0.3% to 0.4% of patients; however, subdural hematomas have occurred exclusively among children and adolescents (384).

CNS Malignancy

Primary malignant neoplasms of the CNS have developed in only a few patients under 20 years of age (344, 389–392); all neoplasms have been lymphomas. The typical clinical picture begins 6 to 9 months postrenal transplantation, and is characterized by headache and focal neurologic deficits that progress rapidly and can be accompanied by evidence of intracranial hypertension. Seizures can occur. The absence of fever and a negative chest radiograph virtually excludes CNS fungal infection, although both conditions can coexist (389). The EEG shows focal slowing over the area of involvement. CT should be performed, and may demonstrate one or more lesions, since these tumors may be multifocal (390–392). However, a normal initial study does not exclude neoplasia. Repeat evaluation should be performed within several days if findings persist or worsen (390). Serologic evidence of recent Epstein-Barr virus (EBV) infection is frequently present (390–392) suggesting that these neoplasms arise as part of an EBV-induced lymphoproliferative disorder resulting from the use of chronic immunosuppression. Radiation therapy has been successful in one patient (389) but in the others death occurred within 2 to 3 weeks from the onset of symptoms.

Other Complications

Progressive multifocal leukoencephalopathy (PML) is an uncommon, subacute demyelinating disease involving white matter of the cerebral and cerebellar hemispheres, and the brainstem (393–395). The disease is caused by the human polyoma viruses JC and SV-40, which have been isolated from the brains of affected patients (396,397). PML has occurred in only nine renal transplant recipients, all adults. The clinical manifestations are those of a slowly progressive dementia, although headaches and focal neurologic deficits may be present. CT can initially be negative and in such cases repeat studies with a double dose of contrast and delayed films can show the characteristic multiple asymmetric areas of abnormal enhancement (397). Concomitant CNS neoplasia can be present and must be ruled out (398). Brain biopsy is sometimes necessary to establish the diagnosis (393). Recently, treatment with cytosine arabinoside has arrested the progression of this formerly fatal disease (397).

Central pontine myelinolysis (CPM) is a fatal disorder of unknown etiology characterized by the development of sharply demarcated, bilaterally symmetric foci of demyelination involving the rostral and central portions of the basis pontis (399). The disease has been identified as a coincidental postmortem finding in two severely debilitated pediatric renal transplant recipients, one of whom died of Pneumocystic carinii pneumonia. Both infection and debility appear to be common antecedents of CPM (76,399). Antemortem diagnosis may be possible in some patients, who present with sensorial clouding, pseudobulbar palsy, facial diplegia, and flaccid quadriparesis (65).

REFERENCES

1. Tyler HR. Neurological complication of dialysis, transplantation, and other forms of treatment in chronic uremia. Neurology 1965;15:1081–1088.
2. Tyler HR. Neurologic disorders in renal failure. Am J Med 1968;44:734–748.
3. Nissensen AR, Levin ML, Klawans HL, et al. Neurological sequelae of end stage renal disease (ESRD). J Chron Dis 1977;30:705–733.
4. Polinsky MS. Neurologic complications of end state renal disease, dialysis, and transplantation. In: Fine RN, Gruskin AB, eds. ESRD in Children. Philadelphia: W.B. Saunders, 1984;307–339.
5. Bergstrom J. Uremia is an intoxication. Kidney Int 1985;28 (suppl 17):S2–S4.
6. Scheinberg P. Effects of uremia on cerebral blood flow and metabolism. Neurology 1954;4:101–105.
7. van den Noort S, Eckel RE, Brine KL, et al. Brain metabolism in experimental uremia. Arch Intern Med 1970;126:831–834.
8. Mahoney CA, Sarnacki P, Arieff AI. Uremic encephalopathy: Role of brain energy metabolism. Am J Physiol 1984;247:F527–F532.
9. Fishman RA, Raskin NH. Experimental uremic encephalopathy, permeability, ion exchange, and brain "spaces." Trans Am Neurol Assoc 1965;90:71–75.
10. Fishman, RA, Raskin NH. Experimental uremic encephalopathy: Permeability and electrolyte metabolism of brain and other tissues. Arch Neurol 1967;17:10–21.
11. Fishman RA. Permeability changes in experimental uremic encephalopathy. Arch Intern Med 1970;126:835–837.
12. Arieff AI, Guisado R, Massry SG. Uremic encephalopathy: Studies on biochemical alterations in the brain. Kidney Int Suppl 1975;7:S194–S200.
13. Mahoney CA, Arieff AI. Central and peripheral nervous system effects of chronic renal failure. Kidney Int 1983;24:170–177.
14. Dettori P, LaGreca G, Biasioli S, et al. Changes of cerebral density in dialyzed patients. Neuroradiology 1982;23:95–99.
15. Minkoff L, Gaertner G, Darab M, et al. Inhibition of brain sodium-potassium ATPase in uremic rats. J Lab Clin Med 1972;80(1):71–78.
16. Fraser CL, Sarnacki P, Arieff AI. Abnormal sodium transport in synaptosomes from brain of uremic rats. J Clin Invest 1985;75:2014–2023.

17. Arieff AI, Massry SG. Calcium metabolism of brain in acute renal failure: Effects of uremia, hemodialysis and parathyroid hormone. J Clin Invest 1974;53:387–392.

18. Akmal M, Goldstein DA, Multani S, et al. Role of uremia, brain calcium, and parathyroid hormone on changes in electroencephalogram in chronic renal failure. J Clin Invest 1984;246:F575–F579.

19. Cogan MG, Covey CM, Arieff AI, et al. Central nervous system manifestations of hyperparathyroidism. Am J Med 1978;65:963–970.

20. Swartz JD, Faerber EN, Singh N, et al. CT demonstration of cerebral subcortical calcifications. J Comput Assist Tomogr 1983;7(3):476–478.

21. Cooper JD, Lazarowitz VC, Arieff AI. Neurodiagnostic abnormalities in patients with acute renal failure. J Clin Invest 1978;61:1448–1455.

22. Arieff AI, Armstrong DK. Parathyroid hormone and uremic neurotoxicity: An unproven association. Contrib Nephrol 1980;20:56–66.

23. Deferrari G, Garibotto G, Robaudo C, et al. Brain metabolism of amino acids and ammonia in patients with chronic renal insufficiency. Kidney Int 1981;10:505–510.

24. Perry TL, Young VW, Kish SJ, et al. Neurochemical abnormalities in brains of renal failure patients treated by repeated hemodialysis. J Neurochem 1985;45(4):1043–1048.

25. Biasioli S, D'Andrea G, Feriani M, et al. Uremic encephalopathy: An updating. Clin Nephrol 1986;25(2):57–63.

26. Olsen S. The brain in uremia. Acta Psychiat Neurol Scand 1961;36:1–122.

27. Passer JA. Cerebral atrophy in end state uremia. Proc Dialysis Transplant Forum 1977;7:91–94.

28. Papageorgiou C, Ziroyannia P, Vathylakis J, et al. The evaluation of cerebral atrophy in renal dialysis patients by computerized tomography. Clin Exper Dialysis and Apheresis 1982;6(2 & 3):97–103.

29. Schnaper HW, Cole BR, Hodges FJ, et al. Cerebral cortical atrophy in pediatric patients with end stage renal disease. Am J Kidney Dis 1983;2(6):645–650.

30. Steinberg A, Afrat R, Pomerantz A, et al. Computerized tomography of the brain in children with chronic renal failure. Int J Pediatr Nephrol 1985;6(2):121–126.

31. Baluarte HJ, Gruskin AB, Hiner LB, et al. Encephalopathy in children with chronic renal failure. Proc Clin Dial Transplant Forum 1977;7:95–98.

32. Bale JF Jr, Siegler RL, Bray PF. Encephalopathy in young children with moderate chronic renal failure. Am J Dis Child 1980;134:581–583.

33. Geary DF, Fennell RS, Andriola M, et al. Encephalopathy in children with chronic renal failure. J Pediatr 1980;96:41–44.

34. Rotundo A, Nevins TE, Lipton M, et al. Progressive encephalopathy in children with chronic renal insufficiency in infancy. Kidney Int 1982;21:486–491.

35. Griswold WR, Reznick V, Mendoza SA, et al. Accumulation of aluminum in a nondialyzed uremic child receiving aluminum hydroxide. Pediatrics 1983;71(1):56–58.

36. Sedman AB, Wilkening GN, Warady BA, et al. Encephalopathy in childhood secondary to aluminum toxicity. J Pediatr 1984;105:836–838.

37. McGraw ME, Haka-Ikse K. Neurologic-developmental sequelae of chronic renal failure in infancy. J Pediatr 1985;106:579–583.

38. Mahoney CA, Arieff AI. Uremic encephalopathies: Clinical, biochemical and experimental features. Am J Kidney Dis 1982;2(3):324–336.

39. Schreiner GE. Mental and personality changes in the uremic syndrome. Medical Annals of the District of Columbia 1959;28(6):316–323, 362.

40. Dinapoli RP, Johnson WJ, Lambert EH. Experience with a combined hemodialysis-renal transplantation program: Neurologic aspects. Mayo Clin Proc 1966;41(12):809–820.

41. Stenback A, Haapanen E. Azotemia and psychosis. Acta Psychiat Scand 1967;43 (Suppl 197):1–65.

42. Plum F, Posner JB. Multifocal, diffuse, and metabolic brain diseases causing stupor or coma. In: Plum F, Posner JB, eds. The Diagnosis of Stupor and Coma. 3rd edition. Philadelphia: F.A. Davis, 1980;225–230.

43. Raskin NA, Fishman RA. Neurologic disorders in renal failure (Part I). N Engl J Med 1976;294(3);143–148.

44. McEnvoy JP. Organic brain syndromes. Ann Intern Med 1981;95:212–220.

45. Swaiman KF. Neurologic complications of renal failure and transplantation. In: Swaiman KF, Wright FS, eds. The Practice of Pediatric Neurology. 3rd Edition. St. Louis: C.V. Mosby, 1975;793–799.

46. Teschan PE, Ginn HE, Bourne JR, et al. Quantitative indices of clinical uremia. Kidney Int 1979;15:676–697.

47. Rasbury WC, Fennell RS III, Morris MK. Cognitive functioning of children with end state renal disease before and after successful renal transplantation. J Pediatr 1983;102(4):589–592.

48. Fennell RS III, Rasbury WC. Cognitive functioning of identical twins discordant for prune belly syndrome and end state renal failure. Int J Pediatr Nephrol 1980;1(4):234–239.

49. Kleinknecht C, Broyer M, Huot D, et al. Growth and development of nondialyzed children with chronic renal failure. Kidney Int Suppl 1983;24 (Suppl 15):S40–S47.

50. Fennell RS III, Rasbury WC, Fennell EB, et al. Effects of kidney transplantation on cognitive performance in a pediatric population. Pediatrics 1984;74(2):273–278.

51. Crittenden MR, Holliday MA, Piel CF, et al. Intellectual development of children with renal insufficiency and end stage disease. Int J Pediatr Nephrol 1985;6(4):275–280.

52. Fennell EB, Fennell RS, Mings E, et al. The effects of various modes of therapy for end stage renal disease on cognitive performance in a pediatric population—A preliminary report. Int J Pediatr Nephrol 1986;7(2):107–112.

53. Fennell RS, Fennell EB, Mings EL, et al. Cognitive performance of children with renal insufficiency. Pediatr Res 1986;20:450A.

54. Polinsky MS, Kaiser BA, Stover JR, et al. Neurologic development of children with severe chronic renal failure from infancy. Pediatr Nephrol 1987;1:157–165.

55. Bird AK, Semmler CJ. The early developmental and neurologic sequelae of children with kidney failure treated by CAPD/CCPD. Pediatr Res 1986;20:446A.

56. So SKS, Chang R, Najarian JS, et al. Growth and development in infants after renal transplantation. J Pediatr 1987;110:343–350.

57. Holliday MA. Calorie deficiency in children with uremia. Effect upon growth. Pediatrics 1972;50:590–597.

58. MacDonnell RC Jr, Buzon MM, Holliday MA. Growth failure in uremic rats: The role of calorie deficiency. Pediatr Res 1973;7:411.

59. Dobbing J, Sands J. Timing of neuroblast multiplication in developing human brain. Nature 1970;226:639–640.

60. Winick M, Rosso P. Head circumference and cellular growth of the brain in normal and marasmic children. J Pediatr 1969;74(5):774–778.

61. Stoch MB, Smyth PM, Moodie AD, et al. Psychosocial outcome and CT findings after gross undernourishment during infancy: A 20-year developmental study. Dev Med Child Neurol 1982;24:419–436.

62. Evans D, Bowie MD, Hansen JDL, et al. Intellectual development and nutrition. J Pediatr 1980;97(3):358–363.

63. Solomon GE, Plum F. General treatment of epilepsy. In: Solomon GE, Plum F, eds. Clinical Management of Seizures: A Guide for the Physician. Philadelphia: W.B. Saunders, 1976;96–123.

64. Tyler HR. Asterixis. J Chron Dis 1965;18:409–411.

65. Raskin NH, Fishman RA. Neurologic disorders in renal failure (Part II). N Engl J Med 1976;294(4):204–210.

66. Stark RJ. Reversible myoclonus with uraemia. Brit Med J 1981;282:1119–1120.

67. Chadwick, D, French AJ. Uraemic myoclonus: An example of reticular reflex myoclonus? J Neurol Neurosurg Psychiatry 1979;42:52–55.

68. Locke S, Merrill JD, Tyler HR. Neurologic complications of acute uremia. Arch Intern Med 1961;108:75–86.

69. Goodhue WW, David JN, Porro RS. Ischemic myopathy in uremic hyperparathyroidism. JAMA 1972;221(8):911–912.

70. Richardson JA, Herron G, Reitz R, et al. Ischemic ulcerations of skin and necrosis of muscle in azotemic hyperparathyroidism. Ann Intern Med 1969;71(1):129–138.

71. Ott SM, Maloney NA, Coburn JW, et al. The prevalence of bone aluminum in renal osteodystrophy and its relation to the response to calcitriol therapy. N Engl J Med 1982; 307(12):709–713.

72. Hodsman AB, Sherrard DJ, Wong EGC, et al. Vitamin D resistant osteomalacia in hemodialysis patients lacking secondary hyperparathyroidism. Ann Intern Med 1981; 94:629–637.

73. Andreoli SP, Bergstein JM, Sherrard DJ. Aluminum intoxication from aluminum-containing phosphate binders in children with azotemia not undergoing dialysis. N Engl J Med 1984;310(7):1079–1084.

74. Chazan JA, Ambler M, Kalderon A, et al. Vascular deposits causing ischemic myopathy in uremia. Ann Intern Med 1970;73:73–79.

75. Berretta JS, Halbrook CT, Haller JS. Chronic renal failure presenting as proximal muscle weakness in a child. J Child Neurol 1986;1:50–52.

76. Lopez RI, Collins GH. Wernicke's Encephalopathy: A complication of chronic hemodialysis. Arch Neurol 1968;18: 248–259.

77. Jacob JC, Gloor P, Elwan CH, et al. Electroencephalographic changes in chronic renal failure. Neurology 1965; 15:419–429.

78. Kiley J. Hines O. Electroencephalographic evaluation of uremia. Arch Intern Med 1965;116:67–73.

79. Engel GL, Romano J, Ferris, EB, et al. A simple method of determining frequency spectra in the electroencephalogram: Observations on effects of physiological variations in dextrose, oxygen, posture, and acid-base balance on the normal electroencephalogram. Arch Neurol Psychiatry 1944;51: 134–146.

80. Guisado R, Arieff AI, Massry SG. Changes in the electroencephalogram in acute uremia. J Clin Invest 1975;55: 738–745.

81. Kiley JE, Pratt KL, Gisser DG, et al. Techniques of EEG frequency analysis for evaluation of uremic encephalopathy. Clin Nephrol 1975;5:279–285.

82. Bourne JR, Ward JW, Teschan PE, et al. Quantitative assessment of the electroencephalogram in renal disease. Electroencephalogr Clin Neurophysiol 1975;39:377–388.

83. John ER, Ahn H, Prichep L, et al. Developmental equations for the electroencephalogram. Science 1980;210(12): 1255–1258.

84. Balzar E, Saltev B, Khass A, et al. Quantitative EEG: Investigation in children with end stage renal disease before and after hemodialysis. Clin Electroencephalogr 1985;17(4): 195–202.

85. John ER, Karmel BZ, Corning WC, et al. Neurometrics. Science 1977;196:1393–1410.

86. Polinsky M, Baird H, Gruskin A, et al. Evaluation of neurologic dysfunction in children with chronic renal disease by neurometrics. Proc Clin Dial Transplant Forum 1980;10: 299–302.

87. Schwartz GJ, Haycoch GB, Edelmann CM Jr, et al. A simple estimate of glomerular filtration rate in children derived from body length and plasma creatinine. Pediatrics 1975;58: 259–263.

88. Cohen SN, Syndulko K, Rever B, et al. Visual evoked potentials and long-latency event-related potentials in chronic renal failure. Neurology (Cleveland) 1983;33:1219–1222.

89. Brown RJ, Sufit R, Sollinger HW. Visual evoked potential changes following renal transplantation. Electroencephalogr Clin Neurophysiol 1987;66:101–107.

90. Rossini PM, DiStefano E, Febro A, et al. Brain stem auditory evoked responses (BAER's) in patients with chronic renal failure. Electroencephalogr Clin Neurophysiol 1984;57: 507–514.

91. Gifford RW Jr, Westbrook E. Hypertensive encephalopathy: Mechanisms, clinical features and treatment. Prog Cardiovasc Dis 1974;17(2):115–124.

92. Healton EB, Brust JCM. Hypertensive encephalopathy and the neurological manifestations of malignant hypertension. Trans Am Neurol Assoc 1979;104:212–214.

93. Dinsdale HB. Hypertensive encephalopathy. Stroke 1983; 13(5):717–719.

94. Still JS, Cottom D. Severe hypertension in childhood. Arch Dis Child 1967;42:34–39.

95. Finnerty FA Jr. Hypertensive encephalopathy. Am J Med 1972;52:672–678.

96. Ingelfinger JR. Hypertension and the central nervous system. In: Ingelfinger JR, ed. Pediatric Hypertension. Philadelphia: W.B. Saunders, 1982;204–217.

97. Healton EB, Brust JC, Feinfeld DA, et al. Hypertensive encephalopathy and the neurologic manifestations of malignant hypertension. Neurology 1982;32:127–132.

98. Trompeter RS, Smith RL, Hoare RD, et al. Neurologic complications of arterial hypertension. Arch Dis Child 1982; 57:913–917.

99. McGregor E, Isles CG, Jay JL, et al. Retinal changes in malignant hypertension. Br Med J 1986;292:233–234.

100. Hulse JA, Dillon MJ, Taylor, DSI. Blindness and paraplegia in severe childhood hypertension. Lancet 1979;2:847.

101. Weingarten KL, Zimmerman RD, Pinto RS, et al. Computed changes of hypertensive encephalopathy. AJNR 1985;6: 395–398.

102. Kwong YL, Yu Yl, Lam KSL, et al. CT appearance in hypertensive encephalopathy. Neuroradiology 1987;29:215.

103. Palmer RF, Lasseter KC. Sodium nitroprusside. N Engl J Med 1975;292(6):294–297.

104. Ingelfinger JR. Hypertensive emergencies and acute hypertension. In: Ingelfinger JR, ed. Pediatric Hypertension. Philadelphia: W.B. Saunders, 1982;218–228.

105. Rudd P, Blaschke TF. Antihypertensive agents and the drug therapy of hypertension. In: Gilman AG, Goodman LS, Rall TW, et al, eds. The Pharmacologic Basis of Therapeutics, 7th edition. New York: Macmillan Publishing Co, 1985; 784–805.

106. Koch-Weser J. Diazoxide. N Engl J Med 1976;294 (23):1271–1273.

107. Anon. Labetalol for hypertension. Med Lett Drugs Ther 1984;26:83–85.

108. Hulse JA, Taylor DSI, Dillon MJ. Blindness and paraplegia in severe childhood hypertension. Lancet 1979;2:553–556.

109. Cove DH, Seddon M, Fletcher RD, et al. Blindness after treatment of malignant hypertension. Br Med J 1979;2:245–246.

110. Pryor JS, Davies PD, Hamilton DV. Blindness and malignant hypertension. Lancet 1979;2:803.

111. Wetherill JH. Blindness after treatment for malignant hypertension. Br Med J 1979;2:500.

112. Brown P, Gross M, Harrison M. Paraplegia following oral hypotensive treatment of malignant hypertension. J Neurol Neurosurg Psychiatry 1987;50:104.

113. Deming QB. Blindness and paraplegia in severe childhood hypertension. Lancet 1979;2:847.

114. Editorial. Thought for autoregulation in the hypertensive patient. Lancet 1979;2:510.

115. Gulliksen G, Hojer-Pederson E, Moller M, et al. Autoregulation of cerebral blood flow in patients with malignant hypertension and hypertensive encephalopathy. Acta Med Scand 1983;678:43–49.

116. Thien TH, Huysmans FTM, Koene RAP. Acute blood pressure reduction in malignant hypertension. Lancet 1979;2: 847.

117. Tyler HR. Neurological aspects of uremia: An overview. Kidney Int Suppl 1975;7(1 Suppl 2):S188–S195.

118. Richet G, Lopez de Noveles E, Verroust P. Drug intoxication and neurologic episodes in chronic renal failure. Br Med J 1979;1:394–395.

119. Bennet WM, Aronoff GR, Golpher TA, et al. Drug prescribing in renal failure: Dosing guidelines for adults. Philadelphia: American College of Physicians, 1987;1–83.

120. Reidenberg MM. The binding of drugs to plasma proteins and the interpretation of measurements of plasma concentrations of drugs in patients with poor renal function. Am J Med 1977;62:466–470.

121. Spector R, Lorenzo AV. The effects of salicylate and probenecid on the cerebrospinal fluid transport of penicillin, aminosalicylic acid and iodide. J Pharm Exper Ther 1974; 188(1):55–65.

122. Fishman RA. Blood-brain and CSF barriers to penicillin and related organic acids. Arch Neurol 1966;15:113–124.

123. Chin DKF, Ho AKC, Tse CY. Neuropsychiatric complications related to use of prazosin in patients with renal failure. Br Med J 1986;293:1347.

124. McAllister CJ, Scowden EB, Stone WJ. Toxic psychosis induced by phenothiazine administration in a patient with chronic renal failure. Clin Nephrol 1978;10(5):191–195.

125. Lieberman JA, Cooper TB, Sockow RF, et al. Tricyclic antidepressant and metabolite levels in chronic renal failure. Clin Pharmacol Ther 1985;37:301–307.

126. Zetin MZ. Letter to the Editor. Clin Nephrol 1979;11: 95–96.

127. Berger M, White J, Travis LB, et al. Toxic psychosis due to cyproheptadine in a child on hemodialysis. Clin Nephrol 1977;7:43–44.

128. El-Housef MK, Janowsky DS, Davis JM, et al. Reversal of antiparkinsonian drug toxicity by physostigmine: A controlled study. Am J Psychiatry 1973;130(2):141–145.

129. Taclob L, Needle M. Drug induced encephalopathy in patients on maintenance hemodialysis. Lancet 1976;1: 704–705.

130. Mandell GL, Sande MA. Antimicrobial agents: Penicillins, cephalosporins and other beta-lactam antibiotics. In: Gilman AG, Goodman LS, Rall TW, et al., eds. The Pharmacologic Basis of Therapeutics. 7th edition. New York: Macmillan Publishing, 1985;1137.

131. Bloomer HA, Burton LJ, Maddock RK Jr. Penicillin-induced encephalopathy in uremic patients. JAMA 1967;200(2): 121–123.

132. Kalloy MC, Tabechian H, Riley GR, et al. Neurotoxicity due to ticarcillin in patients with renal failure. Lancet 1979; 1:608–609.

133. Alfrey AC, Mishell JM, Burks JM, et al. Syndrome of dyspraxia and multifocal seizures associated with chronic hemodialysis. Trans Am Soc Artif Intern Organs 1972;18: 257–261.

134. Burks JS, Alfrey AC, Huddlestone J, et al. A fatal encephalopathy in chronic hemodialysis patients. Lancet 1976;1: 764–768.

135. Alfrey AC, LeGendre GR, Kaehny WD. The dialysis encephalopathy syndrome: Possible aluminum intoxication. N Engl J Med 1976;294:184–188.

136. McDermott JR, Smith AI, Ward MK, et al. Brain aluminum concentration in dialysis encephalopathy. Lancet 1978;1: 901–903.

137. Nathan E, Pedersen SE. Dialysis encephalopathy in a nondialyzed uraemic boy treated with aluminum hydroxide orally. Acta Paediatr Scand 1980;69:793–796.

138. Andreoli SP, Dunn D, DeMyer W, et al. Intraperitoneal deferoxamine therapy for aluminum intoxication in a child undergoing continuous ambulatory peritoneal dialysis. J Pediatr 1985;7(5):760–763.

139. Randall ME. Aluminum toxicity in an infant not on dialysis. Lancet 1983;1:1327–1328.

140. Freundlich M, Zilleruelo G, Abitol C, et al. Infant formula as a cause of aluminum toxicity in neonatal uremia. Lancet 1985;2:527–529.

141. Starkey BJ. Aluminum in renal disease: Current knowledge and future developments. Ann Clin Biochem 1987;24: 337–344.

142. Polinsky MS, Gruskin AB, Balurate HJ, et al. Aluminum in chronic renal failure. In: Strauss J, ed. Pediatric Nephrology Vol 6. Current Concepts in Diagnosis and Management. New York: Plenum Publishing, 1981;315–333.

143. Recker RR, Blotcky AJ, Leffler JA, et al. Evidence for aluminum absorption from the gastrointestinal tract and bone deposition by aluminum carbonate ingestion with normal renal function. J Lab Clin Med 1977;90(5): 810–815.

144. Kaehny WD, Hegg AP, Alfrey AC. Gastrointestinal absorption of aluminum from aluminum-containing antacids. N Engl J Med 1977;296(24):1389–1392.

145. Salusky IB, Coburn JW, Pauneir L, et al. Role of aluminum hydroxide in raising serum aluminum levels in children undergoing continuous ambulatory peritoneal dialysis. J Pediatr 1984;105:717–720.

146. Sedman AB, Miller NL, Warady BA, et al. Aluminum loading in children with chronic renal failure. Kidney Int 1984;26:201–204.

147. Pillion G, Loirat C, Blum C, et al. Aluminum encephalopathy: A potential risk of aluminum gels in children with chronic renal failure. Int J Pediatr Nephrol 1981;2(1):29–32.

148. Polinsky MS, Kaiser BA, Root AW, et al. The effects of phosphate binder dose and parathyroid hormone on serum aluminum levels in pediatric maintenance dialysis patients. Pediatr Res 1986;20(4 Pt 2):456A.

149. Milliner DS, Malekzadeh M, Lieberman E, et al. Plasma aluminum levels in pediatric dialysis patients: Comparison of hemodialysis and continuous ambulatory peritoneal dialysis. Mayo Clin Proc 1987;62:269–74.

150. Graf H, Stummvoll HK, Meisinger V, et al. Aluminum removal by hemodialysis. Kidney Int 1981;19:587–592.

151. Brahm M. Serum aluminum in nondialyzed chronic uremic patients before and during treatment with aluminum-containing phosphate-binding gels. Clin Nephrol 1986;25(5):231–235.

152. Sedman AB, Klein GL, Merritt JR, et al. Evidence of aluminum loading in infants receiving intravenous therapy. N Engl J Med 1985;312(21):1337–1343.

153. Weintraub R, Hams G, Meerking M, et al. High aluminum content of infant milk formulas. Arch Dis Child 1986;61:914–916.

154. McGraw M, Bishop N, Jameson R, et al. Aluminum content of milk formulae and intravenous fluids used in infants. Lancet 1986;1:157.

155. Milliner DS, Shinaberger JH, Shuman P, et al. Inadvertent aluminum administration during plasma exchange due to aluminum contamination of albumin-replacement solutions. N Engl J Med 1985;312:165–168.

156. Fell GS, Maharaj D. Trace metal contamination of albumin solutions used for plasma exchange. Lancet 1986;2:467–468.

157. Klein GL, Alfrey AC, Miller NL, et al. Aluminum loading during total parenteral nutrition. Am J Clin Nutr 1982;35:1425–1429.

158. Mayor GH, Keiser JA, Madani D, et al. Aluminum absorption and distribution: Effect of parathyroid hormone. Science 1977;197:1187–1189.

159. Mayor GH, Sprague SM, Hourani MR, et al. Parathyroid hormone-mediated aluminum deposition and egress in the rat. Kidney Int 1980;17:40–44.

160. Alfrey AC, Sedman A, Chan Y-L. The compartmentalization and metabolism of aluminum in uremic rats. J Lab Clin Med 1985;105:227–233.

161. Cann CE, Prussin SG, Gordan GS. Aluminum uptake by the parathyroid glands. J Clin Endocrinol Metab 1979;49(4):543–545.

162. Morrissey J, Rothstein M, Mayor G, et al. Suppression of parathyroid hormone secretion by aluminum. Kidney Int 1983;23:699–794.

163. Cannata JB, Briggs JD, Junor BJR, et al. Effect of aluminum overload on calcium and parathyroid hormone metabolism. Lancet 1983;1:501–503.

164. Burnatowska-Hledin MA, Doyle TM, Eadie MJ, et al. 1, 25-Dihydroxyvitamin D_3 increases serum and tissue accumulation of aluminum in rats. J Lab Clin Med 1986;108:96–102.

165. Demontis R, Leflon A, Fournier A, et al. 1-alpha (OH) vitamin D_3 increases plasma aluminum in hemodialysed patients taking Al(OH)$_3$. Clin Nephrol 1986;26(3):146–149.

166. Cannata JB, Suarez Suarez C, Cuesta V, et al. Gastrointestinal aluminum absorption: Is it modulated by the iron-absorptive mechanism? Proc Eur Dial Transplant Assoc–Eur Ren Assoc. 1985;21:354–359.

167. Foley CM, Polinsky MS, Gruskin AB, et al. Encephalopathy in infants and children with chronic renal disease. Arch Neurol 1981;38:656–658.

167a. Polinsky MS, Prebis JW, Elzouki AY, et al. A dialysis encephalopathy-like syndrome in childhood: An international survey. Pediatr Res 1980;14:1017.

168. Young JB, Ahmed-Jushuf IH, Browjohn AM, et al. The role of EEG monitoring and immobilization in dialysis encephalopathy. Dial Transplant 1988;17(1):15–17.

169. Platts MM, Anastassiades E. Dialysis encephalopathy: Precipitating factors and improvement in prognosis. Clin Nephrol 1981;15:223–228.

170. Masramon J, Ricart MJ, Caralps A, et al. Dialysis encephalopathy. Lancet 1978;1:1370.

171. Platts M. Dialysis encephalopathy. Lancet 1980;2:1035–1036.

172. Browder AA, Joselow MM, Louria DB. The problem of lead poisoning. Medicine (Baltimore) 1973;52(2):121–139.

173. Hodsman AB, Hood SA, Brown P, et al. Do serum aluminum levels reflect underlying skeletal aluminum accumulation and bone histology before or after chelation by deferoxamine? J Lab Clin Med 1985;106:674–681.

174. Milliner DS, Nebeker HG, Ott SM, et al. Use of the deferoxamine infusion test in the diagnosis of aluminum-related osteodystrophy. Ann Intern Med 1984;101:775–780.

175. Nielsen VK. The peripheral nerve function in chronic renal failure. I. Clinical signs and symptoms. Acta Med Scand 1971;190:105–111.

176. Fine RN, Korsch BM, Grushkin CM, et al. Hemodialysis in children. Am J Dis Child 1970;119:498–504.

177. Romagnoni M. Neuropathy in uremia. N Engl J Med 1970;282(22):1271.

178. McVicar M, Gauthier B, Goodman CT. Uremic Neuropathy: Monitoring of transketolase activity inhibition in a child. Am J Dis Child 1973;125:263–265.

179. Callaghan N. Restless legs syndrome in uremic neuropathy. Neurology (Minn) 1961;16:359–361.

180. Nielsen VK. The peripheral nerve function in uremia: II. Intercorrelation of clinical symptoms and signs and clinical grading of neuropathy. Acta Med Scand 1971;190:113–117.

181. Appenzeller O, Kornfeld M, MacGee J. Neuropathy in chronic renal disease: A microscopic, ultrastructural and biochemical study of sural nerve biopsies. Arch Neurol 1971;24:449–461.

182. Dyck PJ, Johnson WJ, Lambert EH, et al. Segmental demyelination secondary to axonal degeneration in uremic neuropathy. Mayo Clin Proc 1971;46:400–431.

183. Dinn JJ, Crane DL. Schwann cell dysfunction in uremia. J Neurol Neurosurg Psychiatry 1970;33:605–608.

184. Thomas PK, Hollinrake K, Lascelles RG, et al. The polyneuropathy of chronic renal failure. Brain 1971;94:761–780.

185. Savazzi GM, Buzio C, Migone L. Lights and shadows on the pathogenesis of uremic polyneuropathy. Clin Nephrol 1982;18(5):219–229.

186. Arieff AI. Neurologic manifestations of uremia. In: Brenner BM, Rector FC, eds. The Kidney. 3rd edition. Philadelphia: W.B. Saunders, 1985;1747–1751.

187. Hodson AK. Peripheral neuropathy in childhood: An update in diagnosis and management. Pediatr Ann 1983;12(11):814–820.

188. Nielsen VK. The peripheral nerve function in chronic renal failure. VIII. Recovery after renal transplantation. Clinical aspects. Acta Med Scand 1974;195:163–170.

189. Bolton CF, Baltzan MA, Baltzan RB. Effects of renal transplantation on uremic neuropathy: A clinical and electrophysiologic study. N Engl J Med 1971;284(21):1170–1175.

190. Nielsen VK. The peripheral nerve function in chronic renal failure. VI. The relationship between sensory and motor nerve conduction and kidney function, azotemia, age, sex and clinical neuropathy. Acta Med Scand 1973;194:455–462.

191. Avram MM, Feinfeld DA, Huatuco AH. Search for the uremic toxin: Decreased motor nerve conduction velocity and elevated parathyroid hormone in uremia. N Engl J Med 1978;298(18):1000–1003.

192. DiGuilio S, Chkoff N, Lhaste F, et al. Parahormone as a nerve poison in uremia. N Engl J Med 1978;299(20):1134–1135.

193. Mallamaci F, Zoccali C, Ciccarelli M, et al. Autonomic function in uremic patients treated by hemodialysis or CAPD, and in transplant patients. Clin Nephrol 1986;25(4):175–180.

194. Nielsen VK. The peripheral nerve function in renal failure. III. A multivariate statistical analysis of factors presumed to affect the development of clinical neuropathy. Acta Med Scand 1971;190:119–125.

195. Jennekens FGI, Dorhout Mees EJ, van der Most Spijk D. Clinical aspects of uremic polyneuropathy. Nephron 1971;8:414–426.

196. Savazzi GM, Migone L, Cambi V. The influence of glomerular filtration rate on uremic polyneuropathy. Clin Neurol 1980;13:64–72.

197. Tenckhoff HA, Boen FST, Jebsen RH, et al. Polyneuropathy in chronic renal insufficiency. JAMA 1965;192(13):1121–1129.

198. Jebsen RH, Tenckhoff H, Honet, JC. Natural history of uremic polyneuropathy and effects of dialysis. N Engl J Med 1967;277(7):327–333.

199. Versaci AA, Olsen KJ, McMain PB, et al. Uremic polyneuropathy and motor nerve conduction velocities. Trans Amer Soc Artif Int Organs 1964;10:328–331.

200. Lascelles RG, Thomas PG. Changes due to age in internodal length in the sural nerve in man. J Neurol Neurosurg Psychiatry 1966;29:40–44.

201. Nielsen VK. The peripheral nerve function in chronic renal failure. V. Sensory and motor conduction velocity. Acta Med Scand 1973:194:445–454.

202. Bolton CF. Peripheral neuropathies associated with chronic renal failure. J Can Sci Neurol 1980;7(2):89–96.

203. Nielsen VK. The peripheral nerve function in chronic renal failure: A survey. Copenhagen: Christtrev & Petersens, 1974;10.

204. Daniel CR III, Bower JD, Pearson JE, et al. Vibrometry and uremic peripheral neuropathy. South Med J 1977;70(11):1311–1316.

205. Nielsen VK. The peripheral nerve function in chronic renal failure. VII. Longitudinal course during terminal renal failure and regular hemodialysis. Acta Med Scand 1974;195:155–162.

206. Arbus GS, Barnor N-A, Hsu AC, et al. Effect of chronic renal failure, dialysis and transplantation on motor nerve conduction velocity in children. Can Med Assoc J 1975;113:517–520.

207. Mentser MI, Clay S, Malekzadeh MH, et al. Peripheral motor nerve conduction velocities in children undergoing chronic hemodialysis. Nephron 1978;22:337–341.

208. Argov Z, Mastaglia F. Drug-induced peripheral neuropathies. Br Med J 1979;1:663–666.

209. Read DJ, Feest TG, Nassim MA. Clonazepam: Effective treatment for restless leg syndrome in uraemia. Br Med J 1981;283:885–886.

210. Woo GC, Mandelman T, Liu TT, et al. Effect of hemodialysis on contrast sensitivity in renal failure. Am J Optom Physiol Optics 1986;63(5):356–361.

211. Hilton AF, Harrison JD, Lamb AM, et al. Ocular complications in haemodialysis and renal transplant patients. Aust J Ophthalmol 1982;10:247–253.

212. Sverak J, Peregrin J, Hejcmanova D, et al. Long-term observation of retinal electrical activity in dialyzed and renal transplantation patients. Artif Organs 1984;8(3):355–363.

213. Mirahmadi MK, Vaziri ND. Hearing loss in end stage renal disease-effect of dialysis. J Dial 1980;4(4):159–165.

214. Henich WL, Thompson P, Bergstrom L, et al. Effect of dialysis on hearing acuity. Nephron 1977;18:348–351.

215. Bergstrom L, Thompson P. Hearing loss in pediatric renal patients. Int J Pediatr Otorhinolaryngol 1983;5:227–234.

216. Quick CA, Hoppe W. Permanent deafness associated with furosemide administration. Ann Otol 1975;84:94–101.

217. Kanfer A, Stamatakis G, Torlotin JC, et al. Changes in erythromycin pharmacokinetics induced by renal failure. Clin Nephrol 1987;27(3):147–150.

218. Kroboth PD, McNeil MA, Kreeger A, et al. Hearing loss and erythromycin pharmacokinetics in a patient receiving hemodialysis. Arch Intern Med 1983;143:1263–1265.

219. Spinozzi NS, Murray CL, Grupe WE. Altered taste acuity in children with end stage renal disease. Pediatr Res 1978;12:442.

220. Siegler RL, Eggert JV, Udomkesmalee E. Diagnostic indices of zinc deficiency in children with renal diseases. Ann Clin Lab Sci 1981;11(5):428–433.

221. Eggert JV, Siegler RL, Udomkesmalee E. Zinc supplementation in chronic renal failure. Int J Pediatr Nephrol 1982;3(1):21–24.

222. Shapera MR, Moel DI, Kamath SK, et al. Taste perception of children with chronic renal failure. J Am Diet Assoc 1986;86:1359–1365.

223. Ginn HE. Neurobehavioral dysfunction in uremia. Kidney Int 1975;7(1 Suppl 2):S217–S221.

224. Grushkin CM, Korsch BM, Fine RN. Hemodialysis in small children. JAMA 1972;221(8):869–873.

225. Jackson M, Warrington EK, Roe CJ, et al. Cognitive function in hemodialysis patients. Clin Nephrol 1987;27(1):26–30.

226. Teschan PE, Bourne Jr, Reed RB, et al. Electrophysiological and neurobehavioral responses to therapy: The National Cooperative Dialysis Study. Kidney Int 1983;23 Suppl 13:S58–S65.

227. Ratner DP, Adams KM, Lewis NW, et al. Effects of hemodialysis on the cognitive and sensory-motor functioning of the adult chronic hemodialysis patient. J Behav Med 1983;6(3):291–311.

228. Rasbury WC, Fennell RS III, Fennell EB, et al. Cognitive function in children with end stage renal disease pre- and post-dialysis session. Int J Pediatr Nephrol 1986;7(1):45–50.

229. Blumenkrantz M, Lindsay RM. Comparison of hemodialysis and peritoneal dialysis: A review of the literature. Contrib Nephrol 1979;17:20–29.

230. Kennedy AC, Linton AL, Luke RG, et al. Electroencephalographic changes during haemodialysis. Lancet 1963;1:408–411.

231. Foley CM, Dy BO, Polinsky MS. Paroxysmal EEG abnormalities in children with renal failure. Electroencephalogr Clin Neurophysiol 1985.

232. Rizzo PA, Pierelli F, Pozzessere G, et al. Pattern visual evoked potentials and brainstem auditory evoked responses in uremic patients. Acta Neurol Belg 1982;82:72–79.

233. Chan JCM, Eng G. Long-term hemodialysis and nerve conduction in children. Pediatr Res 1979;13:591–593.

234. Caccia MR, Mangili A, Mecca G, et al. Effects of hemodialytic treatment on uremic polyneuropathy: A clinical and electrophysiologic study. J Neurol 1977;217:123–131.

235. Babb A, Popovich RP, Christopher TG. The genesis of the square meter-hour hypothesis. Trans Am Soc Artif Int Organs 1971;17:81–91.

236. Honet JC, Jebsen RH, Tenchkoff HA. Motor nerve conduction velocity in chronic renal insufficiency. Arch Phys Med 1966;47:647–652.

237. Kominami N, Tyler HR, Hampers CL, et al. Variations in motor nerve conduction velocity in normal and uremic patients. Arch Intern Med 1971;128:235–239.

238. Meyrier A, Fardeau M, Richet G. Acute asymmetrical neuritis associated with rapid ultrafiltration dialysis. Br Med J 1972;2:252–254.

239. Teehan BP, Smith LJ, Gilgore GS, et al. Adverse effects of large surface area dialysis on motor nerve conduction velocity. Proc Dial Transplant Forum 1974;4:166–171.

240. Bosl R, Shideman JR, Meyer RM, et al. Effects and complications of high efficiency dialysis. Nephron 1975;15:151–160.

241. Fleming LW, Lenman JAR, Stewart WK. Effect of magnesium on nerve conduction velocity during regular dialysis treatment. J Neurol Neurosurg Psychiatry 1972;35:342–355.

242. Davison AM, Williams IR, Mawdsley C, et al. Neuropathy associated with hepatitis in patients maintained on haemodialysis. Br Med J 1972;1:409–411.

243. Popovtzer MM, Rosenbaum BJ, Gordon A, et al. Relief of uremic polyneuropathy after bilateral nephrectomy. N Engl J Med 1969;281(17):949–950.

244. Kerr DNS. Clinical and pathophysiologic changes in patients on chronic dialysis: The central nervous system. Adv Nephrol 1980;9:109–132.

245. Wakin KG. The pathophysiology of the dialysis disequilibrium syndrome. Mayo Clin Proc 1969;44:406–429.

246. Arieff AI, Massry SG, Barriendos A, et al. Brain water and electrolyte metabolism in uremia: Effects of slow and rapid hemodialysis. Kidney Int 1973;4:177–187.

247. Arieff AI, Guisado R, Massry SG, et al. Central nervous system pH in uremia and the effects of hemodialysis. J Clin Invest 1976;58:306–311.

248. LaGreca G, Dettore P, Biasioli S, et al. Brain density studies during dialysis. Lancet 1980;2:582.

249. Watson AG, Greenwood WR. Studies on the intraocular pressure during dialysis. Can J Ophthalmol 1966;1:301–307.

250. Port FK, Johnson WJ, Klass DW. Prevention of dialysis disequilibrium syndrome by use of high sodium concentration in the dialysate. Kidney Int 1973;3:327–333.

251. Hampers CL, Doak PB, Callaghan MN, et al. The electroencephalogram and spinal fluid during hemodialysis. Arch Intern Med 1966;118:340–346.

252. Wakim KG, Johnson WJ, Klass DW. Role of blood urea and serum sodium concentrations in the pathogenesis of the dialysis disequilibrium syndrome. Trans Amer Soc Artif Int Organs 1968;14:394–401.

253. Arieff AI, Lazarowitz VC, Guisado RG. Experimental dialysis disequilibrium syndrome: Prevention with glycerol. Kidney Int 1978;14:270–278.

254. Moel DI, Kwun YA. Cortical blindness as a complication of hemodialysis. J Pediatr 1978;93(5):890–891.

255. Kennedy AC. Dialysis disequilibrium syndrome. Electroencephlogr Clin Neurophysiol 1970;29:213.

256. Milutinovich J, Warren J, Graefe U. Death caused by brain herniation during hemodialysis. South Med J 1979;72(4):418–420.

257. Mauer SM, Lynch RM. Hemodialysis techniques for infants and children. Pediatr Clin North Am 1976;23(4) 843–856.

258. Borges HF, Hocks J, Kjellstrand CM. Mannitol intoxication in patients with renal failure. Arch Intern Med 1982;142:63–66.

259. Weiner IM, Mudge GH. Diuretics and other agents employed in the mobilization of edema fluid. In: Gilman AG, Goodman LS, Rall TW, et al., eds. The Pharmacologic Basis of Therapeutics. 7th edition. New York: Macmillan Publishing, 1985;889.

260. Bana DS, Graham JR. Renin response during hemodialysis headache. Headache 1976;16:168–172.

261. Quellhorst EA. Ultrafiltration and hemofiltration practical applications. In: Drukker W, Parsons FM, Maher JF, eds. Replacement of Renal Function by Dialysis. 2nd edition. Boston: Martinius Nijhoff, 1985;271.

262. Stewart WR, Fleming LW, Manual MA. Muscle cramps during maintenance dialysis. Lancet 1972;1:1049–1051.

263. Chillar RK, Desforges JF. Muscular cramps during maintenance dialysis. Lancet 1972;2:285.

264. Alvis R, Geheb M, Cox M. Hypo- and hyperosmolar states: Diagnostic approaches. In: Arieff AI, DeFronzo RA, eds. Fluid, Electrolyte and Acid-Base Disorders. New York: Churchill-Livingstone, 1985;209.

265. Blagg CR. Acute complications associated with hemodialysis. In: Drukker W, Parsons FM, Maher JF, eds. Replacement of Renal Function by Dialysis. 2nd edition. Boston: Martinius Nijhoff, 1983;615–17.

266. Nolph KD, Twardowsky ZJ, Popovich RP, et al. Equilibration of peritoneal dialysis solutions during long-dwell exchanges. J Lab Clin Med 1979;93(2):246–256.

267. Ribot S, Jacobs MG, Frankel HJ, et al. Complications of peritoneal dialysis. Am J Med Sci 1966;35:505–517.

268. Smith RJ, Black MR, Arieff AI, et al. Hypernatremic hyperosmolar coma complicating chronic peritoneal dialysis. Proc Dial Transplant Forum 1974;4:96–99.

269. Ayus JC, Krothapalli RK, Arieff AI. Changing concepts in treatment of severe symptomatic hyponatremia: Rapid correction and possible relation to central pontine myelinolysis. Am J Med 1985;78:897–902.

270. Prensky AL, Dodge PR, Barlow CF, et al. Interrelationships between the nervous system and nutritional, electrolyte, and endocrine disorders. In: Swaiman KF, Wright FS, eds. The Practice of Pediatric Neurology. St. Louis: C.V. Mosby, 1982;606–610.

271. Berl T, Anderson RJ, McDonald KM, et al. Clinical disorders of water metabolism. Kidney Int 1976;10:117–132.

272. Whang R, Draney D, Ryan M. Postdialysis convulsions: Treatment with calcium infusion. Rocky Mt Med J 1971;68:41–43.

273. Norman ME. Renal and electrolyte emergencies. In: Fleisher G, Ludwig S, eds. Textbook of Pediatric Emergency Medicine. Baltimore: Williams and Wilkins, 1983;432.

274. David DS. Calcium metabolism in renal failure. Am J Med 1975;48–56.
275. Coburn JW, Massry SG, DePalma R, et al. Rapid appearance of hypercalcemia with initiation of hemodialysis. JAMA 1969;210:2276–2278.
276. Rivera-Vazquez AB, Noriega-Sanchez A, Ramierz-Gonzales R, et al. Acute hypercalcemia in hemodialysis patients: Distinction from dialysis dementia. Nephron 1980;25:243–246.
277. Lotz M, Zisman E, Bartter FC. Evidence for a phosphorus depletion syndrome in man. N Engl J Med 1968;278(8):409–415.
278. Kreisberg RA. Phosphorus deficiency and hypophosphatemia. Hosp Prac 1977;12(3):121–128.
279. Pierides AM, Ward MK, Kerr DNS. Haemodialysis encephalopathy: Possible role of phosphate depletion. Lancet 1976;1:1234–1235.
280. Ward MK, Pierides AM, Fawcett P, et al. Dialysis encephalopathy syndrome. Proc Eur Dial Transplant Assoc 1976;13:348–354.
281. Lentz RD, Brown DM, Kjellstrand CM. Treatment of severe hypophosphatemia. Ann Intern Med 1978;89:941–944.
282. Boyer J, Gill GN, Epstein FH. Hyperglycemia and hyperosmolality complicating peritoneal dialysis. Ann Intern Med 1967;67(3):568–572.
283. Bhatacharjee N, Sharma BK, Kataria PN, et al. Blood glucose changes and hazards of hyperosmolar coma during and after peritoneal dialysis. J Assoc Physicians India 1973;21(6):505–510.
284. Oreopoulos DG. Chronic peritoneal dialysis. Clin Nephrol 1978;9(4):165–173.
285. Leonard CD. Subdural hematoma and dialysis: Survey of reprint requesters. N Engl J Med 1970;282(25):1433–1434.
286. Leonard A, Shapiro FL. Subdural hematoma in regularly hemodialyzed patients. Ann Intern Med 1975;82:650–658.
287. Siddiqui JY, Fitz AE, Lawlor RL, et al. Causes of death in patients receiving long-term hemodialysis. JAMA 1970;212(8):1350.
288. Bechar M, Lakke JPWF, van der Hem GK, et al. Subdural hematoma during long-term dialysis. Arch Neurol 1972;26:513–516.
289. Leonard CD, Weil E, Scribner BH. Subdural haematomas in patients undergoing hemodialysis. Lancet 1969;2:239–240.
290. Del Greco F, Krumlovsky F. Subdural hematoma in the course of haemodialysis. Lancet 1969;2:1009–1010.
291. Sayre MR, Roberge JR, Evans TC. Nontraumatic subdural hematoma in a patient with osteogenesis imperfecta and renal failure. Am J Emerg Med 1987;5(4):298–301.
292. Fine RN, Malekzadeh MH, Pennisi AJ, et al. Long-term results of renal transplantation in children. Pediatrics 1978;61(4):641–650.
293. Mahurkar SD, Dhar SK, Salta R, et al. Dialysis dementia. Lancet 1973;1:1412–1415.
294. Wing AJ. Dialysis dementia in Europe: Report from the registration committee of the European Dialysis and Transplant Association. Lancet 1980;2:190–192.
295. Kaehny WD, Alfrey AC, Holman RE. Aluminum transfer during hemodialysis. Kidney Int 1977;12:361–365.
296. Elliott HL, Dryburgh F, Fell GS, et al. Aluminum toxicity during regular haemodialysis. Br Med J 1978;1:1101–1103.
297. Davison AM, Walker GS, Oli H, et al. Water supply aluminum concentration, dialysis dementia, and effects of reverse osmosis water treatment. Lancet 1982;2:785–787.
298. Cannata JB, Briggs JD, Junor BJR, et al. Aluminum hydroxide intake: Real risk of aluminum toxicity. Br Med J 1983;286:1937–1938.
299. Masselot JP, Adhemar JP, Jaudon MC, et al. Reversible dialysis encephalopathy: Role for aluminum-containing gels. Lancet 1978;2:1386–1387.
300. Buge A, Poisson M, Masson S, et al. Encephalopathie reversible des dialysees apres l'apport d'aluminum. Nouv Presse Med 1979;8(34)2729–2733.
301. Mehta RP. Encephalopathy in chronic renal failure appearing before the start of dialysis. Can Med Assoc J 1979;120:1112–1114.
302. Etheridge WB, O'Neill WM Jr. The "dialysis encephalopathy syndrome" without dialysis. Clin Nephrol 1978;10(6):250–252.
303. Smith DB, Lewis JA, Burks JS, et al. Dialysis encephalopathy in peritoneal dialysis. JAMA 1980;244(4)365–366.
304. Cumming AD, Simpson G, Bell G, et al. Acute aluminum intoxication in patients on continuous ambulatory peritoneal dialysis. Lancet 1982;1:103–104.
305. Rosenbek JC, McNeil MR, Lemme ML, et al. Speech and language findings in a chronic hemodialysis patient: A case report. J Speech Hear Disord 1975;40(2):245–252.
306. Garcia-Bunuel L, Elliott DC, Blank NK. Apneic spells in progressive dialytic encephalopathy. Arch Neurol 1980;37:594–596.
307. Trauner DA, Clayman M. Dialysis encephalopathy treated with clonazepam. Ann Neurol 1979;6(6):555–556.
308. Pascoe MD. Clonazepam in dialysis encephalopathy. Ann Neurol 1981;9(2):200.
309. Sullivan PA, Murnaghan DJ, Callaghan N. Dialysis dementia: Recovery after transplantation. Br Med J 1977;2:740.
310. Mattern WD, Krigman MR, Blythe WB. Failure of successful renal transplantation to reverse the dialysis associated encephalopathy syndrome. Clin Nephrol 1977;7:275–278.
311. Ackrill P, Ralston AJ, Day JP, et al. Successful removal of aluminum from patients with dialysis encephalopathy. Lancet 1980;2:692–693.
312. Pogglitsch H, Petek W, Wawschenek O, et al. Treatment of early stages of dialysis encephalopathy by aluminum depletion. Lancet 1981;2:1344–1345.
313. Arze RS, Parkinson IS, Cartlidge NEF, et al. Reversal of aluminum dialysis encephalopathy after desferrioxamine treatment. Lancet 1987;2:1116.
314. Sprague SM, Corwin HL, Wilson RS, et al. Encephalopathy in chronic renal failure responsive to deferoxamine therapy: Another manifestation of aluminum neurotoxicity. Arch Intern Med 1986;146:2063–2064.
315. Chang TMS, Barre P. Effect of desferrioxamine on removal of aluminum and iron by coated charcoal haemoperfusion and haemodialysis. Lancet 1983;2:1051–1053.
316. Payton DC, Junor BJR, Fell GS. Successful treatment of aluminum encephalopathy by intraperitoneal desferrioxamine. Lancet 1984;1:1132–1133.
317. Andreoli SP, Dunn D, DeMyer W, et al. Intraperitoneal deferoxamine therapy for aluminum intoxication in a child undergoing continuous ambulatory peritoneal dialysis. J Pediatr 1985;107:760–763.
318. Roodhooft AM, van de Vyver FL, D'Haese PC, et al. Aluminum accumulation in children on chronic dialysis: Predictive value of serum aluminum levels and desferrioxamine infusion test. Clin Nephrol 1987;28(3):125–129.

319. Malluche HH, Smith AJ, Abreo K, et al. The use of deferoxamine in the management of aluminum accumulation in bone in patients with renal failure. N Engl J Med 1984; 311(3):140–144.

320. Olivieri NF, Buncic JR, Chew E, et al. Visual and auditory neurotoxicity in patients receiving subcutaneous deferoxamine infusions. N Engl J Med 1986;314:869–873.

321. Davies SC, Marcus RE, Hungerford JL, et al. Ocular toxicity of intravenous high dose deferoxamine. Lancet 1983;2: 181–184.

322. Borgina-Pignatti C, DeStefano P, Broglia AM. Visual loss in patient on high-dose subcutaneous desferrioxamine. Lancet 1984;1:681.

323. Bournerias F, Monnier N, Dufier JL, et al. Toxicite oculaire severe de la desferrioxamine chez l'hemodialyse. Nephrologie 1987;8:27–29.

324. Gallant T, Bayden MH, Gallant LA, et al. Serial studies of auditory neurotoxicity in patients receiving deferoxamine therapy. Am J Med 1987;83:1085–1090.

325. Windus DW, Stokes TJ, Julian BA, et al. Fatal Rhizopus infections in hemodialysis patients receiving deferoxamine. Ann Intern Med 1987;107:678–680.

326. Salusky JB, Coburn JW, Foley J, et al. Effects of oral calcium carbonate on control of serum phosphorus and changes in plasma aluminum levels after discontinuation of aluminum-containing gels in children receiving dialysis. J Pediatr 1986;108(1):767–770.

327. Moriniere PH, Roussel A, Tahiri Y, et al. Substitution of aluminum hydroxide by high doses of calcium carbonate in patients on chronic haemodialysis: Disappearance of hyperaluminaemia and equal control of hyperparathyroidism. Proc Eur Dial Transplant Assoc 1982;19: 784–787.

327a. Salusky IB, Foley J, Nelson P, et al. Aluminum accumulation during treatment with aluminum hydroxide and dialysis in children and young adults with chronic renal disease. N Engl J Med 1991;324:527–531.

328. Guillot A, Hood VL, Runge CF, et al. The use of magnesium-containing phosphate binders in patients with end stage renal disease on maintenance hemodialysis. Nephron 1982;30:114–117.

329. O'Donovan R, Baldwin D, Hammer M, et al. Substitution of aluminum salts by magnesium salts in control of dialysis hyperphosphatemia. Lancet 1986;1:880–882.

330. Graf H, Stummvoll HK, Meisinger V. Dialysate aluminum concentration and aluminum transfer during hemodialysis. Lancet 1982;1:46–47.

331. Joshioka T, Iitaka K, Kasai N, et al. Uncontrollable convulsions responsive to pyridoxal phosphate in a uremic child. Int J Pediatr Nephrol 1984;5(4):221–222.

332. Kopple JD, Swendseid ME. Vitamin nutrition in patients undergoing maintenance hemodialysis. Kidney Int 1975;7(1 suppl 2):S79–S84.

333. Kohaut EC, Whelchel JR, Waldo FB, et al. Living related donor renal transplantation in children presenting with end stage renal disease in the first month of life. Transplantation 1985;40:725–726.

334. Nielsen VK. The peripheral nerve function in chronic renal failure. IX. Recovery after renal transplantation. Electrophysiologic aspects (sensory and motor nerve conduction). Acta Med Scand 1974;195:171–180.

335. Yazbek S, Larbrisseau A, O'Regan S. Femoral neuropathy after renal transplantation. J Urol 1985;134; 720–721.

336. Vogels M, Buskeus F, de Vries J, et al. Femoral neuropathy after renal transplantation. Int J Pediatr Nephrol 1987;8:55–56.

337. Vaziri ND, Barnes J, Mirahmadi K, et al. Compression neuropathy subsequent to renal transplantation. Urology 1976;7:145–147.

338. Probst A, Harder F, Hofer H, et al. Femoral nerve lesions subsequent to renal transplantation. Eur Urol 1982; 8:314–316.

339. Zylicz A, Nuyten FJJ, Notermans SLH, et al. Postoperative ulnar neuropathy after kidney transplantation. Anesthesia 1984;39:1117–1120.

340. Lee M, Lekins J, Gubbay SS, et al. Spinal cord compression by extradural fat after renal transplantation. Med J Aust 1975;1:201–203.

341. Spitzer PG, Tarsy D, Eliopoulos GM. Acute transverse myelitis during disseminated cytomegalovious infection in a renal transplant recipient. Transplantation 1987;44(1): 151–153.

342. Bale JF, Rote NS, Bloomer LC, et al. Guillain-Barré-like polyneuropathy after renal transplant: Possible association with cytomegalovirus infection. Arch Neurol 1980;37:784.

343. Potter D, Feduska N, Melzer J, et al. Twenty years of renal transplantation in children. Pediatrics 1986;77(4): 465–470.

344. Novello AJ, Fine RN. Renal transplantation in children: A review. Int J Pediatr Nephrol 1982;3(2)87–98.

345. Rubin RH, Wofson JS, Cosimi AB, et al. Infection in the renal transplant recipient. Am J Med 1981;70:405–411.

346. Tilney NL, Kohler TR, Strom TB. Cerebromeningitis in immunosuppressed recipients of renal allografts. Ann Surg 1982;195(1);104–109.

347. Lechtenberg R, Sierra MF, Pringle GF, et al. Listeria monocytogenes: Brain abscess or meningoencephalitis? Neurology 1979;29:86–90.

348. Hodson BM, Najarian JS, Kjellstrand CM, et al. Renal transplantation in children ages 1–5 years. Pediatrics 1978;61:458–464.

349. Holden FA, Kaczmer JE, Kinahan CC. Listerial meningitis and renal allografts: A life-threatening affinity. Postgrad Med 1980;68:69–74.

350. Watson GW, Fuller TJ, Elms J, et al. Listeria cerebritis: Relapse of infection in renal transplant patients. Arch Intern Med 1978;138:83–87.

351. Mahoney JF, Manbyah JA, Dalton VC, et al. Pontomedullary Listeriosis in renal allograft recipient. Br Med J 1974;1:705.

352. Peterson LR, Ferguson RM. Fatal central nervous system infection with Varicella-Zoster virus in renal transplant recipients. Transplantation 1984;37(4):366–368.

353. Chow S. Acquisition of donor strains of cytomegalovirus by renal transplant recipients. N Engl J Med 1986; 314(22):1418–1423.

354. Fiala M, Payne JE, Berne TV, et al. Epidemiology of cytomegalovirus infection after transplantation and immunosuppression. J Infect Dis 1975;132:421–433.

355. Schneck SA. Neuropathologic features of human organ transplantation. I. Probable cytomegalovirus infection. J Neuropathol Exp Neurol 1965;24:415–429.

356. Rifkind D, Marchioro TL, Schneck SA, et al. Systemic fungal infections complicating renal transplantation and immunosuppressive therapy: Clinical, microbiologic, neurologic and pathologic features. Am J Med 1967;43:28–38.

357. Gullberg RM, Quintanilla A, Levin ML, et al. Sporotrichosis: Recurrent cutaneous, articular, and central nervous system infection in a renal transplant recipient. Rev Infect Dis 1987;9(2):369–375.

358. Morduchowicz G, Shmueli D, Shapira Z, et al. Rhinocerebral mucormycosis in renal transplant recipients: Report of three cases and review of the literature. Rev Infect Dis 1986; 8(3):441–446.

359. Karalakulasingam R, Arora KK, Adams G, et al. Meningoencephalitis caused by Histoplasma capsulatum. Arch Intern Med 1976;136:217–220.

360. Barmeir E, Mann JH, Marcus RH. Cerebral nocardiosis in transplant patients. Br J Radiol 1981;54:1107–1109.

361. Tsanaclis AMC, de Morais CF. Cerebral Toxoplasmosis after renal transplantation: Case report. Pathol Res Pract 1986;181:339–341.

362. Gordillo-Paniagua G, Munoz-Arizpe R, Ponsa-Molina R. Unusual complication in a patient with renal transplantation: Cerebral Cystircercosis. Nephron 1987;45:65–67.

363. CDC. Aseptic meningitis among kidney transplant recipients receiving a newly marketed murine monoclonal antibody preparation. MMWR 1986;35(34):551–552.

364. Fine RN, Korsch BM, Stiles Q, et al. Renal homotransplantation in children. J Pediatr 1970;75(3):347–357.

365. Fine RN, Korsch BM, Edelbrock HH, et al. Cadaveric renal transplantation in children. Lancet 1971;1:1087–1091.

366. Arbus GS, Galiwango J, DeMaria JE, et al. Transplantation and complications of chronic renal failure. Can Med Assoc J 1980;120:659–664.

367. Rizzoni G, Malekzadeh MH, Pennisi AJ, et al. Renal transplantation in children less than 5 years of age. Arch Dis Child 1980;55:532–536.

368. Bates S, Nathan J, McEnery PT, et al. Epilepsy in childhood renal transplantation: A 20 year experience in 135 patients. Ann Neurol 1986;20(3):426.

369. Prasad KSR, Date A, Chandi SM, et al. Central nervous disease in renal transplant recipients. Nephron 1987;46:395–396.

370. McGonicle RJS, Bewick M, Tafford JAP, et al. Hypertensive encephalopathy complicating transplant renal artery stenosis. Postgrad Med 1984;50:356–358.

371. Gross MLP, Sweny P, Pearson RM, et al. Rejection encephalopathy: An acute neurological syndrome complicating renal transplantation. J Neurol Sci 1982;56:23–34.

372. El-Dahr S, Chevalier RL, Gomez RA, et al. Seizures and blindness following intravenous pulse methylprednisolone in a renal transplant patient. Int J Pediatr Nephrol 1987; 8(2):87–90.

373. The Boston Collaborative Drug Surveillance Program. Acute adverse reactions to prednisone in relation to dosage. Clin Pharmacol Ther 1972;13(5):694–698.

374. Daouk AA, Malek GH, Kauffman HM, et al. Hyperosmolar nonketotic coma in a kidney transplant recipient. J Urol 1972;108:524–525.

375. Shah D, Rylance PB, Rogerson ME, et al. Generalized epileptic fits in renal transplant recipients given cyclosporin A. Br Med J 1984;289:1347–1348.

376. Beaman M, Parvin S, Veitsch PS, et al. Convulsions associated with cyclosporin A in renal transplant recipients. Br Med J 1985;290:139–140.

377. Atkinson K, Biggs J, Darveniza P, et al. Cyclosporine-associated central nervous system toxicity after allogeneic bone-marrow transplantation. N Engl J Med 1984;310(8):527.

378. Hillebrand G, Castro LA, van Scheidt W, et al. Valproate for epilepsy in renal transplant recipients receiving cyclosporine. Transplantation 1987;43(6):915–916.

379. Gruber SA, Pescovitz MD, Simmons RL, et al. Thromboembolic complications in renal allograft recipients: A report from the Prospective Randomized Study of Cyclosporine Versus Azathioprine-Antilymphocyte Globulin. Transplantation 1987;44(6)775–778.

380. Adams HP, Dawson G, Coffman TJ, et al. Stroke in renal transplant recipients. Arch Neurol 1986;43:113–115.

381. Rao KV, Smith EJ, Alexander JW, et al. Thromboembolic disease in renal allograft recipients. Arch Surg 1976;111: 1086–1092.

382. Hulme B, Kenyon JR, Owen K, et al. Renal transplantation in children. Arch Dis Child 1972;486–494.

383. Avner ED, Harmon WE, Grupe WE, et al. Mortality of chronic hemodialysis and renal transplantation in pediatric endstage renal disease. Pediatrics 1981;67(3):412–416.

384. Harris RD, Campbell JK, Howard FM, et al. Neurovascular complications of dialysis and transplantation. Stroke 1974;5:725–729.

385. Dintenfass L, Ibels LS. Blood viscosity factors and occlusive arterial disease in renal transplant recipients. Nephron 1975; 15:456–465.

386. Lieberman E, Heuser E, Gilchrist GS, et al. Thrombosis nephrosis, and corticosteroid therapy. J Pediatr 1968;73:320–328.

387. Vanranterghem Y, Roels L, Lerut T, et al. Thromboembolic complications and haemostatic changes in cyclosporin-treated cadaveric kidney allograft recipients. Lancet 1985;1: 999–1002.

388. Jones JP Jr, Engleman EP, Najarian JS. Systemic fat embolism after renal homotransplantation and treatment with corticosteroids. N Engl J Med 1965;273(27):1453–1458.

389. Schneck SA, Penn I. Cerebral neoplasms associated with renal transplantation. Arch Neurol 1970;22:226–233.

390. Mirra SS, Check IJ, Porter JD, et al. Rapid evolution of central nervous system lymphoma in a renal transplant recipient. Lancet 1981;2:868–869.

391. van Diemen-Steenvoorde R, Donckerwolcke RAMG, Kluin Ph M, et al. Epstein-Barr virus related central nervous system lymphoma in a child after renal transplantation. Int J Pediatr Nephrol 1987;7(1):56–58.

392. Hanevold C. Personal communication (1987).

393. ZuRhein GM, Varakis J. Progressive multifocal leukoencephalopathy in a renal allograft recipient. Lancet 1974; 2:798.

394. McCormick WF, Schochet SS Jr, Sarles HE, et al. Progressive multifocal leukoencephalopathy in renal transplant recipients. Arch Intern Med 1976;136:829–834.

395. Garcia JH, Dismukes WE, Duvall ER. Medical Pathology Conference. Ala J Med Sci 1981;18(1):61–67.

396. Sangalang VE, Embil JA. Recovery of papovavirus in cell culture explants of brain tissue from case of progressive multifocal leukoencephalopathy. Lancet 1982;2:329–330.

397. Saxton CR, Gailiunas P Jr, Helderman JH, et al. Progressive multifocal leukoencephalopathy in a renal transplant recipient: Increased diagnostic sensitivity of computed tomographic scanning by double-dose contrast with delayed films. Am J Med 1984;77:333–337.

398. Egan JD, Ring BL, Reding MJ. Reticulum cell sarcoma and progressive multifocal leukoencephalopathy following renal transplantation. Transplantation 1980;29(1):84–86.

399. Schneck SA. Neuropathological features of human organ transplantation. II. Central pontine myelinolysis and neuro axonal dystrophy. J Neuropathol Exp Neurol 1966;25: 18–39.

Chapter 18
Disorders of Gastrointestinal Tract and Liver

W. Donald Shields

Neurologic disorders are sometimes associated with abnormalities of the gastrointestinal tract and liver. Those diseases primarily affecting the liver are particularly likely to cause signs and symptoms of neurologic impairment. A variety of other neurologic diseases, especially those of childhood as in the case of static encephalopathy, are likely to cause gastrointestinal dysfunction, notably gastroesophageal reflex.

EPISODIC GASTROINTESTINAL DISORDERS

Children with episodic vomiting or abdominal pain are commonly referred for neurologic assessment because of a question of "abdominal migraine" or "abdominal epilepsy." Establishing the correct diagnosis may be difficult because the patient is commonly younger than the age of 5 years and is unable to clearly relate the details of symptoms and signs. Moreover, there is often a lack of typical features of either migraine or epilepsy. Episodic vomiting and abdominal pain are components of a general disorder, the periodic syndrome, reported in 1933 (1); this syndrome also includes episodic headaches, dizziness, or fever.

Cyclic Vomiting

Cyclic vomiting is such a common event in childhood that it would seem difficult to designate it as a "syndrome"; however, the description of Gee (1882) characterized it well: "These cases seem to be all of the same kind, their characteristic being fits of vomiting, which recur after intervals of uncertain length. The intervals themselves are free from signs of disease. The vomiting continues for a few hours or a few days. When it has been severe, the patients are left much exhausted. The patients are children. In most cases, the closest observation fails to discover anything which can be called a cause" (2).

Cyclic vomiting may begin as early as infancy or as late as 8 to 10 years of age; it typically occurs, however, between the ages of 2 and 4 years (1,3). The vomiting can begin at any time of the day or night, and although usually limited to a period of several days, it may last more than a week in some patients (4). In the most severe cases, vomiting leads to dehydration requiring hospitalization. There is a strong association between episodic vomiting occurring in childhood and migraine in the young adult. In the early years of cyclic vomiting, there is little mention of headache; however, in later years, headaches become more prominent and eventually replace vomiting as the predominant symptom. Before presuming that the cyclic vomiting is migrainous in nature, however, other neurologic disorders must be considered and excluded (Table 18.1).

Evaluation

Children who present with cyclic vomiting should have studies to exclude other disorders in which recurrent vomiting may be a notable feature of the disease. The most important part of the evaluation is carrying out a careful, complete history and physical examination. Computed tomographic (CT) or magnetic resonance imaging (MRI) head scans should be obtained if there is any question of increased intracranial pressure or if focal neurologic abnormalities are present. It is always possible that children with recurrent vomiting, particularly when it occurs in the morning, have intracranial space-occupying lesions. In some patients with brain tumors, the usual periodicity of

Table 18.1 Neurologic disorders associated with cyclic vomiting

Migraine

Increased intracranial pressure
   CNS tumors
   Cerebral abscess
   Other space occupying lesions

Metabolic disorders
   Urea-cycle disorders
   Organic acidemias
   Aminoacidopathies
   Hypoglycemia

Epilepsy

Familial dysautonomia

vomiting may not be present, and some patients have vomiting for a few days only to be followed by a period of normalcy for weeks to months. Some of these children have intermittent obstruction of the third or fourth ventricle by a tumor, followed by compensation and clinical recovery. The differentiation can be more difficult to assess because the typical age of presentation of childhood posterior fossa brain tumors is similar to that of children with typical cyclic vomiting.

Most of the remaining disorders can be excluded by electroencephalography (EEG) or by evaluating blood and urine tests, which should include serum ammonia, glucose, lactate and pyruvate levels, as well as amino and organic-acid assays.

There have been reports that cyclic vomiting can be a manifestation of seizures. It is acknowledged that vomiting can be a component of complex partial epilepsy. The vast majority of children with vomiting associated with epilepsy, however, will have other manifestations of a seizure disorder that will make the diagnosis clear. Millichap (5) reported the EEG findings in 33 patients with cyclic vomiting. Seven of the patients had tonic-clonic or complex partial seizures, but the others did not have typical clinical signs of a seizure disorder. The most common EEG abnormalities included atypical spike and wave discharges, paroxysmal high voltage waves, and single spike discharges. The symptoms were improved with phenytoin therapy. It should be remembered, however, that a normal EEG does not rule out epilepsy nor does an abnormal EEG prove the diagnosis. Moreover, phenytoin and other anticonvulsant drugs have been shown to be efficacious in the treatment of migraine. Thus, a beneficial response to anticonvulsant drugs can not be taken as proof of the diagnosis of epilepsy. Epilepsy may be a rare cause of cyclic vomiting, but the patient should have other manifestations of a seizure disorder or a characteristic EEG (or both) to corroborate that diagnosis.

When other etiologies have been excluded, and the features characteristic of migraine are present, then migraine should be seriously entertained as a clinical diagnosis of cyclic vomiting, for there is a strong association between the two. In one study, 40% of children with migraine between the ages of 5 and 18 years of age had episodic vomiting at some time as a part of the symptomatology (6). Eliciting a careful history must include specific questions regarding common symptoms associated with migraine. These symptoms often include pallor, sweatiness, dizziness, photophobia, and abdominal discomfort or cramping. The presence of these associated symptoms supports the diagnosis. Of course, the history of recurrent headache is most persuasive for the diagnosis of migraine if all other disorders that cause increased intracranial pressure have been excluded.

A family history of migraine is important and should be sought in every case. In the studies of Barlow, a positive family history of migraine was obtained in 89% of cases if that history was diligently pursued (7); whereas, if one only cursorily sought a family history of migraine, it was positive in only half of the cases. Because there is a family history of migraine in about 90% of patients with cyclic vomiting, a negative family history makes the diagnosis of migraine less likely. The difficulty in establishing an accurate diagnosis lessens as the child grows older, because migraine headaches become more apparent, and, in retrospect, the diagnosis becomes clear.

Treatment

Appropriate therapy depends on establishing an accurate diagnosis. If a specific neurologic disorder is discovered, treatment is directed to that problem; on the other hand, if the child has cyclic vomiting as a manifestation of migraine, treatment may take one of two directions. The first therapeutic possibility is symptomatic treatment or treating the episode, and the second is prophylactic treatment to prevent recurrence.

Individual episodes of vomiting can be treated with antiemetics. The rectal administration of trimethobenzamide HCl, 100 to 200 mg t.i.d., usually controls the vomiting. Fluid intake and evidence of dehydration must be carefully evaluated and, on occasion, intravenous fluid replacement is required.

If the child has frequent episodes of cyclic vomiting (usually more than 2 episodes per month), and they significantly interfere with school and other activities, prophylactic treatment is appropriate. Most children will respond to the administration of propranolol, 10 mg t.i.d.; older children may require 20 mg t.i.d. If this therapeutic regimen is unsuccessful, other medications can be considered (Table 18.2). The fact that patients with juvenile migraine often respond to prophylactic therapy with anticonvulsant medication further confuses the differentiation of epilepsy and migraine. It must be recognized, however, that a positive response to anticonvulsants is not an indication that the child has epilepsy.

Table 18.2 Prophylactic treatment of migraine (headaches and cyclic vomiting)

Propranolol
   Administer propranolol 10 mg t.i.d. for 2 to 4 weeks to be followed by 20 mg t.i.d. if necessary. Teenagers can be increased up to the maximum adult dosage of 80 mg t.i.d. A period of 3 months may be required to determine drug efficacy.

Anticonvulsant medication

   Phenobarbital
   This drug is often effective, starting with dosages of 15 to 30 mg/day and gradually increasing to 3 to 5 mg/kg/day.

   Carbamazepine
   This drug is administered in doses of 10 to 25 mg/kg/day.

   Phenytoin
   The recommended dosage is 3 to 5 mg/kg/day. A variety of somatic effects may occur including gingival hypertrophy, hirsutism, acneform eruption, and coarsening of facial features; the drug is less commonly used for treatment of migraine.

Cyproheptadine
   A useful drug for younger children when administered in dosage ranging from 2 to 4 mg 2 to 4 times daily.

Calcium-channel blockers
   There is little experience with the use of these drugs in children, although they may be of benefit.

Stress reduction and biofeedback
   Although these measures have been used in the treatment of childhood migraine, no carefully controlled studies are available.

Cyclic Abdominal Pain

Recurrent "stomach ache" is a very common disorder, occurring in at least 1 of 10 children (8). When abdominal pain occurs episodically, without other evidence of illness, it may lead to an extensive gastroenterologic evaluation. In some children, no specific cause for the recurrent pain is discovered, and the child is then referred to a neurologist to rule out "abdominal migraine" or "abdominal epilepsy." In most cases, nonspecific episodic abdominal pain has an underlying psychologic basis. There are, however, cases of migraine or epilepsy that may present in this manner. As in the case of cyclic vomiting, a diagnosis is made by performing a careful history and physical examination. Neither epilepsy nor migraine should be diagnosed by exclusion (9).

The differentiation of abdominal migraine and abdominal epilepsy can be difficult. Prichard (10) described 19 patients with periodic abdominal pain, dividing the patients into two groups on the basis of clinical observation. In one group the pain had a sudden onset, was brief in duration (5 to 10 minutes), and was associated with confusion. The EEGs in this group were abnormal, commonly revealing temporal spike discharges. A diagnosis of complex partial epilepsy/abdominal epilepsy was made. In the second group, the pain had a gradual onset, the duration was longer (1 to 6 hours), and was not associated with alteration of consciousness. Many of these children had pallor, nausea, and vomiting. The EEGs were either normal or nonspecifically abnormal in most patients, but one child had atypical spike-wave discharges. This complex of symptoms led to a diagnosis of abdominal migraine.

Abdominal pain is a common complaint in patients with migraine and occurs more frequently than cyclic vomiting. The pain typically lasts more than 1 hour and is associated with other findings characteristic of migraine such as vomiting, pallor, and photophobia. In older children, the abdominal pain is usually associated with headache. As in the case of patients with cyclic vomiting, the family history is an important part of the assessment, and without identified family members with migraine, that diagnosis is less likely.

Abdominal epilepsy is usually assoicated with other symptoms characteristic of complex partial epilepsy (CPE). Many children with CPE have abdominal pain as part of the "aura," the beginning of the seizure. The pain is usually in the epigastrium and may proceed to a typical "rising epigastric sensation." Some children report an unusual abdominal feeling, but cannot describe it further. The aura is followed by typical manifestations of the complex partial seizure; the patient loses awareness of the environment and may have onset of abnormal motor movements (e.g., chewing, mouthing movements, fumbling with the hands). This may be followed by more complex motor activity such as undressing, walking and running. The patient may interact in a limited way during this phase of the seizure, but has no recollection of the ictal events. After institution of appropriate therapy for epilepsy, occasional abdominal discomfort may persist, and this may be an indication that the seizures are not fully controlled. In this setting, the diagnosis of "abdominal epilepsy" is fully justified. It is the rare epileptic child who has abdominal pain as the only symptom of a seizure disorder. In general, the diagnosis should not be made without associated symptoms of epilepsy and a diagnostic EEG.

DISEASES OF THE GASTROINTESTINAL TRACT

Dysphagia

Because swallowing requires such complex and elegant neurologic control of oronasopharyngeal muscular coordination, it is not surprising that abnormalities of deglutition result from many different neuromuscular disorders. Control of oronasopharyngeal muscular activity is critical for survival. Children with the most serious forms of dysphagia are at risk for recurrent aspiration pneumonia and sudden death from obstruction of the airway.

The differential diagnosis of dysphagia includes virtually all disorders that can affect the neuromuscular system. We will review only the most common conditions or those that must be specifically considered. As in the evaluation of any neurologic problem, neuroanatomic localization of the abnormality is crucial. The lesions causing dysphagia may be upper motor neuron (UMN), lower motor neuron (LMN), cranial or peripheral nerves, at the myoneural junction, or in the muscle itself. Accordingly, the child who presents with dysphagia as the primary symptom must be carefully examined and the lesion localized.

Static encephalopathy is the most common UMN disorder in children causing dysphagia. Other UMN conditions encountered include: developmental (structural) cerebral abnormalities or those affecting the posterior fossa (i.e., Arnold-Chiari malformation), those that affect the autonomic nervous system (i.e., Riley-Day syndrome), and diseases that damage the nervous system (i.e., multiple sclerosis and strokes). Dysphagia is occasionally a component of chromosomal abnormalities such as the "G syndrome," inherited as an autosomal dominant trait, with multiple congenital anomalies. Affected infants have a characteristic facial appearance, and the associated dysphagia is often severe enough to be life threatening (11).

LMN disease may also result in dysphagia. Failure of development of the cranial nerve nuclei can cause dysphagia as in the case of the Moebius syndrome and is often the most threatening abnormality these children encounter. Progressive spinal muscular atrophy (Werdnig-Hoffman disease) may result in severe dysphagia. Guillain-Barré syndrome can be associated with dysphagia, but it virtually never occurs without other characteristic findings of a symmetric polyneuropathy.

Diseases of the neuromuscular junction can present with dysphagia as one of the primary symptoms. Patients with infant botulism present with multiple abnormalities, the most significant of which are related to progressive weakenss (12,13). Most patients have abnormalities of sucking and swallowing as primary symptoms, occasionally preceding the ocular manifestations (12). During the acute phases of infant botulism, patients often require nasogastric feeding, but they usually recover fully with supportive care. Similarly, patients with myasthenia gravis may have dysphagia as one of the most troublesome problems (13).

Dysphagia has also been reported in hyperthyroidism and usually occurs when the disease is well established, appearing to be part of generalized muscle weakness. It may, however, occasionally be the presenting sign of thyrotoxicosis (14,15).

Gastroesophageal Reflux

Gastroesophageal reflux (GER) is a common disorder in children, particularly in those with static encephalopathy. GER occurs when the gastric contents are allowed to flow into the esophagus. It is the result of inadequate sphincter tone at the gastroesophageal junction and when combined with the pressure differential between the abdomen (positive pressure) and the chest cavity (negative pressure, especially during inspiration), the esophagus may become inflamed by the high acidity of the gastric contents, causing severe discomfort. GER usually presents in young infants, but with proper management is self-limited. It occurs in about 1 in 300 infants (16), and it is more common in children with static encephalopathy and other neurologic disorders (17,18). In a study of 136 severely retarded, institutionalized children, Sondheimer (18) observed that 15% had recurrent vomiting, and 3/4 of those had GER. In another study of 29 retarded children with GER (21), a high incidence of kyphoscoliosis (18), dysphagia (17), and "extensor spasms" was noted (19).

Of particular interest is that the converse circumstance may also occur; that is, children with serious GER who appear to have signs and symptoms of neurologic disorders, but in whom those signs and symptoms are secondary to the GER. Apnea is the most common neurologic sequela of reflux; however, it may be associated with more complex neurologic signs and symptoms including disorders of movement, dystonia, torticollis, and "seizures." When these neurologic signs and symptoms occur as a result of reflux, the problem has been designated *Sandifer syndrome*. The seizures are thought to be the result of apnea rather than true epilepsy.

Bray, et al (20), reported 13 children with Sandifer syndrome who were referred to the child neurologist for evaluation of possible neurologic diseases but who proved to have GER. Treatment of the GER led to the resolution of the neurologic symptoms. The children ranged in age from a few months to 5 years at the time of evaluation. Eleven of the children had apparent "dystonia," which was manifested as a head tilt or torticollis in eight patients, increased muscle tone in one, and decreased muscle tone in two patients. Ten children had developmental delay, and six were reported to have had "seizures." The seizures occurred in children younger than 1 year of age and were characterized by apnea, cyanosis, and stiffening. Four patients had been placed on phenobarbital prior to the time of neurologic assessment. None of the patients with "seizures" had any EEG abnormality consistent with epilepsy, although one patient was thought to have infantile spasms. All 13 children had resolution of the neurologic symptoms and signs within a few months following the institution of appropriate treatment for GER. Children with possible Sandifer syndrome should be carefully examined for congenital anomalies. A child with "G" syndrome, inherited as an autosomal dominant trait with multiple congenital anomalies, was reported to have severe GER (21). The boy was initially misdiagnosed as Sandifer syndrome. The characteristic abnormal facies eventually led to the correct diagnosis.

MALABSORPTION DISORDERS

Chronic Cholestasis

A slowly progressive syndrome of neurologic deterioration has been reported in children with chronic liver disease associated with cholestasis (22). The children characteristically have onset of liver disease in infancy. The neurologic abnormalities generally have their onset between 5 and 12 years of age. The first sign of neurologic impairment is the loss of deep-tendon reflexes, and the disease progresses to immobility within a period of months to years in many cases. Characteristic findings include absent deep-tendon reflexes, absent perception of vibration with otherwise normal proprioception, ataxia, ophthalmoplegia (usually impaired upward gaze), distal motor weakness, and unaffected intelligence.

Neuropathologic examination shows abnormalities of the posterior columns, Clarke column, mild degeneration of dorsal and ventral spinocerebellar tracts, and axonal degeneration in peripheral nerves. The changes are similar to those found in animal models of vitamin E deficiency. The children reported also had markedly decreased levels of vitamin E (23,24).

These observations are of great importance to the child with cholestatic liver disease because it appears that the neurologic abnormalities can be prevented by vitamin E administration; when neurologic abnormalities are already apparent, however, treatment is much less effective.

Cystic Fibrosis

Cystic fibrosis is the most common genetic disease in man, and one of its hallmarks is the malabsorption of fat. A milder form of the neurologic syndrome associated with cholestatic jaundice occurs in patients with cystic fibrosis, apparently for the same reasons.

Whipple Disease

Patients with Whipple disease present to the gastroenterologist as having a disorder of malabsorption. The disease is a multisystem disorder, involving not only the intestine, but the brain and spinal cord as well. Although it is generally a disease of middle-aged men, it has been reported in a 3-month-old infant (25) and a 7-year-old child (26). Pathologic examination shows infiltration of the mucosa and lymph nodes by macrophages containing polysaccharide-protein complex. In some cases, Periodic Acid Shiff (PAS) containing histiocytes accumulate in the brain and spinal cord, and patients may have intellectual impairment, ophthalmoplegia, visual impairment, ataxia, and progressive spastic paraparesis. In addition, some patients with Whipple disease have had associated progressive multifocal leukoencephalopathy (27).

INFLAMMATORY BOWEL DISEASES

Crohn disease and ulcerative colitis are only rarely associated with neurologic disorders. Polymyositis has been reported to be associated with inflammatory bowel diseases, but in a series of muscle biopsies in patients with Crohn disease, no evidence of any myopathic process was found. In one review of the extraintestinal complications of 700 patients with inflammatory bowel diseases, including Crohn disease and ulcerative colitis, only one patient was reported who had symptoms that could be referred to a neurologist for evaluation. That patient had diplopia and was found to have orbital myositis (28). Young et al, reported a 14-year-old girl with Crohn disease who presented with bifrontal headaches associated with ocular chemosis, proptosis, and orbital congestion. Following bowel resection and steroid therapy, the ocular symptoms resolved (29).

DISEASES OF THE LIVER

Hepatitis

A variety of neurologic disorders can occur in association with hepatitis. Hepatic encephalopathy, the most common and most severe complication, occurs when the disease has progressed to liver necrosis. Other disorders have been reported including myopathy (30,31), Guillain-Barré syndrome (32), and neuropathy (33). Myalgia, a common problem in patients with hepatitis, is only rarely associated with muscle weakness. If weakness occurs, however, the patient should be evaluated for polymyositis, which usually develops at the onset of the hepatitis and is associated with hepatitis B antigen (30).

Guillain-Barré syndrome has been reported to develop in patients with hepatitis B (32). In most patients, however, progressive weakness began during the recovery phase of the liver infection, but it has preceded or occurred simultaneously with the onset of jaundice in a few cases.

The occurrence of peripheral neuropathy in patients with liver disease is more common than is generally recognized. In one study of patients with hepatic disease, clinical evidence of neuropathy was found in 16.6%, delayed nerve conduction velocities in 41.6%, and segmental demyelination in 75% (33). Thus, peripheral neuropathies, though usually subclinical, are common in this disorder.

Hepatic Coma

Hepatic coma is an infrequent problem in children and is usually the result of acute hepatic necrosis caused by hepatitis. Occasionally, medications such as valproic acid, tetracycline, isoniazid, and acetaminophen can cause liver failure and coma.

In most cases, however, the hepatic disease is readily apparent because the child has obvious jaundice, and a diagnosis of hepatitis has been established. Most children recover uneventfully from hepatitis, but occasionally a child will suffer progressive disease with hepatic necrosis. In such an event, progression to hepatic encephalopathy occurs.

On occasion, a child will have acute deterioration, and in these cases, neurologic impairment may be the result of the hepatic disease with the deterioration secondary to hemorrhage into the gastrointestinal tract, causing a sudden increase in serum ammonia levels. Other factors associated with hepatic disease must be considered, however, including: intracranial hemorrhage resulting from a decrease in clotting factors produced by the liver; hypoglycemia resulting from a loss of available liver glycogen stores; and seizures with a postictal depression.

Clinical Manifestations

The child with hepatic encephalopathy passes through four stages of worsening coma (34).

Stage I. In this earliest stage, the child is only mildly to moderately lethargic. He remains alert and aware of the environment when awake but sleeps more than is usual. The neurologic examination is generally normal at this time, although some children may have asterixis. The EEG is usually normal.

Stage II. As the process develops, the child is increasingly drowsy and when awakened seems inappropriate and disoriented. Agitation often occurs, especially with noxious stimulation. Asterixis is usually present, but the muscle tone and deep tendon reflexes are normal. The EEG is characterized by slow activity.

Stage III. The third stage is characterized by a decreasing level of consciousness and by significant changes in the neurologic examination. The child is difficult to arouse, even with painful stimuli. On arousal, confusion is apparent, and the child may even be incoherent. Painful stimuli may precipitate decorticate or decerebrate posturing. The neurologic examination is markedly abnormal with rigidity (paratonia), increased deep-tendon reflexes, and extensor plantar responses.

Stage IV. In the fourth and deepest stage of coma, the child is unresponsive. The neurologic examination now reveals hypotonia and flaccidity with absent deep-tendon reflexes. The mortality rate is 80% if the coma progresses to stage IV.

Cerebral Edema and Hepatic Coma

One of the major problems that can develop in patients with hepatic encephalopathies is cerebral edema. Though some authorities disagree (35), it has been reported to occur in 30% to 50% of children who reach stage III or IV

coma and to be present in 80% of related autopsies (36). The mechanism of cerebral edema is unknown, but the rapid increase in intracranial pressure caused by cerebral edema may be the cause of death in some patients. In later stages of hepatic encephalopathy, the progression of coma that occurs with increasing intracranial pressure is very similar to the stages of progressive hepatic encephalopathy. Thus, the child must be examined frequently, not only for progression of the hepatic encephalopathy, but for signs of increased intracranial pressure. Clinical signs of cerebral edema with secondary increased intracranial pressure include sudden deterioration in neurologic function, development of focal neurologic signs, or asymmetric pupils. Decreasing pulse rate and increased blood pressure (the Cushing response) may also occur. Although the Cushing response is a good indicator of increasing intracranial pressure, the absence of the response cannot be relied on to indicate that the intracranial pressure is not elevated. The development of papilledema is also a reliable indicator of increased intracranial pressure, but because it may take several days to develop, the absence of papilledema does not mean that the patient has normal intracranial pressure.

Treatment of Neurologic Complications of Hepatic Coma

There is no specific therapy for patients with hepatic encephalopathy. Any treatment is directed toward the correction of the underlying hepatic disease. However, some of the secondary abnormalities can be treated directly; for example, prevention of sudden increases in serum ammonia levels by sterilizing the gut may help prevent progression of coma.

The treatment of increased intracranial pressure is made more difficult than usual because of the underlying disease process. Nearly every therapeutic tool normally used to manage the child with cerebral edema is compromised by one or more of the complications of hepatic encephalopathy. Nevertheless, increased intracranial pressure should be identified and treated promptly.

Often, the first problem encountered is that aggressive and accurate management of increased intracranial pressure usually requires the use of an intracranial pressure monitor. The child with liver failure routinely has decreased clotting factors. Prothrombin time may be increased, and the surgical placement of an intracranial monitor is associated with an increased risk of hemorrhage. The prothrombin time is the most sensitive index of hepatocyte dysfunction and should be monitored throughout the clinical course. It may be necessary to replace the clotting factors with fresh frozen plasma prior to the placement of a monitor.

The usual first therapeutic response to increased pressure is hyperventilation. The goal is to decrease the partial pressure of arterial carbon dioxide ($PaCO_2$) to 22 to 25 $PaCO_2$ mm Hg. The decreased $PaCO_2$ causes cerebral arteriolar vasoconstriction and, thus, reduces the intracranial volume of blood and the intracranial pressure. Patients with liver failure have spontaneous hyperventilation, however, one of the hallmarks of the disease. Thus, patients already have respiratory alkalosis and may have decreased the $PaCO_2$ to 25 mm Hg or below. If the $PaCO_2$ is too low, it may cause excessive arteriolar constriction and lead to secondary brain damage. If the $PaCO_2$ is above 25 mm Hg, hyperventilation is appropriate.

If hyperventilation cannot be done or is unsuccessful, the next step is the administration of an hyperosmolar agent such as mannitol. The usual dose is 0.25 to 1.0 g/kg/dose administered over 20 minutes. It can be repeated every 3 to 4 hours if the increased pressure persists. Mannitol has been shown to improve survival (37). One must be careful, however, that the serum osmolality does not go above 320 mosm. Levels above that point can lead to cardiovascular collapse. Mannitol is excreted via the kidney, and many patients with hepatic failure have an associated renal failure (38). Although most patients with liver failure can excrete the mannitol, the patient's renal state should be assessed prior to the initiation of hyperosmolar therapy.

Hypoglycemia may also contribute to the encephalopathy and to the development of cerebral edema. Gluconeogenesis is impaired by the liver necrosis, leading to a decreased glucose response to the stress of illness. Glucose levels should be carefully monitored and glucose administered to maintain normal blood levels.

Seizures may also occur at any time during the course of the hepatic encephalopathy. When they occur, they should be managed with standard anticonvulsant medications such as lorazepam, (0.1 to 0.2 mg/kg/dose), phenobarbital (10 to 20 mg/kg/dose), or phenytoin (20 mg/kg). Liver metabolism of the anticonvulsants will be decreased, however, so anticonvulsant levels must be carefully monitored to prevent intoxication.

Pathophysiology of Hepatic Encephalopathy

The exact mechanism of hepatic encephalopathy remains controversial. There is little doubt that a direct toxic effect of hyperammonemia exists. Children with urea-cycle defects whose ammonia levels reach very high levels become encephalopathic. Ammonia is normally rapidly detoxified in the astrocytes in the brain by first combining with alpha-ketoglutarate to make glutamate. The glutamate is converted to glutamine by glutamine synthetase. If the brain is unable to detoxify the ammonia, the elevated ammonia levels inhibit membrane chloride conductance and, thereby, reduce postsynaptic inhibitory neurotransmission (39). The loss of inhibition contributes to neuronal excitation and seizures. Ammonia also interferes with energy metabolism of brain cells causing changes similar to hypoxic injury (40). Serum ammonia levels are usually elevated in children with hepatic encephalopathy, but there are cases reported in which the levels were not markedly increased. Thus, other mechanisms may play a role in the encephalopathy. The detoxification of ammonia to glutamine requires alpha-ketoglutarate, a constituent of the tricarboxylic acid (Kreb) cycle. A decrease in alpha-ketoglutarate results in slowing of the tricarboxylic acid cycle and a decrease in available adenosine triphosphate. The lack of available energy stores may play a role in the coma and could also contribute to seizures. Cerebrospinal fluid levels of alpha-ketoglutaramate, a metabolite of glutamine and central nervous system (CNS) depressant, have been shown to be consistently elevated in patients with hepatic encephalopathy (41). The plasma amino acids are consistently altered in patients with hepatic encephalopathy (42). Some of the amino acids undergo beta hydroxylation and become "false" neurotransmitters (43). These "false" neurotransmitters may replace the normal transmitters and impair brain function.

Another possible contributor to hepatic encephalopathies is gamma-aminobutyric acid (GABA), the primary brain inhibitory neurotransmitter. GABA is normally produced by bacteria in the gastrointestinal tract, but is detoxified by the liver. Children with liver disease do not metabolize the GABA produced by the gut flora. This leads to increased serum GABA activity (44). If the GABA crosses the blood-brain barrier, the increased inhibitory activity could augment the coma.

Portal-Systemic Encephalopathy

Portal-systemic encephalopathy may occur in patients who have a fistula between the portal vein and the inferior vena cava. Venous blood from gastrointestinal tract goes into the systemic circulation without passing through the liver, and substances normally detoxified by the liver are consequently allowed into the systemic circulation. The essential difference between the encephalopathy due to liver failure and porto-caval shunts is that the encephalopathy due to liver failure is a relatively acute event with high mortality; whereas, porto-caval shunts cause chronic episodic encephalopathy and has a low mortality rate.

Portal-systemic encephalopathy is generally most evident when there has been distinct increase in serum ammonia from either a high-protein meal or gastrointestinal hemorrhage. Other causes may be the ingestion of medications, such as tranquilizers, which affect the CNS. The serum ammonia levels are higher than normal because the medication does not pass through the liver after absorption from the gastrointestinal tract. Encephalopathy occurs in up to 20% of patients with porto-caval shunts (45). It tends to wax and wane as the circulating toxins rise and fall. Most affected patients are adults who have concomitant liver cirrhosis, but it has been reported in children (46,47).

Porto-systemic encephalopathy clinically presents with waxing-waning neuropsychiatric symptoms including alteration of consciousness, acute psychiatric reactions, chronic cerebellar and basal ganglia signs (48), and spastic paraparesis (49). In adults, these neurologic symptoms have occasionally been severe and irreversible. There has been concern in children that a mild encephalopathy may be present that interferes with development and learning.

In a recent study of portal vein obstruction not associated with liver disease, 42 children were studied up to 24 years after operative shunting (50). The shunting procedure was performed between 2 and 14 years of age. Two control groups composed of children with other abdominal surgeries and children with portal vein obstruction not shunted, were also studied. The serum ammonia levels were higher in the children with portal systemic shunts, but there was little difference in the neuropsychologic testing and no difference in the scholastic achievements. Visual memory and spatial-temporal tests showed slightly worse results in the portal-caval shunt group. The neurologic examinations and the EEG were also unremarkable. Thus, it appears that a portal-caval shunt not associated with liver disease does not cause significant neuropsychologic sequelae.

Neurologic Complications of Liver Transplantation

Liver transplantation is becoming an increasingly common procedure for children with life-threatening liver diseases, and neurologic complications are common. The complications can be divided into three groups: those caused by the underlying disease process; those caused by the transplantation procedure; and finally, complications of the immunosuppressive drugs administered to prevent rejection of the transplanted liver. All of the problems discussed in the section on hepatic coma can occur in the immediate post-transplant periods and may be the result of either decreased function of the liver or of liver failure.

CNS infections are always a concern in the post-transplant patient. The organisms that cause CNS infections are different at different times after the transplant. The postoperative period can be divided into 3 phases; the immediate postoperative period and up to 1 month post transplant; the period between 1 month and 4 to 6 months post transplant; and the time after 4 to 6 months post transplant.

In the immediate postoperative period, the patient is at risk for perioperative infections similar to any other surgical patients; these are the most common infections. Immunosuppression is generally not a concern at this stage.

Infections that were present in the recipient prior to the transplantation, or infections that were present in the donor organ can also occur in the immediate postoperative period. The CNS is rarely involved. In the second phase, after the 1st month, viral infections such as cytomegalovirus, hepatitis virus, and Epstein-Barr virus can develop and may involve the CNS. In the third phase, after 4 to 6 months of immunosuppression, the opportunistic infections begin to appear. Patients who have done well, vis à vis the transplanted liver, and have required only standard immunosuppression are at little risk for opportunistic infection. The patient who has had rejection episodes and has required high levels of antirejection drugs is at great risk, however. As many as 20% of these patients will have opportunistic infections. The most common organisms that affect the CNS are *Listeria monocytogenes, Cryptococcus neoformans,* disseminated *Nocardia,* and disseminated *Aspergillus.*

The immunosuppressed patient may not respond to infection the same as the normal patient. Because immunosuppression prevents the inflammatory response of CNS infections, fever and stiff neck may not occur until late in the disease process. Headaches and lethargy are the most important manifesting signs of CNS infections, and when they occur, a complete evaluation for infection should be performed.

There are four characteristic presentations of CNS infection in the post-liver transplant; acute meningitis, most often (95%) due to *Listeria monocytogenes;* subacute or chronic meningitis, usually from *Cryptococcus neoformans,* Coccidiodomycosis or Histoplasmosis; focal neurologic infections due to Aspergillosis, Toxoplasmosis, *Nocardia,* or *Listeria;* chronic dementia caused by progressive multifocal leukoencephalopathy.

One of the most important contributions to the recent success of liver transplantation has been the use of cyclosporine to prevent rejection. Its use, however, has come at a cost to the nervous system. Cyclosporine frequently causes neurologic complications, primarily seizures, in the immediate postoperative period and has been associated with progressive encephalopathy that may rarely end fatally (51). In one recent report, 13 of 48 patients with liver transplants demonstrated CNS toxicity to cyclosporine. The patients developed confusion, cortical blindness, quadriplegia, seizures, and coma. MRI brain scans showed marked increases in a signal intensity in the cerebral white matter (52).

REFERENCES

1. Wyllie WG, Schlesinger B. The periodic group of disorders in childhood. Br Med J 1933;30:1–21.
2. Gee S. On fitful or recurrent vomiting. St. Bartholomew's Hospital Reports. 1882;18:1–6.
3. Farquhar HG. Abdominal migraine in children. Br Med J 1956;1:1082–1085.
4. Hoyt CS, Stickler GB. A study of 44 children with the syndrome of recurrent (cyclic) vomiting. Pediatrics 1960; 25: 775–779.
5. Millichap JG, Lombroso CT, Lennox WG. Cyclic vomiting as a form of epilepsy in children. Pediatrics 1955;15: 705–714.

6. Lanzi G, Balottin U, Ottolini A, et al. Cyclic vomiting and recurrent abdominal pains as migraine or epileptic equivalents. Cephalalgia 1983;3:115–118.

7. Barlow CF. Headaches and Migraine in Children. London: Spastics International Medical Publications, 1984.

8. Apley J, Naish N. Recurrent abdominal pains: A field survey of 1000 school children. Arch Dis Child 1958;33:165–170.

9. Douglas EF, White PT. Abdominal epilepsy—a reappraisal. J Pediatr 1971;78:59–67.

10. Prichard JS. Abdominal pain of cerebral origin in children. Can Med Assoc J 1958;78:665–667.

11. Einfeld SL, Fairley MJ, Green BF, et al. Brief clinical report: Sudden death in childhood in a case of the G syndrome. Am J Med Genet 1987;28:293–296.

12. Clay SA, Ramseyer JC, Fishman LS, et al. Acute infantile motor unit disorder. Arch Neurol 1977;34:246–249.

13. Dooley JM, Goulden KJ, Gatien JG, et al. Topical therapy for oropharyngeal symptoms of myasthenia gravis. Ann Neurol 1986;19:192–194.

14. Branski D, Levy J, Globus M. et al. Dysphagia as a primary manifestation of hyperthyroidism. J Clin Gastroenterol 1984; 6:437–440.

15. Ming RHC, Dreosti LM, Ou Tim L, et al. Thyrotoxicosis presenting as dysphagia. S Afr Med J 1982;61:554.

16. Carre IJ. Disorders of the oro-pharynx and esophagus. In: Anderson CM, ed. Pediatric Gastroenterology. Oxford: Blackwell Scientific Publications, 1975:33–79.

17. Jolley SD, Herbst JJ, Johnson DG, et al. Surgery in children with gastroesophageal reflux and respiratory symptoms. J Pediatr 1980;96:194–198.

18. Sondheimer JM, Morris BA. Gastroesophageal reflux among severely retarded children. J. Pediatr 1979;94:710–714.

19. Abrahams P, Burkitt BFE. Hiatus hernia and gastro-oesophageal reflux in children and adolescents with cerebral palsy. Aust Pediatr J. 1970;6:41–46.

20. Bray PF, Herbst JJ, Johnson DG, et al. Childhood gastroesophageal reflux. Neurologic and psychiatric syndromes mimicked. JAMA 1977;237:1342–1345.

21. Williams CA, Frias JL. Brief clinical report: Apparent G syndrome presenting as neck and upper limb dystonia and severe gastroesophageal reflux. Am J Med Genet 1987;28:297–302.

22. Rosenblum JL, Keating JP, Prensky AL, et al. A progressive neurologic syndrome in children with chronic liver disease. N Engl J Med 1981;304:503–508.

23. Guggenheim MA, Ringel SP, Silverman A, et al. Progressive neuromuscular disease in children with chronic cholestasis and vitamin E deficiency: Diagnosis and treatment with alpha tocopherol. J Pediatr 1982;100:51–58.

24. Sokol RJ, Heubi JE, Iannaccone ST, et al. Vitamin E deficiency with normal serum vitamin E concentrations in children with chronic cholestasis. N Engl J Med 1984;310: 1209–1212.

25. Aust CH, Smith EB. Whipple's disease in a 3-month-old infant. Am J Clin Pathol 1962;37:66–74.

26. Barakat AY, Bitar J, Nassar VH. Whipple's disease in a seven-year-old child. Am J Proctol 1973;24:312–315.

27. Bale JF, Perlman S. Viral Encephalitis. In: Baker AB, Baker LH, eds. Clinical Neurology. Baltimore: Harper and Row, 1987:26–73.

28. Greenstein AJ, Janowitz HD, Sachar DB. The extra-intestinal complications of Crohn's disease and ulcerative colitis: A study of 700 patients. Medicine 1976;55:401–412.

29. Young RSK, Hodes BL, Cruse RP, et al. Orbital pseudotumor and Crohn disease. J Pediatr 1981;99:250–252.

30. Mihas AA, Kirby JD, Kent SR. Hepatitis B antigen and polymyositis. JAMA 1978;239:221–222.

31. Pittsley RA, Shearn MA, Kaufman L. Acute hepatitis B simulating dermatomyositis. JAMA 1978;239:959.

32. Berger JR, Ayyar R, Sheremata WA. Guillain-Barré syndrome complicating acute hepatitis B. A case with detailed electrophysiological and immunological studies. Arch Neurol 1981; 38:366–368.

33. Chari VR, Katiyar BC, Rastogi BL, et al. Neuropathy in hepatic disorder. A clinical, electrophysiological and histopathological appraisal. J Neurol Sci 1977;31:93–111.

34. Russell GJ, Fitzgerald JF, Clark JH. Fulminant hepatic failure. J Pediatr 1987;111:313–319.

35. Plum F, Posner JB. The Diagnosis of Stupor and Coma. Philadelphia: F.A. Davis, 1980.

36. Silk DBA, Hanid MA, Trewby PN, et al. Treatment of fulminant hepatic failure by polyacrylonitrile membrane haemodialysis. Lancet 1977;2:1–3.

37. Canalese J, Gimson AES, Davis C, et al. Controlled trial of dexamethasone and mannitol for the cerebral oedema of fulminant hepatic failure. Gut 1982;23:625–629.

38. Wilkinson SP, Arroyo A, Moodie H, et al. Abnormalities of sodium excretion and other disorders of renal function in fulminant hepatic failure. Gut 1976;17:501–505.

39. Kvamme E. Ammonia metabolism in the CNS. Prog Neurobiol 1983;20:109–132.

40. Hindfelt B, Blum G, Duffy TE. Effects of acute ammonia intoxication of cerebral metabolism in rats with portacaval shunts. J Clin Invest. 1977;59:386–396.

41. Vergara F, Plum F, Duffy TE. α-ketoglutaramate: Increased concentrations in the cerebrospinal fluid of patients in hepatic coma. Science 1974;183:81–82.

42. Fisher JE, Amino acids in hepatic coma. Dig Dis Sci 1982; 27:97–102.

43. Fischer JE, Baldessarini RJ. False neurotransmitters and hepatic failure. Lancet 1971;2:75–80.

44. Ferenci P, Covell D, Schafer DF, et al. Metabolism of the inhibitory neurotransmitter gamma-aminobutyric acid in a rabbit model of fulminant hepatic failure. Hepatology 1983; 3:507–512.

45. Mutchnick MG, Lerner E, Conn HO. Portosystemic encephalopathy and portocaval shunt: A prospective controlled investigation. Gastroenterol 1974;66:1005–1019.

46. Warren WD, Millikan WJ, Smith RB, et al. Noncirrhotic portal vein thrombosis. Physiology before and after shunt. Ann Surg 1980;192:341–349.

47. Hassall E, Benson L, Hart M, et al. Hepatic encephalopathy after porto-caval shunt in a noncirrhotic child. J Pediatr 1984; 105:439–441.

48. Sherlock S. Hepatic Encephalopathy. Br J Hosp Med 1977; 17:144–159.

49. Pant SS, Rebeiz JJ, Richardson EP. Spastic paraparesis following portacaval shunts. Neurology 1968;18:134–141.

50. Alagille D, Carlier JC, Chiva M, et al. Long-term neuropsychological outcome in children undergoing portal-systemic shunts for portal vein obstruction without liver disease. J Pediatr Gastroenterol Nutr 1986;5:861–866.

51. Adams DH, Gunson B, Honigsberger L, et al. Neurologic complications following liver transplantation. Lancet 1987; 1:949–951.

52. DeGroen PC, Aksamit AJ, Rakela J, et al. Central nervous system toxicity after liver transplantation. The role of cyclosporine and cholesterol. N Engl J Med 1987;317: 861–866.

Carl J. Crosley

The multiple expressions of the diseases of blood and blood forming organs result in neurologic complications in many children. The most apparent complications are hemorrhage and thrombosis in the central and peripheral nervous systems; and in several blood diseases, infections of the central nervous system (CNS) have a significant impact upon morbidity and mortality. In addition, the treatment of many of these diseases is far from innocuous and places children at risk for additional neurologic insults. Several diseases have been described in which associated primary neurologic defects may be present long before the emergence of the hematologic abnormalities.

DISEASES OF HEMOSTASIS AND BLOOD COAGULATION

Blood coagulation is the result of a cascading sequence of many well-controlled enzymatic reactions. The pathway to clot formation is twofold. The intrinsic system includes the participation of factors XII, XI, IX, X, and VIII, ultimately producing activated factor X. In the extrinsic system factor VII and tissue factor, a lipoprotein, form an active complex which also produces activated factor X. In the common pathway, activated factor X permits the conversion of prothrombin to thrombin which then converts fibrinogen to fibrin. Finally the activation of factor XIII permits the covalent bonding of mulitple fibrin monomers.

Inherited Diseases

Deficiencies in one or more of these coagulation factors have been described as hereditary diseases. Although the clinical presentation of most of these diseases is similar, individual family histories may suggest characteristic patterns. Ultimately laboratory studies are needed to determine the precise diagnosis.

Hemophilia

Classic hemophilia results from a deficiency of factor VIII, or antihemophilic factor. This deficiency affects 1 in 10,000 persons, and is the most common inherited bleeding disease (1,2). The severity of the disease is consistent within family members. Christmas disease or Hemophilia B occurs at a frequency about only 1/5 of that of classic hemophilia. The clinical manifestations of these two diseases are essentially indistinguishable. Since both diseases are inherited as sex-linked recessive traits, only boys are affected unless a carrier female is subject to inactivation of an X-chromosome ("lyonization"). Fortunately, only a small minority of boys affected have a severe (<1%) deficiency of factor VIII and subsequent severe bleeding. The most common sites of bleeding are the large joints; however, muscle and other soft tissues can be the sites of hematoma formation, and gastrointestinal hemorrhage and hematuria may occur.

Hemorrhage can occur spontaneously as well as the consequence of direct trauma. Peripheral nerves may be compressed by a clot within a muscle. The most common site for intramuscular hemorrhage is in the iliopsoas (3). Even a small hemorrhage into the iliacus produces considerable pain and discomfort because the muscle is bound by the rigid pelvic wall and the iliacus fascia. In contrast, many other muscles such as the calf, quadriceps, and gluteus are more distensible, and hemorrhage into them produces less discomfort. Muscles affected by hemorrhage rapidly go into spasm, and deformities resulting from intramuscular hemorrhage reflect the consequences of contraction of the involved muscle. Peripheral nerve lesions secondary to intramuscular hemorrhage are relatively frequent. In a study of 153 intramuscular hemorrhages, 42 nerves were compromised (3), including 54% of 48 iliacus hemorrhages but only 24% of hemorrhages into all other muscles. In the arm and forearm, the ulnar, median, and radial nerves were involved; and in the calf and the buttocks, the popliteal and the sciatic nerves, respectively, were affected. It is clear that prolonged neurologic observation is warranted in all cases of intramuscular hemorrhage, for in some instances neurologic symptoms may be delayed for up to 24 hours.

Treatment of an intramuscular hemorrhage includes the replacement of factor VIII or IX and maintaining their levels of at least 30% to 40% of the factor. The damaged muscle should be immobilized in a position of maximal comfort until the hematoma begins to resolve. Relief of pain and diminution in the size of the muscle are signals that resolution is beginning. Active exercise may begin as soon as there is significant lessening of pain. Sensory defects commonly resolve within a few weeks while significant combined motor and sensory loss may require up to 1 year to achieve maximal improvement.

Intraspinal bleeding, either intra- or extramedullary, is an infrequent site of bleeding in hemophilia. In Eyster and colleagues' report (4), 71 cases of CNS hemorrhage occurred in 2,500 hemophiliacs that were followed for 10 years. Six patients had intraspinal bleeding. The presenting signs and symptoms included backache and paralysis. Four of the 6 were operated upon and one of the 6 died.

Intracranial hemorrhage is the most serious neurologic complication in hemophilia. Despite occasional vagaries in defining hemophilia before our current level of understanding of coagulation and the neuroradiologic confirmation of CNS hemorrhage, the incidence of CNS bleeding has remained remarkably constant. Silverstein (5), in a 30-year review of the literature, records an incidence ranging from 2.2% to 7.8%. As other sites of hemorrhage have become more manageable, the relative importance of CNS hemorrhage increases, and at this time it is one of the leading causes of death in hemophiliacs (4,6). Children apparently share disproportionately in the occurrence of CNS hemorrhage. The majority of CNS hemorrhages in Eyster's study occurred in persons under the age of 18 years and many of these patients were infants and toddlers (4). The role of head trauma in CNS hemorrhage is considerable. Trauma of variable severity preceded 54% of CNS hemorrhage in the Hemophilia Study Group summary of 1973 (7). Since the trauma was mild, it was commonly treated as trivial by patients and their families (Figure 19.1). For most patients there was a symptom free interval of up to 4 days (Figure 19.2). Although severe hemophiliacs suffered most of the CNS hemorrhages, their presentation was not disproportionate to their representation in the total population of hemophiliacs. Antibodies to factor VIII occurred in only a small portion of patients in which that status was recorded. The presence or absence of factor VIII antibodies did not appear to affect the prognosis of that subgroup (4,8). In one study (9), the presence of antibodies appeared to

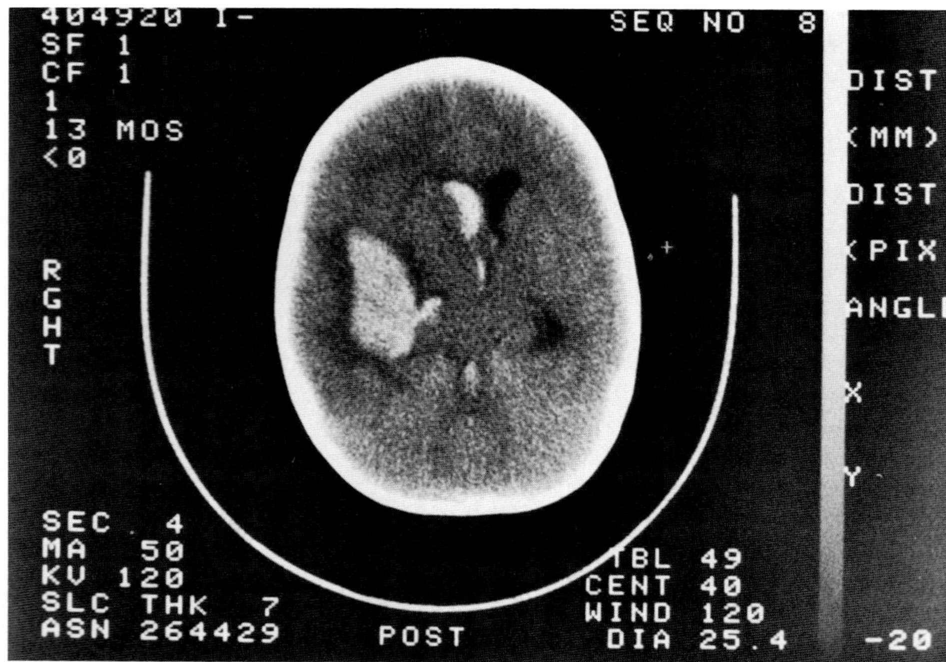

FIGURE 19.1 Unenhanced computed tomographic (CT) scan demonstrating right temporal lobe and basal ganglia hematoma with extension into the ventricles in a 13-month-old boy with factor IX deficiency. He presented with acutely increased intracranial pressure and left hemiparesis. He had lacerated his lip 1 week previously.

FIGURE 19.2 T1-weighted sagittal magnetic resonance image demonstrating a small crescentic subdural fluid collection inferiorly and laterally to the left frontal and temporal lobe. Two weeks prior to presenting with a generalized convulsion, this 17-year-old boy with severe factor VIII deficiency had an apparent minor injury.

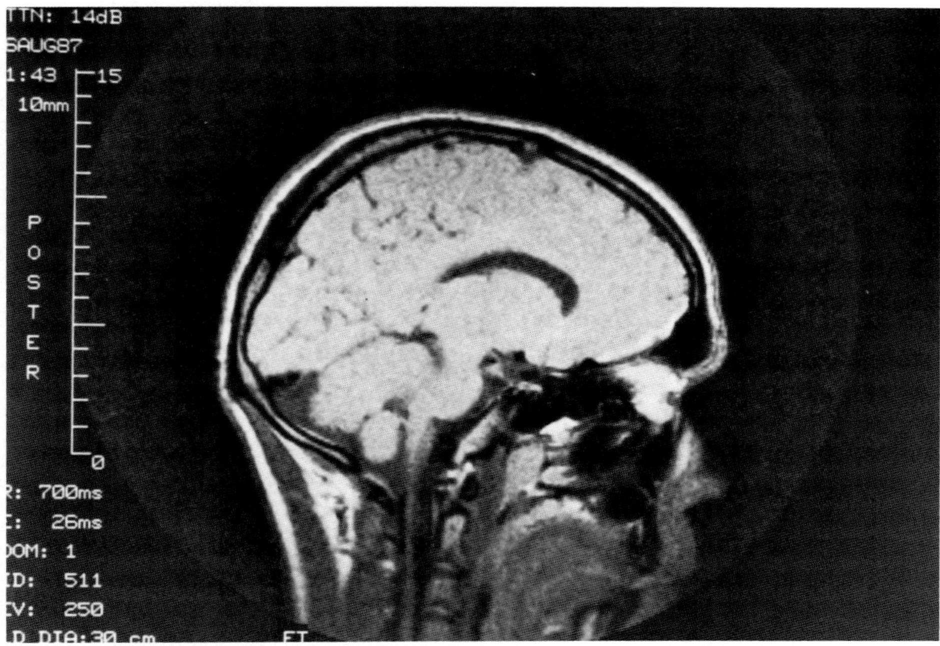

correlate with a higher incidence of intracranial hemorrhage. Recurrent bleeding without trauma was analyzed in the Hemophilia Study Group report, and it was noted that individuals with factor IX deficiency who survived a single intracranial hemorrhage had an increased risk of recurrence. The overall mortality from intracranial hemorrhage in hemophiliacs is about 1/3 with significant morbidity (for example, seizures, mental retardation, and focal neurologic deficits) in almost 1/2 of survivors (4–8). An attempt to prevent intracranial hemorrhage in hemophiliacs with the early use of factor replacement after head trauma has produced some interesting results. Andes et al. (8) described a series of patients in whom 13% of incidents of head trauma were followed by intracranial hemorrhage. However, no patient treated with factor VIII within 6 hours of their injury suffered intracranial hemorrhage. These authors made a strong case for immediate replacement therapy for all hemophiliacs who suffer head trauma. The relatively high mortality in hemophiliacs who have neurologic symptoms after head trauma despite prompt response to such symptoms (4,9–11) further emphasizes the need for immediate action. In contrast to older children, newborns rarely have notable bleeding even with severe disease, but the reason for this phenomenon remains unclear. Transplacental transfer of coagulation factor has not been found and indeed the diagnosis of hemophilia can be made on umbilical cord blood (12).

von Willebrand Disease

The von Willebrand factor is necessary for platelets to adhere to sites of blood vessel injury (1). This disorder is inherited as an autosomal dominant trait, although women are affected more frequently than men. von Willebrand factor and factor VIII normally circulate as a complex protein. In von Willebrand disease the blood concentration of factor VIII is reduced. In contrast to classic hemophilia there is considerable intrafamilial variation in bleeding tendencies. Gastrointestinal bleeding is common but joint hemorrhage is rare; menorrhagia and postpartum bleeding may occur as well. Intracranial hemorrhage is decidedly uncommon, and there are less than 40 cases recorded in the literature (13–17). Moreover, many of these cases preceded our current understanding and definition of the disease. Intracranial hemorrhages occurred shortly after birth in 1 patient, 2 appeared shortly after head trauma, and 4 were spontaneous intracranial hemorrhages. Five patients were over 18 years of age. The diagnosis of von Willebrand disease had been previously recognized in only 1 patient.

Other Inherited Coagulation Diseases

The isolated deficiency of factor VII has been described. Musculoskeletal and gastrointestinal (GI) hemorrhages are most common, although intracranial hemorrhage has occurred in about 10% of affected patients (18,19). A condition even more rare is an isolated factor X deficiency, which may be associated with complicating intracranial hemorrhage (20). Several deficiencies of coagulation factors are associated with thromboembolic disease. Antithrombin III deficiency was found to be the cause of recurrent venous thrombosis in a family in association with trauma, surgery, and pregnancy (21). Two children with thromboembolic disease of the CNS and antithrombin III deficiency have been described. In 1 patient there was a family history of hereditary antithrombin III deficiency (22). Protein C, when activated, functions by inactivating factors V and VIII. Protein C deficiency is inherited as an autosomal dominant trait. In the homozygous form recurrent purpura fulminans leads to death in infancy (23). Individuals who are heterozygous for the condition are subject to recurrent venous thromboembolism that may appear for the first time in adolescence.

Complications of Therapy

Fresh frozen plasma was one of the earliest preparations to be used to replace deficient factors. Moreover, rare hereditary deficiencies of prothrombin and factors V, VII, X, and XII are still relatively easy to treat with fresh frozen plasma. In addition, bleeding in severe liver disease and disseminated intravascular coagulation can be readily treated with fresh frozen plasma. The development of concentrated preparations of specific factors quickly led to their replacement of fresh frozen plasma as the agent for treating bleeding episodes in hemophilia.

Cryoprecipitates, which have been available since the 1960s, are prepared from the plasma of many hundred donors. The use of these preparations, however, exposes the recipient to infections such as hepatitis (24). Consequently, these preparations have largely been replaced as the mainstay of hemophilia treatment by commercially prepared factor concentrates. Nonetheless, the infectious risks have continued.

In 1982 the first case of transfusion-associated acquired immunodeficiency syndrome (AIDS) in a patient with hemophilia was reported, and the number of cases continued to increase through 1984 (25–27). The clinical spectrum of AIDS in hemophilia is not dissimilar from that in AIDS acquired by other means and includes opportunistic infections and subacute encephalopathy (28,29). Given the magnitude of neurologically symptomatic and neuropathologically abnormal persons with AIDS (30), the risks to hemophiliacs and other recipients of blood products is considerable. In response to this calamity, manufacturers of factor VIII concentrates began production of heat-treated concentrates. Heat treatment is effective in decreasing the concentration of human immunodeficiency virus. Unfortunately, this sensitivity is not shared with the hepatitis virus, which may be inactivated only at temperatures that damage or alter the blood coagulants themselves (31).

The use of heat treatment raises the specter of altering the antigenicity of factor VIII so that the problem of inhibitors that is, (antibodies) to factor VIII actually may be increased. Inhibitors develop in 15% of patients with the more severe degrees of factor VIII deficincy. While the presence of inhibitors does not increase the bleeding tendency, it does complicate therapy. Management options in hemophiliacs with inhibitors include high-dose concentrate therapy (32) and the use of prothrombin complex concentrates (29); the latter is of particular value in factor IX deficiency. Earlier preparations of prothrombin complex concentrates have been discovered to have occasional serious and even life-threatening thromboembolic complications (33) and myocardial infarction unrelated to thromboembolism (34). That problem may be the result of activated factor X in some preparations of prothrombin complex concentrates. Epsilon aminocaproic acid is used as an adjunct to prevent the lysis of clot that has formed during specific factor therapy. Generalized seizures have been reported during infusions of epsilon aminocaproic acid (35). Neurologic or potential neurologic complications have not been reported in association with desmopressin acetate (a synthetic analog of vasopressin) and danazol (an attenuated androgen) that are useful therapeutic agents in selected circumstances in hemophilia.

Acquired Diseases

Children with cyanotic congenital heart disease may be polycythemic and have several deficits in hemostasis including coagulation factor deficiencies and thrombocytopenia. In addition, when these children undergo surgical correction with cardiopulmonary bypass, they are prone to another set of coagulation diseases including, disseminated intravascular coagulation (DIC), thrombocytopenia, and coagulation defects (36,37). An important common thread in all children in whom DIC is precipitated is endothelial damage (38). The result of these phenomena is an increased incidence of cerebral thrombotic and embolic events. DIC is a process that may occur in many settings, including severe infections, thermal stress, disseminated malignancies, and major mechanical injuries (30). However, as *Hemophilus influenzae* sepsis, meningococcemia (and meningitis), and severe head injuries are among the leading causes of DIC in children, the incidence, severity, and types of neurologic complications are clouded by the damage to the CNS from these primary processes.

QUALITATIVE AND QUANTITATIVE PLATELET DISEASES

Quantitative platelet abnormalities may result from an increased rate of platelet destruction, reduction of platelet production by the bone marrow, or sequestration of platelets within an increased vascular bed, most often the spleen.

Idiopathic Thrombocytopenic Purpura

The most common destructive thrombocytopenia is idiopathic thrombocytopenic purpura (ITP) of childhood. Its incidence is approximately 4 in 100,000 children (39). It is usually an acute, self-limited disease caused by the binding of immunoglobulin (IgG) to platelets and their subsequent destruction by the reticuloendothelial system (40). More than 90% of children recover uneventfully within a few weeks to months (41–45). Chronic ITP is said to exist when thrombocytopenia lasts longer than 6 months, but even then 10% of children affected will have spontaneous remission. The most serious complication of ITP is intracranial hemorrhage. It is a rare complication occurring in no more than 1% or 2% of all children with ITP, but because of the general frequency of ITP itself it represents a serious hazard to many children. Predisposing factors in a series of about two dozen children with intracranial hemorrhage included mild head trauma, hypertension (possibly secondary to chronic steroid administration), and aspirin ingestion (46,47). Hemorrhage has occurred within 1 month of diagnosis and up to 6 months and even 5 years after diagnosis.

In the acute phase the patient is managed defensively with restriction of injections and activity. Corticosteroids are a part of the primary therapy for ITP for many patients. Corticosteroids are capable of inhibiting macrophage uptake of antibody coated platelets and they decrease capillary permeability (48,49). Despite this reasonable theoretic basis, however, the use of corticosteroids in ITP remains controversial. In the report of Woerner et al. (46), corticosteroids were administered to almost 1/3 of children, and in this study 1/3 of children with intracranial hemorrhage died.

If the endpoint in the efficacy of any treatment for ITP were the prevention of intracranial hemorrhage, the size of any such prospective study would be prohibitive because of the low incidence of intracranial hemorrhage in ITP. It would require from 7,000 to 14,000 children (39); therefore, most trials to date have used normalization of the platelet count as their endpoint. Neither the retrospective (50–53) nor the prospective (54,55) studies have demonstrated an effect on the long-term course of the illness or the frequency of intracranial hemorrhage. The prospective studies seem to indicate that restoration of platelet counts were accomplished more speedily with corticosteroid administration. One can reasonably infer from this fact that the use of corticosteroids in the unavoidably active (younger) child and in those with severe thrombocytopenia or who manifest serious or extensive hemorrhage has merit. Recently sanitized preparations of immune serum globulin have led to the availability of intravenous (IV) IgG as an alternative treatment (56). This product has produced a rapid restoration of platelets counts in some children with ITP. Its efficacy in a selected subset of patients is both rapid and striking; however, it is only this subset that appears to benefit more than if corticosteroids had been administered. Unfortunately, it has not been possible to identify these children in advance.

In emergency situations, such as in the presence of intracranial hemorrhage, large doses of corticosteroids are usually administered. Platelet transfusions also may be used in this setting, although in general the resultant restoration of the platelet count is only transient. Both autologous and homologous platelets are destroyed equally well. Emergency splenectomy produces a return of the platelet count within one or more days (57). Some authors have advocated the use of IV IgG in emergency situations; however, neither the rapidity nor the reliability of this medical management may satisfy all clinicians.

Chronic ITP is characterized by its chronicity (>6 months), a high proportion of older children (over 10 years of age), a higher proportion of girls, and a more insidious less clearly postinfectious history. Splenectomy had been the mainstay of therapy in chronic ITP for many years, but IV IgG has begun to replace splenectomy in selected children with chronic ITP. Many of the reservations applicable to its use in acute ITP are not of as much concern in the chronic disease. In those children in whom splenectomy is still required, the risk of postsplenectomy septicemia is very real. After splenectomy the ability of the patient to limit, much less cure the invasion of the blood stream by encapsulated bacteria, is severely compromised. While pneumococcal vaccine or *Hemophilus influenzae B* vaccine administered prophylactically are helpful in protecting against that bacteria, it offers no protection against meningococcus and other bacteria that also threaten children in the age groups in which ITP is prevalent. Immunosuppressive agents have also been used with some benefit in life-threatening circumstances (58).

Drug-Induced Thrombocytopenia

Drug-induced thrombocytopenia presents similar central nervous system complications to ITP in that a common mechanism for drug-induced thrombocytopenia is immune mediated increased destruction of platelets. Other mechanisms that occur include autoimmune and nonimmune increased destruction and immune mediated underproduction, as well as nonimmune stem cell suppression. Of significant interest in neurologic illnesses of children is the fact that many of the anticonvulsants have been implicated in drug-dependent immune thrombocytopenia. Among these are carbamazepine, clonazepam, diazepam, phenytoin, and valproic acid. Valproic acid deserves special attention in this matter. Although it is associated with a relatively high (>20%) proportion of children with thrombocytopenia, the benign and often transient nature of the condition allows the physician the option of continuing the drug (59). Discontinuation of an offending agent in most cases will lead to a return of the platelet count to normal within days of clearing the drug from the body. Any persistence longer than that should suggest that autoimmune mechanisms or marrow suppression have occurred.

Neonatal Thrombocytopenia

Immune Thrombocytopenia

The neonate who is delivered to a mother with ITP is at special risk for thrombocytopenia. The maternally produced

IgG antibody is transplacentally passed to the fetus and thus subjects the infant to all the risks of thrombocytopenia. Morbidity and mortality in the pregnant woman with ITP is low. Twenty percent of infants and fetuses of these women, however, are either dead or damaged as a consequence of thrombocytopenia (60,61). Mortality in most cases is the consequence of intracranial hemorrhage and occurs during the perinatal period. Corticosteroid therapy for the mother can raise the fetal platelet count (62). Fetal scalp platelet counts can be reliable indicators to predict which infants are safe to deliver vaginally; others are delivered by cesarean section (63–65).

Isoimmune Thrombocytopenia

Isoimmune thrombocytopenia by contrast is more difficult to predict. As in isoimmune erythroblastosis, isoimmune thrombocytopenia occurs when there is a maternal-fetal antigenic incompatibility with the resultant maternal production of antifetal platelet antibodies (66–68). This theoretically places 2% of women at risk. Two percent of women are $P1^{A1}$ negative, therefore, and subject to sensitization. Unlike isoimmune erythroblastosis, the first fetus conceived may be affected. As in maternal ITP the major risk to the fetus is that of intracranial hemorrhage. Once this condition is discovered, all subsequent children are delivered by cesarean section. Intravenous IgG may be beneficial to these children, but unfortunately, even this degree of awareness may not be adequate. In utero intracranial hemorrhage, which is not seen in maternally mediated immune neonatal thrombocytopenia, has been reported several times (66,67,69–71). In these children well-defined intraparenchymal cysts and on occasion intracranial calcifications have been seen (Figure 19.3).

Other Thrombocytopenias

Thrombocytopenia may occur in the newborn as a secondary phenomenon. It has been recognized in association with congenital infections such as toxoplasmosis, syphilis, listeriosis, cytomegalic virus disease, rubella, sepsis, and disseminated intravascular coagulation. A variety of mechanical processes have caused nonimmune microangiopathic thrombocytopenia. Among these are catheters, prostheses, congenital and acquired heart disease (39).

The elements of immunodeficiency, eczema, and thrombocytopenia define the Wiskott-Aldrich syndrome (72). This sex-linked recessive disease presents in early infancy with either hemorrhagic phenomena or opportunistic infections. Many children will survive only a few years as a result of the above complications. A few will develop leukemia or other lymphoreticular malignancies. In a study reviewing the North American experience as of 1979, CNS infections and hemorrhages accounted for 1/4 of all deaths (Figure 19.4). Bone marrow transplantation with prior recipient marrow ablation can correct all of the immunologic defects in this disease (73).

Several syndromes of congenital origin have been described in which thrombocytopenia is an essential part and in which neurologic dysfunction is a concomitant element. Gardner et al. (74) described 3 siblings with unusual facies, redundant skin, megakaryocytic thrombocytopenia, overt spasticity, and delayed development. All 3 children died at birth or within a few months of life. An autosomal dominant pattern of inheritance was seen in a family in whom the affected members had abnormal platelet function, migraine headache, persistent miosis, extreme muscle fatiguability, selected learning disabilities, and mild ichthyosis (75).

Thrombocythemia

The essence of thrombocythemia is the presence of thrombotic and hemorrhagic phenomena and demonstration of selective abnormal increases in platelets and megakaryocytes in peripheral blood and bone marrow, respectively. Secondary thrombocythemia has been recognized in iron deficiency, following mechanical injuries, as part of collagen diseases, and associated with malignancies such as neuroblastoma. Primary thrombocythemia is a myeloproliferative disease in which there is an increase in the absolute number of platelets. Few cases have been reported in childhood (76–79). Neurologic syndromes are the consequences of both arterial and venous hemorrhagic and thrombotic events and as described have included seizures, hemispheric and brainstem infarction, myelopathy, and altered states of consciousness (79,80).

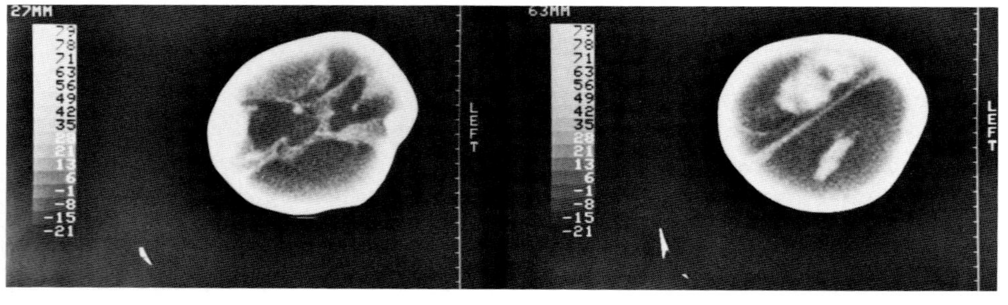

FIGURE 19.3 Isoimmune thrombocytopenia was present in this 1-day-old girl whose CT scan shows unenhancing multiloculated cysts with intra- and extracerebral and intraventricular hemorrhage and massive ventriculomegaly.

FIGURE 19.4 At age 8 weeks this boy with Wiskott-Aldrich syndrome presented with severe thrombocytopenia and cytomegalic virus infection. The CT scan taken at 3 years of age shows a spontaneous right frontal intracerebral hematoma.

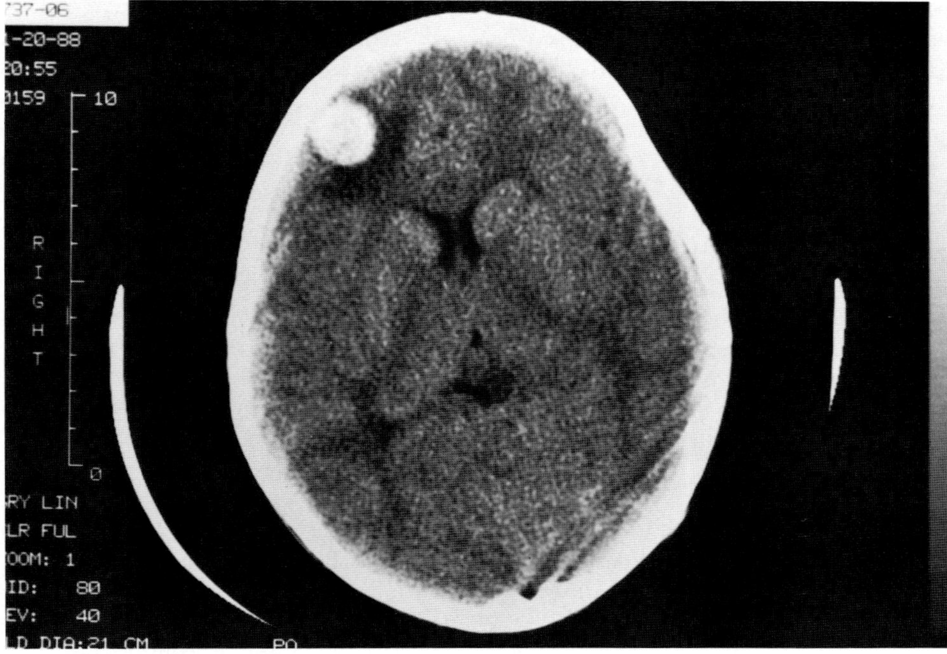

Vascular Purpura

Allergic or anaphylactoid purpura or Henoch-Schönlein purpura is a nonthrombocytopenic purpura characterized by an aseptic vasculitis that affects several target organs. The most commonly affected organs are the skin, joints, GI and renal systems. The heart, respiratory system, and CNS are less often involved. The diagnosis is typically made clinically in a girl between the ages of 3 and 10, a few weeks after an upper respiratory tract (URI) infection with a typical rash developed (81–83). The skin lesion is initially urticarial, but quickly became purpuric and had a predilection for the extensor surfaces of the lower extremities. Joint involvement is characterized by migratory polyarthralgias usually with a prominent arthritis. Colicky abdominal pain is common, but intussusception is frequent enough to produce concern in the presence of any GI symptoms. Hematuria and even transient renal failure are common. Localized swelling of the scalp, hands and feet may also be seen. Chronic renal failure (CRF) occurs in only 10% to 15% of children (78).

Involvement of the nervous system in anaphylactoid purpura is probably under appreciated. Convulsions are a well-recognized complication but for the most part are attributed to concomitant hypertension (84) or renal failure or both (85).

Intracerebral and subarachnoid hemorrhages on the other hand have been postulated to be the result of cerebral arteritis (81). A variety of other defects including common peroneal mononeuropathy (86), altered states of consciousness, and spastic paraplegia have been described (87,88). The basis for each of these signs is at best conjectural. The most clearly defined pathologic study is that of the skin, which is characterized by an aseptic vasculitis prominently involving the corium with a polymorphonuclear perivascular cuff, fibrinoid necrosis, and interstitial edema. Similar lesions have been found in the bowel. The renal lesion is a multifocal glomerulonephritis (78). The nervous system pathology is less well understood. In many studies in which convulsions or other neurologic phenomena are described, there is no pathologic tissue available or the issue of CNS findings is ignored. Circulating IgA and IgG immune complexes are thought to be at the heart of the pathogenesis of anaphylactoid purpura (80). The CNS is unlikely to be exempt from this process.

ANEMIAS

Inherited Diseases of the Red Blood Cell Membrane and Metabolism

Diseases of the red blood cell (RBC) membrane such as hereditary spherocytosis and elliptocytosis (89) and diseases of red blood cell metabolism such as glucose-6-phosphate dehydrogenase (90) and pyruvate kinase deficiency (91) produce neurologic symptoms only in proportion to the degree of hemolytic anemia that each causes. An exception to this is triosephosphate isomerase deficiency in which the CNS is also a primarily affected tissue. This rare condition has been reported in less than 20 children. Each has had a progressive neurologic syndrome described as spasticity and motor retardation (92). The neurologic symptoms are manifest after infancy but actual regression may be delayed for several years. Dystonic movements and tremor appear along with the spasticity. There is electrophysiologic evidence of spinal motor neuron involvement. The children remain intellectually normal. Computed tomography (CT) when done has been normal.

Iron Deficiency Anemia

For over a decade there has been a growing recognition that iron deficiency produces behavioral effects independently of the effect of the anemia itself (93). Several studies have evaluated the hypothesis that children with iron deficiency have impaired cognitive function, are apathetic and inattentive, and have decreased spontaneous daily activities (90,94). It has been further observed that improvement in these symptoms occurs rapidly, within days of initiating treatment, and clearly precedes any significant rise in hemoglobin. Oski et al. (95,96) provide evidence that mean developmental scores as determined by the Bayley Scales of Infant Development improved with 7 days of iron administration in iron deficient anemic children (95,96). Lozoff et al. (97), in a study of Guatemalan children, described developmental deficits in iron-deficient infants but failed to show a clear effect of iron therapy. Other studies in school-aged children have suggested a rapid improvement in attention and performance upon initiation of iron therapy (98). All studies have been criticized as having flaws in methodology including lack of placebo groups, variation in ages of the children tested, and unclear iron status. The pattern of all studies, however, indicates that the effects of iron lack and iron deficiency anemia are realized in lower scores on developmental scales and that in cases of iron deficit or anemia, improvement can be seen within a short time of the initiation of iron therapy.

Megaloblastic Anemia

Megaloblastic anemia is generally the result of folic acid or vitamin B_{12} deficiency. Folate deficiency occurs in instances of inadequate intake, defective absorption, in the presence of drugs that create defective absorption or utilization or both, increased requirements, and specific defects in folate metabolism and increased excretion. Lanzkowsky et al. (99) among others has described children with isolated defects in folic acid absorption and megaloblastic anemia, as well as a coterie of neurologic abnormalities including ataxia, mental retardation, convulsions, and basal ganglia calcification. Congenital defects in folate interconversion and utilization including dihydrofolate reductase methenyl-THF cyclohydrolase and formiminotransferase deficiency have all been associated with varying degrees of mental retardation and cortical atrophy (100). Similarly, defects in absorption, hyposecretion of intrinsic factor, defects in target transportation, and diseases of metabolism can produce the megaloblastic anemia associated with vitamin B_{12}

deficiency. If maternal B_{12} intake is severely deficient, the symptoms may appear in the first few months of life. Children fail to thrive, are pale, hypotonic, listless, and suffer from involuntary movements that resemble ataxia (101). In congenital pernicious anemia, in which there is a failure to secrete intrinsic factor in the child, symptoms usually present within the first 2 years of life (102,103). In contrast, juvenile pernicious anemia is an autoimmune process occasionally associated with various endocrinopathies and with IgA deficiency (98,104,105). It is much more likely to appear in the second decade of life.

Paresthesias are the most common symptoms and may well proceed to objective neuropathy. There may be difficulty walking but the typical subacute combined degeneration is infrequently seen. The neuropathy is a demyelinating process with secondary axis cylinder degeneration. The defects in propionate metabolism that have been described in peripheral nerves of affected children may in part explain the neuropathy (106).

Amyotrophic Chorea-Acanthocytosis

Amyotrophic chorea-acanthocytosis is a hereditary disease characterized by verbal and motor tics, varying dystonic and choreic movements, and a progressive neuropathy or myopathy or both. The hematologic manifestations include both acanthocytosis and a hemolytic anemia (107–109). Although most patients have presented in early and middle adult life, symptoms can be appreciated in later childhood.

Thrombotic Thrombocytopenic Purpura and Hemolytic Uremic Syndrome

Thrombotic thrombocytopenic purpura, Moschcowitz syndrome, is characterized by the triad of hemolytic anemia, thrombocytopenia, and neurologic abnormalities that are characteristically fluctuating. Etiologic factors responsible for thrombotic thrombocytopenic purpura are diverse and no one has adequately explained the genesis of the disease. Moschcowitz in 1925 originally proposed a circulating toxin (110). Other investigators have focused on platelet aggregation factors (111), abnormalities of small blood vessels (112), and possible inherited abnormalities of endothelial function (113). In addition, an association with possible autoimmune diseases (114) and selected infections (115) has been noted. It seems reasonable that this disease is the consequence of endogenous factors and is precipitated by exogenous events or diseases. If hemolysis predominates, the presentation will be anemia or jaundice. Neurologic symptoms are the consequence of occlusive lesions of the microcirculation and have included altered behavior and states of consciousness, seizures (116), and disturbances in sensation as well as cerebral infarction (117) and hemorrhage (118).

Although thrombotic thrombocytopenic purpura may occasionally affect the kidneys, hemolytic-uremic syndrome is defined by renal failure (119). While thrombotic thrombocytopenic purpura is predominatly a disease of adults, hemolytic-uremic syndrome is much more common in children. Precipitating factors in hemolytic-uremic syndrome are infections such as enteroviruses, shigella, other gram-negative bacteria, immunizations, oral contraceptives, antineoplastic agents, and other renal diseases (120).

CNS involvement occurs in 30% to 50% of children (121). Among the symptoms described are alterations in personality and consciousness, status epilepticus, paralysis, and coma (122,123). Because of the absence of discrete neuropathologic features, earlier investigators assumed that CNS changes were secondary to hypertension, uremia, and other metabolic abnormalities. It has become clear with current neuroradiologic imaging techniques that massive hemorrhagic infarction (120) and lacunar infarction (of the basal ganglia) (124), as well as multifocal areas of infarction (125) can and do occur. A favorable outcome can be expected in most children with prompt institution of renal support including dialysis. With such therapy, mortality has fallen from 80% to 10% (118). Several studies have indicated that nonrenal involvement, particularly severe CNS involvement, carries a poor prognosis (118,126). Disequilibrium of breathing presenting either as apnea or as periodic breathing was associated with a fatal outcome in eight out of nine children so affected. On the other hand, total recovery from prolonged coma has also been noted (119).

POLYCYTHEMIA

Polycythemia occurs in children under a variety of circumstances. As polycythemia vera it is a myeloproliferative disease. Polycythemia vera itself is uncommon in children with only 1% of all cases occurring in persons under 25 years of age (127). The secondary polycythemias may occur in the context of appropriate physiologic responses such as cyanotic congenital heart disease, or in circumstances where erythropoietic substances may be inappropriately produced. Examples of inappropriate erythropoietic stimulation are tumors such as Wilms tumor, renal diseases including hydronephrosis, and selected endocrinopathies (for example, pheochromocytoma).

Neonatal polycythemia is of particular interest because of its incidence and acute and chronic neurologic sequelae. The disease is defined as a venous hematocrit over 64%. It is limited for the most part to term or postmature infants. Infants of diabetic mothers (128), small for gestational age infants (129), and newborns with Down syndrome (130) are occasionally affected. The actual incidence is affected by obstetrical practice, and varies from 1.8% with early cord clamping at sea level to 12% with late cord clamping (131). The proposed mechanisms for polycythemia include intrauterine transfusion, intrauterine hypoxia, and increased erythropoietin as in infants of diabetic mothers.

The neurologic complications of polycythemia can be divided into early and late problems. Seizures with or without intracerebral hemorrhage have been seen in the first few hours of life (132). Amit and Camfield (133) described an infant in whom multiple cerebral infarcts presenting with seizures were attributed to the hyperviscosity of polycythemia. One impressive patient is an hydranencephalic infant who had an hematocrit of 78 on the 1st day of life and in whom intrauterine hyperviscosity was proposed as the causal factor in massive cerebral infarction (134). More commonly nonspecific symptoms such as lethargy, poor suck, or jitteriness are seen; however, some infants are completely asymptomatic. It is unclear whether this latter group of children has the same high-risk for late sequelae such as mental retardation, epilepsy, and the varieties of spastic and athetoid static encephalopathy (cerebral palsy) as do those children with severe early symptoms (135–137).

DISEASES OF HEMOGLOBIN

Hemoglobin is the molecule designed to carry oxygen from the lungs to those tissues that depend upon respiration. As the fetus develops and as the child becomes an adult there is an orderly sequence of synthesis of the different polypeptide chains that constitute hemoglobin. Immature fetuses produce zeta and epsilon chains. As the fetus reaches maturity alpha and beta chains that are the components of hemoglobin A of the adult appear. The sequence of hemoglobins we see produced is Portland 1, and Portland 2, Gower 1, Gower 2, F, A, A_2 (138). Diseases of hemoglobin are the consequence of the presence of hemoglobin that incompletely or inefficiently combines with oxygen or is inherently unstable or both. Virtually all of the known hemoglobinopathies are the result of single point abnormalities in the molecule.

Sickle Cell Anemias

The most prevalent and devastating of hemoglobin diseases is sickle cell anemia. Sickle cell disease is the result of the homozygous substitution of valine for glutamic acid in the beta chain at position 6 (139). In the United States there are estimated to be 50,000 persons with sickle cell anemia. Although sickling is initially reversible, cumulative damage to the RBC membrane produces an irreversibly sickled cell. The rate of sickling and in particular the production of sickle crises is determined by a myriad of factors not all of which are completely understood. The sequence of vaso-occlusion and tissue death, however, is probably common to all damage. Children with sickle cell anemia are subject to several different types of crises. There are vaso-occlusive infarctive crises, hemolytic crises, sequestration syndromes, and aplastic or hypoplastic crises (140). In addition, these children have altered reticuloendothelial function including poor opsinization of certain bacteria that predisposes them to pneumococcal and salmonella infections (141). Sickle hemoglobin may occur as a heterozygote in combination with other abnormal hemoglobins. The most common of these, hemoglobin SC disease, occurs somewhat less frequently than homozygous sickle cell anemia; its hemolysis is milder than that of the homozygous sickle S disease. Children with SC disease will have a higher hematocrit but also a higher blood viscosity with its attendant complications. Hemoglobin S-Thalassemia and other combinations have clinical symptoms that vary from mild to severe.

Neurologic symptoms have long been recognized to be a part of sickle cell disease (142). Greer and Schotland (143) found that over 1/3 of their patients with sickle cell anemia had neurologic manifestations most of which occurred during childhood. The most prominent of these were cerebrovascular syndromes. Convulsions, meningeal signs, and impaired visual acuity occurred somewhat less frequently. Uncommon syndromes included radiculopathy, acute mental diseases, and vertigo. Children are at significantly greater risk for cerebral infarction. Adults with sickle cell disease (SS) have a relatively greater risk for intracranial hemorrhage (144,145). Subarachnoid hemorrhage in adults is most commonly the consequence of the rupture of intracranial aneurysms (146). Angiographic studies of apparent infarctions have shown occlusive disease of the circle of Willis and the major branch points of the internal carotid arteries. The phenomenon of moyamoya has also been observed (141,147). Although there had been scattered clinical and pathologic reports prior to 1972, it was the observations of Stockman et al., (148) that first clearly demonstrated that large vessel occlusions were significant in producing the cerebrovascular syndromes in this disease. They hypothesized that ischemic damage to large vessels is produced by occlusion of the vasa vasorum. Prior work had suggested that small vessel occlusion (149) or chronic stasis and diminished blood volume lead to capillary and venous thrombosis (150). Neuropathologic studies have shown exuberant intimal hyperplasia as well as new and old thrombi with evidence of recanalization. Magnetic resonance imaging (MRI) has shown a high percentage of focal abnormalities indicative of arterial border zone infarctions (151). The implication of this finding is that in sickle cell anemia both proximal large vessel disease producing distal insufficiency and distal small vessel disease producing sludging are operative.

If, as some have suggested, susceptible individuals have a defined period of risk after which no additional strokes are seen, then aggressive therapeutic efforts may be justified. Attempts to reduce the recurrence of stroke by hypertransfusion therapy have provided controversial results. Arteriograms have shown clear improvement with 1 to 2 year periods of hypertransfusion (152,153); however, whether this therapy prevents recurrent stroke has not been made clear. In one study, 7 of 10 children had recurrent strokes 5 weeks to 11 months after cessation of a 1 to 2 year hypertransfusion protocol (154). It is unclear whether the duration of therapy was the limiting factor or whether a more complete suppression of hemoglobin S synthesis was necessary to allow healing of damaged cerebral vessels (155).

Infarction of the bone marrow has led to fatal fat embolism (145). The retina is also subject to the ravages of sickle cell disease. A proliferative retinopathy characteristic of sickle cell disease develops in about 20% of persons with the disease (156–158). Blindness occurs in as many as 12% of eyes affected as a result of the retinopathy. Autocoagulation of proliferating vessels that occur in many instances of retinopathy, limiting the extent of the vascular proliferation, may contribute to the relatively low incidence of blindness. Hearing loss is also seen with increased frequency in children with sickle cell disease. Significant sensorineural hearing loss has occurred in 12% of one study of children with sickle cell disease (159). The fact that most affected children also had evidence of other nervous system involvement possibly further defines the population at risk for hearing loss. This hearing loss may be the consequence of temporal bone histopathology including cochlear damage (160). In the presence of opsonization and other defects it is not surprising that both pneumococcal and salmonella meningitis may have fulminant presentations. With these defects being persistent it is also not unexpected that infections such as meningitis may be recurrent (161,162).

Childhood hemoglobin SC disease has a similar, but generally less severe pattern of neurologic complications. Neurologic problems have been reported in 20% of the combined reported series (163–165). In contrast to sickle cell disease, retinopathy is less frequent; however, autocoagulation is less active in SC disease and what retinopathy there is progresses unchecked, leading to more visual loss in those eyes that are affected.

Patients with sickle trait have rarely been reported to have neurologic complications. An individual has been described with complicated migraine and hemoglobin A5 (sickle trait) who developed branch occlusions of his middle cerebral arteries (166). It was hypothesized that platelet abnormalities and neurovascular instability that are known to occur in migraine may have accentuated sickling tendencies.

Thalassemias

The thalassemias are a group of hereditary anemias in which there is decreased synthesis of one or more globin polypeptide chains that combine to form hemoglobin. These hematologic changes result in hypochromia, microcytosis, and anemia.

Alpha Thalassemia

If three of the four alpha-globin loci are abnormal, hemoglobin H disease results. The anemia in this instance is characterized by a striking fragmentation of the RBCs and severe hypochromic microcytosis. Characteristically in patients with intact spleens, there are multiple small inclusions in RBCs which stain with brilliant cresyl blue. In splenectomized patients there are single large Heinz body-like inclusions demonstrated by methyl violet (167). Anemia is usually notable with hemoglobin in the 7 to 10 range and clear development of typical thalassemia facies only occasionally observed. Therapy includes the prevention of exposure to oxidant drugs that can lead to the precipitation of the unstable hemoblobin.

Folic acid may be an effective prophylactic drug for these children. Transfusion and prompt response to infections are also necessary to protect these children (168). In 1981 Weatherall et al. (169) noted the association between hemoglobin H disease and mental retardation in three children from unrelated families. The children were pale, microcephalic, had long inner canthal measurements, club feet, and had intellignece quotients ranging from 50 to 76. Restriction enzyme analysis suggested that there were three different mutations on chromosome 16 that were responsible for the abnormalities. Reports of additional cases followed and have confirmed the existence of the syndrome (170). Although it was initially suspected that intrauterine anemia and hypoxia might have been causal, the presence of mental retardation in other patients with alpha thalassemia alternatively suggested that abnormalities in one or more loci near the alpha-gene loci might produce mental retardation (164).

In the most severe form of alpha thalassemia no alpha chains are made and only hemoglobin H (beta 4) and hemoglobin Barts (gamma 4) are produced. These infants have essentially no useful hemoglobin and severe hydrops fetalis results.

Beta Thalassemia

Although there is only one locus for beta chain synthesis (as opposed to the two for alpha chains), different mutations produce many variations in severity of the disease. In beta thalassemia, trait one beta gene is abnormal and increased amount of hemoglobin A_2 and hemoglobin F are produced. Homozygous beta thalassemia produces a severe anemia and the physical and hematologic consequences of the body's attempts to compensate for the anemia by increased and extramedullary hematopoiesis. In addition to the symptoms of anemia, hepatosplenomegaly, retarded physical growth, diabetes, and heart failure are seen.

The major treatment of beta thalassemia is chronic transfusion therapy in an attempt to maintain hemoglobin at a level that produces adequate oxygenation and suppresses the largely inefficient endogenous hematopoiesis. Hypersplenism and the anemia itself may necessitate splenectomy. Chronic blood transfusions inevitably produce iron overload. Although the major organs affected by iron overload are the heart and liver, many of the endocrine glands also may be damaged. This contributes to the reduction in somatic growth and delay in puberty. In an attempt to reduce the iron load from increased GI absorption of iron and chronic transfusions, chelation therapy has been added to the standard regime for patients with thalassemia major. Deferoxamine is the agent generally used in iron chelation therapy, but when given intravenously an acute cardiovascular collapse may result. In low-dose chronic deferoxamine administration cataracts may appear (171). In more aggressive regimes, visual and auditory loss and aphasia have occurred (172,173). Neuropathologic studies show abnormalities in the retina and optic nerves; auditory damage is sensorineural. Recovery of visual and auditory function upon cessation of deferoxamine has occurred only in some patients.

Other Hemoglobin Diseases

Heinz bodies are inclusions that result from the precipitation of unstable hemoglobin. Heinz body anemia is a hemolytic anemia of varying degree, from severe anemia with splenomegaly and cholelithiasis, precipitation of hemolytic crises by mild viral infection, to a clinically asymptomatic state with incidental hemoglobin instability. Except as a consequence of chronic anemia and its treatment (for example, splenectomy and transfusion), neurologic complications are not seen in Heinz body anemia. In severe cases the calvarium may be distorted and enlarged by marrow expansion.

Methemoglobinemias result from mutations of the hemoglobin molecule near the heme iron. While striking in appearance because of their cyanotic coloration, these patients have few clinical problems. Mutations have also produced hemoglobin with persistently high affinity for oxygen and resultant polycythemia.

BONE-MARROW FAILURE

Bone-marrow failure may be general and affect all cell lines as in aplastic anemia, or selective and affect a single cell line as in neutropenia and red cell aplasia, or simply dysfunctional as in osteopetrosis.

Aplastic Anemia

Aplastic Anemia Syndromes

Acquired aplastic anemia is of idiopathic origin in 1/3 to 1/2 of children affected, but specific drugs, toxins and other factors can be recognized in the remaining majority. The syndrome of paroxysmal nocturnal hemoglobinuria is characterized by aplastic anemia, hemolytic anemia, and venous occlusive disease. Hepatic and more recently cerebral venous thrombosis is a well-recognized and, unfortunately, often fatal complication (174). Anticoagulation with dicumarol as opposed to heparin is recommended to arrest venous thrombosis.

Congenital syndromes producing bone marrow failure include Fanconi anemia, dyskeratosis congenita, and the Shwachman-Diamond syndrome. Dysmorphic characteristics associated with several of these syndromes are likely to bring the affected child to neurologic consultation. In the Shwachman-Diamond syndrome there is exocrine pancreatic insufficiency and growth retardation in addition to marrow failure. Central pontine myelinolysis presenting as coma has been reported (175). The relationship to the central manifestations of the disease, however, remains unexplained. Dyskeratosis congenita is a rare X-linked recessive disease. The most frequently seen dermatologic features of this disease include dystrophic nails and leukoplakia of oral and other mucous membranes. The ectodermal manifestations commonly precede the appearance of bone marrow failure. It is rare for hematologic manifestation to appear first (176). Pre- and postnatal growth retardation and mental retardation are less common features. Although mental retardation occurs in 1/3 of children affected and varies in degree, in most instances it is not severe. The pathophysiology of the retardation is unclear; however, several cases with striking intracranial calcification have been reported (177, 178).

Treatment of Bone-Marrow Failure

Treatment for bone-marrow failure is not innocuous. The infectious complications and hematologic consequences of bone marrow failure leave the clinician few options. However, the aggressive therapies required not uncommonly result in serious complications. Supportive care and replacement of essential blood elements are still the early and primary components of therapy. Androgens as promoters of erythropoietin production and stimulation of erythroid stem cells have long been part of "specific" therapy. An instance of cerebral hemorrhage and infarction has been reported in a boy with aplastic anemia whose hematologic parameters were normalized. He had been treated with androgens for several months (179). Although a causal relationship is difficult to prove, other reasonable and usually causal factors were not present. Other instances of cerebral dysfunction including chorea and acute confusional states lend credence to a direct CNS effect of androgens (180). More recently immunotherapy with cyclophosphamide and antilymphocytic globulin has shown some efficacy in the therapy of aplastic anemia (181,182).

Severe aplastic anemia has been successfully treated with bone-marrow transplantation. The process of bone marrow transplantation gives the patient another possible set of complications (183). The most obvious complication is simple graft rejection. Despite extensive pretransplantation immunosuppression, the host may develop antibody-mediated or cell-mediated nonhuman leukocyte antigen (HLA) transplantation antigens (184). Graft-versus-host disease is the consequence of contamination of the marrow transfusion by mature donor thymocytes. Both the acute and the chronic forms of graft-versus-host disease focus their major effects on the skin, GI system, and the liver although other organs may be involved (185,186). The disabling course of graft-versus-host disease can be modified by methotrexate, cyclophosphamide, and other agents alone or in combinations (180). Graft-versus-host disease rarely affects the nervous system. A myositis has been seen in about 10% of patients with the chronic form of the disease (187). Other than graft-versus-host disease the most significant morbidity and mortality associated with bone-marrow transplantations is the result of opportunistic infections. The agents used to prepare children for transplantation are themselves neurotoxic. Leukoencephalopathies have been documented in children who received bone-marrow transplantation for acute leukemia. In most of these cases the children had received methotrexate or cranial irradiation or both prior to transplantation. Their encephalopathy is probably not different from that which occurs in children with acute leukemia who have not received bone-marrow transplantation. There is no adequate assessment of the effects of bone-marrow transplantation on cognitive function in children. Mechlorethamine, which is used to immunosuppress patients prophylactically, can produce neurotoxicity acutely or many months later, and includes symptoms and signs of confusion, personality changes, diplopia, and paraplegia. Histologic evidence of increased vascularity, gliosis, perivascular fibrosis, and neuronal degeneration have been prominent in the cases examined pathologically (188). A young girl developed myasthenia gravis after bone-marrow transplantation for aplastic anemia. The evidence seemed to implicate the donor as the origin of the myasthenia gravis (189). In a review of 57 children undergoing bone-marrow transplantation almost 1/2 incurred neurologic complications (190). CNS infection and cerebrovascular accidents accounted for the majority of complications. In addition, neuropsychologic sequelae were present in most of the long-term survivors.

Osteopetrosis

Bone-marrow transplantation has been performed with varied success in a variety of inborn errors of metabolism (191). Osteopetrosis or marble bone disease in its severe autosomal recessive form results from defective osteoclastic activity in the presence of normal osteoblastic activity. The chronic form is milder and usually inherited as an autosomal dominant trait (See chapter 22). It is characterized by dense, easily breakable bone. Neurologic symptoms and signs are uncommon, although cerebral embolism from nonbacterial endocarditis (192) and basal ganglia calcifications (193) have been recognized. In the severe form, attempts to compensate for inadequate hematopoiesis result in hepatosplenomegaly and secondary hypersplenism, resulting in thrombocytopenia, leukopenia, and hemolytic anemia. The neurologic manisfestations of osteopetrosis itself are in part the result of the encroachment of sclerotic bone on cranial and other nerves. Deafness (194), blindness (195), and facial palsy (196,197) are well described, and macrocephaly is prominent. Cerebral atrophy and hydrocephalus have also been reported. In at least one study, macrocephaly was not accounted for by the hydrocephalus or the calvarial thickening (191). The onset of the bony sclerosis may be prenatal. The appearance of symptoms in the newborn period has been noted and abnormal radiographs have been obtained in the newborn nursery (192,198). Hydrocephalus has been seen in a stillborn child with osteopetrosis. Neuropathologic studies have demonstrated that the CNS contains neuronal cytoplasmic inclusions composed of lamellar membranes and swollen axons (199). Until recently, therapy for osteopetrosis has been purely supportive, but on occasion prednisone has given a favorable response (191). Bone-marrow transplantation has produced reversal of the hematologic picture and improvement in compressive neuropathies in the few children so treated (200).

DISEASES OF BILIRUBIN METABOLISM

The effects of diseases of bilirubin metabolism upon the nervous system are a consequence of the acute and chronic symptoms of kernicterus. For the most part it is the newborn that suffers from the effects of unconjugated hyperbilirubinemia, although in selected illnesses older children and even adults have been affected. In kernicterus unconjugated bilirubin causes necrosis of neurons most prominently in the hippocampal cortex, basal ganglia, subthalamic nuclei, and the cerebellum (201). There appears to be a direct toxic effect of bilirubin on oxidative processes of neurons that is affected by pH, albumin binding of bilirubin, and the duration of exposure (202,203). The symptoms of kernicterus are evident by the 3rd day of life. Primitive reflexes such as the Moro reflex are suppressed, and the child is hypotonic with depressed startle reflexes. Homeostasis is disturbed as the child becomes apathetic, feeds poorly, and may be febrile (204). Within a few weeks extensor hypertonicity, progressing to opisthotonos and convulsions occur. The chronic encephalopathy of kernicterus develops over several years and is characterized by choreoathetosis, dystonia and even rigidity, upward gaze palsy, and sensorineural hearing loss (205).

Unconjugated hyperbilirubinemia was formerly the consequence of Rhesus factor (Rh) erythroblastosis. The concomitant presence of hemolysis causing the liberation of elements that may compete for bilirubin binding sites and the complications of acidosis and hypoxia make hyperbilirubinemia in this setting especially dangerous (206). With the widespread use of prophylactic Rh antisera, this has become a relatively rare disease. ABO erythroblastosis produces similar signs and symptoms, although rarely as severe. Glucose-6-phosphate dehydrogenase deficiency also produces hemolysis and hyperbilirubinemia. American blacks generally have a milder form than that occurring in Mediterranean and Oriental persons (207).

Crigler-Najjar syndrome is a rare disease with either total or partial deficiency of glucuronyl transferase (208,209). Prior to the advent of phototherapy and exchange transfusion most of the children with total deficiency died as newborns or survived with the full-blown picture of the chronic encephalopathy of kernicterus (204,210). Even with a normal exit from the newborn period, neurologic deterioration has presented itself later in childhood, adolescence, and even in early adulthood (211–214). The clinical presentations later in life have included ataxia, dulling of intellect, and a parkinsonian-like picture. The mechanism for the late deterioration is unknown. Intercurrent viral illnesses have been commonly present. Neuropathologic studies have shown the distribution of the neural damage is similar to that in the neonate, although there is absence of bilirubin pigment (209). In contrast to the autosomal recessive pattern of inheritance in total deficiency of the enzymes, partial glucuronyl transferase appears to be inherited as an autosomal dominant disease (215). In this disease hyperbilirubinemia is less severe, more variable, and exquisitely responsive to phenobarbital therapy. Other than in the immediate neonatal period, kernicterus has not occurred in children with partial deficiency (216).

PORPHYRIAS

The porphyrias are, for the most part, inherited diseases that are the result of deficits in the enzymatic pathway of heme synthesis. The erythropoietic porphyrias are congenital erythropoietic porphyria and congenital erythropoietic protoporphyria. The former is inherited as an autosomal recessive disease and is characterized by neonatal pigmenturia, hemolytic anemia, and extreme photosensitivity of the skin. The latter is inherited as an autosomal dominant and is much more common. It is characterized by significant photosensitivity with only a modest degree of hemolysis. Chronic progressive liver disease is a fatal complication in a few patients. Neurologic disturbances have not been reported in either of these porphyrias (217).

Acute intermittent porphyria, variegate porphyria, coproporphyria, and porphyria cutanea tarda are the hepatic porphyrias. Acute intermittent porphyria is an autosomal dominant disease caused by a deficiency of porphobilinogen deaminase. In latent acute intermittent porphyria the patient has the biochemical defect but no symptoms occur. There is little actual excess of porphobilinogen and, therefore, little photosensitivity occurs. When the disease is expressed, symptoms rarely appear before puberty and are much more common in girls. Attacks occur unpredictably and many drugs including barbiturates, phenytoin, and sulfonamides have been associated with attacks (218).

The clinical symptoms are the result of autonomic neuropathy, peripheral motor neuropathy, and CNS dysfunction. The earliest of autonomic symptoms are episodes of colicky abdominal pain, although constipation, vomiting, and hypertension also can be presenting symptoms. Tests of cardiovascular reflexes are abnormal during an attack and will return to normal in between attacks (219,220). Motor neuropathy is highly variable, fluctuating, and even reversible. Paresis can affect virtually any combination of limbs with absent reflexes and occasionally secondary respiratory insufficiency (215,221). Cortical blindness and cranial neuropathy involving nearly all cranial nerves have been described (222). Coma, inability to swallow, and respiratory dysfunction not attributable to lower motor paralysis suggest that direct involvement of the brainstem occurs. Electromyographic changes have indicated denervation and pathologic examination in one case has confirmed the presence of a dying back axonopathy (223). Although characteristically clinically unaffected, patients with latent acute intermittent porphyria have been shown to have evidence of neuropathy on electrophysiologic testing (224). It is not uncommon for patients with acute intermittent porphyria to present with significant psychiatric diseases (218). The involvement of the hypothalamus is represented by the occurrence of inappropriate antidiuretic hormone syndrome and hyponatremia (225). Abnormalities of adrenocorticotropic hormone (ACTH), thyroid binding globulin, and growth hormone also have been described (226).

These manifestations have been best explained by the depletion of essential substances from the heme biosynthetic pathway and as a result of the accumulation of porphyrin precursors most prominently porphobilinogen and aminolevulinic acid. The majority of drugs that have been associated with attack precipitation alter aminolevulinic acid synthetase activity. There is little support for alternative hypotheses that heme deficiency in neural tissues or abnormal porphyrin precursors play a role (227).

Treatment for acute intermittent porphyria consists of avoiding potential precipitating drugs, supportive therapy, and most recently the infusion of heme. Heme infusion theoretically bypasses the defect and reduces the stimulation of the production of aminolevulinic acid and porphobilinogen (228,229).

Variegate or mixed porphyria contains the features of erythropoietic porphyria and acute intermittent porphyria in varying degrees of expression. The enzymatic defect here is less clearly established, although protoporphyrinogen oxidase appears the most reasonable candidate. In this disease it is again the overproduction of aminolevulinic acid and porphobilinogen that determines the appearance of neurologic symptoms.

Coproporphyria is a third dominantly inherited disease that results in increases in aminolevulinic acid and porphobilinogen and associated neurologic manifestations. Peripheral nerves in individuals with coproporphyria between attacks and even in those who have never had an attack have shown a dying back axonopathy similar to that demonstrated in acute intermittent porphyria (230).

Porphyria cutanea tarda, although hepatic in origin, is a disease of cutaneous manifestations. It is rare in children and is commonly produced by alcoholic liver disease. It also has occurred in association with estrogen administration, uremic patients on hemodialysis, and after hexochlorobenzene exposure (214). Porphyria cutanea tarda has been reported to be inherited as an autosomal dominant disease in a few families.

LEUKOCYTE DISEASES

The Chédiak-Higashi syndrome is a disease of partial oculocutaneous albinism in which giant lysosomal granules are present in the leukocytes. The syndrome is often fatal because of a marked susceptibility to infections and lymphoma (231,232). Very few children survive into adulthood. The neurologic manifestations of this disease are in large part the consequences of a progressive neuropathy. Both stocking glove sensory loss and distally accentuated weakness are described. Evidence for involvement of the CNS is manifest as seizures, mental retardation, and nystagmus. The central and peripheral nervous systems share the characteristic inclusions with the lymphocytes. Inclusions have been seen in most nervous system cells studied including Schwann cells, astrocytes, and cerebral neurons (233).

Neutropenia can be the consequence of a disruption of the proliferation of committed stem cells (as in cyclic neutropenia), a disruption of proliferation of committed myeloid cells (as in benign neutropenia of childhood), or the consequences of an immune process (as in immune neonatal neutropenia). In these and in other causes of neutropenia, however, the clinical symptoms are infections that are usually in proportion to the severity of the neutropenia. Infections are usually bacterial, and most commonly involve the skin or mucous membranes. Pneumonia, septicemia, and meningitis are occasionally more serious infectious complications. Only when the secondary infections involve the CNS are neurologic manifestations noted. Several neutropenias are associated with primary diseases of intermediate metabolism. Children with propionic acidemia and both ketotic and nonketotic hyperglycinemia may have significant neutropenia. Children with these latter diseases are commonly affected by seizures and developmental retardation (234).

Pancytopenia and splenomegaly characterize the syndrome of the sea-blue histiocyte (235). Although these cells rarely can be seen in children with systemic lipidoses, several patients with the primary sea-blue histiocyte syndrome have had a progressive deterioration characterized by ataxia, dementia, and seizures (236).

Leukophilia including both neutrophilia and eosinophilia is most often a secondary phenomenon. The hypereosinophilic syndrome as defined by at least 6 months of an absolute eosinophile count over 1,500 cells per mm^3 without evidence of other causes of eosinophilia and with evidence of constitutional and multiple organ system involvement (237). In this disease the nervous system has been affected by multiple cerebral thrombosis, a demyelinating neuropathy, and dementia (238). Eosinophils induce neuronal damage by direct infiltration, by the release of neurotoxic basic proteins, and by producing an hypercoagulable state. Successful treatment of the hypereosinophilic syndrome has been accomplished with corticosteroids and hydroxyurea (239).

REFERENCES

1. McKee PA. Hemostasis and disorders of blood coagulation. In: Stanbury JB, Wyngaarden JB, Frederickson DS, et al., eds. The Metabolic Basis of Inherited Disease, 5th ed. New York: McGraw-Hill, 1983;1531–1560.
2. Biggs R. Haemophilia treatment in the United Kingdom from 1969 to 1974. Br J Haematol 1977;35:487–504.
3. Hoskinson J, Duthie RB. Management of musculoskeletal problems in the hemophilias. Orthop Clin North Am 1978;9:455–480.
4. Eyester ME, Gill FM, Blatt PM, et al. Central nervous system bleeding in hemophiliacs. Blood 1978;51:1179–1188.
5. Silverstein A. Intracranial Bleeding in Hemophilia. Arch Neurol 1960;3:141–157.
6. Kerr CB. Intracranial hemorrhage in hemophilia. J Neurol Neurosurg Psychiatry 1964;27:166–173.
7. Seeler RA, Imana RB. Intracranial hemorrhage in patients with hemophilia. J Neurosurg 1973;39:1981–185.
8. Andes WA, Wulff K, Smith B. Head trauma in hemophilia. Arch Intern Med 1984;144:1981–1983.
9. Martinowitz U, Heim M, Tadmor R, et al. Intracranial hemorrhage in patients with hemophilia. Neurosurgery 1986;18:538–541.
10. McCarthy JW, Coble LL. Intracranial hemorrhage and subsequent communicating hydrocephalus in a neonate with classical hemophilia. Pediatrics 1973;51:122–123.
11. Penner JA, Kelly PE. Head injury in hemophiliacs. JAMA 1977;237:641.
12. Baehner RL, Strauss HS. Hemophilia in the first year of life. N Engl J Med 1966;275:524–528.
13. Almanni WS, Awidi AS. Spontaneous intracranial hemorrhage secondary to von Willebrand's disease. Surg Neurol 1986;26:457–460.
14. Rice ML. Acute subdural hematoma associated with von Willebrand's disease: A case report. Aust N Z J Surg 1982;52:86–88.
15. Mizoi K, Takehide D, Mori K. Intracranial hemorrhage secondary to von Willebrand's disease and trauma. Surg Neurol 1984;22:495–498.
16. Cooper HA, Bowie EJW, Burgert EO, et al. Hydrocephalus in a child with von Willebrand's disease. Am J Dis Child 1971;121:340–343.
17. Land AE, Meadows JC, Marsden CD. Early onset of the "on-off" phenomenon in children with symptomatic parkinsonism. J Neurol Neurosurg Psychiatry 1982;45:823–825.
18. Marder VJ, Shulman NR. Clinical aspects of congenital factor VII deficiency. Am J Med 1964;37:182–194.
19. Slem GS, Lumi M. Bloody tears due to congenital factor VII deficiency. Ann Ophthalmol 1978;10:593–595.
20. Girolami A, Molaro G, Callagaris A, et al. Severe congenital factor X deficiency in a 5-month-old child. Thromb Diath Haemorrhag 1970;24:175–184.
21. Egeberg O. Inherited antithrombin deeficiency causing thrombophilia. Thromb Diath Haemorrhag 1965:13:516–530.
22. Vomberg PP, Brederveld C, Fleury P, et al. Neuropediatrics 1987;18:42–44.
23. Griffin JH. Clinical studies of protein C. Semin Thromb Hemost 1984;10:162–166.
24. Sugg U, Schnaidt M, Schneider W, et al. Clotting factors and non-A non-B hepatitis. N Engl J Med 1980;303:943.
25. Update: acquired immunodeficiency syndrome (AIDS) in persons with hemophilia. MMWR 1984;33:589–591.
26. Evatt BL, Ramsey Rb, Lawrence DN, et al. The acquired immunodeficiency syndrome in patients with hemophilia. Ann Intern Med 1984;100:499–504.
27. Curran JW, Lawrence DN, Jaffe H, et al. Acquired immunodeficiency syndrome (AIDS) associated with transfusions. N Engl J Med 1984;310:69–75.
28. Rahemtulla A, Durrant STS, Hows JM. Subacute encephalopathy associated with human immunodeficiency virus in haemophilia A. Br Med J 1986;293:993.
29. Elder GA, Sever JL. AIDS and neurological disorders: An overview, Ann Neurol 1988; 23(Suppl):S4–S6.
30. Levy RM, Bredesen DE, Rosenblum ML. Opportunistic central nervous system pathology in patients with AIDS. Ann Neurol 1988:23(Suppl):S7–S12.
31. Lusher JM. Diseases of coagulation: The fluid phase. In: Nathan DG, Oski FA, eds. Hematology of Infancy and Childhood, 3rd ed. Philadelphia: W.B. Saunders, 1987:1293–1342.
32. Mason DY, Ingram GIC. Management of the hereditary coagulation disorders. Semin Hematol 1971;8:158–188.
33. Kasper CK. Postoperative thromboses in hemophilia. B. N Engl J Med 1973;289:160.
34. Agrawal BL, Zelkowitz L, Hletko P. Acute myocardial infarction in a young hemophiliac patient during therapy with factor IX concentrate and epsilon aminocaproic acid. J Pediatr 1981;98:931–933.
35. Feffer SE, Parray HR, Westring DW. Seizure after infusion of aminocaproic acid. JAMA 1978;240:2468.
36. Bahnson HT, Siegler RFA. A consideration of the causes of death following operation for congenital heart disease of the cyanotic type. Surg Gynecol Obstet 1950;90:60–76.
37. Gross S, Keefer V, Lichman J. The platelet in cyanotic congenital heart disease. Pediatrics 1968;42:651–658.

38. Dennis LH, Stewart JL, Conrad ME. Heparin treatment of hemorrhagic diathesis in cyanotic congenital heart disease. Lancet 1967;1:1088–1089.

39. Lilleyman JS. Idiopathic thrombocytopenic purpura—where do we stand? Arch Dis Child 1984;59:701–703.

40. Stuart MJ, Kelton JG. The platelet: quantitative and qualitative abnormalities. In: Nathan DG, Oski FA, eds. Hematology of Infancy and Childhood, 3rd ed. Philadelphia: W.B. Saunders, 1987:1343–1478.

41. Komrower GM, Watson GH. Prognosis in idiopathic thrombocytopenic purpura of childhood. Arch Dis Child 1954;29:502–506.

42. Choi SI, McClure PD. Idiopathic thrombocytopenic purpura in childhood. Can Med Assoc J 1967;97:562–568.

43. Karpatkin S. Autoimmune thrombocytopenic purpura. Blood 1980;56:329–343.

44. Burns TR, Saleem A. Idiopathic thrombocytopenic purpura. Am J Med 1983;75:1001–1007.

45. McClure PD. Idiopathic thrombocytopenic purpura in children: Diagnosis and management. Pediatrics 1975;55:68–74.

46. Woerner SJ, Abildgaard CF, French BN. Intracranial hemorrhage in children with idiopathic thrombocytopenic purpura. Pediatrics 1981;67:453–460.

47. Krivit W, Tate D, White JG, et al. Idiopathic thrombocytopenic purpura and intracranial hemorrhage. Pediatrics 1981;67:570–571.

48. Faloon WW, Greene RW, Lozner EL. The hemostatic defect in thrombocytopenia as studied by the use of ACTH and cortisone. Am J Med 1952;13:12–20.

49. Robson HN, Duthie JKJ. Capillary resistance and adrenocortical activity. Br Med J 1950;2:971–973.

50. Lammi AT, Lovric VA. Idiopathic thrombocytopenic purpura: An epidemiologic study. J Pediatr 1973;83:31–36.

51. Lusher JM, Emami A, Ravindranath Y, et al. Idiopathic thrombocytopenic purpura in children. Am J Pediatr Hematol Oncol 1984;6:149–157.

52. Benham ES, Taft LI. Idiopathic thrombocytopenic purpura in children: Results of steroid therapy and splenectomy. Aust Paediatr J 1972;8:311–317.

53. Walker JH, Walker W. Idiopathic thrombocytopenic purpura in childhood. Arch Dis Child 1981;36:649–657.

54. Sartorius JA. Steroid treatment of idiopathic thrombocytopenic purpura in children. Preliminary results of a randomized cooperative study. Am J Pediatr Hematol Oncol 1984;6:165–169.

55. Buchanan CR, Holtkamp CA. Prednisone therapy for children with newly diagnosed idiopathic thrombocytopenic purpura of childhood. Am J Pediatr Hematol Oncol 1984;6:355–361.

56. Imbach P, Wagner HP, Berchtold W, et al. Intravenous immunoglobulin versus oral corticosteroids in acute immune thrombocytopenic purpura in childhood. Lancet 1985;2:464–448.

57. Zerella JT, Martin LW, Lampkin BC. Emergency splenectomy for idiopathic thrombocytopenic purpura in children. J Pediatr Surg 1978;13:243–246.

58. Lightsey AL, McMillan R, Koenig HM. Childhood idiopathic thrombocytopenic purpura. Aggressive management of life-threatening complications. JAMA 1975;232:734–736.

59. Barr RD, Copeland SA, Stockwell ML, et al. Valproic acid and immune thrombocytopenia. Arch Dis Child 1982;57:681–684.

60. Pearson HA, McIntosh S. Neonatal thrombocytopenia. Clin Hematol 1978;7:111–122.

61. Krye JJ, Corrigan JJ. Idiopathic thrombocytopenic purpura during pregnancy. A pediatric viewpoint. Am J Pediatr Hematol Oncol 1983:5:21–25.

62. Kelton JG. Management of the pregnant patient with idiopathic thrombocytopenic purpura. Ann Intern Med 1983;99:796–800.

63. Scott JR, Cruikshank DP, Kochenour NK, et al. Fetal platelet counts in the obstetric management of immunologic thrombocytopenic purpura. Am J Obstet Gynecol 1980;136:495–499.

64. Ayromlooi J. A new approach to the management of immunologic thrombocytopenic purpura in pregnancy. Am J Obstet Gynecol 1978;130:235–236.

65. Carloss HW, McMillan R, Crosby WH. Management of pregnancy in women with immune thrombocytopenic purpura. JAMA 1980;244:2756–2758.

66. Galea P, Patrick MJK, Goel KM. Isoimmune neonatal thrombocytopenic purpura. Arch Dis Child 1981;56:112–115.

67. Morales WJ, Stroup M. Intracranial hemorrhage in utero due to isoimmune neonatal thrombocytopenia. Obstet Gynecol 1985;65(Suppl):S20–S21.

68. Sandowitz PD, Balcom R. Intrauterine intracranial hemorrhage in an infant with isoimmune thrombocytopenia. Clin Pediatr 1985;24:655–657.

69. Zalneraitis EL, Young RK, Krishnamoorthy KS. Intracranial hemorrhage in utero as a complication of isoimmune thrombocytopenia. J Pediatr 1979;95:611–614.

70. Pochedly C. Thrombocytopenic purpura of the newborn. Obstet Gynecol Survey 1971;26:63–103.

71. Jesurun CA, Levin GS, Sullivan WR, et al. Intracranial hemorrhage in utero re thrombocytopenia. J Pediatr 1980;97:695–696.

72. Perry GS, Spector BD, Schuman LM, et al. The Wiskott-Aldrich syndrome in the United States and Canada (1892–1979). J Pediatr 1980;97:72–78.

73. Parkman R, Rappaport J, Geha R, et al. Complete correction of the Wiskott-Aldrich syndrome by allogenic bone marrow transplantation. N Engl J Med 1978;298:921–927.

74. Gardner RJM, Morrison PS, Abbott GD. A syndrome of congenital thrombocytopenia with multiple malformations and neurologic dysfunction. J Pediatr 1983;102:600–602.

75. Stormorken H, Sjaastad O, Langslet A, et al. A new syndrome: Thrombocytopathia, muscle fatigue, asplenia, miosis, migraine, dyslexia and ichthyosis. Clin Genet 1985;28:367–374.

76. Sceats DJ, Baiton D. Primary thrombocythemia in a child. Clin Pediatr 1980;19:298–300.

77. Freedman MH. Olivares RS, McClure PD, et al. Primary thrombocythemia in a child. J Pediatr 1973;83:163–164.

78. Sanyal SK, Yules RB, Eidelman AL, et al. Thrombocytosis, central nervous system disease and myocardial infarction pattern in infancy. Pediatrics 1966;38:629–636.

79. Huttenlocher PR, Smith DB. Acute infantile hemiplegia associated with thrombocytosis. Dev Med Child Neurol 1968;10:621–625.

80. Korenman G. Neurologic syndromes associated with primary thrombocythemia. J Mt Sinai Hosp NY 1969;36:317–323.

81. Van LA, Kauffmann RH, Valentijn RM. Renal manifestations of systemic disease. In: Holliday MA, Barratt TM, Vernier RL, eds. Pediatric Nephrology. 2nd ed. Baltimore: Williams and Wilkins, 1987;28:492–498.

82. Borges WH. Anaphylactoid purpura. Med Clin North Am 1972;56:201–206.

83. Gottlieb AJ. Allergic purpura. In: Williams WJ, Buetler E, Ersleve AJ, et al., eds 3rd ed. Hematology. New York: McGraw-Hill, 1983;150:1371–1377.

84. Lewis IC, Philipott MG. Neurological complications in the Schönlein-Henoch syndrome. Arch Dis Child 1956;31:369–371.

85. Norkin S, Weiner J. Henoch-Schönlein syndrome. Am J Clin Pathol 1960;33:55–65.

86. Ritter FJ, Seay AR, Lahey ME. Peripheral mononeuropathy complicating anaphylactoid purpura. J Pediatr 1983;103:77–78.

87. Turpin JC, Duc JP, Larget-Piet L, et al. Les manifestations neurologiques du purpura rhumatoide. Rev Pediatr Obstet Gynecol 1973;28:185–192.

88. Ryder HG, Marcus J. Henoch-Schönlein purpura. S Afr Med J 1976;50:2005–2006.

89. Lux Se. Disorders of the red cell membrane skeleton: hereditary spherocytosis and hereditary elliptocytosis. In: Stanbury JB, Wyngaarden JB, Frederickson DS, et al., eds. The Metabolic Basis of Inherited Disease, 5th ed. New York: McGraw-Hill, 1983:1573–1605.

90. Beutler E. Glucose-6-phosphate dehydrogenase deficiency. In: Stanbury JB, Wyngaarden JB, Frederickson DS, et al., eds. The Metabolic Basis of Inherited Disease, 5th ed. New York: McGraw-Hill, 1983:1629–1653.

91. Valentine WN, Tanaka KR, Paglia DE. Pyruvate kinase and other enzyme deficiency disorders of the erythrocyte. In: Stanbury JB, Wyngaarden JB, Frederickson DS, Goldstein JL, et al., eds. The Metabolic Basis of Inherited Disease, 5th ed. New York: McGraw-Hill, 1983:1606–1628.

92. Poll-The BT, Aicardi J, Girot R, et al. Neurological findings in triosephosphate isomerase deficiency. Ann Neurol 1985;17:439–443.

93. Lozoff B, Brittenham GM. Behavioral aspects of iron deficiency. Prog Hematol 1986;14:23–53.

94. Oski FA. The non hematologic manifestations of iron deficiency. Am J Dis Child 1979;133:315–322.

95. Oski FA, Honig AS, Helu B, et al. Effect of iron therapy on behavior performance in nonanemic, iron-deficient infants. Pediatrics 1983;71:877–880.

96. Oski FA, Honig AS. The effects of therapy on the developmental scores of iron deficient infants. J Pediatr 1978;92:21–25.

97. Lozoff B, Brittenham GM, Viteri PE, et al. Developmental deficits in iron-deficient infants: effects of age and severity of iron lack. J Pediatr 1982;101:948–952.

98. Pollit E, Soemantri AG, Yunis F, et al. Cognitive effects of iron deficiency anemia. Lancet 1985;1:158.

99. Lanzkowsky P, Erlandson ME, Bezan AI. Isolated defect of folic acid absorption associated with mental retardation and cerebral calcification. Blood 1969;34:452–465.

100. Lanzkowsky P. Clinical, pathogenetic, and diagnostic considerations in folate deficiency. In: Nathan DG, Oski FA, eds. Hematology of Infancy and Childhood, 3rd ed. Philadelphia: W.B. Saunders, 1987:321–338.

101. Lanzkowsky P. Clinical, pathogenetic, and diagnostic considerations of vitamin B_{12} (cobalamin) deficiency and other congenital and acquired disorders. In: Nathan DG, Oski FA, eds. Hematology of Infancy and Childhood, 3rd ed. Philadephia: W.B. Saunders, 1987:344–362.

102. Heisel MA, Siegel SE, Falk RE, et al. Congenital pernicious anemia: Report of seven patients, with studies of the extended family. J Pediatr 1984:105:564–568.

103. Miller DR, Bloom GE, Streiff RR, et al. Juvenile "congenital" pernicious anemia. N Engl J Med 1966:275:978–983.

104. Spurling CL, Sacks MS, Jiji RM. Juvenile pernicious anemia. N Engl J Med 1964;271:995–1003.

105. Reisner EH, Wolff JA, McKay RJ, et al. Juvenile pernicious anemia. Pediatrics 1951;8:88–106.

106. Frenkel EP. Abnormal fatty acid metabolism in peripheral nerves of patients with pernicious anemia. J Clin Invest 1973:53:1237–1245.

107. Spencer SE, Walker FO, Moore SA. Chorea-amyotrophy with chronic hemolytic anemia. Neurology 1987;37:645–649.

108. Villegas A, Moscat J, Vasquez A, et al. A new family with hereditary choreo-acanthocytosis. Acta Haematol 1987;77:2125–2129.

109. Serra S, Xerra A, Arena A. Amyotrophic choreo-acanthocytosis: A new observation in southern Europe. Acta Neurol Scand 1986;73:481–486.

110. Moschcowitz E. An acute febrile poliochromic anemia with hyaline thrombosis of terminal arteries and capillaries: An undescribed disease. Arch Intern Med 1925;36:89–93.

111. Lian ECY. The role of increased platelet aggregation in TTP. Semin Thromb Hemost 1980;6:401–415.

112. Altschule MD. A rare type of acute thrombocytopenic purpura: A morphological study of its histogenesis. Am J Pathol 1950;26:155–167.

113. Remuzzi G, Marchesi D, Misiani R, et al. Familial deficiency of a plasma factor stimulating vascular prostacyclin activity. Thromb Res 1979;17:517–525.

114. Amorosi EL, Ultmann JE. Thrombotic thrombocytopenic purpura: Report of 16 cases and review of the literature. Medicine (Baltimore) 1966;45:139–159.

115. Berberich FR, Cuene SA, Chad RL, et al. Thrombotic thrombocytopenic purpura: Three cases with platelet and fibrinogen survival studies. J Pediatr 1974;84:503–509.

116. Pilz P. Moschcowitz syndrome with involvement of the central nervous system. Virchows Arch (A) 1975;366:59–66.

117. Vilanova Jr, Norenberg MD, Stuard ID. Thrombotic thrombocytopenic purpura. NY State J Med 1975;75:2246–2248.

118. Jacobsen BM. Case records of the Massachusetts General Hospital. Case 1–1968. N Engl J Med 1968;278:36–43.

119. Milkler K, Kim Y. Hemolytic uremic syndrome. In: Holliday MA, Barratt TM, Vernier RL, eds. Pediatric Nephrology, 2nd ed., Baltimore: Williams and Wilkins, 1987;28:482–491.

120. Aster RH, Hemolytic-uremic syndrome. In: Williams WJ, Buetler E, Erslev AJ, et al., eds. Hematology, 3rd ed. New York: McGraw-Hill, 1983;150:1308–1331.

121. Upadhyaya K, Barwick K, Fishaut M, et al. The importance of nonrenal involvement in hemolytic-uremic syndrome. Pediatrics 1980;65:115–120.

122. Steele BT, Murphey N, Chuang SH, et al. Recovery from prolonged coma in hemolytic uremic syndrome. J Pediatr 1983;102:402–404.

123. Crisp De, Siegler RL, Thompson JA. Hemorrhagic cerebral infarction in the hemolytic-uremic syndrome. J Pediatr 1981;99:273–276.

124. DiMario FJ, Bronte-Stewart K, Sherbotie J, et al. Lacunar infarction of the basal ganglia as a complication of hemolytic-uremic syndrome. Clin Pediatr 1987;26:586–590.

125. Mendelsohn DB, Hertzanu Y, Chaitowitz B, et al. Cranial CT in the haemolytic-uraemic syndrome. J Neurol Neurosurg Psychiatry 1984;47:876–878.

126. Bos AP, Donckerwolcke RA, van Vught AJ. The hemolytic-uremic syndrome: Prognostic significance of neurological abnormalities. Helv Paediat Acta 1985;40:381–389.

127. Danish EH, Rasch CA, Harris JW. Polycythemia vera in childhood: Case report and review of the literature. Am J Hematol 1980;9:421–428.

128. Gamsu HR. Neonatal morbidity in infants of diabetic mothers. J R Soc Med 1978; 71:273–279.

129. Hakanson DO, Oh W. Hyperviscosity in the small-for-gestational age infant. Biol Neonate 1980; 37:109–112.

130. Miller M, Cosgriff JM. Hematological abnormalities in newborn infants with Down's syndrome. Am J Genet 1983; 16:173–177.

131. Reisner SH, Mor N, Levy Y et al. Incidence of neonatal polycythemia. Isr J Med Sci 1983;19:848–849.

132. Miller GM, Black VD, Lubchenco LO. Intracerebral hemorrhage in a term newborn with hyperviscosity. Am J Dis Child 1981;135:377–378.

133. Amit M, Camfield PR. Neonatal polycythemia causing multiple cerebral infarcts. Arch Neurol 1980;37:109–110.

134. Koffler H, Keenan WJ, Sutherland JM. Hydranencephaly following elevated hematocrit values in a newly born infant. Pediatrics 1974;54:770–772.

135. Baum RS. Hyperviscous blood and perinatal pathology. Pediatr Res 1967;1:288–290.

136. Gatti RA, Muster AJ, Cole RB, et al. Neonatal polycythemia with transient cyanosis and cardiorespiratory abnormalities. J Pediatr 1966;69:1063–1072.

137. Danish EH. Neonatal polycythemia. Prog Hematol 1986;14:55–98.

138. Winslow RM, Anderson WF. The hemoglobinopathies. In: Stanbury JB, Wyngaarden JB, Frederickson DS, et al., eds. The Metabolic Basis of Inherited Disease, 5th ed. New York: McGraw-Hill, 1983:1666–1710.

139. Baglioni C. An improvement method for the fingerprinting of human hemoglobin. Biochim Biophys Acta 1961;48: 392–396.

140. Konotey-Ahulu FLD. The sickle cell diseases. Arch Intern Med 1974;133:611–619.

141. Winkelstein JA, Shin HS, Smith MR. Pneumococcal infection in sickle cell disease. Deficiency of heat labile opsonin activity. In: Hercules JI, Schechter AN, Eaton WA, et al., eds. Proceedings of the 1st National Symposium on Sickle Cell Disease. Bethesda: DHEW Publication (NIH) 75–723, 1974;1:71–72.

142. Anderson WW, Ware RL. Sickle cell anemia. Am J Dis Child 1932;44:1055–1072.

143. Greer M, Schotland D. Abnormal hemoglobin as a cause of neurologic disease. Neurology 1962;121:114–123.

144. Powars D, Wilson B, Imbus C, et al. The natural history of stroke in sickle cell disease. Am J Med 1978;65:461–471.

145. Portnoy BA, Herion JC. Neurological manifestations in sickle cell disease with a review of the literature and emphasis on the prevalence of hemiplegia. Ann Intern Med 1972;76:643–652.

146. Hitchcock ER, Tsementzis SA, Richardson SGN, et al. Subarachnoid hemorrhage in sickle-cell anemia. Surg Neurol 1983;19:251–254.

147. Merkel KH, Ginsberg PL, Parker JC, et al. Cerebrovascular disease in sickle cell anemia: A clinical, pathological and radiological correlation. Stroke 1978;9:45–52.

148. Stockman J, Nigro MA, Mishkin MM, et al. Occlusion of large cerebral vessels in sickle-cell anemia. N Engl J Med 1972;287:846–849.

149. Baird RL, Weiss DL, Ferguson AD, et al. Studies in sickle cell anemia XXI. Clinico-pathologic aspects of neurological manifestations. Pediatrics 1964;34:92–100.

150. Hughes JG, Diggs LW, Gillespie CE. The involvement of the nervous system in sickle cell anemia. J Pediatr 1940;17: 166–184.

151. Pavlakis SG, Bello J, Prohovnik, et al. Brain infarction in sickle cell anemia: Magnetic resonance imaging correlates. Ann Neurol 1988;23:125–130.

152. Russell MO, Goldberg HI, Hodson A, et al. Effect of transfusion therapy on arteriographic abnormalities and on recurrence of stroke in sickle cell disease. Blood 1984; 63:162–169.

153. Russell M, Goldberg H, Reis L, et al. Transfusion therapy for cerebrovascular abnormalities in sickle cell disease. J Pediatr 1976;88:382–387.

154. Wilmas J, Goff JR, Anderson MA, et al. Efficacy of transfusion therapy for one to two years in patients with sickle cell disease and cerebrovascular accidents. J Pediatr 1980; 96:205–208.

155. Buchanan GR, Bowman WP, Smith SJ. Recurrent cerebral ischemia during hypertransfusion therapy in sickle cell anemia. J Pediatr 1983;103:921–923.

156. Goldberg MF. Natural history of untreated proliferative sickle retinopathy. Arch Ophthalmol 1971;85:428–437.

157. Stevens TS, Busse B, Lee C, et al. Sickling hemoglobinopathies macular and perimacular vascular abnormalities. Arch Ophthalmol 1974;92:455–463.

158. Condon PI, Serjeant GR. Behavior of untreated proliferative sickle retinopathy. Br J Ophthalmol 1980;64:404–411.

159. Friedman EM, Lubvan NLC, Herer GR, et al. Sickle cell anemia and hearing. Ann Otol Rhinol Laryngol 1980;89: 342–347.

160. Morgenstein KM, Manace ED. Temporal bone histopathology in sickle cell disease. Laryngoscope 1969;79:2172–2180.

161. Kabions SA, Lerner C. Fulminant pneumococcemia and sickle cell anemia. JAMA 1970;211:467–471.

162. Sachs JM, Pacin M, Counts GW. Sickle hemoglobinopathy and Edwardsiella tarda meningitis. Am J Dis Child 1974; 128:387–388.

163. Fabian RH, Peters BH. Neurological complications of hemoglobin SC disease. Arch Neurol 1984;41:289–292.

164. Chambers J, Publisi J, Kernitsky R. Iris atrophy in hemoglobin SC disease. Am J Ophthalmol 1974;77: 247–249.

165. Shaw HE, Osher RH, Smith JL. Amaurosis fugax associated with SC hemoglobinopathy and lupus erythematosus. Am J Ophthalmol 1979;87:281–285.

166. Bussone G, LaMantia L, Boiardi A, et al. Complicated migraine in AS hemoglobinopathy. Eur Neurol 1984; 23:22–25.

167. Nienhuis AW, Wolfe L. The thalassemias. In: Nathan DG, Oski FA, eds. Hematology of Infancy and Childhood, 3rd ed. Philadelphia: W.B. Saunders, 1987:699–778.

168. Kan Y. The thalassemias. In: Stanbury JB, Wyngaarden JB, Frederickson DS, et al., eds. The Metabolic Basis of Inherited Disease, 5th ed. New York: McGraw-Hill, 1983: 1711–1725.

169. Weatherall DJ, Higgs Dr, Bunch C, et al. Hemoglobin H disease and mental retardation. N Engl J Med 1981;305: 607–612.

170. Bowcock AM, van Tonder S, Kenkins T. The haemoglobin H disease mental retardation syndrome: Molecular studies on the South African case. Br J Haematol 1984;56:69–78.

171. Modell B, Berdoukas V. The Clinical Approach to Thalassemia. New York: Grune and Statton, 1984:229.

172. Olivieri NF, Buncic JR, Chew E, et al. Visual and auditory neurotoxicity in patients receiving subcutaneous deferoxamine infusions. N Engl J Med 1986;314:869–873.

173. Dickeroff R. Acute aphasia and loss of vision with deferoxamine overdose. Am J Pediatr Hematol Oncol 1987; 9:287–288.

174. Johnson RV, Kaplan SR, Blailock ZR. Cerebral venous thrombosis in paroxysmal nocturnal hemoglobinuria. Neurology 1970;20:681–686.

175. Steinsapir KD, Vinters HV. Central pontine myelinolysis in a child with Shwachman-Diamond syndrome. Hum Pathol 1985;16:741–743.

176. DeBoeck K, Degreef H, Verwilghen R, et al. Thrombocytopenia: First symptom in a patient with dyskeratosis congenita. Pediatrics 1981;67:898–903.

177. Womer R, Clark JE, Wood P, et al. Dyskeratosis congenita: Two examples of this multisystem disorder. Pediatrics 1983;71:603–609.

178. Steler W, VanVoolen A, Selmanowitz VJ. Dyskeratosis congenita: Relationship to Fanconi's anemia. Blood 1972; 39:510–521.

179. Shiozawa Z, Tsunoda S, Noda A, et al. Cerebral hemorrhagic infarction associated with anabolic steroid therapy for hypoplastic anemia. Angiology 1986;37:725–729.

180. Tilzey A, Heptonstall J, Hamblin T. Toxic confusional state and choreiform movements after treatment with anabolic steroids. Br Med J 1981;283:349–350.

181. Baran DT, Griner PF, Klemperer MR. Recovery from aplastic anemic after treatment with cyclophosphamide. N Engl J Med 1976;295:1512–1526.

182. Gluckman E, Devergie A, Poros A, et al. Results of immunosuppression in 170 cases of severe aplastic anemia. Br J Haematol 1982;51:541–550.

183. Rappaport JM. Bone marrow transplantation. In: Nathan DG, Oski FA, eds. Hematology of Infancy and Childhood, 3rd ed. Philadelphia: W.B. Saunders 1987:242–264.

184. Parkamn R, Rappaport JM, Camita B, et al. Successful use of multiagent immunosuppression in the bone marrow transplantation of sensitized patients. Blood 1978;52: 1163–1169.

185. Sullivan KM. Graft-versus-host disease. In: Petz LD, Blume KG, eds. Clinical Bone Marrow Transplantation. New York: Churchill Livingstone, 1983:91–123.

186. Schubert MM. Sullivan KM, Morton TH et al. Oral manifestations of chronic graft-v-host disease. Arch Intern Med 1984;144:1591–1595.

187. Deeg HJ, Storb R, Thomas ED. Bone marrow transplantation: A review of delayed complications. Br J Haematol 1984;57:185–208.

188. Sullivan KM, Storb R, Shulman HM et al. Immediate and delayed neurotoxicity after mechlorethamine preparation for bone marrow transplantation. Ann Intern Med 1982;97:182–189.

189. Smith CIE, Aarli JA, Biberfeld P, et al. Myasthenia gravis after bone-marrow transplantation. Evidence for a donor origin. N Engl J Med 1983;309:1565–1568.

190. Wiznitzer M, Packer RJ, August CS, et al. Neurological complications of bone marrow transplantation in childhood. Ann Neurol 1984;16:569–576.

191. Krivit W. Correction of inborn errors of metabolism by bone marrow transplantation. Basic Life Sci 1983;25:63–76.

192. Sand JJ, Biller J, Aschenbrener CA. Nonbacterial thrombotic endocarditis and nondisseminated malignancy associated with osteopetrosis. Eur Neurol 1987;27:167–172.

193. Whyte MP, Murphy WA, Fallon MG, et al. Osteopetrosis, renal tubular acidosis and basal ganglia calcification in three sisters. Am J Med 1980;69:64–74.

194. Lehman RAW, Reeves JD, Wilson WB, et al. Neurological complications of infantile osteopetrosis. Ann Neurol 1977; 2:378–384.

195. Keith CG. Retinal atrophy in osteopetrosis. Arch Ophthalmol 1968;79:234–241.

196. Miyamoto RT, House WF, Brackmann DE. Neurologic manifestations of the osteopetrosis. Arch Otolaryngol Head Neck Surg 1980;106:210–214.

197. Moe PJ, Sklaeveland A. Therapeutic studies in osteopetrosis. Acta Paediatr Scand 1969;58:593–600.

198. Fitch N, Carpenter S, Lachance RC. Prenatal axonal dystrophy and osteopetrosis. Arch Pathol 1973;95:298–301.

199. Ambler MW, Trice J, Gauerholz J, et al. Infantile osteopetrosis and neuronal storage disease. Neurology 1983; 33:437–441.

200. Coccia PF, Krivit W, Cervenka J, et al. Successful bone-marrow transplantation for infantile malignant osteopetrosis. N Engl J Med 1980;302:702–708.

201. Haymaker W, Margoles C, Pentschew A, et al. Pathology of kernicterus and posticteric encephalopathy. In: Kernicterus and its Importance in Cerebral Palsy. American Academy for Cerebral Palsy. Springfield: Charles C Thomas, 1961:21–228.

202. Claireaux AE, Cole PG, Lathe GH. Icterus of the brain in the newborn. Lancet 1953;2:1226–1230.

203. Silverberg DH, Johnson L, Ritter L. Factors influencing toxicity of bilirubin in cerebellum tissue culture. J Pediatr 1970; 77:386–396.

204. Van Praagh R. Diagnosis of kernicterus in the neonatal period. Pediatrics 1961;28:870–876.

205. Perlstein MA. The late syndrome of posticteric encephalopathy. Pediatr Clin North Am 1960;7:665–687.

206. Maisels MJ. Bilirubin: On understanding and influencing its metabolism in the newborn infant. Pediatr Clin North Am 1972;19:447–501.

207. Luzzato L. Genetic heterogeneity and pathophysiology of G6PD deficiency. Br J Haematol 1974;28:151–155.

208. Wolkoff AW, Chowdhury JR, Arias IM. Hereditary jaundice and disorders of bilirubin metabolism. In: Stanbury JB, Wyngaarden JB, Frederickson DS, et al., eds. The Metabolic Basis of Inherited Disease, 5th ed. New York: McGraw-Hill, 1983:1385–1417.

209. Familial unconjugated hyperbilirubinemias. In: Silverman A, Roy CC, ed. Pediatric Clinical Gastroenterology. St Louis: C.V. Mosby, 1983:567–570.

210. Huang PW, Rozdilsky B, Gerrard JW, et al. Crigler-Najjar syndrome in four of five siblings with postmortem findings in one. Arch Pathol 1970;90:536–542.

211. Rosenthal IM, Zimmerman JH, Hardy N. Congenital nonhemolytic jaundice with disease of the central nervous system. Pediatrics 1956;18:378–386.

212. Gardner WA, Konigsmark BW. Familial nonhemolytic jaundice: Bilirubinosis and encephalopathy. Pediatrics 1969;43: 365–376.

213. Blumenschein SD, Kallen RJ, Storey B, et al. Familial nonhemolytic jaundice with late onset of neurological damage. Pediatrics 1968;42:786–792.

214. Wolkoff AW, Chowdhury JR, Gartner LA, et al. Crigler-Najjar syndrome (type I) in an adult male. Gastroenterology 1979;76:840–848.

215. Arias IM, Gartner LM, Cohen M, et al. Chronic non-hemolytic unconjugated hyperbilirubinemia with glucuronyl transferase deficiency. Am J Med 1969;47:395–409.

216. Gartner LM, Whitington PF. Disorders of bilirubin metabolism. In: Nathan DG, Oski FA, eds. Hematology of Infancy and Childhood, 3rd ed. Philadelphia: W.B. Saunders, 1987:74–103.

217. Kappas A, Sassa S, Anderson KE. The porphyrias. In: Stanbury JB, Wyngaarden JB, Frederickson DS, eds. The Metabolic Basis of Inherited Disease, 5th ed. New York: McGraw-Hill, 1983:1325–1384.

218. Stein JA, Tschundy DP. Acute intermittent porphyria. Medicine 1970;49:1–16.

219. Gupta GL, Saksena HC, Bupta BD. Cardiac dysautonomia in acute intermittent porphyria. Indian J Med Res 1983;78:253–256.

220. Laiwah AY, Macphee G, Boule P, et al. J Neurol Neurosurg Psychiatry 1985;48:1025–1030.

221. Goldberg A. Acute intermittent porphyria. A study of 50 cases. Q J Med 1959;28:183–209.

222. Lai C, Hung T, Lin WSJ. Blindness of cerebral origin in acute intermittent porphyria. Arch Neurol 1977;34:310–312.

223. Thorner PS, Bilbao JM, Sima AAF et al. Porphyric Neuropathy: An untrastructural and quantitative case study. Can J Neurol Sci 1981;8:281–287.

224. Mustajoki P, Seppalainen AM. Neuropathy in latent hereditary hepatic porphyria. Br Med J 1975;2:310–312.

225. Ludwig GD, Goldberg M. Hyponatremia in acute intermittent porphyria probably resulting from inappropriate secretion of antidiuretic hormone. Ann N Y Acad Sci 1963;104:710–734.

226. Glass J, Robinson SH. Disorders of heme metabolism: Sideroblastic anemia and the porphyrias. In: Nathan DG, Oski FA, eds. Hematology of Infancy and Childhood, 3rd ed. Philadelphia: W.B. Saunders, 1987:1363–1388.

227. Laiwah ACY, Moore MR, Goldberg A. Pathogenesis of acute porphyria. Q J Med Sci 1987;63:377–392.

228. Samuels MA. Case records of the Massachusetts General Hospital. Case 39–1984. N Engl J Med 1984;311:839–847.

229. Lamon JM, Frykholm BC, Hess RA, et al. Hematin therapy. Medicine 1979;58:252–259.

230. Di Trapani G, Casali C, Tonali P, et al. Peripheral nerve findings in hereditary coproporphyria. Acta Neuropathol 1984;63:96–107.

231. Blume RS, Wolff SM. The Chédiak-Higashi syndrome: Studies in four patients and a review of the literature. Medicine 1972;51:247–280.

232. Witkop CJ, Quevedo WC, Fitzpatrick TB. Albinism and other disorders of pigment metabolism. In: Stanbury JB, Wyngaarden JB, Frederickson DS, et al., eds. The Metabolic Basis of Inherited Disease, 5th ed. New York: McGraw-Hill, 1983:301–343.

233. Lockman LA, Kennedy WA, White JG. The Chediak-Higashi syndrome: Electrophysiologic and electron microscopic observation in the peripheral neuropathology. J Pediatr 1967;70:942–951.

234. Tanaka K, Rosenberg LE. Disorders of branched chain amino acid and organic acid metabolism. In: Stanbury JB, Wyngaarden JB, Frederickson DS, et al., eds. The Metabolic Basis of Inherited Disease, 5th ed. New York: McGraw-Hill, 1983:440–473.

235. Silverstein MN, Ellefson RD, Ahern EJ. The syndrome of the sea-blue histiocyte. N Engl J Med 1970;282:1–4.

236. Lake BD, Stephens R, Neville BGR. Syndrome of the sea-blue histiocyte. Lancet 1970;2:309.

237. Chusid MF, Dale DC, West BC, et al. The hypereosinophilic syndromes: Analysis of fourteen cases with review of the literature. Medicine 1975;54:1–27.

238. Weaver DF, Heffernan LP, Purdy RA, et al. Eosinophil-induced neurotoxicity: Axonal neuropathy, cerebral infarction, and dementia. N Engl J Med 1988;38:144–146.

239. Parrillo JF, Fauci AS, Wolff SM. Therapy of the hypereosinophilic syndrome. Ann Intern Med 1978;89:167–172.

Chapter 20
Neurologic Manifestations of Systemic Cancer

Jeffrey C. Allen

This chapter addresses the clinical neurologic syndromes related to primary or metastatic childhood cancer that arise outside the central nervous system (CNS). The natural history of CNS metastases has been characterized more extenisvely in adult than in pediatric cancers. Although the types of systemic cancers arising in adults are usually different from those in children (that is carcinomas vs. sarcomas), the biology of CNS metastasis is similar.

CNS metastases from solid tumors appear to be increasing in incidence, not only as a function of greater awareness and more sophisticated neurodiagnostic instrumentation, but also as a function of treatment effects. In a prior era of relative ineffective therapies, patients died early and primarily from the effects of uncontrolled local disease. As newer, more effective treatments emerged, the primary tumor and the systemic metastases were put in temporary remission. Disease sanctuaries such as the CNS, where chemotherapy drugs distribute poorly, became a more frequent site of recurrence. This phenomenon appears to be evident in children as well as in adults with solid and hematopoietic cancer in the terminal phases of their illnesses. As the natural history of a disease is better appreciated and more effective therapies are discovered, the prospect of curative therapy emerges. Treatment strategies must address not only local disease control but also the eradication of micrometastases in the body and CNS.

There also exists a number of specific neurologic syndromes that are indirect manifestations of systemic cancer. Remote effects of cancer are rare in adults but are more rare in children. The best described is the opsoclonus-myoclonus syndrome associated with neuroblastoma (NB). Occasionally, certain biologic aspects of the systemic cancer place the CNS at high risk for injury, such as the predisposition for spontaneous brain hemorrhage in acute promyelocytic leukemia or the encephalopathy associated with high intravascular white-blood-cell (WBC) counts and leukostasis in leukemia.

PATTERNS OF CENTRAL NERVOUS SYSTEM METASTASIS

Neurologic signs and symptoms are one of the most commonly recognized manifestations of metastatic cancer; that is, the CNS is a sentinel organ. This relates in part to its unique sensitivity but also to its lengthy confinement within the bony structures of the cranium and vertebral canal. Neurologic syndromes arise most commonly in patients with widespread recurrent systemic disease. Less commonly, patients present with CNS metastases at the time of diagnosis, or the initial localized solid tumor is in close proximity to a neurologically sensitive structure like the head or paravertebral region.

Systemic cancer can spread to the CNS in several ways. Brain or intracerebral metastases probably arise from intravascular tumor seedlings. Leptomeningeal metastases probably have a similar origin. Occasionally, leptomeningeal metastases invade the brain or spinal cord and produce a lesion that behaves clinically as a focal brain metastasis.

The most common form of CNS injury in solid tumors is epidural metastasis in which symptoms are produced by external compression rather than by direct invasion. This brain or spinal cord syndrome can arise from two conditions; viz, an intraosseus metastasis extending from a vertebral body or cranial bone, or a paravertebral tumor or base of skull metastasis can insinuate itself through a bony foramen and reach the epidural space. Rarely, a blood-born metastasis may lodge directly in the epidural space (Figure 20.1).

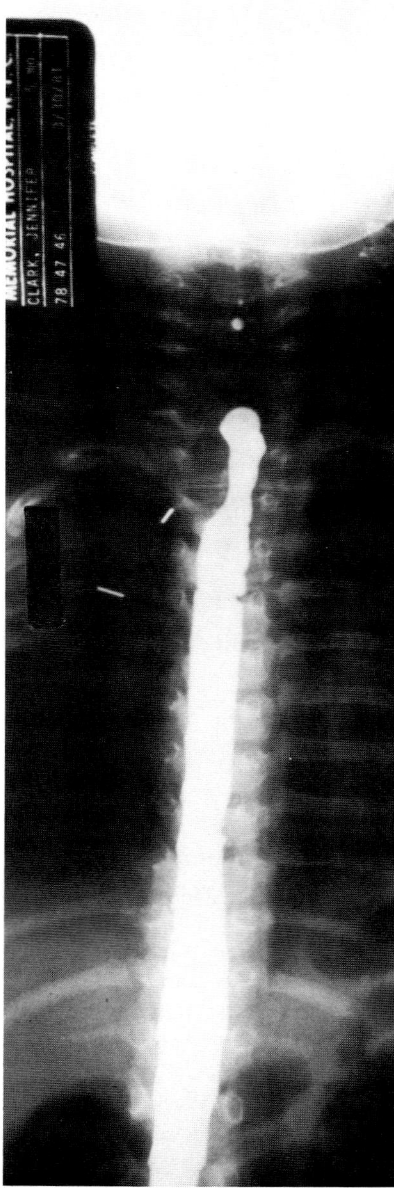

FIGURE 20.1   Epidural cord compression in the right upper thoracic region from disseminated neuroblastoma.

The spinal epidural space, as opposed to its cranial counterpart, is a genuine anatomic structure. It lies between the bony periosteum and the dura mater, covering the spinal cord and cauda equina. The dura serves as a major impediment to the extension of tumor into the CNS. The space contains areolar connective tissue and an extensive paravertebral venous plexus of Batsen. These veins contain no valves and connect freely with the veins draining the adjacent vertebral bodies, retroperitoneum, peritoneum, thoracic organs, and the dural venous sinuses within the skull (1).

The pattern of CNS metastasis is relatively disease or cancer specific, because certain tumors have characteristic patterns of spread. These patterns are reviewed.

Epidural Metastasis

The spinal cord is at greatest risk for serious and irreparable injury from epidural metastases because of its relatively intolerant location within a bony canal, a predisposition to edema formation, and a vulnerable blood supply. Thus, epidural cord compression is a neurologic emergency. Solid tumors that are associated with epidural cord compression include NB, embryonal rhabdomyosarcoma, osteosarcoma (OS), Ewing sarcoma (ES), and lymphoma. In a recent review from St. Jude Children's Research Hospital (2), epidural metastases arose in 81 of 2,967 children treated for all forms of cancer over a 17-year period. Cord compression was one of the initial signs of disease at presentation in 29 of 81 (36%) of the patients and was much more commonly diagnosed in children with solid tumors. For example, considering only patients with solid tumors, cord compression was present in 16% of patients with ES, 8.1% of those with OS, 6.9% of those with NB, and 5.3% of those with embryonal rhabdomyosarcoma during the course of their illnesses. The patients with lymphomas and leukemias had a much lower incidence of cord compression; that is, those with non-Hodgkin lymphoma, 4.1%; Hodgkin lymphoma, 1.7%; the leukemias-acute myelogenous, 0.7%; and acute lymphocytic leukemia, 0.2%.

Back pain is usually the first symptom of impending cord compression and may antedate neurologic signs of cord compression by weeks to months. The pain is usually gradual in onset and initially localized to the midline. It is often related to invasion or collapse of bone or stretching of periosteum. Subsequently, radicular pain can emerge and is usually exacerbated by mechanical factors such as movement, coughing, and straining. The pain is usually worse in recumbency, especially at night. Radicular symptoms in the lower cervical and upper thoracic region will produce paresthesias in the upper extremities, radicular symptoms in the thorax produce unilateral or bilateral radiating pain in a band-like distribution, and in the lumbar region a "sciatica" syndrome may emerge. Motor symptoms are unusual during this period, although subtle signs, such as mild weakness, hyperreflexia, or an extensor plantar response, may be apparent on neurologic examination.

If the syndrome is not recognized at the radicular stage, signs and symptoms of myelopathy will soon emerge as cord compression progresses. Symptoms include weakness and sphincteric dysfunction, and signs include a partial or complete Brown-Séquard syndrome. Recognition of a cord compression syndrome at an early age is paramount, because the likelihood of preservation or recovery of function is inversely related to the duration and severity of signs of spinal cord dysfunction at diagnosis. Signs of mild weakness related to corticospinal tract injury may progress to quadriplegia or paraplegia in a matter of hours.

The clinical syndrome of spinal cord compression can be divided into three clinical presentations related to the area of spinal cord primarily involved; that is, the spinal cord, conus medullaris, and cauda equina. The spinal cord syndrome includes the region below C2 and above T10. When the tumor affects predominantly one side, there are frequently localizing segmental sensory symptoms with a contralateral pain and temperature loss and ispilateral loss of position sense. The motor findings relate to two types of injury: segmental, root deficits secondary to perineural compression; and ipsilateral corticospinal tract injury causing ipsilateral weakness, clonus, hyperreflexia, and an extensor plantar response. Sphincteric symptoms occur late, usually when there is bilateral involvement, and the bladder becomes spastic; that is, frequent voids with small volumes and urinary urgency.

The cauda equina syndrome occurs with involvement below L2; that is, below the level of the conus medullaris. Frequently, significant radicular pain occurs either in a sciatic (below L4) or upper lumbar distribution (L1 to 4) that is usually asymmetric, and the straight leg raising manuevers are positive. There may be a segmental sensory loss, but it is rarely complete. The deep-tendon reflexes are reduced, and the Babinski sign is negative. Segmental motor loss is rarely severe and infrequently symptomatic. Sphincteric disturbances arise late when other signs are severe. The bladder becomes atonic and large, and overflow incontinence, frequently without perception, occurs. The conus medullaris syndrome combines signs and symptoms of the two syndromes above except that sphincteric symptoms are usually early and there may be a saddle-type sensory loss (S2 to 5)(3).

Intracranial epidural metastases are frequently asymptomatic, but cause symptoms when they are very large or invade the large venous sinuses such as the transverse or sagittal sinuses. This occurs most commonly in patients with NB. Focal seizures or raised intracranial pressure can also occur.

Until recently, a complete myelogram was the diagnostic test of choice for epidural spinal cord compression. Most centers use water-soluble contrast media, which can flow more readily beyond partial obstructions and is completely eliminated by renal excretion. Some centers use oil-based dye, which in complete blocks is left in the subarachnoid space and is used to follow the progress of treatment. Radiographs of the spine and bone scans are frequently adjunctive in localizing diseased vertebral bodies. If a complete block is encountered from below, intracisternal dye is introduced to delineate the upper level of the block or the presence of multiple lesions (or both). The need to determine the upper and lower extensions of the epidural metastasis is a prerequisite for radiotherapy treatment planning. Presently, magnetic resonance imaging (MRI) with and without gadolinium has become the diagnostic procedure of choice. It is sensitive, noninvasive, and can be repeated without clinical morbidity. MRI also reveals more of the adjacent anatomy.

The treatment of epidural cord compression deserves urgent attention if there are signs of long tract (corticospinal, spinothalamic, posterior column) injury. High-dose steroids, that is 10 mg of dexamethasone given by intravenous push, followed by 4 to 6 mg q6h is the first treatment administered. Steroids are used primarily for treatment of cord compression rather than the cauda equina syndrome. Peripheral nerves are more resistant to compression. Steroids often alleviate the radicular pain in either syndrome, however. When confronted with progressive neurologic deterioration, the dose should always be increased.

Radiotherapy is the treatment of choice for most patients with histologically determined epidural disease that is reasonably radiosensitive. The usual radiotherapy plan includes a port to extend two vertebral bodies above and below the level of the radiographically designated lesion with a daily dose of 180 to 200 cGy to 3000 to 4000 cGy. The ultimate dose depends on the anticipated radiosensitivity of the tumor and the use of supplementary chemotherapy. Not infrequently, myelography/MRI discloses multiple, subclinical lesions. It is usually not desirable to administer total spine irradiation. However, because of the difficulty of treating contiguous fields at a later time and creating "hot spots" at overlapping ports, subclinical epidural lesions in close proximity to the symptomatic lesion are usually included in the initial field. The goal of radiotherapy is to prevent progression to paraplegia and to relieve the pain of vertebral body collapse and radicular compression. In most cases, these goals can be achieved without surgery (4).

Surgery should be considered for newly diagnosed patients who present with epidural disease of undiagnosed etiology or for those patients with highly radioresistant disease; that is previously irradiated tumors. There are several problems with a surgical approach to epidural disease. The epidural tumor tends to grow circumferentially around the cord, and only the posterior portion can be removed using the conventional approach with a decompressive laminectomy. Because the vertebral body is frequently involved, the spine can be rendered unstable after removal of the posterior spinal elements. In newly diagnosed patients, long-term morbidity such as scoliosis and kyphosis can arise following curative therapy. Radiotherapy may produce similar effects as well.

The ideal therapy for patients with newly diagnosed epidural disease that has been previously histologically characterized would be chemotherapy because it has the least long-term effects on surrounding soft and bony tissues. Unfortunately, only a few cancers are exquisitely sensitive and potentially curable with chemotherapy alone. This approach has been tried with some measure of success in NB of infancy, ES, and lymphoma (5).

There are numerous studies of children and adults to document the value of early recognition and intervention in spinal cord compression. In the St. Jude study (1), only 4 (18%) of 22 children who were paraplegic longer than 48 hours prior to therapy recovered some degree of motor function, compared with 33 (81%) of 49 who were treated within 48 hours of recognition of a myelopathy. In a randomized trial in adults with epidural spinal cord compression comparing radiotherapy alone vs. surgery followed by radiotherapy, no significant difference was found with regard to pain relief, improved ambulation, or sphincteric function (6). Treatment of cranial epidural disease usually involves radiotherapy alone. Frequently, whole brain radiotherapy is administered. Occasionally, for metastases recurring after radiotherapy, radioresistant tumors or newly diagnosed lesions, surgery is utilized. Metastases at the base of the skull can cause characteristic neurologic syndromes involving the hypoglossal, facial, or trigeminal nerves.

Leptomeningeal Metastasis

Leptomeningeal metastasis usually implies a widespread invasion of the spinal and intracranial subarachnoid space by cancer. Solid tumors can grow in diffuse sheets in the subarachnoid space, and clusters can detach and spread elsewhere. The most viable tumor cells are probably those that attach and acquire a blood supply. Only a small minority of viable cells are able to survive in the cerebrospinal fluid (CSF). In fact, in the presence of diffuse or multifocal clinical involvement, the CSF cytologic examination can be negative. Leukemic cells appear to be able to survive and perhaps multiply in the CSF slowly as single cell suspensions, although leptomeningeal spread is invariably accompanied by arachnoidal and superficial parenchymal invasion in both solid and hematopoietic malignancies. (7).

The signs and symptoms of leptomeningeal metastasis can be subtle and confusing. Focal cerebral deficits and seizures may arise as the tumor invades adjacent brain. Perineural invasion can cause multifocal cranial and peripheral neuropathies. Certain cranial nerves, such as the facial and abducens nerves, appear to be especially vulnerable. Hydrocephalus can occur as the tumor occludes the subarachnoid space. The neurologic examination frequently reveals more widespread neurologic deficits than the patient recognizes. The deep-tendon reflexes are frequently depressed throughout (8).

The diagnosis is confirmed by the identification of clumps of malignant cells on the CSF cytologic examination. The yield for this test in solid tumors is usually low with a single examination. Therefore, multiple samplings of large volumes (5 to 10 ml) are desirable. An inferential diagnosis can be made by the documentation of relatively low CSF concentrations of glucose and high protein, the identification of nerve root thickening on myelography, or diffuse meningeal enhancement on brain computed tomography (CT), or MRI. These signs may develop relatively late in the course of the syndrome. Occasionally, a meningeal biopsy at the time of ventricular shunt or Ommaya placement will confirm the diagnosis. The frequency of leptomeningeal metastases in adults with disseminated cancer is 8%. The incidence varies considerably with the disease and the location of the primary tumor in both adults and children (9).

Leptomeningeal disease has been characterized best in head and neck rhabdomyosarcoma (Figure 20.2). A clinical incidence of 50% has been reported in some series and constitutes the major treatment challenge for these patients (10). Approximately 5% of children with acute lymphocytic leukemia (ALL) will present with CNS leukemia. Prior

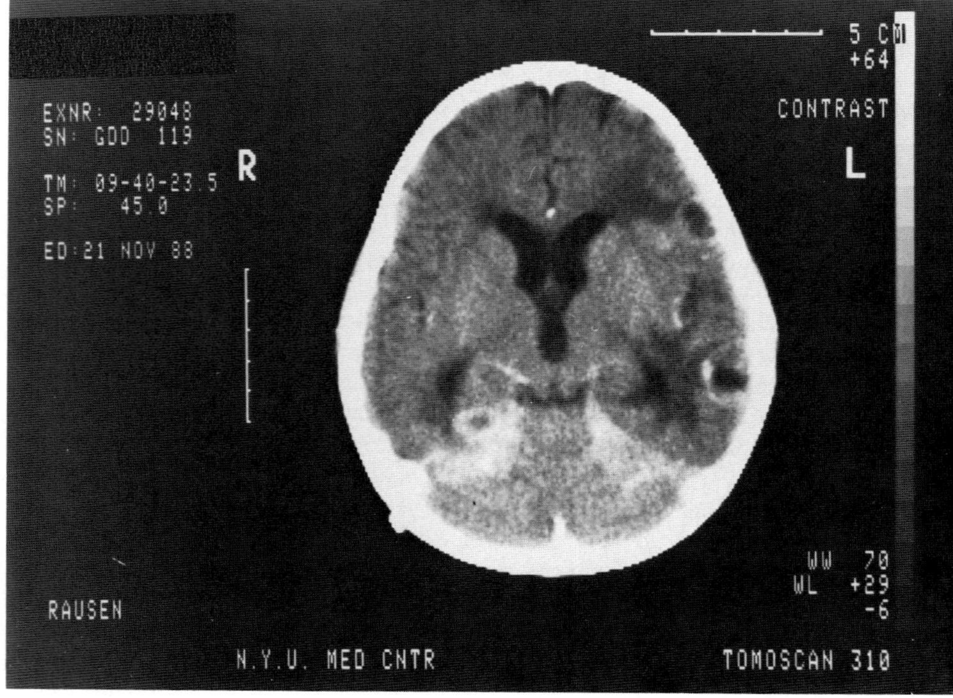

FIGURE 20.2 A noncontrast computed tomographic head scan of an 8-year-old child with disseminated systemic embryonal rhabdomyosarcoma with meningeal sarcomatosis manifested as a seizure disorder, headache, nuchal rigidity, and obtundation. Note the diffuse enhancement of the tentorium and multiple lesions in the cerebral cortex.

to the introduction of CNS prophylaxis with cranial irradiation and intrathecal methotrexate, leptomeningeal leukemia was the most important cause of treatment failure.

The treatment of leptomeningeal metastases in solid tumors is controversial and of limited success. For hematopoietic disease, intrathecal and intraventricular chemotherapy (methotrexate + / − cytosine arabinoside and hydrocortisone) has induced enduring remissions alone or in conjunction with cranial irradiation. Patients with an isolated CNS leukemia relapse, or those who present with CNS leukemia, are still potentially curable. Chemotherapy is usually administered via an Ommaya reservoir connected to an intraventricular catheter (11).

With this experience as an encouraging example, neurooncologists have utilized a similar approach for adult patients with solid tumors with leptomeningeal disease. The results have been disappointing. Left untreated, adult patients usually succumb within 6 to 8 weeks after diagnosis. In diseases responsive to the available intrathecal chemotherapy drugs, the median survival may be extended several months.

Intraventricular drug administration is superior to lumbar intrathecal administration for several reasons. The drug travels with the CSF flow and achieves cytotoxic levels within and without the ventricles. In addition, the lumbar injection fails to deliver drug to the subarachnoid space in 5% to 10% of occasions when an inadvertent subdural injection occurs. Moreover, only a few drugs can be safely administered by this route (12).

Treatment failure utilizing this technique occurs for several reasons. The subarachnoid space is frequently obliterated by sheets of tumor in a sporadic fashion, and cytotoxic drugs in the CSF cannot penetrate loculated tumor masses in effective concentrations.

The solid tumors that typically cause leptomeningeal disease are highly resistant to treatment and are not likely to respond to monotherapy. Theoretically, intravenous chemotherapy should be more effective because the blood–brain barrier is usually markedly impaired by widespread leptomeningeal invasion. This approach has not been widely applied because most of the patients have developed leptomeningeal metastases while receiving the conventional, parenteral chemotherapy. Leptomeningeal metastases usually emerge in patients with solid tumors in the context of persistent or recurrent systemic disease or when parenteral chemotherapy is already being administered.

Radiotherapy has limited application in leptomeningeal disease because craniospinal irradiation is rarely curative and would severely impair the ability to deliver parenteral chemotherapy. Retaining this ability is important because most patients require chemotherapy to control concomitant systemic disease. Rather, radiotherapy is administered focally to relieve pain or serious neurologic deficits. Cranial irradiation may also increase the likehood of producing leukoencephalopathy following intrathecal/intraventricular methotrexate therapy. Thus, the management of leptomeningeal metastases leaves much to be desired.

Brain Metastasis

Brain metastases from systemic solid tumors (sarcomas) are uncommon in children. They are more prevalent in adults with various types of malignancies, and more is known about their natural history in older patients. Large autopsy series have documented a prevalence of 15%, and in approximately 2/3 of these adult patients, the brain metastases produce clinical symptoms (9). Multiple brain metastases are found in 2/3 of cases. The incidence varies widely in adults depending on the type of primary tumor and is most common in patients with melanoma (40%) and lung carcinoma (21%) (9).

Brain metastases in adults arise as the initial manifestation of systemic cancer in 10% to 20% of cases and are thought to arise most commonly from hematogenous dissemination via the arterial circulation. Thus, either primary or metastatic pulmonary cancer usually precedes brain metastases. Alternative pathways of parenchymal spread include Batson venous plexus, the epidural venous structure that connects pelvic and CNS circulation, as well as parenchymal invasion from leptomeningeal deposits.

Symptoms from brain metastases are similar to those from a primary brain tumor and are related to their location, rapidity of growth, multiplicity, and predispostion to spontaneous hemorrhage. Thus seizures, focal neurologic deficits, and signs and symptoms of raised intracranial pressure are common in patients with cerebral lesions.

There appears to be a rising incidence of brain metastases in adult and pediatric patients with sarcomas. Espana et al. (13) reviewed a six-year experience (1971 to 1977) from the Baltimore Cancer Center. Eleven (10%) of 114 patients with sarcoma developed clinically manifest brain metastases. Prior studies reported a clinical incidence of 3%. The authors postulated that chemotherapy resulted in prolonged survival due to control of systemic metastases, but was relatively ineffective for CNS metastases.

There is a paucity of published information on this condition in children. Brain metastases were discovered in 10 (2.2%) of 445 patients entered in a cooperative ES group protocol (14). Two retrospective, predominantly postmortem reviews were reported from Memorial Sloan-Kettering Cancer Center over a 10-year interval. Vannucci and Baten (15) reported a 6% incidence (13 of 217) of brain metastases in children who underwent a complete postmortem examination from 1951 to 1972. The metastases were encountered in the brain in 12 patients and cerebellum in one. Pulmonary metastases occurred in 9 of these patients. The incidence varied considerably according to histology, arising in 13% of 31 patients with Wilms tumor and 6.6% of 45 patients with rhabdomyosarcoma, yet only in 2.7% of 75 patients with NB. The brain metastases produced clinical symptoms in 8 of 11 patients.

Graus et al. (16) reported 13 clinically (CT scans) and 18 postmortem determined cases from the same institution from 1973 to 1982. In the autopsy series, the incidence of brain metastases was 13% for patients with solid tumor. Osteosarcoma and rhabdomyosarcoma were the most common diagnoses in children younger than 15 years, and testicular germ-cell tumors were the most common in those from 15 to 21 years of age. The disease-specific incidence in patients younger than 15 years of age included OS—14%; rhabdomyosarcoma—13%; and NB—0 of 37 cases. It is of interest that no patient with Wilms tumor and brain metastases was encountered in this series, reflecting the dramatic improvement in cure rates with chemotherapy and radiotherapy over the 10-year period since the first survey. Pulmonary metastases were apparent in 28 (90%) of 31 patients, and no patients presented with brain metastases. Evidence of intratumoral hemorrhage was found in 50% of patients.

The treatment of brain metastases depends on their location, multiplicity, anticipated radio- or chemosensitivity, and overall prognosis of the patient. Single brain metastasis should be resected and adjuvant whole brain radiotherapy (3000 cGy over 2 to 3 weeks) provided thereafter. Because systemic disease usually prevails, systemic chemotherapy is also administered. Single metastases that are very chemosensitive, such as germ-cell tumors, may be controlled with chemotherapy and radiotherapy alone.

The prognosis of patients with brain metastases overall is poor. For adults with solid tumors, the median survival after diagnosis of brain metastases in a series of 191 patients was 3.7 months, but for those who received surgery, radiotherapy, and/or chemotherapy, it was 9.7 months (17). Brain metastases contributed to death in 50% of cases.

Graus et al. (16), reported the survival of 25 pediatric sarcoma patients treated for brain metastases. The median survival of 6 patients with single brain metastases who received surgery and radiotherapy with or without chemotherapy was 7 months, and only 1 of the patients died of recurrent brain metastases. Fifteen patients, the majority with multiple brain lesions, received whole brain irradiation and chemotherapy. The median survival was 4 months, and 27% died of neurologic causes. Thus, for children, aggressive management of brain metastases appears useful and prolongs survival in patients with single brain lesions.

Peripheral and Cranial Nerve Syndromes

A number of neurologic syndromes can arise from bone metastases as they encroach upon or infiltrate adjacent peripheral or cranial nerves. The most common sites of encroachment are related to metastases at the base of the skull. Childhood tumors that frequently invade the skull include NB, rhabdomyosarcoma, ES, and less commonly,

OS. At least five clinical syndromes have been well characterized in adults with predominantly metastatic breast, prostate, lung, head, and neck carcinomas (18).

The *orbital syndrome* is most common in patients with NB. Typical signs and symptoms include exophthalmos, diplopia, periorbital swelling, pain, and, rarely, impaired vision. On examination, there may be mild proptosis and unilateral restriction of eye movements. The CT scan usually reveals destruction of the orbital wall with an intraorbital mass.

The *parasellar syndrome* emanates from bony metastases to either the petrous apex or the sella turcica as revealed by CT. The patients usually present with unilateral frontal headache, impaired function of cranial nerves III, IV or VI, and less commonly, a sensory deficit in the ophthalmic division of the trigeminal nerve.

The *middle fossa* syndrome is somewhat less easy to characterize but usually consists of unilateral facial numbness occasionally associated with extraocular palsies. The site of the base of skull metastases is the petrous ridge lateral to the sella. Radiographic changes develop late in this syndrome, and the diagnosis must be suspected clinically. Metastasis on the anterior surface of the petrous ridge may cause an abducens palsy, and those on the posterior surface may cause a facial nerve paresis. Occasionally the middle fossa syndrome blurs with the parasellar syndrome.

The *jugular foramen* syndrome consists of unilateral occipital or postauricular pain and hoarseness and dysphagia as the IX and X nerves become entrapped. Less commonly, the function of cranial nerve XII can be impaired.

The *occipital condyle* syndrome is anatomically closely related. The headache is usually more severe, and the hypoglossal nerve function becomes impaired as the nerve is compressed in the adjacent hypoglossal foramen.

The management of these cranial nerve syndromes in a patient who carries a diagnosis of cancer includes the early clinical suspicion of metastatic disease. CT scanning, radionuclide bone scans and, less often, plain radiographs or tomograms should identify a bony abnormality. In a recent study of adult patients, objective documentation of base of skull metastases could only be made in 77% of 40 patients, but all patients received a course (3600 cGy) of focal irradiation (18). Because leptomeningeal metastases can also cause cranial neuropathies, a CSF cytologic examination is indicated if the neurodiagnostic scans are normal. Radiotherapy, and in some cases chemotherapy, may provide excellent palliation in the short term.

Another unusual entrapment neuropathy can arise in the mandible, where the patient complains of unilateral numbness in the chin including the lip, in the distribution of the mental nerve. A distal twig of the inferior alveolar branch of the mandibular division of the trigeminal nerve is usually entrapped in the mandible.

The brachial and lumbar plexuses can become invaded by metastatic disease. A brachial plexus neuropathy can evolve from an adjacent apical lung metastasis or axillary lymph node. The patient usually complains of relatively severe shoulder pain that radiates down the medial aspect of the arm, occasionally to the fourth and fifth fingers. The tumor usually invades the lower roots initially involving (C7, C8, & T1). Muscle weakness and atrophy as well as Horner syndrome become apparent later in the disease course (19).

The lumbar plexus is less commonly involved, usually from retroperitoneal pelvic tumors such as rhabdomyosarcoma, ES or NB. The syndrome is variable, but most frequently involves the upper roots of the plexus (L1–3) with sensory and eventually motor deficits. The syndrome must be carefully distinguished from an epidural or intradural spinal cord syndrome, which would be managed differently. Thus, pelvic MRI and CT, myelography, and CSF cytologic examination may be necessary.

NEUROLOGIC COMPLICATIONS OF SPECIFIC SOLID TUMORS

The most common solid tumors of childhood include NB rhabdomyosarcoma, OS, ES, Hodgkin lymphoma, non-Hodgkin lymphoma, and Wilms tumor. Because most neurologic complications arise from metastatic lesions, the cancers that require neurologic consultation are most frequently those with the least favorable prognosis. This situation is ever changing because major improvements in prognosis are occurring in the majority of patients with these diseases. For example, the cure rate in patients with Wilms tumor now exceeds 80%, and neurologic complications from this disease have virtually disappeared over the past 15 years. To optimize patient care as a neurooncology consultant, it is essential to have a general understanding of the unique natural histories of the more common solid tumors.

Neuroblastoma

NB is one of the 4 small round-cell tumors of childhood that must be carefully distinguished from ES, rhabdomyosarcoma, and non-Hodgkin lymphoma. It comprises 8% of childhood cancer with an annual incidence of 16 cases/million children. The tumor is derived from peripheral neural crest tissue that was destined to form the sympathetic nervous system. Although primary tumors may develop anywhere along the paravertebral sympathetic chain, the adrenal medulla is the most common locus.

NB manifests most commonly as a congenital tumor in that 50% of the cases arise in infants younger than 2 years of age and 2/3 of cases arise in children younger than 5 years (20). NB has the unique propensity among congenital tumors to be capable of spontaneous involution. It is suspected from autopsy data derived from asymptomatic infants who die of other causes, that without this phe-

nomenon, the incidence of neuroblastoma would be 40 to 50 times higher (21). This involuting tendency occurs not only in localized congenital disease (stages I & II) but also in a peculiar metastatic form (IV-S) with widespread metastases to liver, skin, and bone marrow, but not to bone. Often minimal therapy will steer this disease toward spontaneous involution.

The diagnosis of NB is suspected by palpation of a large abdominal mass in an infant or young child. The local tumor is usually quite extensive, and more then 2/3 of patients present with metastatic disease at diagnosis (22). Elevated serum and urine catecholamines are present in more than 90% of patients. Aggresive multimodality therapy in older children can induce remissions, but resistance to therapy usually emerges so that the majority of children will succumb to their disease.

Primary tumors arising in the posterior mediastinum, although potentially capable of malignant behavior, may occasionally behave in a more indolent fashion, with histologic evidence of differentiation toward a ganglioneuroblastoma, and grow to considerable size, often compressing vital mediastinal structures. Primary tumors arising in this paravertebral location can also cause spinal cord compression. Such "dumbell" tumors insinuate themselves through an intervertebral foramen and initially cause radicular and then myelopathic deficits (23).

Any child presenting with a large paravertebral mass should have a staging myelogram or MRI study prior to therapy because a number of children will have subclinical intraspinal extension. Although radical surgical resections combining thoracic, retroperitoneal, and spinal approaches are practiced in some centers, there is a growing willingness to use chemotherapy alone in infants with NB to avoid the long-term consequences of radical surgery.

NB characteristically metastasizes to specific organs, especially bone, and often in a bilateral, diffuse manner. Bone marrow metastases are present in more than 50% of patients at diagnosis. Both the local and metastatic tumors often respond completely to combinations of radiotherapy and chemotherapy, but more than 95% of children older then 1 year of age will develop widespread metastases within 1 to 2 years of therapy (24).

Metastatic bone lesions tend to produce characteristic clinical syndromes. Retroorbital metastases (orbital syndrome—vide supra) can produce proptosis, periorbital edema, ecchymosis, and an impaired visual acuity and ocular motility. Epidural skull metastases, in addition to causing focal neurologic deficits and seizures, can cause raised intracranial pressure if they obstruct the large venous sinuses. Paravertebral metastases can cause epidural cord compression at multiple levels. These extraneural lesions cause neurologic symptoms by compression and displacement.

Much less commonly, intra-CNS metastases occur. This phenomenon appears to be related to prolonged survival and widespread extra-CNS metastases, especially in the head and neck. In one autopsy series of 31 patients with NB, 15 had dural lesions, 9 of which had, in addition, leptomeningeal invasion (25). In 3 of the latter patients, local extension into superficial cortical gray matter was seen. In only 1 patient was a brain metastasis distinct from overlying meninges observed.

The rarity of parenchymal brain metastasis is unique to NB and probably reflects the rarity of pulmonary metastasis. There is a case report of an infant with congenital NB diagnosed on the 3rd day of life who presented with widespread retroperitonal disease and intraspinal, extradural extension (26). She died at 3 months of age, and at autopsy widespread leptomeningeal and intracerebral metastases were observed.

In a clinical and pathologic review of 36 patients with neurologic manifestations of the tumor, 5 had brain invasion from leptomeningeal lesions; whereas, 1 appeared to have an isolated brain metastasis (27). Fourteen patients had leptomeningeal invasion, and 13 had extradural spinal metatases.

The management of neurologic syndromes related to metastatic NB is problematic. In most cases, at the time of neurologic complications the disease is highly resistant, having recurred after intensive chemotherapy. Timely irradiation usually prevents the development of myelopathy due to epidural metastases. Analgesics should be used liberally because severe pain occurs with bony metastases, and relatively high doses of radiotherapy (3000 to 4000 cGy) are usually required to control local disease. For cerebral disease, whole brain irradiation is usually administered.

Rhabdomyosarcoma

Rhabdomyosarcoma, a soft tissue sarcoma, arises in children with an annual incidence of 3.7 cases/million. The majority of cases appear in infancy and early childhood, with a peak age of occurrence between 2 and 6 years of age and a secondary peak in late adolesence (28). The tumor is highly malignant and has a mesenchymal derivation; there are two histologic subtypes. The embryonal subtype accounts for 50% to 65% of cases, especially those arising in younger children. Although a muscle origin is implied by the terminology, striations typical of skeletal muscle are present in only 1/2 of cases. Apparently, the majority of tumors are too primitive to show terminal differentiation, but they stain positively for the cytoskeletal component, desmin. The alveolar subtype occurs predominantly in older children (29).

Rhabdomyosarcoma can arise in any part of the body where mesenchymal tissues exist in ontogeny, including the CNS, but there are more typical sites of occurrence. The most common region is the head and neck (41%), followed by genitourinary areas (21%), intraabdominal areas (10%), and truncal sites (7%). Younger children tend to have primary tumors in the head and neck or genitourinary areas; whereas, adolescents are more predisposed to truncal, extremity, or paratesticular locations (29).

A number of staging schema have been developed, but the most important factors in terms of prognosis appear to be whether the tumor is localized at diagnosis or is widely metastatic. In only 16% of patients can the tumor be resected with disease-free margins: 28% have resectable disease but with microscopic residual disease following surgery; 36% have unresectable tumors; and 20% present with metastatic disease at diagnosis. Some of the primary tumors are unresectable except for mutilating operations (30) because of their location in the genitourinary tract or head and neck regions.

The present therapeutic modalities include surgery for diagnosis with wide excision and in some cases staging procedures, regional high dose radiotherapy (5000 to 6000 cGy), and adjuvant chemotherapy. Although local control can be achieved in at least 80% of patients with surgery and radiotherapy, only 10% to 20% of patients will experience long-term survival (31). Disease failure occurs primarily from widespread systemic metastases. With the addition of adjuvant chemotherapy to include such agents as vincristine, actinomycin D, and cyclophosphamide (VAC) with or without doxorubicin, the 5-year disease-free survival is at leat 40% to 50% (32). Thus, major improvement in outcome will relate to the development of more effective multidrug chemotherapy regimens and the control of sanctuary (CNS) disease. Improvement in the quality of life will follow as less radical surgery and lower doses or smaller radiotherapy fields are utilized.

The neurologic complications of rhabdomyosarcoma fall into two categories; that is, those related to widely metastatic systemic disease either at diagnosis or relapse, like epidural cord compression, and those related to "sanctuary" disease. The incidence of leptomeningeal dissemination is extraordinarily high (50% to 65%) in patients with rhabdomyosarcoma arising in the "parameningeal" locations at the base of the skull. Head and neck rhabdomyosarcomas arising in the orbit, middle ear, paranasal sinuses, and nasopharynx often erode the base of skull early in their growth. They probably gain local access to the leptomeninges by invasion of venous plexuses, which have direct continuity with the leptomeninges. When the leptomeninges are involved, the entire CNS can become contaminated as the tumor cells are widely dispersed via the CSF.

Once the tumor has gained access to the CNS, conventional treatment modalities (surgery, focal irradiation, and parenteral chemotherapy) are relatively ineffective. The use of craniospinal irradiation is limited often by: the young age of the patients; the radiotherapy tolerance of the spinal cord when curative doses are considered in excess of 5000 cGY; the poor tolerance to systematic chemotherapy if craniospinal radiotherapy is administered; the exclusion of chemotherapy drugs into the CNS by a partially intact blood–brain barrier; and the absence of drugs effective against rhabdomyosarcoma that can be administered intrathecally or intraventricularly. Thus, once a diagnosis of leptomeningeal infiltration is made, the prognosis for curative therapy in several studies appears nil (29).

Tefft et al. (33), reviewed a series of 141 patients with head and neck rhabdomyosarcoma enrolled in the Intergroup Rhabdomyosarcoma Study (IRS). This study evaluated among other parameters, the effects of extent of disease at presentation, tumor histology, radiotherapy dose and volume, and chemotherapy on survival. This study was completed in a period prior to the general availability of CT scanning. Meningeal involvement was diagnosed according to the following criteria: cranial neuropathy; myelopathy probably due to intradural disease; radiographic evidence of erosion of bone at the base of skull; and evidence of raised intracranial pressure. All patients received surgery, regional radiotherapy, and parenteral chemotherapy. Of the 141 patients, 57 had primary tumors in a parameningeal site. These sites included the nasopharynx (29), paranasal sinuses (15), and middle ear (13). Residual disease remained following surgery in all cases. Forty had regional disease, and 17 had metastatic disease at diagnosis.

Meningeal involvement was detected in 10 (17.5%) patients at diagnosis and another 10 at recurrence, for an incidence of 35% (20 of 57). This diagnosis was made in all patients within 12 months of entry in the study, at a median interval of 5 months. Analysis of the radiotherapy data indicated that the radiotherapy volume was too small (i.e., < 2 cm margins around tumor) in 11 of 19 (58%) and the dose insufficient (< 5000 rads) in 13 of 19 (68%). The median survival was 9 months in this group of 20 patients; 18 patients had already died at the time of reporting, and 2 were alive with meningeal disease.

Although many of these children received inadequate radiotherapy by the study requirements, the authors were not optimistic that larger regional volumes and higher doses would control known meningeal disease at diagnosis; they believed that the tumor most probably had already spread beyond the local radiotherapy field within the CNS. They considered for future studies the use of "prophylactic" craniospinal irradiation or intrathecal chemotherapy (or both). Of interest in this study was that meningeal seeding developed in none of the 24 patients with orbital primary tumor.

A more recent large retrospective institutional review included 40 patients with head and neck rhabdomyosarcoma treated at the Princess Margaret Hospital from 1960 to 1977 (34). Surgery and radiotherapy alone were administered to 24 children, and the remaining 16 received in addition, adjuvant chemotherapy. The initial tumor arose in the orbit (13), nasopharynx (7), middle ear (8), paranasal sinuses (5), orapharynx (2), and base of the skull (1). All but 4 patients had either residual disease following surgery (33) or metastatic disease (3) at diagnosis.

The criteria for meningeal involvement in this study included: cranial neuropathy, erosion of base of the skull, abnormal CSF cytology examination or myelogram, or raised intracranial pressure. In neither the Intergroup nor the institutional studies were routine pretreatment myelography or CSF cytologic examination performed; hence, patients with subclinical CNS metastases may have been missed. Nevertheless, in the Toronto study, 20 (50%) children had meningeal spread at initial diagnosis, another 2 had disease at this site develop at recurrence, and 2 more had subclinical meningeal involvement at autopsy for a total incidence of 65% (24 of 40) (34).

The overall 5-year survival of this group of 40 patients was 35%. Two unexpected observations emerged. Thirty percent of the patients were in continuous remission at 5 years compared with none of 20 patients in the IRS study. Although 41% of the 18 patients without meningeal disease from the Toronto study remained in continuous remission at 5 years, the difference (41% to 30%) was not statistically significant at the time of reporting, negating any survival disadvantage to the presence of meningeal involvement at diagnosis. Although the conclusions of the two studies differ, the Toronto group believed that the greater adherence to radiotherapy guidelines; namely, 5000 cGy with 2 to 3 cm margins improved not only local control but also stopped local meningeal invasion from spreading. This improvement was manifested despite the fact that only 40% of the patients received adjuvant chemotherapy.

A greater understanding of the impact of meningeal involvement on prognosis in this and other soft-tissue sarcomas will await definitive prospective trials that use newer more sensitive neurodiagnostic instruments such as CT and MRI scanning as well as routine CSF cytologic and spinal staging studies at diagnosis and at regular intervals thereafter. The management of patients with clinical leptomeningeal invasion at any time in the course of their illness remains a formidable challenge. No large clinical pediatric trials are addressing this issue despite the fact that leptomeningeal invasion has been described with all of the soft-tissue sarcomas to a greater or lesser extent, but not with as high an incidence as in head and neck rhabdomyosarcoma.

Ewing Sarcoma

There are two soft tissue sarcomas that arise in bone in children, ES and OS. They have much different natural histories and responses to therapy, and they are managed differently. ES is 1 of the 4 small round-cell tumors of childhood (rhabdomyosarcoma, NB, and non-Hodgkin lymphoma) with an annual incidence of 2.1/million children. As opposed to OS, it arises principally in the midshaft of the long bones, most commonly, the femur, as well as the pelvis. Although the tumor can arise in any bone or adjacent to it, involvement of bones below the umbilicus is the usual circumstance, affecting predominantly older children and adolescents. The presence of periodic acid Schiff material on light microscopy, consistent with intracellular glycogen, confirms the diagnosis. The precise derivative tissue of ES has not been determined (35).

Prior to the use of chemotherapy, patients were managed with surgical resection and focal irradiation, and they had a poor prognosis—fewer than 15% survived beyond 5 years. The primary tumor was usually radiosensitive, and local control could be achieved with conventional high doses (> 5000 rads). Subclinical micrometastases as in other soft-tissue sarcomas was the major treatment challenge.

Wilkins et al. (36), reviewed a large institutional series (140 patients) from the Mayo Clinic collected from 1969 to 1982. The mean age of the patients was 16.9 years. The disease was metastatic at diagnosis in 25% (35 of 140) of patients; sites of metastases included the lungs in 25 and other bones, like the vertebral column, in 16 patients. Three factors contributed to an unfavorable prognosis: the presence of metastases at diagnosis; a pelvic primary tumor; an elevated erythrocyte sedimentation rate at diagnosis. The overall 5 year survival rate was 38%, but those patients with localized disease who had a complete surgical excision, some form of chemotherapy, usually including VAC, and local + / − prophylactic lung irradiation, had a 74% 5-year survival rate.

Advanced experimental protocols have been designed to control micrometastases, not only in the lungs, the most common site, but also in other bones. Thus, pilot studies have included high-dose chemotherapy and total body irradiation followed by autologous bone marrow rescue after marrow purging (37). The neurologic complications of ES are rather predictable. Patients with widespread metastases at initial diagnosis or at relapse are at high risk for epidural cord compression. Isolated intradural CNS metastases (meningeal, brain) are unusual. In a review of 445 patients from the Intergroup Ewing Sarcoma Study (IESS) I, only 10 patients (2.2%) had CNS lesions, 2 with meningeal and 8 with brain metastases (14). Although the brain was considered a disease sanctuary in a National Cancer Institute study, further analysis of a larger data base has dissuaded investigators from initiating prophylactic cranial irradiation. There is one case report of an unusual method of intradural spread, via perineural extension (38). As in other soft-tissue sarcomas, as systemic chemotherapy becomes more effective and survival is prolonged, CNS metastases will become more prevalent.

A relatively small percentage of patients develop primary ES in the bones of the head and neck. In a review of data from the IESS, approximately 4% of tumors arose in these areas (39). As opposed to rhabdomyosarcoma arising in the same region, the prognosis for patients with head and neck ES is quite favorable, with a 5-year survival of 80% following multimodality therapy. The relative rarity of meningeal invasion appears to be the event most likely to contribute to this favorable outcome.

Osteosarcoma

OS is the most common form of primary bone cancer in children arising in 1.3/million children per year. As opposed to ES, it tends to arise in the growth plates at the end of long bones, especially during the 2nd and 3rd decades of life when osteoblastic activity is normally at its peak. More than 1/2 of the primary tumors arise in close proximity to the knee; that is the distal femur and proximal tibia. Central axis bone tumors comprise fewer than 10% of cases (39).

The majority of patients (75%) appear to present with localized disease. The most common area of metastasis is the lungs and then to other bones. The more sensitive the screening test for pulmonary metastases, the higher the frequency of detection. In an era when amputation was the sole therapy, the overall 5-year survival was 20%, and 50% of patients developed overt pulmonary metastases. The median survival was 12 to 15 months and pulmonary metastases were usually apparent by 6 to 10 months, suggesting that microscopic disease had been present for a long time. OS is a relatively radioresistant tumor, and radiotherapy doses in excess of 5000 rads are required for local control. The late effects of this type of radiotherapy are significant.

Several controversies have prevailed in the management of patients with OS but most are becoming resolved. For a period of time there was doubt that adjuvant chemotherapy improved survival, but several pilot institutional and randomized clinical trials have unequivocally confirmed the role of neoadjuvant (presurgical) and adjuvant (postsurgical) chemotherapy with drugs including high-dose methotrexate with leucovorin rescue, bleomycin, cyclophosphamide, doxorubicin, and cisplatin (40). At present, the 5-year relapse-free survival in patients presenting with localized disease is a least 60%.

Another major advance has been the use of *en bloc* resection of the distal femur or proximal tibial primaries with prosthetic replacement and joint reconstruction (41). Usually, neoadjuvant chemotherapy is given for several months prior to surgery to determine the chemosensitivity of the tumor, to reduce the bulk of the tumor, and thereby increasing the likelihood of surgical resection and removal of systemic micrometastases. Postoperative adjuvant chemotherapy is administered thereafter. Even with isolated pulmonary metastases, aggressive surgical management with gross total resections may promote long-term survival and even cures (42).

Neurologic complications of osteosarcoma at the time of diagnosis are unusual. Occasionally, a patient presents with epidural cord compression related to primary or metastatic disease involving a vertebral body. In relapsed patients, brain metastases may arise in fewer than 1% of cases and usually in those with long-standing pulmonary metastases (43). The metastases usually contain osteoid material and are detectable on plain skull radiographs or unenhanced CT scans.

The incidence of brain metastases rises in autopsy series. In a study from Memorial Sloan Kettering Cancer Center of 28 patients with OS who had a complete autopsy, 5 (13.5%) had evidence of brain metastases (16). All patients eventually died with lung metastases. There is a tendency for these brain metastases to undergo spontaneous hemorrhage. Four of these patients had clinical symptoms from the brain metastases. The median interval from initial diagnosis to the detection of lung metastases was 8 months and to the detection of brain metastases was 22 months. Because osteosarcoma is so radioresistant, single brain metastases are usually resected. Subsequently, whole brain radiotherapy or chemotherapy (or both) should be given to control micrometastases.

The management of epidural cord compression in OS is problematic. When it occurs in relapsed patients, it is relatively resistant to radiotherapy and chemotherapy. Radical surgery may offer the best form of palliation and prevention of myelopathy in the short term. The side effects of surgery beyond a simple laminectomy are considerable, however. Attempts have been made to resect the epidural disease anterior to the cord as well as the diseased vertebral bodies (44). Unfortunately, the spine is rendered unstable, and another surgical procedure must be performed to stabilize the spine. The rehabilitation may be long.

Paraneoplastic Syndromes

Paraneoplastic neurologic syndromes or "remote effects" have been extensively characterized in the adult literature. A variety of cognitive, cerebellar, myelopathic, peripheral nerve, and myopathic entities that usually evolve in a subacute fasion and often precede the overt manifestations of a cancer have been described in adults (45). There is usually no obvious explanation for these neurologic deficits in terms of direct involvement by the cancer, and etiologic hypotheses have included immunologic (autoantibodies) and toxic effects (46).

One paraneoplastic syndrome has been well characterized in pediatric oncology; viz., the opsoclonus–myoclonus; syndrome of NB. Although the first case was probably described by Cushing and Wolbach (47) in 1927 in a 2-year-old child with cerebellar ataxia and ganglioneuroblastoma, Solomon and Chutorian (48) have more recently crystallized the clinical syndrome and led others to subsequently present a number of case reports.

The neurologic syndrome is distinctive. In an otherwise healthy toddler or young child, a subacute syndrome evolves including irritability, ataxia, myoclonic jerks, and opsoclonus; that is, random, chaotic, irregular, multidirectional, conjugate eye movements. Because of the growing awareness of the association with occult NB, a diagnostic survey should include chest radiographs, intravenous pyelography, and serum and urine catecholamine determinations. Not infrequently, a calcified localized, partially differentiated ganglioneuroblastoma is discovered.

From an oncology perspective, the group of children so diagnosed has several unusual features. Altman and Baehner (49) reported 2 cases and reviewed 26 others from the literature. Patients presenting with the opsoclonus syndrome had a more favorable prognosis with a 2-year survival of 89% compared with 30% for the larger group of children with NB. Although such patients tend to present with more favorable tumor stages, that is, localized stage I or II or the special IV-S syndrome, 5 of 7 patients with stages III and IV had long-term survival. Fewer than 30% would be expected to survive beyond 2 years. The overall survival for patients younger then 2 years of age was 91% (25% to 29% expected) and beyond 2 years was 84% (< 10% expected) with this neurologic syndrome.

The primary NB appeared to arise in unusual locations like the mediastinum (53% compared with 15% expected). A larger proportion of these patients than expected had differentiated ganglioneuroblastomas.

The clinical course of the opsoclonus syndrome is unpredictable. It is not unusual for the neurologic signs to persist for months or years, despite the apparent curative state of the child following surgery and other therapeutic modalities. Senalick et al. (50), reviewed a large number of cases of this syndrome as well. In 48% (11 of 23), the neurologic syndrome was noted months to years before the tumor was detected, and some form of residual neurologic impairment was present in 82% of patients months to years following therapy. Long-lasting mental retardation was identified in 36% and ataxia in 64%.

The etiology of the opsoclonus syndrome remains obscure. The severity of the syndrome is not directly related to the bulk or the presence of the tumor and not all of the patients have elevated catecholamines. Autopsies of the brain have been reported in 2 cases (50). In one child, the brain was normal, and in the other mild demyelinative changes surrounding the dentate nucleus was noted. No tumor deposits were detected.

NEUROLOGIC COMPLICATIONS OF THE LEUKEMIAS AND LYMPHOMAS

Acute Leukemia

The acute leukemias (lymphocytic and nonlymphocytic) are the most common form of childhood cancer, comprising 40% of all diagnoses. Their overall annual incidence is 38 per million children, and acute lymphocytic leukemia

(ALL) comprises more than 3/4 of cases. The remarkable recent improvement in survival in children with ALL relates primarily to the prevention and treatment of meningeal disease. The insights gained in understanding the pathogenesis and control of meningeal leukemia have also been widely applied to other hematopoietic and solid cancers that tend to invade the meninges.

The prognosis in patients with ALL is related primarily to the age of the patient at diagnosis and the magnitude of the peripheral WBC at diagnosis. Children of intermediate age (4 to 6 years) have the best prognosis, and cure is inversely proportional to the initial WBC at diagnosis (51). The typical presentation of a child with ALL includes nonspecific symptoms such as fever, irritability, anorexia, malaise, purpura, and diffuse bone pain, most commonly in the legs.

The initial hemoglobin (Hgb) and platelet count are usually depressed, and the WBC may range from abnormally low (< 500/uL) to extremely high (> 500,000/uL). Although lymphoblasts may be observed in peripheral blood, the diagnosis is confirmed at bone marrow examination when more than 5% of the cells are lymphoblasts.

The concern that the CNS is a pharmacologic sanctuary has become an increasing focus over the past 30 years in direct relation to the successes incurred with the use of multiagent chemotherapy for the control of systemic disease. In earlier studies of the 1950s, when treatment regimens served to prolong survival, the incidence of clinically asymptomatic CNS leukemia was approximately 10%. As the chemotherapy regimens improved, the incidence rose to 40% in the later part of that decade and to 80% in the late 1960s (52). Thus, the notion evolved that the CNS is contaminated subclinically with leukemic cells in the majority of cases at diagnosis. With the administration of effective systemic chemotherapy alone, the CNS will become the most important disease sanctuary. For example, there is a linear relationship between the incidence of CNS leukemia at diagnosis and the magnitude of the initial WBC. In an earlier study, 43.5% of children with an initial WBC less than 10,000/uL and 83.3% of children with an initial WBC greater than 10,000/uL eventually acquired CNS leukemia (51).

Thus, eventual cure of ALL is primarily dependent on two factors; viz., the eradication of systemic disease using multiagent chemotherapy and an effective and safe means of treating subclinical CNS leukemia at diagnosis.

The chemotherapy management of meningeal leukemia is limited. The drugs that are routinely administered intrathecally include only methotrexate, cytosine arabinoside (Ara C), and hydrocortisone. In the past, CNS leukemia was difficult to eradicate with intrathecal methotrexate alone, and the addition of other drugs did not prolong the CNS remission. Although short-term remissions could be induced with regularity, CNS relapse, and more importantly, systematic relapse occurred with alarming regularity. Patients had to be maintained for long periods of time with intrathecal methotrexate, increasing the likelihood of leukoencephalopathy. Furthermore, lumbar intrathecal administration resulted in inadvertent subdural or epidural injections, making the methotrexate unavailable to the subarachnoid compartment. It was presumed that the best way to cure CNS leukemia was to prevent it.

Frei et al. (53) in 1965 were the first to report the use of CNS prophylaxis when intrathecal methotrexate was given during induction early in treatment. The value of prophylactic CNS irradiation was established in a series of studies from 1962 to 1971. A dose of 2400 rads to the whole brain with or without short-term-induction intrathecal methotrexate was found to be optimum. Craniospinal therapy was less effective overall because it impaired the ability to deliver systemic chemotherapy. Combined cranial irradiation and intrathecal methotrexate was found to be more effective in a group of patients considered to be at high risk for CNS relapse.

When intrathecal methotrexate was given throughout the induction and maintenance phase of therapy, it alone was as effective as cranial irradiation in preventing CNS relapse (54). A current series of clinical trials is designed to maintain the intensity of CNS prophylaxis while diminishing late effects. For example, children receiving cranial radiotherapy may have a 2% to 5% chance of developing a second primary neoplasm of the brain (55). The late effects of cranial radiotherapy also include learning and cognitive deficits and hormonal deficiencies. These sequelae are becoming increasingly important because currently more than 70% of children will survive ALL.

The clinical signs and symptoms of meningeal leukemia relate to raised intracranial pressure—lethargy, headache, nausea, vomiting, and nuchal rigidity; perineural infiltration resulting in cranial or peripheral neuropathies; and brain or spinal infiltration causing hypothalmic dysfunction such as hyperphagia and obesity, behavior alterations, seizures, and focal neurologic dysfunction. Occasionally, subdural or spinal epidural deposits can cause external brain or cord compression, and rarely, a focal tumor expansion within the brain or cord (chloroma) may cause signs and symptoms of an intramedullary tumor.

Careful funduscopic examination may reveal papilledema. The assessment of visual acuity may help differentiate papilledema from papillitis due to optic nerve infiltration. The blindness secondary to the latter diagnosis may be reversible with focal eye irradiation.

The diagnosis of meningeal leukemia is made by detecting lymphoblasts in the CSF using the cytocentrifuge technique. Although there is frequently a CSF pleocytosis, this may not always be the case. In most circumstances, the diagnosis of meningeal leukemia is made in the preclinical stage. CSF hypoglycorrhachia prevails in more than 50% of patients, and the protein concentration is usually elevated (56). Because intrathecal chemotherapy alone may transiently cause a CSF pleocytosis and elevated protein concentration, the morphology of the cytospin preparation must be carefully examined to distinguish reactive from malignant lymphocytes.

The management of overt meningeal leukemia has not changed greatly over the past 15 years. Once it was determined that intrathecal methotrexate, an antifolinic agent, was well tolerated and effective in the short term, it remained to determine the optimum dose, dose schedule, and duration of therapy that would ensure a prolonged CNS remission. Clinicians were slow to appreciate the neurotoxic potential of chronic methotrexate administration, and the early cases of leukoencephalopathy were managed as CNS leukemia.

More recently, because of the concern for leukoencephalopathy, especially in children who had prior CNS relapses, there has been an active search for other intrathecal cytotoxic agents that could be administered intrathecally. Ara C and thiotepa are newer agents that are relatively safe and effective, but they have not proved themselves capable of replacing methotrexate.

The issues of drug distribution are a growing concern. An intraventricular cannula connected to a subcutaneous Ommaya reservoir allows chemotherapy to be administered with less effort, painlessly, and safely "downstream" into the ventricle and eventually to the subarachnoid space. Lumbar injection is more uncomfortable, and the drug distribution is more unpredictable (57).

Several authors have reported encouraging results with intra-Ommaya chemotherapy. Bleyer et al. (58), conducted a study using either lumbar or intra-Ommaya therapy (2.94 vs. 0.93 relapses/months), and the median duration of remission was longer with intra-Ommaya therapy (475 + vs. 286 days). The major complications of intra-Ommaya therapy included, in addition to the risk of leukoencephalopathy, ventriculitis and Ommaya dysfunction. If cytotoxic drugs are inadvertently injected directly into brain parenchyma because of a wandering or malpositioned ventricular catheter, local tissue necrosis can occur.

Several other well-defined neurologic syndromes affect patients with acute leukemia either at initial diagnosis or relapse including cerebral leukostasis secondary to a very high peripheral blood blast count and sagittal sinus or cerebral venous thrombosis due to a hypercoaguable state.

The leukostasis syndrome is more common in acute nonlymphocytic leukemia. Leucocytosis (> 100,000/uL) is present in more than 20% of patients at initial diagnosis. When the peripheral blood count exceeds 200,000/uL, a significant risk of spontaneous and fatal intracerebral hemorrhage prevails. Cerebral leukostasis can cause symptoms of a diffuse encephalopathy and raised intracranial pressure. Small petechial brain hemorrhages are usually present. If this syndrome cannot be rapidly controlled, death due to intracerebral hemorrhage or hemorrhage into other vital organs such as the lungs will ensue, and this may happen in 10% to 15% of patients. Approximately 3% to 6% of patients with ALL and 12% to 14% with ANLL will die from this syndrome at initial diagnosis (59).

Early symptoms of cerebral leukostasis are vague and include headache, delirum, visual obscurations, and tinnitus. Examination may reveal papilledema with retinal venous distension. The diagnosis can only be confirmed at autopsy.

In recent review (60), 10% of 294 patients with ANLL died as a result of hemorrhage or leukostasis (or both) within the first 12 days of diagnosis. Patients with hyperleukocytosis and acute monocytic leukemia (French–American–British classification M5) had the greatest predisposition to this syndrome, and there was a 72% early mortality when these 2 conditions prevailed. Eleven of the 30 patients died prior to the initiation of therapy. Ten of 11 had acute monocytic leukemia, and 7 died of a CNS hemorrhage. Leukostasis, either alone or with CNS hemorrhage, was the probable cause of death in 11 children. Ten of the 30 children came to autopsy. Cerebral leukostasis, that is, the accumulation of intravascular blast forms, was found in 5 of the patients.

The treatment for cerebral leukostasis is an oncologic emergency. Leukostasis causes a hyperviscosity state, thereby decreasing cerebral perfusion and promoting petechial hemorrhages. The spontaneous destruction of leukemic cells, especially in promyelocytic leukemia causes disseminated intravascular coagulation. The peripheral WBC may be lowered by leukophoresis or exchange blood transfusions; cytostatic therapy—hydroxyurea and Ara C; and cranial irradiation.

Malignant Lymphomas

The classification of malignant lymphomas in children is complex and is evolving as more sophisticated cellular and molecular tumor markers are applied. From a clinical perspective, one needs principally to distinguish among Hodgkin, non-Hodgkin, or diffuse lymphoma.

Hodgkin Lymphoma

Hodgkin lymphoma is a discrete, indolent lymphoma affecting 7.5 per million children each year. It arises in lymph nodes and remains confined to the nodes and spleen in 90% of patients. The cervical and supraclavicular lymph nodes are most commonly involved, and with more advanced disease, mediastinal, paraaortic, and iliac lymph nodes may become involved. The disease appears to spread by contigous extension to adjacent nodal regions.

When therapy is limited to regional modalities like surgery and radiotherapy, careful and precise staging of the disease is a prerequisite for curative therapy; hence, the use of a staging exploratory laparatomy. Radiotherapy in the range of 3500 to 4000 rads provides a high probability of local control (< 95%), and treatment failures are related primarily to the inability to ascertain the full extent of disease (61).

Multimodality therapy including radiotherapy and chemotherapy with regimens such as MOPP (nitrogen mustard, vincristine, procarbazine, and prednisone) have been reserved for patients presenting with advanced disease. The 5-year disease-free survival for all patients is in excess of 65%.

Neurologic complications of Hodgkin disease are relatively uncommon and usually related to epidural cord compression at the time of diagnosis or at relapse. Clinical suspicion of cord compression is critical. The prevention of a permanent myelopathy is usually possible with the timely use of high-dose steroids, in itself, lymphocytotoxic, and radiotherapy. Occasionally, epidural disease regrows in a previously irradiated site, and the treatment options may be limited. Several cases have been described in which Hodgkin disease can cause intradural CNS metastasis (62).

Diffuse Non-Hodgkin Lymphomas

There are predominantly two forms of diffuse childhood lymphomas—those of either B-cell (Burkitt lymphoma) or T-cell origin. Thus, lymphomas in childhood tend to express some degree of cytodifferentiation. Cancer of the stem cell or some more primitive precursor bone marrow tissue is usually manifest as acute lymphocytic leukemia. There are many similarities between some forms of leukemia and T-cell lymphomas, however.

The B-cell lymphomas are rare in the United States but are common in Africa. The annual incidence in the United States is 2 cases per/million children. The African and American diseases are probably different. The African form, for example, is almost always associated with Epstein-Barr virus; it commonly produces jaw tumors, is curable occasionally with single drug chemotherapy (cyclophosphamide), and relapses frequently within the CNS (33%). In the American form, the contrary prevails. At the time of diagnosis approximately 20% of patients with Burkitt lymphoma as compared with < 10% of patients with American B-cell lymphoma have CNS involvement. The primary tumor in patients with American B-cell lymphoma tends to arise in the abdomen, usually the ileum or cecum, rather than in the jaw (63).

Prior to the use of chemotherapy, bone marrow relapse would occur in 15% to 70% of patients after resection of the primary tumor, and the 5-year survival was less than 20% in patients of either continent. With single drug chemotherapy, 90% of patients with African Burkitt lymphoma experienced prolonged survival. At this time in the United States, with multidrug chemotherapy and intrathecal methotrexate prophylaxis, more than 50% of patients will survive beyond a year and will probably be cured. It is becoming increasingly apparent that patients with B-cell lymphoma require different combinations of drugs than those that have proved curative for patients with ALL and T-cell lymphoma. CNS prophylaxis in both the African and American forms appears useful (63).

Although randomized trials of short-term intrathecal chemotherapy prophylaxis or craniospinal radiotherapy (or both) in patients without CNS disease at diagnosis have failed to reduce the CNS relapse rate, intrathecal chemotherapy when given more intensively, clearly results in prolonged CNS remissions in patients with recurrent CNS Burkitt lymphoma. As opposed to ALL and T-cell lymphoma, isolated recurrent CNS Burkitt lymphoma is not commonly followed by systemic bone marrow relapse, the primary cause of mortality for patients with ALL.

The most common type of non-Hodgkin lymphoma in American children is the T-cell lymphoblastic lymphoma comprising approximately 2/3 of cases. This tumor appears to arise from thymocytes because it contains the thymocyte enzyme marker, TdT. The malignant cells tend to involve the thymus, peripheral nodes, and bone marrow. Anterior mediastinal masses are usually present in 50% to 80% of patients at diagnosis and may be large enough to cause respiratory symptoms.

T-cell lymphoma is also exquisitely sensitive to chemotherapy, which is, in fact, the same chemotherapy used to treat patients with ALL. In current therapeutic regimens, surgery and radiotherapy have a diminishing, if negligible, role. It is also apparent that some form of CNS prophylaxis is necessary in that CNS relapse can occur in as many as 50% of children unprotected by intrathecal chemotherapy (64). Because the non-Hodgkin lymphomas are extremely sensitive to chemotherapy, this modality has been used instead of radiotherapy for the treatment of epidural cord compression.

Primary CNS lymphoma is extremely rare in children. It tends to arise in immunocompromised hosts, such as those with AIDS or those who have received renal transplants. The B-cell type appears to be the predominant variant in adults. The disease carries a poor prognosis when either radiotherapy alone, or radiotherapy and chemotherapy, is used (65).

REFERENCES

1. Rodriguez M, Dinapoli R. Spinal cord compression, with special reference to metastatic epidural tumors. Mayo Clin Proc 1980;55:442–448.
2. Ch'ien L, Kalwinsky D, Peterson G, et al. Metastatic epidural tumors in children. Med Pediatr Oncol 1982;10:455–462.
3. Baten M, Vannucci R. Intraspinal metastatic disease in childhood. J Pediatr 1977;90:207–212.
4. Greenberg H, Kim J, Posner J. Epidural spinal cord compression for metastatic tumor: Results with a new treatment protocol. Ann Neurol 1980;8:361–362.

5. Hayes F, Thompson E, Hvizdala E, et al. Chemotherapy as an alternative to laminectomy and radiation in the management of epidural tumor. J Pediatr 1984;104:221–224.

6. Young R, Post E, King G. Treatment of spinal epidural metastases. J Neurosurg 1980;53:741–746.

7. Huli-mei Juo A, Yataganoa X, Galicich J, et al. Proliferative kinetics of CNS leukemia. Cancer 1975;36:232–239.

8. Wasserstrom W, Glass P, Posner J. Diagnosis and treatment of leptomeningeal metastases for solid tumors: Experience with 90 patients. Cancer 1982;49:759–772.

9. Posner J, Chernik N. Intracranial metastases from systemic cancer. In: Schomberg B, ed. Advances in Neurology, Vol. 19. New York: Raven Press, 1978,579–592.

10. Berry M, Jenkin R. Parameningeal rhabdomyosarcoma in the young. Cancer 1981;48:281–288.

11. Green D, West C, Brecher M. The use of subcutaneous cerebrospinal fluid reservoirs for the prevention and treatment of meningeal relapse of acute lymphoblastic leukemia. Am J Pediatr Hematol Oncol 1982;4:147–154.

12. Edwards M, Levin V, Wilson C. Brain tumor chemotherapy: An evaluation of agents in current use in phase II and III trials. Cancer Treat Rep 1980;64:1179–1205.

13. Espana P, Chang P, Wiernik P. Increased incidence of brain metastases in sarcoma patients. Cancer 1980;45:377–380.

14. Trigg M, Gloubiger D, Nesbit M. The frequency of isolated CNS involvement in Ewing's sarcoma. Cancer 1982; 49: 2404–2409.

15. Vannucci R, Baten M. Cerebral metastatic disease in childhood. Neurology 1974;24:981–985.

16. Graus F, Walker R, Allen J. Brain metastases in children. J Pediatr 1983;103:558–561.

17. Zimm S, Galen W, Stablein D, et al. Intracerebral metastases in solid tumor patients: Natural history and result of treatment. Cancer 1981;48:384–394.

18. Greenberg H, Deck M, Vikram B, et al. Metastasis to the base of skull: Clinical findings in 43 patients. Neurology 1981; 31:530–537.

19. Lederman R, Wilbourn A. Bracheal plexopathy: Recurrent cancer or radiation? Neurology 1984;34:1331–1335.

20. Gross R, Farber S, Martin L. American Academy of Pediatrics proceedings on neuroblastoma: A study and report of 217 cases. Pediatrics 1959;23:1179–1191.

21. Beckwith J, Perrin E. In situ neuroblastoma: A contribution to the natural history of neurol crest tumor. Am J Pathol 1963; 43:1089–1104.

22. Evans A, D'Angio G, Propert K, et al. Prognostic factors in neuroblastoma. Cancer 1987;59:1853–1859.

23. Akwari O, Payne W, Onofrio B. Dumbell neurogenic tumors of the mediastinum: Diagnosis and management. Mayo Clin Proc 1978;53:353–358.

24. Poplack D, Blatt J. Neuroblastoma. In: Levin A, ed. Cancer in the Young. New York: Masson Publishers, 1982;663–682.

25. Monte S, Moore G, Hutchins G. Non-random distribution of metastases in neuroblastic tumors. Cancer 1983;52:915–925.

26. Dressler S, Harvey D, Levisohn P. Retroperitoneal neuroblastoma widely metastatic to the central nervous system. Ann Neurol 1979;5:296–298.

27. Alpert J, Mones R. Neurologic manifestations of neuroblastoma. J Mt Sinai Hosp 1969;36:37–47.

28. Young J, Miller R. Incidence of malignant tumors in US children. J Pediatr 1975;86:254–259.

29. Maurer H, Ragab A. Rhabdomyosarcoma. In: Sutow W, Fernbach D, Vietti T, eds. Clinical Pediatric Oncology. St. Louis: Mosby, 1984;622–651.

30. Donaldson S, Belli J. A rational clinical staging system of childhood rhabdomyosarcoma. J Clin Oncol 1984:135–141.

31. Tefft M. Radiation of rhabdomyosarcoma in children: Local control in patients enrolled in the Intergroup Rhabdomyosarcoma Study. Natl Cancer Inst Monogr 1981;56:75–81.

32. Mourer H, Donaldson M, Gehan E, et al. The Intergroup Rhabdomyosarcoma Study: Update November 1978. Natl Cancer Inst Monogr 1981;56:61–68.

33. Tefft M, Fernandez C, Donaldson M, et al. Incidence of meningeal involvement by rhabdomyosarcoma of the head and neck in children. A report of the Intergroup Rhabdomyosarcoma Study. Cancer 1978;42:253–258.

34. Berry M, Jenkin R. Parameningeal rhabdomyosarcoma in the young. Cancer 1981;48:281–288.

35. Chan R, Sutow W, Lindberg R, et al. Management and results of localized Ewing's sarcoma. Cancer 1979;43:1001–1006.

36. Wilkins R, Pritchard D, Burgert E. Ewing's sarcoma of bone experience with 140 patients. Cancer 1986;58:2551–2555.

37. Glaubiger D, Tepper J, Makuch R. Ewing's sarcoma. In: Levin A, ed. Cancer in the Young. New York: Masson Publishers, 1982;603–614.

38. Wald S, Rolant T. Intradural spinal metastasis in Ewing's sarcoma: Case report and review of the literature. Neurosurgery 1984;15:873–877.

39. Dahlin D, Coventry M. Osteogenic sarcoma: A study of 600 cases. J Bone Joint Surg 1967;49:101–110.

40. Winkler K, Beron G, Katz R, et al. Neoadjuvant chemotherapy for osteogenic sarcoma: Results of a cooperative German/Austrian Study. J Clin Oncol 1984;2:617–624.

41. Rosen G, Marcove R, Caparros B, et al. Primary osteogenic sarcoma. The rationale for preoperative chemotherapy and delayed surgery. Cancer 1979;43:2163–2177.

42. Rosenberg S, Flye M, Conkle D, et al. Treatment of osteogenic sarcoma II aggressive resection of pulmonary metastases. Cancer Treat Rep 1979;63:753–756.

43. Danziger J, Wallace S, Handel S, et al. Metastatic osteogenic sarcoma to the brain. Cancer 1979;43:707–710.

44. Perrin R, McBroom, J. Spinal fixation after anterior decompression for symptomatic spinal metastasis. Neurosurgery, 1988;22:324–327.

45. Anderson W, Cunningham J, Posner J. Autoimmune pathogenesis of paraneoplastic neurological syndromes. CRC Neurobiology 1987;3:245–299.

46. Kimmel D, O'Neill B, Lennan V. Subacute sensory neuronopathy associated with small cell lung carcinoma: Diagnosis aided by autoimmune serology. Mayo Clin Proc 1988; 63:29–32.

47. Cushing H, Wolback S. The transformation of a malignant paravertebral sympathicoblastoma into a benign ganglneuroma. Am J Pathol 1927;3:203–210.

48. Solomon G, Chutorian A. Opsoclonus and occult neuroblastoma. N Engl J Med 1968;279:475–477.

49. Altman A, Baehner R. Favorable prognosis for survival in children with coincident opso-myoclonus and neuroblastoma. Cancer 1976;37:846–852.

50. Senelick R, Bary P, Lahey M, et al. Neuroblastoma and myoclonic encephalopathy: Two cases and a review of the literature. J Pediatr Surg 1973;8:623–632.

51. George S, Fernback D, Vietti T, et al. Factors influencing survival in pediatric acute leukemia: The SW CCSG experience 1958–70. Cancer 1973;32:1542–1553.

52. Aur R, Simone J, Hustu H. Central nervous system therapy and combination chemotherapy of childhood lymphocytic leukemia. Blood 1971;37:272–281.

53. Frei E, Saller S. Acute lymphoblastic leukemia treatment. Cancer 1978;42:828–838.

54. Haghbin M, Cunningham-Rundles S, Thaler H, et al. A long term follow-up of children with ALL treated with intensive chemotherapy regimens. Cancer 1980;46:241–252.

55. Meadows A, Baum E, Fassati-Bellani F, et al. Second malignant neoplasms children: An update from the Late Effects Study Group. J Clin Oncol 1985;3:532–537.

56. Aaronson A, Hayden S, Melomed M. Spinal fluid cytology during chemotherapy of leukemia of the CNS in children. Am J Clin Path 1975;63:528.

57. Green D, West C, Brecher M, et al. The use of subcutaneous cerebrospinal fluid reservoirs for the prevention and treatment of meningeal relapse of acute lymphoblastic leukemia. Am J Pediatr Hematol Oncol 1982;4:147–154.

58. Bleyer W, Poplock D, Simon R. Intraventricular vs. intralumbar methotrexate for central nervous system leukemia: Prolonged remission with the Ommaya reservoir. Med Pediatr Oncol 1979;6:207–213.

59. Walk B, Heisel M, Ortega J. Frequency of early death in children with acute leukemia presenting with hyperleukocytosis. Cancer 1982;50:150–153.

60. Creutzig U, Ritter J, Budde M, et al. Early deaths due to hemorrhage and leukostasis in children acute myelogenous leukemia. Cancer 1987;60:3071–3079.

61. Peters M, Brown T, Rideout D. Hodgkin's disease: Prognostic influences and radiation therapy according to pattern of disease. JAMA 1973;223:53–59.

62. Lyding J, Tseng A, Newman, A, et al. Intramedullary spinal cord metastasis in Hodgkin's disease. Cancer 1987;60:1741–1744.

63. White L, Siegel S. Non-Hodgkin's lymphoma in childhood. In: Sutow WW, Fernbach DG, Vietti TJ, eds. Clinical Pediatric Oncology. St. Louis: Mosby, 1984;452–497.

64. Hilter J, Favora B, Nelson M, et al. Non-Hodgkin's lymphoma in children: Correlation of CNS disease with initial presentation. Cancer 1975;36:2132–2137.

65. Loeffler J, Ervin, Mauch P. Primary lymphomas of the CNS: Patterns of failure and factors that influence survival. J Clin Oncol 1985;3:490–494.

Chapter 21

Neurologic Manifestations of Endocrine Diseases

Dennis M. Styne

Endocrine disorders may manifest neurologic signs and symptoms, but there is a larger group of neurologic diseases that cause endocrine abnormalities. Both types of conditions are considered in this chapter as well as those caused by agents used in treating neurologic and endocrine disorders.

FACTORS AFFECTING GROWTH

Growth hormone is a 191 amino acid peptide that is produced, stored in, and released from the anterior pituitary gland. The release of growth hormone is controlled by hypophysiotropic factors which are released from the median eminence of the hypothalamus into the pituitary-portal system; growth hormone is stimulated by growth hormone releasing factor (GHRH) and inhibited by somatostatin, or somatotropin-release-inhibiting factor (SRIF). The growth promoting action of growth hormone is postulated to primarily occur through somatomedin C, or insulin-like growth factor 1 (IGF-1), a peptide which rises and falls in growth hormone excess and deficiency, respectively. Growth hormone concentrations are low throughout most of the day in normal patients, but during the 24-hour period rise several times, especially during electroencephalographic stages 3 or 4 of sleep. Random growth hormone measurements cannot reveal adequate secretion except in the fortuitous occasion of sampling during a spontaneous peak. Only sequential measurements taken every 10 to 20 minutes throughout a 12- or 24-hour period, or measurements performed after the administration of a secretagogue will help in diagnosis, unless the goal is the diagnosis of states of increased growth hormone secretion (1,2).

In growth hormone deficiency, the bone-age development (assessed by radiographs of the left hand and wrist) is delayed; whereas, the upper to lower segment ratio (the length from the symphysis pubis to the top of the head divided by the length from the symphysis pubis to the floor) is normal for bone age. This contrasts with hypothyroidism where bone age is severely delayed, and the upper to lower segment ratio is increased due to lack of appropriate growth of the limbs. Patients with untreated isolated growth hormone deficiency have delayed onset of puberty;

of course those with additional gonadotropin deficiency will have permanent hypogonadism.

The major source of IGF-1 is the liver, although IGF-1 is produced in mesenchymal tissue throughout the body. IGF-1 has mitogenic effects in most dividing cells and is thought to cause growth by attaching to receptors in the cartilage.

IGF-1 is the somatomedin most closely correlated with growth (3). Plasma IGF-1 is age dependent, being low in the neonate with a slow rise through childhood until a peak is reached during the pubertal period. Such changes in plasma levels of IGF-1 confuse their interpretation if the age of the patient, or stage of physiologic development, as reflected by the bone age is not taken into consideration. In contrast to the changes in IGF-1, concentrations of insulin-like growth factor 2 (IGF-2) are decreased in growth hormone deficiency but do not rise above normal in growth hormone excess.

Thyroid hormone is essential for postnatal growth, although it has no effect upon prenatal growth. Adequate thyroid hormone is necessary for the normal secretion of growth hormone as hypothyroid patients may not respond to growth hormone stimulation tests. Bone-age development is also retarded in hypothyroidism. Usually puberty is delayed if thyroid hormone is decreased, but with profound hypothyroidism puberty may occur prematurely.

Sex steroids exert stimulatory effects upon growth, skeletal, and pubertal development. Sex steroids are essential for the pubertal growth spurt and account for approximately 1/2 of the growth achieved during puberty. When sex steroid concentrations are elevated during a long period, as in sexual precocity, the epiphyses of the long bones will fuse prematurely and, paradoxically, the tall child will cease growing and become a short adult.

Glucocorticoids exert impressive growth suppressive effects when in excess. Cushing syndrome, whether due to endogenous or exogenous glucocorticoids, will cause the cessation of growth and lead to short stature. A decrease or absence of glucocorticoids will not affect growth rate.

Insulin is also important in the maintenance of normal growth. When found in excess, as in the case of an infant of a diabetic mother, insulin will increase growth rate in the fetus or in postnatal life (e.g., in patients with insulinomas or islet cell hypertrophy). Insulin deficiency will decrease growth and fetal and postnatal growth will be poor in the absence of insulin receptors, as demonstrated in the leprechaun syndrome.

Adequate nutrition is the most essential factor for growth and reproductive development, and world-wide malnutrition accounts for the majority of growth deficiency. Voluntary decrease in nutrient intake or chronic diseases can exert the same effect as economic malnutrition due to poverty on decreasing growth. Neurologic diseases in which there is decreased nutritional intake can have similar devastating effects on growth. Psychologic problems may also affect growth either from a nutritional standpoint or through an endocrine effect. Psychosocial dwarfism is a functional form of hypopituitarism precipitated by abnormal parent–child interaction. Thus, socioeconomic and psychosocial factors, as well as nutritional factors, are important considerations in the interpretation of growth rate.

Growth Hormone Deficiency

Congenital growth hormone deficiency is not rare, and acquired growth hormone deficiency is becoming more common with increasingly successful treatment methods available for various types of cancers (as in the case of growth hormone deficiency in children with cancer treated by head and neck irradiation). Characteristic growth hormone deficiency has been found in approximately 1 in 4,000 children in Scotland; while the incidence in the United States (US) may be lower, it is not a rare disease. Growth hormone deficiency must always be considered as a cause of growth failure.

Decreased hypothalamic GHRH accounts for the majority of cases of idiopathic growth hormone deficiency, although rare patients are found without pituitary glands or somatotropes. The dividing line between growth hormone deficiency and normal growth hormone secretion is becoming increasingly blurred by the increasing incidence of patients with partial growth hormone deficiency.

Since growth hormone deficiency does not affect prenatal growth, a child with congenital growth hormone deficiency has a normal birth weight and length. After birth, even in the 1st year of life, careful observation will suggest an abnormally slow growth rate in affected children, and usually, extremely short stature with normal head circumference will be noted by 2 to 4 years of age. Typical growth hormone deficient patients have a "cherubic" appearance of chubbiness and a high pitched voice (Figure 21.1). They may seem precocious because their appearance will suggest a younger age, but their speech and abilities are that of an older child. Newborn males may have microphallus (stretched penis length less than 2.5 cm), especially if there is associated gonadotropin deficiency (4). Hypoglycemia may occur in the absence of growth hormone, and more profound hypoglycemia will occur if adrenocorticotropin (ACTH) is also absent; hypoglycemic seizures occur in either situation. The combination of hypoglycemic seizures and normal birth length should alert the observer to a possible diagnosis of neonatal hypopituitarism. If the patient is a male with microphallus or if there is optic hypoplasia, the diagnosis must be ruled out before any other condition is considered (5).

Midline cerebral defects ranging from cleft palate to holoprosencephaly may be associated with congenital hypopituitarism. Patients with optic nerve hypoplasia may manifest visual impairment, pendular nystagmus, as well as associated anterior and posterior pituitary deficiency (5).

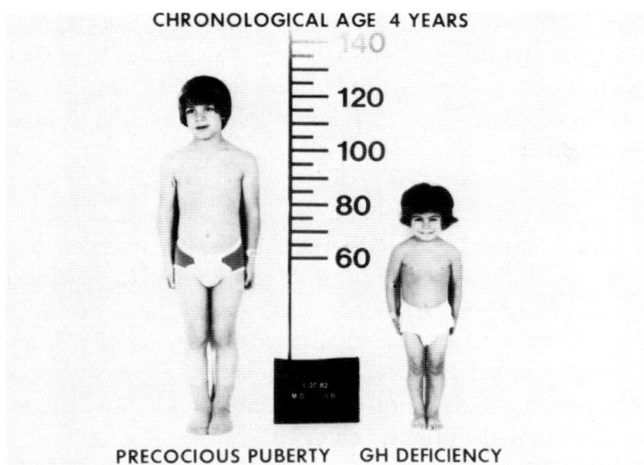

FIGURE 21.1 Comparative heights of two patients of the same chronologic age of 4 years, one with precocious puberty and the other with growth hormone deficiency. Note the "cherubic" appearance of the child with growth hormone deficiency (right). (Courtesy of Dr. Selna Kaplan, University of California Medical Center, San Francisco).

Fifty percent of patients with optic nerve hypoplasia and pituitary impairment will also have absence of the septum pellucidum (septo-optic dysplasia). Complications such as vaginal bleeding at various times during gestation, unusually short labors, intrapartum distress and aysphyxia, and breech delivery are frequently associated with historical features of patients with congenital hypopituitarism.

Since most cases are sporadic, familial growth hormone deficiency is rare. However, growth hormone deficiency may occur as an autosomal recessive, autosomal dominant, or in an X-linked pattern of inheritance. Relatives are described who lack a 7.6 Kb portion of DNA as the etiology of growth hormone deficiency (6).

Diagnosis

Growth hormone deficiency should be suspected in a variety of circumstances including: a patient who is exceptionally short for age according to growth charts; a child who is short for family heights [charts are available to correct a child's height for midparental height (7)]; and one who is growing poorly for age and without historic or physical finding or laboratory evidence for another disorder (8). Growth hormone deficient children with central nervous system (CNS) tumors or other acquired disorders may not fit the typical appearance of a chubby, cherubic child, but growth hormone deficiency should be considered in the diagnosis of a child with any signs or symptoms of CNS abnormality and short stature.

Establishing the diagnosis of growth hormone deficiency has become more complex with increased knowledge of growth hormone physiology. Typical growth hormone deficiency is defined as the inability to raise growth hor-

mone concentration above an accepted limit (generally 7 to 10 ng/mL in most laboratories) after two stimulatory tests. Unfortunately, it has become clear that GH measurements on the same sample may vary up to 60% among different commercial laboratories; a patient may be diagnosed as normal by one laboratory and GH deficient in another. The measurement of basal growth hormone concentration is useless unless the timing is perfect (by chance) and the sample is taken just as the patient is experiencing a spontaneous peak of growth hormone. Exercise may be used as a physiologic stimulatory test, for after 10 minutes of vigorous exercise, almost to the point of exhaustion, normal children will raise their growth hormone in 80% of trials. Sequential samples at night may be taken with the hope that the peak in serum GH is captured as it occurs approximately 90 minutes after the onset of sleep, but few physicians can efficiently perform this test in a busy clinical practice. One way to determine if there is a normal circadian rhythm of growth hormone secretion involves sampling for growth hormone levels every 10 to 20 minutes for a 12- or 24-hour period, but the facilities or personnel for such a study are generally unavailable and the actual benefit over customary secretagogue administration in diagnosis is not yet established.

The most common types of diagnostic procedures used to determine growth hormone deficiency are pharmacologic stimulation tests. Secretagogues invoked in the testing for growth hormone deficiency are given the first thing in the morning after an overnight fast. Because any normal child may fail to raise growth hormone concentration after one test, two tests of growth hormone secretory ability are usually performed. L-Dopa in doses of 125 mg for body weight up to 15 kg, 250 mg for weight up to 35 kg, and 500 mg for body weight over 35 kg is given in one protocol; samples are taken at 0, 30, 60, and 90 minutes. Possible side effects include nausea and vomiting for several hours. The alpha adrenergic agent, clonidine, can be given in a dose of 0.1 to 0.15 mg/m² and sample obtained at the same time sequence; side effects in this case may include hypotension and lethargy, lasting for several hours. Intravenous arginine infusion of 0.5 g/kg body weight up to 20 g over a period of 20 minutes can be given with blood samples taken at the same time periods noted above; no side effects are likely. Insulin-induced hypoglycemia [after intravenous (IV) administration of 0.075 to 0.1 units/kg of insulin] is an effective but dangerous test. The patient must be shown to have a normal fasting blood sugar just before the test and must not have a known tendency toward hypoglycemia. A patent intravenous line must be available to infuse dextrose should a hypoglycemic seizure occur, and the patient must be watched carefully by a physician during the test. Glucose and growth hormone should be measured at 0, 15, 20, 30, 60, and 90 minutes, and cortisol reserve may be tested at 60 and 90 minutes. If severe hypoglycemia occurs, dextrose must be administered immediately; no more than 25% dextrose at 1 mL/kg, and preferably

12.5% dextrose at 1 to 2 mL/kg should be infused so that blood sugar will rise but no severe change in osmolality is precipitated.

GHRH is presently in use in clinical research settings but is not commercially available. Growth hormone deficient patients demonstrate either no rise in GH or a blunted rise after a dose of 5 to 10 µg/kg of GHRH is administered (9).

Plasma somatomedin concentrations are often used to assist in the diagnosis of growth hormone deficiency, but this test must always be used with caution. Low values of somatomedin may indicate malnutrition as well as growth hormone deficiency. A differentiating factor is that in malnutrition, growth hormone values usually rise and somatomedin values fall. In delayed puberty, somatomedin values are more appropriate for bone age than chronologic age and may be incorrectly interpreted as abnormally low in such a situation. The measurement of IGF-2, in addition to IGF-1, has been suggested to add accuracy to the diagnosis of growth hormone deficiency. Recently, measurements of IGF binding proteins have become available and are thought to increase the accuracy of diagnosis. In addition, in some cases the need for growth hormone in a poorly growing child is compatible with a normal somatomedin concentration. Thus, IGF-1 measurements cannot be used as the only criterion for the diagnosis of growth hormone deficiency, but may confirm growth hormone secretory test results.

Treatment

The treatment of growth hormone deficiency is presently accomplished by the administration of biosynthetic recombinant DNA-derived growth hormone. Previously, cadaver-donated pituitary-derived growth hormone was administered, but the possibility that some batches were contaminated with the prions (proteinaceous infectious particles) of Jakob-Creutzfeld disease led to the discontinuation of such therapy in April 1985. At present, there are several proved or suspected cases of Jacob-Creutzfeld disease in young adults who were previously treated with human cadaver growth hormone. Their clinical courses were similar in that cerebellar and extrapyramidal signs initially appeared with little or no mental deterioration, myoclonus, or the characteristic EEG findings of typical, older patients with the disease (10–12).

Biosynthetic growth hormone is available with an N terminal methionyl group in a 192 amino acid form (Somatrem, given at 0.05 to 0.1 mg/kg per dose, three times per week) from Genentech or in the 191 amino acid form (Somatropin, given at 0.06 mg/kg three times per week) from Eli Lilly Co. Previously, GH was given intramuscularly, but it has been proved acceptable to inject GH subcutaneously. Recent evidence suggests that daily injections may be more effective than the usual three times per week regimen, even if the total weekly dose is kept constant. There are patients who do not have growth hormone defi-

ciency on careful testing, but who improve their growth rate with growth hormone therapy. The incidence of these patients is unknown, but they are characterized by extremely short stature, poor growth rate, and delayed bone ages.

If growth hormone therapy in adequate dosage is begun early, patients with idiopathic growth hormone deficiency can reach their appropriate final height. However, a study of the final growth pattern of 27 children who developed growth hormone deficiency after the treatment of an intracranial tumor other than craniopharyngioma, found that no patient achieved their genetic height potential, although 12 patients attained an adult height above the 3rd percentile for the population (13).

Clinical research trials have demonstrated a role for the hypothalamic peptide GHRH in the treatment of growth hormone deficiency (14). As the defect in the patient appears to be a lack of GHRH in most cases, the administration of GHRH can often reverse the growth hormone deficiency. Up to now, most studies utilized a portable, pulsatile pump for GHRH administration, but new methods of administering GHRH (such as intranasal or depot preparations) which do not require such a pump are now under study. Insulin-like growth factor has just entered clinical trials for Laron dwarfism (patients who lack growth hormone receptors).

Although concern may be raised by parents, growth hormone treatment is not felt to cause recurrence or increased size of brain tumors (15). Tumor recurrence rates (medulloblastoma-14 patients, glioma-8, ependymoma-2, leukemia-6, and T-cell lymphoma-1) of patients who received growth hormone treatment for growth failure secondary to cranial irradiation, when compared with recurrence rates of patients treated with radical radiation therapy for the same tumor types but who did not receive GH, demonstrated that GH therapy did not increase the relapse rates of medulloblastoma, glioma, and leukemia. In this study there were only 2 patients with ependymoma, but it is recognized that the prognosis in these patients is poor. Other evidence suggests there is no increase in the rate of relapse for craniopharyngiomas with growth hormone therapy.

Prader-Labhart-Willi Syndrome

There are several syndromes of obesity and short stature that are diagnosed by their typical physical findings. The Prader-Labhart-Willi syndrome (16) is characterized by mental retardation, short stature, obesity, insatiable hunger, infantile hypotonia, small hands and feet, and a typical facial appearance with almond-shaped eyes. Behavioral modification has been increasingly successful in controlling weight gain in these patients. Puberty is often delayed. We are aware of several cases in which the patients grew well in childhood as would be expected in exogenous obesity, but due to advanced bone age had early epiphyseal fusion and attained a short adult stature. Fifty percent of patients have a deletion of chromosome 15.

Patients with Prader-Labhart-Willi syndrome have varying degrees of pubertal dysfunction, ranging from delayed to absent onset of puberty due to inadequate secretion of gonadotropic hormones. The testes and ovaries are reportedly slow to respond to exogenous stimulation, possibly indicating primary gonadal failure, but this may be a result of the inadequate priming they have had from endogenous pituitary hormones (17). There are also several reports of precocious adrenarche or full precocious puberty in these patients; the clinical variation is therefore extremely wide (18,19).

The short stature of patients with Prader-Labhart-Willi syndrome is not usually due to typical growth hormone deficiency, and the massive obesity of the children could fallaciously decrease the response of GH to secretogogue. Nonetheless, patients with Prader-Labhart-Willi syndrome have been treated with growth hormone to increase their stature with at least some initial success; long-term studies are needed to confirm the ultimate benefit of such studies (20).

Laurence-Moon-Biedl Syndrome

The Laurence-Moon-Biedl syndrome (21), inherited as an autosomal recessive trait, consists of short stature, mental retardation, obesity, retinitis pigmentosa and visual impairment, and polydactyly. Puberty may be delayed, presumably secondary to hypothalamic hypogonadism. However, primary hypogonadism has also been reported (22).

Growth Hormone Excess

Pituitary gigantism denotes the presence of a growth hormone secreting pituitary adenoma in childhood; acromegaly is the result of the same type of tumor in adults. Since the epiphyses of the long bones are not closed in an affected child, height velocity and stature are increased; the coarse features of an acromegalic appearance may also be noted even in childhood. As in acromegaly, organomegaly, glucose intolerance, or diabetes mellitus may result. Other related features of growth hormone excess include proximal muscle weakness and carpal tunnel syndrome. Elevated fasting growth hormone concentrations or IGF-1 levels confirm the diagnosis of excessive GH secretion. If the tumor is small, treatment may be accomplished by transsphenoidal micro-adenomectomy.

The diencephalic syndrome of infancy can be associated with either normal or increased growth hormone (GH)

(23). Patients are emaciated but happy, exhibit hyperactivity, and grow quickly (Figure 21.2). Other associated symptoms and signs may include vomiting, nystagmus, occasionally poor temperature regulation, and later neurologic symptoms and signs of increased intracranial pressure occur. The syndrome is secondary to a tumor of the floor of the 3rd ventricle or optic chiasm which involves the hypothalamus. Usually astrocytic tumors are found, but ependymomas and oligodendrogliomas have also been reported.

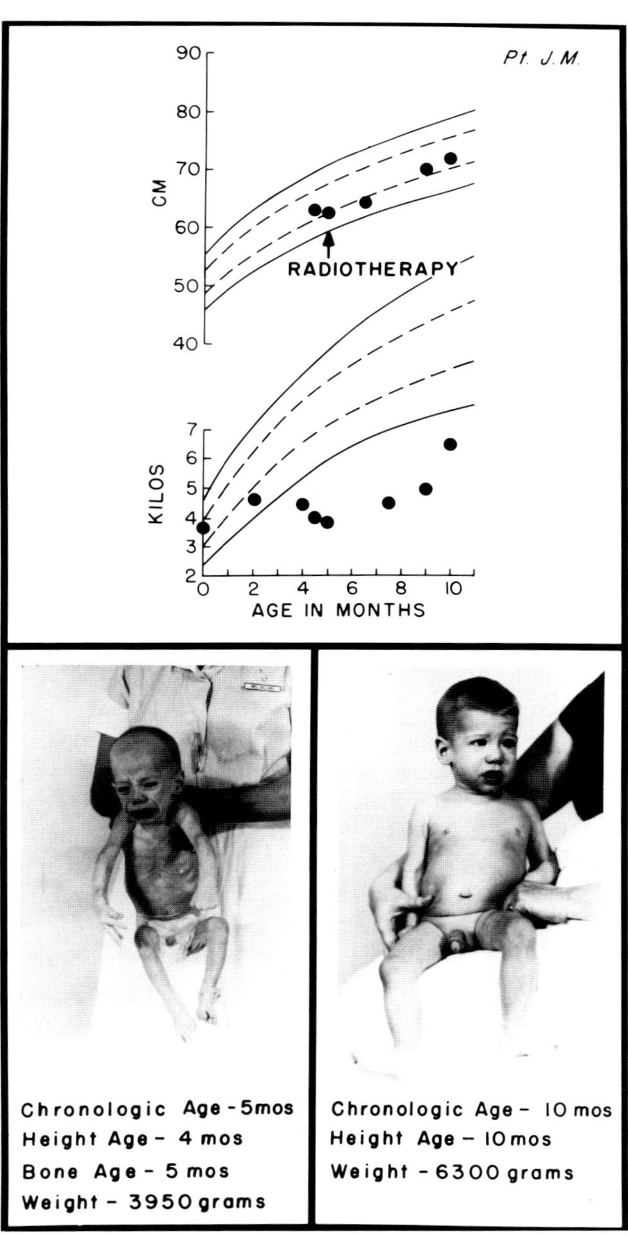

FIGURE 21.2   A 4-month-old infant with the diencephalic syndrome of infancy prior to, and 5 months after completion of radiation treatment directed to a glioma in the anterior 3rd ventricular floor. Note (lower inset) that linear growth is within normal limits; whereas, the weight is notably below the 3rd percentile at the time of diagnosis. (Courtesy of Dr. Selna Kaplan, University of California Medical Center, San Francisco).

Excess Growth With Normal Growth Hormone Secretion

Cerebral gigantism (Soto syndrome) is notable for large size at birth and infancy, decreased intelligence, characteristic facies with a sharp chin and broad forehead, and normal growth hormone (24). Rapid growth is most characteristic of infancy but height velocity decreases by midchildhood.

These patients have decreased body fat, advanced bone age, rapid growth, large hands and feet, hypertrichosis, and brownish pigmentation; girls may have clitoromegaly (25). There is an autosomal-recessive pattern of inheritance. Muscles may be hypertrophic and histologic study of biopsies may show increased or normal glycogen. This syndrome is extremely rare. Precocious puberty or hyperthyroidism are two other causes of excess growth.

DISORDERS OF PUBERTY

Disturbances of pubertal development (26,27) are often caused by neurologic disease. The complex endocrine changes that cause the striking physical characteristics of puberty actually begin in the fetus. Shortly after birth, the pubertal hormones are suppressed and remain so for about a decade. The reawakening of gonadal function that follows is known as gonadarche, and the increased adrenal androgen secretion is known as adrenarche; the two components are associated in the process known as puberty.

Gonadarche

The secretion of the pituitary gonadotropins, luteinizing hormone (LH) and follicle-stimulating hormone (FSH), is stimulated by the release of hypothalamic gonadotropin-releasing hormone (GnRH). GnRH is secreted episodically into the pituitary portal system in varying amplitudes and frequencies during different stages of development (and different stages of the menstrual cycle in females). If GnRH secretion is continuous rather than pulsatile, the pituitary gonadotrope decreases its affinity for GnRH and its quantity of GnRH receptors; this leads to decreased gonadotropin secretion (down regulation).

A feedback loop controls gonadotropin secretion. Thus, LH stimulates Leydig cell secretion of testosterone (T) in boys, and testosterone then exerts negative feedback inhibition of LH secretion. FSH stimulates follicle formation and estrogen secretion in girls, and estradiol (E2) then exerts negative feedback inhibition of FSH secretion. FSH has little effect in boys until spermarche (the onset of maturation of spermatozoa), when it supports the development of sperm.

In the peripubertal period just before the physical changes of puberty occur, there are quantitative changes in gonadotropin secretion. Gonadotropin concentrations rise during sleep due to increased amplitude of pulsatile secre-

tion every 60 to 90 minutes. With the progression of puberty, the episodes of gonadotropin secretion occur throughout the day until no diurnal variation remains in the adult. While gonadotropin values are higher in the adult than in the prepubertal child, the pulsatility of gonadotropin secretion makes the interpretation of single values inaccurate. If a nadir in gonadotropin secretion occurs during sampling, a different interpretation will be reached than if a peak is captured. The rise in pituitary storage of readily releasable gonadotropin is reflected in the gonadotropin response to a bolus of exogenous GnRH. A 100 µg bolus of GnRH will cause a rise of LH greater than 16 mIU/mL in pubertal or adult subjects; whereas, a far smaller rise is found in prepubertal subjects. Thus, the rise in LH after administration of GnRH is a useful reflection of pubertal status in a patient not yet exhibiting physical changes, and this GnRH test is diagnostically useful.

Sex-steroid secretion is more constant throughout the day than is gonadotropin secretion and is, therefore, more clinically useful. There is a stepwise increase in sex steroid concentration as puberty progresses. More than 97% of sex steroids are noncovalently bound to sex hormone binding globulin (SHBG) and presumably inactivated by this process.

Adrenarche

An increase in adrenal androgens is noted several years before the onset of rising gonadotropin secretion and before the onset of physical pubertal development. A rise in the weak androgen dihydroepiandrosterone (DHA) and its sulfate (DHAS) occurs at 6 to 7 years in girls and 7 to 8 years in boys with a continuation of the rise through midpuberty. It seems clear that control of adrenarche is separate from the mechanism of gonadotropin stimulation. Although ACTH must be present for adrenarche to occur, another as yet unknown factor must also be operative as well.

PHYSICAL PUBERTAL DEVELOPMENT

The Tanner method of describing the stages of pubertal development is widely accepted (28,29). Objective description of physical development is essential to observe clinical progress. Note that prepubertal is stage 1; there is no stage 0 (Tables 21.1–21.4).

Sexual Precocity

A child has sexual precocity if a boy develops secondary sexual characteristics before the age of 9 years, or a girl before the age of 8 years (30). The condition is true, or central precocious puberty if the etiology is premature

Table 21.1   Breast development

B1	Prepubertal: elevation of the papilla only.
B2	Breast buds are noted or palpable with enlargement of the areola.
B3	Further enlargement of the breast and areola with no separation of their contours.
B4	Projection of areola and papilla to form a secondary mound over the rest of the breast.
B5	Mature breast with projection of papilla only.

Modified with permission from Archives of Diseases in Childhood 1969;44:291–303.[28]

Table 21.2   Female pubic hair development

PH1	Prepubertal: no pubic hair.
PH2	Sparse growth of long, straight or slightly curly, minimally pigmented hair, mainly on the labia.
PH3	Considerably darker and coarser hair spreading over the mons pubis.
PH4	Thick adult type hair which does not yet spread to the medial surface of the thighs.
PH5	Hair is adult in type and is distributed in the classic inverse triangle.

Table 21.3   Male genital development

G1	Prepubertal.
G2	The testes are over 2.5 cm in the longest diameter and the scrotum is thinning and reddening.
G3	Growth of the penis occurs in width and length and further growth of the testes is noted.
G4	Penis is further enlarged and testes are larger with a darker scrotal skin color.
G5	Genitalia are adult in size and shape.

Modified with permission from Archives of Diseases in Childhood 1970;45:13–23.[29]

Table 21.4   Male pubic hair development

P1	Prepubertal: no pubic hair.
P2	Sparse growth of slightly pigmented, slightly curved pubic hair mainly at the base of the penis.
P3	Thicker, curlier hair spread to the mons pubis.
P4	Adult type hair which does not yet spread to the medial thighs.
P5	Adult type hair spread to the medial thighs.

maturation of the hypothalamic-pituitary axis. Incomplete precocious puberty occurs if the etiology is autonomous secretion of sex steroids or in boys, the autonomous secretion of human chorionic gonadotropin (hCG). Precocious puberty will cause rapid growth and skeletal maturation, and a child who does not receive treatment will be a paradoxically tall child who ceases growing early and becomes a short adult.

True or Complete Precocious Puberty

If no tumor or other definitive diagnosis to explain precocious puberty is found, the diagnosis of exclusion is idio-pathic precocious puberty. These patients manifest all of the endocrine findings of normal puberty, albeit at an early age. Their progress may be rapid and continuous or slow, waxing and waning. Boys with this condition will first demonstrate testicular enlargement. Girls are brought for evaluation of idiopathic precocious puberty more often than boys (Figure 21.1).

Central Nervous System Disorders.   Central nervous system (CNS) tumors are found more often in boys with precocious puberty than in girls, but because precocious puberty is more common in girls, the actual number of cases of CNS tumors is greater in girls with precocious puberty. Associated hamartomas of the tuber cinereum are found more frequently in patients since the advent of computed tomography (CT) and magnetic resonance imaging (MRI) (31). Prior to these neuroimaging techniques, some patients would have otherwise had the diagnosis of "idiopathic precocious puberty" (32). Hamartomas are not progressive tumors, but rather congenital lesions where GnRH containing hypothalamic tissue is ectopic. Although hamartomas of the tuber cinereum are amenable to surgical removal, due to their sensitive location the morbidity and mortality may be prohibitive. Medical therapy with GnRH agonists is the treatment of choice.

Gliomas of the hypothalamus or optic nerve that involve the hypothalamus may also cause precocious puberty. Other tumor types that may cause precocious puberty include astrocytomas, ependymomas, and teratomas. Germinomas may secrete hCG and cause incomplete precocious puberty in boys by stimulating the Leydig cells, or they may activate the whole hypothalamic-pituitary axis and cause true precocious puberty in boys and girls by causing maturation of the hypothalamic-pituitary axis.

Additional CNS causes of precocious puberty include other space occupying lesions or causes of increased intracranial pressure, including hydrocephalus. Head trauma has long been known to be associated with precocious puberty. One study demonstrated a higher incidence of precocious puberty in girls than boys after head injury; cerebral atrophy and focal encephalomalacia were present in all patients with and 69% of children without precocious puberty. There was, however, no difference in the incidence of motor or cognitive impairment or epilepsy between children suffering head injury with precocious puberty compared to those without pubertal development (33).

Androgen exposure for prolonged periods due to exogenous administration or endogenous secretion from the testes or adrenal gland can mature the hypothalamic-pituitary axis and cause central precocious puberty. The triad of café au lait spots, polyostotic fibrous dysplasia of the long bones with notable cystic changes on radiographs, and usually incomplete precocious puberty defines the McCune Albright syndrome (34). This syndrome can also be associated with other conditions exhibiting increased endocrine activity such as Cushing syndrome, hyperthyroidism, and gigantism. Remarkably, though septo-optic dysplasia is usually associated with decreased anterior pituitary activity, patients with this disorder have been reported with early pubertal development (35).

Diagnosis of Central Precocious Puberty.   Central precocious puberty is associated with all endocrine changes found in normal gonadarche. Affected patients demonstrate increased pulsatile release of gonadotropins, a pubertal response of LH to GnRH administration, and pubertal concentration of gonadal steroids. Children under 6 years of age may lack the adrenarche, while older children may develop adrenarche as well as gonadarche in the normal pubertal pattern. Ultrasonography of the uterus will reveal enlargement and attainment of a more mature uterine shape than is found in the prepubertal girl. Thus, the length will exceed 3 cm and the fundus to cervix size ratio will increase (36).

Treatment of Central Precocious Puberty.   Superactive GnRH agonists act as a constant infusion of GnRH and by desensitizing the pituitary gonadotropes and decreasing gonadotropin secretion, are used to reverse the manifestations of precocious puberty. This treatment is not effective in incomplete precocious puberty where there is no activation of the hypothalamic-pituitary-gonadal axis. Patients with hamartomas of the tuber cinereum, other brain tumors, post androgen therapy precocious puberty, or idiopathic central precocious puberty have been all reported to respond to GnRH analogues given subcutaneously or by intranasal insufflation. The long-acting GnRH analogue D-Trp6-Pro9-NEt-LHRH was one of the first agents used, but several others have been successfully employed for therapy in precocious puberty (37). The GnRH analogues successfully reduce the rate of pubertal development, reverse some of the signs of puberty, decrease the rapid progression of bone age advancement, and improve the final height prognosis of affected patients (38).

Incomplete Precocious Puberty in Boys

Some neurologic diseases can cause pubertal development in boys independently from the hypothalamic-pituitary axis. Hypothalamic germinomas, or germinomas and teratomas of other locations can secrete hCG, which will stimulate Leydig cell testosterone production in boys. Hepatoblastomas and hepatomas can also stimulate Leydig cell function via hCG secretion. The hCG will cause the testes to be enlarged, but due to the absence of concomitant FSH secretion and lack of Sertoli cell and seminiferous tubule stimulation, the testes will not grow as large as seen in later normal puberty.

A primary intracranial hCG-producing tumor was found in an 8-year-old boy with congenital adrenal hyperplasia. This rare association shows that precocious puberty in any child, even one with a known disorder involving excess androgens such as congenital adrenal hyperplasia, warrants thorough investigation to determine whether another potential cause of the findings of advanced sexual development is operative (39).

Diagnosis and Treatment of Incomplete Precocious Puberty in Boys with Neurologic Disease.   Neurologic disorders can also cause incomplete precocious puberty in boys by causing increased secretion of hCG. The hCG will cross-react in LH radioimmunoassays, leading to the report of exceptionally high levels of LH or a positive pregnancy test. If a beta hCG determination is performed the result will be low as hCG does not cross-react in the assay. Treatment is directed to removing or inactivating the primary lesion.

Large Testes Without Precocious Puberty

Four 46 XY siblings with congenital bilateral megalo-orchidia, macrogenitosomia, and severe mental deficiency were investigated (40). The testicular size was significantly larger than age-matched normal males. Normal hypothalamic-pituitary gonadotropin function was demonstrated by finding normal levels of luteininizing and follicle-stimulating hormones in the basal state and by normal responses to gonadotropin-releasing hormone and testosterone administration. Normal testicular function was demonstrated by normal plasma testosterone and estradiol levels, normal testosterone response to human chorionic gonadotropin (hCG), normal sperm analysis, and normal testicular morphology and cell architecture. Adrenal function was within normal limits. These patients, therefore, have normal functional testicular hyperplasia. Family studies have suggested this distinct congenital disorder is inherited as an X-linked recessive trait, and is recognized as the fragile-X syndrome.

Delayed Puberty

A boy who has not initiated secondary sexual development by 14 years of age or a girl who has not done so by 13 years of age has delayed puberty. Even at those ages, 0.6% of the normal population enter puberty spontaneously at a later time; it is prudent to avoid unnecessary evaluations until these age limits are attained (41). Abnormalities of the hypothalamic-pituitary-gonadal axis may follow a normal age of onset of puberty only to be followed by later cessation of progressing secondary sexual development.

Central Nervous System Abnormalities

Gonadotropic secretion may be affected by hypothalamic-pituitary tumors, although this generally occurs less commonly than effects on growth hormone secretion. Late onset, as opposed to congenital pituitary deficiency, and particularly the combination of anterior and posterior pituitary defects should suggest the diagnosis of a tumor of the CNS.

Craniopharyngiomas and other tumors of the CNS outside the sella turcicia such as germinomas of the pineal gland, astrocytomas, and gliomas may also cause hypopituitarism. Intrasellar adenomas are rare but they may also impair pituitary function. Histiocytosis-X (Hand-Schuller-Christian disease) may infiltrate the areas of vasopressin production and secretion and cause diabetes insipidus, but the disorder may also affect other hypothalamic hormones (42). Granulomas of tuberculosis or sarcoid, post infectious processes, and vascular lesions of the CNS have been reported to impair hypothalamic-pituitary function. CNS trauma from accidents or child abuse, increased intracranial pressure associated with hydrocephalus or, in fact, surgery can all affect hypothalamic-pituitary function.

Kallmann syndrome, characterized by deficiency of gonadotropins, is often associated with hyposmia or anosmia. It is generally thought to be an X-linked recessive trait, but the occurrence of this syndrome in a father-to-son transmission is consistent with an autosomal dominant inheritance (43). It is important to realize that anosmia need not be a sign of tumor in these patients but rather an indication of congenital defect. Associated hypogonadism and cerebellar ataxia have also been described (44). Vision can also influence pubertal development as blind girls have an earlier onset of menarche than sighted girls, but blind boys have been reported to have delayed onset of puberty (45).

Children and young adults with ataxia–telangiectasia have been found to have elevated basal levels of FSH and LH and a markedly increased response of FSH to LHRH (46). In pubertal and adult females the basal levels of estradiol were low. The clinical and laboratory findings in these patients suggest that primary gonadal failure is an integral part of ataxia–telangiectasis (Chapter 24).

Central Nervous System Tumors Associated With Endocrine Disease

Virtually any tumor of the CNS can exert pressure on the hypothalamic-pituitary area by enlarging or by metastatic deposits and may provoke signs and symptoms of endocrine abnormalities (Figure 21.3). Craniopharyngiomas are rare tumors, but when compared with other types of CNS neoplasms in the pediatric age group, they are most commonly associated with signs and symptoms of endocrine deficiencies such as short stature, hypogonadism, and thyroid or adrenal insufficiency (Figure 21.4). Other tumors can also lead to impaired endocrine function; for example, hypothalamic tumors can cause precocious puberty, may disrupt normal eating patterns, temperature regulation, and the state of attentiveness.

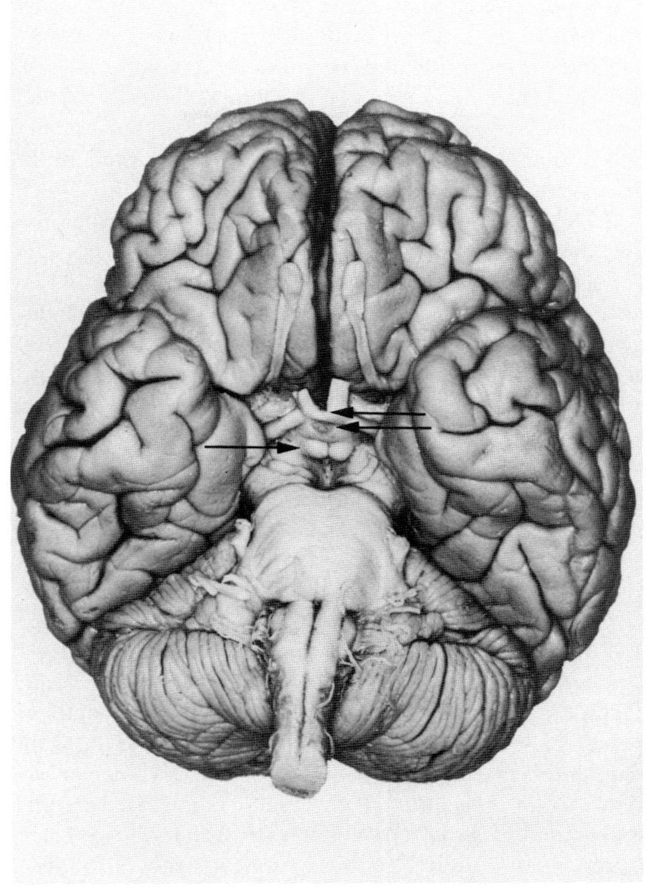

FIGURE 21.3   Basilar aspect of the brain showing the close proximity of the infundibulum (lower right arrow), optic chiasm and nerves (upper right arrow), and the mammillary body (left arrow). (Courtesy of Dr. Stephen DeArmond, University of California Medical Center, San Francisco).

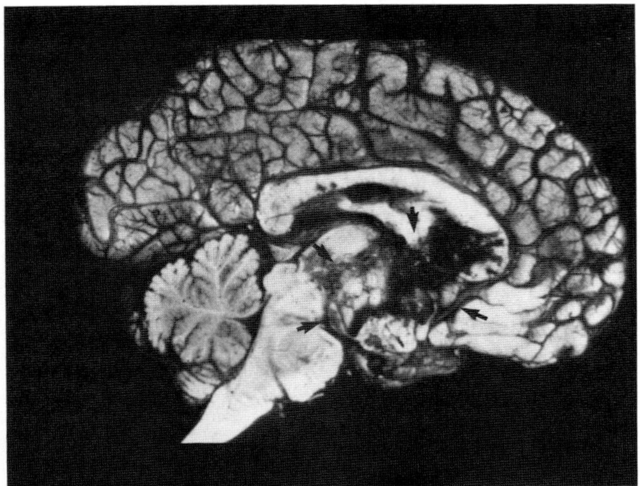

FIGURE 21.4   A sagittal section of a craniopharyngioma in situ, demonstrating the close relationship of the tumor to the hypothalamus. (Courtesy of Dr. Robert Karnei, Director, Armed Forces Institute of Pathology, Washington, DC).

Craniopharyngiomas are derived from Rathke pouch and arise in the pituitary stalk (47). They can grow superiorly into the hypothalamus or inferiorly to involve the sella turcica. Often cystic, they can contain cholesterol-laden fluid which resembles motor oil. They are often calcified and about 80% show flecks of calcium on skull radiographs and CT scans. (Figure 21.4).

A child of any age may develop a craniopharyngioma, but the peak incidence is during the early teen years. Patients may complain of headache, poor vision, and may have polyuria and polydipsia of diabetes insipidus. In addition, their growth charts will demonstrate decreased growth velocity (growth failure is the most common sign), and delayed puberty can occur. However, some patients with craniopharyngiomas are reported to have precocious puberty.

The physical examination is usually characterized by short stature, the chubbiness of hypopituitarism, pale atrophic optic discs, or less commonly papilledema with visual field defects. Subtle findings of hypothyroidism may be present. Commonly, patients have a prepubertal appearance or a cessation of progressing secondary sexual development, even in adolescence. These clinical findings characterize a typical patient with craniopharyngioma; however, some tumors are accidentally found on skull radiographics obtained following head trauma or for orthodontic procedures. If the tumor is intrasellar, transsphenoidal surgical removal is carried out; however, in larger tumors, radical subtotal surgical removal followed by radiation therapy is recommended since the tumor is radiosensitive (48).

Germinomas of the hypothalamus are also rare tumors and have their peak incidence in the early teen years (49). The tumor location can cause any hypothalamic-pituitary deficiency possible, and patients may be asymptomatic except for endocrine effects such as diabetes insipidus, growth failure, and delayed puberty. Visual defects are less commonly found in patients with germinomas than with craniopharyngiomas. HCG has been histologically localized to syncytiotrophoblastic giant cells in germinomas, as well as other germ cell tumors such as choriocarcinomas and embryonal carcinomas. Germinomas may secrete hCG and cause incomplete precocious puberty in affected boys; the majority of cases have other endocrine deficiencies at the time of diagnosis. The syndrome of profound muscle weakness, polyuria, adipsia, hypernatremia and hyperlipidemia is reported to occur with some germinomas. This tumor is also radiosensitive but it should be remembered that other additional endocrine deficiencies may occur following radiation therapy directed to the brain (50,51).

Neurofibromatosis, inherited as an autosomal-dominant trait, is characterized by neurofibromas, café au lait spots, and axillary and inguinal freckling. There is an increased incidence of brain tumors in neurofibromatosis, including those that interfere with normal hypothalamic-pituitary

function, such as growth hormone deficiency, hypogonadotropic hypogonadism, and precocious puberty (52). Pheochromocytomas occur more frequently in neurofibromatosis than in the general population (Chapter 23).

Tumors or congenital anomalies of the ventromedial hypothalamus are rare, but they can impair the sense of satiety and lead to obesity. If control of hypothalamic factors and pituitary function is not affected, tall stature may occur, but if growth hormone release is decreased, short stature will result. Episodic uncontrolled rage in addition to massive obesity has been reported to occur in rare patients with hypothalamic disease.

Pituitary adenomas rarely occur during childhood, but prolactinomas, corticotropic adenomas (previously called basophilic adenomas), and most rarely of all, somatotropic adenomas (previously called eosinophilic adenomas) are reported. Prolactinomas are surgically removed if possible, and bromocriptine suppression is utilized if the tumor is not amenable to surgical extirpation. Corticotropic and somatotropic adenomas are removed by trans-sphenoidal microadenomectomy, if possible.

Patients with any hypothalamic-pituitary tumor may develop growth hormone, thyroid, and gonadotropin deficiencies, or any combination of these endocrinopathies. Patients are generally obese, but obesity may also occur following surgical or radiation therapy. The archaic term "Froelich syndrome" or adipiso-genito-dystrophy, refers to a hypothalamic-pituitary tumor associated with obesity; it was first applied to a patient who was ultimately shown to have a tuberculous granuloma in the hypothalamic-pituitary region. The term is less than descriptive and no longer serves any function. One group of patients grows well after craniopharyngioma removal, and in spite of their growth hormone deficiency, their IGF-1 concentrations are normal. Some have elevated prolactin concentrations as well but all patients are obese (53).

Congenital defects of the CNS should be manifest in the neonatal period. Optic nerve hypoplasia, the appearance of a small pale optic disc usually surrounded by a dark margin, is associated with impaired vision and pendular nystagmus. This condition should not be confused with acquired optic atrophy (54). Approximately 50% of patients with optic nerve hypoplasia have absence of the septum pellucidum (septo-optic dysplasia). These patients may be normal with respect to endocrine function but any combination of anterior or posterior pituitary deficiencies can occur, with GH deficiency occurring most commonly. Other midline cranial defects such as cleft palate associated with CNS anomalies, may be found with endocrine defects (55). Children are rarely reported with agenesis of the pituitary gland and a shallow sella turcica, but this is a devastating condition leading to hypoglycemia and shock soon after birth.

The "empty sella" syndrome is so-named because a cerebrospinal fluid filled arachnoid hernia fills the pituitary fossa and compresses the pituitary gland, creating the illusion of an empty sella on neuroimaging studies but an enlarged pituitary fossa on skull radiographs. This condition is rare in children and up to 1984 only 27 cases had been reported. Children with an empty sella do not exhibit the higher female incidence that is reported in the adult population, and they have a higher incidence of associated endocrine and visual abnormalities. Newer neuroimaging techniques including CT and MRI brain scans have increased the number of reports of variants of the empty sella syndrome; however, some of these patients do not have an enlarged pituitary fossa and, therefore, do not strictly conform to the definition of the syndrome (56).

Radiation therapy, commonly used to treat brain tumors and as prophylaxis in CNS leukemia, can cause hypothalamic-pituitary deficiencies (57). The effects are dose dependent and appear more frequently in children treated at younger ages. Growth hormone is affected first and most often, and 9 to 18 months after completion of therapy, decreased GH secretion and growth failure may be noted. Thyrotropin (TSH), ACTH, and gonadotropins have also been reported as deficient in some cases. Because of the increasing incidence of successfully treated brain tumors in childhood; (e.g., leukemia with bone marrow transplants requiring CNS radiation therapy during their course of therapy), patients should be watched prospectively for the development of such endocrinopathies. Endocrine abnormalities following radiation therapy appear to originate in the hypothalamus more often than in the pituitary gland, and growth hormone response to insulin induced hypoglycemia appears to be more affected by irradiation than the response to arginine. There is wide variation, however, in patient responses (58).

There is clear evidence of psychologic impairment in some children following cranial irradiation therapy, particularly in younger children. Lack of head growth as determined by serial head measurements has also been shown to occur in some children who have received radiation therapy directed to the skull. Since the field of irradiation may include the thyroid gland, a search for primary hypothyroidism is in order, and replacement with exogenous thyroxine in doses appropriate to decrease TSH concentrations is a method of minimizing the likelihood of a thyroid neoplasm developing from TSH stimulation (59). In some cases where the spine is included in the radiation field, there may be inhibition of upper body growth, leading to decreased height velocity in association with a high upper to lower segment ratio (60–63). When the gonads are included in the radiation field, gonadal failure may result.

CNS trauma may also impair hypothalamic-pituitary function, but in some cases it may promote premature pubertal development. Children of abusive families should be considered at risk for psychosocial dwarfism, but they must also be considered as vulnerable to head trauma

which is a known cause of hypopituitarism and poor growth (64).

Hypothalamic Involvement

The Shapiro syndrome, characterized by intermittent hypothermia and agenesis of the corpus callosum, can also be manifested by intermittent mutism or coma (65). Chronic hypothermia or poikilothermia can occur with any disturbance of the hypothalamus and should awaken concern about hypothalamic tumor. Hyperthermia is more common than hypothermia as a manifestation of a hypothalamic lesion.

Hyperprolactinomas

Prolactin (PRL) is an anterior pituitary hormone which shares similarities to the growth hormone molecule. It is required for milk production. Elevated plasma prolactin levels can cause infertility, amenorrhea, or delayed pubertal development. Plasma levels may be elevated because of a pituitary micro- or macroadenoma, or the empty sella syndrome, while a destructive lesion of the pituitary gland would decrease prolactin secretion. Since prolactin is one pituitary hormone that is constantly suppressed (primarily by dopamine), a functional or anatomic defect in the hypothalamus will often increase prolactin secretion; thus, hypothalamic tumors or congenital hypopituitarism are often but not always associated with increased plasma prolactin concentrations. Stalk section from surgery or other trauma is usually associated with elevated prolactin concentrations. Many psychoactive drugs such as the phenothiazines, thioxanthenes, benzamides, butyrophenones, reserpine, or methyl-dopa will cause an increase in prolactin secretion. Trauma, inflammation, or stimulation of the chest wall or nipple will also increase prolactin secretion (66). The intravenous administration of TRH stimulates prolactin secretion.

Seizure disorders are another cause of elevated plasma prolactin (67). In one study, prolactin secretion was increased in complex partial seizures without secondary generalization. Secondary generalization to nontemporal lobe areas was also associated with increased PRL plasma levels, and stimulation of the amygdala resulted in similar increases of PRL. No significant elevation of PRL was determined in nonepileptic (pseudoseizures) types of seizure disorders (68). The elevated plasma PRL levels were suggested to have 72% accuracy in differentiating seizures from pseudoseizures.

The basal level of plasma PRL is elevated in patients with following severe head injuries, but those patients exhibited a lower PRL response to TRH. The basal values for TSH and the response to TRH, however, remained in the normal range (69).

DISORDERS OF VASOPRESSIN METABOLISM

Diabetes insipidus (DI) is characterized by polyurea and polydipsia and occurs in two forms: true or central DI and a familial nephrogenic type. Central DI is generally responsive to the administration of antidiuretic hormone (ADH); whereas, nephrogenic DI is recalcitrant to treatment (70).

Arginine vasopressin is synthesized in the paraventricular and supraoptic nuclei and stored, for the most part, in the posterior pituitary gland. Vasopressin is released from the posterior pituitary gland in response to hyperosmolality, blood volume contraction, or hypotension. Regulation is accomplished by an intrahypothalamic osmostat, carotid baroreceptors, and intraatrial volume sensors. Vasopressin can increase water retention at the collecting duct of the nephron and thereby increase blood pressure. Some neurologic diseases are notable for causing disturbances of normal vasopressin physiology and, in turn, disturbances of normal vasopressin secretion can shift fluid and electrolyte balance to such extent that neurologic signs and symptoms are provoked.

Central Diabetes Insipidus

Central diabetes insipidus is the inability to release adequate arginine vasopressin in the face of increased serum osmolality. CNS tumors, congenital defects, trauma, infection, or granulomas precipitate central diabetes insipidus. Even if some vasopressin secretion is maintained but the amount is not commensurate with the need for water conservation, excessive urination will occur. The sense of thirst may or may not remain intact, depending upon the location of the defect; a patient with diabetes insipidus who lacks the normal sense of thirst in accordance with the degree of dehydration is difficult to manage.

The most common tumors causing DI in the pediatric age group are craniopharyngiomas or germinomas. Histiocytosis-X, characterized by infiltrative lesions in or around the basilar aspect of the brain, may also result in diabetes insipidus. When late onset posterior pituitary disease as manifested by DI is associated with any anterior pituitary deficiency, one should make every effort to rule out a tumor or infiltrative lesion. The late onset of isolated DI is itself an ominous sign in this regard. CNS trauma such as a fall from a horse or following surgery for craniopharyngioma, for example, can lead to diabetes insipidus. Hydrocephalus can also result in vasopressin deficiency.

Idiopathic, congenital central diabetes insipidus without recognized anatomic abnormalities can occur sporadically or in a dominantly inherited pattern. Anatomic congenital midline defects of the CNS can lead to diabetes insipidus, often in combination with anterior pituitary deficiencies. Optic nerve hypoplasia is often associated with hypothalamic abnormalities, visual impairment, and endocrine disorder, including DI.

Histiocytosis-X and craniopharyngiomas, though usually occurring at a later age, can be found in infants. The early onset of anterior and posterior pituitary disorders usually suggests a more benign prognosis of congenital hypopituitarism and DI; however, an evaluation for potential tumors should be carried out even in the youngest cases of combined anterior and posterior pituitary deficiency.

There is some evidence to suggest an autoimmune etiology of idiopathic DI. In one study, 28% of patients with idiopathic DI had other autoimmune diseases; whereas, those with DI secondary to hypothalamic lesions had no such association. Moreover, 30% of the idiopathic group had auto-antibodies to vasopressin secretory cells; whereas, none were found in secondary cases (71).

Essential hypernatremia is characterized by a variety of findings including: recurrent hypernatremia, adipsia/polydipsia, obesity, inability to excrete a water load, lack of growth hormone release in response to provocative stimuli, blunted thyrotropic releasing hormone responses, and in some cases hypothyroidism and hyperlipemia. It is characteristically found without an associated anatomic lesion. In one patient, the syndrome was tentatively attributed to a disturbance of the opioid-peptide system, but the overall etiology remains unknown (72).

Diagnosis of Diabetes Insipidus

It is essential that before an evaluation for DI is undertaken, patients are proven not to have chronic renal disease or urinary tract infection that could explain the symptoms. A random urine sample should be dilute and free of sugar to suggest a diagnosis of DI. The history should reveal whether the patient is really urinating frequently and in large quantities throughout the day and night, or if there is merely increased frequency of urination. The first step toward confirmation of polyuria and polydipsia is to obtain intake and output volumes in hospital, or under the supervision of reliable parents. As the first voided urine sample in the morning is the most concentrated over a 24-hour period, a sample should be analyzed for specific gravity and osmolality. In DI the values for serum osmolality and sodium will be normal if the patient has free access to water and a normal thirst mechanism. In contrast, patients with psychogenic polydipsia will have low to normal values due to the dilutional effect of water drinking. A patient without a thirst mechanism will have a high osmolality and sodium because of the lack of a normal drive to increase water intake with contraction of the blood volume. If no CNS anatomic abnormality is present, this condition is called primary or essential hypernatremia in some reports.

A water deprivation test should be performed if the above tests still suggest the patient has DI (73). The child must be constantly observed for signs of dehydration as well as for "cheating" and taking water surreptitiously. It is essential that the test is done with only full staff and that no part of the thirst should occur without careful observation.

The night before the test the child should have a normal dinner and the usual nighttime routine. The first voided urine should be analyzed for osmolality on the morning of the test, the patient's weight and blood pressure determined, and a serum sodium and hematocrit obtained. A normal breakfast can be given with normal fluid intake, but then all oral intake should cease. The weight and blood pressure are taken hourly, the serum osmolality and hematocrit determined every two hours, and all urine volumes monitored and osmolality measured at every void. If the weight drops 5%, the blood pressure falls, or the osmolality rises above 300 mOsm/L, the test must be discontinued.

After 8 hours, the serum and urine osmolality should be compared and a serum vasopressin obtained to match with the osmolalities (although the vasopressin value will not return from the laboratory for weeks, it may prove useful if the diagnosis is still in doubt at that time). The standardized test is interpreted that a patient with DI cannot concentrate the urine to more than 1.5 times the serum osmolality. Thus, if the serum osmolality rises to 300 mOsm/L or higher, the urine should be more than 450 mOsm/L in a normal person.

Patients with partial DI may just pass one test with adequate urinary concentration while, if the test is repeated the next day, the patient may be totally unable to concentrate the urine because of the exhaustion of the patient's meager supply of vasopressin. If the serum osmolality has risen without concentration of the urine osmolality, a dose of aqueous vasopressin is administered of 0.3 mL/m^2 of 20 units/mL aqueous vasopressin subcutaneously or 0.1 mL of D-arginine-D-amino-vasopressin (DDAVP) in each nostril. In the next 30 to 60 minutes the volume of urine and the concentration is compared to the values before the administration of exogenous vasopressin or DDAVP. If the patient has central DI, at the end of the thirst, maximal but inadequate vasopressin will further concentrate the urine. In psychogenic polydipsia, because of the excess water load the patient has taken in prior to the onset of the test, the serum osmolality will not rise above normal during the thirst. If the patient has maintained an adequate medullary interstitial gradient in spite of high urine flow, the exogenous vasopressin will cause further concentration. A patient with nephrogenic diabetes insipidus will not be able to concentrate urine in spite of rising serum osmolality, and with the addition of exogenous vasopressin, will not further raise urine osmolality or reduce urine volume.

Treatment of Diabetes Insipidus

The treatment of choice for central diabetes insipidus is DDAVP, an altered vasopressin molecule that has 140 times the urine concentrating ability, but almost none of the vasoactive effects of arginine vasopressin. A dose of DDAVP will usually last approximately 12 hours but there is individual variation. DDAVP is administered in measured doses by inhalation through the nostrils or by parenteral injection. A dose of 0.05 to 0.15 mL per nasal spray is given and repeated when the child complains of increasing thirst or an infant begins to increase urinary frequency again. Ideally DDAVP is given twice daily to make administration easier in school aged children. It is generally advisable, however, to allow the patient to experience a phase of urination before the next dose is given, so a standing order of bid dosage is not advisable. In the presence of an intact thirst mechanism, the patient should maintain a normal sodium concentration by taking in water when thirst is experienced.

Patients without thirst mechanism due to trauma or surgery, for example, are extremely difficult to treat. A regimen of the correct number of glasses of water per day to keep the serum sodium normal should be determined under close observation of the patient's intake, output, and serum electrolytes. An extra glass of water or so is given for moderately increased activity or exposure to extremes of temperature. Every week or two the serum sodium should be determined, and more often if a stable state has not been reached. The consequences of dehydration or overhydration can be quite severe in this complex condition. Hyponatremia may cause cerebral edema while hypernatremia may lead to brain shrinkage and rupture of bridging vessels. Vasopressin treatment has been shown to affect memory in lower animals and humans, and it has been suggested to improve learning ability in attention and learning disorders as well as in Down syndrome.

Syndrome of Inappropriate Antidiuretic Hormone Secretion

The syndrome of inappropriate antidiuretic hormone secretion (SIADH) exists when there is hyposmolality of the serum with hyponatremia, urine hyperosmolality with existent excretion of sodium. This clinical condition will improve if there is normal renal and adrenal function and if water intake is restricted. The expansion of intravascular volume of SIADH will cause a lowering of serum sodium and osmolality, as well as a sodium diuresis and some degree of urine concentration (physiologically paradoxical because low serum sodium and osmolality could be corrected if the urine is maximally diluted and maximal urinary sodium reabsorption is accomplished). Atrial naturetic peptide is elevated in SIADH and probably accounts for the sodium diuresis. SIADH is often iatrogenic and its incidence would notably decrease if fluid therapy in the treatment of conditions predisposing to SIADH were appropriately regulated and serum sodium concentrations routinely monitored.

Any disorder of the lungs, including those requiring respirator care, can cause the release of vasopressin mediated by the volume receptor in the right atrium. Thus, the commonly prescribed increased fluids in pneumonia can precipitate an episode of SIADH. Most neurologic conditions, including meningitis, brain tumors, post operative states, and trauma can increase vasopressin secretion. These potential complications are well recognized and account for the usual orders for reduced fluid administration in neurologic diseases (74). Plasma concentrations of arginine vasopressin in patients with bacterial meningitis are significantly greater than those noted in normal children with other febrile illnesses, accounting for the tendency toward SIADH in these patients. Infant botulism, especially during the respiratory dependent phase can lead to SIADH.

There is increased vasopressin secretion following any type of surgery and the patient is susceptible to SIADH; thus, the orders to push fluids after surgery can precipitate an episode of SIADH. Any condition causing nausea and vomiting, including malignancies or administration of chemotherapeutic agents, can increase vasopressin secretion. Many of the drugs used in cancer therapy, such as vancomycin, vincristine, and cytoxan can, in addition to their own tendency to cause nausea, increase vasopressin secretion. Ectopic hormone secretion is found with many types of cancers so that a patient with cancer may be susceptible to SIADH from the cancer, from nausea of cancer therapy, and from the chemotherapeutic agent itself.

Prevention is the most important consideration in these circumstances. SIADH is primarily an iatrogenic disease, so that monitoring the patient's fluid therapy by performing frequent serum sodium concentrations virtually eliminates the possibility of encountering severe shifts of sodium. Fluid restriction to the minimum possible volume is the recommended treatment once SIADH develops, and maintaining IV fluids at a level to keep the IV line open may be appropriate. Patients with less severe hyponatremia can be managed by replacing their volume of urine output with an equal amount of IV fluid determined every 2 to 4 hours. The patient with SIADH may be confused with a dehydrated patient because the urine flow is low and the specific gravity high in SIADH, and there is a tendency to administer boluses of fluid to increase urinary output. If oliguria is due to dehydration, the boluses are appropriate, but if SIADH is present, the boluses of fluid will only intensify the SIADH. If careful records of fluid intake and output are maintained, the diagnosis should be evident.

There are other methods to control SIADH and allow some urination and volume contraction. Lithium and demeclocycline interfere with ADH action on the collecting duct, but the side effects inherent in their use eliminates them as viable choices. If hyponatremia is severe and seizures have occurred, furosemide may be administered to initiate diuresis; replacement of part of the volume diuressis with 3% saline will help correct the hyponatremia. This procedure is dangerous, however, and can cause rapid fluid shifts and a patent IV line must be maintained to administer fluids as necessary.

The sodium diuresis characteristic of SIADH is continuous during the active phase of the disorder, and sodium administered orally or intravenously will only be passed out in the urine. The use of intravenous hypertonic saline will likewise only temporarily raise serum sodium, but it has been suggested as one method of stopping a hyponatremic seizure. The only effective treatment for seizures caused by hyponatremia is raising sodium concentration. The intravenous administration of 3% saline has been suggested as helpful on a very temporary basis, but if seizures are intractable, the combination of furosemide and hypertonic saline may be the only possibility while awaiting volume contraction to occur as fluid intake is being decreased.

Diabetes Insipidus and SIADH After Craniopharyngioma Surgery

Patients with craniopharyngiomas often have diabetes insipidus before surgery, but if not, DI may occur when the pituitary stalk is cut and the patient is yet on the operating table. A few days later, there may be unrestrained release of vasopressin as the damaged nerve cells regenerate; if the high level of fluid replacement necessary for the DI is continued during vasopressin secretion phase, SIADH will develop. A 3rd phase can occur in the following days in which permanent diabetes insipidus or, in patients where the surgical cut is low on the pituitary stalk, normal vasopressin secretion can resume. Fluid output must be carefully monitored so that intake is matched to output, and fluid overloading does not occur.

ADRENAL GLAND

Glucocorticoid Excess States

An abnormal regulation of the pituitary–adrenal axis leads to the specific diagnosis of Cushing disease (known as bilateral adrenal hyperplasia because of the enlarged appearance of the adrenal glands, even though the etiology lies in the hypothalamic-pituitary axis) (75). The original report by Cushing describes a patient with a basophilic (corticotropic) adenoma and physical signs of hypercortisolism, but it was not until 50 years later that the primary importance of the pituitary microadenomas in these patients was proved by the technique of transsphenoidal microadenomectomy. Selective removal of the microadenoma alleviated the disease (76). The fact that some patients appropriately treated with microadenomectomy have recurrences suggests that hypothalamic corticotropic releasing factor (CRF) may be the cause of microadenoma, although others have suggested that pituitary cells are primarily responsible for the development of the adenoma. ACTH secreting pituitary micro- and macroadenomas as well as intrahemispheric tumors have been responsible for Cushing syndrome. Cushing syndrome refers to any cause of increased glucocorticoid effects and includes the specific case of Cushing disease. Thus, adrenal adenomas or carcinomas can precipitate the same clinical symptoms as ACTH secreting pituitary adenomas.

The first manifestation of Cushing disease in childhood is growth failure which is quickly followed by weight gain in a truncal or centripetal pattern and muscle wasting with thin and weak extremities. Steroid myopathy in this disorder, or any state of increased glucocorticoid dosage, is progressive and primarily affects proximal limb muscles. Stretch reflexes are decreased and electrophysiologic studies show normal or low amplitude, short-duration motor unit potentials. Muscle biopsy is characterized by type 2 fiber atrophy and muscle fiber vacuolation and mitochondrial aggregation; increased lipid content in type 2 fibers has been described (77).

The typical Cushingoid appearance of adipose tissue on the back of the neck (buffalo hump) may develop as well as purple striae on the trunk from thinning of skin and exposure of the capillaries. Sometimes weakness and lack of energy, an increased pigmentation of the flexor skin surfaces, gingiva, and the early appearance of acne or pubic hair in a child may be present. The personality of patients with Cushing disease may be bizarre and some are described as obsessive. The systolic and diastolic blood pressures may be elevated (Figure 21.5).

Because of the usually small size of the pituitary lesion in Cushing disease, signs and symptoms of neurologic abnormality may not be present. Diagnosis is established by measuring cortisol, ACTH, and their metabolites before and after dexamethasone suppression. A biochemical diagnosis is mandatory because neuroimaging studies are generally of little help in establishing a diagnosis. Removal of the adenoma is curative; however, there is a risk of recurrence from regrowth of unremoved cells or the development of a new tumor in the pituitary gland, possibly resulting from hypothalamic corticotropic stimulating factor. Glucocorticoids must be administered to guard against adrenal crisis after surgery.

Partial or total adrenalectomy had been earlier suggested for treatment of Cushing syndrome as well as chemical adrenal ablation with mitotane (OPDDD) or aminoglutethimide. The latter treatment methods did not address the primary etiology of the disorder, that is, the pituitary adenoma. Without elevated concentrations of serum ACTH to exert feedback suppression, the tumor is able to enlarge and cause local pressure effects. This is referred to as the Nelson syndrome and is characterized by hyperpigmentation (resulting from extremely high elevations of ACTH concentrations), and an enlarging pituitary tumor (78). Local extension makes surgical removal difficult.

Pharmacologic Use of Glucocorticoids

Although glucocorticoids are often administered in an attempt to reduce brain edema secondary to head injury, their use is controversial. A recent study has demonstrated that children with severe head injury that were not given

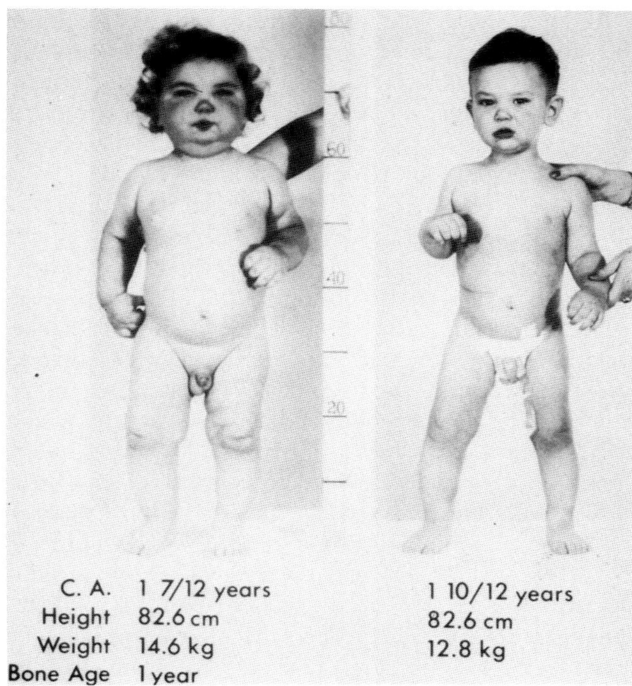

FIGURE 21.5 Cushing syndrome secondary to an adrenal adenoma before and after treatment. (Courtesy of Dr. Selna Kaplan, University of California Medical Center, San Francisco).

dexamethasone showed up to a twentyfold increase in urinary cortisol excretion, suggesting that endogenous cortisol secretion increases to such degree that exogenous glucocorticoids may be superfluous (79).

Pseudotumor cerebri, or benign increased intracranial pressure, is characterized by headache and bilateral papilledema in the absence of a space occupying lesion. CT brain scans show small ventricles. This syndrome is known to occur with glucocorticoid therapy, withdrawal of exogenous glucocorticoids, chronic hypocalcemia, primary adrenal insufficiency, among other nonendocrine disorders. Several cases of pseudotumor cerebri have also been reported after the onset of thyroxine therapy for Hashimoto thyroiditis or hypothalamic hypothyroidism (80–82). Pseudotumor cerebri should be considered as a potential complication during abrupt withdrawal of glucocorticoids or the initiation of thyroxine therapy in patients with hypothyroidism.

It is well recognized that psychiatric symptoms can develop during the administration of corticosteroids (83). One study reported that severe psychiatric reactions occurred in approximately 5% of steroid-treated patients, and that a large proportion of these patients had affective or other psychotic symptoms that usually presented early in the course of steroid treatment. The female sex, systemic lupus erythematosis, and high doses of prednisone may be risk factors for the development of steroid-induced psychiatric symptoms. Most patients recover within several weeks of symptom onset.

ACTH has been used for over thirty years as a treatment for intractable seizures; including, infantile spasms and other types of myoclonic epilepsies. The mechanism of action is unknown, but large doses appear to be necessary; the same effects may occur during adrenal gland suppression with exogenous glucocorticoids (84,85). One controlled study of changes in CT brain scan in children with different generalized epilepsies treated with ACTH and dexamethasone demonstrated enlargement of the ventricles and subarachnoid spaces during the initial phase of treatment with Depot-ACTH. Similar but less severe changes were noted with dexamethasone treatment. The changes were reversed when the treatment was discontinued (86). Another CT study of infants and children with intractable epilepsy who were treated with synthetic ACTH-Z, showed brain shrinkage in all cases after seven weeks of daily doses of ACTH, the maximum changes present within 4 weeks of treatment. Almost all of these changes reversed within 1 to 3 months after ACTH was discontinued. More striking changes were observed in the younger patients. Since the administration of ACTH reduces the internal carotid blood flow, as demonstrated on CT, it has been postulated that this factor may affect the brain (87).

The withdrawal of ACTH therapy in infantile spasms and other types of myoclonic epilepsies would be expected to cause fewer complications than withdrawal of glucocorticoid therapy, because it is the suppression of endogenous ACTH by exogenous glucocorticoid therapy that leads to long term glucocorticoid insufficiency. Although most children appear to have adequate response after discontinuing ACTH, ACTH release is transiently suppressed in some children after exogenous ACTH treatment. Tapered withdrawal and stress coverage is recommended temporarily following discontinuation of ACTH (88,89).

Glucocorticoid Deficiency States

Addison disease, a condition in which there is both glucocorticoid and mineralocorticoid deficiency, is caused by hypoplastic or destructive changes of the adrenal gland. The initial process such as an adrenal hemorrhage may leave residual tissue, and patients may not manifest signs or symptoms of adrenal insufficiency until some future period of stress such as an infectious process; by this time calcification of the gland may be apparent on abdominal radiographs. Original reports described the tuberculous destruction of the gland, but other infectious processes or metastatic tumor may be responsible for injury to the adrenals. In some patients no cause can be determined for the adrenal insufficiency. More recently it has been determined that the adrenals may be affected by some autoimmune process; moreover, some patients may have associated hypothyroidism, hypoparathyroidism, and diabetus mellitus.

Patients with Addison disease characteristically have increased skin pigmentation (due to excess ACTH secretion) that is commonly observed in the flexor creases, mucous membranes, and the gingiva. Other signs and symptoms of the disease include apathy, weakness, anorexia, vomiting, hypotension, and weight loss. Disorientation, irritability, and personality changes have been reported, and psychoses rarely occur. A metabolic encephalopathy can be present with symptoms of confusion and delirium that may progress to coma and seizures.

Adrenoleukodystrophy

Schilder described the neuropathologic findings in 3 patients with abnormalities of the central white matter, and terms such as "encephalitis periaxialis diffusa," diffuse sclerosis, and Schilder disease were applied (90–92). Later studies, however, suggested that each of these patients had different diseases of the cerebral white matter, and there is a question whether Schilder disease (diffuse sclerosis) as initially described, actually exists (93–95).

Patients with a degeneration of the white matter associated with melanoderma, "bronzed sclerosing encephalomyelitis" was described in 1923 (96). Then in 1970, Blaw introduced the term "adrenoleukodystrophy" (ALD), which has been used to the present time (97). ALD is inherited as an X-linked recessive trait and has been mapped to the distal end of the long arm of X-chromosome (Xq27–28), near the locus for red–green color blindness and hemophilia. Powers and Schaumburg (1974) demonstrated that both the brain and adrenal cortex were involved in this disease process, showing characteristic lamellar inclusions in the Schwann cells as well as the cells of the adrenal zona fasciculata and reticularis. The inclusions were shown to consist of cholesterol, esterified (98,99) with abnormally long-chain fatty acids (VLCFAs) (C_{24}–C_{30}). The cerebral white matter and the adrenal cortex of all patients with ALD have been shown to have an excess of VLCFAs in the cholesterol esters and ganglioside fraction; more recent studies have shown elevated levels of VLCFAs in all lipid moieties, tissue, and body fluids of all affected patients (100–107). Various forms of ALD have been recognized and classified as peroxisomal disorders, generally on the basis of single or multiple peroxisomal function(s) (108,109).

Schaumburg and associates described the clinical and neuropathologic features of 17 patients. The onset of signs and symptoms of childhood ALD is about 8 years of age but can be as early as 3 years and as late as 12 years of age. The child shows behavioral changes with less interest in the environment, decreased school performance with memory impairment, emotional lability, and progressive dementia. Motor signs and symptoms (corticospinal tract), either unilateral or bilateral, become apparent as manifested by progressive gait disturbance. Vision becomes impaired with loss of acuity, field defects, and optic atrophy is ultimately present. Auditory agnosia may be present early, with deafness demonstrated later in the disease course. Seizures are usually observed later in the disease but may occur early. About 20% of patients have typical findings of adrenal insufficiency at the time of neurologic deterioration with apathy, weakness, vomiting, and melanoderma, particularly in the skin creases; whereas, others have only mild adrenal involvement that is determined by adrenal function tests, especially by ACTH stimulation. The disease is relentlessly progressive and within months to years the child becomes vegetative and decorticate, expiring either from adrenal crisis or other causes such as pulmonary infections (110–113).

CT brain scans show diminished white matter attenuation, primarily in a parieto-occipital distribution with caudorostral progression (114). MRI studies show white matter changes with increased signal intensity on T-2 weighted spin-echo sequences.

Although there is no specific treatment for ALD, steroid replacement therapy must be carefully monitored particularly during times of stress, as in the case of infection. Thus far, there has been no successful treatment including diet management for this peroxisomal abnormality that results in the accumulation of VLCFAs in a variety of tissues. Whether bone marrow transplantation is of benefit remains to be determined.

Adrenomyeloneuropathy

Patients with adrenomyeloneuropathy (AMN) have onset of signs and symptoms of neurologic impairment usually between the ages of 20 and 30 years, although it may be earlier or later. The disease is inherited as an X-linked recessive trait. Adrenal insufficiency is commonly present in childhood and hypogonadism occurs in variable degrees. Neurologic findings are those of myelopathy with progressive weakness and sensory loss in the legs. Associated neurologic findings include involvement of the peripheral and autonomic nervous systems, with sphincteric disturbances and impotence. Cerebellar ataxia and progressive dementia occur later in the course of the disease (115,116). Diagnostic methods and recommendations for treatment are similar to those of childhood adrenoleukodystrophy.

Neonatal Adrenoleukodystrophy

Ulrich and associates (117) described a hypotonic infant with severe neonatal seizures and psychomotor retardation who died at 5 months of age. Pathologic studies showed bilateral adrenal cortical atrophy and cerebral demyelination with inclusions similar to those observed in ALD (117). This neonatal form of ALD (NALD), inherited as an autosomal recessive trait, is different from the childhood form of ALD not only in clinical manifestations and inheritance but its generalized, or multiple, peroxisomal deficiencies. The clinical features include severe hypotonia, seizures, and very poor growth and development; whereas, patients with the childhood form of ALD have normal infancy and early childhood. Additional features of NALD include macrocephaly with large fontanelle, nystagmus, optic atrophy, and occasionally a pigmentary retinopathy (118). Hepatosplenomegaly is commonly present as well as nonspecific dysmorphic features. Most patients with NALD expire before 5 years of age though some patients have survived as long as 10 years (119,120).

Heterozygous Female Carriers of Adrenoleukodystrophy

The identification of heterozygous female carriers of ALD and AMN is of particular importance since the prenatal diagnosis of these forms of adrenoleukodystrophy is now possible (121). Moser and colleagues have shown that measurement of VLCFAs in plasma and cultured skin fibroblasts is an effective method of not only identifying patients with ALD and AMN but also the female obligate heterozygous carriers of the disease.

In some kindreds there are varying degrees of neurologic impairment in these patients, usually manifested as mild spastic paraparesis beginning in the 3rd decade. Other patients noted symptoms only when specifically asked about their presence, such as urinary urgency, muscle tightness, clumsiness, or weakness of the legs. Peripheral neuropathy was generally mild and noted by delayed conduction velocities. Patient response to the administration of ACTH was generally normal. The incidence of obligate heterozygous female carriers is not well established although it has been thought to be about 10%, a figure based on the reporting of clinical symptoms. However, 1 study suggests an incidence of about 40% when careful neurologic examinations are carried out (109,121).

Adrenal Medullary Disorders

The chromaffin cells of the adrenal medulla or extra adrenal tissue give rise to pheochromocytomas. These tumors are rare in childhood but are important because they represent a curable cause of hypertension and must be considered in the differential diagnosis of high blood pressure. Pheochromocytomas occur more frequently in multiple endocrine neoplasia syndromes, neurofibromatosis, and Von Hippel-Lindau disease than in the general population (Chapter 23) (122,123).

The usual signs and symptoms of pheochromocytomas include hypertension (occurring more often in a constant than episodic pattern in children), weight loss, headache, vomiting, and more rarely in children than in adults, paroxysmal episodes of tachycardia, flushing, sweating, and palpitations, or anxiety. Pheochromocytomas are diagnosed by the demonstration of elevated urinary catecholamines, vanillylmandelic acid (VMA), or total metanephrine excretion, in a 24-hour urine collection. Plasma catecholamine concentrations may not add any information to the urinary collections which serve as a reflection of the integrated catecholamine production over the day. Spot urine analyses are now available and simplify the monitoring process. Provocative pharmacologic tests are no longer employed because of the specificity of the urine and plasma collections and the danger of precipitating a hypertensive crisis.

Multiple endocrine neoplasia type 2 encompasses thyroid medullary carcinoma, pheochromocytoma, and parathyroid chief cell hyperplasia or tumor. It is inherited as an autosomal dominant trait with medullary carcinoma of the thyroid gland exhibiting the greatest degree of penetrance.

Patients with multiple endocrine neoplasia, type 3 (previously called MEN 2b) are characterized by a Marfan-like body type with full, fleshy lips, white–yellow nodules (neuromas) on the tip and edges of the tongue, buccal mucosa, conjunctiva, and hyperplastic corneal nerves. Intestinal ganglioneuromas and megacolon are sometimes associated findings, as well as peroneal muscular atrophy and pes cavus. The disease is inherited as an autosomal dominant trait (124). Other neurologic manifestations include neurogenic constipation, impaired vision, and facial disfigurement. Somatic motor and sensory as well as autonomic nerves may be affected. Autopsy findings indicate that symptoms can be derived from neuroma formation with characteristic plaques composed of hyperplastic interlacing bands of Schwann cells and myelinated fibers overlying the posterior columns of the spinal cord.

DIABETES MELLITUS

Diabetes mellitus is the most common endocrine disorder in childhood. This disturbance of glucose metabolism can lead to acute disorders of mentation and chronic diseases of the peripheral nerves, eyes, and kidneys. In childhood, however, the majority of problems are acute. Type 1 diabetes mellitus or insulin-dependent diabetes mellitus (IDDM) is the most common type of diabetes encountered in the pediatric population; it is characterized by inadequate insulin production, a tendency to ketosis which may extend to ketoacidosis, an association with other autoimmune diseases, and the presence of circulating antibodies to cytoplasmic and cell-surface components of pancreatic cells.

The autosomal recessive DIDMOAD syndrome is characterized by diabetes insipidus, diabetes mellitus, optic atrophy, and high-tone deafness (125). The Alström-Hallgren syndrome includes retinal degeneration, nerve deafness, and occasionally, diabetes mellitus and acanthosis nigricans.

Ataxia–telangiectasia and myotonic dystrophy have associated insulin resistance without a tendency toward ketosis. Muscular dystrophies of the Duchenne and Facioscapulohumeral types have glucose intolerance, possibly due to decreased muscle utilization of glucose, and Friedreich ataxia is also frequently associated with insulin-dependent diabetes mellitus. Several other syndromes of obesity such as Alström-Hallgren, Laurence-Moon-Biedl, and Prader-Labhart-Willi syndromes may also exhibit glucose intolerance, possibly due to the effects of the obesity itself; these are nonketotic types of diabetes mellitus.

Clinically apparent cerebral edema is a rare but an often fatal complication of diabetic ketoacidosis. Numerous studies have not revealed the cause of this condition nor are specific recommendations available to avoid its occurrence. The onset of cerebral edema may be suggested by the absence of improvement in mental status as the blood chemistry values improve, or a decline in neurologic status after an initial improvement. It is generally suggested that a slower rate of fluid administration and decrease in blood sugar concentration is safer than rapid corrections, but these factors are only generally related to the occurrence of cerebral edema. A study of CT brain scans suggests that subclinical brain swelling may be a common finding during treatment of diabetic ketoacidosis in children. Hyperosmolar nonketotic coma is rare in childhood but has been reported; cerebral edema has also been observed in this condition (126).

Peripheral neuropathy is the most common neurologic complication of diabetes mellitus (127). While the patient may not complain about weakness, careful examination may reveal distal weakness of the lower extremities, diminished stretch reflexes, and wasting of the interosseous muscles. Peroneal nerve conduction velocity is slowed in 11% of neurologically asymptomatic juvenile diabetic patients from 8 to 15 years of age, and many will have abnormal bilateral peroneal somatosensory evoked potentials (128). The duration and level of control of diabetes mellitus correlates with the severity of the neuropathy and retinopathy. Autonomic neuropathy is increasingly recognized in patients with IDDM, and becomes more apparent with increasing duration of the disease. Acute left hemiparesis was reported in three insulin-dependent children with headache and concomitant respiratory tract infection but without hypoglycemia. There were no abnormalities demonstrated at cerebral angiography and CT brain scans; there was complete resolution of neurologic abnormalities within 8 to 24 hours (129). Visual changes may occur in patients with diabetes mellitus because of changes in osmolality within the lens and varying glucose concentrations, hemorrhages, exudates, and neovascularization.

HYPOGLYCEMIA

Glucose is the major fuel for brain function, although ketone bodies can be used as an alternative source of energy. When glucose concentrations drop sufficiently, especially when the drop is sudden, adrenergic signs and symptoms including sweating, tremor, flushing, palpitations, headaches, nausea, and weakness occur. When serum glucose levels drop below 20 to 30 mg/dL, seizures are common. Lower levels can precipitate coma. Dysarthria, paresis, and ataxia are among the consequences of hypoglycemia, and progressive hypoglycemia is said to cause progressively impaired neural function (130).

THYROID DISORDERS

Thyroxine, or T_4, is produced by the thyroid gland in response to stimulation by TSH. The secretion of TSH is regulated by hypothalamic thyrotropic releasing factor (TRF). In states of primary hypothyroidism, T_4 falls while TSH rises in attempt to increase T_4 secretion. Secondary hypothyroidism is due to inadequate TSH production, and tertiary hypothyroidism is caused by inadequate TRF production and secretion (131).

Hypothyroidism

Inadequate thyroid hormone can cause temporary or permanent neurologic abnormalities. If hypothyroidism is congenital, brain development can be permanently impaired; whereas, if the deficiency of thyroid hormone is acquired, changes are readily reversed with thyroxine replacement.

Congenital hypothyroidism is a common disease with a frequency of 1 in 4000 live births in the US. Because of the paucity of signs of hypothyroidism in the newborn and the likelihood of permanent mental retardation if treatment is not started in the neonatal period, statewide screening programs were instituted in all of the US and most other countries. Ideally, a heelstick blood sample is obtained at 1 to 3 days of age and sent to a centralized laboratory for analysis of thyroid hormones and often for phenylalanine and galactose as well, to screen for hypothyroidism, phenylketonuria, and galactosemia, respectively. In a representative program, serum T_4 is assessed and if lower than a predetermined limit, TSH is measured; in some areas only TSH is monitored. If the T_4 is low and the TSH is high, the child is presumptively positive for primary hypothyroidism. If the T_4 is low and the TSH is low, further screening is necessary to determine whether there is low serum thyroid protein binding capacity or whether the child has hypothalamic or pituitary deficiency, resulting in hypothyroidism. Due to early discharge from hospital as well as home deliveries, some children are missed in the screening programs, even though there are procedures to attempt to guard against such a possibility. Even more distressing is the possibility that a premature infant may spend months in an intensive care nursery before the discharge blood sample is obtained, and if that infant is hypothyroid, the diagnosis may be made too late for adequate therapy to begin. Moreover, a premature baby or one who is small for gestational age may have low serum thyroid binding proteins. In most cases, however, the diagnosis is made and treatment begun before the infant is 3 weeks old.

The majority of patients with congenital hypothyroidism have anatomic abnormality of the gland which may be ectopic, hypoplastic, or both. These types of congenital hypothyroidism are sporadic in occurrence. Biochemical defects in iodine trapping, organification of iodine, and coupling of monoiodotyrosine and diiodotyrosine are possible abnormalities inherited as an autosomal recessive traits. The Pendred syndrome combines an organification defect and congenital deafness and is inherited as an autosomal recessive trait. Endemic cretinism was formerly found in areas of low iodine availability, but since the advent of iodine supplementation to food, it occurs uncommonly. Deaf-mutism, mental retardation, and spasticity were also found in patients with endemic cretinism; postnatally deaf-mutism may be the only obvious clinical sign.

Untreated congenital hypothyroidism is a well known cause of severe mental retardation (132). The cerebrum and cerebellum are developmentally immature on gross examination, and microscopic studies show disordered synaptic connections. Spasticity and cerebellar ataxia are frequent concomitants. The low intelligence is generally thought to be permanent, although one study has suggested the possibility of improvement after a period of 10 to 15 years. This outcome has not been reported by others; however, such long-term follow-up is rarely available in most centers. It has been demonstrated that intelligence was lower the longer the treatment was delayed after birth. Recent studies have shown that with treatment initiated in the first few weeks after birth, mental development can be within normal limits. Reports from Canada showed some minor motor abnormalities remaining 5 to 6 years after early treatment, but other studies do not suggest neurologic impairment.

The almost universal screening programs for congenital hypothyroidism have virtually eliminated the possibility of mental retardation. At the same time, it is important to be familiar with the clinical characteristics of congenital hypothyroidism in case neonatal screening fails. The infants are often "post dates" and large at birth; they have temperature instability and hypothermia, mottled skin, late onset of stooling (longer than 24 hours after birth), prolonged jaundice, and decreased activity. Within several months there is coarsening of facial features, thickening of the tongue, brittle hair formation, abdominal distention, poor limb growth, irritability, and a hoarse cry (Figures 21.6, 21.7).

Acquired hypothyroidism after 2 years of age leads to inactivity and apathy, both of which are reversible with thyroxine treatment. Speech is slow, the voice becomes hoarse, mentation is slow, and memory is impaired. Remarkably, the increased attention span noted in such

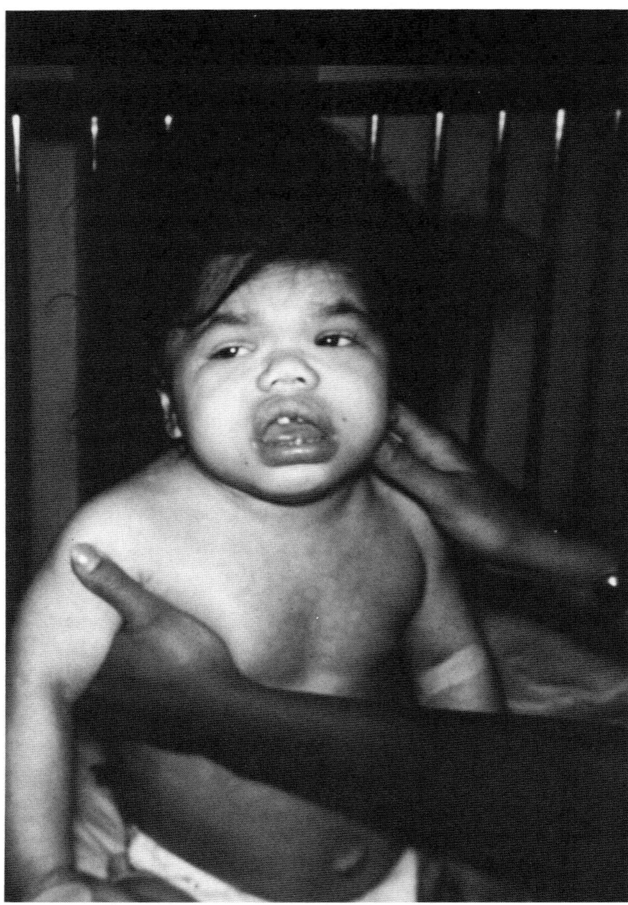

FIGURE 21.6   Cretinism in a 5-month-old infant demonstrating coarsening of facial features, large thickened tongue, and umbilical hernia. The child, though apathetic, was irritable and had a hoarse cry. (Courtesy of Dr. Selna Kaplan, University of California Medical Center, San Francisco).

hemianopsia. Appropriate treatment with thyroxine will reduce the size of the pituitary gland, sometimes resulting in an empty sella. Optic nerve infiltration and pseudotumor with papilledema have been reported.

Physical features of acquired hypothyroidism include short stature with impaired growth of limbs that is greater than upper body growth. This results in a higher upper to lower segment ratio than appropriate for age. Facial features may become coarse with thickened eyelids, dull and coarse dry hair (loss of the outer 3rd of the eyebrows is frequently described), and the pulse may be slow. Other findings include cold intolerance, coarsening of the hair, constipation, disturbances of menstruation, and fertility. Myxedema coma with bradycardia, hypotension, and severe hypothermia occurs rarely in childhood. General supportive care as well as thyroxine replacement is required.

Before cytogenetic testing was readily available, some patients with Down syndrome were confused with hypothyroid patients. There is, in fact, an increased incidence of thyroid dysfunction in patients with Down syndrome, particularly with advancing age. Intellectual impairment is worse in the hypothyroid Down syndrome patient than in those who are euthyroid (137).

Thyroid function tests were studied in epileptic children who received long term anticonvulsant treatment with phenobarbital, primidone, or phenytoin. Serum T_4 was decreased in all three treated groups, and serum T_3 was diminished only in those treated with phenytoin and primidone. FT_4 was also significantly decreased while serum TSH and thyroid binding globulin (TBG) were not affected in the treated patients. The effect of anticonvulsant drugs on thyroid hormone catabolism and peripheral conversion of T_4 seems to be important in these alterations (138).

children may enable them to earn good grades, and when treated their attention span may decrease, resulting in lower grades.

Other symptoms of hypothyroidism at any age include delayed relaxation of stretch reflexes, particularly the ankle jerks. The Kocher-Debre-Semelaigne syndrome ("infant Hercules") is characterized by congenital hypothyroidism and muscular hypertrophy (133). A deposition of mucopolysaccharides in muscle fibers has been observed in some cases but not in others. Afifi and associates found no abnormality of muscle at light and electron-microscopy (134). Electromyographic studies have been within normal limits (135,136). Myoedema has been noted in some patients with hypothyroidism. Myasthenia gravis has also been noted to occur in some patients, more commonly in adults than children.

Primary hypothyroidism causes increased TSH secretion. The thyrotropic hyperplasia may be so severe that the pituitary gland is enlarged and associated with a bitemporal

Hyperthyroidism

Hyperthyroidism is almost universally due to autonomous thyroid stimulation by thyroid stimulating immunoglobulin. It is a hypermetabolic state which influences much of body function. Tachycardia, increased systolic blood pressure and widened pulse pressure are found. Weight loss occurs in the face of increased appetite; increased sweating, tachycardia, and diarrhea are typical findings. Exophthalmos due to intraorbital (extraocular muscle) infiltration, may result in a staring expression. Lid lag, diplopia, difficulty or inability to converge (Moebius sign), infrequent and incomplete blinking (Stellwag sign), the appearance of constant staring (Dalrymple sign), and the absence of wrinkling the forehead in upward gaze (Joffroy sign) are other associated findings (139). Neurologic symptoms include hyperactivity, emotional lability, tremulousness, and insomnia. Neuromuscular signs and symptoms including exophthalmic ophthalmoplegia, thyrotoxic myopathy,

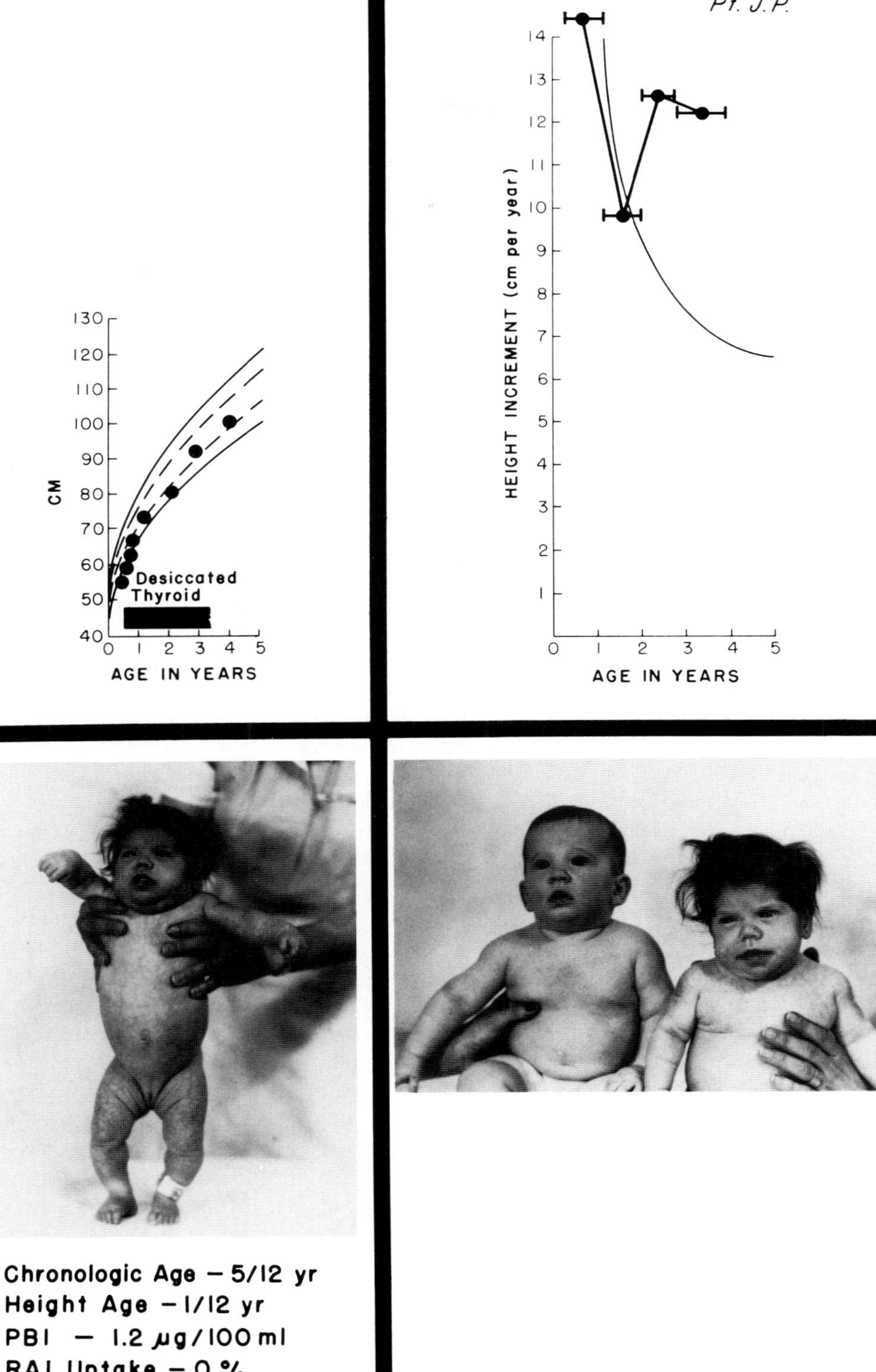

FIGURE 21.7 Comparative facial features of a 5-month-old cretin (lower right inset) and a normal infant of same age. The upper insets demonstrate linear growth of the patient in relation to treatment period with dessicated thyroid. The upper right inset shows height increment in centimeters per year.

myasthenia gravis, and periodic paralysis may occur. Neuromuscular abnormalities are more commonly found in girls than boys in a 6:1 ratio (140).

Thyrotoxic myopathy may occur with mild to moderate weakness of muscles of the shoulder girdle and upper arms; the lower limbs are less affected. Muscle atrophy is commonly present and fasciculations are often observed; the muscle stretch reflexes are normal to hyperactive in contrast with other myopathic processes. Creatine kinase is usually normal and sometimes low; electromyographic studies show typical myopathic changes with reduced numbers of small amplitude polyphasic potentials. These abnormalities are more commonly noted in the proximal muscles (141).

Clinical findings of typical myasthenia gravis can be associated with hyperthyroidism. The pathophysiology of this association, however, is not well understood. It has been suggested that the neuromuscular transmission abnormality is secondary to a desensitization block at the postsynaptic membrane or to a conduction block at motor nerve terminals. Symptoms usually follow the onset of hyperthyroidism and sometimes thyroid storm. It does not necessarily follow that appropriate treatment of this thyroid disorder results in reversal of signs and symptoms of myasthenia, for some patients have worsening of symptoms when the hyperthyroidism has been controlled.

Typical clinical and laboratory findings of familial hypokalemic periodic paralysis rarely occurs in hyperthyroid children. The attacks, usually appearing during sleep or when at rest, are generally provoked by strenuous exercise, eating a meal rich in carbohydrates and salt, anesthesia, surgery, and menstruation. Serum potassium concentration falls below normal during the episode. With appropriate treatment, the hyperthyroid patient becomes euthyroid and there is cessation of the periodic paralytic episodes. If, however, hyperthyroidism recurs, the attacks may recur as well.

Episodic chorea or choreoathetosis are sometimes observed in hyperthyroidism; headaches are common and seizures sometimes occur.

CALCIUM DISORDERS

Serum calcium concentration is maintained within narrow limits by absorption of calcium from the small intestine, mediated by 1,25 $(OH)_2$ vitamin D (D), the reabsorption of calcium from the renal tubules, increased by 1,25 $(OH)_2D$, and by reabsorption of bone by osteoclasts stimulated by 1,25 $(OH)_2D$ and parathyroid hormone. Ionized calcium is the active factor in calcium metabolism, and a fall in ionized calcium stimulates the secretion of parathyroid hormone which increases the 1-alpha-hydroxylation of 25 (OH) D (142).

Hypocalcemia

Symptoms and signs of hypocalcemia are secondary to decreased stability of neural membranes including muscle cramps, weakness, lethargy, paresthesias of the extremities, and tetany. Laryngospasm and seizures can also occur. Three prominent signs indicating hypocalcemia include the

following: the Chvostek sign, a twitching of facial muscles at the angle of the mouth following a brisk tap over the area of the facial nerve; Trousseau sign, carpopedal spasms resulting from inflation of blood pressure cuff to at least 15 mm Hg above the systolic pressure; and the peroneal sign, a plantar flexion following tapping the peroneal nerve over the tibial prominence. Spasms of muscles ennervated by the autonomic nervous system can occur in the gastrointestinal tract, urinary bladder, and in cardiac muscle, resulting in prolongation of the QT interval on ECG. Convulsions and loss of consciousness may occur often without prior recognition of tetany. Seizures are commonly associated with generalized EEG abnormalities which usually revert to normal after hypocalcemia has been corrected. While tetany is a typical sign of hypocalcemia, it may also occur in hypokalemia, hypomagnesemia, and in respiratory alkalosis, when the ionized fraction of calcium falls because of enhanced protein binding. Other manifestations of hypocalcemia include intracranial calcification chiefly affecting the basal ganglia and dentate nuclei of the cerebellum, lenticular cataracts, brittleness of the nails, and poor dental enamel formation, particularly if hypocalcemia has been present from infancy. Pseudotumor cerebri is a recognized complication of hypocalcemia, as well as a variety of metabolic disorders.

Hypoparathyroidism

Hypocalcemia is a characteristic finding of hypoparathyroidism and results from either decreased parathyroid hormone (PTH) or lack of responsiveness of end organs to PTH (pseudohypoparathyroidism). Deficiency of the PTH may result from injury or the inadvertent removal of the parathyroid gland(s) during thyroid surgery or other surgical procedures involving the neck. Parathyroid abnormalities are commonly secondary to autoimmune disorders. Other causes include infection, glandular infiltration by granulomatous processes (that is, tuberculosis, sarcoid), or heavy metals (143). Congenital hypoparathyroidism has been described in defects of embryogenesis (DiGeorge syndrome) in which parathyroid hypoplasia is associated with thymic hypoplasia or aplasia and abnormalities of the heart and great vessels. One other congenital form of hypoparathyroidism is a genetically determined failure to secrete PTH, which is not associated with other anomalies.

Pseudohypoparathyroidism

This disorder is due to end-organ unresponsiveness to parathyroid hormone (PTH), and is inherited as an autosomal X-linked trait. In spite of elevated PTH serum concentrations, patients have hypocalcemia and may also develop hyperphosphatemia and calcification of the basal ganglia. These patients are typically short in stature, obese, and have round faces, short necks, cataracts, and brachydactyly. Metacarpal and metatarsal hypoplasia resulting in shortened 4th and 5th fingers and toes as well as subcutaneous calcifications can occur. The presence of elevated PTH concentrations (usually greater than 2 to 3 times normal) in the face of hypocalcemia should suggest the appropriate diagnosis; the lack of cAMP excretion after PTH administration is also a useful sign. As in hypoparathyroidism, the treatment includes the administration of high doses of vitamin D or an analogue, with additional calcium administration as needed.

Pseudopseudohypoparathyroidism shares the same phenotype as pseudohypoparathyroidism but the biochemical abnormalities are not present. Wilson disease can be associated with hypocalcemia and hyperphosphaturia due to parathyroid insufficiency, possibly secondary to copper deposition in the parathyroid glands (143).

Hypocalcemia Associated With Anticonvulsant Medication

It is well recognized that institutionalized children who receive long term administration of antiepileptic drugs (AED) have an increased incidence of osteomalacia with decreased bone width, bone pattern density, and bone salt density, resulting in an increased incidence of bony fractures. These patients have decreased serum calcium (total and ionized), 25 hydroxy vitamin D, but elevated parathyroid hormone and alkaline phosphatase. The defects characteristic of hypoparathyroidism are found in bed bound children who have not received AED, but the administration of these medications appears to emphasize the problem.

Anti-epileptic drugs, especially phenobarbital and the phenytoins, increase the metabolism of 25 (OH) D to more inactive, more highly polar metabolites, thereby reducing the supply of the substrate for 1-α-hydroxylase. There appears to be no difference in age, sex, physical activity, sunshine exposure, or dietary intake of vitamin D in both the osteomalacic and nonosteomalacic groups, but the length of time that the AED were administered was important, with 75% of institutionalized children having osteomalcia after 10 years of AED therapy (144,145). Treatment with 800 IU (20 μg) of vitamin D will assure correction of hypocalcemia and hypophosphatemia in these children, especially if calcium intake is safeguarded. Ambulation, when possible, also decreases the incidence of osteomalacia.

Hypercalcemic Disorders

Hypercalcemia is less common in children than in adults, primarily because the humoral hypercalcemia of malignancy is very rare in children. Hypercalcemia stabilizes neural membranes. The symptoms of hypercalcemia depend upon the serum calcium concentration since most patients with serum calcium levels below 11.55 to 12 mg/dL are asymptomatic. However, when serum calcium concentrations are higher, symptoms such as nausea, vomiting, anorexia, constipation (if the condition is chronic), weight loss, lethargy, weakness, inattentiveness, and depression become manifest. Hypercalcemia causes polyuria due to the inability to concentrate the urine. Stupor and coma may develop if serum calcium rises to more than 16 mg/dL.

Major clinical manifestations of hypercalcemia include dehydration, band keratopathy of the medial and lateral margins of the cornea, shortening of the QT interval of the ECG, hypercalciuria and nephrolithiasis, pancreatitis, peptic ulcer disease, and azotemia, which is related to polyuria, dehydration, nephrocalcinosis, and renal stones. Malaise and weakness, with electromyographic changes of myopathy have been reported. Stretch reflexes are increased.

Hypercalcinosis of Malignancy

Leukemia may cause hypercalcemia and erosion of bone. Children with Burkitt lymphoma have hypercalcemia due to the release of lymphokines which increase osteoclastic bony erosion and release of mineral from bone. Hypercalcemia lessens with the treatment of the malignancy.

Other Endocrine Disorders Causing Hypercalcemia

Patients with hyperthyroidism have an active bone turnover and enhanced resorption with the development of mild hypercalcemia. Adrenal insufficiency is associated with hypercalcemia which may be caused by increased intestinal calcium absorption. Glucocorticoid therapy reverses the hypercalcemia.

Familial hypocalciuric hypercalcemia is a rare autosomal dominant trait associated with benign symptoms even though serum calcium values rise to 15.0 mg/dL. Affected children have inappropriately decreased urine excretion for the level of hypercalcemia.

Miscellaneous

Immobilization hypercalcemia occurs in patients who are confined to bed and are not weight bearing, when there is enhanced bone resorption and diminished bone formation. William syndrome is characterized by transient hypercalcemia of fetal life or infancy, elfin facies, short stature, cocktail patter conversation, combined with mental deficiency and supravalvular aortic stenosis (146). At the time of diagnosis, the period of hypercalcemia may already have passed.

ANTIEPILEPTIC DRUG EFFECTS ON ENDOCRINE FUNCTION

Valproic acid has been reported to decrease gonadotropin secretion in the basal state and after gonadotropin releasing factor administration, but to have no effect on pubertal development. There is also a suggestion that growth hormone secretion and growth may be affected by valproate therapy, but follow-up studies are needed to confirm or deny this.

Phenytoin can lower T_4 into the hypothyroid range, possibly by increasing conversion of T_4 to T_3 and, thereby, maintaining normal T_3 and TSH concentrations. Phenytoin also competes with T_4 for binding to thyroid binding globulin.

Phenobarbital also inhibits the binding of T_4 to its TBG in vitro, but probably does not exert such an effect in vivo. However, it is capable of increasing the metabolic clearance rate of T_4 and thereby worsening, in hypothyroid patients, serum T_4 concentrations.

Carbamazepine lowers serum thyroxine and triiodothyronine in previously euthyroid patients, but does not change TSH concentrations; patients remain clinically euthyroid so that thyroid treatment does not appear warranted unless TSH increases. Hypothyroid patients, however, may need a larger replacement dose of thyroxine after the onset of carbamazepine therapy (147,148). The findings observed might be due to accelerated T_4 metabolic clearance together with augmented T_4 to T_3 conversion rate, as previously demonstrated for phenytoin.

Vasopressin secretion can be decreased by phenytoin and increased by phenobarbital and carbamazepine. Phenytoin also decreases ACTH release and insulin secretion.

STIMULANT DRUGS AND GROWTH

Dextroamphetamine, methylphenidate, and pemoline can inhibit linear growth in a dose-dependent manner. The etiology is not known. One method of minimizing the effect is taking "vacations" from therapy on weekends or during the summer. Some catch-up growth is possible but there will likely be permanent impairment of height after long-term treatment.

REFERENCES

1. Styne DM. Growth. In: Styne DM. Pediatric Endocrinology for the House Officer. Baltimore: Williams & Wilkins, 1988;1–28.
2. Styne DM. Growth. In: Greenspan FS, ed. Basic and Clinical Endocrinology. Los Altos: Lange Medical Publications, 1991;147–176.
3. Preece MA. The insulin-like growth factors. In: Styne DM, Brook CGD, eds. Current Concepts in Pediatric Endocrinology. New York: Elsevier, 1987;155–183.
4. Lovinger RD, Kaplan SL, Grumbach MM. Congenital hypopituitarism associated with neonatal hypoglycemia and microphallus: Four cases secondary to hypothalamic hormone deficiences. J Pediatr 1975;87:1171–1181.
5. Patel H, Tze WJ, Crichton JU, et al. Optic nerve hypoplasia with hypopituitarism. Am J Dis Child 1975;129:175–180.
6. Braga S, Phillips JA III, Joss E, et al. Familial growth hormone deficiency resulting from 7.6 kb deletion within the growth hormone cluster. Am J Med Genet 1986; 25:443–452.
7. Roche AF, Wainer H, Thissen D. The RWT method for the prediction of adult stature. Pediatrics 1975;56:1026–1033.
8. Kaplan SA. Growth and Growth Hormone: Disorders of the Anterior Pituitary. In: Kaplan SA, ed. Clinical Pediatric Endocrinology. Philadelphia: WB Saunders, 1990;1–62.
9. Rosenthal SM. Synthetic human pancreas growth hormone releasing factor (hpGRF[1–44]-NH₂) stimulates growth hormone secretion in normal men. J Clin Endocrinol Metab 1983;57:677–679.
10. Koch TK, Berg BO, DeArmond SJ, et al. Creutzfeldt-Jacob disease in a young adult with idiopathic hypopituitarism: Possible relationship to administration of cadaveric human growth hormone. N Engl J Med 1985;313:731–733.
11. Brown P. Growth hormone therapy and Creutzfeldt-Jacob disease: A drama in three acts. Pediatrics 1988;81:85–92.
12. Tinter R, Brown P, Hedley-White ET, et al. Neuropathologic verification of Creutzfeld-Jacob disease in the exhumed American recipient of human pituitary growth hormone: Epidemiologic and pathogenetic implications. Neurology 1986;36:932–936.
13. Herber SM, Dunsmore IR, Milner RD. Final stature in brain tumors other than craniopharyngioma: Effect of growth hormone. Horm Res 1985;22:63–67.
14. Thorner MO, Reschke J, Chitwood J, et al. Acceleration of growth in two children treated with human growth hormone releasing factor. N Engl J Med 1985;312:4–9.
15. Clayton PE, Shalet SM, Gattamaneni HR, et al. Does growth hormone cause relapse of brain tumors? Lancet 1987; 1(8535):711–713.
16. Prader A, Labhart A, Willi H. Ein Syndrom von Adipositas: Kleinwuchs, Kryptorchismus und Oligophrenie nach myatonieartigem Zustand in Neugeborenenalter. Schweiz Med Wochenschr 1956;86:1260–1261.
17. Jeffcoate WJ, Laurance BM, Edwards CR, et al. Endocrine function in the Prader-Willi syndrome. Clin Endocrinol 1980;12:81–89.
18. Kauli R, Prager-Lewin R, Laron Z. Pubertal development in the Prader-Labhart-Willi syndrome. Acta Paediatr Scand 1978;67:763–767.
19. Wannarachue N, Ruvalcaba RH. Hypogonadism in Prader-Willi syndrome. Am J Ment Defic 1975;79: 592–603.
20. Lee PD, Wilson DM, Rountree L, et al. Linear growth response to exogenous growth hormone in Prader-Willi syndrome. Am J Med Genet 1987;28:865–871.
21. Laurenc JZ, Moon RC. Four cases of retinitis pigmentosa occurring in the same family and accompanied by general imperfections of development. Ophthamol Rev 1966;2:32.

22. Perez-Palacios G, Uribe M, Scaglia H, et al. Pituitary and gonadal function in patients with the Laurence-Moon-Biedl Syndrome. Acta Endocrinol 1977;84:191–199.

23. Russell A. A diencephalic syndrome of emaciation in infancy and childhood. Arch Dis Child 1951;26:274.

24. Sotos JF, Dodge PR, Muirhead D, et al. Cerebral gigantism in childhood. N Engl J Med 1964;271:109–116.

25. Senior B. Lipodystrophic muscular hypertrophy. Arch Dis Child 1961;36:426–431.

26. Grumbach MM, Styne DM. Puberty. In: Wilson JD, Foster D, eds. Williams Textbook of Endocrinology. Philadelphia: W.B. Saunders (in press).

27. Styne DM, Grumbach MM. Puberty in the male and female: Its physiology and disorders. In: Yen SSC, Jaffe RB, eds. Reproductive Endocrinology: Physiology, Pathophysiology, and Clinical Management. Philadelphia: WB Saunders, 1991;511–554.

28. Marshall WA, Tanner JM. Variations in the pattern of pubertal changes in girls. Arch Dis Child 1969;44:291–303.

29. Marshall WA, Tanner JM. Variations in the pattern of pubertal changes in boys. Arch Dis Child 1970;45:13–23.

30. Styne DM. Puberty. In: Greenspan FS, ed. Basic and Clinical Endocrinology, third edition. Los Altos: Lange Medical Publications, 1991;519–542.

31. Rieth KG, Comite F, Dwyer AJ, et al. CT of cerebral abnormalities in precocious puberty. AJR 1987;148:1231–1238.

32. Cacciari E, Frejaville E, Cicognani A, et al. How many cases of true precocious puberty in girls are idiopathic? J Pediatr 1983;102:357–360.

33. Sockalosky JJ, Kriel RL, Krach LE, et al. Precocious puberty after traumatic brain injury. J Pediatr 1987;110:373–377.

34. DiGeorge AM. Albright's syndrome: Is it coming of age? J Pediatr 1975;87:1018–1020.

35. Huseman CA, Kelch RP, Hopwood NJ, et al. Sexual precocity in association with septo-optic dysplasia and hypothalamic hypopituitarism. J Pediatr 1978;92:748–753.

36. Styne DM, Harris DA, Egli CA, et al. Treatment of true precocious puberty with a potent luteinizing hormone releasing factor agonist: Effect on growth, sexual maturation, pelvic sonography, and the hypothalamic-pituitary-gonadal axis. J Clin Endocrinol Metab 1985;61:142–151.

37. Pescovitz OH, Comite F, Hench K, et al. The NIH experience with precocious puberty: Diagnostic subgroups and response to short-term luteinizing hormone releasing hormone analogue therapy. J Pediatr 1986;108:47–54.

38. Grumbach MM, Kaplan SL. Recent advances in the diagnosis and management of sexual precocity. Acta Ped Japonica 1988; 30 (suppl):155–175.

39. Levine LS, Novogroder M, Saxena B, et al. Primary intracranial HCG-producing germinoma in a boy with congenital adrenal hyperplasia. Acta Endocrinol (Copenh) 1978; 88:122–131.

40. Cantu JM, Scaglia HE, Medina M, et al. Inherited congenital normofunctional testicular hyperplasia and mental deficiency. Hum Genet 1976;33:23–33.

41. Styne DM. Puberty. In: Styne DM, ed. Pediatric Endocrinology for the House Officer. Baltimore: Williams & Wilkins, 1988;49–70.

42. Dean HJ, Bishop A, Winter JS. Growth hormone deficiency in patients with histiocytosis X. Acta Endocrinol 1986; 113:145–152.

43. Merriam GR, Beitins IZ, Bode HH. Father-to-son transmission of hypogonadism with anosmia: Kallman's syndrome. Am J Dis Child 1977;131:1216–1219.

44. Matthews WB, Rundle RT. Familial cerebellar ataxia and hypogonadism. Brain 1964;87:463–468.

45. Bellastella A, Criscuolo T, Sinisi AA, et al. Influence of blindness on plasma luteinizing hormone, follicle-stimulating hormone, prolactin, and testosterone levels in prepubertal boys. J Clin Endocrinol Metab 1987;64:862–864.

46. Zadik Z, Levin S, Prager-Lewin R, et al. Gonadal dysfunction in patients with ataxia telangiectasia. Acta Paediatr Scand 1978;67:477–479.

47. Thomsett MJ, Conte FA, Kaplan SL, et al. Endocrine and neurologic outcome in childhood craniopharyngioma: Review of effect of treatment in 42 patients. J Pediatr 1980; 97:728–735.

48. Baskin DS, Wilson CB. Surgical management of craniopharyngioma: Review of effect of treatment in 42 patients. J Neurosurg 1986;65:22–27.

49. Dayan AD, Marshall AHE, Miller AA, et al. Atypical teratomas of the pineal gland and hypothalamus. J Pathol Bacteriol 1966;92:1.

50. Sklar CA, Grumbach MM, Kaplan SL, et al. Hormonal and metabolic abnormalities associated with central nervous system germinoma in children and adolescents and the effect of therapy: Report of 10 patients. J Clin Endocrinol Metab 1981;52:9–16.

51. Pomarede R, Czernichow P, Finidori J, et al. Endocrine aspects and tumoral markers in intracranial germinoma: An attempt to delineate the diagnostic procedure in 14 patients. J Pediatr 1982; 101:374–378.

52. Pasztor E, Remenar L. Optic nerve gliomas. Acta Neurochir 1978;41:191–203.

53. Gluckman PD, Holdaway IM. Prolactin and somatomedin studies in the syndrome of growth hormone-independent growth. Clin Endocrinol 1976;5:545–549.

54. Hoyt WF, Kaplan SL, Grumbach MM, et al. Septo-optic dysplasia with pituitary dwarfism. Lancet 1970;1:893–894.

55. Arslanian SA, Rothfus WE, Foley TP Jr, et al. Hormonal, metabolic, and neuroradiologic abnormalities associated with septo-optic dysplasia. Acta Endocrinol 1984; 107: 282–288.

56. Costigan DC, Daneman D, Harwood-Nash D, et al. The empty sella in childhood. Clin Pediatr 1984;23:437–440.

57. Richards GE, Wara WM, Grumbach MM, et al. Delayed onset of hypopituitarism: Sequelae of the therapeutic irradiation of central nervous system tumors. J Pediatr 1976; 89:553–559.

58. Oberfield SE, Kirkland JL, Frantz A, et al. Growth hormone response to GRF 1–44 in children following cranial irradiation for central nervous system tumors. Am J Pediatr Hematol Oncol 1987;9:233–238.

59. Oberfield SE, Allen JC, Pollack J, et al. Long-term endocrine sequelae after treatment of medulloblastoma: Prospective study of growth and thyroid function. J Pediatr 1986; 108: 219–223.

60. Winter RJ, Green OC. Irradiation induced growth hormone deficiency: Blunted growth response and accelerated skeletal maturation to growth hormone therapy. J Pediatr 1985;106: 609–612.

61. Lustig RH, Schriock EA, Kaplan SL, et al. Effect of growth hormone-releasing factor on growth hormone release in children with radiation-induced growth hormone deficiency. Pediatrics 1985;76:274–279.

62. Clayton PE, Shalet SM, Price DA, et al. The role of growth hormone in stunted head growth after cranial irradiation. Pediatr Res 1987;22:402–404.

63. Shalet S. Irradiation-induced growth failure. Clin Endocrinol Metab 1986;15:591–606.

64. Miller WL, Kaplan SL, Grumbach MM. Child abuse as a cause of post-traumatic hypopituitarism. N Engl J Med 1980;302:724–728.

65. Shapiro WR, Williams GH Jr, Plum F. Spontaneous recurrent hypothermia accompanying agenesis of the corpus callosum. Brain 1969;92:423–436.

66. Bongiovanni AM. Prolactin: A review with pediatric clinical implications. Adv Pediatr 1985;32:349–368.

67. Bye AM, Nunn KP, Wilson J. Prolactin and seizure activity. Arch Dis Child 1985; 60:848–851.

68. Laxer KD, Mullooly JP, Howell B. Prolactin changes after seizures classified by EEG monitoring. Neurology 1985; 35:31–35.

69. Matsumura H, Nakazawa S, Wakabayashi I. Thyrotropin-releasing hormone provocative release of prolactin and thyrotropin in acute head injury. Neurosurgery 1985; 16:791–795.

70. Styne DM. Vasopressin metabolism. In: Styne DM, ed. Pediatric Endocrinology for the House Officer. Baltimore: Williams & Wilkins, 1988;82–91.

71. Scherbaum WA, Wass JA, Besser GM, et al. Autoimmune cranial diabetes insipidus: Its association with other endocrine diseases and with histiocytosis X. Clin Endocrinol 1986;4:411–420.

72. Hayek A, Peake GT. Hypothalamic adipsia without demonstrable structural lesion. Pediatrics 1982;70:275–278.

73. Frasier SD, Kutnik LA, Schmidt RT, et al. A water deprivation test for the diagnosis of diabetes insipidus in children. Am J Dis Child 1967;114:157–160.

74. Kaplan SL, Feigin RD. The syndrome of inappropriate secretion of antidiuretic hormone in children with bacterial meningitis. J Pediatr 1978;82:758–761.

75. Styne DM. Adrenal Gland. In: Styne DM, ed. Pediatric Endocrinology for the House Officer. Baltimore: Williams & Wilkins, 1988;71–81.

76. Styne DM. Treatment of Cushing's Disease in childhood and adolescence by transsphenoidal microadenomectomy. N Engl J Med 1984;309:889–893.

77. Afifi A, Bergman RA, Harvey JC. Steroid myopathy. Clinical, histologic and cytologic observations. Johns Hopkins Med J 1968;123:158–174.

78. Hapwood NJ, Kenny FM. Incidence of Nelson's syndrome after adrenalectomy for Cushing disease in children. Am J Dis Child 1977;131:1353.

79. Kloti J, Fanconi S, Zachmann M, et al. Dexamethasone therapy and cortisol excretion in severe pediatric head injury. Childs Nerv Syst 1987;3:103–105.

80. Van Dop C, Conte FA, Koch TK, et al. Pseudotumor cerebri associated with initiation of levothyroxine therapy for juvenile hypothyroidism. N Engl J Med 1983;308:1076–1080.

81. Zadik Z, Barak Y, Stager D, et al. Pseudotumor cerebri in a boy with 11-beta-hydroxylase deficiency—A possible relation to rapid steroid withdrawal. Childs Nerv Syst 1985;1:179–181.

82. Weissman MN, Page LK, Bejar RL. Cushing's disease in childhood: Benign intracranial hypertension after transsphenoidal adenomectomy. Neurosurgery 1983;13:195–198.

83. Lewis DA, Smith RE. Steroid-induced psychiatric syndromes. A report of 14 cases and a review of the literature. J Affective Disord 1983;5:319–332.

84. Robinson RO. Seizures and steroids. Arch Dis Childhood 1985;60:94–95.

85. Lagenstein I, Willig RP, Kuhne D. Cranial computed tomography (CCT) findings in children treated with ACTH and dexamethasone: First results. Neuropaediatrie 1979; 10:370–384.

86. Satoh J, Takeshige H, Hara H, et al. Brain shrinkage and subdural effusion associated with ACTH administration. Brain Dev 1982;4:13–20.

87. Futagi Y, Abe J, Kawahigashi K. Cerebral blood flow and brain shrinkage seen on CT during ACTH therapy. Brain Dev 1984;8:566–600.

88. Ross DL. Suppressed pituitary ACTH response after ACTH treatment of infantile spasms. J Child Neurol 1986;1:34–37.

89. Matsumoto A, Kumagi T, Takeuchi T, et al. Clinical effects of thyrotropin-releasing hormone for severe epilepsy in childhood: A comparative study with ACTH therapy. Epilepsia 1987;28:49–55.

90. Schilder P. Zur Kenntnis der sogennanten diffusen Sklerose. Z Gesamte Neurol Psychiatr 1912;10:1–60.

91. Schilder P. Zur Frage der Encephalitis periaxialis diffusa. Z Gesamte Neurol Psychiatr 1913;15:359–376.

92. Schilder P. Die Encephalitis periaxialis diffusa. Arch Psychiatr Nervenkr 1924;71:327–356.

93. Lumsden C. Fundamental problems in the pathology of multiple sclerosis and allied demyelinating diseases. Br Med J 1951;1:1035–1043.

94. Poser CM, van Bogaert L. The natural history and evolution of the concept of Schilder's diffuse sclerosis. Acta Neuropathol Scand 1956;31:285–331.

95. Poser C, Goutieres F, Carpentier M, et al. Schilder's myelinoclastic diffuse sclerosis. Pediatrics 1986;77:107–112.

96. Siemerling E, Creutzfeldt HC. Bronzekrankheit und sklerorierende Encephalomyelitis (diffuse Sclerose). Arch Psychiatr 1923;668:217–244.

97. Blaw ME. Melanodermic type leukodystrophy (Adrenoleukodystrophy). In: Vinken PJ, Bruyn GW, eds. Handbook of Clinical Neurology. New York: American Elsevier, 1970; 10:128–133.

98. Powers JM, Schaumburg HH. Adrenoleukodystrophy: Similar ultrastructural changes in adrenal cortex cells and Schwann cells. Arch Neurol 1974;30:406–408.

99. Aubourg PR, Sack GH, Moser HW. Frequent alterations of visual pigment genes in adrenoleukodystrophy. Am J Hum Genet 1988;42:408–414.

100. Igarashi M, Schaumburg HH, Powers JM, et al. Fatty acid abnormality in adrenoleukodystrophy. J Neurochem 1976;26:851–860.

101. Menkes JH, Corbo LM. Adrenoleukodystrophy: Accumulation of cholesterol esters with very long chain fatty acids. Neurology 1977;27:929–932.

102. Molzer B, Bernheimer H, Budka H, et al. Accumulation of very long chain fatty acids is common to 3 variants of adrenoleukodystrophy (ALD): Classical ALD, atypical ALD (female patient) and adrenomyeloneuropathy. J Neurol Sci 1981;51:301–310.

103. Ramsey RB, Banik NL, Davison AN. Adrenoleukodystrophy; brain cholesterol esters and other neutral lipids. J Neurol Sci 1977;32:69–77.

104. Kobayashi T, Katayama M, Suzuki S, et al. Adrenoleukodystrophy: Detection of increased very long chain fatty acids by high-performance liquid chromatography. J Neurol 1983;230:209–215.

105. Molzer B, Bernheimer H, Heller R, et al. Detection of adrenoleukodystrophy by increased C 26:0 fatty acid levels in leukocytes. Clin Chim Acta 1982;125:299–305.

106. Moser HW, Moser AE, Frayer KK, et al. Adrenoleukodystrophy: Increased plasma content of saturated very long chain fatty acids. Neurology 1981;31:1241–1249.

107. Moser HW, Moser AE, Kawamura N, et al. Adrenoleukodystrophy: Elevated C 26 fatty acid in cultured skin fibroblasts. Ann Neurol 1980;7:542–549.

108. Tolbert E. Metabolic pathways in peroxisomes and glyoxysomes. Annu Rev Biochem 1981;50:133–157.

109. Moser HW. Peroxisomal disorders. J Pediatr 1986;108:89–91.

110. Schaumburg HH, Powers JH, Raine CS, et al. Adrenoleukodystrophy: A clinical and pathological study of 17 cases. Arch Neurol 1975;32:577–591.

111. Chemke J, Lieberman E, Carmi R, et al. Adrenoleukodystrophy in Israel: A genetic, clinical, and biochemical study. Isr J Med Sci 1984;20:1123–1132.

112. Moser HW, Moser AE, Kawamura AN, et al. Adrenoleukodystrophy. Studies of the phenotype, genetics, and biochemistry. Johns Hopkins Med J 1980;147:217–224.

113. Moser HW, Moser AE, Singh I, et al. Adrenoleukodystrophy: Survey of 303 cases: biochemistry, diagnosis, and therapy. Ann Neurol 1984;16:628–641.

114. Aubourg P, Chaussain JL, Dulac O, et al. Adrenoleukodystrophy; its diverse CT appearances and an evolutive or phenotypic variant: The leukodystrophy without adrenal insufficiency. Neuroradiology 1982;24:33–42.

115. Griffin JW, Goren E, Schaumburg HH, et al. Adrenomyeloneuropathy: A probably variant of adrenoleukodystrophy; clinical and endocrinological aspects. Neurology 1977;27:1107–1113.

116. O'Neill BP, Marmion LC, Feringa ER. The adrenomyeloneuropathy complex; expression in four generations. Neurology 1981;31:151–156.

117. Ulrich J, Herschkowitz N, Heitz P, et al. Adrenoleukodystrophy: Preliminary report of a connatal case. Acta Neuropathol 1978;43:77–83.

118. Jaffe R. Crumrine, Hassida Y, et al. Neonatal adrenoleukodystrophy: Clinical, pathological, and biochemical delineation of a syndrome affecting both male and females. Am J Pathol 1982;108:100–111.

119. Aubourg P, Chaussain JL, Dulac O, et al. Adrenoleucodystrophie chez l'enfant: A propos de 20 observations. Arch Fr Pediatr 1982;39:663–669.

120. Kelley RI, Datta NS, Dobyns WB, et al. Neonatal adrenoleukodystrophy: New cases, biochemical studies and differentiation from Zellweger and related peroxisomal polydystrophy syndromes. Am J Med Genet 1986;23:869–901.

121. O'Neill BP, Moser HW, Saxena KM, et al. Adrenoleukodystrophy: Clinical and biochemical manifestations in carriers. Neurology 1984;34:798–801.

122. Ehrich E, Aranoff G, Johnson WG. Familial achalasia associated with adrenocorticol insufficiency, alacrima, and neurological abnormalities. Am J Med Genet 1987;26:637–644.

123. Voorhess ML. Adrenal medulla, sympathetic nervous system, and multiple endocrine adenomatosis. In: Rudolph AM, ed. Pediatrics. Los Altos: Appleton & Lange, 1991;1614–1620.

124. Dyck PJ, Carney JA, Sizemore GW, et al. Multiple endocrine neoplasia, type 2b: Phenotype recognition; neurological features and their pathological basis. Ann Neurol 1979;6:302–314.

125. Richardson JE, Hamilton W. Diabetes insipidus, diabetes mellitus, optic atrophy, and deafness. 3 cases of 'DIDMOAD' syndrome. Arch Dis Child 1977;52:796–798.

126. Krane EJ, Rockoff MA, Wallman JK, et al. Subclinical brain swelling in children during treatment of diabetic ketoacidosis. N Engl J Med 1985;312:1147–1151.

127. Eeg-Olofsson O, Petersen I. Childhood diabetic neuropathy. Acta Paediatr Scand 1966;53:163–167.

128. Cracco J, Castrella S, Mark E. Spinal somatosensory evoked potentials in juvenile diabetics. Ann Neurol 1984;15:545–558.

129. MacDonald JT, Brown BR. Acute hemiparesis in juvenile insulin-dependent mellitus (JIDDM). Neurology 1979;29:893–896.

130. Pleet AB, Saphier DJ, O'Doherty DS. Neurologic manifestations of endocrine disturbances. In: Baker AB, Baker LH, eds. Clinical Neurology. Philadelphia: Harper & Row, 1985.

131. Styne DM. Thyroid Gland. In: Styne DM, ed. Pediatric Endocrinology for the House Officer. Baltimore: Williams & Wilkins, 1988;92–107.

132. Smith DW, Blizzard RM, Wilkins L. The mental prognosis in hypothyroidism of infancy and childhood. Pediatrics 1957;91:1011–1022.

133. Debre R, Semelaigne G. Syndrome of diffuse muscular hypertrophy in infants causing an athletic appearance: Its connection with congenital myxedema. Am J Dis Child 1935;50:1351–1361.

134. Afifi AK, Najjar SS, Mire-Salman J, et al. The myopathy of Kocher-Debre-Semelaigne syndrome. J Neurol Sci 1974;22:445–470.

135. Ramsay ID. Thyroid Diseases and Muscle Dysfunction. Chicago: Year Book, 1974.

136. Scarpalezos S, Lygidakis C, Papageorgiou C, et al. Neural and muscular manifestations of hypothyroidism. Arch Neurol 1973;29:140–144.

137. Pueschel SM, Pezzullo JC. Thyroid dysfunction in Down syndrome. Am J Dis Child 1985;139:307–310.

138. Ilyes I, Tornai A, Kirilina S, et al. Influence of anticonvulsant drugs on thyroid hormones in epileptic children. Acta Paediatr Hung 1985;26:307–310.

139. Bender MB, Rudolph SH, Stacy CGB. The neurology of the visual and oculomotor systems. In: Baker AB, Baker LH, eds. Clinical Neurology. Philadelphia: Harper & Row, 1985;102.

140. Mosier HD. Hyperthyroidism. In: Gardner LI, ed. Endocrine and Genetic Diseases of Childhood. Baltimore: W.B. Saunders, 1975.

141. Fenichel GM, Swaiman KF, Wright FS. Neuromuscular disease. In: Swaiman KF, Wright FS, eds. The Practice of Pediatric Neurology. St. Louis: CV Mosby, 1982;1139.

142. Chesney RW. Calcium metabolism. In: Styne DM, ed. Pediatric Endocrinology for the House Officer. Baltimore: Williams & Wilkins, 1988;108–121.

143. Carpenter TO, Carnes DL Jr, Anast CS. Hypoparathyroidism in Wilson's disease. N Engl J Med 1983;309:873–877.

144. Tolman KG, Jubiz W, Sannella JJ, et al. Osteomalacia associated with anticonvulsant drug therapy in mentally retarded children. Pediatrics 1975;56:45–50.

145. Nishiyama S, Kuwahara T, Matsuda I. Decreased bone density in severely handicapped children and adults, with reference to the influence of limited mobility and anticonvulsant medication. Eur J Pediatr 1986;144:457–463.

146. Friedman WF, Mills LF. The relationship between vitamin D and the craniofacial and central anomalies of the supravalvular aortic stenosis syndrome. Pediatrics 1969;43:12–18.

147. Strandjord RE, Aanderud S, Myking OL, et al. Influence of carbamazepine on serum thyroxine and triiodothyronine in patients with epilepsy. Acta Neurol Scand 1981;63: 111–121.

148. De Luca F, Arrigo T, Pandullo E, et al. Changes in thyroid function tests induced by 2 month carbamazepine treatment in L-thyroxine-substituted hypothyroid children. Eur J Pediatr 1986;145:77–79.

Chapter 22
Disorders of Connective Tissue and Bone

Ian J. Butler

Connective tissue and bone are of mesodermal origin and are closely related anatomically to the central and peripheral nervous systems. In the central nervous system (CNS), these mesodermal elements have a supportive and protective role; thus, the brain is surrounded by the bony cranium and the spinal cord and nerve roots by the vertebral column. These bones are joined together by internal and external ligaments. Flexibility of the articulated, neural-related skeleton is enabled by the fibrocartilaginous intervertebral disks and by movement at joints. Although the supportive and protective roles of connective tissue and bone are not as obvious for the peripheral nervous system as the CNS, nerves exit through various bony and fibrous foramina before their termination. Finally, the other tissue components of mesodermal origin important in nervous system function are the vascular conduits, both arteries and veins.

In any discussion of the impact of disorders of connective tissue and bone on the nervous system, it is of practical significance to decide whether bone, connective tissue, or both elements are primarily involved in causing the neurologic deficit. Encroachment on nervous tissue by bone may be treated by surgical removal of the compressing structure; whereas, spinal instability due to ligamentous laxity may be managed best by fusion of bones. In many conditions both elements are affected and a combination of surgical excision and stabilization may be necessary.

Simply stated the neural skeleton is externally and internally surrounded by periosteum. Internally and intimately apposed to periosteum is the dura mater, which surrounds the brain and continues into the spinal canal as the dural sac, ending in the upper sacral region. Furthermore, the dura mater gives rise to dural sheaths of nerve roots exiting from the CNS as cranial and spinal nerves. Within the dura, and separated by the subdural space, lie the leptomeninges, the arachnoid and pia mater. The leptomeninges surround the brain and spinal cord and permit circulation of cerebrospinal fluid (CSF) around nervous tissue in the subarachnoid spaces.

For many of the conditions to be discussed, the diagnosis is based on clinical criteria; however, for an increasing number of the syndromes there are specific enzymatic or molecular and genetic defects that have been identified (1). Bone disorders usually present with shortness of stature (dwarfism), skeletal deformities, or both. Shortness of stature is usually due to shortened limbs and sometimes a short trunk due to flattened vertebrae (platyspondyly). Vertebral abnormalities lead to a bent (lordosis, kyphosis) or twisted (scoliosis) spine, and limb deformities secondary to bowing (for example, genu varus or valgum). Other significant bony anomalies in these patients include a large head (macrocranium), frontal bossing, prominent nasal bridge, high palate, chest deformities (pectus carinatum or excavatum) and abnormally shaped joints and bones. Radiographic studies are frequently of diagnostic importance in these disorders.

Connective tissue disorders may present with a wide spectrum of symptoms and signs given the ubiquitous nature of this mesodermal tissue. Pathologic processes include increased ligamentous length (ligamentous laxity, joint dislocation, mitral valve prolapse, and lens dislocation), connective tissue thinning (blue sclerae, diaphragmatic and abdominal hernia), and connective tissue weakness (spontaneous pneumothorax, subarachnoid, and extradural spinal arachnoid cysts). Blood vessels, including arteries, veins, and venous sinuses are of mesodermal origin and anatomically closely related to bones, joints, and nervous tissue and can be involved in pathologic processes (compression, aneurysmal dilatation).

Although cognitive changes may be present clinically, the primary or secondary relationship to the underlying defects of mesenchymal tissue (bone or connective tissue) is sometimes difficult to assess (2).

ACHONDROPLASIA

The skeletal dysplasia known as achondroplasia is the best known and commonest form of congenital short-limbed dwarfism. The disorder has been recognized for some 5,000 years and achondroplasts are represented in Egyptian statues in museums, in paintings by Valasquez, and in the literature of Charles Dickens. Achondroplasts were gladiators in Roman times, court jesters in medieval history, and wrestlers or circus clowns in modern times (3).

Achondroplasia, a disorder of endochondral bone formation that is apparent at birth, affects 1 in 26,000 liveborn infants (4). The disorder is inherited as an autosomal dominant trait, although in most patients achondroplasia occurs sporadically as a new mutation. Dwarfs frequently marry other dwarfs and should both have achondroplasia, there will be a 25% risk of a homozygous offspring having a severe and lethal form of achondroplasia (5).

The neurologic complications of achondroplasia have been recognized in adults for more than half a century (6–8), and can usually be attributed to a defect in bone formation, connective tissue structures, or in both tissues. More recently similar neurologic complications have been recognized in infants, young children, and teenagers with achondroplasia (9,10). Defective endochondral bone ossification leads to a small, abnormally shaped foramen magnum and a vertebral skeleton with short vertebral pedicles and narrow spinal canal. The narrowing of the spinal canal may be particularly apparent due to the relative increase in size of the spinal cord at the cervical and lumbar enlargements. Various foramina may be narrowed and compress structures passing through the bone. The internal jugular vein can be compressed in the jugular foramen at the base of the skull, and exiting spinal nerves compressed by narrowing at the intervertebral neural foramina. Occasionally defective vertebral column alignment leads to scoliosis, kyphoscoliosis, lumbar gibbus deformity, and severe lordosis that can compress the spinal canal contents including the spinal cord and cauda equina. Defective connective tissue elements in achondroplasia frequently lead to ligamentous laxity and subsequent joint dislocation. In peripheral joints, this instability and malalignment can contribute to delayed motor development so frequently observed in

achondroplasia (11). Within the CNS the ligamentous laxity at the atlantooccipital and atlantoaxial joints of the craniocervical junction can cause sufficient joint instability to compromise the medulla oblongata and upper cervical cord. Instant death, apnea, acute, subacute and chronic spastic quadriparesis can be a complication of joint instability at the craniocervical junction. The combination of joint instability with excessive movement in an area already narrowed by abnormal bone formation can lead to devastating compression of the medulla and upper cervical cord.

Achondroplasia is a prototypic disorder to study since both bone and connective tissue are affected. Advances in our understanding of the disease during the last decade have depended in part on advances in neuroradiology (computed tomography [CT] and magnetic resonance imaging [MRI]) and diagnostic electrophysiology (sleep studies using polysomnography and cortical evoked responses). As the result of a multidisciplinary approach to this multisystem disorder, several groups have proposed and documented mechanistic explanations for complications of achondroplasia and particularly those related to the nervous system (9,10). This pragmatic approach has permitted management directed at the altered physiology and includes surgical decompression, spine stabilization, respiratory airway enlargement, and treatment of cor pulmonale. Specific treatments will be discussed in more detail in an order that approximates the chronologic presentation of symptoms and signs to the physician (Table 22.1).

Developmental Delay

Psychomotor delays in infants with achondroplasia have been frequently observed (11) and are usually attributed to a relatively large head for body size, causing head lag, and skeletal abnormalities, including ligamentous laxity at various joints, causing delayed sitting and standing. Although these explanations may be generally acceptable to explain failure to walk until the age of two years, neurologic factors may be operative and hypotonia can be secondary to myelopathy rather than ligamentous laxity.

Table 22.1   Neurologic complications of achondroplasia

Developmental delay	Large head, ligamentous laxity, myelopathy
Craniovertebral junction	Small foramen magnum, abnormal atlantoaxial joint
Vertebral canal stenosis	Abnormal vertebral skeleton
Hydrocephalus	Communicating and non-communicating types
Vertebral column misalignment	Scoliosis, kyphosis, lordosis, gibbus deformity
Nerve root compression	Occipital nerve, spinal nerve compression

In order to detect an underlying neurologic cause for the motor delay, centers evaluating many achondroplasts have initiated a multidisciplinary approach to follow patients with achondroplasia once the diagnosis has been confirmed genetically and radiologically (9,10). Frequent evaluations every 6 months during the first few years of life by a child neurologist or developmental pediatrician will assist in the identification of those patients who develop a high cervical myelopathy with quadriparesis, contributing to the motor impairment. Neurologic findings may be subtle and the detection of motor problems difficult to discern during these first few years of life. The neurologic assessment at this age can be supplemented after the age of 3 months by routine studies of somatosensory evoked responses (13).

On occasion there is concern that psychomotor delay of the achondroplast may be secondary to impaired intelligence (12). These children, however, usually have a normal range of intelligence unless there are neurologic complications related to hydrocephalus, head injury from falling readily, or impaired respiratory function such as sleep apnea with hypoxemia. Impaired receptive language skills have been attributed to the increased frequency of serous otitis media. Hearing impairment and articulation problems in young achondroplasts may be related to the mid-face hypoplasia of the disease.

Vertebral Canal Stenosis

Vertebrae of the spinal canal are also involved in the disordered endochondral bone ossification observed in achondroplasia. Although there are defects of the vertebral bodies, including wedged vertebrae and a posterior central bony spur, most of the problems are secondary to the short pedicles and narrowing of the interpediculate distances, with canal stenosis at all levels of the vertebral column. At the levels of the cervical and lumbar enlargement of the cord, this bony narrowing can potentially compress the spinal cord and nerve roots of the cauda equina. In general, compression of the cervical region is apparent in childhood, whereas lumbar stenosis appears in adulthood. The reverse, however, can occur and not infrequently symptoms and signs due to cord compression at multiple levels may be apparent (that is, craniocervical junction, cervical, and lumbar region stenosis).

Clinical symptoms and signs will depend on the level of maximal involvement and range from quadriparesis or quadriplegia from cervical cord stenosis to paraparesis or paraplegia from thoracolumbar region stenosis. There is a gradual impairment of gait with ataxia, spasticity, and excessive falling. At times the ready tendency for achondroplasts to fall impacts the spinal column, and there is a temporary deterioration in spinal function closely related to minor closed trauma, such as a blow to the spine or suddenly sitting down on the buttocks. Any deterioration in bladder or bowel function in an achondroplast may be an indication of spinal compression. In young children evaluation of bladder and bowel dysfunction can be problematic, but of notable clinical significance. Frequently in lower spinal compression there are symptoms of intermittent claudication of the conus medullaris and cauda equina (14). There are complaints of pain radiating from the buttocks down one or both legs and associated back pain. The pain, paresthesias or dysesthesias, frequently become apparent after exercise such as walking a defined distance. Persistent pain with weakness of the legs and falling occurs unless the achondroplast sits down and rests for a number of minutes or assumes a squatting position with the back to a vertical support such as a wall. These postures and maneuvers are thought to improve impaired blood supply to the conus medullaris and cauda equina by reducing the lumbar lordosis and decompressing the spinal cord and roots. This clinical picture is often dramatic and is a sure indication of progressive and potentially permanent loss of motor and sensory function of the lower spinal cord.

Compression of the spinal cord at any level eventually produces a central cord syndrome that can be acute, subacute, or chronic. Compressive myelopathy produces central necrosis of the cord with subsequent atrophy, narrowing, or occasionally widening due to formation of a traumatic syrinx that may be bilateral (15). Compression may affect the blood supply to the cord since spinal segmental blood vessels arise from the anterior spinal artery and supply 1/2 of the cord. Segmental or anterior spinal artery compression can thus produce a central cord necrosis (15,16) or unilateral ischemia (Brown-Séquard syndrome), and both entities can be acute, transient, or permanent.

The clinical examination may assist in defining the extent and level of myelopathy. Dorsal column compression may affect vibration and proprioception; however, in young children demonstration of posterior cord compression may require careful evaluation of somatosensory-evoked responses with stimulation both of upper and lower limbs (13). Pain and electric sensations up and down the cervical spinal cord (Lhermitte sign) can occur with neck flexion in achondroplasts with cervical cord stenosis. Deep tendon reflexes may be absent, depressed, or inverted, particularly in the upper arm, indicative of cervical or lumbar radiculomyelopathy.

Modern investigations for suspected myelopathy in achondroplasia have depended on the combination of CT to determine the level of bone compression and MRI to observe the level of cord compression as determined by narrowing, gliosis, or cystic changes apparent in the spinal cord. Although myelography was previously performed, this is usually technically difficult because of the generalized canal stenosis and severe, persistent back pain that is frequently observed postmyelography. Similar problems were also apparent with water-soluble contrast medium injected intrathecally and subsequent examination by CT. Somatosensory-evoked responses can assist in localizing the spinal level of impaired function and, more recently, percutaneous cranial magnetic stimulation of corticospinal tracts have been utilized to examine the anterior spinal cord (17).

Various forms of treatment for compressive myelopathy have been used including external truncal support corsets or cervical collars, weight loss to remove excessive spinal canal fatty tissue, and physical therapy. Long-term arrest of progression or clinical improvement, however, is usually seen only with surgical decompression by laminectomy at the appropriate level with preservation of the posterior facet joints to maintain stability of the spine. Removal of the dura and replacement by a dural graft is necessary to complete the decompression of the cord and cauda equina. Although there is frequently improvement in limb function or bladder control, the improvement may only persist for several years before deterioration at another spinal level adjacent to or remote from the area of surgery occurs.

Hydrocephalus

Macrocephaly or an enlarged head is an easily recognizable phenotypic feature of achondroplasia. The etiology of the head enlargement has been of concern, particularly in young children under 2 years of age with delayed motor development (11), and demonstrating impaired head control, rolling over, sitting, and walking skills. Earlier studies emphasized that head enlargement, as indicated by head circumference measurements or skull radiographs, was on the basis of hydrocephalus (7). Other studies, however, showed that on many occasions the enlarged head was due to an enlarged brain (megalencephaly) and that the ventricles were normal or only mildly dilated (18). Subsequently, investigators developed standard growth curves for achondroplasts (obtained in 400 patients) that included height, weight, and head circumference measurements (19). These growth curves indicated that achondroplasts have a larger head size than the normal population although there is some overlap. The charts should be used routinely to assess achondroplasts and particularly any variation in head circumference over a period of time that could suggest progressive hydrocephalus. Similarly, the depressed nasal bridge with relative frontal bone protuberance can give the impression of an enlarged head until the circumference is plotted on the achondroplastic growth curves. Although previously a thickened cranial vault was considered a cause of macrocephaly in achondroplasia, this is not apparent on CT. There is no evidence that megalencephaly of achondroplasia is associated with impaired cognitive skills (11,12).

Hydrocephalus with dilated ventricles has been recognized for many decades in achondroplasia; however, the exact mechanism in any individual is not always certain and remains controversial (20). Noncommunicating hydrocephalus due to stenosis of the aqueduct of Sylvius has been recognized (21) and has been attributed to kinking of the aqueduct and compressive obliteration of the basal cisterns related to the small cranial base (basis cranii). Communicating hydrocephalus is seen more frequently in achondroplasia and frequently diagnosed as hydrocephalus ex vacuo. However, there is usually no evidence of brain atrophy or impaired mental development in such achondroplasts. Occasionally after posterior fossa decompressive surgery we have observed decompensation of moderate hydrocephalus with leaking of CSF at the operative site. Milder degrees of communicating hydrocephalus may be difficult to distinguish from mild ventricular dilation frequently observed in achondroplasia using CT (22).

The communicating hydrocephalus, including prominent subarachnoid spaces over the cortex, has been attributed to impaired absorption of CSF via the arachnoid villi of the superior sagittal sinus. The pressure in the venous drainage of the brain, including the sagittal sinus, can be elevated by constriction of the jugular veins in the jugular foramina at the deformed base of the achondroplastic skull (18,23). More recently investigators have shown that there may be a further constriction of venous return to the heart at the level of the superior thoracic opening due to the small chest of the achondroplast. A recent study of achondroplasts showed reversal of blood flow in the emissary veins connecting the intracranial and extracranial venous systems and indicated that this was due to raised venous pressure in the jugular veins (24). Clinically this increased venous pressure may appear as a prominence of scalp veins in the achondroplast. Hydrocephalus in achondroplasia may not be obvious clinically and is frequently discovered during routine evaluation of macrocephaly or neurologic signs such as gait impairment or limb weakness. Often during the 1st year of life, hydrocephalus may be suspected in an achondroplast with a bulging anterior fontanelle. Although CT will often demonstrate the degree of ventricular dilatation (22), MRI will show more detailed anatomy (for example, aqueductal stenosis) and also the presence of subependymal fluid indicating decompensation of the hydrocephalus and probable need for surgical shunting. It is usually possible to serially monitor with CT those achondroplasts with mild-to-moderate ventricular dilatation of the communicating type and surgery can often be avoided. Neuropsychologic testing and evaluation by a neurosurgeon are usually indicated before deciding to perform a shunting procedure for clinically significant ventricular dilatation (20). Rarely the ventricular dilatation is due to such severe jugular venous outflow obstruction that venous angiography with venous pressure gradient evaluations may be necessary prior to venous graft anastomosis of an internal venous sinus to an external vein in order to improve collateral circulation and decrease venous backflow pressure (25). There is evidence that raised jugular venous pressure can produce dilated ventricles in young children due to communicating hydrocephalus; whereas, in older subjects pseudotumor cerebri occurs with small ventricles (25). This may depend on the ability of the skull to expand in the young child prior to fusion of the sutures.

Vertebral Column Malalignment

Scoliosis and kyphosis are infrequent in achondroplasia and usually do not contribute to the neurologic problems of achondroplasts. Two conditions that may cause neurologic complications in achondroplasia, however, are lumbar lordosis and thoracolumbar gibbus formation.

The marked angulation of the sacrum has been noted as a common malformation of the spine in achondroplasia (7). The reasons for the sacral angulation to almost a right angle to the lumbar vertebrae are not well established, but the degree of lordosis does appear to increase with age. This angulation seems to contribute to compression of nerve roots of the cauda equina. Clinicians have observed that symptoms and signs of intermittent claudication of the cauda equina are relieved by squatting and resting against a firm wall. These measures reduce the degree of lordosis at the lumbosacral junction. Furthermore, claudication symptoms are unusual following exercise on a bicycle in which the lumbosacral spine curvature is reduced by postural changes. Achondroplasts usually have claudication of the cauda equina while standing or walking upright with maximum tendency to lumbosacral lordosis.

A gibbus deformity of the thoracolumbar vertebrae is not uncommon in achondroplasia and should be investigated by lateral radiographs of these vertebrae. Early documentation of anterior wedging of one or more vertebral bodies is important since angulation at this level can compress the conus medullaris and cauda equina. In the younger achondroplast wedging of the vertebrae should be carefully followed radiologically since the angulation may be progressive, and optimum management must be determined by orthopedic techniques to anteriorly reduce the vertebral angulation with bone struts. In older patients with established angulation and neurologic symptoms of paraparesis or intermittent claudication of the cauda equina, a combined orthopedic approach of laminectomy and angle reduction may be necessary.

Nerve Root Compression

Compression of the nerve roots as they exit the spinal cord is common in achondroplasia. The abnormal shortening of the pedicles of the vertebrae appears to contribute to the small size of the neural foramina. Narrowing of neural foramina can occur at multiple levels but is clinically significant in the cervical and lumbar regions. The patients complain of dysesthesias and paresthesias in the upper and lower limbs, particularly distally. Subsequently, there may be a loss of tendon reflexes and focal muscle wasting. We have frequently noticed a depressed triceps reflex unilaterally or bilaterally with an inverted reflex (flexion at the elbow) as an early sign of nerve root compression in achondroplasts. Loss of multiple reflexes, either in the arms or legs, is associated with progressive neurologic deficits in manipulating fingers and hands as well as walking.

Occipital neuralgia due to compression of the occipital nerve or nerves exiting through the posterior atlantooccipital membrane, is not uncommon in achondroplasia. Presumably the nerve is entrapped by the fibrous membrane or by the proximity of the posterior lip of the foramen magnum and posterior arch of the atlas (which may be fused in achondroplasia). These patients complain of paresthesias or headache in the occipital region of the scalp and may have an area of analgesia in the distribution of the occipital nerve. These symptoms may be difficult to distinguish clinically from those due to narrowing of the foramen magnum and compression of the cervicomedullary junction.

Electromyographic examination of specific muscle groups will help to localize particular nerve roots that are functionally compressed. Often there is improved function following enlargement of the neural foramina surgically, either at the time of laminectomy or occasionally as an isolated procedure at one or more foramina. Occipital neuralgia can be treated by occipital neurectomy provided that significant craniocervical junction compression has been excluded.

Craniovertebral Junction Anomalies

Anomalies of the craniovertebral junction are frequent in achondroplasia and may occur as single or one of several defects. The defect in endochondral ossification that is integral to achondroplasia has a particular effect on bones making up the foramen magnum and the atlantoaxial joints. The various components of the craniovertebral junction that are involved in achondroplasia and can lead to neurologic complications include the following: foramen magnum stenosis, upper cervical vertebral canal stenosis (C1, C2), abnormal odontoid shape or position, ligamentous laxity, and jugular foramen stenosis.

The reduced growth of the occipital bones produces a small foramen magnum in most achondroplasts (26). This reduction in growth leads to an abnormally shaped foramen magnum and a reduction in the foramen diameter, particularly in the transverse plane as determined by CT (27). Neurologic complications appear more commonly associated with a very small transverse diameter. At birth the achondroplastic foramen magnum is smaller than the nonachondroplast, particularly in the transverse diameter. Neither dimension shows the dramatic increase in size demonstrated in the nonachondroplast during the initial 18 months of life (12). Although symptomatic and asymptomatic achondroplastic subjects had similar foramen magnum dimensions at birth, the symptomatic individuals showed a decreased mean rate of growth in both dimensions; however, this was not statistically significant due to overlap. The mean transverse diameter of an adult achondroplastic foramen magnum is equivalent to a nonachondroplastic newborn such that growth in this diameter is negligible during life. Failure of foramen magnum growth has been attributed to premature fusion and aberrant development of the posterior synchondrosis, in addition to a defect in bone development. The posterior fusion defect may also contribute to the shelving defect of the posterior margin of the foramen magnum. This hypertrophied margin can be observed radiologically to project into the posterior brainstem and has been implicated in the severe angulation and pressure necrosis of the brainstem at this level.

The two vertebrae making up the atlantoaxial complex are also involved in the achondroplastic process and contribute to the narrowing of the vertebral canal in the upper cervical region. Initially this contribution to compression at the medullary level was not appreciated as investigators had concentrated on the obvious stenosis at the foramen magnum. Routine evaluation with multiplanar (axial, coronal, and sagittal) reconstruction by CT of the upper cervical vertebrae increased our understanding of the multiple levels of upper cervical canal stenosis. Furthermore, in achondroplasia the posterior neural arch of the atlas may fuse with the posterior margin of the foramen magnum and contribute to the posterior, protruding shelf.

In addition to the previously mentioned anomalies of the neural arches in achondroplasia there may be defects in the odontoid process. The odontoid tends to project posteriorly and superiorly into the foramen magnum, and the medulla oblongata is anatomically draped over this protuberance. Projection of the odontoid into the anterior aspects of the medulla can lead to compression necrosis particularly affecting the corticospinal tracts (10). Furthermore this protuberance may damage the arterial supply (anterior spinal artery) to the medulla and cervical cord leading to more widespread neurologic damage.

The ligaments that contribute to the craniocervical junction, including in particular those of the anterior atlantoaxial joint (odontoid), can be involved in the ligamentous laxity seen in achondroplasia. This ligamentous laxity could potentially contribute to joint instability and excessive movement in the presence of severe canal stenosis can produce a traumatic myelopathy.

As the result of the above anomalies there is frequently a tendency for bony stenosis and instability at the craniocervical junction that can compress the cervicomedullary cord and upper nerve roots. Various syndromes have been described in achondroplasts due to damage of the spinal cord at this high level and include the following: sudden infant death, sleep apnea syndrome, disorders of respiration, myelopathy, syringobulbia-myelia, and hydrocephalus.

Sudden Infant Death

The unexpected death of an infant is often unexplained and has been the subject of considerable investigation and speculation. Similar events have been described in infants with achondroplasia and a recent study documented sudden

unexpected death or unexplained apnea in 13 such infants (28). As a result of this and other studies (10,29), investigators have postulated that constriction at the level of the foramen magnum interferes with respiratory control centers with cessation of respiration that may result in death of the infant achondroplast. This often occurs during sleep since at this time the respiratory control centers are particulary sensitive either to postural effects at the craniovertebral junction (neck flexion) or changes in carbon dioxide and oxygen levels in blood during sleep. In a few younger children there are recurrent diurnal apneic episodes (10,30), some of which may be alarmingly prolonged and lead to evaluation as a possible seizure disorder. Recognition that these episodes are nonepileptic in nature is important in management. Postmortem changes, including gliosis, edema, and cystic myelomalacia at the level of the medulla appear to be the basis for the damage to respiratory control centers. This injury is due to acute or chronic compression of the spinal cord by constriction at the foramen magnum.

Sleep Apnea Syndrome

In the older child with achondroplasia there is increasing recognition of the various sleep apnea syndromes that have been observed in nonachondroplastic adults (9,10). Commonly achondroplastic children will have a history of excessive snoring at night and this symptom may be a valuable clue to the need for further studies. As a result of the recurrent apneic episodes during sleep, mixed with the startles and arousals that follow prolonged apnea, there is a lack of nocturnal sleep and these children may present with excessive daytime somnolence. Some children with achondroplasia have excessive weight gain, poor linear growth, fluid retention, headache, and dyspnea. Such problems are due to cor pulmonale with carbon dioxide retention and hypoxia during apneic episodes causing reactive constriction of pulmonary vasculature. These systemic complications will resolve with appropriate management of the sleep apnea.

In the past sleep apnea syndromes in achondroplasia have been considered secondary to obstruction of the airway due to enlarged tonsils, glossoptosis, and pharyngolaryngeal wall laxity requiring direct surgical management; however, recent studies have emphasized the neural basis for some cases of sleep apnea. As a consequence of detailed studies on achondroplasts using polysomnography, we and others (9,10) have demonstrated the presence of obstructive, central, and mixed (obstructive and central) forms of apnea during sleep. Following decompression of the medulla oblongata by enlargement of the foramen magnum, we have observed improvement in the apnea, whether of the obstructive or central type. This is consistent with other neurologic conditions having obstructive apnea as a symptom and including syringomyelia, poliomyelitis, and lateral medullary syndrome (31). Presumably there is damage to the medulla by constriction at the foramen magnum in achondroplasia that impairs respiratory control mechanisms, leading to apnea either during wakefulness or sleep. In addition, there is injury to the motor nuclei of the brainstem that control the reflex movements of the larynx and pharynx during respiration, and discoordinated movements of the upper airway muscle wall during inspiration cause airway obstruction severe enough to produce apnea.

Disorders of Respiration

In addition to the dramatic manifestations of sudden death and sleep apnea in young achondroplasts, there may be other factors as a basis for impaired respiration and dyspnea. Physicians caring for these patients need to determine whether limitations in walking are due to spinal cord claudication or actual dyspnea on a respiratory basis. Achondroplasts have a relatively small chest circumference that could restrict respirations; however, this does not appear to be a factor in the sleep apnea syndrome (10). Following progressive cervical myelopathy or as a complication after surgical decompression of the cervical cord, there may be impairment of phrenic nerve control of the diaphragm or spinal tracts to the intercostal nerves. The effect on respiration would depend on the degree of involvement and in particular whether there was unilateral or bilateral spinal cord injury.

Myelopathy

Traumatic myelopathy of the medulla due to constriction at the foramen magnum is well recognized in achondroplasia at all ages, although in our experience this appears more frequent in young achondroplasts and is presumably due to growth limitations of the foramen magnum in the early years of life (10,26). Clinically these youngsters have gait disturbances progressing to quadriparesis and quadriplegia. In the infant there may be extreme hypotonia progressing to hypertonia with increased reflexes and extensor plantar responses. Older children may have impaired dorsal column sensation with a positive Romberg sign. The changes at autopsy of gliosis, edema, and cystic formation in the spinal cord (cystic myelomalacia) are thought to be secondary to a traumatic myelopathy. Changes above or below the level of the foramen magnum are believed to be related to thrombosis and occlusion of the anteriorly placed vertebrobasilar arterial system.

Syringobulbia-Myelia

In our series of achondroplasts we have on several occasions observed the apparent progression of the cystic myelomalacia to syringomyelia. This also appears to be on the basis of local compression of the spinal cord by the constricted foramen magnum (15). In one child there was an associated subependymal glioma with a cyst, in another

there were two cysts (double-barrelled shotgun appearance), and in another there was an elongated central calcified lesion. These elongated cystic lesions were observed as an incidental finding on CT and sagittal reconstruction to evaluate the size of the foramen magnum. The cystic changes appear to be due to a traumatic cystic necrosis of the spinal cord since similar findings have been observed in accidental cervical spinal trauma. The subependymal glioma associated with cystic changes in one patient may be more than a chance finding and could represent the late manifestations of gliosis secondary to the traumatic myelomalacia of prolonged compression.

Hydrocephalus

Hydrocephalus may have many causes in achondroplasia and can be associated with foramen magnum compression. Some authors have implicated compression of the outlet foramina of the fourth ventricle by the foramen magnum as a basis for the ventricular enlargement. Some degree of cerebellar tonsillar herniation and basilar impression may also contribute to compression of ventricular outflow foramina and impaired subarachnoid absorption. Since most of our achondroplasts with hydrocephalus had aqueductal stenosis or dilated cortical subarachnoid spaces, we doubt a major role of the foramen magnum constriction in producing hydrocephalus.

Homozygous Achondroplasia

Homozygous achondroplasia can theoretically occur in a quarter of offspring of a union between two heterozygous achondroplasts; however, few of these infants have been reported and most die in the early months of life of respiratory complications. Recently, with the recognition that some of the respiratory complications could be related to medullary and cervical spinal cord compression, there has been a more aggressive approach to treatment and prolonged survival (5,28). The physical characteristics of these infants are similar to but more severe than patients with heterozygous achondroplasia.

Initially the respiratory complications, including cor pulmonale, were attributed to the extremely small chest size and restrictive pulmonary disease. The severe bone dysplasia, however, affects not only long bones but also the foramen magnum, which may be extremely small, and the bones of the vertebral column. As a result of the stenosis at the craniocervical junction there may be marked compression of the medullary respiratory centers and outflow pathways and subsequent apnea and respiratory insufficiency. Motor delay and hypotonic quadriparesis or quadriplegia are complications of the homozygous achondroplastic state. Hydrocephalus may be evident on CT and require shunting procedures. Unfortunately, despite surgical decompression at the bony craniocervical junction, these infants do not appear to survive more than a few years because of the severity of the bone dysplasia (5).

Hypochondroplasia

In studies of dwarfism, hypochondroplasia has received less attention than the more common condition of achondroplasia. Hypochondroplasia is usually defined by similar but less severe clinical and radiographic features of achondroplasia and with normal facial features (4,32). Hypochondroplasia is dominantly inherited; however, as in achondroplasia, most cases appear to be sporadic. There may be considerable overlap clinically and radiographically between achondroplasia and hypochondroplasia, and neurologic complications have been observed in the latter category. In particular, spinal canal stenosis occurs in a minority of patients with hypochondroplasia (4), but in our experience spinal canal stenosis can occur in hypochondroplasia and symptoms, signs, and management are similar to those in achondroplasia.

MANAGEMENT OF ACHONDROPLASIA

The comprehensive management of the child with achondroplasia involves many physicians and disciplines. Following the initial diagnosis, these infants should be followed carefully, particularly during the first few years of life. In addition to orthopedic and otorhinolaryngologic assessments, the pediatric neurologist has a very definite role in this team approach to childhood achondroplasia (9,10). The hypotonia and delayed motor development should not be dismissed as related only to ligamentous laxity, since this may well be an early manifestation of spinal paralysis. After 3 months of age, we have found that somatosensory-evoked responses in both upper and lower limbs can be helpful in evaluating the dorsal columns in these infants or young children in which neurologic assessment of this aspect of spinal cord function can be difficult (13). Furthermore somatosensory evoked responses can be assessed serially and before, during, and after surgical decompression. Abnormalities of somatosensory-evoked responses may also have some localizing value in assessing the level of cord dysfunction since the neurologic examination and routine radiographs may not be informative.

In the past, radiologic investigations of the achondroplast have relied upon plain radiographs and myelography. More recently CT, with particular attention to the posterior fossa, has been utilized. In addition to the foramen magnum, CT also permits evaluation of the brain and ventricles, along with sagittal reconstruction of the posterior fossa and upper cervical canal, allowing a more detailed assessment of the relationship of bones of the craniocervical junction and soft tissue structures. These sagittal views enable visualization of the odontoid process in addition to

the posterior neural arches of the atlas and axis and may indicate multiple levels of cord compression in addition to the small foramen magnum (5). Similar studies can be performed at the cervical and lumbar levels to demonstrate canal stenosis at these potentially significant sites. More recently we have utilized MRI of the brain and spinal cord in an attempt to define the anatomic level of hydrocephalus and the degree of ventricular compensation (that is, the presence or absence of subependymal CSF extravasation) or compression of the spinal cord. Gliosis, edema, and narrowing are readily apparent on MRI of the cord, and an area of cystic necrosis or syringomyelia can be visualized at the level of compression. MRI appears helpful in the assessment of children requiring surgical decompression; however, CT scanning remains the basis of our assessments.

In children with clinical respiratory problems, we have frequently consulted with pediatric pulmonologists and otorhinolaryngologists in order to define the relative contribution of peripheral (small chest cage, enlarged tonsils) and central (neurologic) mechanisms producing stridor, apnea, snoring, repeated pneumonia, or respiratory distress. Moreover, in addition to chest radiographs and direct visualization of the upper airways, polysomnography can be utilized to investigate the nature of the respiratory disorder and particularly whether sleep apnea is present (9,10). Achondroplasts with abnormal polysomnograms may need further evaluation for cor pulmonale by a pediatric cardiologist, to include an electrocardiogram (ECG) and echocardiogram.

Following this detailed clinical evaluation by multiple physicians and the assessment of pertinent studies, members of the multidisciplinary team, to include an experienced neurosurgeon, present the indications for or against surgical decompression to the patient and family. On occasion this decision may be delayed to evaluate further natural progress of the achondroplastic patient. The risks and benefits of surgical decompression are outlined and relevant radiographs should be demonstrated to the patient and family.

The surgical approach depends on the level of the nervous system that appears to have the greatest functional impairment, even in situations where there may be documented multiple levels of involvement. In the younger patient this dysfunction has usually been related to the level of the foramen magnum and upper cervical vertebrae. After careful placement in the sitting position, a portion of the occipital bone is removed to enlarge the foramen magnum. The sitting position helps to minimize hemorrhage from enlarged venous plexuses surrounding the foramen magnum. The dura mater is removed and this often includes a thickened area of dura at the level of the foramen magnum posteriorly. In addition, the upper two or three posterior neural arches are also removed without disturbance of the lateral facet joints. The medulla and spinal cord are observed, cord ultrasonography is performed, and intraoperative somatosensory-evoked responses may be utilized to assess the spinal cord at the level of the foramen magnum and upper cervical region. A dural graft is inserted and the dorsal cervical muscles replaced. In patients with moderately dilated ventricles, a ventricular reservoir is established since some patients have had CSF leakage postoperatively, which is believed to be caused by transient decompensation of the hydrocephalus. Careful suturing of the dural graft and daily removal of ventricular CSF enables rapid healing of the operative site.

Other surgical procedures include lower cervical or lower thoracolumbar laminectomy. Enlargement of neural foramina may improve compressive radiculopathy and occipital neurectomy may occasionally be necessary. In general, we have avoided ventriculoperitoneal shunting for hydrocephalus unless this appeared significant in a particular patient. CT brain scanning has permitted serial assessment of ventricular size, and in most patients, the mild or moderate ventricular dilatation does not appear symptomatic. Serial neuropyschologic evaluations are necessary to evaluate cognitive functions. Achondroplasts rarely have significant hydrocephalus due to jugular foramen obstruction; and a large surgically produced venous anastomosis may be necessary to control the ventricular dilatation. Lesser degrees of increased pressure due to venous obstruction may, however, have a role in the milder forms of communicating hydrocephalus observed in achondroplasia.

Long-term evaluation of achondroplasts requiring surgery is particularly necessary since vertebral canal stenosis will often appear at other levels as the patient becomes a teenager or adult. We have seen children requiring posterior fossa decompression who subsequently develop compression at the cervical or lumbar region, and it is suspected that these patients have a particularly severe congenital skeletal abnormality at multiple levels. In a few patients, despite successful surgical decompression of the posterior fossa, we have observed central and obstructive sleep apnea several years later that responded dramatically to continuous positive airway pressure (CPAP) administered by a nasal mask adapted for the midface hypoplasia of the achondroplast. This approach may avoid reconstructive surgery of the upper airway or the need for tracheostomy. On occasions such approaches may be necessary to avoid serious consequences of repeated apnea.

It is believed that the recognition and management of this group of disorders is important since there are successful surgical and medical therapies of these potentially crippling and life-threatening neurologic complications of achondroplasia in children (10).

MUCOPOLYSACCHARIDOSES

The mucopolysaccharidoses (MPS) are heritable multisystem lysosomal storage disorders in which there is a defective enzymatic degradation of complex carbohydrate molecules. There are six distinct types and several subtypes described based on enzymatic, clinical, and genetic characteristics. The accumulation of mucopolysaccharides in lysosomes affects numerous tissues, including bone, connective tissue, and the CNS. Recent advances in enzymology have permitted more definitive diagnosis of the enzymatic deficiency and correlation with the clinical syndrome. For example, in Hurler syndrome, one of the best described MPS, there is a severe deficiency of α-iduronidase and patients may have mental retardation, hydrocephalus (acute and chronic), and soft tissue thickening of the nasopharynx, meninges, and dura mater due to deposition of mucopolysaccharide. Scheie syndrome is a less severe form of the same enzyme defect and is slowly progressive with similar complications appearing in adulthood. Compound disorders in which the patient is a double heterozygote and has two different alleles (Hurler-Scheie syndrome), may present with an intermediate enzyme deficiency and clinical disorder (33). In contrast, Morquio syndrome due to a deficiency of galactosamine-6-sulfate sulfatase, primarily involves bone and connective tissue with odontoid hypoplasia, ligamentous laxity, and the possibility of atlantoaxial dislocation (34).

Advances in radiology, particularly the application of CT (34,35) and MRI (36), to study patients with MPS have permitted a greater understanding of the underlying pathogenesis of the neurologic complications, and in certain circumstances, have indicated specific decompressive surgical therapy. Further advances in MRI, such as cardiac gating and high resolution scans using surface coils, minimize CSF movement artifact and permit improved definition of the distorted anatomy of the craniocervical junction, meninges, and nasopharynx (Table 22.2).

Mental Retardation

Mental retardation in MPS is generally assumed to be progressive, mild, or moderate to severe, depending on the enzyme defect, and related to the storage of mucopolysaccharides and gangliosides in brain parenchyma (including

Table 22.2 Neurologic complications in mucopolysaccharidoses

Mental retardation	Neuronal storage
Hydrocephalus acute/chronic	Thickened meninges
Compressive myelopathy	Thickened dura mater
Craniocervical junction syndrome	Atlantoaxial dislocation Odontoid hypoplasia Thickened meninges Ligamentous laxity
Compressive peripheral neuropathy	Thickened carpal and tarsal ligaments
Sleep apnea	Compression of cervicomedullary junction Pharyngeal soft tissue enlargement
CNS embolization	Abnormal thickened cardiac valves

neurons). Recently high resolution MRI has shown increased signal intensity on T2-weighted images in the periventricular white matter (36) of patients with α-iduronidase and iduronide sulphatase deficiency. These periventricular changes are seen in the absence of hydrocephalus, and probably represent the expanded, fluid-filled periadventitial spaces and loose connective tissue observed pathologically in MPS (37,38). The extent of white matter involvement appeared to correlate with intellectual impairment; whereas, the periventricular abnormalities were not seen in the Morquio syndrome in which intelligence is normal or minimally reduced. Chronic hydrocephalus can lead to mental retardation and be readily demonstrated by CT or MRI prior to ventricular decompression by ventriculoperitoneal shunting.

Hydrocephalus

Hydrocephalus with clinically significant dilatation of all ventricles (communicating hydrocephalus) has been described as an acute or chronic complication of MPS (39). The enlarging head circumference due to hydrocephalus must be distinguished in patients with MPS from that due to thickened cranial bones (macrocranium) and an enlarged brain without ventricular dilatation (megalencephaly). Potentially all three causes could coexist in the same patient, and careful neuroradiologic studies are necessary to identify those patients that would benefit from surgical decompression of dilated ventricles. Acute hydrocephalus is suspected clinically by a rapid neurologic deterioration, as distinct from a more gradual decline in MPS patients, including vomiting, ataxia, headache, and impaired cognition or level of consciousness. Chronic hydrocephalus may be more difficult to distinguish from the natural decline in neurologic function of the particular MPS, and an increased clinical suspicion should lead to screening evaluations of the brain using CT to determine the ventricular size.

Communicating hydrocephalus has been observed in various MPS including Hurler, Hunter, Sanfilippo, and Maroteux-Lamy syndromes (40) and is presumably due to thickening of the leptomeninges by mucopolysaccharide deposition and impaired absorption of CSF over the superior surfaces of the brain.

Compressive Myelopathy

The MPS affect bone and connective tissue to varying degrees. Potential encroachment of the spinal canal at various levels (craniocervical junction, cervical, and lumbar) could result from bone and joint abnormalities, thickening of the leptomeninges by infiltration with mucopolysaccharides, or a combination of these complications. Definition of the relative contributions to the narrowed spinal canal causing cord compression will be necessary to determine appropriate therapy.

Clinical findings will depend on the level of cord compression, rate of compression, and whether multiple levels are involved. At the level of the craniocervical junction there is clinically progressive spastic paraparesis or quadriparesis with ataxia, impaired neck mobility, and abnormal posturing (torticollis, retrocollis) together with pain in the neck and occiput. Impaired speech, continence, control of respiration, sleep apnea, and localized sensory impairments are usually delayed findings and may be due to development of a traumatic cystic myelopathy (syringobulbia and syringomyelia). In part, the foramen magnum may be narrowed by thickening of the dura mater surrounding the medulla oblongata. In Morquio syndrome, however, there may be odontoid hypoplasia and ligamentous laxity leading to vertebral displacement and cord compression due to atlantoaxial dislocation (34). Often the restraining ligaments surrounding the odontoid process are thickened by infiltration with mucopolysaccharide material (balloon cells) and contribute to the canal narrowing (41).

Compressive myelopathy may occur at other levels of the spinal cord due to canal stenosis from thickening of the spinal ligaments (posterior vertebral ligament and ligamentum flavum), leptomeninges, and the dura mater surrounding the spinal cord at the cervical and lumbar regions. Compression in the cervical region may be difficult to distinguish clinically from compression at the craniocervical junction unless bulbar symptoms are present in the latter. Careful investigations using upper and lower limb somatosensory-evoked responses, respiratory function (polysomnography), and extensive neuroradiologic studies with CT or MRI, may be necessary to define the extent and clinically significant localized compression of the spinal cord (33). Localized levels of compression should be sought since these can be approached surgically by dural resection; whereas, generalized stenosis would require extensive laminectomy and may be contraindicated since spinal instability would occur without subsequent stabilization by vertebral fusion. In addition to thickened ligaments and leptomeninges, patients with MPS may have flattened and distorted vertebrae leading to dwarfing, scoliosis, gibbus deformity, subluxation, and subsequent spinal canal stenosis. Orthopedic alignment and stabilization of the spinal vertebrae can be useful in management together with local dural resection.

Peripheral Nerve Compression

Connective tissue involvement in MPS may be widespread and the infiltration and thickening affects various ligaments and tissues surrounding peripheral nerves and roots. A radiculopathy may be present due to neural foramen stenosis by thickening of the dural extension surrounding nerve roots. Loss of sensation and decreased reflexes are clinically detectable. Thickening of peripheral ligaments in the wrist or foot lead to the carpal or tarsal tunnel syndromes. At times the connective tissue claw deformity seen in the hands of patients with MPS may obscure an underlying contribution from compression of the median nerve beneath the thickened carpal ligament. Electrophysiologic studies of median nerve function should be routinely examined in MPS patients since surgical decompression of the carpal tunnel by ligament resection can lead to improved hand function.

Sleep Apnea

Pulmonary function in MPS can be affected by restriction of mechanical chest function, upper airway obstruction due to mucopolysaccharide infiltration of soft tissues of the upper pharynx, or damage to central neurologic pathways of respiratory control. Neuronal damage can be at the level of the respiratory centers in the medulla oblongata or outflow pathways to intercostal and diaphragmatic musculature and depends on the site of compression of the spinal cord. Compromise of these centers and pathways can eventually lead to nocturnal snoring and sleep apnea from airway obstruction, or central apnea, or mixed mechanisms (42). Diagnosis will depend on careful pulmonary function studies, including polysomnography, and soft-tissue radiologic studies of nasopharynx, larynx, and cervicomedullary junction by CT or MRI (36). Treatment depends on whether the upper airway obstruction can be bypassed (tracheostomy) or reconstituted surgically, or the nervous system can be decompressed; various approaches may be necessary in individuals (33).

OSTEOPETROSIS

Osteopetrosis (osteosclerosis, marble bone, Albers-Schönberg disease) is a rare disorder of bone in which recent studies have demonstrated lysosomal dysfunction of the monocyctic-macrophage cell line and abnormalities of osteoclast function (43). Defective osteoclast function leads to impaired bone resorption and excessive bone growth. The osteoclasts may be either reduced or increased in number and in the latter, the osteoclasts are assumed to be functionally defective. The bony overgrowth leads to an encroachment of the bone marrow, and extramedullary hematopoiesis occurs with hepatosplenomegaly, anemia, and thrombocytopenia. Osteopetrosis occurs in two predominant forms: a milder autosomal dominant or tarda form with childhood onset and usually lacking neurologic sequelae, and a congenital, malignant, autosomal recessive form with marked neurologic sequelae (44). In addition to increased density of the long bones, ribs, sternum, and spine, there is enlargement of the skull and increased density of bones of the base of the skull. These changes are readily demonstrated radiographically and more recently

CT has been used to examine the underlying brain and ventricles. Radiographic studies may demonstrate constriction of the various cranial nerve foramina, including optic and auditory canals.

As a result of the bony encroachment of the various foramina of the cranial nerves exiting from the osteosclerotic skull base, there is severe compression and loss of function of these nerves in the early onset malignant form of the disorder. Anosmia, blindness, facial palsy, deafness, and trigeminal paralysis may occur in varying combinations. Cranial nerve palsies may be a presenting feature in these children. Blindness with optic atrophy can be caused by optic nerve compression (with abnormal visual-evoked responses) or of retinal origin (with abnormal electroretinography). Macrocephaly is often prominent and is due to a number of causes including a thickened skull (osteopetrosis and dural extramedullary hematopoiesis) and hydrocephalus with dilatation of the ventricles and cortical subarachnoid spaces. The reason for hydrocephalus is debated; however, there are indications that abnormalities around the sagittal sinuses or compression of jugular veins at the skull base increase pressure in the superior sagittal sinus and impair uptake of CSF. This could explain dilatation of the ventricles and subarachnoid spaces in younger patients with nonfused skull sutures and reports of benign intracranial hypertension (pseudotumor cerebri) in older subjects with fused sutures. The box-like macrocephaly may be accompanied by enlarged scalp veins representing anastomotic diploic veins.

Developmental delay, particularly in motor skills, has been frequently reported in the severe form of osteopetrosis and has been attributed to the relatively enlarged head. Hypotonia is seen early and hypertonia with spasticity and long tract neurologic findings becomes apparent (44). There are varying explanations for motor impairment but this has not been investigated by modern techniques of CT and MRI as utilized for investigation of the achondroplast with similar problems. There are reports of strabismus, vertical nystagmus, screaming episodes, in addition to the onset of spasticity; detailed studies of potential involvement of another basal foramen, the foramen magnum, will be necessary in the future.

Intracranial hemorrhage in the brain parenchyma or subarachnoid spaces from thrombocytopenia appears rare. Extramedullary hematopoiesis in the dura and related to the brain or spinal cord can occasionally compress underlying nervous tissue and lead to paresis. There have been two cases associated with the rare neurologic disorder of infantile neuraxonal dystrophy.

The management of the neurologic complications of osteopetrosis has been directed at surgical decompression of the entrapped cranial nerves in the thickened skull base and particularly directed at enlarging the optic and auditory canals. Such approaches have been of varying success. Clinically significant hydrocephalus may require ventriculoperitoneal shunting. Recently, due to an understanding of the cellular basis for the disorder, several centers have performed bone marrow transplants in appropriate subjects (45) with improved hematopoietic and radiographic findings. Following surgical decompression of the cranial nerves, a bone marrow transplant may stabilize this inexorable condition.

OSTEOGENESIS IMPERFECTA

Osteogenesis imperfecta occurs in 1 in 40,000 to 60,000 live births and is a genetically heterogenous group of disorders of connective tissue. The current classification into four types is based on the clinical and radiologic changes. There is also genetic heterogeneity with autosomal dominant and recessive traits. Clinical characteristics include bone fragility, laxity of joints and occasionally skin, blue sclerae, hearing loss, dentinogenesis imperfecta, and macrocephaly.

Neurologic manifestations in osteogenesis imperfecta are in general related to basilar impression and subsequent compression of brainstem structures and cerebellum. There is invagination of the upper cervical vertebrae and margins of the foramen magnum with stenosis at the foramen magnum level and compression of the medulla oblongata and spinal cord. As a result the cranium is malformed with overhanging of the occipital region giving a mushroom shape to the skull. Macrocephaly is frequent with frontal bossing and there may be an underlying dilatation of the ventricles. Delayed development with hypotonia in patients with osteogenesis imperfecta may be attributed to the enlarged head, ligamentous laxity, or frequent fractures of the long bones. Slowly progressive compression of the medulla and spinal cord at the foramen magnum, however, may present as hypotonia, and later hypertonicity and quadriparesis may become clinically apparent. Radiographic studies, including CT, will demonstrate the basilar invagination into the posterior fossa and the degree of spinal canal stenosis. Hydrocephalus as a basis for macrocephaly will also be apparent and frequently with dilatation of the cortical subarachnoid spaces (46). Similar explanations for hydrocephalus as discussed in the section on achondroplasia may be operative in osteogenesis imperfecta. Recurrent apnea or respiratory rhythm irregularities can occur as a result of the basilar invagination and compression of the medullary respiratory centers (47).

Other neurologic complications in osteogenesis imperfecta involve intrauterine and intrapartum trauma with stillbirth and intracranial hemorrhage occurring in the severe congenital form (48). Gait disturbances can be due to fractures or laxity of ligaments; however, platyspondyly and scoliosis can also lead to spinal cord compression and paralysis. Rarely, there is neural compression due to exuberant callus formation in fractured bones adjacent to peripheral nerves or by hemorrhage into or adjacent to nerves (for example, femoral neuropathy). Abnormal capillary fragility and platelet dysfunction have been reported as part of osteogenesis imperfecta and may contribute to this hemorrhagic tendency.

In patients with clinically significant basilar invagination, surgical decompression at the level of the foramen magnum is necessary to reverse the progressive compression of the brainstem and medulla and possibly lead to neurologic improvement. Several approaches are utilized including posterior decompression of the foramen magnum and upper cervical canal or anterior resection of the invaginated odontoid process (48,49). Subsequent fusion of the skull and spine will be necessary following either approach.

EHLERS-DANLOS SYNDROME

Ehlers-Danlos syndrome is a genetically and clinically heterogenous disorder of connective tissue with 11 different subtypes currently recognized (50). Autosomal dominant, recessive, and X-linked traits have been described. Cardinal manifestations include hyperextensible skin, dystrophic scarring, and easy bruising with joint hypermobility and connective tissue fragility. Phenotypic variability accounts for the clinical manifestations and neurologic manifestations are rare (2).

The defects in collagen in Ehlers-Danlos syndrome can affect various structures in anatomic relationship to the central and peripheral nervous systems and lead to neurologic compromise. Ligamentous laxity at the atlanto-occipital and atlantoaxial joints can produce progressive instability at the craniovertebral junction with medullary and spinal cord compression and subsequent quadriparesis. Abnormal collagen of the annulus fibrosis of the intervertebral disk can lead to disk bulging into the spinal canal at many levels and even spontaneous or traumatic rupture and herniation of nucleus pulposus with cord or root compression. Brachial and lumbosacral plexus neuropathies may explain sudden onset of pain and weakness in the limbs of patients with Ehlers-Danlos syndrome (51). This neuropathy has been attributed to compression of nerve roots by ectasia of the dura and ligaments of the spinal canal. Painful muscle cramps beginning in childhood are common in the calves of Ehlers-Danlos patients. These cramps occur mainly at night and resolve later in life or respond to quinine and quinidine. Thus, there may be various explanations for pain and weakness in the limbs of these subjects and only after careful evaluation may a readily correctable cause be determined, such as a herniated disk fragment compressing a spinal root or spinal cord (2).

The abnormal collagen in blood vessels in Ehlers-Danlos syndrome appears responsible for the defects in small and large blood vessels. Aortic aneurysms can dissect, rupture, and occlude spinal arteries with ischemic myelopathy. Single or multiple intracranial aneurysms have also been reported and spontaneous rupture produces a catastrophic intracranial hemorrhage with subarachnoid hemorrhage and hematoma formation. Abnormal collagen in peripheral vessels may be responsible for the tendency to bruise readily in Ehlers-Danlos syndrome and, in addition, there may be abnormal platelet function and platelet-collagen interaction in subtypes of the disorder. Rupture of a peripheral artery with hematoma formation can compress a closely related peripheral nerve and this has been reported with the brachial artery and median nerve (52).

Congenital intracranial abnormalities in Ehlers-Danlos syndrome are rare and include vascular malformations and abnormal, heterotopic grey matter. Hemiparesis and mental retardation are rare problems and probably only indirectly related to the collagen disorder. There is evidence, however, that collagen may act as a matrix for neuronal migration, and defective collagen could thus lead to abnormal cerebral embryogenesis (for example, neuronal heterotopia).

SUBARACHNOID OR LEPTOMENINGEAL CYSTS

Surrounding the spinal cord and nerve roots and within the thick connective tissue layer of dura mater of the vertebral canal are the leptomeninges. Disorders of these mesodermal elements impacting anatomically on brain, spinal cord, and roots have been observed as an isolated defect or part of a generalized connective tissue disorder such as Ehlers-Danlos and Marfan syndromes. In these isolated conditions, defects of the cranial and spinal leptomeninges may lead to intracranial subarachnoid cysts, or intradural and extradural spinal arachnoid cysts. Although many cases are sporadic, some occur as an autosomal dominant trait.

Intracranial subarachnoid or leptomeningeal cysts occur at many sites within the cranium but particularly in the posterior fossa, anterior temporal aspect of the middle fossa, and adjacent to the sylvian fissure (53). These cysts may or may not communicate with the subarachnoid spaces and have a tendency to behave as space-occupying lesions compressing the underlying brain and leading to ataxia, seizures, hemiparesis, and hydrocephalus.

Within the spinal canal the enlarging leptomeningeal cyst or cysts will compress the spinal cord with onset of subacute or chronic spastic myelopathy, particularly of the lower limbs since most cysts occur in the thoracic region (54). On occasion the cyst will expand into the cervical region producing quadriparesis or quadriplegia. Localized pain and spinal tenderness may occur due to nerve root irritation. A sensory level may be apparent on careful examination of the back using hot-cold and pinprick sensations. Kyphoscoliosis may be present and loss of bladder and bowel continence is a serious consequence of progressive cord compression. In some subjects, there is herniation of the leptomeningeal cyst through a defect in the dura with subsequent cephalad and caudad extension of the cyst in the epidural space (55). Usually the extradural extension is

posteriorly placed near the posterior septum or laterally near the exiting spinal roots. This cyst may be multiloculated and communicate with the subarachnoid space. CSF accumulates and eventually the extradural cyst will compress the spinal cord. There may be an association (56,57) with a double row of eyelashes (distichiasis) and acquired lymphedema of the legs (Milroy disease) in several members of the family as a dominantly inherited condition. An extradural arachnoid cyst rarely occurs in the sacral region with erosion and enlargement of the sacral canal (58,59). The dural sac normally ends at the S1 level and the extradural leptomeningeal cyst may erode anteriorly through neural foramina and produce a scimitar-shaped sacrum with compression of the bladder and bowel in the pelvis (60). Rupture of the cyst spontaneously or iatrogenically can lead to an ascending meningitis as a result of CSF contamination (58).

Radiologic studies include plain radiographs showing scoliosis, erosion of vertebral bodies posteriorly, and increased interpediculate distance. Myelography with water-soluble contrast medium may be helpful, particularly if followed by a delayed CT scan and patient repositioning, since contrast material may only enter the narrow valvular neck of the cyst after some time delay and in a supine position. MRI in multiple planes (59) is sensitive and noninvasive and shows the anatomic relationships necessary for complete surgical removal, particularly if there are multiple subarachnoid cysts. Postoperative studies are necessary and MRI is ideal for long-term neuroimaging follow-up.

MARFAN SYNDROME

Marfan syndrome is a systemic genetic disorder attributed to a defect in connective tissue formation. It is inherited as an autosomal dominant trait and cardinal features include ocular, cardiovascular, and skeletal changes. The ocular abnormality is ectopic lentis and is present early. It is usually bilateral and the lens is displaced upward. The mesodermal defect of bones and ligaments are manifest as scoliosis, kyphosis, lordosis, and posterior scalloping of vertebral bodies. Hypotonia is frequent and related to the ligamentous laxity observed in Marfan syndrome.

Neurologic complications of Marfan syndrome are rare and usually related to abnormalities of the spinal canal. Presumably, as a result of the mesodermal defect affecting the dura mater, there may be progressive enlargement of the dural sac in the spinal canal with subsequent herniation through various foramina, including those of the intervertebral and sacral neural foramina. Dural ectasia can be seen in other disorders affecting mesoderm, including Ehlers-Danlos syndrome and neurofibromatosis. Progressive dural ectasia with herniation (anterolateral meningocele) into the thoracic cage, abdomen or pelvis can present as a paraspinous mass communicating with the subarachnoid space and filled with CSF. While rare, the cyst can spontaneously rupture into the rectum or bladder and contaminate the subarachnoid fluid, which can lead to acute or recurrent ascending meningitis. A valve-like action at the narrowed entrance to the cyst neck can produce progressive enlargement and compression upon anatomically related structures. Neurologically an anterior sacral meningocele can compress nerves of the lumbosacral plexus with pain and leg weakness (61).

Although it is rare, a myelopathy can complicate Marfan syndrome causing progressive paraparesis, paraplegia and incontinence (62). Arachnoid cysts have been described in association with this myelopathy and can internally compress the spinal cord. Recently we observed a child with Marfan syndrome with a progressive myelopathy and enlarged abdominal cysts that were palpated and demonstrated radiologically. Decompression of the largest cyst with internal drainage of CSF into the peritoneal cavity resulted in reduced size of the cyst and improved strength in the legs. Dissection of an aortic aneurysm with involvement of the arteries to the spinal cord could also produce spinal cord paralysis in Marfan syndrome. Dissection of the aorta at the base of the heart could involve internal carotid vessels and produce a cerebrovascular accident. Embolization from abnormal cardiac valves (mitral valve prolapse) or endocarditis could infarct the brain in Marfan subjects.

LARSEN SYNDROME

A genetic syndrome of multiple congenital dislocations at various joints, together with facial and other bony abnormalities, was described by Larsen et al. in 1950 (63). Both dominant (64) and recessive (65) inheritance patterns have been described; and in addition to ligamentous laxity of many joints, particularly the craniocervical junction, there may be other connective tissue defects including hernias, chest deformities, and cardiac valve defects (65).

Ligamentous laxity at the craniovertebral junction may be clinically important since instability of the atlantooccipital and atlantoaxial joints can lead to dislocation and symptomatic (potentially lethal) compression of the cervicomedullary junction. Symptoms and signs should be carefully sought in these patients and appropriate radiologic and neuroradiologic studies performed. Detailed neurophysiologic studies (for example, polysomnography and somatosensory-evoked responses) may be necessary to document impaired spinal cord function. Stabilization of the craniocervical junction by fusion techniques is generally performed before neurologic compression occurs. There is a report of focal glial proliferation similar to that seen in tuberous sclerosis in one patient (66) and reminiscent of the parenchymal brain defects observed in Ehlers-Danlos syndrome (2).

CUTIS LAXA SYNDROMES

Cutis laxa conditions appear to be a heterogenous group of disorders in which the skin is lax with multiple redundant folds but not hyperelastic. Several genetic conditions with cutis laxa have been observed, including a dominant form usually apparent in adulthood, a recessive form presenting early in life with lethal emphysema, and an X-linked recessive form with defective copper transport and lysyl oxidase function. Another intermediate form of cutis laxa begins early in childhood and is associated with delayed mental and growth development (67,68). Disorders with cutis laxa may have ligamentous laxity in addition to the skin defect, making patients prone to joint deformities and dislocations at various sites (hips, knees, ankles), similar to other connective tissue disorders. In addition, diverticula of the gastrointestinal and urinary tracts as well as diaphragmatic and inguinal hernias may be seen in this group of disorders. Although the cause for the developmental delay and hypotonia in these children may not be readily apparent, we suspect that the ligamentous laxity and resultant joint instability impairs motor development similarly to that seen in achondroplasia and other ligamentous laxity syndromes. In some children there was improved motor function with age (68). There is a report of congenital cutis laxa with athetosis, mental retardation, and cloudy corneas as a distinct entity (69).

CONGENITAL ODONTOID ANOMALIES

Dysgenesis of the odontoid process of the second cervical vertebra is a rare disorder affecting children, and recognition of this cause of atlantoaxial instability can lead to successful treatment by surgical stabilization of the craniocervical junction (70). Neurologically, there is onset of progressive quadriparesis with cervical and occipital pain. Initially, symptoms and signs may be transient but they eventually become permanent. As a result of either absence of the odontoid or failure of fusion of the odontoid process, there is a subluxation of C1 on the C2 vertebra with medullary compression and, on occasion, vascular occlusion of the vertebrobasilar system (71). Posterior fusion of the occiput and upper cervical neural arches prevents excessive movement and may lead to arrest or improvement of the neurologic defects.

MISCELLANEOUS CONDITIONS

Spondyloepimetaphyseal dysplasia is a rare recessive connective tissue disorder characterized by ligamentous laxity and dislocations at many joints. Dwarfism is present and spinal malalignment with scoliosis may be severe enough to produce paraplegia (72).

Hereditary chondrodysplasia punctata is characterized by macrocephaly and a depressed nasal bridge, icthyosis and proximal shortening of the limbs. Radiographic features include deformities of the vertebral bodies and punctate calcifications of distal long bones, vertebrae, and pubis. The recessive form is more severe than the dominant form and death occurs in the early years of life. Gibbus deformity from the vertebral bone abnormality and congenital paraparesis has been reported, but it is rare (73).

The familial joint instability or hypermobility syndrome is believed to be a mild, dominantly inherited disorder of collagen synthesis (74,75). Familial joint laxity with recurrent dislocations of the hip and other joints has been recognized as an autosomal dominant trait. Some of these families become circus performers as a result of their abilities to assume grossly distorted postures (pretzel or India-rubber people). In addition to limb pain, probably due to traumatic osteoarthrosis (76), we have observed delayed onset of motor skills in infancy and impaired motor abilities in youngsters with this disorder. There may be improvement in motor skills with decreased ligamentous laxity in adulthood. We believe that milder forms of this disorder may be a relatively common cause for mild-to-moderate delays in motor development in children.

Asymptomatic atlantoaxial instability has been observed in about 10% to 15% of individuals with Down syndrome. Only about 10% of these patients, however, were clinically symptomatic and required surgical stabilization of the craniovertebral junction to prevent progressive spinal cord compression (77).

Progressive facial hemiatrophy (Parry-Romberg disease) is a rare disorder of unknown etiology that affects the subcutaneous tissues of the face, although skin, muscle, and bone may also be involved. Neurologic deficits observed in these patients have included trigeminal neuralgia, epilepsy, hemiparkinsonism, thalamic pain, and cerebral atrophy with hemiatrophy of the body (78).

Disorders of connective tissue occur secondary to metabolic defects and include the recessive disorder of homocystinuria and X-linked Menkes syndrome due to systemic copper deficiency (79). Both disorders frequently have severe neurologic deficits.

Disorders of bone and connective tissue clearly impact on the nervous system and the clinical syndromes range in severity from trivial to life-threatening. There is considerable overlap between the disorders as to the type of neurologic complications likely to be observed. Given an understanding of the pathogenesis of the bony or collagen disorder, the clinician should be able to predict the neurologic complications. Thus, a clinician encountering one of these relatively rare conditions for the first time should confidently be able to predict and, subsequently, examine and investigate logically any patient presenting with a neurologic complication.

REFERENCES

1. Pope FM, Nicholls AC. Molecular abnormalities of collagen in human disease. Arch Dis Child 1987;62:523–528.
2. Pretorius ME, Butler IJ. Neurologic manifestations of Ehlers-Danlos syndrome. Neurology 1983;33:1087–1089.
3. Scott CI. Achondroplastic and hypochondroplastic dwarfism. Clin Orthoped 1976;114:18–30.
4. Oberklaid F, Danks DM, et al. Achondroplasia and hypochondroplasia. J Med Genet 1979;16:140–146.
5. Hecht JT, Horton WA, Butler IJ, et al. Foramen magnum stenosis in homozygous achondroplasia. Eur J Pediatr 1986;145:545–547.
6. Vogl A, Osborne RL. Lesions of the spinal cord (transverse myelopathy) in achondroplasia. Arch Neurol Psychiatr 1949;61:644–662.
7. Spillane JD. Three cases of achondroplasia with neurological complications. J Neurol Neurosurg Psychiatry 1952;15:246–252.
8. Vogl A. The fate of the achondroplastic dwarf (neurologic complications of achondroplasia). Exp Med Surg 1962;20:108–117.
9. Reid CS, Pyeritz RE, Kopits SE, et al. Cervicomedullary compression in young patients with achondroplasia: Value of comprehensive neurologic and respiratory evaluation. J Pediatr 1987;110:522–530.
10. Nelson FW, Hecht JT, Horton WA, et al. Neurological basis of respiratory complications in achondroplasia. Ann Neurol 1988;24:89–93.
11. Todorov AB, Scott CI, Warren AE, et al. Developmental screening tests in achondroplastic children. Am J Med Genet 1981;9:19–23.
12. Hecht J. Personal communication.
13. Nelson FW, Goldie WD, Hecht JT, et al. Short-latency somatosensory evoked potentials in the management of patients with achondroplasia. Neurology 1984;34:1053–1058.
14. Blau JN, Logue V. Intermittent claudication of the cauda equina. Lancet 1961;1:1081–1086.
15. Hecht JT, Butler IJ, Scott CI. Long term neurological sequelae in achondroplasia. Eur J Pediatr 1984;143:58–60.
16. Szymanski D, Collier R, Orr S. Central cord syndrome. Ann Emerg Med 1983;12:45–47.
17. Hess CW, Mills KR, Murray NMF. Measurement of central motor conduction in multiple sclerosis by magnetic brain stimulation. Lancet 1986;2:355–358.
18. Dennis JP, Rosenberg HS, Alvord EC. Megalencephaly, internal hydrocephalus and other neurological aspects of achondroplasia. Brain 1961;84:427–445.
19. Horton WA, Rotter JI, Rimoin DL, et al. Standard growth curves for achondroplasia. J Pediatr 1978;93:435–438.
20. Pierre-Kahn A, Hirsch JF, Renier D, et al. Hydrocephalus and achondroplasia. Child's Brain 1980;7:205–219.
21. Cohn S, Weinberg A. Identical hydrocephalic achondroplastic twins: Subsequent delivery of single sibling with same abnormalities. Am J Obstet Gynecol 1956;72:1346–1348.

22. Mueller SM, Bell W, Cornell S, et al. Achondroplasia and hydrocephalus. Neurology 1977;27:430–434.

23. Yamada H, Nakamura S, Tajima M, et al. Neurological manifestations of pediatric achondroplasia. J Neurosurg 1981; 54:49–57.

24. Mueller SM, Reinertson JE. Reversal of emissary vein blood flow in achondroplastic dwarfs. Neurology 1980;30:769–772.

25. Sainte-Rose C, LaCombe J, Pierre-Kahn A, et al. Intracranial venous sinus hypertension: Cause or consequence of hydrocephalus in infants? J Neurosurg 1984;60:727–736.

26. Hecht JT, Nelson FW, Butler IJ, et al. Computerized tomography of the foramen magnum: Achondroplastic values compared to normal standards. Am J Genet 1985;20: 355–360.

27. Wang H, Rosenbaum AE, Reid CS, et al. Pediatric patients with achondroplasia: CT evaluation of the craniocervical junction. Radiology 1987;164:515–519.

28. Pauli RM, Scott CI, Wassman ER, et al. Apnea and sudden unexplained death in infants with achondroplasia. J Pediatr 1984;104:342–348.

29. Stokes DC, Phillips JA, Leonard CO, et al. Respiratory complications of achondroplasia. J Pediatr 1983;102:534–541.

30. Fremion AS, Garg BP, Kalsbeck J. Apnea as the sole manifestation of cord compression in achondroplasia. J Pediatr 1984;104:398–401.

31. Haponik EF, Givens D, Angelo J. Syringobulbia-myelia with obstructive sleep apnea. Neurology 1983;33:1046–1049.

32. Walker BA, Murdoch JL, McKusick VA, et al. Hypochondroplasia. Am J Dis Child 1971;122:95–104.

33. Kaufman HH, Rosenberg HS, Scott CI, et al. Cervical myelopathy due to dural compression in mucopolysaccharidosis. Surg Neurol 1982;17:404–410.

34. Edwards MK, Harwood-Nash DC, Fitz CR, et al. CT metrizamide myelography of the cervical cord in Morquio syndrome. AJNR 1982;3:666–669.

35. Watts RW, Spellacy E, Kendall BE, et al. Computed tomography studies on patients with mucopolysaccharidosis. Neuroradiology 1981;21:9–23.

36. Kulkarni MV, Williams JC, Yeakley JW, et al. Magnetic resonance imaging in the diagnosis of the cranio-cervical manifestations of the mucopolysaccharidoses. Magn Reson Imaging 1987;5:317–323.

37. Dekaban AS, Constantopoulos G. Mucopolysaccharidosis Types I, II, IIIA and V: Pathological and biochemical abnormalities in the neural and mesenchymal elements of the brain. Acta Neuropathol (Berl) 1977;39:1–7.

38. Wassman ER, Johnson K, Shapiro LJ, et al. Postmortem findings in the Hurler-Scheie syndrome (Mucopolysaccharidosis I-H/S). Birth Defects 1982;18:13–18.

39. Shinnar S, Singer HS, Valle D. Acute hydrocephalus in Hurler's syndrome. Am J Dis Child 1982;136:556–557.

40. Young R, Kleinman G, Ojemann RG, et al. Compressive myelopathy in Maroteux-Lamy syndrome: Clinical and pathological findings. Ann Neurol 1980;8:336–340.

41. Sze G, Brant-Zawadzki MN, Wilson CR, et al. Pseudotumor of the craniovertebral junction associated with chronic subluxation: MR imaging studies. Radiology 1986;161: 391–394.

42. Verma NP, Kapen S, King SD, et al. Bimodality electrophysiologic evaluation of brainstem in sleep apnea syndrome. Neurology 1987;37:1036–1039.

43. Case records of the Massachusetts General Hospital: Weekly clinicopathological exercises. Case 37-1982. N Engl J Med 1982;307:735–743.

44. Lehrman RAW, Reeves JD, Wilson WB, et al. Neurological complications of infantile osteopetrosis. Ann Neurol 1977; 2:378–384.

45. Coccia PF, Krivit W, Cervenka J, et al. Successful bone marrow transplantation for infantile malignant osteopetrosis. N Engl J Med 1980;302:701–708.

46. Tsipouras P, Barabas G, Mathews WS. Neurologic correlates of osteogenesis imperfecta. Arch Neurol 1986;43:150–152.

47. Pozo JL, Crockard HA, Ransford AO. Basilar impression in osteogenesis imperfecta. J Bone Joint Surg 1984;66-B: 233–238.

48. Pozzati E, Poppi M, Gaist G. Acute bilateral extradural hematomas in a case of osteogenesis imperfecta congenita. Neurosurgery 1983;13:66–68.

49. Frank E, Berger T, Tew JM. Basilar impression and platybasia in osteogenesis imperfecta tarda. Surg Neurol 1982;17: 116–119.

50. Beighton P, de Paepe A, Danks D, et al. International nosology of heritable disorders of connective tissue, (Berlin) 1986. Am J Med Genet 1988;29:581–594.

51. Kayed K, Kåss B. Acute multiple brachial neuropathy and Ehlers-Danlos syndrome. Neurology 1979;29:1620–1621.

52. Bowers WH, Spencer JB, McDevitt NB. Brachial-artery rupture in Ehlers-Danlos syndromes: An unusual cause of high median-nerve palsy. J Bone Joint Surg 1976;58-A: 1025–1026.

53. Rock JP, Zimmerman R, Bell WO, et al. Arachnoid cysts of the posterior fossa. Neurosurgery 1986;18:176–179.

54. Kim JH, Shucart WA, Haimovici H. Symptomatic arachnoid diverticula. Arch Neurol 1974;31:35–37.

55. Kendall BE, Valentine AR, Keis B. Spinal arachnoid cysts: Clinical and radiological correlation with prognosis. Neuroradiology 1982;22:225–234.

56. Bergland RM. Congenital intraspinal extradural cyst. Report of three cases in one family. J Neurosurg, 1968;38: 495–499.

57. Schwartz JR, O'Brien MS, Hoffman JC. Hereditary spinal arachnoid cysts, distichiasis, and lymphedema. Ann Neurol 1980;7:340–343.

58. Rengachary SS, O'Boynick P, Karlin CA, et al. Intrasacral extradural communicating arachnoid cyst: Case report. Neurosurgery 1981;8:236–240.

59. Sundaram M, Awwad EE. Magnetic resonance imaging of arachnoid cysts destroying the sacrum. Am J Radiol 1986; 146:359–360.

60. Ivamato HS, Wallman LJ. Anterior sacral meningocele. Arch Neurol 1974;31:345–346.

61. Fishman EK, Zinreich SJ, Kumar AJ, et al. Sacral abnormalities in Marfan syndrome. J Comput Assist Tomogr 1983; 7:851–856.

62. Newman PK, Tilley JB. Myelopathy in Marfan's syndrome. J Neurol Neurosurg Psychiatry 1979;42:176–178.

63. Larsen LJ, Schottstaedt ER, Bost FC. Multiple congenital dislocations associated with characteristic facial abnormality. J Pediatr 1950;37:574–581.

64. Stanley D, Seymour N. The Larsen syndrome occurring in four generations of one family. Int Orthop (SICOT) 1985; 8:267–272.

65. Strisciuglio P, Sebastio G, Andria G, et al. Severe cardiac anomalies in sibs with Larsen syndrome. J Med Genet 1983; 20:422–424.

66. Henriksson P, Ivarsson S, Theander G. The Larsen syndrome and glial proliferation in brain. Acta Paediatr Scand 1977;66:653–657.

67. Sakati NO, Nyhan WL, Shear CS, et al. Syndrome of cutis laxa ligamentous laxity and delayed development. Pediatrics 1983;72:850–856.
68. Rogers JG, Danks DM. Cutis laxa with delayed development. Aust Paediatr J 1985;21:281–283.
69. DeBarsy AM, Moens E, Dierckx L. Dwarfism, oligophrenia and degeneration of the elastic tissue in skin and cornea. A new syndrome? Helv Paediatr Acta 1968;23: 305–313.
70. Davis D, Gutierrez FA. Congenital anomaly of the odontoid in children. Child's Brain 1977;3:219–229.
71. Phillips PC, Lorentsen KJ, Shropshire LC, et al. Congenital odontoid aplasia and posterior circulation stroke in childhood. Ann Neurol 1988;23:410–413.
72. Beighton P, Gericke G, Kozlowski K, et al. The manifestations and natural history of spondylo-epimetaphyseal dysplasia with joint laxity. Clin Genet 1984;26:308–317.
73. Curless RG. Dominant chondrodysplasia punctata with neurologic symptoms. Neurology 1983;33:1095–1097.
74. Horton WA, Collins DL, DeSmet AA, et al. Familial joint instability syndrome. Am J Med Genet 1980;6:221–228.
75. Child AH. Joint hypermobility syndrome: Inherited disorder of collagen synthesis. J Rheumatol 1986;13:239–243.
76. Bird HA. A clinical review of the hyperlaxity of joints with particular reference to osteoarthrosis. Eng Med 1986;15: 81–85.
77. Pueschel SM, Scola FH. Atlantoaxial instability in individuals with Down syndrome: Epidemiologic, radiographic and clinical studies. Pediatrics 1987;80:555–560.
78. Lakhani PK, David TJ. Progressive hemifacial atrophy with scleroderma and ipsilateral limb wasting. J Roy Soc Med 1984;77:138–139.
79. Danks DM. Of mice and men, metals and mutations. J Med Genet 1986;23:99–106.

Chapter 23
Neurocutaneous Disorders

Bruce O. Berg

NEUROCUTANEOUS SYNDROMES

The neurocutaneous syndromes are comprised of a variety of clinical entities generally characterized by abnormalities of the skin and nervous system. Because these abnormalities are primarily but not entirely derived from ectoderm, they have been variously called "congenital ectodermoses" (1), "congenital neuroectodermal dysplasias" (2), and "geno-neuroectodermoses" (3).

Bielschowsky (1919) believed that neurofibromatosis and tuberous sclerosis were similar in nature because of their dysplastic nature and tendency to form tumors (4,5). Van der Hoeve considered the occasional retinal plaques of tuberous sclerosis to be similar in nature to the retinal lesions of neurofibromatosis and coined the inappropriate term "phakomatosis" (Greek *phakos*: lentil, mole, birthmark) to characterize these diseases (6) and as noted by Critchley, "muddying the waters." He later added Sturge-Weber syndrome and von Hippel-Lindau disease to the group (7,8). Moreover, Louis-Bar described the clinical features of another disease currently recognized as ataxia-telangiectasia and thought that this, too, belonged in the group of phakomatoses (9).

Since that time a variety of other syndromes, all of which are unusual and many lacking the typical features of neurocutaneous syndromes, have been added to this list of disorders. The major syndromes are considered in depth in the text; other less common disorders are also described (Table 23.1).

TUBEROUS SCLEROSIS

Tuberous sclerosis (TS), inherited as an autosomal dominant trait, is characterized by cutaneous lesions, seizures, and varying degrees of mental subnormality. Although initially described by von Recklinghausen (10) in his report of a newborn who died shortly after birth and who was found to have cardiac ventricular "myomata" and cerebral "scleroses," Bourneville is credited with the first clinical description of the disease (11). He documented the neuropathologic findings of a 15-year-old hemiplegic, mentally retarded, epileptic female who died in status epilepticus, noting focal areas of firm cerebral cortex (tubers). When sectioning the brain he also found nodules protruding into the ventricle and small areas of glial tissue in the striatum. Though he noted the patient had erythematous facial papules, he paid little attention to their presence, labeling them "acne rosacea." The patient also had multiple small tumors of both kidneys.

During the next 2 decades Bourneville and colleagues described additional patients with similar findings, emphasizing the association of the cerebral tubers and renal tumors (12,13). The facial lesions were described more fully by other authors and became known as "adenoma sebaceum" (14,15). Vogt (1908) noted a triad of findings in tuberous sclerosis, including adenoma sebaceum, seizures, and mental retardation (16). Sherlock (1911) introduced the term "epiloia" to indicate "epilepsy" and "mindlessness" (17). Critchley and Earl suggested the term "tuberous sclerosis" should be used for the fully manifested form of the disease (18).

The clinical expression of the disease depends upon the age of the patient and the extent of organ involvement. Seizures, the most common presenting symptom of the disease (90%), can occur any time after birth and are most commonly generalized in type (84%), though partial seizures can occur (29%) (19–22). Of the generalized epilepsies, infantile spasms and myoclonic fits are the most common; absence spells only rarely occur. The early onset and the severity of the convulsive disorder are correlated with mental subnormality, but there is notable variability of mental function of patients with tuberous sclerosis.

At the present time it is believed that 1/2 to 2/3 of affected patients are mentally subnormal (23). However, it must be emphasized that with the utilization of newer neuroimaging techniques, a greater number of asymptomatic patients have been identified. Clinical studies to date, therefore, may represent a higher incidence of mental retardation than is the fact of the matter. Moreover, some patients can have normal early development, only to show deterioration of mental function later in the 1st or 2nd decades of life. Notable, sometimes autisic-like behavioral changes,

Table 23.1   Selected neurocutaneous syndromes

Disease	Clinical Manifestations
Autosomal dominant	
Waardenberg syndrome I	Wide nasal bridge with lateral displacement of nasal canthus of both eyes; pigmentation abnormality (frontal patch of white hair, heterochromia irides, white eye lashes, leukoderma); cochlear deafness of varying severity (some patients are not deaf).
Waardenberg syndrome II	Similar findings to WWI without lateral displacement of nasal canthus but with higher incidence of deafness.
Autosomal recessive	
Chediak-Higashi	Partial oculocutaneous albinism (skin, hair, eyes); recurrent infection; neurologic (headache peripheral neuropathy, ataxia, and seizures) and ophthalmologic (photophobia, squint, nystagmus) disturbances. Giant cytoplasmic organelles are observed; associated immunologic and bleeding disorders.
Giant axonal neuropathy	Hypotonia with sensorimotor polyneuropathy; notably frizzly hair without pili torti. Dysarthria with varying degrees of mental subnormality. There is segmental axonal enlargement which at EM show closely packed swirls of neurofilaments.
Refsum syndrome	Retinal pigmentary degeneration (retinitis pigmentosa), polyneuropathy, ataxia, with increased CSF protein. Most patients have sensorineural hearing impairment, anosmia, and cardiopathy.
Rothman-Thomson syndrome	Erythematous skin lesions in early life followed by telangiectasis, atrophy, hypo- or hyperpigmentation, and ectodermal dysplasia. Cataracts, hypogonadism, bony abnormalities, and short stature. Body hair is sparse or absent; intelligence is usually normal.
Rud syndrome	Ichthyosis, hypogonadism, hypoplastic teeth and nails, peripheral neuropathy, sensorineural deafness, and seizures.
Sjögren-Larsson syndrome	Congenital ichthyosis with mental retardation and corticospinal tract dysfunction. Other features can include dental abnormalities, short stature, and fits.
Werner syndrome	Sclerodermoid skin changes with premature graying and alopecia. Cataracts, muscle atrophy, with leg ulcers, soft tissue calcification, and osteoporosis. There is an increased incidence of malignancies.
Xeroderma pigmentosa	Defect of DNA repair with premature aging of tissues exposed to sunlight. Microcephaly, mental subnormality, ocular changes, corticospinal tract dysfunction, ataxia, and movement disorders can be present.

particularly in those patients who had onset of seizures early in life, can occur.

Occasional patients have corticospinal tract dysfunction manifested by various patterns of weakness such as hemiplegia or spastic diplegic. Truncal or limb ataxia, however, is seldom observed despite the demonstration of cerebellar hamartomatous lesions or extensive cerebellar calcification.

Skin lesions are the most common sign of tuberous sclerosis and are represented by hypomelanotic macules, adenoma sebaceum, periungual fibromas, and shagreen patches. Additional cutaneous changes include fibromas, hyperpigmented macules, fibroma molluscum, and pigmented naevi. The hypopigmented macules are generally oval, or leaf (ash leaf) shaped, measuring 1 to 2 cm in length and affecting 80% to 90% of patients (24,25). Some hypopigmented lesions are smaller and some larger, but they rarely exceed 5 cm in length (Figure 23.1). They can occur singly or as multiple lesions and are often present at birth. When present in patients of fair complexion, they are more readily demonstrated when viewed under a Wood light (360 nm wave length) in a darkened room (26,27).

Adenoma sebaceum are angiofibromatous lesions that usually have a symmetric distribution, involving the nasolabial folds and the nose, and are sometimes found on the chin (16,24). They are initially present as erythematous papules during the first several years of life, gradually increasing in size with time and affecting about one half of patients (Figure 23.2). They are reported to have first appeared during the neonatal period or as late as 20 years

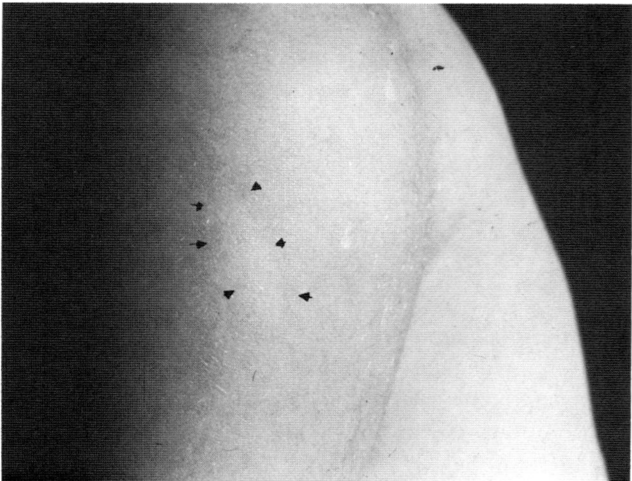

FIGURE 23.1 Typical leaf-shaped hypopigmented spot (arrows) on the lateral aspect of the right arm.

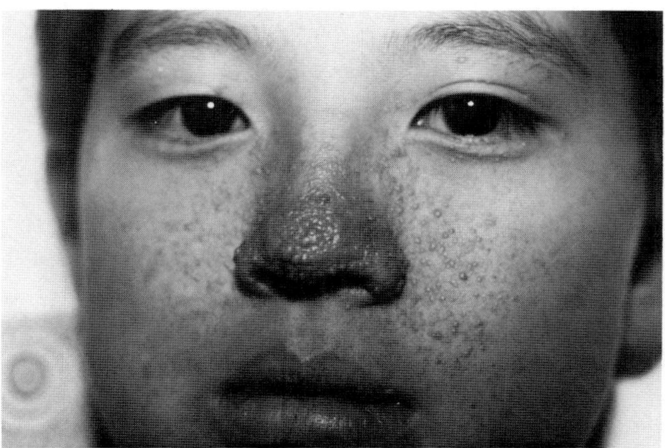

FIGURE 23.2 A 9-year-old mentally retarded male who had seizures and adenoma sebaceum affecting the nose, cheeks, and nasolabial folds.

of age. They are usually identified clinically and seldom require biopsy confirmation.

Fibromas are usually located on the forehead, the temporal fossae, scalp, or gingivae; they are firm, smooth, and only slightly elevated, enlarging only slowly (28). Koenen tumors are sub- or periungual fibromas, present in about one fifth of patients, that affect the toes more often than the fingers and are usually apparent during or after the second decade of life (Figure 23.3). Females are affected more often than males (29,30,31).

Shagreen patches are hamartomatous skin lesions usually found on the skin of the lumbosacral region and appear during the second decade, though they can appear earlier (Figure 23.4). They have an irregular surface likened to that of an orange peel (French: *peau de chagrin*) with either no color change or a faint yellow-brown discoloration. The lesions are present in about 20% of patients with tuberous sclerosis.

Other organs that can be involved in tuberous sclerosis include the eyes, heart, kidneys, and lungs. Retinal hamartomas have been observed in about one half of patients, but they are seldom the cause of visual symptoms (32,33).

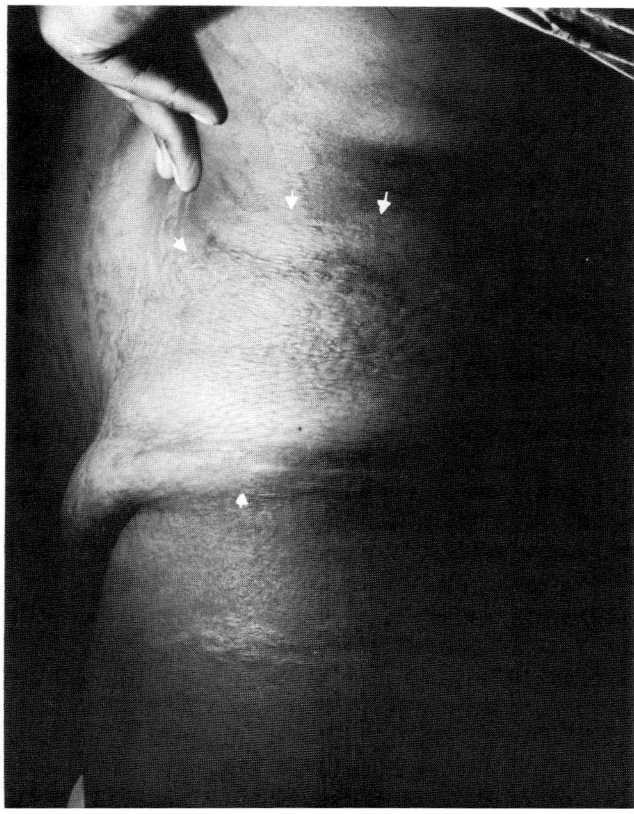

FIGURE 23.4 Shagreen patch overlying the lumbosacral region and extending over the lateral aspect of the hip (arrows).

These lesions are single or multiple and involve one or both eyes (Figure 23.5). They are commonly found in the retinal periphery and are best visualized by indirect ophthalmoscopy. Additional ocular lesions observed in the disease include retinal glial patches, iritic hypomelanotic spots,

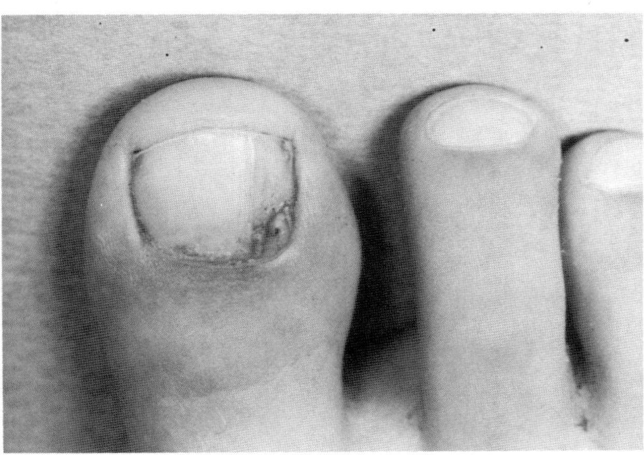

FIGURE 23.3 Typical periungual fibroma (Koenen tumor) found in about 20% of patients with tuberous sclerosis.

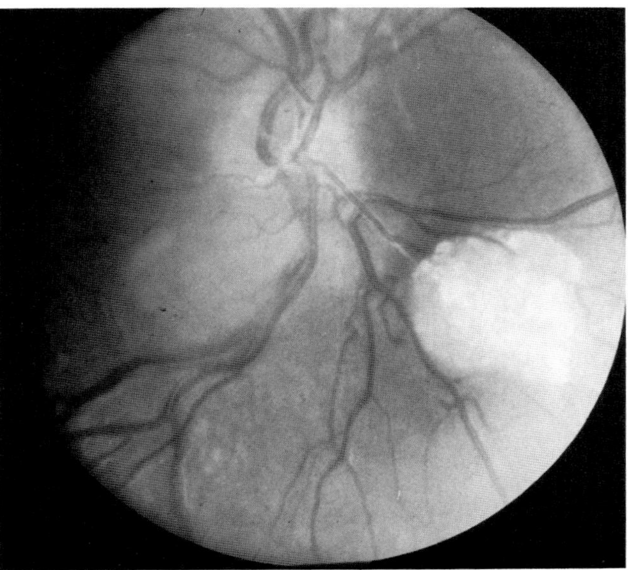

FIGURE 23.5 Retinal astrocytic hamartoma (mulberry lesion) in tuberous sclerosis.

cataracts, and colobomas affecting the iris, lens, and/or the choroid (34).

Cardiac rhabdomyomas are present in at least one half of patients and are manifested as single, multiple, or diffuse tumors that infiltrate the myocardium. These tumors, readily demonstrated by cardiac echocardiography, can be responsible for ventricular outflow obstruction and arrythmias or as abnormalities of the conducting system. Cardiac rhabdomyomas can also be demonstrated by other imaging techniques, including computed tomography (CT) and magnetic resonance imaging (MRI) (35–38).

About one half of patients have renal involvement, manifested as angiomyolipomas or cystic lesions. The lesions are often asymptomatic but can be manifested as hematuria, renal failure, or hypertension (39). Renal cysts are also generally asymptomatic and can occur independently or associated with angiomyolipomas.

The lung is occasionally affected in patients with TS and is observed almost entirely in females. There can be interstitial fibrosis as well as cystic changes of the lung. Patients can have progressive dyspnea with decreased vital capacity and pulmonary hypertension (pulmonary fibrosis), and those patients with cystic pulmonary changes can have, in addition, spontaneous pneumothorax and/or hemoptysis (40–42). The lung has a characteristic radiographic appearance. Other rare abnormalities of the liver, spleen, and endocrine glands have been reported.

Radiographic studies are important to confirm the diagnosis of tuberous sclerosis. About 60% of patients have intracranial calcifications, commonly observed in the periventricular region or in the area of the interventricular foramina of Monro. With newer neuroimaging techniques available, notably CT and MRI, plain skull radiographs are only rarely obtained (Figure 23.6). CT head scans can show cerebral hamartomas, subependymal nodules or giant cell tumors, and areas of diffuse demyelination. The most reliable finding, however, is the mineralized subependymal nodule (43–46). MRI readily demonstrates uncalcified nodules as well as the distortion of cerebral cytoarchitectonics (Figure 23.7) (47). Other abnormal radiographic findings in TS can include cystic changes of the phalanges, the metacarpals, and metatarsals; sclerotic changes of the long bones; and areas of increased or decreased density of the skull bones.

The tuber is the most striking neuropathologic feature of the disease and can be found within the cortical gyri or anywhere in the cerebral hemisphere. Smaller subependymal nodular tubers are often observed in the region of the sulcus terminalis or the basal ganglia, protruding into the ventricle. Giant cell tumors develop in the same region as the subependymal nodule and can grow within the ventricle, obstructing the flow of cerebrospinal fluid and resulting in hydrocephalus (48).

At microscopy the tuber is characterized by decreased numbers of neurons with scattered large, bizarre-shaped vacuolated "monster" neurons. Commonly, there is fibril-

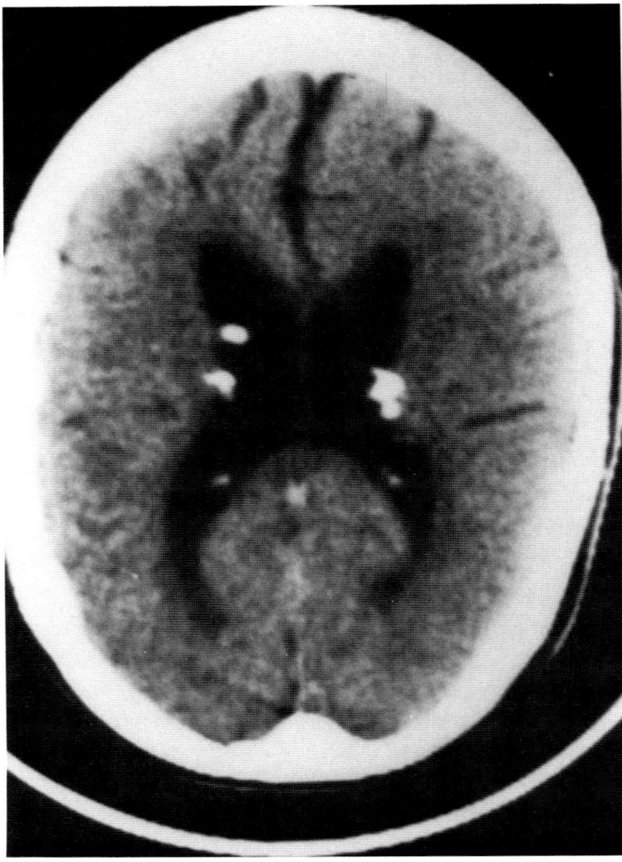

FIGURE 23.6 An axial noncontrast CT scan demonstrates subependymal calcific densities in the region of the foramen of Monro.

lary astrocytic proliferation, demyelination, and abnormalities of cortical cytoarchitectonics. The subependymal tubers are fibrocellular in nature with round or oval cells and whorls of fibrillary glial tissue. Giant cell tumors consist of large cells resembling gemistocytic astrocytes. At electron microscopy the giant cells have astrocytic features and contain large mitochondria. The ependymal lining is intact, overlying the glial cells and processes. Amyloid and/or calcium can be deposited within the tuber, and calcification of the cerebellum has been reported (49–51).

Tuberous sclerosis is inherited as an autosomal dominant trait with an estimated disease frequency of 1 in 29,000 (52,53). In order to address the heterogeneity of the disease, genetic linkage studies have been carried out; data have supported a locus on the distal 9q chromosome. There is evidence that more than one gene is involved in these family studies (54). Some authors have provided evidence for a TS gene on chromosome 11, but they had no data to support the view that more than one gene was involved (55).

Treatment of patients with TS depends on which organs are involved and the severity of that involvement. Convulsive disorders are managed by the administration of anticonvulsant drugs, but their control cannot always be

FIGURE 23.7 An axial MRI head scan shows multiple cortical and subcortical tubers, abnormal cortical cytoarchectonics, and cerebral atrophy.

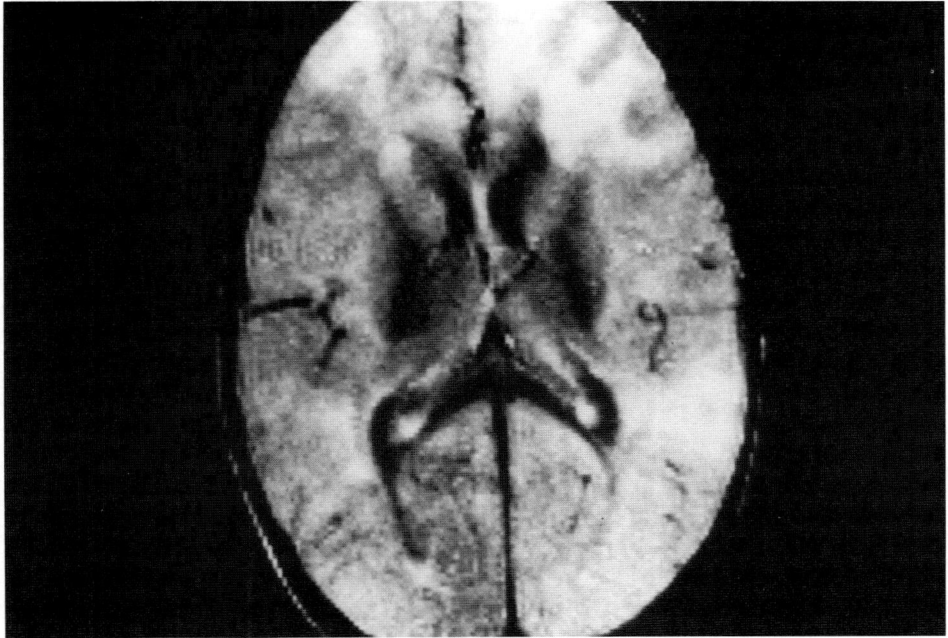

ensured. There is no specific treatment for the wide variety of skin lesions unless they are subjected to frequent irritation; selected lesions may require surgical removal. All patients with tuberous sclerosis must be provided long-term medical management, emotional support and guidance. Genetic counseling is required for all patients and family members.

NEUROFIBROMATOSIS

Neurofibromatosis (NF), inherited as an autosomal dominant trait, is characterized by tumor formation of the peripheral and central nervous systems and a variety of abnormalities of the skin, bone, gastrointestinal, endocrine, and vascular systems. The disease is notable for the heterogeneity of its clinical expression. Although von Recklinghausen is credited for the first description of the disease, it had been described earlier (55–59).

There are two recognized forms of neurofibromatosis: NF-1, the more common type, is generally known as von Recklinghausen disease and is characterized by multiple peripheral neurofibromas and hyperpigmented macules; NF-2 was earlier considered a central form of NF and is characterized by 8th nerve tumors, although other intracranial and intraspinal tumors often occur. The criteria for establishing the diagnosis of both types of the disease have been outlined by an NINCDS Consensus Committee on Neurofibromatosis (60) (Table 23.2).

Skin lesions found in the disease are varied and can be focal or diffuse and are often present before any manifestation of neurologic abnormality. Typical skin lesions include café au lait spots (CAL) or hyperpigmented macules of

Table 23.2   Diagnostic criteria for neurofibromatosis

Neurofibromatosis type 1

The diagnostic criteria for NF–1 are met in an individual if two or more of the following are found:

Two or more neurofibromas of any type or one plexiform neuroma

Freckling in the axillary or inguinal regions

Optic glioma

Two or more Lisch nodules (iris hamartomas)

A distinctive osseous lesion such as sphenoid dysplasia or thinning of long bone cortex with or without pseudoarthroses

A first-degree relative (parent, sibling, or offspring) with NF–1 by the above criteria

Neurofibromatosis type 2

The diagnostic criteria for NF–2 are met by an individual who has the following:

Bilateral eighth nerve masses seen with appropriate imaging techniques (e.g., CT or MRI)

or

A first-degree relative with NF–2 and either

   a. unilateral eighth nerve mass, or

   b. two of the following:

      neurofibroma
      meningioma
      glioma
      Schwannoma
      juvenile posterior subcapsular lenticular opacity

NIH Consenus Development Conference on Neurofibromatosis 1987 (60).

varying sizes, patchy or diffuse areas of hyperpigmentation, fibroma molluscum, hypopigmented spots, and angiomas.

CAL spots are usually present at birth; their number and degree of hyperpigmentation tend to increase during the first year or so of life, but thereafter the number of CAL spots remains relatively stable (Figure 23.8). They can involve any part of the body except probably the scalp, palms, and soles. The lesions are characteristically flat with discrete margins, and they vary in size from millimeters to centimeters. Crowe and colleagues observed that patients with six or more CAL spots with diameters greater than 1.5 cm had the presumptive diagnosis of neurofibromatosis (61) (Table 23.2). He later noted that axillary freckling was another important feature of the disease (62). Freckling can also occur in other intertriginous areas. More diffuse areas of hyperpigmentation can be the earliest sign of an underlying plexiform neuroma. It should be noted that the presence of CAL spots does not necessarily establish a diagnosis of NF, for about 10% of the population have one or more hyperpigmented macules.

Fibroma molluscum are found in the dermis or adjacent to it and are discrete soft or firm papules that range in size from millimeters to several centimeters. These lesions are flat, sessile, or pedunculated and are easily impressed into the underlying skin. Focal areas of hypopigmentation as well as focal areas of skin hypoplasia, lymphangiomas, and angiomas can also be present (63,64).

Lisch nodules, iritic melanocytic hamartomas, are age dependent and bilateral. They are present in about 10% of patients younger than 6 years old, 50% of patients under 30 years, and almost all patients over 50 years of age (65).

Neurofibromas can occur anywhere from the dorsal root ganglion to the terminal peripheral nerve branches, as well as the sensory and autonomic ganglia. They vary in size and are more commonly found on the trunk than limbs (Figure 23.9). Any organ system can be affected. In one study of 68 patients, the authors concluded that spinal nerve sheath tumors in patients with NF-1 were neurofibromas, whereas spinal nerve sheath tumors in NF-2 were more frequently schwannomas (66). Plexiform neuromas are comprised of interwoven elements of tumor and connective tissue that infiltrate normal tissue (Figure 23.10). They can be superficial or deep, affecting viscera and adjacent tissues. The incidence of sarcomatous changes in these tumors is generally accepted as ranging from 2% to 7% (67–69). The most common malignancy in NF-1 is neurofibrosarcoma, and embryonal malignancies, including rhabdomyosarcoma

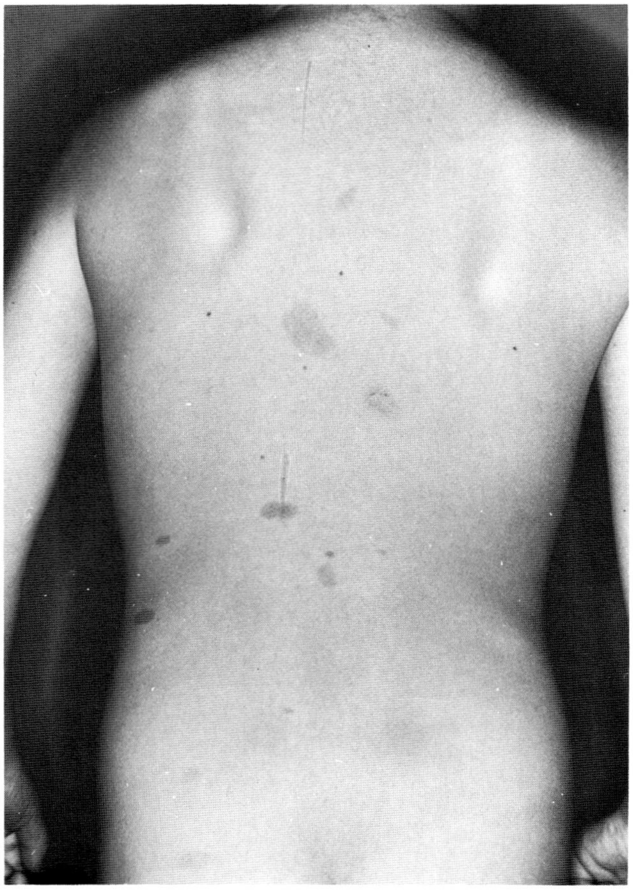

FIGURE 23.8   Multiple café au lait spots of varying sizes on the trunk of a 9-year-old child.

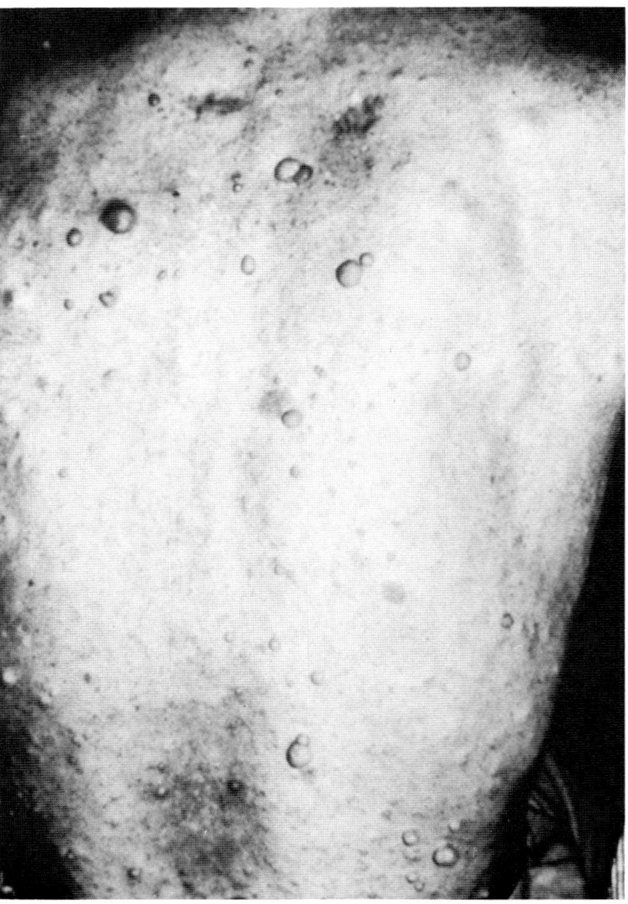

FIGURE 23.9   Numerous peripheral neurofibromas on the back of a young adult.

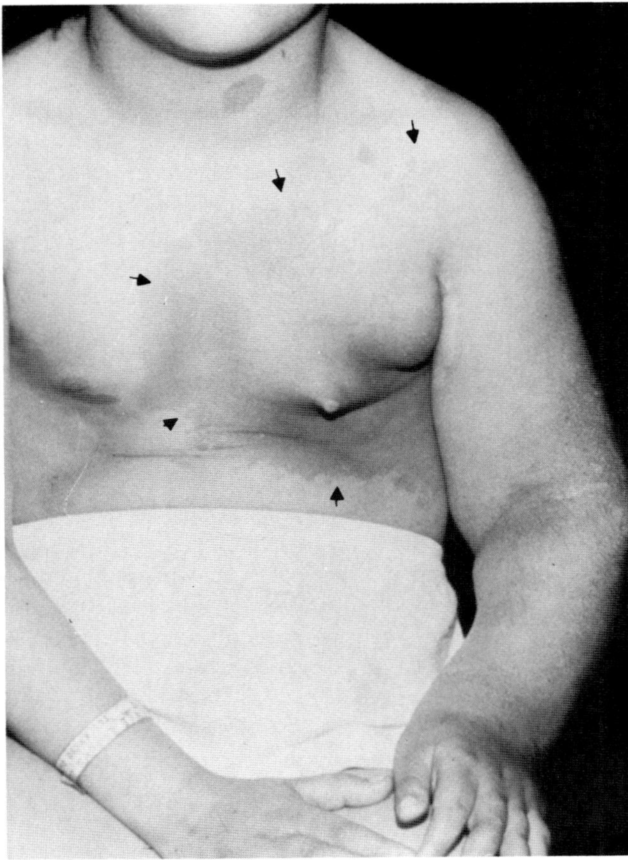

FIGURE 23.10 Multiple café au lait spots and a large hyperpigmented patch (arrows) overlying a plexiform neuroma affecting the left arm and hemithorax.

and Wilms tumor, occur with increased frequency in neurofibromatosis (70–74).

Intracranial tumors are primarily astrocytomas that can affect the cerebrum and cerebellum (65). There is an increased incidence of optic nerve gliomas, and other cranial nerves can be affected by schwannomas. Bilateral acoustic neuromas are a characteristic feature of NF-2, and meningiomas are also found with increased frequency in neurofibromatosis type 2. Medulloblastomas, ependymomas, and hamartomas occur more often in patients with neurofibromatosis than in the general population (75). There is also an increased incidence of pheochromocytomas.

Intraspinal tumors can be single or multiple and are located in the intradural or extradural space(s). They can be associated with spinal anomalies such as syringomyelia. Some intraspinal tumors extend through the intervertebral foramina, assuming a dumbbell shape.

Ocular abnormalities in neurofibromatosis, in addition to Lisch nodules, include optic nerve gliomas and congenital glaucoma (76). Optic nerve gliomas occur in about 15% of patients and usually present with symptoms of decreased visual acuity or visual field defects (75). Occasionally, patients present with signs and symptoms of increased

intracranial pressure. The tumor can involve the optic chiasm or hypothalamus and is rarely manifested as the diencephalic syndrome of infancy (77–79). Optic gliomas of childhood are probably hamartomatous in nature, indolent, and slow growing (80).

Congenital glaucoma (buphthalmous) is often associated with a neurofibroma of the superior eyelid (Figure 23.11). It is usually secondary to angle obstruction from neurofibromatous thickening of the ciliary body and choroid, fibrovascularization and synechial narrowing of the angle, or developmental abnormalities of the angle (76).

A variety of bony changes in neurofibromatosis highlight the dysplastic nature of the disease. The skull is particularly vulnerable to these abnormalities, and bony defects of the orbit, the occipital bones, and other cranial bones are common. Dysplasia of the sphenoid wing and the orbit can be associated with a plexiform neuroma, but there is generally no evidence of bony erosion from tumor. The reasons for these bony changes is not understood (81–84).

Other skeletal abnormalities include dysplastic changes of the spine such as scalloping of the vertebrae that can be unrelated to the presence of neurofibromas, scoliosis,

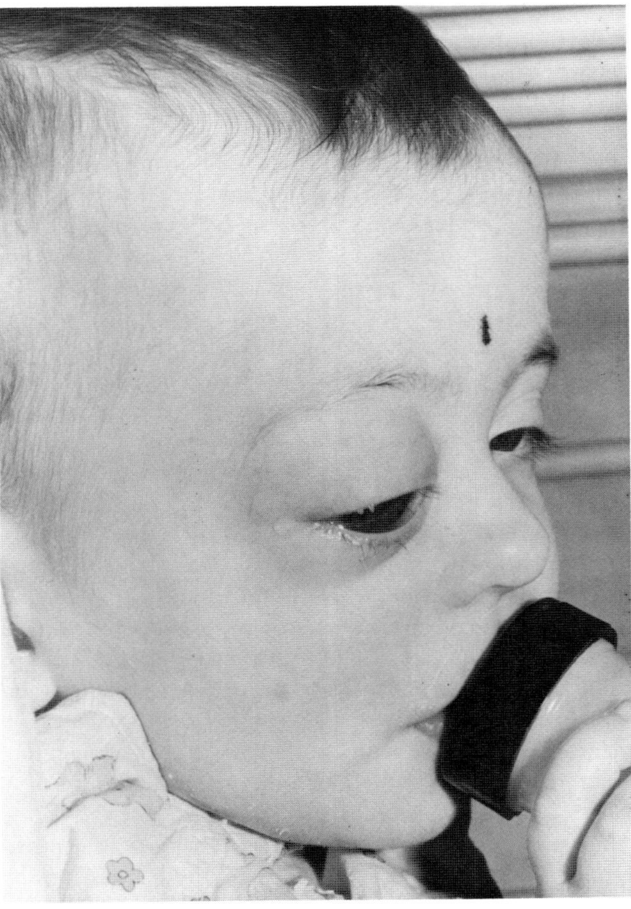

FIGURE 23.11 Congenital glaucoma (buphthalmos) in a 14-month-old male who also had an optic glioma and multiple café au lait spots.

kyphosis, anterior meningocele, enlarged intervertebral foramina, bony overgrowth, and bowing of the tibia and fibula. Pseudarthrosis is a characteristic feature of NF and usually involves the distal tibia, though other tubular bones can also be affected.

Additional features of the disease include macrocephaly and short stature that is not related to growth hormone deficiency. Mental retardation and seizures, though not necessarily related, occur in about 10% of patients and about 40% of patients have specific learning disabilities and hyperactivity (85,86). Precocious puberty has been observed in patients with hypothalamic gliomas, hamartomas, and in some patients with gliomas of the optic chiasm that involve the hypothalamus. Ganglioneuromas can involve the intestines, resulting in varying degrees of functional abnormalities of bowel motility (87). Hypertension can also occur, secondary to intimal proliferation and fibromuscular changes of the media of small renal arteries (88).

Other tumors occur in neurofibromatosis more frequently than in the general population, inluding pheochromocytoma, leukemia, neuroblastoma, and Wilms tumor. Moreover, there is an increased incidence of multiple endocrine neoplasia and medullary thyroid carcinoma. Of patients with pheochromocytomas, 4% to 23% have neurofibromatosis; whereas, fewer than 1% of patients with neurofibromatosis have been found to have pheochromocytomas (89).

NF-1, inherited as an autosomal dominant trait, has an estimated prevalence of 1 in 3,000, about half of which are new mutations. Linkage studies with characterized probes have identified the gene for NF-1 near the centromere on chromosome 17. Though linkage to the nerve growth factor receptor gene on 17q12–17q22 has been shown, crossovers occurred suggesting that the NF-1 gene is not coincident with the nerve growth receptor gene itself (90–91). NF-2 has been linked to chromosome 22 (92).

The treatment of patients with neurofibromatosis is generally symptomatic. Peripheral neurofibromas are usually indolent, and no surgical treatment is required unless the lesions are subjected to frequent trauma or there is inordinate tumor growth. Plexiform neuromas are sometimes removed for cosmetic reasons. Intracranial tumors and intraspinal tumors are treated by appropriate neurosurgical measures, radiation, or chemotherapy. Optic gliomas of childhood are generally thought to be hamartomas, and some investigators have recommended their conservative manangement by carefully following and documenting visual function rather than by surgery or radiation therapy (80–93).

It is important to realize that most patients with neurofibromatosis have full, functional lives without requiring any invasive therapeutic measures. Patients should receive thoughtful and complete medical and emotional supportive care.

VON HIPPEL-LINDAU DISEASE

Inherited as an autosomal dominant trait with variable penetrance, von Hippel-Lindau disease is characterized by retinal and cerebellar hemangioblastomas. Additional manifestations of the disease include cystic lesions of the kidney, pancreas, and epididymis; malignant tumors, and other cystic lesions of the liver, spleen, and lung may occur.

Panas and Remy first described the retinal lesions but were unaware that they were hemangioblastomas (94). Fuchs thought the retinal lesions were arteriovenous malformations (95), and Collins believed they were heritable capillary abnormalities (96). Von Hippel thought the retinal lesions were hemangioblastomas but labeled them "angiomatosis retinae" (97). One patient followed by von Hippel was found at autopsy to also have a cerebellar tumor, hypernephroma, as well as cystic lesions of the pancreas, kidney, and epididymis.

Lindau realized the similarity of tissue type of the retinal and cerebellar tumors and, moreover, observed that the same type of tumor was sometimes found in the medulla and spinal cord (98). The associated retinal and cerebellar tumors became recognized as the von Hippel complex, and Van Der Hoeve considered the syndrome as another phakomatosis, despite the fact that cutaneous lesions were not part of the clinical findings.

The retinal lesion, though reported to have occurred during the first decade of life, is usually initially diagnosed at some time during the third decade. It can first appear as an aneursymal dilation of a retinal capillary, but as it increases in size it appears flat or as a slightly elevated gray-white disc and only later assumes the appearance of a round, red tumor. Characteristically there is a dilated arteriole–venule pair of tortuous vessels coursing from the disc to the lesion, which is commonly found in the periphery of the retina (Figure 23.12). If careful ophthalmoscopy is not carried out, the lesion(s) can be easily overlooked. Flourescein

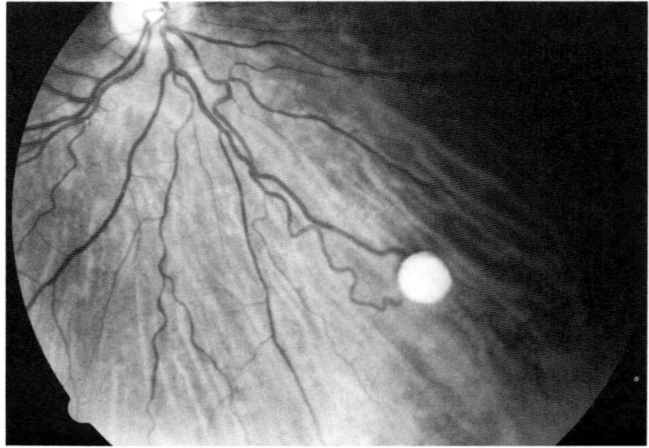

FIGURE 23.12   Typical elevated round white-red retinal hemangioblastoma of von Hippel-Lindau disease.

angiography is helpful in demonstrating the lesion (99–101). The accumulation of fluid within or beneath the retina may occur, and retinal detachment with progressive visual loss is commonly observed as the first suggestion of retinal abnormality (102–105).

Hemangioblastomas of the CNS usually affect the cerebellum but are sometimes found in the medulla and spinal cord; they rarely occur in the cerebral hemispheres. The cerebellar hemangioblastoma as in the case of the retinal tumor can rarely occur in childhood but is usually found in patients during or after the fourth decade. The initial signs and symptoms can be those of a posterior fossa space occupying lesion and manifested by cerebellar dysfunction and/ or signs of increased intracranial pressure. Hemangioblastomas of the spinal cord are associated with syringomyelia in about 80% of cases. In a report of 50 patients with VHL studied with gadolinium-enhanced MRI, 36 (72%) had one or more CNS tumors with the most frequently affected sites, excluding the retina, including the cerebellum (52%), spinal cord (44%), and brain stem (18%). Forty-one percent of all VHL patients with CNS tumors were asymptomatic. The tumor is reported to occur rarely in the supratentorial region and has been observed in the pituitary, the third ventricle, or cerebral hemispheres (frontal, temporal, parietal, and parieto-occipital lobes) (106).

A variety of renal lesions has been found in VHL including benign cysts, hemangiomas, adenomas, and malignant hypernephromas. The cystic lesions vary in size from a few millimeters to several centimeters, and though the lesions can be unilateral, they are often bilateral and multiple (107). In some VHL patients, renal cysts are so numerous that an incorrect diagnosis of polycystic renal disease has been made. A prominent cause of morbidity and mortality is the malignant hypernephroma, occurring with a frequency next to that of retinal and cerebellar hemangioblastomas. Because there are few controlled longitudinal studies of patients with VHL, and particularly those in which newer imaging studies have been utilized to the fullest extent, it is unclear how frequent the occurrence of renal cystic lesions is (108–111).

Additional cystic lesions can also be found in the pancreas, adrenal gland, and epididymis. Other organs reported less commonly to have cystic changes include the liver, spleen, and lung. Pheochromocytomas occur more frequently in patients with VHL than in the general population, with an incidence reported to vary from 3.5% to 17% of VHL patients (100).

The diagnosis of retinal hemangioblastoma is established by careful ophthalmoscopy with fluorescein retinal angiography demonstrating the characteristic lesion. CT and gadolinium-enhanced MRI will demonstrate the cerebellar or other CNS hemangioblastomas. Intra-abdominal cystic lesions of the viscera are well vizualized by CT, MRI, or ultrasonography.

Laboratory studies that can assist in diagnosis include the red blood cell count, which can be elevated in patients with cerebellar hemangioblastoma or malignant hypernephroma because of the increased erythropoietin activity of the cyst fluid. It must be emphasized, however, that the absence of polycythemia does not exclude the diagnosis of the tumor. Patients with CNS tumors commonly have increased protein concentration of the cerebrospinal fluid. The urine assay for epinephrine, norepinephrine, and vanillylmandelic acid should be carried out to screen for the presence of pheochromocytoma (112,113).

Cerebellar hemangioblastomas are usually found in the paramedial aspect of the cerebellar cortex and can be surgically removed with good results in about 90% of cases. The recurrence rate varies from 8% to 15%. There is little place for radiation therapy except in those cases where the lesion is surgically inaccessible. The retinal hemangioblastoma should be carefully followed by serial ophthalmologic evaluations if the lesion is small; however, as in case of visual loss or retinal detachment, the lesion can be treated by either laser photocoagulation or cryotherapy.

STURGE-WEBER SYNDROME

Sturge-Weber syndrome (SWS) is characterized by a facial angioma (nevus, port-wine stain) associated with a leptomeningeal angioma. In 1860 Schirmer described a patient with a facial vascular nevus and associated buphthalmos but he did not mention any central nervous system (CNS) abnormality (114). Sturge (1879) is credited with the first clinical description of this syndrome by his report of a 6 1/2-year-old girl with a facial nevus that also affected the lips, gingiva, palate, the floor of the mouth as well as uvula, and pharynx; the patient had congenital glaucoma and was hemiparetic. Sturge believed that she also had a vascular nevus of the underlying brain (115). It was not until 1897, however, that the first neuropathologic study of a similar patient was reported (116).

It is commonly accepted that the facial nevus conforms to the first or second, and sometimes third sensory divisions of the trigeminal nerve. However, other investigators have suggested that the distribution of the facial angioma is determined by the embryologic development of the facial clefts (117). The tendency to involve the forehead and superior eyelid can be related to the persistence of the primitive vascular plexus in the human embryo.

Intracranial calcifications observed in skull radiographs were initially reported by Weber, and Dimitri described the serpentine intracerebral calcific densities or "tram sign" (118,119). Van der Hoeve inappropriately considered the SWS as the "fourth phakomatosis," and only by virtue of time and tradition is it included in the category of neurocutaneous syndromes.

The Sturge-Weber syndrome is characterized by a congenital facial angioma that can be unilateral or bilateral and involves at least the upper face and periorbital region as well as the ipsilateral choroid (Figure 23.13). It can also involve other facial areas as well as the lips, gingiva, palate, tongue, pharynx, and larynx. On occasion, the ipsilateral or contralateral neck, trunk, and extremities can also be affected. An associated ipsilateral leptomeningeal angioma overlies the parietal, temporal, and/or occipital lobes; both hemispheres are sometimes affected. Leptomeningeal venous angiomas can occur unassociated with facial angioma, and although the related neurologic signs and symptoms are similar to those of SWS, these patients are more appropriately considered to have leptomeningeal angiomatosis rather than SWS (120–122).

In earlier reports, the incidence of convulsive disorders in SWS has varied from 70% to 90%. Seizures are primarily partial motor in type, although some patients have primary or secondarily generalized tonic-clonic fits. Other seizure activity includes infantile spasms, and myoclonic seizures; atonic fits occur less frequently. There can be a relentless progression of seizures with increasing frequency and severity. Postictal paralysis (Todd paralysis) can require

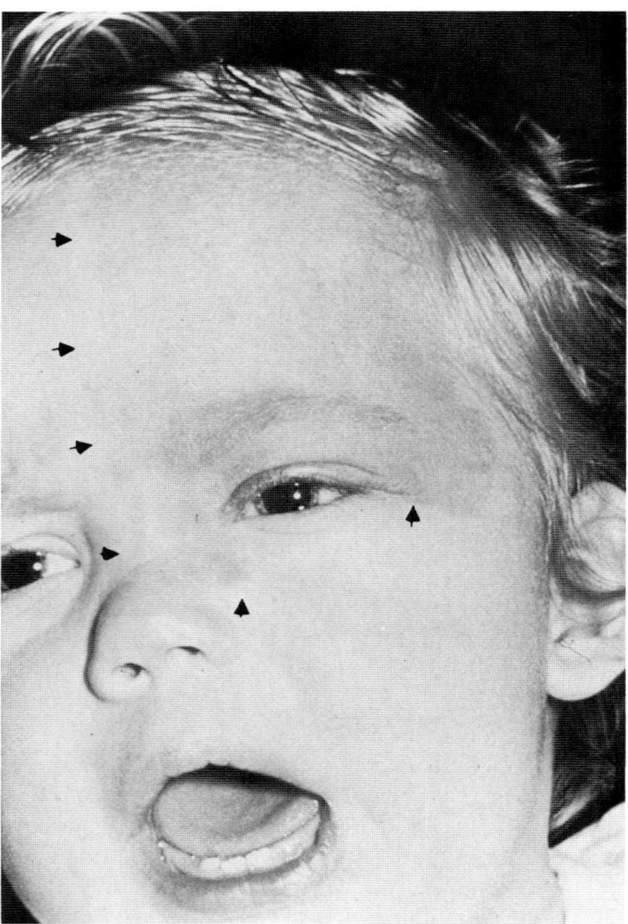

FIGURE 23.13 Facial angioma (port-wine stain) affecting the left upper face (arrows) in Sturge-Weber syndrome.

longer periods of time to resolve until there is a permanent hemiparesis. It has been suggested that hypoxic injury to the cerebral cortex results from venous congestion secondary to failure of cortical vein development (117,123,124).

In a retrospective study of SWS from the Mayo Clinic, 102 patients were studied during the period of 1942 to 1986. Eighty-eight patients had one cerebral hemisphere affected and 14 patients had bilateral involvement. Seizures occurred in 75% of patients. Of the 88 patients with unilateral hemispheric disease, 63 patients had seizures with the mean age of seizure onset of 24 months. Thirteen of 14 patients with bilateral hemispheric involvement had seizure disorders with a mean age of seizure onset of 6 months (125).

Electroencephalographic studies commonly show decreased amplitude and frequency of electrocerebral activity over the affected hemisphere. Diffuse multiple and independent spike foci are commonly present (126).

The neurologic status of patients is often dependent on their age and the severity of convulsive disorder. About 1/4 to 1/2 of patients are hemiparetic and hemiatrophy is present in about 1/3 of patients. Bilateral hemipareses are usually present in patients with facial angiomas affecting both sides of the face, but they are occasionally present in those with unilateral facial angioma. The sensory status of young patients is sometimes difficult to determine, particularly if they are mentally subnormal. However, sensory deficits associated with hemiatrophy are often demonstrated in later childhood (122–123).

Hemianopia is sometimes difficult to determine, particularly in young children, but it is thought that about 1/4 of patients have some defect of the visual fields. Glaucoma is present in about 1/3 of patients, and about 1/2 of these have buphthalmos ipsilateral to the facial angioma. Glaucoma can be unilateral or bilateral whether or not the facial angioma is bilateral.

Although intracranial calcification is seldom observed on skull radiographs of young children, it has been observed in the neonate and is present in most patients by the end of the second decade. About 90% of adult patients have intracranial calcification that is readily apparent in skull radiographs. The calcification is usually observed in the occipital or parieto-occipital regions but can be found in the temporal and less often the frontal regions (Figure 23.14). The calcifications are generally linear, serpentine, or have a parallel configuration (tram sign) (116,124). CT head scans demonstrate more readily the calcifications and cerebral atrophy than plain skull radiography. MRI demonstrates thickened cortex, decreased convolutions, and abnormal white matter. The two studies, therefore, CT and MRI, complement each other in that CT demonstrates more definitively the typical cortical calcifications; whereas, the T2-weighted MRI images show smaller, nonspecific foci of hypointense signals (127).

Cerebral angiography often demonstrates decreased cerebral venous drainage with dilated deep cerebral veins.

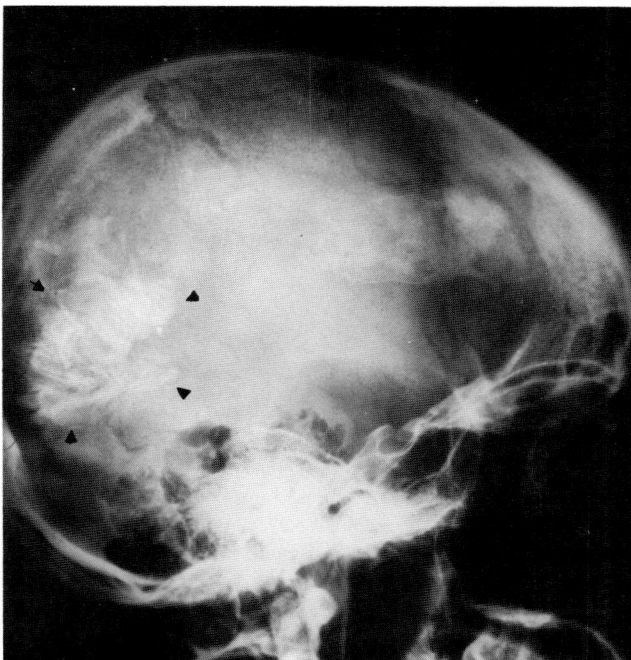

FIGURE 23.14 Skull radiograph of patient with Sturge-Weber syndrome showing linear parallel calcifications (tram sign).

Other vascular abnormalities reported in about 1/3 of patients include thrombotic lesions, dural venous sinus abnormalities, and arteriovenous malformations (128).

Positron emission tomography (PET) has provided a sensitive measure of the extent of cerebral metabolic impairment. Serial PET scanning in children with SWS can be of particular value in documenting the progression of the disease (129).

Neuropathologic studies have shown thickened hypervascularized leptomeninges primarily affecting the occipital, parietal, or temporoparietal regions. The meningeal vessels are generally small and tortuous and rarely enter the underlying cerebral tissue. Calcific deposits can be found in the walls of some small cerebral vessels but are primarily found in the outer pyramidal and molecular cortical layers. There is increased calcium content in the gray and white matter with normal concentrations of iron. The pathophys-

iologic mechanisms for deposition of intracerebral calcium are not well understood (118,130,131).

There has been no well-controlled, long-term study of patients with SWS, but in a recent Mayo Clinic retrospective study of 102 patients evaluated between 1942 and 1986, 47 patients (46%) had subnormal intelligence; of this group 17 were severely mentally retarded. The relationship of the convulsive disorder and mental function has been speculative thus far, but of the 25 patients with unihemispheric leptomeningeal involvement who did not have seizures, all were of average intelligence (125). Moreover, one patient with bihemispheric lesions was unaffected by seizures and that patient also had average intelligence. It would appear from these data that seizures have some role in either failure of mental development or in causing deterioration of mental function.

Patients with SWS require thoughtful medical and emotional support. Convulsive disorders should be managed by the appropriate administration of anticonvulsant drugs. Those patients with progressive seizure disorders that are recalcitrant to treatment should be carefully evaluated with reference to the surgical removal of affected lobe(s) or hemispherectomy. Rochkind and associates have demonstrated that seizure control following surgery was higher than in those patients who received only anticonvulsant medications. Moreover, the incidence of normal or borderline intelligence was higher than in patients who were treated conservatively (132,133). The management of patients with behavioral problems and mental subnormality requires the skill of the attentive physician, psychologist, and social worker.

ATAXIA-TELANGIECTASIA

Ataxia-telangiectasia is a multisystem disease process characterized by neurologic dysfunction, notably a progressive ataxia, proclivity to sinopulmonary infections, and immunoincompetence associated with lymphoreticular and other types of tumors. The disease is inherited as an autosomal recessive trait (see Chapter 24).

REFERENCES

1. Yakovlev PI, Guthrie RH. Congenital ectodermosis (neurocutaneous syndromes) in epileptic patients: Bourneville tuberous sclerosis (epiloia). Arch Neurol Psychiatry 1931; 26:1145–1194.
2. Van Boegart L. Les dysplasies neuroectodemiques congenitales. Rev Neurol (Paris) 1935;63:354–398.
3. Kissel P, Beurey J. Les geno-neuro-dermatoses. VIII Congr Dermatol Syphilol. Langue française, Nancy-Vittel 1953; 3:273–320.
4. Bielschowsky M. Uber tuberose Sklerose und ihre Beziehungen nur Recklinghausen Krankheit. Z Gesamte Neurol Psychiatr 1914;26:133–153.
5. Bielschowsky M. Entwurf eines Systems der Heredodegenerationen des Zentralnervensystems einschliesslich der Zugerhoren Striatumerkrankungen. J Psychol Neurol 1919;24:48.
6. Van der Hoeve J. Eye diseases in tuberous sclerosis of the brain and in Recklinghausen disease. Trans Ophthalmol Soc UK 1923;43:534–540.
7. Van der Hoeve J. The Doyne Memorial Lecture; eye symptoms in phakomatoses. Trans Ophthalmol Soc UK 1932;52: 380–401.
8. Van der Hoeve J. Les phacomatoses de Bourneville de Recklinghausen et de von Hippel-Lindau. J Belge Neurol Psychiatr 1933;33:752.

9. Louis-Bar D. Sur un syndrome progressif comprenant des telangiectasies capillaires cutanée et conjunctivales symmetriques a disposition naevoide et des troubles cerebelleux. Confin Neurol 1941;4:32–42.

10. Von Recklinghausen F. Ein Herz von einem Neugeboren welches mehrer Theils nach aussen, Theils nach den hohlen prominiernde tumoren (Myomen) trug. Verh Ges Geburtssh 25 Marz. Monatsschr Geburtskd 1862;220:1–2.

11. Bourneville DM. Sklerose tubéreuse des circonvolutions cérébrales: Idiotie et épilepsie hémiplégique. Arch Neurol (Paris) 1880;1:81–91.

12. Bourneville DM, Brissaud E. Encéphalite ou sklérose tubéreuse des circonvolutions cérébrales. Arch Neurol (Paris) 1881;1:390–412.

13. Bourneville DM, Brissaud E. Idiote et épilepsie symptomatique de sclérose tubéreuse ou hypertrophique. Arch Neurol (Paris) 1980;10:29–39.

14. Balzer F, Menetrier P. Étude sur un cas d'adénomes sébacés de la face et du cuir chevelu. Arch Physiol Norm Pathol (serie III) 1885;6:564–576.

15. Pringle JJ. A case of congential adenoma sebaceum. Br J Dermatol 1890;2:1–14.

16. Vogt H. Zur Diagnostik der tuberösen Sklerose. Z Erforsch Behandl Jugendl Schwachsinns 1908;2:1–12.

17. Sherlock FB. The Feeble-Minded. London: MacMillan 1911.

18. Critchley M, Earl CJC. Tuberous sclerosis and allied conditions. Brain 1932;55:311–346.

19. Gomez MR. Tuberous sclerosis. In: Gomez MR, ed. Neurocutaneous Diseases: A Practical Approach. Boston: Butterworths, 1987;30–52.

20. Gastaut H, Roger J, Soulayrol R, et al. Encéphalopathie myoclonique infantile avec hypsarythmie (syndrome de West) et sclérose tubéreuse de Bourneville. J Neurol Sci 1965;2:140–160.

21. Pampiglione G, Moynahan EF. The tuberous sclerosis syndrome: clinical and EEG studies in 100 children. J Neurol Neurosurg Psychiatry 1976;39:666–673.

22. Lagos, JC, Gomez MR. Tuberous sclerosis: Reappraisal of a clinical entity. Mayo Clin Proc 1967;42:26–49.

23. Borberg A. Clinical and genetic investigation into tuberous sclerosis and Recklinghausen's neurofibromatosis: Contributions to elucidation of interrelationship and eugenics of the syndrome. Acta Psychiatr Neurol Scand 1951;3 (Suppl 71) 11–239.

24. Alper JC, Holmes LB. The incidence and significance of birthmarks in a cohort of 4,641 newborns. J Pediatr Dermatol 1983;1:58–68.

25. Gomez MR. Neurologic and psychiatric symptoms. In: Gomez MR, ed. Tuberous Sclerosis. New York: Raven Press, 1979;85–93.

26. Chao DHC. Congenital neurocutaneous syndromes in childhood. II. Tuberous sclerosis. J Pediatr 1959;55:447–459.

27. Gold AP, Freeman JM. Depigmented nevi: The earliest sign of tuberous sclerosis. Pediatrics 1965;35:1003–1005.

28. Papanayotou P, Vezirtzi E. Tuberous sclerosis with gingival lesions. Oral Surg 1975;39:578–582.

29. Barroeta S, Grinspan-Bozza N. Tumor de Koenen sin otras manifestaciones clinicas de epiloia. Arch Argent Dermatol 1962;12:290–292.

30. Nickel WR, Reed WB. Tuberous sclerosis. Arch Dermatol 1962;85:209–226.

31. Kiun TP. A propos de deuz caz de tumeurs de Koenen isolae. Bull Soc Fr Dermatol Syphilol 1964;71:586.

32. Messinger HC, Clark BE. Retinal tumors in tuberous sclerosis. Review of the literature and report of a case with special attention to microscopic structure. Arch Ophthalmol 1937;18:1–11.

33. Walsh FB, Hoyt WF. Clinical Neuro-Ophthalmology, 3rd ed. Baltimore: Williams and Wilkins, 1969;1962–1965.

34. Gomez MR, ed. Neurocutaneous Diseases: A Practical Approach. Boston: Butterworths, 1987.

35. Mair DD. Cardiac manifestations. In: Gomes MR, ed. Tuberous Sclerosis. New York:Raven Press 1979;155–169.

36. Ostor AG, Fortune DW. Tuberous sclerosis initially seen as hydrops fetalis. Arch Pathol Lab Med 1978;102:34–39.

37. Crawford DC, Garrett C, Tynan M, et al. Cardiac rhabdomyomata as a marker for the antenatal detection of tuberous sclerosis. J Med Genet 1983;20:303–304.

38. Konkol RJ, Walsh EP, Power T, et al. Cerebral embolism resulting from an intracardiac tumor in tuberous sclerosis. Pediatr Neurol 1986;2:1108–1110.

39. Robbins TO, Bernstein J. Renal involvement. In: Gomez MR, ed. Tuberous Sclerosis. New York:Raven Press 1979;143–154.

40. Dawson J. Pulmonary tuberous sclerosis. Q J Med 1954;47:113–145.

41. Dwyer JM, Hickie JB, Garvan J. Pulmonary tuberous sclerosis: report of three patients and review of the literature. Q J Med 1971;157:115–125.

42. Lie JT, Miller RD, Williams DE. Cystic disease of the lungs in tuberous sclerosis: Clinicopathologic correlation, including body plethysmographic lung function tests. Mayo Clin Proc 1980;55:547–553.

43. Fitz CR, Harwood-Nash DCF, Thompson JR. Neuroradiology of tuberous sclerosis in children. Radiology 1974;110:635–642.

44. Martin GL, Kaiserman D, Wegler D, et al. Computer assisted cranial tomography in early diagnosis of tuberous sclerosis. JAMA 1976;235:2323–2328.

45. Garrick R, Gomez MR, Houser OW. Demyelination of the brain in tuberous sclerosis: Computed assisted tomography evidence. Mayo Clin Proc 1979;54:685–689.

46. Maki Y, Enomoto T, Maruyama H, et al. Computed tomography in tuberous sclerosis: with special reference to relations between clinical manifestations and CT findings. Brain Dev 1979;1:38–42.

47. McMurdo SK, Moor SG, Brant-Zawadski M, et al. Magnetic imaging of intracranial tuberous sclerosis. AJNR 1987;887–883.

48. Kapp JP, Paulson GW, Odom GL. Brain tumors with tuberous sclerosis. J Neurosurg 1967;26:1191–2022.

49. Russell DS, Rubenstein LJ. Pathology of tumors of the nervous system, 4th ed. London: Edward Arnold, 1977.

50. Trombley IK, Mira SS. Ultrastructure of tuberous sclerosis: Cortical tuber and subependymal tumor. Ann Neurol 1981;9:174–181.

51. Schafer J, Berg BO. Cerebellar calcification in tuberous sclerosis. Arch Neurol 1975;32:642–643.

52. Bundey S, Evans K. Tuberous sclerosis: A genetic study. J Neurol Neurosurg Psychiatry 1969;32:591–603.

53. Berberich MS, Hall BD. Penetrability and variability in tuberous sclerosis. Birth Defects 1979;15:297–304.

54. Sampson JR, Yates JRW, Pirrit LA, et al. Evidence for genetic heterogeneity in tuberous sclerosis. J Med Genet 1989;26:511–516.

55. Smith M, Smalley S, Cantor R, et al. Mapping of a gene determining tuberous sclerosis to human chromosome 11q14–11q23. Genomics 1990;6:105–114.

56. Tilesius WG. Historia pathologica singularis cutis turpitudinus. Leipzig, 1793.

57. Smith RW. A treatise on the pathology, diagnosis, and treatment of neuroma. Dublin: Hodges and Smith, 1849.

58. Fulton JF. Robert Smith's description of generalized neurofibromatosis (1849). N Engl J Med 1929;200:1315–1317.

59. Von Recklinghausen F. Uber die multiplen Fibrome der Haut und ihre Beziehung zu den multiplen Neuromen. Berlin: Hirschwald, 1882.

60. Neurofibromatosis: National Institutes of Health Consensus Development Conference Statement (NINCDS) 6.1987; 12:1.

61. Crowe FW, Schull WJ, Neil JW. A clinical, pathological and genetic study of multiple neurofibromatosis. Springfield: Charles C. Thomas, 1956.

62. Crowe FW. Axillary freckling as a diagnostic aid in neurofibromatosis. Ann Intern Med 1964;61:1142–1143.

63. Westerhof, Delleman JW, Wolters E, et al. Blue-red macules and pseudoatrophic macules: Additional cutaneous signs in neurofibromatosis. Arch Dermatol 1982;118:577–581.

64. Wertelecki W, Superneau DW, Blackburn WR, et al. Neurofibromatosis: Skin hemangiomas and arterial disease. Birth Defects 1982;18:29–41.

65. Riccardi VM. Neurofibromatosis. In: Gomez MR, ed. Neurocutaneous Diseases: A Practical Approach. Boston: Butterworths, 1987:11–29.

66. Halliday AL, Sobel RA, Martuza RL. Benign spinal nerve sheath tumors: Their occurrence sporadically and in neurofibromatosis types 1 and 2. J Neurosurg 1991;74:248–253.

67. Canale DJ, Bebin J, Knighton RS. Neurologic manifestations of von Recklinghausen's disease of the nervous system. Confin Neurol 1964;24:359–403.

68. Pearce J. The central nervous system pathology in multiple neurofibromatosis. Neurology 1967;17:691–697.

69. Riccardi VM, Eichner JE. Neurofibromatosis-Phenotype Natural History, and Pathogenesis. Baltimore: Johns Hopkins University Press, 1986.

70. Hope DG, Mulvihill JJ. Malignancy in neurofibromatosis. Adv Neurol 1981;29:33–35.

71. Herrera GA, deMoreaes HP. Neurogenic sarcomas in patients with neurofibromatosis (von Recklinghausens's disease) Virchows Arch [A] 1984;403:361–376.

72. Riccardi VM, Wheeler TM, Pickard LR, et al. The pathophysiology of neurofibromatosis II. Angiosarcoma as a complication. Cancer Genet Cytogenet 1984;12:275–280.

73. Riccardi VM, Elder DW. Multiple cytogenetic aberrations in neurofibrosarcomas complicating neurofibromatosis. Cancer Genet Cytogenet 1986;23:199–209.

74. Clark RD, Hutter JJ, Jr. Familial neurofibromatosis and juvenile chronic myelogenous leukemia. Hum Genet 1982; 60:230–232.

75. Wander JV, Das Gupta TK. Neurofibromatosis. Curr Probl Surg 1977;14:1–81.

76. Grant WM, Dalton DS. Distinctive gonioscopic findings in glaucoma due to neurofibromatosis. Arch Ophthalmol 1968;79:1127–1134.

77. Adornato BT, Berg BO. Diencephalic syndrome in von Recklinghausen disease. Arch Neurol 1977;2:159–160.

78. Holt JF. Neurofibromatosis in children. Am J Radiol 1978; 130:615–639.

79. Saxena KM. Endocrine manifestations of neurofibromatosis in children. Am J Dis Child 1970;120:265–271.

80. Hoyt WF, Baghdassarian SA. Optic gliomas of childhood: Natural history for rationale for conservative management. Br J Ophthalmol 1969;53:793–798.

81. Rubenstein AE, Mytilineoau C, Yahr MD, et al. Neurologic aspects of neurofibromatosis. In: Riccardi VM, Mulvihill JJ, eds. Advances in Neurology, Vol. 29: Neurofibromatosis (von Recklinghausen disease). New York: Raven Press, 1981.

82. Hunt JC, Pugh DG. Skeletal lesions in neurofibromatosis. Radiology 1961;76:1–19.

83. Taveras JM, Wood EH. Diagnostic Neuroradiology. Baltimore: Williams and Wilkins, 1964.

84. Ozonoff MB. Angiography. In: Newton TH, Potts DG, eds. Radiology of the Skull and Brain. St. Louis: CV Mosby, 1974;2749.

85. Fienman NF, Yakovac WC. Neurofibromatosis in childhood. J Pediatr 1970;76:339–346.

86. Dunn D. Neurofibromatosis in children. Ann Neurol 1988;24:306.

87. Hochberg FH, Dasilva AB, Galdabini J, et al. Gastrointestinal involvement in von Recklinghausen's neurofibromatosis. Neurology 1974;24:1144–1151.

88. Smith CJ, Hatch FE, Johnson JG. Renal artery dysplasia as a cause of hypertension in neurofibromatosis. Arch Int Med 1971;125:1022–1024.

89. Bravo EL, Gifford RW, Jr. Pheochromocytoma: Diagnosis, localization, and management. N Engl J Med 1984;311: 1298–1303.

90. Barker D, Wright E, Nguyen K, et al. Gene for von Recklinghausen neurofibromatosis is in the pericentromeric region of chromosome 17. Science 1987;236:110–1102.

91. Seizinger BR, Rouleau G, Ozelius L, et al. Genetic linkage of von Recklinghausen neurofibromatosis to the nerve growth factor receptor gene. Cell 1987;49:589–594.

92. Martuza RL, Eldridge R. Neurofibromatosis 2 (Bilateral acoustic neurofibromatosis) N Engl J Med 1988;318: 684–688.

93. Imes RK, Hoyt WF. Childhood chiasmal gliomas: Update on the fate of patients in 1969 San Francisco study. Br J Ophthalmol 1986;70:179–182.

94. Panas F, Remy DA. Anatomie Pathologique de l'Oeil. Paris: Delahaye. 1879;88.

95. Fuchs E. Aneurysm arterio-vensosum retinae. Arch Augenheilk 1882;11:440.

96. Collins ET. Intra-ocular growths. I. Two cases, brother and sister, with peculiar vascular new growth, probably retinal, affecting both eyes. Trans Ophthalmol Soc UK 1894;14: 141–149.

97. Von Hippel E. Die anatomische Grundlage der von mir beschreiben "sehr seltene Erkrankung der Netzhaut." Albrecht von Graefes Arch Ophthalmol 11911;79:350.

98. Lindau A. Studien uber Kleinhirncysten: Bau, Pathogenese und Bieziehungen zur angiomatosis retinae. Acta Pathol Microbiol Scand 1926;1 Suppl: 1–128.

99. Ausburger JJ, Shields JA, Goldberg RE. Classification and management of hereditary retinal angiomas. Int Ophthalmol 1981;4:93–106.

100. Atuk NO, McDonald T, Wood T, et al. Familial pheochromocytomas, hypercalcemia, and von Hippel-Lindau disease: A ten year study of a large family. Medicine 1979;58: 209–218.

101. Greenwald MJ, Weiss A. Ocular manifestations of the neurocutaneous syndromes. Pediatr Dermatol 1984;2:98–117.

102. Palmer JJ. Haemangioblastomas: A review of 81 cases. Acta Neurochir 1972;27:125–148.

103. Kupersmith MJ, Berenstein W. Visual disturbances in von Hippel-Lindau disease. Ann Ophthalmol 1981;13:195–197.

104. Goldberg MF, Duke JR. Von Hippel-Lindau disease: Case report with histopathological findings in a treated and untreated eye. Am J Ophthalmol 1968;66:693–705.

105. Salazar FG, Lamiell JM. Early identification of retinal angiomas in a large kindred with von Hippel-Lindau disease. Am J Ophthalmol 1980;89:540–545.

106. Filling-Katz MR, Choyke PL, Oldfield E, et al. Central nervous system involvement in von Hippel-Lindau disease. Neurology 1991;41:41–46.

107. Melmon KL, Rosen SW. Lindau's disease: A review of the literature and study of a large kindred. Am J Med 1964;36:595–617.

108. Horton WA, Wong V, Eldridge R. Von Hippel-Lindau disease: clinical and pathological manifestations in nine families with 50 affected members. Arch Int Med 1976;136:769–777.

109. Fill WL, Lamiell JM, Polk NO. The radiographic manifestations of von Hippel-Lindau disease. Diagn Radiol 1979;133:289–295.

110. Ludmerer KM, Kissane JH. Renal mass in a man with von Hippel-Lindau disease. Am J Med 1981;71:287–297.

111. Christenson PJ, Craig JP, Bibro MC, et al. Cysts containing renal cell carcinoma in von Hippel-Lindau disease. J Urol 1982;71:798–800.

112. Scully RE, Sarin LK, MacNeely BU. Case records of the Massachusetts General Hospital. N Engl J Med 1978;298:95–101.

113. Jeffreys R. Clinical and surgical aspects of posterior fossa haemangioblatoma. J Neurol Neurosurg Psychiatry 1975;38:105–111.

114. Schirmer R. Ein Fall von Telangiektasie. Graefes Arch Ophthalmol 1860;7:119–121.

115. Sturge WA. A case of partial epilepsy, apparently due to a lesion of one of the vaso-motor centres of the brain. Trans Clin Soc London 1879;12:162–167.

116. Kalischer S. Demonstration des Gehirns eines kindes mit Telangiectasie der linksseitigen Gesichts-Kopfhaut and Hirnoberflache. Berl Klin Wochenschr 1897;34:1059.

117. Alexander GL, Norman RM. The Sturge-Weber Syndrome. Bristol: John Wright and Son, 1960:73.

118. Weber FP. Right-sided hemihypotrophy resulting from right-sided congenital spastic hemiplegia, with a morbid condition of the left side of the brain revealed by radiograms. J Neurol Neurosurg Psychiatry 1922;3:134–139.

119. Dimitri V. Tumor cerebral congenito (angio cavernoso). Rev Assoc Med Argent 1923;36:1029–1037.

120. McKusick VA. Mendelian Inheritance in Man; 7th ed. Baltimore: Johns Hopkins University Press, 1986;691.

121. Jacobs AH, Walton RG. The incidence of birthmarks in the neonate. Pediatrics 1976;58:218–222.

122. Alexander GL. Sturge-Weber syndrome. In: Vinken PJ, Bruyn GW, eds. Handbook of Clinical Neurology. New York: American Elsevier, 1972;14:223–240.

123. Chao DHC. Congenital neurocutaneous syndromes of childhood. III. Sturge-Weber disease. J Pediatr 1959;55:635–649.

124. Hebold O. Haemangiom der weichen Hirnhaut bei Naevus vasculosos des Gesichts. Arch Psychiatr Nervenkr 1913;51:445–457.

125. Bebin EM, Gomez MR. Prognosis in Sturge-Weber disease: Comparison of unihemispheric and bihemispheric involvement. J Child Neurol 1988;3:181–184.

126. Aminoff MJ. Electrodiagnosis in clinical neurology. New York: Churchill-Livingstone 1986;58–59.

127. Chamberlain MC, Press GA, Hesselink JR. MR imaging and CT in three cases of Sturge-Weber syndrome: Prospective comparison. AJNR 1989;110:491–496.

128. Bentson JR, Wilson GH, Newton TH. Cerebral venous drainage pattern in the Sturge-Weber syndrome. Radiology 1957;68:327–336.

129. Chugani HT, Mazziotta JC, Phelps ME. Sturge-Weber syndrome: A study of cerebral glucose utilization with positron emission tomography. J Pediatr 1989;114:244–253.

130. Wachswulth N, Lowenthal A. Determination chimique d'elements mineraux dans les calcifications intracerebrales de la maladie Sturge-Weber. Acta Neurol Psychiatr Belg 1950;50:305–313.

131. Tinghey AH. Iron and calcium in Sturge-Weber disease. J Ment Sci 1956;102:178–180.

132. Hoffman HJ, Hendrick EB, Dennis M, et al. Hemispherectomy for Sturge-Weber syndrome. Child's Brain 1979;5:233–248.

133. Rochkind S, Hoffman HJ, Hendrick EB. Sturge-Weber syndrome: Natural history and prognosis. J Epilepsy (in press).

Part IV

Neurologic Manifestations of Immunologic Disorders

Chapter 24
Disorders of Immunologic Dysfunction

Alfred J. Spiro and
Daniel R. Pack

EXPERIMENTAL MODELS OF DISEASES OF PUTATIVE AUTOIMMUNITY

The acquired autoimmune inflammatory disorders represent an extensive group of diseases which may afflict nearly any portion of the neuraxis. They are characterized by both acute and chronic syndromes and may be monophasic, relapsing and remitting, or relentlessly progressive in their destructive effects. Characteristically their etiology is unknown, but they are often considered to be a consequence of viral infection and may be more frequently encountered in persons of particular tissue types, implying that certain major histocompatibility complex (MHC) gene products may play a role in their pathogenesis.

Among the more frequently encountered neurologic diseases putatively attributed to disorders of autoimmunity are multiple sclerosis, the inflammatory demyelinating polyradiculoneuropathies, and the inflammatory myopathies. Attempts to characterize these disorders have provoked a search for representative animal models. Spontaneously occurring animal analogs are lacking many features considered essential when making a diagnosis in humans, leaving investigators to turn to laboratory facsimiles. Experimental allergic encephalomyelitis (EAE), experimental allergic neuritis (EAN), and experimental autoimmune inflammatory myopathy (EAM) are all diseases of autoimmunity that may be produced in naive animals by the injection of tissue-specific antigens in combination with immune adjuvants or by injection of antigen-sensitized syngeneic T lymphocytes (1–4). Factors determining vascular permeability and the access of circulating constituents (immune effector cells, specific antibodies, and immune complexes, for example) to the specific tissues attacked appear to have a crucial role in the symptomatic expression of these diseases (2,5,6).

Experimental Allergic Encephalomyelitis

EAE is an inflammatory and demyelinating disease of the central nervous system caused by class 2 MHC-restricted T cell-dependent delayed hypersensitivity to central nervous system (CNS) antigens. It is easily induced in a number of laboratory species with a single injection of either purified myelin-basic protein (MBP), whole myelin, white matter, or spinal cord in combination with Freund adjuvant, a method referred to as active sensitization. Acute EAE manifests approximately 10 to 14 days following the injection and runs a typically monophasic and fatal course. Chronic relapsing EAE has a delayed onset and an exacerbating-remitting course that is limited by the life span of the animal. Passive or adoptive transfer of the disease is accomplished by the injection of sensitized lymphoid cells from donor animal actively sensitized for EAE into syngeneic or immunologically compromised naive recipients (7). Induction and dose-dependent clinical expression of EAE by passive transfer of class 2 MHC-restricted helper/inducer T-cell clones (1,8) supports a T cell-mediated mechanism for EAE, as does the finding that injected monoclonal antibodies reactive to T helper cell surface antigens may prevent or reverse the effects of the disease (9,10). Evidence exists, however, for a contributing role played by B cells and antibodies against myelin lipids (11–14).

The histologic picture of EAE in its early stages is characterized by lymphocyte perivascular cuffing. Large mononuclear cells then exit small vessels and invade parenchymal tissues, at which time demyelination and clinical signs become evident. In the SJL/J mouse, 7 days postinoculation, an abundance of infiltrating T cells may be found in meningeal, perivascular, and parenchymal areas throughout the CNS. Class 2 MHC gene products (Ia antigen) can be demonstrated on some endothelial cells within the brain

and actrocytes in the spinal cord. Albumin and Ig deposits (evidence of vascular permeability) are present in brain and, to a lesser extent, spinal cord. During chronic stages, some restoration of blood-brain barrier (BBB) integrity occurs. Galactocerebroside may be found on vascular endothelium throughout the neuraxis while MBP has a more limited distribution (15). The presence of class 2 MHC and myelin antigens on CNS vascular endothelium in animals with chronic relapsing EAE might fulfill requirements for local antigen presentation and proliferation of encephalitogenic T cell clones (16), and might also provoke interactions with circulating white blood cells that alter vascular permeability and induce inflammatory cell migration into the parenchyma. Astrocytes have also been shown to present MBP antigen and stimulate encephalitogenic T cell lines, suggesting a role consistent with accessory cell function (17). Astrocytes can perform this function only after being induced to express class 2 MHC antigens. This occurs during interaction with stimulated T lymphocytes (18), and is probably mediated by interferon (19–20).

During the latent period and first episode of clinical signs, lesions contain diffuse, unstructured infiltrates in which all types of hematogenous cells are intermixed. Lesions found during chronic stages of the disease present with a distinct distribution pattern of inflammatory cells in which L3T4 + cells predominated within the parenchyma while Lyt2 + cells were more common in perivascular and meningeal areas. L3T4 + cells were even more numerous and widespread in chronic progressive than in exacerbating-remitting disease, where they were found in the lesion only (15). At 10 days post-inoculation, B cells and macrophages appear and remain in perivascular regions (21). Thickening or hydration of the outer myelin lamellae is the first visible indicator of demyelination, followed by vesiculation and dissolution of myelin. Antibody and hydrolytic enzymes appear requisite to this process (22–23). Myelin stripping is then provided by macrophages via receptor-mediated phagocytosis; the myelin droplets are seen associated with coated pits on the macrophage cell surfaces (24). Astrocytes also participate in the uptake of myelin, but whether they process myelin antigens for presentation to T cells is unknown. Groups of naked axons are left as the attack on the CNS subsides and the macrophages depart via the Virchow-Robin space of blood vessels (7). Gliosis and remyelination have been described in chronic demyelinated plaques of chronic relapsing EAE (25) and some oligodendrocytes are known to survive within these plaques. Investigation of factors stimulating oligodendrocyte proliferation and remyelination of stripped axons may provide future avenues for therapeutic intervention (26).

Experimental Allergic Neuritis

EAN is an inflammatory demyelinating disease of the peripheral nervous system inducible in many species by intradermal inoculation with peripheral nerve, peripheral nerve myelin, or P_2 basic protein in Freund adjuvant. Like EAE, it is an organ specific, T helper cell dependent delayed-type hypersensitivity reaction. It is, however, ostensibly directed against P_2 of peripheral myelin (27), a cationic/adherent protein that holds the inner cytoplasmic membranes of the Schwann cell myelin lamellae together. EAN is considered to be an appropriate animal model for Guillain-Barré syndrome (GBS) because of the striking clinical and histologic similarities. Both diseases appear to follow a monophasic, self-limited course occasionally terminating in death, and chronic variants occur both in animals (28) and humans. Onset is typically acute, occurring approximately 10 to 14 days following inoculation (or infection in GBS), and is characterized by weakness (often progressing to paralysis), loss of deep tendon reflexes, ataxia, and sensory disturbances. Nerve conduction abnormalities, such as early perturbation of late responses, decreased nerve conduction velocity, and conduction failure paralleling that seen in human disease have been documented (29). Elevated cerebrospinal fluid (CSF) protein without marked pleocytosis reflects radicular involvement and is common to both.

The active sensitization techniques for inducing EAN are extensions of methods developed for EAE. Passive transfer has been accomplished utilizing P_2-reactive T helper cell clones (3,4,29). The lesions of EAN are morphologically indistinguishable from those of GBS. They first appear approximately 11 days after inoculation as cuffing of endoneurial vessels by small lymphocytes and mononuclear cells with accompanying demyelination (30). Mononuclear cells attach to vessel walls, then enter the endoneurium, invading nerve fibers and pushing Schwann cell bodies aside. Macrophage cytoplasmic processes separate myelin lamellae from the main sheath and proceed to strip the axon. Myelin may then be either phagocytosed or lysed into vesicular masses (7). Axonal diameter decreases during the acute demyelination and axonal dimensions are not restored with remyelination (31). In regions of intense inflammation, axonal degeneration may be evident (32). The disappearance of T cells from the intraneural compartment is associated with clinical recovery (32).

Early morphologic features of EAN include alterations in nerve blood vessel permeability (33). Significant changes in both the number and extent of degranulation of mast cells in rat sciatic nerve has been observed during the course of the disease. Mast cell degranulation in EAN precedes the onset of clinical symptoms and may be mediated by antibody or by factors released by sensitized T cells (6). The blood-nerve barrier (BNB) prevents access of circulating antibodies to nerve until inflammation compromises BNB integrity. Vasoactive amines (VAA) probably facilitate access of circulating elements (for example, inflammatory cells, immunoglobulins, complement) to the neural compartment. VAA depletion has been shown to delay or suppress the expression of both EAN (34) and EAE (5).

Coonhound paralysis and Marek disease are two spontaneously occurring animal analogs of Guillain-Barré syndrome. Both are associated with viral infection and produce lesions of the peripheral nerves indistinguishable from those of EAN. It is postulated that the viral infection in these diseases compromises the blood-nerve barrier, allowing autosensitization to myelin antigens (7). Chronic variants of EAN or GBS may be due to continued or recurrent compromise of the blood-nerve barrier, producing repeated exposure of myelin antigens to circulating T cells and leakage of antibodies into peripheral nerve. The role of antibodies in the development of EAN (and GBS) is at present controversial. EAN sera will destroy myelinated peripheral nerves in cultures in the presence of complement (35). GBS serum will produce some demyelination but it is milder than that of EAN serum. It has been demonstrated that GBS serum injected into nerves produces conduction block, myelin breakdown and phagocytic infiltration (36). Antibodies of the IgM type appear to be responsible. IgM antibodies are especially effective in fixing complement; the best IgM responses are initiated by sugar moieties, and IgM responses are relatively acute and short-lived. The role of these antigens in the pathogenesis of human disease is unclear. Antibodies to P_2 are rarely found in acute and chronic GBS, and when they are seen, it is likely their presence is an epiphenomenon. The antigens responsible for human disease are unknown, but the list of candidates includes galactocerebroside and ganglioside, among many others.

Experimental Autoimmune Inflammatory Myopathy

Inflammatory muscle disease has been induced experimentally in animals and bares some resemblance to human syndromes. Active sensitization is accomplished with injections of muscle homogenates and complete Freund adjuvant. As occurs in EAE and EAN, clinical symptoms appear approximately 10 days after innoculation. The observed pathologic alterations include cellular infiltration of perivascular, perimysial and endomysial tissues, and muscle fiber necrosis. Ultracentrifugation of the muscle homogenate revealed the myofibrillary fraction to be most active. Creatine kinase elevations and lesion frequency both reached a maximum at 4 to 5 weeks postinjection. Antibodies directed against A-band myosin were present throughout the period of active disease (37). Anti-muscle antibodies are found in strains of mice in which active sensitization is attempted but fail to develop EAM (38). Anti-muscle antibodies are also infrequently found in human disease. Passive transfer of EAM has been successful using splenocytes co-cultured with skeletal muscle and injecting the cells into naive, syngeneic animals. A high percentage of mice from a strain sensitive to the effects of vasoactive amines (SJL/L) developed the disease. In contrast, injection of muscle-sensitized lymphocytes into mice genetically insensitive to vasoactive amines (BALB/c) failed to induce EAM in any animal. The lesions produced in this model were not organ specific. Lymphocytes co-cultured with smooth muscle cells produced inflammatory infiltration in skeletal muscle in 50% of the animals injected (2). EAM has been produced by intraperitoneal injection of coxsackie virus Bl, Tucson strain, in CDl Swiss mice. Weakness was evident 7 days after injection and lasted more than 10 weeks, despite inability to detect virus after 14 days (39). This suggests that persistent myositis may be immunologically mediated and triggered by an initial viral infection. Further support for this concept comes from protein sequencing studies that have found homology between some muscle and viral proteins and *Escherichia coli t*RNA synthetases. The *E. coli* proteins have been identified as autoantigens in some human inflammatory myopathies (40).

To date, there have been no reports of a chronic variant of EAM that more closely resembles the human inflammatory myopathies. EAM is a self-limited, monophasic reaction to an administered precipitant. Human inflammatory myopathies typically run a protracted course and are not infrequently accompanied by more widespread tissue involvement. The relevance of the animal models, particularly as regards potential immunologic modulation and therapeutic modalities, remains to be demonstrated.

CHILDHOOD DERMATOMYOSITIS AND POLYMYOSITIS

Childhood dermatomyositis (CDM) and childhood polymyositis (CPM) are autoimmune disorders falling under the broad category of inflammatory myopathies, with inflammation of skeletal muscle being a major pathologic feature. In CDM inflammatory changes occur in the skin as well as in muscle. Inflammatory myopathies also include viral (41) and parasitic myositides (42), inclusion body myositis (43) (this has not been identified in children), dermatomyositis and polymyositis associated with connective tissue disorders, and dermatomyositis and polymyositis associated with malignancy (this has not been clearly identified to occur in children).

CDM, CPM, and CPM associated with connective tissue disorders appear to be distinct diseases, but they are linked by several features: their clinical and pathologic involvement of skeletal muscle with weakness as a major sign, an unknown etiology, a positive therapeutic response to prednisone, abnormalities of electrodiagnostic studies, and abnormalities of serum muscle enzyme values.

Incidence

CDM and CPM are uncommon disorders, but the exact annual incidence of new cases is unclear. Most epidemiologic studies have included adult and childhood cases of polymyositis and dermatomyositis syndromes; the annual incidence of all combined cases varied from 0.1 to 7.7 per 100,000 persons (44). Most reports of CDM, which is more frequent than CPM, have demonstrated a preponderence of girls, with onset of signs and symptoms occurring most often during school age. However, CDM has been documented in late infancy.

Pathogenesis

Genetic Factors

With rare exceptions, neither CDM nor CPM occurs in more than one member of a family. However, in some reports there is an increased incidence of other autoimmune disorders in first-degree relatives of patients with adult type polymyositis or dermatomyositis syndromes (45).

Reports of histocompatability leukocyte antigen (HLA) types in CDM have revealed HLA-B8 in 72% of white patients with that disorder, compared to 21% in a controlled population and 64% in patients with adult type polymyositis (46). However, other studies have failed to demonstrate consistent confirmation of these findings, and HLA types cannot, at this time, be used as specific markers in CDM or CPM.

Immune-Mediated Tissue Damage

Immunofluorescence studies of biopsies of skeletal muscle and results of a search for immune complexes in blood revealed that CDM may result from an immune complex-induced vasculopathy. Deposits of IgG, IgM, and C-3, individually or in combination, occur within the walls of intramuscular blood vessels in CDM more frequently than CPM and adult inflammatory myopathies (47). Endomysial and perimysial blood vessels are severely affected and may represent the target of the autoimmune response. The antigenic factor that initiated self-sensitization, however, has not been defined.

Mononuclear cells are observed in muscle biopsies of patients with CDM and CPM, and have been suspected of playing a role in the production of muscle damage. Whether these cells are the cause of the muscle cell damage or whether their presence is an effect of an immunologic response to antigens released as a result of muscle damage is not completely understood. In one reported study, peripheral blood lymphocytes of five children with active inflammatory myopathy were shown to release a lymphotoxin that caused necrosis or impaired protein synthesis in human fetal muscle monolayers in tissue culture. This process could be reversed with methylprednisolone (48).

Monoclonal Antibody Studies

Results of recent studies of monoclonal antibodies in inflammatory myopathies, including CDM and CPM, have increased our knowledge of the immune mechanisms in these disorders (49–50). It is probable that mast cells, granulocytes, B and T lymphocytes, macrophages, and accessory cells, for example, interact at various anatomic locations (endothelial cells, sarcolemma, for example) to produce the spectrum of autoimmune inflammatory myopathies. Identification of the specific muscle surface antigens provoking these inflammatory responses remains an elusive, although realistic goal which, if accomplished, would possibly result in the development of more specific therapeutic modalities.

Infectious Agents

There are no definitive data to support a viral etiology for CDM or CPM, a view based on the finding of alleged viral particles in muscle biopsies of patients with these disorders. However, the possibility exists that a viral infection could react with antigens in muscle resulting in an altered immune state which produces muscle damage, or by some other mechanism resulting in changes in the immunoregulatory mechanisms.

Acute infection with toxoplasmosis has also been identified in association with a syndrome with the same clinical features as CDM (51). Acquired immune deficiency syndrome and Lyme disease have been associated with polymyositis in adults (See Chapters 12 and 25) but no documentation in children has been reported. In a study of the prevalence of Coxsackie B virus antibodies in patients with CDM, 83% of 12 children with this disease had detectable titers of complement-fixing antibody to one or more Coxsackie B viral antigens within 4 months of onset of the muscle disease (52–54). Only about 25% of normal controls had detectable titers. These data were interpreted by the authors to suggest that host response to Coxsackie B virus might be related to the pathophysiology of CDM. However, there has been no unequivocal identification of a specific pathogenic organism using rigorous microbiologic methods, such as isolation, repeated animal passage, or tissue culture.

Association With Malignancy

Although there is as yet an unclear relationship of malignancy and polymyositis or dermatomyositis in adults, only extremely rare examples of such a relationship have occurred with CDM or CPM.

Association With Connective Tissue Disorders (Overlap Group)

CPM and CDM may be associated with disorders of connective tissue, such as systemic lupus erythematosus (SLE), Sjögren syndrome, mixed connective tissue disease, scleroderma, and rheumatoid arthritis. To substantiate the diagnosis of overlap syndrome the criteria for diagnosis of both CDM or CPM and one or more of these disorders must be fulfilled. Varying degrees of muscular weakness may be a prominent feature in each of these disorders.

Clinical Features of CDM and CPM (53, 55–57)

The onset of both disorders is usually subacute or subchronic over a period of weeks or a few months, but may less commonly be acute. Muscular weakness, the most common presenting complaint, is generally proximal and symmetric and more pronounced in the legs than in the arms. Manifestations of weakness include difficulty in walking up stairs, rising from a seated position, carrying packages, or in combing one's hair. Muscle pain is a presenting symptom in less than a third of patients with CDM or CPM, and is not a necessary feature for diagnosis. The intensity of the pain is variable, but may be marked, sometimes making functional or manual motor testing difficult and not reproducably reliable. Facial and extraocular muscles are uninvolved in CDM or CPM, but the flexors of the neck and proximal muscles of the pelvic and shoulder girdle are selectively vulnerable. Weakness of the anterior tibialis muscles is also common, manifested by easy tripping and inability to walk on one's heels. At the time of initial presentation, neither enlargement of the muscles, as commonly seen in X-linked muscular dystrophy, nor atrophy of muscles is observed.

Skin manifestations are present in all patients with CDM and in some patients with CPM. These lesions may be very subtle, especially in CPM, and may not be recognized by the patient or parents as being abnormal. Erythema, sometimes accompanied by subcutaneous tissue edema, is common in the periorbital and malar regions, anterior neck, and extensor surfaces of the arms and legs (Figure 24.1A–B). Another commonly affected region, especially in CDM, is the skin over the metacarpophalangeal and interphalangeal joints of the fingers, including the skin immediately proximal to the fingernails. The rash may be violaceous and is often scaley or lichenified. In CDM fine telangiectases may reflect the underlying vasculitis. The severity of the skin lesions may vary greatly in the course of the disease and may be present prior to onset of muscle weakness. They may also be followed by increased or decreased pigmentation. Arthralgias, but no overt arthritis, are present in approximately 25% of patients. The course of CDM is generally categorized as monocyclic or limited, polycyclic, or continuous (58).

Clinical Features of the Overlap Group

The proximal muscle weakness which occurs in these disorders is generally indistinguishable from the weakness which occurs in CPM or CDM. See other sections for clinical patterns of the underlying disorders; namely, SLE,

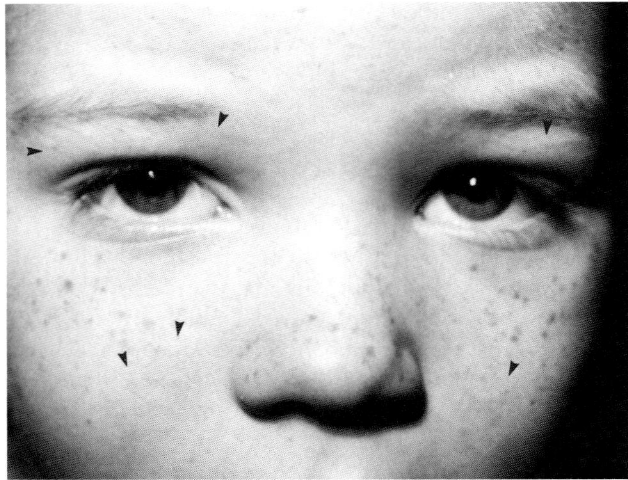

A

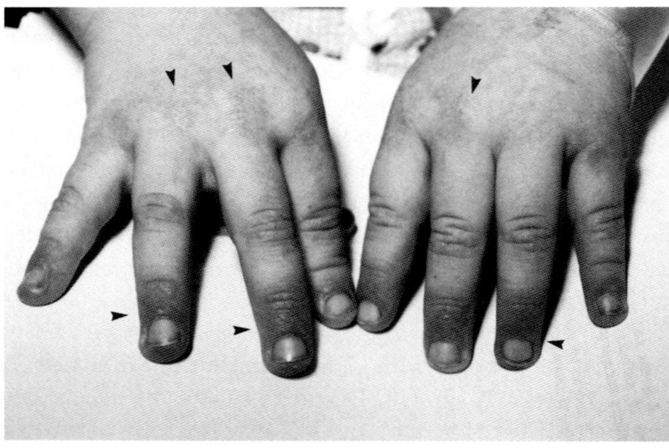

B

FIGURE 24.1   Childhood dermatomyositis in a 5-year-old boy. Note the periorbital edema and violaceous rash with subcutaneous edema (**A**) in the malar regions (arrows). **B:** A typical violaceous, somewhat scaley rash affecting the dorsal surfaces (arrows) of the metacarpophalangeal and interphalangeal joints. (Courtesy of Dr. Bruce O. Berg, University of California Medical Center, San Francisco).

scleroderma, juvenile rheumatoid arthritis, mixed connective tissue disease, and Sjögren syndrome.

Diagnosis (57)

Dermatomyositis or polymyositis should be suspected in any patient whose presenting symptoms and signs include symmetric weakness of the pelvic and shoulder girdle muscles which has been present for a period of weeks or months, whether a characteristic rash is present or not. The conventional guidelines in evaluating a patient with weakness, that is incorporation of signs and symptoms, genetic studies, levels of skeletal muscle enzymes, electrodiagnostic

tests, pathologic studies and ancillary clinical or laboratory examinations, will usually result in confirmation or elimination of the suspected diagnosis.

CDM and CPM are not in the usual sense genetically determined disorders. If an additional family member is found to have manifestations similar to the index case, the diagnosis with very rare exception (59) can be eliminated.

Serum muscle enzymes, including creatine kinase (CK), lactic dehydrogenase (LDH), and serum glutamic oxaloacetic and pyruvic transaminase (SGOT and SGPT) are useful in the diagnosis of CPM and CDM in that they are generally elevated in these disorders. Elevations of CK are probably most sensitive and one or more of these enzymes may be elevated rather than the entire group. The presence of normal enzyme values despite active disease, however, does not exclude the diagnosis of CPM or CDM, since these values may be normal in a small percentage of cases.

Electrodiagnostic studies can be very useful in substantiating the diagnosis of CDM or CPM. As with serum enzyme determinations, a normal electromyogram (EMG) does not exclude the diagnosis since the EMG can be normal in a small percentage of cases. Nerve conduction velocity (NCV) studies are generally normal, since peripheral nerves are not primarily involved. EMGs should preferably be limited to one side of the body to enable a muscle biopsy to be performed on the opposite side. This will eliminate the possibility of producing a so-called "needle myopathy," changes produced by the EMG needle which are occasionally confused with disease-related abnormalities. The triad of fibrillation potentials and positive sharp waves at rest, short duration and abundant single motor unit potentials on minimal volitional movement, and high frequency bizarre discharges, is highly suggestive of CDM or CPM. These findings, however, are not pathognomonic of the diseases. Clinicians must remember that electrodiagnostic studies are quite uncomfortable; they should be performed and interpreted by electromyographers experienced with children.

Muscle biopsy has been very useful in the diagnosis of CDM and CPM. If possible, a moderately weak proximal muscle should be selected for biopsy, most commonly the quadriceps, biceps, or deltoid. The tissue should be processed using histochemical and ultrastructural studies in addition to conventional fixed tissue studies. Biopsy findings have been abnormal and diagnostic in the large majority of cases, when processing is done using state-of-the-art methods (57).

In CPM inflammatory exudates are present frequently around blood vessels in the endomysial and perimysial connective tissue, as well as focally around necrotic, degenerating, or even normal, muscle fibers. The exudates consist of a high percentage of T cells and a small percentage of B cells (49). Variation of fiber size, scattered, randomly occurring necrosis and phagocytosis, and increased amounts of endomysial connective tissue may also be noted.

In CDM perifascicular atrophy, that is atrophy of muscle fibers in the periphery of fascicles, is a characteristic diagnostic feature. Intramuscular blood vessels demonstrate endomysial hyperplasia, and deposits of immunoglobulin complexes are noted with immunofluorescent studies. These latter deposits, however, do not have to be observed to establish the diagnosis. Ultrastructural alterations in intramuscular blood vessels are numerous. Inflammatory cells are seen as in CPM, but they are primarily perivascular. A positive alkaline phosphatase reaction is also frequently observed both with CDM and CPM.

Biopsy of the skin is not a routine procedure in establishing the diagnosis of CDM; skin lesions vary greatly according to the stage of the disease and the region of the biopsy. If a biopsy is done, changes consist of perivascular infiltrates as well as edema of the superficial layers. Caution should be exercised if a skin biopsy is performed to avoid artifactual changes induced by the biopsy procedure itself. Biopsy findings of skeletal muscle in patients in which CPM or CDM is present as part of an overlap syndrome are similar to the above descriptions (57).

Ancillary studies may be helpful in the diagnosis of CDM or CPM. Erythrocyte sedimentation rate is abnormal in only approximately 1/3 of patients. Nonspecific electrocardiographic changes are seen in over 1/2 of patients. Pulmonary function assessment will document restrictive ventilatory defects in many patients.

When CPM or CDM are suspected to be associated with an overlap syndrome, appropriate confirmatory laboratory studies should be performed. Evaluations for an underlying malignancy do not have to be performed in CDM or CPM unless there is an unusual compelling reason to do so.

Differential Diagnosis

CDM can usually be readily differentiated from other disorders in which a rash is a major feature, since muscle weakness is virtually always present in CDM and it is not a feature of primary dermatologic disorders. Recognition of the characteristic topography of the rash associated with CDM should lessen errors in the diagnosis; however, the rash associated with CDM is frequently very subtle and may be atypically located.

When muscle weakness is the presenting symptom or sign of CDM or CPM, the differential diagnosis includes a wide array of disorders varying from genetically determined or metabolic disorders of skeletal muscle or anterior horn cells to sporadically occurring disorders (56). The former group includes muscular dystrophy, juvenile progressive spinal muscular strophy, and acid maltase deficiency, for example. The latter group includes acute viral myositis, "growing pains," conversion reactions, Guillain-Barré syndrome, and toxic myopathies.

Careful analysis of the history in conjunction with the clinical examination, negative genetic history, serum muscle enzyme values, electrodiagnostic studies, muscle biopsy results and ancillary studies will generally provide a correct diagnosis to enable the patient to be treated appropriately.

Therapy

Despite the lack of double blinded conclusive prospective studies, prednisone is generally considered to be the preferential agent in the treatment of CDM or CPM because of its anti-inflammatory and immunosuppressive effects (60). Its therapeutic efficacy must be balanced against its deleterious side effects. Alternate day regimens usually result in fewer and less severe side effects. A single morning dose on alternate days ostensibly interferes less with the normal pituitary-adrenal cycle, but may not result in as adequate suppression of the inflammatory response as does daily therapy. In some cases, the sustained suppression provided by a divided daily dose regimen may be required; unfortunately, this frequently results in increased numbers and severity of side effects of the drug. Once activity of the disease is suppressed, however, alternate day therapy may be adequate. The conversion from daily to alternate day therapy is generally accomplished by doubling the total daily dose of prednisone on the "on" day; this amount is prescribed as a single morning dose. Individual patients may require a varying, but usually small, dose of prednisone on the "off" day. This "off" day dose may be tapered depending on the response. The obvious goal is to maximize therapeutic efficacy and minimize side effects.

Several varying dosage regimens have been advocated in the treatment of CDM and CPM, but none are based on a statistically validated prospective study. Many authors advocate an initial high single daily dose of prednisone (1.5 to 2 mg/kg) followed by an alternate day schedule when clinical improvement is documented (60). The alternate day schedule is continued for a minimum of 2 to 6 months until there is sustained improvement in strength. Improvement in functional muscle strength in children under 5 years of age or in manual muscle testing results in children over that age, is the primary determinant of efficacy of therapy. Reduction of serum muscle enzyme values generally precedes clinical improvement and may suggest a trend; that is, lack of response or response to treatment. However, neither these values nor the erythrocyte sedimentation rate can be used alone as a gauge of improvement. When clinical improvement has been sustained, the dose of the high alternate day prednisone may be tapered; this should be done slowly, by as little as 2.5 mg decrements weekly. The rate at which tapering is accomplished is gauged on the maintenance of strength measured by manual or functional muscle testing. If the patient becomes weaker or more easily fatigued after tapering, the larger dose should be maintained for a period of time before an attempt at tapering is reinstituted. If the patient's strength remains normal after the alternate day dose is down to 5 to 10 mg, it is our practice to maintain this dose for a prolonged period, occasionally 2 to 3 years or more, if necessary. In principle, treatment of CDM is directed at the weakness and not at the rash which generally requires no specific therapy.

There are several alternate regimens, especially for milder cases of CDM or CPM. Some investigators suggest that the use of high dose prednisone at the onset of therapy and maintenance of a relatively high dose when remission has occurred will result in the need for a more prolonged course of treatment. Thus, an initial moderate dose of prednisone (1 to 1.5 mg/kg/day) for approximately 2 weeks is favored by those investigators (61). After clinical improvement has begun the dosage is gradually reduced by about 2.5 mg per week. If regression occurs, the prior week's dose is maintained for a further week. Other regimens include high dose pulse intravenous methylprednisolone administration (62,63), especially in early and mild CDM. It seems obvious that every patient's treatment plan must be tailor made and governed by the severity and course of the illness.

In the event the patient does not have a beneficial response after the initial period of corticosteroid therapy, or if the patient experiences intolerable side effects related to the therapy, immunosuppressive agents such as azathioprine (64), methotrexate, cyclophosphamide, or cyclosporine may be added or substituted (53,65). As with prednisone therapy, there have been no prospective controlled studies with these agents in the treatment of CDM or CPM. Azathioprine has certain advantages in that it can be used orally, and side effects are generally fewer and less severe. Although plasmapheresis has been used in selected cases of CDM or CPM, no conclusions can be made concerning its efficacy at this time (66). Rigorous evaluation of the efficacy of intravenous gamma globulin therapy, purportedly beneficial in selected examples of chronic polymyositis, also has to be done (67).

In the event that toxoplasmosis is demonstrated to be the causative agent in CDM, therapy with pyrimethamine and sulfadiazine may be successful (51). A program of physical therapy is generally part of the overall treatment plan. Contractures of joints occur frequently and are generally avoided if treated with passive range of motion exercises if the patient is too ill for an active program. When there is dysphagia or respiratory muscle involvement, patients must be observed very carefully and treated appropriately in a timely fashion when indicated. Intensive care unit observation may be warranted.

Complications

Very severe complications can occur in treated or untreated cases of CDM or CPM including respiratory involvement, gastrointestinal bleeding, severe muscle wasting, subcutaneous calcinosis, and even death. Calcinosis may occur in varying degrees in an appreciable percentage of patients with CDM or CPM, and can be readily visualized with computed tomographic (CT) scanning (68,69). These deposits may be represented by small nodules, subcutaneous calcified masses occurring near joints, or sheet-like deposits in the fascial planes, and may occur concurrently with the active disease or months to years after the activity has ceased. In some cases the deposits are more disabling than the disease itself. In addition to pain, limitation of adjacent joints, skin ulcerations, and abscess formation may occur. Although some deposits disappear spontaneously, some symptomatic calcifications must be surgically removed. Use of chelating agents has not generally been successful; in individual reports oral colchicine therapy (1 mg/day) was said to be followed within 2 months by significant regression of local inflammation and healing of skin ulcers (70). It has been suggested by some long term follow-up studies that the best predictor of good functional recovery and minimal calcinosis is treatment early after onset of the symptoms, but this remains to be proven.

Less frequently occurring complications include chronic interstitial pulmonary fibrosis, pneumothorax, cardiac arrythmias, pericarditis, retinopathy, and pneumatosis intestinalis (53,56,57).

In an isolated instance CDM has been associated with cerebral vasculitis in a patient with agammaglobulinemia (71); CPM has been described in association with immunoglobulin A deficiency and intestinal malabsorption, and also with acne fulminans (72). In the latter case IgA was moderately increased. Relapses in CDM may occur several years after successful treatment with any regimen (58).

Complications of corticosteroid therapy (56), although minimized by single dose alternate day administration, include cushingoid appearance, gastrointestinal tract ulcerations, behavioral disturbances, growth retardation, hypertension, steroid induced weakness, diabetes, osteoporosis with compression fractures of the vertebrae, cataracts, increased susceptibility to infection, and aseptic necrosis of the femur. In some instances steroid induced weakness is difficult to differentiate from weakness related to the disease itself.

Prognosis

Mortality in CDM or CPM has been significantly reduced with corticosteroid therapy, and the prognosis is generally good (55). Despite the uncertainty of the relationship of adult onset dermatomyositis with malignancy, the relationship does not exist in children, with extremely rare exceptions (73). However, complications of the disease and various treatment methods may be significant and there appears to be a subgroup of patients who do not respond to any treatment mode. The ultimate outcome for an individual patient with respect to functional recovery, does not appear to correlate well with age, sex, or severity at the onset of the disease.

CONNECTIVE TISSUE DISEASES: SYSTEMIC LUPUS ERYTHEMATOSUS

Systemic lupus erythematosus (SLE) is an immunologically mediated syndrome in which antigen-antibody complexes are found in various body tissues resulting in multiorgan involvement. Neurologic events commonly occur in SLE, but are frequently difficult to assess, because although they may be related to the illness, per se, they may be related to therapy, infection, complications, or to functional problems related to the underlying disorder (74).

Pathology and Pathogenesis

Several varying pathologic abnormalities (75) have been observed in the CNS in patients with SLE with neurologic involvement. CNS lesions include cerebral atrophy, multiple infarcts due to emboli, vasculitis (76,77), petechial hemorrhages, areas of demyelination, all most likely related to cytotoxic antibodies that vary in their composition and antigenicity, and, thus, selectively attacking vulnerable regions of the nervous system. The skeletal muscles may also be involved as described in the section on CDM/CPM.

Clinical Features

Nonneurologic Involvement

Although renal disease, sometimes very acute in onset, is observed in many patients with SLE, other varied clinical signs and symptoms may be present (78). Criteria for the diagnosis have been established by the American Rheumatism Association (79). Signs and symptoms include facial erythema, fever, weight loss, anorexia, pleuritis, pericarditis, myocarditis, anemia, and thrombocytopenia (78).

Neurologic Involvement

Some, probably the majority of neurologic events occurring in patients with SLE, can be explained by metabolic, pharmacologic, and vascular abnormalities (74). According to some studies only a small fraction of neurologic complications in SLE are due solely to immunologically mediated nervous system lesions. Thus, when confronted with a patient with SLE who experiences an abnormality of neurologic function, trauma, neoplasm, or other independent neurologic disorders must be excluded. Then the clinician can attempt to decide if the nervous system event is related to: high temperature, focal vascular abnormalities, marked hypertension, drug toxicity, coagulopathy, metabolic imbalance, etc., all of which are frequently associated with SLE; to the SLE itself; or to a combination of these factors. Imaging techniques such as computerized tomography or

magnetic resonance imaging (MRI) may be useful in attempting to clarify some of these problems.

There is a large diversity of neurologic complications associated with SLE. Seizures, either generalized or less commonly focal, occur in up to 1/2 of children with SLE and may herald the onset of the disease. Seizures in children with SLE may occur in association with complications related to SLE, such as severe renal disease, hypertension, or CNS infection.

A smaller number of children with SLE experience cerebrovascular disease based on small vessel occlusion and/or arteritis (80) which may result in aphasia, visual field defects, blindness, hemiparesis, or other focal events. These generally occur rather late in the course of SLE, and may be related to severe hypertension or thrombocytopenia. Personality disorders, depression, acute psychosis (81), or dementia may occur in approximately 1/4 of children with SLE and as in the case with seizures, psychiatric manifestations may herald the onset of SLE. In children with SLE taking corticosteroids, psychiatric abnormalities may be related to that drug rather than to CNS involvement; these frequently are difficult to distinguish, and judgement as to increasing or decreasing the dose of steroids based on criteria which assess the activity of the SLE, such as serial C4 measurements or antinuclear antibody titers, are not always reliable.

Chorea may occur in SLE early in the course of the disease, and may be the heralding symptom (75). Chorea occurs equally in both sexes and may last from several days to 3 years. There is no definite relationship between chorea and other SLE manifestations, either neurologic or non-neurologic, and there is no known specific etiology. It is of interest that chorea in SLE most frequently is manifest between the ages of 10 and 40 years in females, with the majority falling in the age group between 15 and 25 years; it essentially does not occur in males after the age of 20 years. Chorea may be episodic like SLE itself, and the abnormal movements may be generalized or limited to one side of the body (hemichorea).

Other regions of the CNS may be involved less commonly in children with SLE. Brain stem, cranial nerves, and spinal cord abnormalities may result in signs and symptoms referable to these regions, such as external ophthalmoplegia, facial paresthesias or numbness, and myelopathy, manifested by paraplegia and sensory loss below the level of the lesion. Retinal hemorrhages may result in blindness or blurred vision (76). Papilledema associated with increased intracranial pressure may also be observed. Ataxia, dysarthria, and pseudotumor cerebri have also been noted as well as various combinations of neurologic signs and symptoms (82). A self-limiting aseptic meningitis with meningismus, headache, fever, and pleocytosis has been described in children with SLE, usually occurring early in the disease.

Lumbosacral plexus, peripheral nerves, and muscle may also be affected in children with SLE. The neuropathy may result in sensory and motor disturbances such as weakness and numbness or paresthesias. A symmetric polyradiculoneuropathy simulating Guillain-Barré syndrome can also be seen. Inflammatory myopathy (polymyositis) occurs infrequently in children with SLE and weakness is usually mild. Myasthenia gravis has also been associated with SLE in children.

Diagnosis and Differential Diagnosis

The diagnosis of SLE can be made by utilizing clinical, laboratory, and biopsy criteria established for this purpose (77–79). Laboratory abnormalities include leukopenia, lymphopenia, anemia, thrombocytopenia, and an elevated erythrocyte sedimentation rate. Circulating antinuclear antibodies detected by immunofluorescence are seen in all patients. Lowering of complement level can serve as a sensitive measure of tissue deposition. Rheumatoid factor, prolonged partial thromboplastin time, and false positive serologic tests for syphilis can also be seen. Renal biopsy can be very helpful in the diagnosis.

In the presence of seizures, electroencephalographic, cerebrospinal fluid, and imaging studies can be useful (83,84); however, as noted seizures may be related to non-SLE events such as hypertension, metabolic disturbances, and CNS infection, and it may be difficult to determine an etiology. Similar differential diagnostic problems may arise in children with SLE who experience cerebrovascular events.

When chorea (75) is a single presenting neurologic manifestation, other etiologies for chorea (Sydenham chorea, for example, among many others) might be considered in the differential diagnosis; the presence of antinuclear antibody titers and the frequent coexistence of SLE chorea with other neurologic deficits can readily establish the diagnosis. Similarly, the various motor unit disorders which occur with SLE in children can generally be documented by appropriate studies. These include electrodiagnostic tests (in peripheral neuropathies or Guillain-Barré syndrome); CSF studies (increased protein in Guillain-Barré syndrome, for example); muscle biopsy (CDM or CPM); and pharmacologic tests (edrophonium test in myasthenia gravis).

A lupus-like syndrome and/or elevated antinuclear antibody titers in asymptomatic children, may be induced by numerous pharmacologic agents (85), the most common being phenytoin, ethosuximide, and procainamide. Loss of prior adequate seizure control in epileptic patients should alert the clinician to a possibility of a drug-induced lupus-like syndrome. Substituting another anticonvulsant might produce a rapid improvement in such a case.

Treatment

The general management of a child with SLE, which is a multidisciplinary effort, is beyond the scope of this section.

Since many of the neurologic events noted in children with SLE are related to severe hypertension, infection, metabolic abnormalities, vascular abnormalities, drug toxicity, coagulopathy or combinations of the above, therapy (antihypertensive agents, antibiotics, renal dialysis, steroids, for example) has to be directed to control or ameliorate these events. In conjunction with this, therapy is also directed at the active SLE itself.

In the event of seizures, as well as directing therapy toward correcting an underlying systemic abnormality, anticonvulsants should be used. In the face of renal failure and/or dialysis, careful serial assessments of serum anticonvulsant drug levels must be done. Loading doses of phenobarbital or phenytoin should be about 1/2 (or even less) of conventional doses in children with renal failure.

Chorea, when observed as an isolated manifestation of SLE, can be treated with a variety of drugs including diazepam, haloperidol (86), or valproic acid. However, chorea is frequently associated with seizures and psychiatric disturbances, and additional treatment has to be provided. In the presence of psychiatric manifestations, steroid-induced psychiatric problems are difficult to distinguish from those caused by the SLE itself. Antidepressant drugs are sometimes useful in the presence of depression.

In the presence of cerebrovascular events, increased intracranial pressure, or retinal artery occlusion in active SLE, corticosteroids given either as high intravenous pulse doses, or high daily oral doses, can be very beneficial (87). Immunosuppressant agents may also be very useful. In hemiplegia or paraplegia, physical therapy should be instituted. Central nervous system infections are treated with appropriate antibiotic therapy.

Inflammatory myopathy (polymyositis) can be treated with corticosteroids. Myasthenia gravis when associated with SLE, may be successfully treated with pyridostigmine, but prednisone or immunosuppressive agents may be supplemented when necessary.

Complications and Prognosis

With improved renal management and the cautious use of corticosteroids and immunosuppressants, the life expectancy of children with SLE has improved, but treatment is difficult. Despite therapy the mortality is significant, and quality of life may be impaired because of multiple manifestations of the disease affecting many organ systems.

OTHER CONNECTIVE TISSUE DISEASES

Mixed Connective Tissue Disease

Mixed connective tissue disease is rare in children and as the name suggests has features of SLE, scleroderma, rheumatoid arthritis, Sjögren syndrome and dermato-myositis (88–89). Diagnosis of this disease in which symptoms can include many of those seen in the other connective tissue disorders, may be confirmed by the presence of high titers of extractable nuclear antigen. In addition, abnormal rheumatoid factor and antinuclear antibody titers may be found, and the erythrocyte sedimentation rate may be elevated (90).

Neurologic Manifestations

A proximal muscle weakness syndrome may be observed; this is coupled with elevations of serum muscle enzymes, a myopathic electromyogram, and muscle biopsy evidence of an inflammatory myopathy. Treatment is with prednisone (See Childhood Polymyositis), and if needed, other immuno-suppressant agents. Headaches and seizures have also been described in mixed connective tissue disease.

Sjögren Syndrome

Although Sjögren syndrome (SS) occurs most commonly between the 4th and 6th decades of life, it has been described in childhood and adolescence, with a higher frequency in girls than in boys (91). It is a chronic autoim-mune disorder. In primary SS the sicca complex (dryness of eyes, mouth, mucous membranes, and skin) occurs in the absence of another connective tissue disease; whereas, in secondary SS sicca syndrome occurs in the presence of rheumatoid arthritis, SLE, or systemic sclerosis. Diagnosis is based on the clinical pattern coupled with the detection of the RO (SS–A) antibody (92).

Neurologic Manifestations

Many adults with SS, especially when cutaneous vasculitis is present, have evidence of central or peripheral nervous system disease, but this is undoubtedly extremely rare in children. CNS manifestations (93) include subcortical dementia, seizures, focal deficits, movement disorders, dif-fuse encephalopathy, recurrent aseptic meningitis (94), and a multiple sclerosis-like picture (95). With reference to the peripheral nervous system (96), a symmetric sensory or motor neuropathy, entrapment syndromes, mononeuritis multiplex, and cranial neuropathies have been described. Psychiatric disorders have also been reported in adults. The pathogenesis of the nervous system involvement appears to be the result of immunologically mediated insults. Increased protein, oligoclonal bands, and atypical mononuclear cells may be present in the cerebrospinal fluid. It has been suggested that corticosteroids and/or immunosuppressant therapy may ameliorate some of the nervous system manifestations.

Scleroderma

In scleroderma a progressive hardening of the skin and subcutaneous tissue may be accompanied by gastrointesti-nal tract, cardiac, lung, and joint involvement. In general-ized scleroderma, which affects adults only, there is diffuse involvement; whereas, in focal scleroderma, the lesions are discreet and associated with atrophy and hyperpigmenta-tion. The focal form of scleroderma, morphea, primarily affects children (97,98). Diagnosis can be substantiated with a skin biopsy in which increased thickness and density of collagen is seen, by radiographic or computed tomo-graphic studies of subcutaneous tissue showing calcinosis, diminished esophageal motility during a barium swallow, and with laboratory studies to exclude other disorders of connective tissue.

Neurologic Manifestations of Focal Scleroderma (Morphea)

Focal scleroderma occurs more commonly in girls; this disease occurs at any age, but in one series the mean age was 8 years. The most common skin lesions are plaques which are discrete and waxy colored, and sometimes sur-rounded by a violaceous halo. They may be associated with hemiatrophy and scoliosis. Underlying skeletal muscle may be affected. Neurologic manifestations (98) are commonly found (68% in one series). These include psychomotor retardation, dyslexia, seizures, hemiparesis (with accompa-nying cerebral atrophy), neuropathy, synkinesias, optic atrophy, and anisocoria. Electroencephalographic abnor-malities are more common when compared to age-matched controls.

Acute Rheumatic Fever

Acute rheumatic fever (RF) is a diverse disorder which is related to a group A beta-hemolytic streptococcal infection in an immunologically compromised individual. The signs and symptoms are variable, and cardiac, joint, dermato-logic and/or neurologic abnormalities may predominate. Diagnosis is generally made using the modified Jones crite-ria (99), established as a guideline for that purpose. Major criteria include carditis, erythema marginatum, migratory polyarthritis, subcutaneous nodules, and chorea. Minor criteria include fever, arthralgia, electrocardiographic abnormalities, elevation of phase reactants, and elevation of streptoccal antibodies.

Neurologic Involvement

Sydenham chorea is (100) by far the most common neuro-logic manifestation of RF, and in some patients it is the only sign of the disease. In many children with chorea, how-ever, laboratory evidence for a recent streptoccal infection is lacking. Chorea generally involves purposeless distal rapid movements, primarily affecting the hands. The movements may be accentuated by asking a child to bring a glass of water to his mouth, for example, or by asking the child to hold his hands above his head, at which time a peculiar "spooning" (a dystonic movement) may be noted. The feet may also be involved, resulting in bizarre dance-like movements (Saint Vitus dance). The movements may be limited to one side of the body (hemichorea) or may be generalized. Onset may be acute or insidious, and may be accompanied by an emotional disorder, with diminished attention span, irritability, personality changes, and poor school performance. Delayed relaxation of the deep tendon reflexes may be noted as well as hypotonia. Although Sydenham chorea is the most common form of chorea in children, there is a large differential diagnosis (101), including chorea associated with degenerative, genetic, infectious, vascular, metabolic, and other diseases.

In searching for a cause of acquired chorea, throat cultures for beta-hemolytic streptoccus have a very low yield, and antistreptolysin-O titers are not universally elevated. The coexistence of a rheumatic cardiac involvement supports the diagnosis of RF. If no alternative diagnosis for the chorea is available, prophylaxis against RF should be instituted in the form of intramuscular or oral penicillin given indefinitely, since rheumatic heart disease is associated with Sydenham chorea (102). The movement disorder varies in intensity and may be very mild to severe; improvement may be seen in several weeks to a few months, although in some instances recovery is incomplete (103). Several agents can be used to control the chorea including phenobarbital, diazepam, haloperidol, and chlorpromazine; but carbamazepine (104) and valproic acid (105) are probably more effective. Any of these drugs can be used in the lowest dosage to control symptoms; the duration for which a drug will be required can be ascertained by periodically tapering the dosage and observing the child for redevelopment of symptoms.

Other neurologic manifestations in RF have been reported but occur infrequently. These include seizures (106), pseudotumor cerebri, papilledema, retinal artery occlusion, and meningoencephalitis.

Juvenile Rheumatoid Arthritis

Juvenile rheumatoid arthritis (JRA), based on clinical characteristics, has been classified into three major subgroups (107): pauciarticular, polyarticular, and systemic onset. The pauciarticular type has been further subcharacterized into three subtypes. All of these have different clinical presentations, joint involvement, radiographic and laboratory findings.

JRA patients rarely have clinically significant central nervous system disease, but drowziness, seizures, irritability, stupor, and meningismus have been described (108). Similarly, some JRA patients have nonspecific abnormalities of the electroencephalogram. Muscle aches and pains are not uncommon, but weakness simulating inflammatory myopathy is very rare.

MYASTHENIA GRAVIS

Myasthenia gravis (MG) is an acquired autoimmune disorder of neuromuscular transmission. Acetylcholine receptor (AChR) deficiency (109) at the neuromuscular junction (NMJ) results in weakness and excessive fatigability on exertion, with improvement on rest or after administration of anticholinesterase drugs. Circulating antibodies against AChR are present in over 80% of the cases (110); in addition, immune complexes are deposited on the postsynaptic membrane of the myoneural junction (MNJ). Clinical classifications proposed over 2 decades ago divided MG into adult and pediatric forms and subdivided each of these into several subgroups. Thus, adult MG was divided into the following (111): group 1, which is limited to extraocular muscle involvement; group 2A, mild generalized disease, in which respiratory muscles are spared, and response to anticholinesterase drugs is good with low mortality; group 2B, in which generalized disease is moderately severe; group 3, in which the disease begins suddenly and is fulminating and severe with early respiratory involvement and in which response to anticholinesterase drugs is poor; and group 4, in which patients develop severe disease after having had mild disease for at least 2 years. Pediatric forms of MG include transient neonatal MG which develops in approximately one in seven newborns born to myasthenic mothers, and other childhood forms. However, acquired autoimmune MG can occur at virtually any age in childhood and can be mild or severe. Since the nonautoimmune pathogenesis has become better understood, the so-called congenital myasthenic syndromes can be considered as different entities from MG (112). These disorders, in the past, had generally been considered as a subgroup of MG.

Incidence

The incidence of MG is approximately 2 to 5 cases per million population per year. The disease may be present at any age, and approximately 10% of all cases are children. In children and young adults, females are affected more frequently than males.

Pathogenesis

Investigation in experimental autoimmune MG in animals has provided researchers with a great deal of information how pathogenic AChR antibodies reduce postsynaptic AChR in MG in humans (109). Experimental allergic myasthenia gravis (EAMG) has been induced in many species of animals with purified AChR. Susceptibility to experimental allergic MG is affected by several factors including genetic influences that affect the immune responses to AChR, and the safety margin of neuromuscular transmission. AChR immunization results in acute and then chronic EAMG; this resembles human MG electrophysiologically and morphologically. During chronic EAMG, the decrease in the postsynaptic membrane resembles the ultrastructural alterations seen in human MG; the electrophysiologic changes in EAMG also resemble those observed in human MG.

The underlying mechanism which initiates sensitization to AChR in MG is not completely understood. A genetic control is suggested (113) since there is an association of different types of MG in various HLA genotypes, including the HLA complex on chromosome 6 and the GM (immunoglobulin allotype) complex on chromosome 14. There is a high concordance for MG in identical twins and a low concordance for siblings; these features suggest a polygenic pattern of inherited susceptibility.

The thymus plays a significant role in MG. Hyperplasia is found in about 65% of cases and thymoma in 15%; thymectomy is beneficial in a high proportion of cases (114,115). The thymus from patients with MG contains increased numbers of B cells (116). Thymic cells (antigen-specific T-helper cells) have been demonstrated to increase AChR antibody production by autologous peripheral blood lymphocytes. This is probably the explanation for a beneficial affect of thymectomy in MG; however, the role of the thymus is not completely understood. The mechanism why sensitivity to AChR occurs is also not completely understood.

AChR antibodies are polyclonal, although the majority recognize one immunogenic region of AChR. Specific features of the AChR antibody which correlate with the various clinically delineated types of MG have been looked for; and although there are some differences, these do not appear to be definitive (117). To be sure, characteristics of the AChR may vary and change with the duration of the MG. AChR antibodies have been demonstrated to be present at the myoneural junction in MG; the presence of the antibody results in complement-mediated destruction of the junctional folds and accelerates the internalization and degradation of AChR. Humoral factors may also influence the pathogenesis of MG; these are also incompletely understood (109).

Approximately 10% to 15% of patients with typical acquired MG have no detectable AChR antibodies using sensitive conventional methods of measurement (113). Although in many patients with no detectable antibodies the clinical manifestations are mild, in some the manifestations may be generalized and severe. Some investigators have concluded that the pathogenesis in these cases is similar to other patients with acquired autoimmune MG, with the basic abnormality involving an antibody-mediated reduction of the number of AChRs at the myoneural junc-

tions. Immunoglobulin is thought to be the most likely affector mechanism.

Clinical Presentation (118,119)

All voluntary muscles can be affected by weakness and fatigability, but the extraocular muscles are initially involved in about 1/2 of patients and eventually in nearly all. The muscles of mastication as well as the facial, lingual, and pharyngeal muscles may also be weakened. If weakness is present in the limbs, the proximal muscles are generally more affected than the distal ones.

Ptosis is unilateral or bilateral as is weakness of other extraocular muscles which may result in diplopia. Signs and symptoms can vary greatly even in the course of a single examination, but they are generally more pronounced late in the day. Mimetic musculature may be weakened, resulting in an expressionless face, and the mouth and jaw may hang open. Palatal muscle weakness may result in hypernasal speech and regurgitation of liquids. Chewing and swallowing may be difficult and associated with choking. Speech may become difficult to understand and the patient may become breathless in the middle of a phrase. The myasthenic tongue may show a triple longitudinal furrow.

Symptoms may be variable, may fluctuate greatly, and may be worsened by emotional upset, exertion, or infection. The association with emotional upset can result in the confusion of MG with conversion reaction. The deep tendon reflexes are generally normal or brisk, but may become reduced if elicited repeatedly.

In neonates with transient neonatal MG (120–122), symptoms generally appear shortly after delivery, and include feeding difficulty, generalized weakness and hypotonia, respiratory difficulty, weak cry, and facial and eyelid weakness. These symptoms in milder cases, may resolve spontaneously; however, they will more frequently persist for approximately 2 to 3 weeks prior to resolution. The severity of the symptoms of MG in the mother or the status of her treatment does not necessarily reflect the degree of involvement in the neonate. In some affected women MG improves during pregnancy (the opposite may also be true) and the diagnosis in the mother may be overlooked or not made at all, resulting in difficulty in establishing the diagnosis of the affected newborn. Some mothers who deliver babies with transient neonatal MG might report diminished fetal movements in the latter portion of pregnancy.

Diagnosis

In characteristic cases, especially those in which the extraocular muscles are clearly involved, diagnosis can be confirmed by finding a positive edrophonium (Tensilon) test (123), a decremental response to repetitive nerve stimulation (124) and/or abnormal AChR antibodies (110,117). In atypical situations, for example in patients in whom there is no extraocular muscle weakness, or in whom there is no weakness on examination although the complaints of the mother or patient are consistent with MG, or in patients who have an equivocal response to the edrophonium test, and in those who have negative AChR antibodies, more refined electrophysiologic and morphologic studies might be necessary to confirm or exclude the diagnosis of MG.

Edrophonium (Tensilon)(123) is an acetylcholinesterase inhibitor, and acts positively within a few seconds; the effect lasts only for a few minutes. In infants 0.05 to 0.1 mL can be given subcutaneously; in children up 34 kg in weight 0.1 mL can be given intravenously. In older children 0.1 mL of edrophonium is given intravenously, and if there is no response within 30 seconds an additional 0.5 mL of the drug is injected. In order for the test to be considered as positive, an objective endpoint must be chosen such as elimination of ptosis, correction of an extraocular muscle paresis in older children, or a change in tone, breathing or degree of movement in a newborn. If necessary, a placebo injection may be used or the test can be done double blind. Where an objective endpoint may be difficult to determine, a commonly encountered problem in infants and children, a trial of prostigmine given subcutaneously or intramuscularly may be used; since the effect may last up to 2 hours, this might allow a more appropriate evaluation.

The edrophonium test may be positive in both congenital myasthenic syndromes associated with AChR deficiency at the MNJ or with diminished acetylcholine synthesis (nonautoimmune MG)(112). It does not, therefore, necessarily serve to differentiate these disorders which may have many other clinical similarities.

Electrodiagnostic tests in infants and children must always be interpreted with caution because of technical difficulties so frequently encountered. In MG a decremental response of the compound muscle action potential evoked by supramaximal stimuli applied to a motor nerve can frequently be recorded. The test is most reliable at slow repetitive stimulation (2 to 3 Hz) but it is not positive in all muscles of all patients, especially in those individuals with ocular or mild generalized MG. Testing for "jitter" with single fiber electromyography may produce a higher yield of diagnosis but is difficult to perform in young children, and like the edrophonium tests is not necessarily specific for MG.

The AChR antibody test is positive in approximately 80% of patients with MG. The level of antibody only correlates loosely with the severity of the disease. Levels of antibody may change with treatment, again correlating loosely with the type of therapy. The great majority of infants born to myasthenic mothers have AChR antibodies (120); only a fraction are clinically associated with transient neonatal MG. Striated muscle antibodies may also be found in some patients with MG, but the role of these antibodies is not completely understood.

Differential Diagnosis

Infants with transient neonatal MG can occasionally have a similar clinical picture as observed in other "floppy baby" syndromes. The history that the mother has MG (which may not be immediately available), the positive response to edrophonium and/or prostigmine, the preservation of deep tendon reflexes, and the finding of AChR antibodies should readily allow the diagnosis to be made. In infants, botulism must be distinguished from MG (125). Infant botulism is usually associated with constipation, multiple cranial nerve involvement, hypotonia, muscle weakness, and respiratory depression. An incremental response is detected in repetitive nerve stimulation at high (40 to 50 Hz) frequencies. Confirmation of the diagnosis is made by finding clostridium botulinum organisms or toxin in the feces.

Differentiation of the more common acquired autoimmune MG in childhood from the less common nonimmune mediated congenital myasthenic syndromes may be difficult and may require sophisticated electrophysiologic, morphologic, cytochemical and immunochemical studies available in specialized centers (112). These familial syndromes, contrary to acquired autoimmune MG, may be related to defects in acetylcholine synthesis or mobilization, endplate acetylcholinesterase deficiency, slow channel abnormalities, or endplate AChR deficiency. They may be observed at birth or in some cases, later in childhood, and are frequently associated with diminished deep tendon reflexes. AChR antibodies are absent.

Conversion reactions can generally be differentiated by the lack of objective findings. Genetically determined neuromuscular disorders can be differentiated by the lack of varying extraocular involvement and by appropriate clinical, electrophysiologic, and morphologic studies. Mitochondrial myopathies, some congenital myopathies in which extraocular muscles are involved, and progressive bulbar palsies can be differentiated by morphologic, pharmacologic, and biochemical studies. AChR antibodies are not found in any of these disorders. Dysthyroid states associated with MG are very rare in children.

Therapy

Anticholinesterase drugs, prednisone, immunosuppressants, plasmapheresis, and thymectomy are the major therapeutic modalities in MG. Anticholinesterase drugs are useful in all clinical forms of MG, including transient neonatal MG, and are the drugs of choice in ocular MG. Plasmapheresis is generally limited to patients with severe MG, and this therapy has only temporary beneficial effects. There are no universally acceptable criteria for thymectomy in adults, and there is less agreement in children.

Anticholinesterase Drugs (111,118,119)

Pyridostigmine (Mestinon) is the most frequently used drug and, if needed for small children, it is available as a syrup (12 mg/mL) in addition to the usual 60 mg tablet. It acts within one hour, and its effect lasts from 4 to 6 hours. In older children the dose ranges from 30 mg to 60 mg taken every 4 to 6 hours. In younger children proportionately smaller doses are used. The drug is available in an injectable (intramuscular) form, which contains 5 mg/mL; approximately 1/30 of the oral dose provides the equivalent effect intramuscularly.

Neonatal transient MG may be self limiting and may improve spontaneously (120,121); the symptoms generally can be relieved with pyridostigmine given orally or parenterally, if needed. Since the symptoms in untreated cases last usually less than 3 weeks, tapering the dose (slowly) can be attempted when the baby has stabilized. If the infant has side effects from the drug, the dose can be lowered. Some neonates require respiratory support.

Some patients might require the more rapid onset of effect (30 minutes) but shorter duration (2 to 3 hours) of neostigmine, but this drug has more muscarinic side effects than pyridostigmine; namely, abdominal cramps and diarrhea. The dose ranges from 7.5 to 30 mg taken every 2 to 3 hours. Neostigmine is also available for subcutaneous or intramuscular use; 1 mg of the injectable drug is equivalent to 15 mg of the oral preparation.

Anticholinesterase drugs provide symptomatic relief of MG, and some older children can titrate these drugs on a demand basis. With younger children, the caretaker has to provide this dose regulation, which is frequently difficult. If patients require more than average doses of anticholinesterase drugs, or if side effects are intolerable, other forms of treatment should be considered.

Prednisone (111,118,119)

If ocular MG is refractory to anticholinesterase drugs in conventional doses, and if the patient is disturbed by the symptoms and bothered by use of an eye patch used to eliminate diplopia (the patch can be changed from eye to eye), therapy with prednisone might be considered. Prednisone is indicated primarily for patients with disabling disease whose symptoms are not satisfactorily relieved with anticholinesterase drugs. There are several acceptable regimens, including high single dose (100 mg for older children and adults) alternate day therapy for a period of up to 8 months followed by tapering after an improvement period. Another regimen suggests use of alternate day 25 mg dosage with increments of 12.5 mg every 6 days until maximum benefit or 100 mg is reached. It may take from several weeks to months before significant improvement is noted. A lowering of AChR antibody values may signify a positive trend in treatment. Obviously the potential side effects of long-term high alternate day steroids have to be considered.

High pulse doses of intravenous methylprednisolone have also been used (126).

Immunosuppressive and Immunologic Agents

Azathioprine given in doses of 1.5 to 2.5 mg/kg or more, if necessary to lower the white blood cell count, has also been demonstrated to be effective in some cases of generalized MG (127–129). The effect, however, is delayed after starting this drug, and benefits may not become apparent for 3 to 5 months. Some patients experience gastrointestinal irritation and abnormal liver function tests with this drug.

Cyclosporine has recently been used in the management of MG, with beneficial results similar to those reported with azathioprine (130). Nephrotoxicity is the major side effect of cyclosporine. Intramuscular and intravenous gamma globulin administration has in some patients with MG produced beneficial results, but further investigation is needed in this type of therapy (131,132).

Plasmapheresis (133)

Plasmapheresis can be very effective in severe generalized MG when anticholinesterase drugs and/or steroids are not effective. Improvement generally appears after 1 or 2 days, and can be correlated with a drop in the AChR antibody titer. However, when plasmapheresis is stopped, the symptoms may reappear unless other forms of treatment are used concurrently. Use of plasmapheresis is generally limited to its being a life saving procedure, but it is not generally used as a long-term treatment in most cases.

Thymectomy (114,115)

There is a growing consensus that all adult generalized MG patients should have a thymectomy. In children there have been many reports of improvement in generalized MG, but these are not based on a controlled trial. Thymectomy is generally not recommended in ocular MG and in some centers is only used in generalized MG if the patient is not controlled with corticosteroid therapy. The transsternal approach is generally more efficacious than the transcervical approach although the latter is a more readily tolerated procedure (134). In most centers, patients scheduled for thymectomy are prepared with steroids or with plasmapheresis prior to surgery. Thymectomy may result in a temporary improvement in the immediate postoperative period, but the lasting and permanent results, if any, are not necessarily observed for several years.

Crisis (118,135)

Unrelenting and progressive weakness associated with the administration of increasing amounts of anticholinesterase drugs frequently indicates the onset of myasthenic or cholinergic crisis. Cholinergic and myasthenic crisis can coexist, since different muscle groups respond differently. Because of difficulties encountered in distinguishing the two types of crisis, myasthenic patients who experience increasing difficulty with respiration, handling secretions, and feeding are most successfully treated in an intensive care unit by withdrawing anticholinesterase drugs, intubation or tracheostomy, respiratory support, and parenteral feeding. Crisis is generally transient, and drug therapy can usually be restarted in a few days after the refractory period subsides. Plasmapheresis can sometimes be very beneficial during the crisis period.

Complications

Despite all therapeutic possibilities, some children with MG experience respiratory and swallowing problems which are generally managed by aggressive intervention. Drugs which can worsen the neuromuscular transmission defect or interfere with acetylcholine release should be avoided in children with MG since their administration can result in increasing weakness. These drugs include aminoglycoside antibiotics, morphine, quinine, quinidine, procainamide, propranolol and chlorpromazine (136). When corticosteroid therapy is used, the patient may experience side effects induced by that class of drugs. The coexistence of MG with thymoma and other autoimmune diseases such as Grave disease, rheumatoid arthritis, Hashimoto disease, systemic lupus erythematosus, pemphigus, and multiple sclerosis, is far less common in children with MG than in adults.

Prognosis (118,119,137)

In recent years the morbidity and mortality from MG has been markedly reduced. This is most probably related to corticosteroid therapy and improved respiratory management. Despite the severity of respiratory failure when it occurs in MG, appropriate mechanical ventilation, prevention and treatment of pneumonia, and tracheal toilet should insure survival. If patients with severe MG can be kept alive for the first 2 to 3 years, the course of the disease is often one of gradual improvement with fewer periods of exacerbations.

MULTIPLE SCLEROSIS

Multiple sclerosis (MS) is a chronic and remitting disorder characterized by white matter lesions in the CNS, disseminated in space and time. The most current view is that MS is an autoimmune disease in some way related to a viral infection (138,139).

Incidence

MS is common in temperate zones of the Northern and Southern Hemispheres; the prevalence in these areas varies from 50 to 100 per 100,000 population (140,141). Although the majority of cases are found in the 30- to 50-year-old age group, approximately 10% to 15% are found in the adolescent age range, and a small percentage, 0.2% to 2% of all cases are reported with onset in children less than 10 years old. Girls are affected more frequently than boys (142), and MS has been documented in a 2-year-old child (143), the youngest patient on record. A small percentage of all cases are familial (144).

Pathogenesis

Experimental allergic encephalomyelitis (EAE) is the most commonly studied animal model of MS. EAE has been shown to be a T cell-mediated autoimmune disease in which there is inflammation and in chronic animals, demyelination. In MS there is an inflammatory response in the central nervous system consisting mainly of activated T lymphocytes and macrophages (145). This is accompanied by a local immune reaction with interleukin secretion, which results in the synthesis of oligoclonal immunoglobulin by plasma cells. An "imbalance" in the immune system may play a major role in the pathophysiology of MS (138,139). The lesions in the CNS are patchy and plaque-like and are generally perivenular. Myelin sheaths degenerate with less involvement of axis cylinders. Glial overgrowth leads to a sclerotic plaque which, at autopsy, appears grayish and translucent. These lesions are similar to those seen in EAE.

Clinical Presentation (142,146–149)

As expected in a CNS disorder in which the lesions are characteristically disseminated, the symptoms are variable and may even be those of a single focal lesion. A common presenting complaint, for example, is a rapid deterioration in central vision which may progress to optic neuritis and total loss of vision in one eye. The patient may complain of pain on eye movement, and the eye is often tender to pressure. The ophthalmoscopic appearance may be virtually indistinguishable from early papilledema associated with increased intracranial pressure, but vision is preserved in early papilledema. If the optic neuritis involves the portion of the optic nerve behind the globe the optic disc may appear normal, and the term retrobulbar neuritis is applicable. Optic neuritis (unilateral or bilateral) may occur simultaneously with transverse myelopathy. The latter lesion is most often at the thoracic level, resulting in lower extremity weakness, sensory abnormalities up to the level involved, and bowel and bladder disturbances. Hyperreflexia in the legs and extensor plantar responses are the rule.

Other common symptoms include incoordination or weakness of one or more extremities, paresthesia or numbness, headache which may be severe, diplopia, vertigo, or slurred speech. Less commonly the patient may experience an encephalopathy, with a diminished level of consciousness and fever, and even convulsions as the presenting symptoms.

Characteristically, the initial symptoms and signs may diminish over a period of days, weeks or months; they may also remit completely, or relapse even years or decades after the initial attack. Because of this, the findings on examination will depend to a great degree on the stage of the disease at which time the patient is examined. Common signs observed in MS include optic atrophy or pallor of the temporal portions of one or both optic discs, intention tremor, extensor plantar responses, hyperreflexia, diminished or absent abdominal reflexes, nystagmus, long-tract weakness and proprioceptive or other sensory deficits.

Diagnosis

The diagnosis of MS should be entertained if the basis of neurologic abnormalities can be explained only by the presence of more than one CNS lesion. There is no single confirmatory laboratory test or procedure which will document the disease in every case. The CSF (150) may have a normal or moderately elevated protein content, but a more reliable abnormality is the finding of oligoclonal bands. Oligoclonal bands (151), however, are not necessarily pathognomonic for MS, and can be seen in other CNS disorders. Visual evoked responses are also very useful, and can be abnormal in patients in whom visual acuity and conventional ophthalmoscopic examinations are completely normal (152). Similarly, brain stem auditory evoked response abnormalities can be useful in documenting a brain stem lesion in MS (153,154). Sensory evoked response abnormalities may also demonstrate objective evidence of the presence of lesions of the spinal cord. Multiple lesions with characteristic but not pathognomonic appearance may be seen with enhanced computerized tomography (CT) studies or with magnetic resonance imaging (MRI)(150). MRI is probably the best method for demonstrating dissemination in the CNS (150).

When clinical and laboratory results are incorporated, patients can generally be placed into one of several classes of diagnosis: clinically definite MS; laboratory supported definite MS; clinically probable MS; and laboratory supported probable MS (148).

Differential Diagnosis

Space occupying lesions in the spinal cord and brain can in some instances be confused initially with MS, but neuroimaging techniques can usually provide the correct diagnosis. Some neurologic complications of Lyme disease can simulate the neurologic abnormalities associated with MS, but they are generally differentiated with appropriate studies and the history of a tick bite. Conversion reactions sometimes simulate MS, but the lack of neurologic abnormalities can usually serve to differentiate these from MS.

Diplopia associated with myasthenia gravis or diabetes mellitus, for example, can usually be quickly differentiated from the diplopia noted with MS. Numbness and paresthesias can occasionally simulate those findings seen in peripheral neuropathies; however, the sensory changes resulting from MS tend to be asymmetric and tend to occur quite suddenly.

Therapy

Therapeutic goals in MS differ widely and include the following: improving recovery from acute attacks; preventing or diminishing the number of relapses; holding the disease in its chronic progressive stage; and caring for the patient as a human being in the context of his family. Many patients recover from an acute attack without any treatment. Because of this and because of the remitting exacerbating natural course, the efficacy of any treatment regimen has been difficult to assess. Many questions concerning the nature of the acute attack and what stops it remain unanswered. In a therapy plan designed to prevent or decrease the number of relapses, efficacy becomes even more difficult to prove because of the variable nature of the relapse rate and the variable natural history of the disease itself.

Adrenocorticosteroid hormone (ACTH)(155) or corticosteroids (156) have been the most widely used types of treatment in MS during the past (157) 2 to 3 decades. High dose intravenous methylprednisolone has also been reported to be beneficial. In general, these drugs should not be used for more than a month, since steroid dependency may be induced. Short and intensive courses of steroids appear to speed recovery from attacks. They probably have negligible effects on the progression of MS and produce no major alteration of the natural course of the disease.

Azathioprine may offer some benefit to patients with MS, but its effect is not immediate or dramatic (158–160). It can be used in a dose which will lower the white blood cell count to approximately $4,000/mL^3$, either with or without corticosteroids. Other drugs (158,159) or treatment modalities used in MS include cyclophosphamide (161), plasma exchange (162,163), lymphocytopheresis, interferon (164,165), total lymphoid irradiation (166,167), cyclosporine (168,169) and copolymer 1 (170,171). Future therapy might be directed specifically to immunologically activated cells (172,173).

Baclofen may be used to treat flexor spasms or spasticity. Since a multidisciplinary approach to this disease may be most efficacious because of the potential need for intervention by psychologists, physiatrists, urologists, ophthalmologists, and other professional personnel, patients might receive optimum treatment in a specialized center designed for MS patients.

Complications

As MS progresses, increased CNS scarring and fixed disability, such as joint contractures may occur. If drug therapy for spasticity with baclofen or dantrium is unsuccessful, some patients may benefit from local peripheral nerve blocking procedures. In the event that a neurogenic bladder results from MS, vigorous attention has to be paid to preventing and treating urinary tract infection, and in some cases surgical urinary diversion techniques can be very beneficial. Psychologic depression as with any other chronic disease has to be treated vigorously.

Prognosis

Generally, MS in children is a serious disease (142,146, 147), and its course is similar to that seen in adults (174). The follow-up in many studies of childhood MS, however, is incomplete, because these studies must be continued for many years after the initial attack to determine the outcome.

BEHÇET SYNDROME

Behçet syndrome (BS), a multisystem disorder rarely reported in the pediatric age group (175), is characterized by mucocutaneous, ocular, articular, vascular, gastrointestinal, and neurologic abnormalities. The diagnosis is difficult to establish and must be based on clinical criteria, since there is no pathognomonic clinical feature or laboratory test.

Incidence

BS is much more common in some areas of Japan and in Eastern Mediterranean countries than it appears to be in the United States (US), Northern Europe, or the United Kingdom. In the US it is unusual in the adult population and is probably very rare in childhood.

Pathogenesis

Recent light and electron-microscopic as well as immunofluorescent data support an underlying neutrophilic vasculitis in the early mucocutaneous lesions (176). Genetic, viral, and environmental factors have been implicated in the pathogenesis. There is evidence to suggest that at least some clinical aspects of BS are related to autoimmune abnormalities (177), including elevated levels of immunoglobulin, immune complexes, immunoglobulin binding to oral mucosa, and antibodies that react with fetal oral mucosal tissue. There is evidence that unresponsiveness of T cells to interleukin-2 may contribute to immunologic alterations in BS (178).

Clinical Presentation and Diagnosis

There is no unanimity of opinion as to what constitutes the major diagnostic criteria and there is no pathognomonic laboratory test. One author selected six clinical manifestations for diagnosis including recurrent oral aphthosis, recurrent genital aphthosis, uveitis, synovitis, cutaneous pustular vasculitis (pathergy), and meningoencephalitis (177). Oral aphthosis and at least two additional features must be present for a definite diagnosis. Gastrointestinal symptoms and a tendency for thrombosis of large veins and arteries may also be present.

Neurologic Manifestations

In one series of 25 patients with BS, 7 had evidence of meningoencephalitis (headache, fever, neck stiffness, and CSF pleocytosis)(179). Neurologic manifestations may be more common than noted because they may occur 1 to 10 years after onset of the other manifestations of BS. In addition to meningoencephalitis, neurologic manifestations (177,180) may include benign increased intracranial pressure (181) (possibly related to dural sinus thrombosis), brain stem lesions, cranial nerve palsies, pyramidal, extrapyramidal and cerebellar signs, spinal cord, and peripheral nerve lesions. There may be subtle involvement such as headache which may mimic migraine, mild confusion, or memory loss. Psychiatric signs and symptoms are also common in some series (176). In an American report describing BS in 6 pediatric patients (2 months to 11 years) 2 had neurologic involvement with mental status changes and CSF pleocytosis, for which no other cause was found (175). Three neonates with transplacentally acquired BS have been reported (182), probably through passage of immune complexes or antibodies. Severe mucosal and skin lesions were observed in those babies, but they healed with scarring and the disease resolved spontaneously after the 1st 6 to 8 weeks of life. No neurologic abnormalities were noted.

The clinical course is variable. The nonneurologic features are usually those noted initially, whereas the neurologic involvement may be delayed for several years.

Therapy

Assessment of various modes of therapy is difficult because of the unpredictable course of the disease (176). Topical agents, including triamcinalone and local anesthetics can be used as palliative measures for the mucosal lesions. Mild ocular disease can be treated with topical corticosteroids. Oral aphthae can be treated with orally administered colchicine, although this mode of treatment has been questioned. In some reports oral thalidomide has been stated to be very effective in the treatment of the mucocutaneous, rheumatologic and ocular manifestations. Systemic corticosteroids appear to be the major mode of therapy in all forms of BS, although this drug may not prevent blindness or neurologic sequelae. Azathioprine and cyclophosphamide have also been used.

Both oral chlorambucil and cyclosporin have been used in severe ocular and neurologic manifestations. In the presence of papilledema, conventional methods aimed at reducing increased intracranial pressure can be used.

ATAXIA-TELANGIECTASIA

Ataxia-Telangiectasia (A-T) is inherited as an autosomal recessive trait, the salient features of which include progressive cerebellar ataxia, recurrent sinopulmonary infections, oculocutaneous telangiectasis, immunodeficiencies, a propensity to develop malignancies, x-ray hypersensitivity, and impaired organ maturation (183–184). The incidence in the US is reported to be approximately 1 in 40,000 births. The gene frequency is said to be 1 per 100 of the population (185). The gene has been localized to chromosome 11 q22–23 (186).

Pathology

The major autopsy features concern the neurologic and immunologic systems. The neuropathologic findings are found primarily in the cerebellum (187–189). In addition to atrophy of the cerebellar vermis which may be marked, there is also loss of Purkinje, granular, and basket cells; the dentate and olivary nuclei also have degenerative changes. The cerebral hemispheres and basal ganglia are generally not significantly involved. Older A-T patients may have degeneration of the anterior horn cells, the posterior and lateral columns, as well as gliovascular malformations. Other regions of the central nervous system may be involved especially in older A-T patients, but this involvement is generally less severe than cerebellar abnormalities. Neurochemical abnormalities, primarily in the cerebellum, have also been described (190).

Other pathologic abnormalities include the absence or notably limited amounts of thymus tissue, with absence of cortical lymphoid tissue and Hassall corpuscles. Abnormalities of other organs in the lymphoreticular system may also be present. The lymph nodes contain reduced numbers of lymphoid follicles and show reticular cell hyperplasia and loss of the follicular pattern. Ovaries and testes may be atrophied, and the liver may show fatty deposits. The telangiectatic skin shows dilated venules.

Etiology

The cause of A-T remains unknown. Based on the results of experimental studies, several mechanisms have been suggested to explain the multiple defects observed in this disorder (184). Synthesis of antibodies and selected immunoglobulin subclasses are disrupted in A-T due to disorders of B-cell and helper T-cell function (191). Disorders of cell-mediated immunity are also found in A-T (192) including the inability to produce antigen-specific cytoxic lymphocytes to viral pathogens. Disorders of chromosomal integrity and cell growth are also present (193). There is an increased sensitivity to ionizing radiation and to selected chemical and physical agents (184). Abnormalities in DNA repair mechanisms may also be present. A generalized disorder of tissue differentiation, suggested by the findings of an embryonic-appearing thymus and persistent production of alpha-fetoprotein, is also present (184,194).

Clinical Features

Neurologic and Ophthalmologic

Ataxia is the first signal of a neurologic abnormality (183,185). An unusual gait manifested by frequent falling is noted soon after the child learns to walk, and although this is mild at the onset, it worsens as the child gets older with progressive development of hypotonia, diminished deep tendon reflexes, and dysmetria. By 8 to 10 years of age the child often becomes wheelchair bound; dysarthria may also become prominent. In early adolescence there is increased evidence of extrapyramidal signs including mask-like parkinsonian facies, slowed and rigid purposeful movements, and drooling. Choreoathetoid movements are present in the majority of older patients (183–185).

Deep tendon reflexes may become absent with advancing age, and wasting of muscles may be observed. Sensory perception and cranial nerve function except for the ophthalmologic manifestations are generally perserved. Cognitive function is generally normal at the onset, but a progressive decline in intelligence testing scores is common with advancing age.

Ophthalmologic manifestations are prominent. Conjunctival telangiectasis, which generally appears between 3 to 5 years of age, are symmetric and most prominent in the canthal regions (Figure 24.2). They do not extend beyond the limbic region and are found in all patients with A-T.

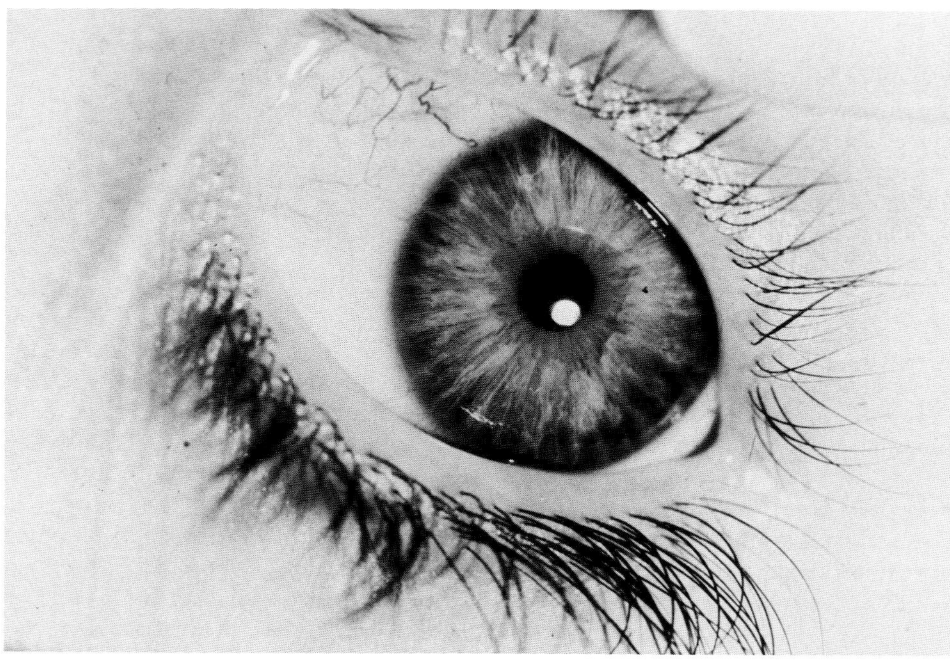

FIGURE 24.2 Early telangiectasia affecting the bulbar conjunctiva of a 4-year-old boy with ataxia-telangiectasia. (Courtesy of Dr. Bruce O. Berg, University of California, San Francisco).

Nystagmus, absence of optokinetic nystagmus, oculomotor apraxia, other abnormal ocular movements, and frequent blinking are common. However, visual acuity is preserved, and funduscopic examination reveals normal findings (195). Strabismus is also common.

Dermatologic

Cutaneous telangiectasis usually develops before 10 years of age, appearing in a butterfly distribution of the face, the external ears, and periorbital regions (183,185,186). As the child ages, telangiectasis appears on the neck, the dorsal surfaces of the hands and feet, the popliteal, and antecubital fossae. Café au lait spots are also common as well as seborrheic dermatitis, eczema, and atopic dermatitis. With advancing age there may be loss of subcutaneous fat and diffuse graying of the scalp hair.

Other Organ Involvement

Recurrent viral and bacterial infections occur in the majority of patients and are the most common cause of death. Growth retardation and endocrine disorders (insulin-resistent diabetes, testicular hypoplasia, and ovarian agenesis) are frequent in A-T. Generalized lymphadenopathy with or without splenomegaly is common.

Diagnosis

In the presence of progressive ataxia and ocular and cutaneous telangiectasia, the diagnosis is readily apparent. CT head scans may reveal symmetric enlargement of the cisterns surrounding the cerebellum and pons, dilatation of the fourth ventricle, and a prominent cerebellar folial pattern (196). Radiographs of the chest may show signs of chronic obstructive pulmonary disease.

A variety of cellular (abnormal responses to skin testing and graft rejection studies) and humoral immunologic defects are commonly seen in A-T (192). The majority of patients have deficient or absent IgA_2, and many have circulating anti-IgA antibodies; absent or low levels of IgE are also commonly found. IgG_2 and IgG_4 levels are frequently low, and a low molecular weight form of IgM is found commonly.

Almost all patients with A-T have elevated levels of alpha-fetoprotein and carcinoembryonic antigen (194). Elevated hepatic transaminases and glucose intolerance are seen in about one half of patients with A-T, and lymphocytopenia is also common. Chromosomal abnormalities occur much more commonly in A-T patients as compared to the normal population (193). Nerve conduction velocity studies may also be indicative of a peripheral neuropathy (185,197).

Differential Diagnosis

Neurologic differential diagnosis is limited to those disorders in which chronic progressive ataxia is present. Congenital disorders of the cerebellum, spinocerebellar degenerative disorders, or posterior fossa neoplasms do not demonstrate the typical skin lesions that are always present in A-T and the immunologic defects so commonly seen in this disorder. A syndrome mimicking A-T in which ataxia and oculomotor apraxia are present but in which there is no multisystem involvement has recently been described (198).

Therapy

There is no specific treatment available. Appropriate antibiotics are used during active infection, and physical therapy can be used to treat the neurologic dysfunction. Conventional methods of management of the respiratory problems are also useful. Prenatal diagnosis has been accomplished by measurement of alpha-fetoprotein in amniotic fluids and other studies.

Complications and Prognosis

Death frequently occurs in late childhood and is related to respiratory infections or insufficiency, or to malignant tumors which are commonly seen in patients with A-T. The types of neoplasms seen in A-T are similar to those seen in other immunodeficiency diseases. Family members carrying the A-T gene lack the clinical findings of the homozygotes, but they are a cancer prone segment of the population, with a significantly elevated incidence of malignancy (199). A-T families also have an increased incidence of idiopathic scoliosis and vertebral anomalies, though this is not striking (200).

GUILLAIN-BARRÉ SYNDROME

Guillain-Barré syndrome (GBS) is an immunologically mediated acute acquired demyelinating neuropathy which occurs in adults and children (201). A history of prior minor illness is commonly elicited in a majority of patients. The clinical and electrophysiologic pattern is generally distinct and the course is usually monophasic. Prognosis is usually favorable. The annual incidence of GBS per 100,000 people ranges from 0.6 to 1.9 in different populations in widely scattered regions of the world (202).

Pathogenesis

Inflammatory lesions occur throughout the peripheral nervous system in GBS (203). These are focal areas in which demyelination has taken place in the presence of lymphocytes and macrophages. Myelin appears essentially to be stripped away from the Schwann cell body and from the axon. There is good experimental evidence to indicate that this activity is immune mediated, but the precise mechanism remains unexplained (204–206). There is a strong resemblance of GBS to an experimentally produced allergic neuritis which is an animal model of human demyelinating neuropathy produced by sensitization to various peripheral nerve components (207).

Clinical Pattern

GBS is characterized by rapidly developing motor weakness which varies in degree from minor involvement of the legs to total paralysis of all limb and trunk muscles (201). Weakness may be preceded by ataxia and by a nonspecific viral infection. The weakness is usually accompanied by areflexia, although early in the onset, the deep tendon reflexes may be normal or hypoactive. Weakness is generally symmetric, and although it may develop rapidly and wax and wane, the course is monophasic; the progression of signs and symptoms usually ends by 4 weeks into the illness. Fever is lacking during this phase. Signs and symptoms of sensory involvement are generally mild and overshadowed by the motor weakness, although it is not unusual for a child with GBS to complain of muscular or limb pain early in the illness. Bilateral facial muscle weakness is common in GBS, but less commonly other cranial nerves may be involved. Even less commonly, the disease may begin with extraocular muscle involvement (Miller-Fisher syndrome)(208). The tongue and muscles involved in swallowing may also be affected. Autonomic dysfunction manifested by tachycardia, fluctuating hypotension and hypertension, and cardiac arrhythmias are common. Recovery frequently begins a few weeks after progression ceases, although in milder cases this may occur earlier. In other patients recovery may be delayed for a prolonged period of time, even many months. Rarely there is no recovery with permanent deficits. Bowel and bladder functions are not characteristically involved, but bladder dysfunction may be transient. Similarly, some patients will demonstrate some degree of CNS involvement as manifest by extensor plantar responses and a sensory level.

Diagnosis

Examination of the CSF can provide strong support for the diagnosis when this examination is coupled with the clinical findings. The CSF is generally acellular or contains fewer than 10 mononuclear leukocytes per cubic millimeter, although uncommonly up to 50 such cells may be seen. CSF protein values are almost always elevated; if they are not elevated initially they may become elevated on serial lumbar punctures.

Electrophysiologic studies may be extremely helpful in supporting the diagnosis (209,210). Abnormalities of motor and sensory conduction velocity are present in the vast majority of patients, but in some instances since the pathology is focal, several nerves have to be studied. On routine conduction velocity determinations, abnormalities may be absent in the early stage of the illness (initial 2 weeks) but become apparent later. Application of F-wave responses provide a better indication of slowing related to demyelination in proximal portions of nerve trunks and roots. These abnormalities are present early in the course of GBS, but a small minority of patients with GBS will have normal studies.

There are certain clinical features which should make the diagnosis very suspicious including persistent marked asymmetry and persistent bowel and bladder dysfunction. Similarly, a sharp sensory level is not seen in GBS, and should point to spinal cord involvement.

GBS may be associated with acute Epstein-Barr virus, cytomegalovirus, and other infections such as mycoplasma (211,212), Lyme disease (213), AIDS, childhood exanthema and mumps (214). When indicated appropriate studies can be done to include or exclude these entities.

Differential Diagnosis

In addition to the tick of Lyme disease, a bite of the tick *Dermacentor andersoni,* can produce a clinical picture indistinguishable from GBS (215). Thus, the skin should always be scrupulously examined for the presence of this tick; recovery of weakness follows its removal. The neuropathy associated with acute intermittent porphyria can also simulate GBS (216). This can be diagnosed by measuring the urinary porphobilinogen and delta-aminolevulinic acid. A pattern of muscle weakness can be observed with volatile solvents such as n-hexane and methyl n-butyl ketone or with organophosphorus compounds; careful history can usually elicit this type of intoxication (217).

Paralysis associated with poliomyelitis is more commonly asymmetrical and/or focal and occurs at the time of a very high fever, contrary to the paralysis in GBS which is symmetric, and occurs when the patient is fever free. The CSF profile in acute poliomyelitis also differs from that of GBS in that there is an abundance of cells in polio, frequently with a high percentage of polymorphonuclear cells at the onset. Paralysis associated with a conversion reaction can usually be diagnosed by the lack of objective neurologic abnormalities. In botulism in older children, a history of eating tainted food or of another family member being similarly involved may be elicited; weakness can be sudden and severe, but extraocular muscles are frequently involved early in the disease contrary to GBS (125). Electrodiagnostic studies can also serve to assist in differentiation where this may be troublesome clinically. In acute fulminating MG the weakness may be severe but extraocular muscles are generally involved early and the deep tendon reflexes are most often preserved. In MG no CSF abnormalities are noted, the edrophonium test is positive, and electrodiagnostic studies (repetitive stimulation and F-wave determinations) can readily differentiate the two entities.

The first episode of autosomal dominant hypokalemic periodic paralysis may initially be mistaken for GBS until the family history and the hypokalemia are noted. In patients with chronic relapsing polyneuropathy the onset is usually slow (over several months) differing from the acute or subacute onset in GBS (218).

In diphtheritic polyneuropathy palatal weakness and blurring of vision due to paralysis of accomodation are generally the first symptoms. These are followed by evidence of involvement of other cranial and pharyngial nerves. These early symptoms can distinguish this form of polyneuropathy from GBS.

Therapy

Since children with GBS can have a rapidly progressive course within the initial 3 to 4 weeks after the onset of the disease, even following a period in which the disease appears to be quiescent, patients need scrupulous observation, preferably in an intensive care unit. Ventilation is the major problem, and patients will require elective intubation and respiratory assistance if their vital capacity, which should be determined frequently, falls below acceptable values (219). Similarly, if the patient becomes breathless or if the blood gas values deteriorate, elective ventilatory assistance should be undertaken. If it appears that ventilatory support is needed for a prolonged period of time, elective tracheostomy should be considered. Careful pulmonary and/or tracheostomy care is mandatory.

Because of the possibility of autonomic nervous system dysfunction (such as blood pressure changes or arrhythmias) monitoring is crucial, and conventional therapy for these problems should be instituted if and when they arise. Nutritional requirements and electrolyte balance have to be maintained carefully in all patients.

Cautious physical therapy, including passive range of motion exercises, turning of the patient, scrupulous care of pressure areas and avoidance of joint contractures are crucial in a paralyzed patient. Constant reassurance by family and medical personnel is also mandatory in weakened patients. In patients who are severely paralyzed and/or intubated ingenious methods to allow the patient to communicate his needs have to be devised.

Based on several studies designed to investigate the value of corticosteroids in the treatment of GBS, it has generally been concluded that steroids have no beneficial value in this disease (220). Similarly, there is no conclusive evidence that gamma globulin or conventional immunosuppressive agents such as azathioprine and cyclophosphamide are beneficial in GBS (221). However, it must be remembered that due to the variability of the course of this disease, large numbers of patients are needed to assess the effects of treatment.

There have been several reports of studies on the efficacy of plasmapheresis in GBS (222–226). The results generally conclude that plasmapheresis hastens recovery and may prevent progression in patients already unable to walk unassisted. Plasmapheresis therapy also results in a significant reduction in the number of GBS patients who require ventilatory assistance. In one study, the equal efficacy of albumin as a replacement fluid as compared to fresh frozen plasma was documented.

As a result of these studies of plasmapheresis in GBS, several guidelines can be formulated at the time of this writing, obviously subject to modifications as more information becomes available (225). Patients with mild involvement related to GBS can be observed carefully in the hospital, preferably in a center experienced in managing this type of patient. Pheresis can be begun if the patient has appreciable reduction in respiratory capacity or if the patient begins to lose the ability to walk unassisted. If the patient's weakness worsens after completion of a course of pharesis, an additional course might be indicated.

Prognosis

Although the majority of patients with GBS recover, significant numbers of children with GBS have varying degrees of permanent motor and/or sensory impairment. When various electrodiagnostic study results are assessed with reference to their value to predict outcome, it has been ascertained that a distal compound motor action potential amplitude value at 0% to 20% of the lower limit of normal was associated with a poor prognosis and incomplete recovery (209–210). Ventilator dependence and rapid evolution of weakness are also more common in patients with a poor prognosis. Scrupulous control of respiratory problems, infection, and autonomic dysfunction should diminish the mortality to a very low value.

CHRONIC RELAPSING POLYNEUROPATHY

Chronic relapsing polyneuropathy (CRP) is an unusual demyelinating disorder with similar clinical, pathologic and electrophysiologic features as GBS; however, the onset is slower and the course is either remitting or chronic (218,227). The treatment is also different. Several terms have been applied to this disorder, including chronic relapsing GBS, relapsing corticosteroid-dependent polyneuritis, and chronic inflammatory demyelinating polyradiculoneuropathy.

Pathogenesis

The segmental demyelination in nerve biopsies from patients with CRP are similar to those observed in GBS (228). There is experimental evidence that abnormal immune mechanisms play an important role in the pathogenesis, but the exact mechanism remains unknown.

Clinical Pattern (218,227)

This disease affects persons of both sexes and involves children as well as adults. Distal limb weakness and paresthesias are the most common presenting symptoms; progression is slow, usually over several months, resulting in a maximum involvement (severe weakness and sensory findings) in 6 to 12 months although in some cases onset is subacute. Progression then stops. A preceding minor illness observed so commonly in GBS, is not seen in CRP. Cranial nerves are involved less frequently than in GBS, but deep tendon reflexes are generally absent, and remain so even in the recovery period. Respiratory problems are very uncommon as are signs of autonomic involvement. An irregular tremor, observed best in the outstretched hands, is common; in many patients it occurs at the time of a relapse, but in one of our patients it was the presenting problem prior to the onset of any demonstrable weakness. The course may be either steadily progressive or relapsing and remitting.

Diagnosis

The CSF protein is always elevated in CRP, generally with levels above 100 mg/dL, but the fluid is acellular (218). The CSF protein is highest during exacerbations and is decreased during remission or treatment. Motor nerve conduction velocities are characteristically markedly slowed and sensory potentials are absent in CRP. Conventional blood studies are unrevealing; serum protein electrophoresis and immunoelectrophoresis are normal.

Differential Diagnosis

In patients with CRP a family history of a similar disorder is absent. Care should be taken to examine family members when the diagnosis of CRP is entertained to exclude the presence of hereditary sensory-motor neuropathies; in this group of disorders progression is usually insidious over years, contrary to CRP. In toxic neuropathies, the history of intoxication can usually be elicited and signs of systemic illness, such as weight loss can be frequently noted. The peripheral neuropathies associated with systemic illnesses or gammopathies can be excluded by appropriate studies. In a case report, recurrent polyneuropathy in a child was associated with a cytomegalovirus infection and recurrence was associated with an Epstein-Barr reinfection (229).

Therapy

CRP is a treatable disorder, and functional recovery can be predicted in almost every patient treated. Corticosteroids are the drugs of first choice (218,230,231). Therapy is usually begun with 1.5 mg/kg of prednisone in young children and up to 100 mg in older children or adults, as a single daily dose. After a period of three to four weeks the dose is tapered to an alternate day schedule by reducing an alternate "off day" dose slowly over several weeks. If the dose is diminished too rapidly a relapse can appear, sometimes requiring restarting of a higher steroid dose. After reinstitution of a tapering schedule the patient may be kept on a minimum single alternate day dose which will prevent relapse. The clinical picture is the most sensitive monitor of improvement, but the CSF protein will frequently become normal in remission. The deep tendon reflexes will remain absent, and to the nerve conduction velocity studies will generally remain abnormally slow. The irregular tremor may remain, but become diminished, or disappear. Other modalities of treatment, such as azathioprine, (232), cyclophosphamide, intravenous gamma globulin (233) and plasmapheresis (234) may be useful, but controlled documentation is lacking.

Prognosis

Therapy will provide functional recovery in the majority of patients. However, in some patients, response to therapy is lost after several relapses, and permanent weakness and/or ventilatory problems, both of which may be severe, remain.

REFERENCES

1. Zamvil SS, Nelson PA, Mitchell DJ, et al. Encephalitogenic T-cell clones specific for myelin basic protein. J Exp Med 1985;162:2107–2124.
2. Hart MN, Linthicum DS, Waldschmidt MM, et al. Experimental autoimmune inflammatory myopathy. J Neuropathol Exp Neurol 1987;46:511–521.
3. Rostami A, Burns JB, Brown MJ, et al. Transfer of experimental allergic neuritis with Pz-reactive T-cell lines. Cellular Immunol 1985;91:354–361.
4. Linington C, Izumo S, Suzuki M, et al. A permanent rat T cell line that mediates experimental allergic neuritis in the Lewis rat in vivo. J Immunol 1984;133:1946–1950.
5. Linthicum DS, Frelinger JA. Acute autoimmune encephalitis in mice. J Exp Med 1982;155:31–40.
6. Brosnan CF, Lyman WD, Tansey FA, et al. Quantitation of mast cells in experimental allergic neuritis. J Neuropathol Exp Neurol 1985;44:196–203.
7. Raine CS. Experimental allergic encephalomyelitis and neuritis. In: Vinken PJ, Bruyn GW, Klawans HL, et al., eds. Handbook of Clinical Neurology. Amsterdam: Elsevier Science 1985;47 (Revised series 3): 429–466.
8. Zamvil S, Nelson P, Trotter J, et al. T-cell clones specific for myelin basic protein induce chronic relapsing paralysis and demyelination. Nature 1985;317:355–358.
9. Waldor MK, Sriram S, Hardy R, et al. Reversal of experimental allergic encephalitis with a monoclonal antibody to a T-cell subset marker. Science 1985;227:415–417.
10. Brostoff SW, Mason DW. Experimental allergic encephalomyelitis: Successful treatment in vivo with a monoclonal antibody that recognizes T helper cells. J Immunol 1984;133:1938–1942.
11. Raine CS, Johnson AB, Marins M, et al. Demyelination in vitro. Absorption studies demonstrate that galactocerebroside is a major target. J Neurol Sci 1981;52:117–131.
12. Brosnan CF, Traugott U, Raine CS. Analysis of humoral and cellular events and the role of lipid haptens during CNS demyelination. Acta Neuropathol 1983;9:59–70.
13. Gausas J, Paterson P, Day ED, et al. Intact B-cell activity is essential for complete expression of experimental allergic encephalomyelitis in Lewis rats. Cell Immunol 1982;72:360–366.
14. Willenborg DO, Prowse SJ. Immunoglobulin-deficient rats fail to develop experimental allergic encephalomyelitis. J Neuroimmunol 1983;5:99–109.
15. Traugott U, McFarlin DE, Raine CS. Immunopathology of the lesion in chronic relapsing experimental autoimmune encephalitis in the mouse. Cell Immunol 1986;99:395–410.
16. McCarron RM, Kempski O, Spatz M, et al. Presentation of myelin basic protein by murine cerebral vascular endothelial cells. J Immunol 1985;134:3100–3103.
17. Fontana A, Fierz W, Wekerle H. Astrocytes present myelin basic protein to encephalitogenic T-cell lines. Nature 1984;307:273–276.
18. Fierz W, Endler B, Reske K, et al. Astrocytes as antigen-presenting cells. J Immunol 1985;134:3785–3793.
19. Fontana A, Otz U, DeWeck AL, et al. Glia cell stimulating factor (GSF): A new lymphokine: Part 2. Cellular sources and partial purification of human GSF. J Neuroimmunol 1981;2:73–81.
20. Wong GHW, Bartlett PF, Clark-Lewis I, et al. Induction of H-2 and Ia antigens on cultured brain cells by an interferon-γ-like molecule [abstract]. Neuroscience Letters 1983;36 Suppl 11:S84.
21. Sobel RA, Blanchette BW, Bhan AK, et al. The immunopathology of experimental allergic encephalomyelitis. J Immunol 1984;132:2393–2401.
22. Brosnan CF, Stoner DL, Bloom BR, et al. Studies on demyelination by activated lymphocytes in the rabbit eye. II. Antibody-dependent cell-mediated demyelination. J Immunol 1977;118:2103–2110.
23. Brosnan CF, Cammer W, Norton WT, et al. Proteinase inhibitors suppress the development of experimental allergic encephalomyelitis. Nature 1980;285:235–237.
24. Epstein LG, Prineas JW, Raine CS. Attachment of myelin to coated pits on macrophages in experimental allergic encephalomyelitis. J Neurol Sci 1983;61:341–348.
25. Raine CS, Snyder DH, Valsamis MP, et al. Chronic experimental allergic encephalomyelitis in inbred guinea pigs. Lab Invest 1974;31:369–380.
26. Moore GRW, Traugott U, Raine CS. Survival of oligodendrocytes in chronic relapsing experimental autoimmune encephalomyelitis. J Neurol Sci 1984;65:137–145.
27. Brostoff S, Burnet P, Lampert P, et al. Experimental allergic neuritis. Isolation and characterization of a protein from sciatic nerve myelin responsible for experimental allergic neuritis. Nature 1972;235:210.

28. Pollard JD, King RHM, Thomas PK. Recurrent experimental allergic neuritis. An electron microscope study. J Neurol Sci 1975;24:365–383.

29. Heininger K, Stoll G, Linington C, et al. Conduction failure and nerve conduction slowing in experimental allergic neuritis induced by P2-specific T-cell lines. Ann Neurol 1986; 19:44–49.

30. Astrom KE, Webster HdeF, Arnason BG. The initial lesion in experimental allergic neuritis. A phase and electron microscope study. J Exp Med 1968;128:469–495.

31. Raine CS. Schwann cell responses during recurrent demyelination and their relevance to onion-bulb formation. Neuropathol Appl Neurobiol 1977;3:453–470.

32. Olsson T, Holmdahl R, Klareskog L, et al. Dynamics of 1a-expressing cells and T lymphocytes of different subsets during experimental allergic neuritis in Lewis rats. J Neurol Sci 1984;66:141–149.

33. Powell HC, Braheny SL, Myers RR, et al. Early changes in experimental allergic neuritis. Lab Invest 1983;48:332–338.

34. Brosnan CF, Tansey FA. Delayed onset of experimental allergic neuritis in rats treated with reserpine. J Neuropathol Exp Neurol 1984;43:84–93.

35. Raine CS, Bornstein MB. Experimental allergic neuritis. Ultrastructure of serum-induced myelin aberrations in peripheral nervous system cultures. Lab Invest 1979;40: 423–432.

36. Sumner AJ. The physiological basis for symptoms in Guillain-Barré syndrome. Ann Neurol 1981;9 Suppl:28–30.

37. Manghani D, Partridge TA, Sloper JC. The role of myofibrillar fraction of skeletal muscle in the production of experimental polymyositis. J Neurol Sci 1974;23:489–503.

38. Rosenberg NL, Ringel SP, Kotzin BL. Experimental autoimmune myositis in SJL/J mice. Clin Exp Immunol 1987;68:117–129.

39. Strongwater SL, Dorovini-Zis K, Ball RD, et al. A murine model of polymyositis induced by coxsackievirus B1 (Tucson strain). Arthritis Rheum 1984;27:433–442.

40. Walker EJ, Jeffrey PD. Polymyositis and molecular mimicry. A mechanism of autoimmunity. Lancet 1986;2:605–607.

41. Hays AP, Gamboa ET. Acute viral myositis. In: Engel AG, Banker BQ, eds. Myology, Vol. 2. New York: McGraw-Hill, 1986;1439–1466.

42. Banker BQ. Parasitic myositis. In: Engel AG, Banker BQ, eds. Myology, Vol. 2. New York: McGraw-Hill, 1986; 1467–1499.

43. Mikol J. Inclusion body myositis. In: Engel AG, Banker BQ, eds. Myology, Vol. 2. New York: McGraw-Hill, 1986; 1423–1438.

44. Medsger TA Jr, Dawson WN, Masi AT. The epidemiology of polymyositis. Am J Med 1970;48:715–723.

45. Walker GL, Mastaglia FL, Roberts DF. A search for genetic influence in idiopathic inflammatory myopathies. Acta Neurol Scand 1982;66:432–443.

46. Pachman LM, Cooke N. Juvenile dermatomyositis: A clinical and immunologic study. J Pediatr 1980;96:226–234.

47. Kissel JT, Mendell JR, Rammohan KW. Microvascular deposition of complement membrane attack complex in dermatomyositis. N Engl J Med 1986;314:329–334.

48. Currie S. Destruction of muscle cultures by lymphocytes from cases of polymyositis. Acta Neuropathol 1970; 15:11–19.

49. Arahata K, Engel AG. Monoclonal antibody analysis of mononuclear cells in myopathies. I: Quantitation of subsets according to diagnosis and sites of accumulation and demonstration and counts of muscle fibers invaded by T cells. Ann Neurol 1984;16:193–208.

50. Engel AG, Arahata K: Monoclonal antibody analysis of mononuclear cells in myopathies. II. Phenotypes of auto-invasive cells in polymyositis and inclusion body myositis. Ann Neurol 1984;16:209–215.

51. Schroter HM, Sarnat HB, Matheson OS, et al. Juvenile dermatomyositis induced by toxoplasmosis. J Child Neurol 1987;2:101–104.

52. Christensen ML, Pachman LM, Schneiderman R, et al. Prevalence of coxsackie B virus antibodies in patients with juvenile dermatomyositis. Arthritis Rheum 1986;29:1365–1370.

53. Pachman LM. Juvenile dermatomyositis. Pediatr Clin North Am 1986;33:1097–1117.

54. Bowles NE, Dubowitz V, Sewry CA, et al. Dermatomyositis, polymyositis, and coxsackie-B-virus infection. Lancet 1987; 1:1004–1007.

55. Goel KM, King M. Dermatomyositis-polymyositis in children. Scott Med J 1986;31:15–19.

56. Spiro AJ. Childhood dermatomyositis and polymyositis. Pediatr Rev 1984;6:163–172.

57. Banker BQ, Engel AG. The polymyositis and dermatomyositis syndromes. In: Engel AG, Banker BQ, eds. Myology, Vol. 2. New York: McGraw-Hill, 1986;1385–1422.

58. Lovell HB, Lindsley CB. Late recurrence of childhood dermatomyositis. J Rheumatol 1986;13:821–822.

59. Harati Y, Niakan E, Bergman EW. Childhood dermatomyositis in monozygotic twins. Neurology 1986;36: 721–723.

60. Cook JD, Fink CW, Henderson-Tilton AC. Comparison of the initial response of childhood dermatopolymyositis to daily versus alternate day corticosteroid administration: A retrospective study [abstract]. Ann Neurol 1984;16: 400–401.

61. Dubowitz V. Treatment of dermatomyositis in childhood. Arch Dis Child 1976;51:494–500.

62. Laxer RM, Stein LF, Petty RE. Intravenous pulse methylprednisolone treatment of juvenile dermatomyositis. Arthritis Rheum 1987;30:328–334.

63. Castro-Gago M, Alvez-Gonzalez F, Pena-Guitian J. High-dose intravenous methyl-prednisolone in chronic polymyositis/dermatomyositis [letter]. Brain Dev 1986;8:570.

64. Bunch TW, Worthington JW, Combs JJ, et al. Azathioprine with prednisone for polymyositis. A controlled, clinical trial. Ann Intern Med 1980;92:365–369.

65. Niakan E, Pitner SE, Whitaker JN, et al. Immunosuppressive agents in corticosteroid-refractory childhood dermatomyositis. Neurology 1980;30:286–291.

66. Dau PC, Bennington JL. Plasmapheresis in childhood dermatomyositis. J Pediatr 1981;98:237–240.

67. Roifman CM, Schaffer FM, Wachsmuth SE, et al. Reversal of chronic polymyositis following intravenous serum globulin therapy. JAMA 1987;258:513–515.

68. Fishel B, Diamant S, Papo I, et al. CT assessment of calcinosis in a patient with dermatomyositis. Clin Rheumatol 1986;5:242–244.

69. Randle HW, Sander HM, Howard K. Early diagnosis of calcinosis cutis in childhood dermatomyositis using computed tomography. JAMA 1986;256:1137–1138.

70. Fuchs D, Fruchter L, Fishel B, et al. Colchicine suppression of local inflammation due to calcinosis in dermatomyositis and progressive systemic sclerosis. Clin Rheumatol 1986; 5:527–530.

71. Gotoff SP, Smith RD, Sugar O. Dermatomyositis with cerebral vasculitis in a patient with agammaglobulinemia. Am J Dis Child 1972;123:53–56.

72. Noseworthy JH, Heffernan LP, Ross JB, et al. Acne fulminans with inflammatory myopathy. Ann Neurol 1980; 8:67–69.

73. Eckardt JJ, Ivins JC, Perry HO, et al. Osteosarcoma arising in heterotopic ossification of dermatomyositis: Case report and review of the literature. Cancer 1981;48:1256–1261.

74. Kaell AT, Shetty M, Lee BCP, et al. The diversity of neurologic events in systemic lupus erythematosus: Prospective clinical and computed tomographic classification of 82 events in 71 patients. Arch Neurol 1986;43:273–276.

75. Bruyn GW, Padberg G. Chorea and systemic lupus erythematosus. A critical review. Eur Neurol 1984;23:435–448.

76. Graham EM, Spalton DJ, Barnard RO, et al. Cerebral and retinal vascular changes in systemic lupus erythematosus. Ophthalmology 1985;92:444–448.

77. Moskowitz N. Systemic lupus erythematosus of the central nervous system: Classification, epidemiology, pathology, diagnosis and therapy. Mt Sinai J Med 1988;55:147–153.

78. Szer IS. The diagnosis and management of systemic lupus erythematosus in childhood. Pediatr Ann 1986;15:596–604.

79. Tan EM, Cohen AS, Fries JF, et al. The 1982 revised criteria for the classification of systemic lupus erythematosus. Arthritis Rheum 1982;25:1271–1277.

80. Hart RG, Miller VI, Coull BM, et al. Cerebral infarction associated with lupus anticoagulants—Preliminary report. Stroke 1984;15:114–118.

81. Futrell N, Millikan C. Causes and treatment of altered consciousness or acute psychosis in systemic lupus erythematosus [abstract]. Ann Neurol 1988;24:170–171.

82. Kaplan RE, Springate JE, Feld LG, et al. Pseudotumor cerebri associated with cerebral venous sinus thrombosis, internal jugular vein thrombosis, and systemic lupus erythematosus. J Pediatr 1985;107:266–268.

83. Verness M, Bernstein RM, Bydder M, et al. Nuclear magnetic resonance (NMR) imaging of brain in systemic lupus erythematosus. J Comput Assist Tomogr 1983;7:461–467.

84. Weisberg LA. Cranial computed tomographic findings in patients with neurologic manifestations of systemic lupus erythematosus. Comput Radiol 1986;10:63–68.

85. Miller JJ. Drug-induced lupus-like syndromes in children. Arthritis Rheum 1977;20:308–311.

86. Heilman KM, Kohler WC. Haloperidol treatment of chorea associated with systemic lupus erythematosus. Neurology 1971;21:963–965.

87. Austin HA III, Klippel J, Balow JE, et al. Therapy of lupus nephritis: Controlled trial of prednisone and cytotoxic drugs. N Engl J Med 1986;314:614–619.

88. Fraga A, Gudino J, Ramos-Niembro F, et al. Mixed connective tissue disease in childhood: relationship with Sjögren's syndrome. Am J Dis Child 1978;32:263–265.

89. Singsen BH, Bernstein BH, Kornreich HK, et al. Mixed connective tissue disease in childhood. A clinical and serologic survey. J Pediatr 1977;90:893–900.

90. Sharp GC, Irwin WS, Tan E, et al. Mixed connective tissue disease—An apparently distinct rheumatic disease syndrome associated with a specific antibody to an extractable nuclear antigen (ENA). Am J Med 1972;52:148–159.

91. Athreya BH, Norman ME, Myers AR, et al. Sjögren's syndrome in children. Pediatrics 1977;59:931–938.

92. Provost TT, Vasily D, Alexander E. Sjögren's syndrome: Cutaneous, immunologic, and nervous system manifestations. Neurol Clin 1987;5:405–426.

93. Alexander EL, Provost TT, Stevens MB, et al. Neurologic complications of primary Sjögren's syndrome. Medicine 1982;61:247–257.

94. Alexander EL, Alexander GE. Aseptic meningoencephalitis in primary Sjögren's syndrome. Neurology 1983;33:593–599.

95. Alexander EL, Malinow K, Lejewski JE, et al. Primary Sjögren's syndrome with central nervous system disease mimicking multiple sclerosis. Ann Intern Med 1986;104:323–330.

96. Moline R, Provost TT, Alexander EL. Peripheral inflammatory vascular disease in Sjögren's syndrome: Association with nervous system complications. Arthritis Rheum 1985;28:1341–1347.

97. Kass H, Hanson V, Patrick J. Scleroderma in childhood. J Pediatr 1966;68:243–256.

98. Hwang P, Watters GV, Metrakos K, et al. Neurological complications of scleroderma [abstract]. Ann Neurol 1983;378.

99. Ad hoc committee of the council on rheumatic fever and congenital heart disease: Jone's criteria (revised) for guidance in the diagnosis of rheumatic fever. Circulation 1965;32:664–668.

100. Nausieda PA, Grossman BJ, Koller WC, et al. Sydenham chorea: An update. Neurology 1980;30:331–334.

101. Barbeau A. The nosology of extrapyramidal disorders. Birth Defects 1971;7:156–166.

102. Markowitz M. The decline of rheumatic fever: Role of medical intervention. J Pediatr 1985;106:545–550.

103. Aron AM, Freeman JM, Carter S. The natural history of Sydenham's chorea. Am J Med 1965;38:83–95.

104. Roig M, Montserrat L, Gallart A. Carbamazepine: An alternative drug for the treatment of nonhereditary chorea. Pediatrics 1988;82:492–495.

105. Dhanaraj M, Radhadrishnan AR, Srinivas K, et al. Sodium valproate in Sydenham's chorea. Neurology 1985;35:114–115.

106. Ch'ien LT, Economides AN, Lemmi H: Sydenham's chorea and seizures. Arch Neurol 1978;35:382–385.

107. Brewer EJ, Giannini EH, Person DA. Juvenile rheumatoid arthritis. Philadelphia: WB Saunders, 1982, 1–53.

108. Brewer EJ, Giannini EH, Person DA. Juvenile rheumatoid arthritis. Philadelphia: WB Saunders, 1982, 36–37.

109. Drachman DB, DeSilva S, Ramsay D, et al. Humoral pathogenesis of myasthenia gravis. Ann NY Acad Sci 1987;505:90–104.

110. Vincent A, Newsom-Davis J. Acetylcholine receptor antibody as a diagnostic test for myasthenia gravis: Results in 153 validated cases and 2967 diagnostic assays. J Neurol Neurosurg Psychiatry 1985;48:1246–1252.

111. Osserman KE, Genkins G. Studies in myasthenia gravis: Review of a twenty-year experience in over 1200 patients. Mt Sinai J Med 1971;38:497–537.

112. Engel AG. Myasthenic syndromes In: Engel AG, Banker BQ, eds. Myology. New York: McGraw-Hill, 1986;1955–1990.

113. Compston DA, Vincent A, Newsom-Davis J, et al. Clinical, pathological, HLA antigen and immunological evidence for disease heterogeneity in myasthenia gravis. Brain 1980;103:579–601.

114. Jaretzki A III, Penn AS, Younger DS, et al. "Maximal" thymectomy for myasthenia gravis: Results. J Thorac Cardiovasc Surg 1988;95:747–757.

115. Papatestas AE, Genkins G, Kornfeld P, et al. Effects of thymectomy in myasthenia gravis. Ann Surg 1987;206:79–88.

116. Lisak RP, Abdou NI, Zweiman B, et al. Aspects of lymphocyte function in myasthenia gravis. Ann NY Acad Sci 1976;274:402–410.

117. Vincent A, Newsom-Davis J. Anti-acetylcholine receptor antibodies. J Neurol Neurosurg Psychiatry 1980;43:590–600.

118. Grob D, Arsura EL, Brunner NG, et al. The course of myasthenia gravis and therapies affecting outcome. Ann NY Acad Sci 1987;505:472–499.

119. Genkins G, Kornfeld P, Papatestas AE, et al. Clinical experience in more than 2000 patients with myasthenia gravis. Ann NY Acad Sci 1987;505:500–513.

120. Morel E, Eymard B, Vernet-der Garadedian B, et al. Neonatal myasthenia gravis: A new clinical and immunologic appraisal on 30 cases. Neurology 1988;38:138–142.

121. Bartoccioni E, Evoli A, Casali C, et al. Neonatal myasthenia gravis: Clinical and immunological study of seven mothers and their newborn infants. J Neuroimmunol 1986;12:155–161.

122. Lefvert AK, Osterman PO. Newborn infants to myasthenic mothers: a clinical study and investigation of acetylcholine receptor antibodies in 17 children. Neurology 1983;33:133–138.

123. Osserman KE, Teng P. Studies in myasthenia gravis—A rapid diagnostic test. Further progress with edrophonium (tensilon) chloride. JAMA 1956;160:153.

124. Elmqvist D, Hofmann WW, Kugelberg J, et al. An electrophysiological investigation of neuromuscular transmission in myasthenia gravis. J Physiol 1964;174:417–434.

125. Brown LW. Infant botulism. Pediatr Ann 1984;13:135–148.

126. Arsura E, Brunner NG, Namba T, et al. High-dose intravenous methylprednisolone in myasthenia gravis. Arch Neurol 1985;42:1149–1153.

127. Niakan E, Harati Y, Rolak LA. Immunosuppressive drug therapy in myasthenia gravis. Arch Neurol 1986;43:155–156.

128. Witte AS, Cornblath DR, Schatz NJ, et al. Monitoring azathioprine therapy in myasthenia gravis. Neurology 1986;36:1533–1534.

129. Hohlfeld R, Michels M, Heininger K, et al. Azathioprine toxicity during long-term immunosuppression of generalized myasthenia gravis. Neurology 1988;38:258–261.

130. Tindall RS, Rollins JA, Phillips JT, et al. Preliminary results of a double-blind, randomized, placebo-controlled trial of cyclosporine in myasthenia gravis. N Engl J Med 1987;316:719–724.

131. Arsura EL, Bick A, Brunner NG, et al. High-dose intravenous immunoglobulin in the management of myasthenia gravis. Arch Intern Med 1986;146:1365–1368.

132. Arsura EL, Bick A, Brunner NG, et al. Effects of repeated doses of intravenous immunoglobulin in myasthenia gravis. Am J Med Sci 1988;295:438–443.

133. Dau PC, Lindstrom JM, Cassel CK, et al. Plasmapheresis and immunosuppressive therapy in myasthenia gravis. N Engl J Med 1977;297:1134–1140.

134. Cooper JD, Al Jilaihawa AN, Pearson FG, et al. An improved technique to facilitate transcervical thymectomy for myasthenia gravis. Ann Thorac Surg 1988;45:242–247.

135. Sellman MS, Mayer RF. Treatment of myasthenic crisis in late life. South Med J 1985;78:1208–1210.

136. Adams SL, Mathews J, Grammer LC. Drugs that may exacerbate myasthenia gravis. Ann Emerg Med 1984;13:532–538.

137. Descamps H, Bataille J, Estournet B, et al. Long-term evolution of childhood myasthenia. Ann Med Interne 1987;138:615–619.

138. Waksman BH, Reynolds WE. Multiple sclerosis as a disease of immune regulation. Proc Soc Exp Biol Med 1984;294:175–282.

139. Freedman MS, Antel JP. Immunoregulatory circuits in multiple sclerosis: Is there a "short?" (editorial). Ann Neurol 1988;24:183–184.

140. Baum HM, Rothschild BB. The incidence and prevalence of reported multiple sclerosis. Ann Neurol 1981;10:420–428.

141. Kurtzke JF: Epidemiologic contributions to multiple sclerosis: An overview. Neurology 1980;30:61–79.

142. Duquette P, Murray TJ, Pleines J, et al. Multiple sclerosis in childhood: clinical profile in 125 patients. J Pediatr 1987;111:359–363.

143. Bejar JM, Ziegler DK. Onset of multiple sclerosis in a 24-month old child. Arch Neurol 1984;41:881–882.

144. Ebers GC, Bulman DE, Sadovnick AD, et al. A population-based study of multiple sclerosis in twins. N Engl J Med 1986;315:1638–1642.

145. Hafler DA, Weiner HL. T-cells in multiple sclerosis and inflammatory central nervous system disease. Immunol Rev 1987;100:307–333.

146. Bye AME, Kendall B, Wilson J. Multiple sclerosis in childhood: A new look. Dev Med Child Neurol 1985;27:215–222.

147. Haslam RH. Multiple sclerosis: Experience at the Hospital for Sick Children. Int Pediatr 1987;2:163–167.

148. Poser C, Paty D, Scheinberg L, et al. New diagnostic criteria for multiple sclerosis. Ann Neurol 1983;13:227–231.

149. Kurtzke JK. Clinical manifestations of multiple sclerosis. In: Vinken PJ, Bruyn GW, eds. Handbook of Clinical Neurology, Vol. 9. Amsterdam: North-Holland, 1970:160–216.

150. Johnson, KP, Nelson BJ. Multiple sclerosis: Diagnostic usefulness of cerebrospinal fluid. Ann Neurol 1977;2:425–431.

151. Paty DW, Oger JJF, Kastrukuff LF, et al. MRI in the diagnosis of MS: A prospective study with comparison of clinical evaluation, evoked potentials, oligoclonal banding, and CT. Neurology 1988;38:180–185.

152. Cohen S, Syndulko K, Tourtellotte W. Visual evoked potentials in the diagnosis of multiple sclerosis. In: Poser C, Paty D, Scheinberg L, et al., eds. The Diagnosis of Multiple Sclerosis. New York: Thieme-Stratton, 1984, 103–119.

153. Robinson K, Rudge P. The use of the auditory evoked potential in the diagnosis of multiple sclerosis. J Neurol Sci 1980;45:235–244.

154. Chiappa KH, Harrison JL, Brooks EB, et al. Brainstem auditory evoked responses in 200 patients with multiple sclerosis. Ann Neurol 1980;7:135–143.

155. Carter JL, Hafler DA, Dawson DM, et al. Immunosuppression with high dose IV cyclophosphamide and ACTH in progressive multiple sclerosis: cumulative 6-year experience in 164 patients. Neurology 1988;38(suppl 2):9–14.

156. Troiano R, Cook SD, Dowling PC. Steroid therapy in multiple sclerosis: point of view. Arch Neurol 1987;44:803–807.

157. Warren KG, Catz I, Verona MJ, et al. Effect of methylprednisolone on CSF IgG parameters, myelin basic protein and anti-myelin basic protein in multiple sclerosis exacerbations. Can J Neurol Sci 1986;13:25–30.

158. Weiner HL, Hafler DA. Immunotherapy of multiple sclerosis. Ann Neurol 1988;23:211–222.

159. Lisak RP. Overview of the rationale for immunomodulating therapies in multiple sclerosis. Neurology 1988;38(suppl 2): 5–8.

160. Ellison GW, Myers LW, Mickey MR, et al. Clinical experience with azathioprine: The pros, Neurology 1988;38 Suppl 2:20–23.

161. Likosky WH. Experience with cyclophosphamide in multiple sclerosis: The cons. Neurology 1988;38 Suppl 2: 14–18.

162. Tindall R. A closer look at plasmapheresis in multiple sclerosis: The cons. Neurology 1988;38 Suppl 2:53–56.

163. Khatri BO. Experience with the use of plasmapheresis in chronic progressive multiple sclerosis: The pros. Neurology 1988;38(suppl 2):50–52.

164. Johnson KP. Treatment of multiple sclerosis with various interferons: The cons. Neurology 1988;38 Suppl 2: 62–64.

165. Knobler RL. Systemic interferon therapy of multiple sclerosis: The pros. Neurology 1988;38 Suppl 2:58–61.

166. Devereux C, Troiano R, Zito G, et al. Effect of total lymphoid irradiation on functional status in chronic multiple sclerosis: Importance of lymphopenia early after treatment—the pros. Neurology 1988;38 (suppl 2):32–37.

167. Myers LW, Ellison GW, Fahey JL, et al. Clinical drawbacks of total lymphoid irradiation: The cons. Neurology 1988; 38 Suppl 2:38–40.

168. Rudge P. Cyclosporine and multiple sclerosis: The cons. Neurology 1988;38 Suppl 2:29–30.

169. Dommasch D. Comparative clinical trial of cyclosporine in multiple sclerosis: The pros. Neurology 1988; 38 Suppl 2:28–29.

170. Baumhefner RW, Tourtellotte WW, Syndulko K, et al. Copolymer 1 as therapy for multiple sclerosis: The cons. Neurology 1988;38 Suppl 2:69–71.

171. Bornstein MB, Miller A, Slagle S. et al. Clinical experience with COP-1 in multiple sclerosis. Neurology 1988;38 Suppl 2:66–69.

172. Champlin RE. Treating multiple sclerosis with monooclonal antibodies: The cons. Neurology 1988;38 Suppl 2: 47–49.

173. Hafler DA, Weiner HL. Immunosuppression with monoclonal antibodies in multiple sclerosis. Neurology 1988;38 Suppl 2:42–47.

174. Confavreux C, Aimard G, Devic M. Course and prognosis in multiple sclerosis assessed by the computerized data processing of 349 patients. Brain 1980;103:281–300.

175. Ammann AJ, Johnson A, Fyfe GA, et al. Behçet syndrome. J Pediatr 1985;107:41–43.

176. Jorizzo JL. Behçet's disease. Neurol Clin 1987;5:427–440.

177. Jorizzo JL, Solomon AR, Cavallo T. Behçet's syndrome: Immunopathologic and histopathologic assessment of pathergy lesions is useful in diagnosis and followup. Arch Pathol Lab Med 1985;109:747–751.

178. Sakane T, Suzuki N, Ueda Y, et al. Analysis of interleukin-2 activity in patients with Behçet's disease: ability of T-cells to produce and respond to interleukin-2. Arthritis Rheum 1986;29:371–378.

179. O'Duffy JD, Goldstein NP. Neurologic involvement in seven patients with Behçet's disease. Am J Med 1976;61:170–178.

180. Jorizzo JL. Behçet's disease: An update based on the 1985 International Conference in London. Arch Dermatol 1986; 122:556–558.

181. Pamir MN, Kansu T, Erbengi A, et al. Papilledema in Behçet's syndrome. Arch Neurol 1981;38:643–645.

182. Lewis MA, Priestly BL. Transient neonatal Behçet's disease. Arch Dis Child 1986;61:805–806.

183. Boder E. Ataxia telangiectasia: An overview. KROC Found Ser 1985;19:1–63.

184. Waldmann TA, Misiti J, Nelson DL, et al. Ataxia-telangiectasia: A multisystem hereditary disease with immunodeficiency, impaired organ maturation, x-ray hypersensitivity, and a high incidence of neoplasia. Ann Intern Med 1983; 99:367–379.

185. Smith LL, Conerly SL. Ataxia-telangiectasia or Louis-Bar syndrome. J Am Acad Dermatol 1985;12:681–696.

186. Gatti RA, Berkel I, Boder E, et al. Localization of ataxia-telangiectasia to chromosome 11q22–23. Nature 1988;336: 577–580.

187. Leon GA, Grover WD, Huff DS. Neuropathologic changes in ataxia-telangiectasia. Neurology 1976;26:947–951.

188. Paula-Barbosa MM, Ruela C, Taveres MA, Pontes C, Saraiva A, Cruz C. Cerebellar cortex ultrastructure in ataxia-telangiectasia. Ann Neurol 1983;13:297–302.

189. Aguilar MJ, Kamoshita S, Landing BH, et al. Pathological observations in ataxia-telangiectasia: A report of five cases. J Neuropathol Exp Neurol 1986;27:659–676.

190. Perry TL, Kish SJ, Hinton D, et al. Neurochemical abnormalities in a patient with ataxia-telangiectasia. Neurology 1984;34:187–191.

191. Waldman TA, Broder S, Goldman CK, et al. Disorders of B cells and helper T cells in the pathogenesis of the immunoglobulin deficiency of patients with ataxia-telangiectasia. J Clin Invest 1983;71:282–295.

192. Waldman TA. Immunological abnormalities in ataxia-telangiectasia. In: Bridges BA, Harnden DG, eds. Ataxia-Telangiectasia. New York: John Wiley, 1982, 37–51.

193. Schroeder TM. Genetically determined chromosome instability syndromes. Cytogenet Cell Genet 1982;33:119–132.

194. Sugimoto T, Sawada T, Tozawa M, et al. Plasma levels of carcinoembryonic antigen in patients with ataxia-telangiectasia. J Pediatr 1978;92:436–439.

195. Baloh RW. Eye movements in ataxia-telangiectasia. Neurology 1978;28:1099–1104.

196. Nemet P, Godel V, Reider-Growasser L, Lazar M. Ataxia-telangiectasia. Ophthalmologica 1980;181:330–333.

197. Agamanolis DP, Greenstein JI. Ataxia-telangiectasia: Report of a case with Lewy bodies and vascular abnormalities within cerebral tissue. J Neuropathol Exp Neurol 1979;38:475–489.

198. Aicardi J, Barbosa C, Andermann E, et al. Ataxia-ocular motor apraxia: A syndrome mimicking ataxia-telangiectasia. Ann Neurol 1988;24:497–502.

199. Swift M, Sholman L, Perry M, et al. Malignant neoplasms in the families of patients with ataxia-telangiectasia. Cancer Res 1976;36:209–215.

200. Welshimer K, Swift M. Congenital malformations and developmental disabilities in ataxia-telangiectasia, Fanconi anemia and xeroderma pigmentosum families. Am J Hum Genet 1982;34:781–793.

201. Asbury AK. Diagnostic considerations in Guillain-Barré syndrome. Ann Neurol 1981;9 Suppl:1–5.

202. Schonberger LB, Hurwitz ES, Katona P, et al. Guillain-Barré syndrome: Its epidemiology and associations with influenza vaccination. Ann Neurol 1981;9 Suppl:31–38.

203. Prineas JW. Pathology of the Guillain-Barré syndrome. Ann Neurol 1981;9 Suppl:6–19.

204. Rostami AM, Burns JB, Eccleston PA, et al. Search for antibodies to galactocerebroside in the serum and cerebrospinal fluid in human demyelinating disorders. Ann Neurol 1987; 22:381–383.

205. Hartung H-P, Schwenke C, Bitter-Suermann D, et al. Guillain-Barré syndrome: Activated complement components C3a and C5a in CSF. Neurology 1987;37:1106–1109.

206. van Doorn PA, Brand A, Vermeulen M. Clinical significance of antibodies against peripheral nerve tissue in inflammatory polyneuropathy. Neurology 1987;37:1798–1802.

207. Waksman BH, Adams RD. Allergic neuritis: An experimental disease of rabbits induced by the injection of peripheral nervous tissue and adjuvants. J Exp Med 1955;102: 213–235.

208. Fisher M. An unusual variant of acute idiopathic polyneuritis (syndrome of ophthalmoplegia, ataxia and areflexia). N Engl J Med 1956;255:57–65.

209. Cornblath DR, Mellits ED, Griffen JW, et al. Motor conduction studies in Guillain-Barré syndrome: Description and prognostic value. Ann Neurol 1988;23:354–359.

210. Miller RG, Peterson GW, Daube JR, et al. Prognostic value of electrodiagnosis in Guillain-Barré syndrome. Muscle Nerve 1988;11:769–774.

211. Dowling PC, Cook SD. Role of infection in Guillain-Barré syndrome: Laboratory confirmation of herpes virus in 41 cases. Ann Neurol 1981;9 Suppl:44–55.

212. Goldschmidt B, Menonna J, Fortunato J, et al. Mycoplasma antibody in Guillain-Barré syndrome and other neurological disorders. Ann Neurol 1980;7:108–112.

213. Reik L, Steere AC, Hartenhagen NH, et al. Neurologic abnormalities of Lyme disease. Medicine 1979;58:281–294.

214. de la Monte SM, Gabuzda DH, Ho DD, et al. Peripheral neuropathy in the acquired immunodeficiency syndrome. Ann Neurol 1988;23:485–492.

215. Henderson FW. Tick paralysis. JAMA 1961;175:615–617.

216. Ridley A. The neuropathy of acute intermittent porphyria. Q J Med 1969;38:307–333.

217. Hopkins A. Toxic neuropathy due to industrial agents. In: Dyck PJ, Thomas PK, Lambert EH (eds). Peripheral neuropathy, Vol. 2. Philadelphia: WB Saunders 1975, 1207–1226.

218. Dalakas MC, Engel WK. Chronic relapsing (dysimmune) polyneuropathy: Pathogenesis and treatment. Ann Neurol 1981;9 Suppl:134–145.

219. Hughes RAC, Kadlubowski M, Hufschmidt A. Treatment of acute inflammatory polyneuropathy. Ann Neurol 1981;9 Suppl:125–133.

220. Hughes RAC, Newsom-Davis J, Perkin GD, et al. Controlled trial of prednisolone in acute polyneuropathy. Lancet 1978;2:750–753.

221. Kleyweg RP, van der Meche FGA, Meulstee J. Treatment of Guillain-Barré syndrome with high-dose gammaglobulin. Neurology 1988;38:1639–1641.

222. The Guillain-Barré syndrome study group. Plasmapheresis and acute Guillain-Barré syndrome. Neurology 1985;35: 1096–1104.

223. Dyck PJ, Kurtzke JF. Plasmapheresis in Guillain-Barré syndrome (editorial). Neurology 1985;35:1105–1107.

224. McKhann GM, Griffen JW. Plasmapheresis and the Guillain-Barré syndrome (ed). Ann Neurol 1987;22:762–763.

225. French Cooperative Group on Plasma Exchange in Guillain-Barré Syndrome. Efficiency of plasma exchange in Guillain-Barré syndrome: Role of replacement fluids. Ann Neurol 1987;22:753–761.

226. McKhann GM, Griffen JW, Cornblatt DR, et al. Plasmapheresis and Guillain-Barré syndrome: Analysis of prognostic factors and the effect of plasmapheresis. Ann Neurol 1988;23:347–353.

227. Thomas PK, LaScelles RG, Hallpike JF, et al. Recurrent and chronic relapsing Guillain-Barré polyneuritis. Brain 1969;92:589–606.

228. Prineas JW, McLeod JG. Chronic relapsing polyneuritis. J Neurol Sci 1976;27:427–458.

229. Crisp DE, Bray PF, Bloomer LC. Recurrent polyneuropathy with multiple herpesvirus infections. Pediatrics 1983;71: 163–165.

230. Oh SJ. Subacute demyelinating polyneuropathy responding to corticosteroid treatment. Arch Neurol 1978;35:509–516.

231. DeVivo DC, Engel WK. Remarkable recovery of a steroid-responsive recurrent polyneuropathy. J Neurol Neurosurg Psychiatry 1970;33:330–337.

232. Dyck PJ, O'Brien P, Swanson C, et al. Combined azathioprine and prednisone in chronic inflammatory-demyelinating polyneuropathy. Neurology 1985;38:1173–1176.

233. Curro-Dossi B, Tezzon F. High-dose intravenous gammaglobulin for chronic inflammatory demyelinating polyneuropathy. Ital J Neurol Sci 1987;8:321–326.

234. Server AC, Lefkowith J, Braine H, et al. Treatment of chronic relapsing inflammatory polyradiculoneuropathy by plasma exchange. Ann Neurol 1979;6:256–261.

Chapter 25
AIDS in Children

Thomas K. Koch

Since 1981 when the acquired immunodeficiency syndrome (AIDS) was first recognized, it has become pandemic with extraordinary morbidity and mortality (1–4). Initially, it was believed to be a disease limited to one nation and one group of patients characterized by sexual orientation. Other populations, however, including intravenous drug abusers, Haitians, hemophiliacs, heterosexual prostitutes, and female sexual partners of patients with AIDS were soon identified as high-risk groups (5–10). The cause of the disease was unknown, but the explosive increase in incidence and the groups at risk suggested an infectious agent that was transmitted sexually or by blood and blood products. Two years after its original recognition, AIDS was seen in infants and children who had been transfusion recipients or who were born to women at risk for AIDS (11–15).

In 1983, it was speculated that AIDS may be related to a new human retrovirus that was initially called T-lymphotropic retrovirus (16) and later lymphadenopathy-associated virus (17). By 1984, Gallo et al. had published several reports characterizing the human T-cell lymphotropic virus type III (HTLV-III) and its association with AIDS (18–22). The development of a T4–lymphocyte cell line that was permissive for viral replication yet also partially resistant to its cytopathic effect led to further biochemical and serologic studies on HTLV-III. In 1985, a commercial antibody test became available that permitted mass screening of potentially infected individuals as well as the world's blood supply (23). In an attempt to simplify and unify the numerous previous designations for the AIDS virus, the International Committee on Taxonomy of Viruses rendered the name human imunodeficiency virus (HIV) in May 1986 (24).

In October 1987, the United Nations General Assembly approved a resolution calling for international cooperation to combat AIDS. They recognized that AIDS was not strictly a medical problem; rather it has far-reaching economic, social, cultural, and political ramifications. By November 1987, more than 62,000 cases of AIDS were reported to the World Health Organization (WHO) from 127 countries. Current estimates indicate that HIV has infected 5 to 10 million people worldwide and that 1 to 2 million cases of AIDS can be expected in the early 1990s (25). Despite the rapid accumulation of knowledge regarding HIV and improved patient care, AIDS still remains a fatal disease without a cure.

EPIDEMIOLOGY

AIDS in children and adults is a disease primarily found in urban populations. The majority of childhood cases (73%) is reported from New York, New Jersey, California, and Florida, although nearly every state has reported cases of pediatric AIDS (26,27). The ethnic distribution of pediatric AIDS is composed of approximately 53% black, 23% Hispanic, 23% white, and 1% other.

Detailed epidemiologic studies have documented three basic modes of transmission for HIV: sexual, parenteral, and perinatal. Sexual transmission has occurred predominantly among homosexual and bisexual men and accounts for 63% of the cases nationwide (28). Although heterosexual transmission is currently associated with 4% of total cases nationwide, it accounts for 29% of cases in women (28). Heterosexual transmission correlates with high-risk contacts (prostitutes or intravenous drug abusers), the number of sexual partners, and use of condoms (28–30).

Parenteral transmission accounts for approximately 23% of the cases of AIDS nationwide. It originally occurred with transfusion of infected blood and blood products (1979–1985) and continues to occur at an increasing rate with intravenous drug abuse (28). In studies of single parenteral exposure to HIV, the risk of infection appears to be related to the volume of injected inoculum. Recipients of a single unit of HIV-infected blood have an approximate 90% risk of infection (31). This may be even higher in infants (32). Hemophiliacs who had received untreated factor VIII concentrate prior to 1985 have a positive HIV seroprevalence rate as high as 74% to 86%; rates are somewhat lower in those who received only cryoprecipitate (33). Among parenteral drug abusers, the cumulative risk of HIV infection after multiple exposures to infected individuals is 51% to 87% (4). Although the inoculum is small, similar to that of a hospital-acquired needle stick, the parenteral drug abuser is injecting the inoculum directly into the vein and thus increasing the efficiency of transmission. Studies of health-care workers who have sustained needle-stick injuries while working with patients with AIDS appear to have an approximate risk of 0.5% (34). When needle-stick injuries have resulted in HIV transmission, a significant volume of blood has usually been injected.

Although pediatric AIDS currently accounts for a small percentage of AIDS nationwide, unfortunately it is rapidly increasing. Perinatal transmission (mother to infant) accounts for approximately 80% of all cases of pediatric AIDS (15,27,35). These children are born to mothers who are HIV infected. Seventy-five percent of these children have at least one parent who is a parenteral drug abuser. Many of the HIV-infected mothers are asymptomatic at the time of birth, although they frequently have subtle immunologic abnormalities (12,15). The overall risk of transmission of HIV from an infected mother to her infant ranges from 30% to 40% (36–42); women who have a previously HIV-infected infant appear to have a subsequent transmission rate of 65% (41). Although controversial, recent reports suggest a possible relationship between the clinical and immunologic status of the infected mother, viral antigenemia, and the risk of perinatal transmission (43,44).

Although perinatal transmission of HIV may occur before, during, or after birth, in-utero transplacental transmission is an important route of infection. In-utero transmission of HIV has been documented with viral isolation from fetal tissue as early as 15 weeks' gestation (45–48). In a recent study of six fetuses obtained from HIV seropositive women (14 to 23 weeks' gestation), HIV infection could be demonstrated by culture and DNA hybridization techniques in multiple tissues including brain (47). HIV has also been isolated from amniotic fluid and cord blood (48–50). As might be expected with transplacental transmission, cesarean section does not appear to have any protective effect (51). Transplacental transmission has been supported by reports of an HIV embryopathy characterized by a distinct dysmorphic syndrome (52,53). The features of this embryopathy include failure to thrive, microcephaly, hypertelorism, a prominent box-like forehead, flattened nasal bridge, obliquity of the eyes, long palpebral fissures, blue sclera, short nose with a flattened columella, triangular philtrum, and patulous lips with a prominent vermillion border. There is significant controversy regarding the existence of this syndrome because it has not been uniformly observed (54). Most investigators now doubt its existence.

Despite observations supporting transplacental transmission of the infection, the mechanism by which it occurs and the factors controlling infectivity are unknown. Monozygotic twins discordant for HIV have been reported (55). Postnatal transmission of HIV has also been reported in breast-fed infants whose mothers acquired HIV after delivery (56). HIV can be isolated from cell-free breast milk (57).

Transfusion/hemophilia-acquired AIDS accounts for nearly 20% of pediatric cases (27,35). Most have been infants transfused in the neonatal period or children with coagulopathy requiring replacement therapy. Approximately 75% of hemophiliac children in the United States who received blood products between 1979 and 1985 are HIV-antibody positive. The risk of HIV infection from blood or blood products has been dramatically reduced since March 1985, when blood banks in the United States began to routinely screen all donated blood for HIV antibody. Despite this fact, there is still a small but identifiable risk of HIV transmission from blood transfusions screened as HIV-antibody negative (58). The hemophiliac population is no longer at significant risk for contracting HIV because of routine blood screening and the current method of heat treating all transfusable clotting factors that inactivate the HIV virus.

CLASSIFICATION

The Centers for Disease Control (CDC) has defined AIDS as a "reliably diagnosed disease that is at least moderately indicative of an underlying cellular immunodeficiency in a person who has no known underlying cause of cellular immunodeficiency nor any other cause of reduced resistance reported to be associated with that disease" (59). A classification system for HIV infections in the adult was proposed in 1986, clarifying the previously used descriptive system of persistent generalized lymphadenopathy, AIDS-related complex (ARC), and AIDS (60). A similar classification for children younger than 13 years of age appeared in April 1987 (Table 25.1)(61). In August 1987, the CDC revised the case definition of AIDS to include HIV encephalopathy, HIV wasting syndrome, and a broader range of specific AIDS-indicative diseases in patients with laboratory evidence of HIV infection (62). AIDS is now defined "as an illness characterized by one or more of the

Table 25.1 Classification of HIV infection in children younger than 13 years of age

Class P–0: Indeterminate infection

Class P–1: Asymptomatic infection

  Subclass A: Normal immune function
  Subclass B: Abnormal immune function
  Subclass C: Immune function not tested

Class P–2 Symptomatic infection

  Subclass A: Nonspecific findings
  Subclass B: Progressive neurologic disease
  Subclass C: Lymphoid interstitial pneumonitis
  Subclass D: Secondary infectious disease

    Category D–1: CDC-defined AIDS-associated[a]
    Category D–2: Recurrent serious bacterial infections
    Category D–3: Other specified secondary infections[b]

  Subclass E. Secondary cancers

    Category E–1: CDC-defined AIDS-associated[c]
    Category E–2: Other cancers possibly secondary to HIV infection

  Subclass F: Other diseases possibly due to HIV infection[d]

[a]*Pneumocystis carinii* pneumonia, chronic cryptosporidiosis, disseminated toxoplasmosis with onset after 1 month of age, extraintestinal strongyloidiasis, chronic isosporiasis, candidiasis (esophageal, bronchial, or pulmonary), extrapulmonary cryptococcosis, disseminated histoplasmosis, noncutaneous extrapulmonary, or disseminated mycobacterial infection, cytomegalovirus infection with onset after 1 month of age, chronic mucocutaneous or disseminated herpes simplex virus infection with onset after 1 month of age, extrapulmonary or disseminated coccidioidomycosis, nocardiosis, and progressive multifocal leukoencephalopathy.

[b]Oral candidiasis persisting for 2 or more months, 2 or more episodes of herpes stomatitis within a year, multidermatomal or disseminated herpes zoster infection.

[c]Kaposi sarcoma, B-cell non-Hodgkin lymphoma, or primary lymphoma of the brain.

[d]Hepatitis, cardiomyopathy, nephropathy, anemia, thrombocytopenia, and dermatologic diseases.

following 'indicator' diseases, depending on the status of laboratory evidence of HIV infection" (Tables 25.2 and 25.3)(62). It is now clear that AIDS consists of a variety of clinical syndromes that include primary infections caused by HIV as well as opportunistic infections and neoplasms secondary to the underlying immunodeficiency state.

CLINICAL SYNDROMES

Systemic Involvement

Many infants with perinatally acquired HIV infection manifest signs of clinical disease during the first year of life with failure to thrive, developmental delay, hepatosplenomegaly, lymphadenopathy, thrush, chronic diarrhea, recurrent bacterial infections, and chronic interstitial pneumonitis

Table 25.2 AIDS indicator diseases* with questionable HIV status

Pneumocystis carinii pneumonia

Candidiasis of the esophagus, trachea, bronchi, or lungs

Lymphoid interstitial pneumonitis/pulmonary lymphoid hyperplasia in a child < 13 years

Cryptococcosis, extrapulmonary

Cryptosporidiosis with diarrhea for > 1 month

Cytomegalovirus disease of an organ other than liver, spleen, or lymphoid node in a patient > 1 month of age

Herpes simplex infection causing a mucocutaneous ulcer that persists > 1 month, or bronchitis, pneumonitis, or esophagitis in a patient > 1 month of age

Primary central nervous system lymphoma in patients < 60 years

Kaposi sarcoma in patients < 60 years

Mycobacterium avium complex or *M. kansasii,* disseminated

Toxoplasmosis of the brain in a patient > 1 month of age

*Definitively diagnosed diseases.

(12–15,35–37,63,64). The disease often progresses rapidly, with the demise of the child by two years of age (Table 25.4). Although acute HIV infection is often asymptomatic, in some adolescents and adults early HIV disease may manifest as a "mononucleosis-like" illness with fever, lymphadenopathy, headache, cough, and night sweats (65). These initial symptoms of acute infection occur about 6 to 8 weeks after exposure to the virus. The disease then enters an asymptomatic state that may last years. One report of the natural history of HIV infection in homosexual and bisexual men showed that AIDS developed in 42% within 9 years after seroconversion (66). In a cohort of neonatal transfusion recipients, 44% remained asymptomatic at

Table 25.3 AIDS indicator diseases* with + HIV status

Bacterial infections, multiple or recurrent (at least two in a 2-year period in children < 13 years)
  Septicemia, pneumonia, meningitis, bone or joint infection, or internal abscess caused by *Haemophilus, Streptococcus* (including pneumococcus), or other pyogenic bacteria

HIV encephalopathy (AIDS dementia complex)

Coccidioidomycosis, disseminated

Histoplasmosis, disseminated

Isosporiasis with diarrhea persisting > 1 month

Kaposi sarcoma at any age

Primary CNS lymphoma at any age

Non-Hodgkin lymphoma of B-cell or unknown immunologic phenotype and the following histologic types
  Small noncleaved lymphoma (either Burkitt or non-Burkitt type)
  Immunoblastic sarcoma

Any mycobacterial disease other than *M. tuberculosis,* disseminated

M. tuberculosis, extrapulmonary

Salmonella (nontyphoid) septicemia, recurrent

HIV wasting syndrome

*Definitively diagnosed diseases.

Table 25.4 Clinical manifestations of pediatric HIV infection

Recurrent bacterial infections
    pneumonia, sepsis, otitis, meningitis, lymphadenitis

Failure to thrive

Oral candidiasis

Hepatosplenomegaly

Lymphadenopathy

Pneumonitis
    Acute—*Pneumocystis carinii*
    Chronic—Lymphoid interstitial

Developmental delay/encephalopathy

Opportunistic infections
    Cytomegalovirus, Epstein-Barr virus, Herpes
    Cryptosporidiosis, *M. avium intracellulare*

Parotitis

Cardiomyopathy

Nephropathy

Pancytopenia

Eczemoid rash

Malignancy

6 years of age (67). Although the asymptomatic interval tends to be shorter with perinatally acquired HIV, periods as long as 10 years have been observed (68).

Pediatric HIV disease is characterized by several unique features rarely seen in the adult (Table 25.5). Recurrent bacterial infections are often the cause of presenting symptoms and are a major source of morbidity and mortality (63,64,69,70). The pathogens of these infections include *Streptococcus pneumoniae, Haemophilius influenzae* type b, *Staphylococcus,* and *Salmonella,* as well as other enteric organisms (gram-negative rods). These bacteria may cause chronic and recurrent otitis media, mastoiditis, lymphadenitis, pneumonia, bacteremia, meningitis, diarrhea, and skin infections.

Another unique feature of pediatric HIV disease is chronic lymphoid interstitial pneumonitis, which may be the initial manifestation of AIDS in 40% to 60% of children (63,70). Lymphoid interstitial pneumonitis (LIP) is histologically characterized by diffuse infiltration of the alveolar septa and peribronchiolar areas with lymphocytes and plasma cells (71). Clinical and radiologic features can distinguish to some extent LIP from the interstitial involvement of *Pneumocystis carinii* pneumonia (PCP)(72). LIP does not manifest with acute respiratory distress and does not require immediate therapy although later, severe hypoxemia and respiratory failure can develop. Children

Table 25.5 Unique features characteristic of pediatric AIDS

        Recurrent bacterial infections
        Lymphoid interstitial pneumonitis
        Parotitis
        Absence of toxoplasmosis

with LIP have an overall better long-term prognosis than have children with PCP (73). Some medical centers are now treating progressive LIP with steroids and have encouraging preliminary results. Although no consistent pathogen has been isolated from the lungs of patients with LIP, some evidence suggests that Epstein-Barr virus (EBV) may be the responsible agent (74).

Acute and chronic parotid involvement is observed in 10% of children with AIDS (63). Although the etiology remains unknown, it has been postulated that EBV may be responsible, because there appears to be an association between the occurrence of parotitis and LIP (64).

Opportunistic infections are common in children and adult patients with AIDS. PCP is the most common and life-threatening infection, occurring in 53% of children with AIDS (70,73). *Candida* esophagitis and disseminated cytomegalovirus (CMV) each occur in approximately 20% of children with HIV (70,73). Other infections include *Mycobacterium avium intracellulare,* cryptosporidium, herpes simplex, and herpes varicella-zoster. Unlike the adult with AIDS in whom *Toxoplasma gondii* is a common central nervous system (CNS) pathogen, toxoplasmosis has rarely been reported (75).

Although malignancies in general appear to be less common in children than in adults with HIV, primary lymphomas of the CNS occur in 3% of children with AIDS (76). Kaposi sarcoma has been reported only rarely. Other important, though less common manifestations of HIV infection include hematologic disease with thrombocytopenia, anemia and neutropenia, renal disease presenting as the nephrotic syndrome, cardiomyopathy, and hepatitis (64,77–81).

Neurologic Involvement

Neurologic disease occurs in approximately 40% to 66% of adult patients with AIDS, and may be the presenting manifestation of AIDS in 10% (82–85). Postmortem studies have shown that 80% of patients with AIDS have evidence of CNS involvement (86–89). The initial neurologic manifestations of AIDS were believed to be caused by opportunistic diseases; it is now clear, however, that direct HIV infection of the nervous system is a major cause of neurologic morbidity. The spectrum of neurologic involvement with HIV infection includes primary HIV-related disease, opportunistic diseases, and cerebrovascular and peripheral nervous sysstem disease (Table 25.6). Primary HIV-related disease includes AIDS dementia complex or HIV encephalopathy, HIV myelopathy, and HIV meningitis (82–85,90,91). Fifty-five percent to 90% of children may have clinical evidence of nervous system dysfunction, and as is true for systemic manifestations, there are unique features characteristic of childhood neurologic disease (92–97).

Table 25.6 HIV-related neurologic disease

Primary HIV disease
  HIV encephalopathy (AIDS dementia complex)
  Vacuolar myelopathy
  Aseptic meningitis

Opportunistic disease/neoplasms
  Viral infections
  Bacterial infections
  Fungal infections
  Protozoan infections
  Neoplasms

Cerebrovascular disease
  Hemorrhage
  Infarction

Peripheral nervous system disease
  Peripheral neuropathy
    Inflammatory demyelinating neuropathy
    Mononeuropathy multiplex
    Distal symmetric polyneuropathy
  Cranial neuropathies
  Myopathy

Human Immunodeficiency Virus Encephalopathy

HIV encephalopathy is the most common form of neurologic involvement in infected children (95–97). It is a progressive subacute disorder that often begins insidiously. It is characterized by a loss of developmental milestones, deterioration of play, intellectual impairment, apathy, and development of bilateral corticospinal tract signs with a spastic quadriparesis. Often there is impaired brain growth with acquired microcephaly (Table 25.7)(92–97). Other less common manifestations include movement disorders, tremor, rigidity, dystonia, or bradykinesia, ataxia, and seizures (95–97). Except for myoclonus, seizures are often isolated events provoked by fever. Recurrent seizures may be the first sign of focal neurologic disease suggesting a possible CNS lymphoma or stroke (76). Infants may initially present with hypotonia and pathologic reflexes. The earliest sign of the HIV encephalopathy in children appears to be neurodevelopmental delay, arrest, or regression in an otherwise asymptomatic infant or child (96–101). Psychometric testing often reveals abnormalities in motor and language function (93–99). Although the clinical course is generally progressive, there may be plateaus of relative stability lasting months and, rarely, periods of mild improvement (95–97). In general, the appearance of a progressive

Table 25.7 Clinical features of HIV encephalopathy in children

Loss of developmental milestones
Deterioration of play
Apathy
Intellectual impairment
Spasticity
Acquired microcephaly
Movement disorder
Ataxia
Myoclonus

Table 25.8 HIV encephalopathy in children* (2 or more criteria required)

Impaired head growth by serial measurement > 3 months' duration, or
Advancing cerebral atrophy by CT or MRI > 3 months' duration

Developmental/intellectual regression by formal testing > 3 months' duration

Progressive motor deficits persistent for at least 3 months

CSF HIV-Ag > 25 pg/mL

*Proposed definition by Drs. L. Epstein and E. Connor, UMDNJ, Newark, NJ.

encephalopathy is associated with a poor prognosis, and most children die within a year (94–96)(Table 25.8).

Computed tomography (CT) of the brain in children with HIV encephalopathy may demonstrate cerebral atrophy with enlargement of subarachnoid spaces and ventricles and may show attenuation of the white matter. Another common finding unique to the childhood HIV encephalopathy is calcification of the basal ganglia and frontal white matter which is usually bilateral (Figure 25.1)(93–96,102,103). Early in the disease, contrast

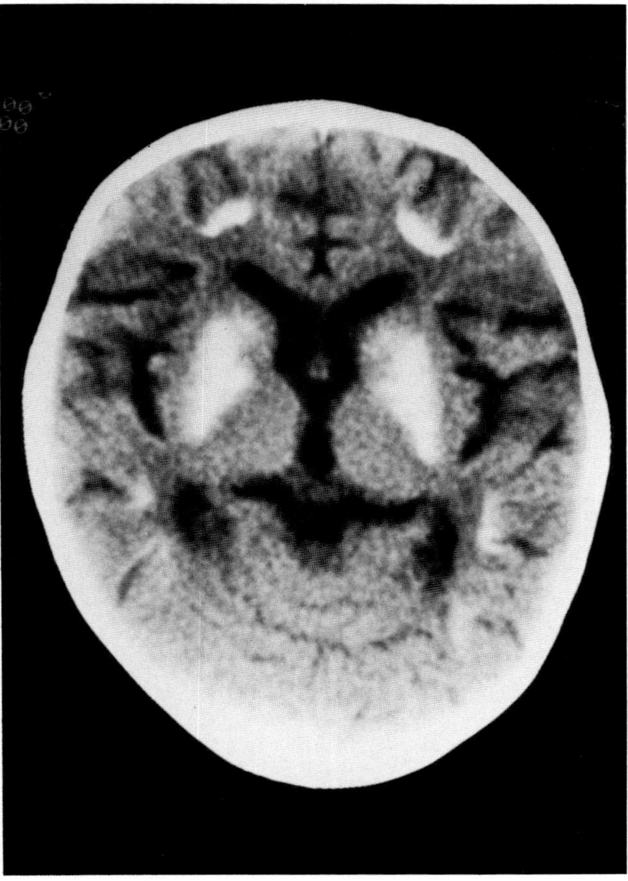

FIGURE 25.1 Noncontrast computed tomographic scan of a child with human immunodeficiency encephalopathy shows mild cortical atrophy with bilateral calcification of the basal ganglia and frontal posterior periventricular white matter.

enhancement of the basal ganglia may precede its eventual calcification (102,103). Serial CT head scans can show progressive atrophic and calcific changes that often correspond to the patient's clinical deterioration (93,94). Magnetic resonance imaging (MRI) also shows cerebral atrophy as well as changes of the white matter. On T2-weighted images, bilateral patchy to confluent abnormalities of the white matter are seen as high-signal areas (Figure 25.2)(104). The diffuse changes seen on both CT and MRI appear to be related to primary HIV involvement. The calcific vasculopathy involving the basal ganglia may be an end-stage phenomenon indicating previous endothelial cell injury by HIV (97,102–104).

The cerebrospinal fluid (CSF) in children with HIV encephalopathy is often normal, but there may be a mild lymphocytic pleocytosis (up to 50 white blood cells/mL) and mild elevation of CSF protein (up to 80 mg/dL) (93–97). These abnormalities when present are usually transient, occurring early in the course of infection. HIV can be isolated from CSF; there is no correlation, however, with the patient's clinical status (105). In adults with clinical signs of AIDS, the frequency of HIV isolation from the

CSF is less than from HIV seropositive patients without clinical signs of the disease (5% and 28%, respectively) (106). Although the intra-blood-brain barrier synthesis of HIV-specific antibody (HIV-Ab) probably indicates a host response to HIV invasion of the CNS, it is not a specific indicator of HIV encephalopathy. The intra-blood-brain barrier synthesis of HIV-Ab can usually be tested in children with a progressive encephalopathy, but may also be found in asymptomatic individuals (94). An HIV-specific p24 antigen (HIV-Ag) can be detected in serum and CSF shortly after infection, but then frequently becomes undetectable for a variable period of time (95,96,107). This disappearance of HIV-Ag corresponds to a time of HIV-antibody production and is most likely accounted for by antigen-antibody complexes. The subsequent reappearance of HIV-Ag in the CSF of children often heralds relentless neurologic deterioration and impending demise (94–96,108).

Electroencephalograms (EEGs) may be abnormal but nonspecific with diffuse mild to moderate background slowing (93,94). The EEG does not appear to be an early marker for CNS disease. In both symptomatic and asymptomatic HIV-infected adults, abnormalities of brain stem and sensory evoked potentials have been reported (109). Brainstem auditory evoked responses (BSER) may demonstrate prolongation of the wave I-V interpeak latency, suggesting incipient conduction defect within the brain stem (109). With tibial nerve sensory evoked potentials (SEPs), the mean latency of the spinal cord potential at T12 may be increased, indicating a conduction defect at or near the spinal root ganglion or lumbar spinal cord (109).

In children with AIDS, BSER abnormalities consisting of prolongation of waves I-V latencies have been reported (93), whereas, in infants we have observed only elevated hearing thresholds or a delayed wave I or both. Brainstem interpeak latencies in infants have been normal (110). Tympanograms are often abnormal indicating a peripheral hearing loss, presumably due to chronic serous otitis from repeated infections. In children, abnormalities of median nerve SEPs have been observed early in the course of the HIV encephalopathy with absence or marked attenuation of the N_{18} potential (111). Further studies are needed to delineate the possible usefulness of median nerve SEPs for following disease progression in infants and children as well as disease response to a variety of therapeutic modalities. A standardized operational definition of the HIV encephalopathy in children has been formulated (Table 25.8).

Human Immunodeficiency Virus Myelopathy

A vacuolar myelopathy is present in approximately 25% of adult patients with AIDS at autopsy (86,112). Pathologic findings are characterized by loss of myelin and spongy degeneration of the lateral and posterior columns of the spinal cord, closely resembling the abnormalities found in subacute combined degeneration of vitamin-B_{12} deficiency

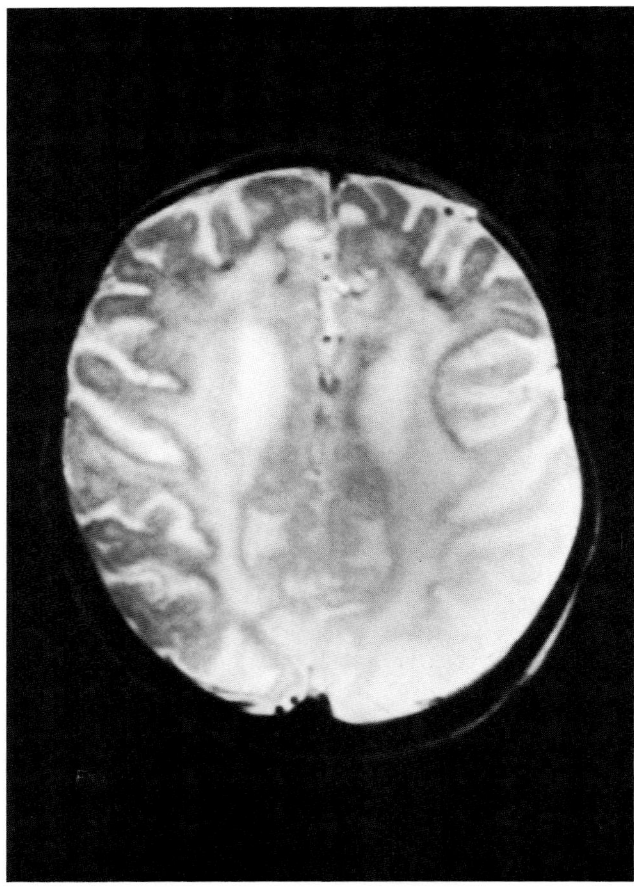

FIGURE 25.2 T2-weighted (TR 2.5, TE 80) magnetic resonance image of a child with human immunodeficiency virus encephalopathy shows mild cortical atrophy with a diffuse high-signal abnormality of the white matter in both cerebral hemispheres.

(112). Although abnormalities of the spinal cord are common in autopsy series of children with AIDS, the myelopathy differs from that of adult patients (113,114). The pathologic findings consist of corticospinal tract degeneration with myelin pallor and sparing of the posterior columns (113). Inflammatory cell infiltrates with multinucleated cells can be seen, and in-situ hybridization demonstrates HIV genomes in both gray and white matter (114). Unlike the myelopathy in adult patients, vacuolar changes are rarely seen (114). In children, there are prominent signs of spasticity, and the majority of patients have evidence of concomitant encephalopathy.

Human Immunodeficiency Virus Meningitis

In 1983, 15 homosexual patients were reported to have an atypical aseptic meningitis characterized by prolonged and recurrent bouts of headache, fever, meningeal signs, cranial neuropathies, and long tract signs (115). It has been recognized that this is not an uncommon occurrence, and HIV can be cultured from the CSF in the majority of these patients (105,116). CSF analysis reveals a mild to moderate lymphocytic pleocytosis and a mild elevation of CSF protein (90). The illness can range from acute meningitis to a more chronic headache syndrome (117). The acute illness tends to occur early in the course of HIV infection, near the time of seroconversion; whereas, chronic syndrome tends to occur late in the disease, along with ADC. The occurrence of HIV meningitis does not necessarily predict the development of other HIV-related neurologic disease (117). Neither the acute nor the chronic syndrome has been clearly observed in infants or children.

OPPORTUNISTIC DISEASES

Infection

CNS infections in patients with AIDS were among the first recognized complications of AIDS: they include diseases caused by viral, bacterial, fungal, and protozoan agents (Table 25.9) (82–84,90,118–124) Opportunistic CNS infections are less common in children (95–97), which is thought to be due to the lower incidence of primary infections in early childhood with less reactiviation of latent infections. In the report of Belman et al. (97), 11.6% of 68 children had CNS infections caused by conventional and opportunistic pathogens. Three infants had bacterial meningitis (*Streptococcus pneumoniae, Escherichia coli, Haemophilus influenzae*); in one a *Candida albicans* meningitis developed later. Two children had CMV encephalitis, one had a varicella-zoster arteritis, and another had Epstein-Barr meningitis. Toxoplasma encephalitis has been reported in an infant with AIDS (75), and one child with AIDS has been treated for cerebral mucormycosis (90).

Table 25.9 HIV-related opportunistic disease/neoplasm

Viral infections (encephalitis, myelitis vasculitis, retinitis)
  Cytomegalovirus
  Herpes varicella-zoster virus
  Herpes simplex virus types I and II
  Epstein-Barr virus

Bacterial infections
  Streptococcus pneumoniae
  Escherichia coli
  Haemophilus influenzae
  Mycobacterium avium-intracellulare
  Mycobacterium turberculosis hominis
  Mycobacterium kansasii
  Listeria monocytogenes
  Nocardia asteroides

Fungal infections
  Candida albicans
  Cryptococcus neoformans
  Aspergillus fumigatus
  Coccidioides immitis
  Mucor

Protozoan infections
  Toxoplasma gondii

Neoplasms
  Primary CNS lymphoma
  Metastatic systemic lymphoma
  Metastatic Kaposi sarcoma (adult)

Neoplasms

In the early history of the AIDS epidemic, neoplasms were recognized as frequent complications of HIV infection in adults. Among the original criteria for the diagnosis of AIDS was Kaposi sarcoma and primary lymphoma of the CNS. Primary CNS lymphomas are extremely rare in the general population, with an estimated incidence of 0.0001% (125). This risk increases to approximately 2% to 10% in adults with AIDS, making it the most common neoplasm involving the CNS in this population (82–84, 90,126,127). Metastases to the CNS from systemic lymphomas also occur with a high incidence in patients with AIDS (128,129). Similarly, both primary CNS and metastatic lymphomas seem to occur with a higher frequency in children with AIDS. Belman et al. (97) reported three patients, two with systemic lymphomas metastatic to the CNS and one with primary CNS lymphoma. Epstein et al. (76) reported an incidence of 3% for primary CNS lymphoma in children with AIDS. It appears that CNS lymphoma is the most common focal or multifocal mass lesion in pediatric AIDS. These lymphomas tend to manifest with acute or subacute progressive focal neurologic signs and seizures (76,97). Although Kaposi sarcoma is a common feature of adult AIDS, it rarely metastasizes to the CNS (83,90). In children, Karposi sarcoma is distinctly unusual and has not been reported in the CNS.

Cerebrovascular Complications

Cerebrovascular disease is a common neurologic complication of HIV infection (82,83,90,130,131). One neuropathologic study reported that 19% of 94 unselected patients with AIDS had cerebral infarctions (130). Both hemorrhagic and ischemic infarcts have been noted. While hemorrhage has often occurred in the setting of CNS neoplasm or thrombocytopenia, ischemic infarcts may be related to meningeal infection, cerebral vasculitis, marantic endocarditis, or a hypercoagulable state. Recently, lupus anticoagulant, a serum factor with hypercoagulant properties, has been found in some HIV-infected individuals (132). In one series of 68 symptomatic HIV-infected children, 8.8% or six children had strokes (133). Two had hemorrhagic infarctions, and one had both hemorrhagic and ischemic infarcts. Two of the hemorrhagic infarcts were associated with thrombocytopenia. Of the children with ischemic infarctions, one had an arteritis thought to be due to varicella-zoster virus, and another had vascular ectasia with segmental aneurysmal dilatation of most of the major intracerebral arteries. One child had periventricular infarcts, multiple petechial hemorrhages, and abnormal mitochondria suggesting an acquired mitochondrial cytopathy. Multiple ischemic infarcts and persistent varicella-zoster skin lesions have been reported in a child with AIDS. At autopsy, a granulomatous angiitis was found associated with areas of ischemic infarction (134).

Peripheral Nervous System Disease

Peripheral nervous system involvement is becoming a well recognized complicaton of HIV infection in adults, with an incidence ranging between 9% and 35% (82,83, 135–142). One study reported subclinical abnormalities, as determined by electrophysiologic studies and muscle biopsy, in 60% of patients with AIDS (141).

Although the etiology remains largely unkown, there appear to be three distinct types of peripheral nerve involvement in adult patients (142). The first is an inflammatory demyelinating polyneuropathy, both acute and chronic forms, which tends to be present with HIV seroconversion, in HIV seropositive asymptomatic individuals, and in patients with ARC (135–137,142–144). It may respond to plasmapheresis, similar to non-HIV inflammatory demyelinating polyneuropathies (136,138,142). The second type is mononeuropathy multiplex, which usually occurs in patients with ARC. Nerve biopsy may reveal active vasculitis suggesting an autoimmune disorder (138,142). The most common neuropathy described, however, is a distal symmetric polyneuropathy that is predominantly sensory, and may manifest with symptoms of painful dysesthesias (137–139,142). Pathologic studies suggest this is a dorsal root ganglionopathy possibly due to HIV or some opportunistic virus such as CMV (138,142).

This AIDS-related neuropathy does not respond to plasmapheresis. There is one report of improvement in a patient being treated with zidovudine (145). The efficacy of this form of therapy remains to be proved (146).

Recently, neuropathologic evidence of ganglioneuritis has been recognized in children (147). In one patient, CMV inclusions were seen in adjacent peripheral nerve. Thus far, there has been no evidence of a clinical or subclinical peripheral neuropathy occurring in children.

In adults, HIV may be associated with muscle involvement, usually in the form of a polymyositis-like illness called HIV-associated myopathy (137,148–150). Patients have a subacute onset of progressive proximal muscle weakness that may precede the onset of AIDS or ARC by several months. The creatine kinase is elevated. Muscle biopsy specimens show fiber necrosis, variable inflammatory cell infiltrate, and nemaline rod bodies (149–150). Corticosteroid therapy (148,149) or plasmapheresis (150) may be of benefit. This myopathy has not yet been recognized in children.

NEUROPATHOLOGY

Neuropathologic changes are found in approximately 80% of patients with AIDS at autopsy (86–89). Many of these changes in adults are associated with opportunistic infections and neoplasms. Neuropathologic studies of children, however, show an infrequent occurrence of opportunistic CNS disease (96,151).

The AIDS dementia complex in adults is characterized histologically by macrophage and multinucleated giant-cell infiltration, initially in the cerebral white matter and then later in subcortical gray structures (86,87,152,153). Diffuse myelin pallor is observed in the majority of patients and is associated with mild vacuolation of the white matter and mild perivascular lymphocytic reaction (86,153). With disease progression, there is widespread loss of white matter with reactive astrocytosis and the appearance of abundant macrophages, multinucleated cells, and glial nodules (86,153). Neuronal loss and rod cell infiltration are observed in subcortical structures, especially the basal ganglia.

In one series of 14 children who died of AIDS, all had small brains by weight (96). A variety of neuropathologic findings were found, many of which were similar to those seen in adults; a typical feature, present in 85% of patients, was white-matter pallor with diffuse myelin loss and astrocytosis. The white-matter degeneration was often more severe than that observed in adults and involved the centrum semiovale, corpus callosum, and descending corticospinal tracts. Inflammatory cell infiltrates with microglial nodules and multinucleated giant cells were seen in 72% of patients (151). A feature unique to children was vascular mineralization, which occurred in 93% of patients. Calcification was present within or adjacent to small vessel walls in the basal ganglia and frontal white matter, corresponding to the radiographic abnormalities noted on CT scans. In general, the severity of pathologic change appears to correlate with the severity of the clinical dementia (153,154). One reported infant who died with a severe encephalopathy, however, had few inflammatory changes, yet large amounts of viral-specific genome were present by hybridization techniques (151,155).

The presence of HIV in the brains of patients with AIDS was first demonstrated by direct passage of HIV from brain tissue obtained postmortem from chimpanzees (156). Subsequently, HIV has been demonstrated by in-situ hybridization (96,151,155,157–159), direct viral isolation from both CSF and brain (105,116,160), immunohistochemistry (161–163), and electron microscopy, where both mature and immature forms of HIV viral particles have been found (151,164). Using these varied techniques, the cells of the CNS most frequently infected include macrophages, multinucleated giant cells, and pleomorphic microglia. Other, less frequently involved cells include astrocytes and endothelial cells (159–163). The involvement of neurons rarely occurs; when present, however, it appears in patients with severe CNS involvement (159–163). It is clear from these studies that HIV is responsible for a number of neurologic conditions, but the mechanism by which this occurs remains unknown. Cellular localization of HIV in brain suggests that clinical CNS dysfunction may not be caused by direct infection of neurons or glia, but is more likely related to inflammatory cell involvement and possible indirect effects on neuronal and glial function (159).

HUMAN IMMUNODEFICIENCY VIRUS BIOLOGY

HIV is an RNA virus possessing reverse transcriptase belonging to the family of retroviruses. It has been further classified to the subfamily Lentivirinae, in accordance with its morphology and morphogenetic characteristics (165, 166). Visna, a well-recognized neurotropic retrovirus responsible for a chronic degenerative neurologic disease in sheep (167), is also a member of this group of viruses.

Viral Structure

HIV is a spherical virus measuring 100 nm in diameter that has an outer membrane envelope studded with knobs and a viral core containing a dense eccentric inner core (Figure 25.3)(165–169). The outer membrane knobs consist of two highly glycosylated proteins, gp41, which spans the membrane, and gp120, which is attached to gp41 and extends beyond the membrane forming the outer knob component. The viral core consists of an outer core shell composed of the protein p18 and a tubular inner or central core consisting of protein p24 (165,166,168,169). Within the central core are two identical strands of viral RNA as

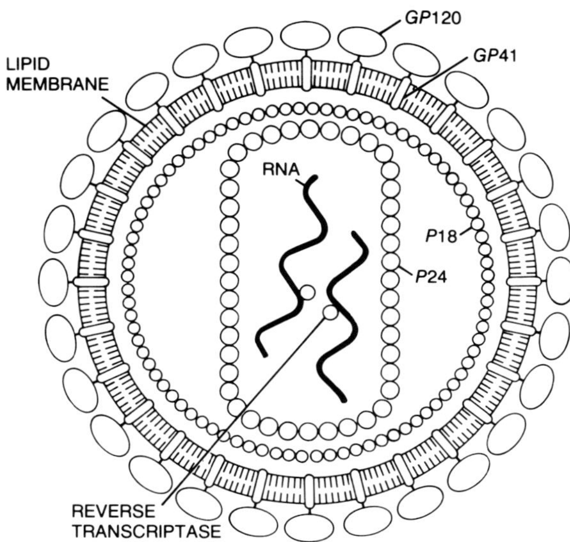

FIGURE 25.3   Human immunodeficiency virus Virion is a sphere that consists of an outer lipid membrane envelope studded by glycoprotein knobs. These knobs contain two glycoprotein components: gp41, which spans the membrane, and gp120, which is attached to gp41 and forms the outer knob. The viral core consists of an outer core protein, p18, and an inner core, p24. Within the inner core is contained the viral RNA genome and the enzyme reverse transcriptase.

well as structural proteins (p7/9), reverse transcriptase and integrase , the latter being responsible for splicing the HIV provirus genome into the host cell's DNA (169).

Molecular Biology

Despite its mere 9,749 nucleotides, HIV is genetically extremely complex. It appears that HIV has an array of regulatory genes that allow it to regulate its own expression. Thus far, nine genes have been identified (169–171). Three of the nine are the major structural genes: *gag* for the viral core proteins, *pol* for reverse transcriptase, and *env* for the envelope glycoproteins. The remaining genes (*tat, rev, nef, vif, vpu,* and *vpr*) serve to regulate expression of the major structural genes (168–173). At either end of the viral genome are redundant sequences called long terminal repeats, which do not code for protein but rather have a regulatory function by initiating the expression of other viral genes and appear to be triggered by host cell activation (168,169).

In addition to this complex genetic structure and the ability to regulate its own self-expression, HIV is extremely pleomorphic and has significant genetic variability (165, 169,172). Isolates of HIV from the brain appear to represent a distinct subtype possessing different biologic and serologic properties than isolates from peripheral blood (160,173,174). The most substantial genomic differences among the various strains of HIV occur in the *env* gene. Both of the envelope glycoproteins have regions that are highly variable with differences in up to 22% of the amino-acid constituents (170,175). The majority of these changes are clustered around the exterior portion of the envelope glycoproteins. Based on secondary structure, glycosylation pattern and hydrophilicity, these regions appear to be antigenic sites (176). This genetic variability, with corresponding antigenic variability, is a significant problem in designing a vaccine against HIV. In addition, this variability may be important for virus-host cell interactions and accounts for the preferential infection of certain types of cells by HIV.

Viral Infection/Replication

The entry of HIV into the host cell depends on the interaction of one or more of the constant regions of the envelope glycoprotein gp120 and host cell membrane receptors (168, 169,172). Although the major attachment site appears to be the DC4 complex proteins found on the surface of helper T cells (T4-lymphocyte) and to a lesser extent on monocytes and macrophages (177,178), cells lacking this cell surface protein complex or expressing it at low levels may still be infected by HIV and replicate the virus at low titers (179). In tissue culture, glial cells lacking CD4 protein have been successfully infected by HIV (180). Once viral attachment has occurred, there is fusion of the viral membrane with the host cell membrane allowing the inner core of the virus to enter the cell (Figure 25.4). Next, viral uncoating takes place with release of the viral RNA genome. Reverse transcriptase then copies the RNA to a single strand of DNA, which is duplicated to a double-strand DNA provirus. This DNA provirus migrates to the nucleus of the cell and is integrated into the host cell DNA by the enzyme integrase (169). This integrated DNA remains part of the host cell's genetic material for the lifetime of the cell. The provirus may then remain latent or alternatively direct its own transcription into RNA and eventual translation into viral components (165,168,169). The viral components are assembled into new virions at the cell membrane and are released by a process of budding. This process may proceed slowly in a controlled fashion or rapidly with host cell lysis (169).

Pathophysiology

Although HIV is capable of infecting several different cell types, it preferentially destroys the T4-lymphocytes and is capable of near elimination of the T4-population. Its cytopathic effects, which include cell fusion, the formation of multinucleated giant cells, and cell death, are highly dependent on the properties of the viral envelope proteins (168,169,172). Once viral envelope proteins are present in the infected host cell membrane, these cells express an avidity for other cells possessing the CD4 complex. The infected

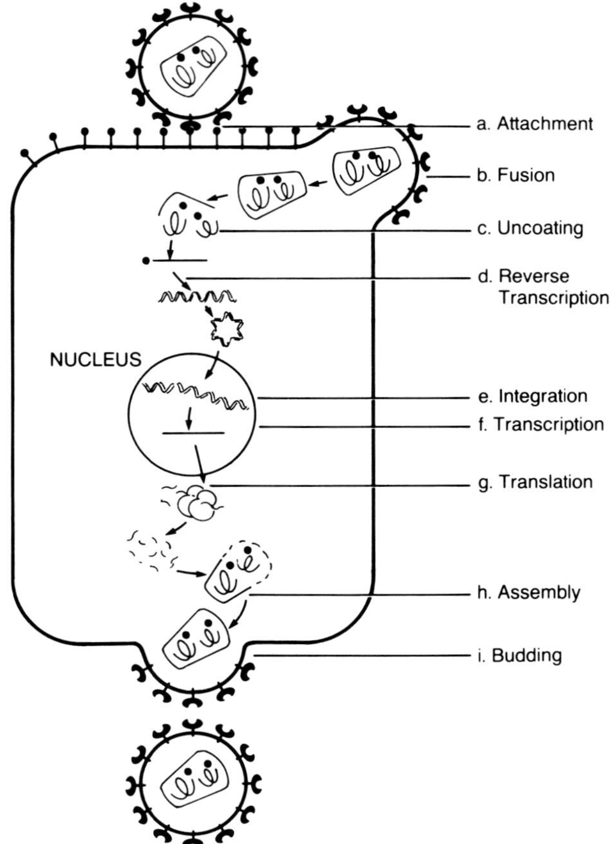

FIGURE 25.4   Human immunodeficiency virus life cycle. Viral attachment to the host cell occurs through the interaction between the viral envelope glycoprotein, gp120, and the host cell CD4 receptors (**A**). The virion then fuses with the host cell allowing the viral core to enter (**B**). Next, there is viral uncoating (**C**), followed by viral RNA transcription by reverse transcriptase (**D**). The newly formed DNA provirus enters the nucleus where it integrates into the host cell genome (**E**). The provirus may then direct the transcription of viral RNA (**F**), of which some is translated into new viral protein components (**G**). These viral components and viral RNA are then assembled at the host cell membrane (**H**) with eventual viral budding (**I**).

cells may then bind and fuse with those cells, forming syncytia (181). Cell death can result from syncytial formation or during the process of viral budding. As virus is shed from host cells, the viral membrane protein (gp120) may bind to surrounding CD4 cells, distorting and disrupting their membrane integrity and eventually leading to cellular death (169). Alternatively, T4-lymphocyte death can be mediated immunologically by antibodies directed against shed viral envelope protein (gp120), which is free to bind to the CD4 receptors of uninfected cells (182,183).

The pathophysiology of HIV-related brain dysfunction is less clear, although direct neuronal infection appears to be rare (159–163). Considerable indirect effects on neuronal function may occur as a result of the release of toxic factors by other infected cells within the CNS or by other immunologic means. Possible toxic factors could include viral-coded molecules or host cell gene products that have been released as a result of infection, such as immune mediators or trophic factors. Recently, the neurotrophic factor neuroleukin has been found to have homology with the HIV envelope glycoprotein gp120, and gp120 appears to be able to compete with the neuronal survival effects of neuroleukin in cell culture systems (184). Thus, neurologic disease may result from disturbed neurochemical interactions within the CNS (172,184).

IMMUNOLOGY/DIAGNOSIS

Immune-System Evaluation

In adults, a low T-helper/T-suppressor (T4/T8) ratio has been documented in high-risk groups, individuals with prodromal symptoms, and in patients with AIDS (185). Lymphopenia, hypergammaglobulinemia, and skin test anergy have also been associated with AIDS related conditions (185,186). Some children may have similar laboratory evidence of marked T cell dysfunction; whereas, others, especially early in the course of infection, may have normal absolute lymphocyte counts, normal percentages of T cells and T cell subsets, and normal nonspecific mitogen responses (37,64). Delayed hypersensitivity skin tests are of limited value in diagnosing T cell immunodeficiency in young children (187). As in adult patients, B cell dysfunction is manifested by a polyclonal hypergammaglobulinemia, yet there is poor response to new antigenic challenges (35,36,64,87,187,188). This lack of ability to form antibody to newly encountered antigen may account for the difference in the frequency of bacterial infections in adult and childhood AIDS. Because of the polyclonal hypergammaglobulinemia, adult patients will produce antibody to a variety of antigens that they have previously encountered. In contrast, infants and children have a more limited repertoire of previous antigen exposure; so, despite the hypergammaglobulinemia, their antibodies are not directed at as great a number of antigens (64).

Human Immunodeficiency Virus Diagnostic Testing

The development of antiviral antibody testing has allowed for the identification of patients infected with HIV. Routine screening is performed using a commercially available enzyme-linked immunosorbent assay (ELISA) for antibody directed against HIV in which the patient's serum is reacted with a lysate of HIV (19). This test is designed for screening purposes with good sensitivity but less specificity. All ELISA-positive sera need confirmation by the Western blot assay. With this test, lysates of HIV are electrophoresed to separate viral proteins. These proteins are then transferred to nitrocellulose strips, and the patient's serum is allowed to react with them. The sites of reaction are visualized on roentgenographic film using radioactive labeling. This test is more cumbersome than is the ELISA, but is highly reliable and specific for anti-HIV antibody.

In older children and adults, the sensitivity of HIV antibody detection as an indicator of HIV infection is 97%, whereas the specificty is 99% (189). Testing for the presence of HIV antibody in infants is much less reliable, however. First, maternal transplacental antibodies are present in all infants of HIV seropositive mothers, and this maternal immunoglobulin G may persist for up to 15 months (49). Sequential antibody testing is therefore necessary in all infants to determine the presence of persistent or increasing HIV antibody, indicating primary infection. Second, as many as 10% of infants and children may not produce antibody to HIV (37,190). Once these HIV-infected infants lose their maternal antibody, they convert to a seronegative state. Despite this fact, they are infected, are usually symptomatic, and have either positive cultures or HIV antigen in their serum (190). It is speculated that this may be the result of early in utero infection leading to immune tolerance. Recently, five HIV-infected infants were observed to have intervals lasting 3 to 6 months in which they became seronegative by ELISA and Western blot techniques before reverting to a seropositive state (191). As is true in adult patients, some terminally ill children may lose antibody to several HIV components, resulting in a negative ELISA premortem.

Although the recovery and culture of HIV from peripheral blood mononuclear cells is the definitive means to positively identify HIV infection, culture methods are costly, tedious, slow, variable, and are not readily accessible. Several commercially available HIV core protein (p24) antigen capture enzyme immunoassays (EIAs) are now available. Unfortunately, there is some variability among these assays in terms of specificity and sensitivity (192).

In children, the prevalence of antigenemia appears to be somewhat higher than reported in adults. Antigenemia may be important in determining HIV infection in young infants when maternal antibody obscures the interpretation of the serology; the absence of HIV antigen, however, does not preclude the presence of infection (193,194). Persistent antigenemia in children, especially in high titers, appears to be associated with poor clinical prognosis (193–195). HIV p24 antigen when found in CSF often correlates with a progressive encephalopathy (108). A p14 titer greater than 25 pg/mL has been proposed as a criterion for defining the HIV encephalopathy in children (Table 25.7).

MANAGEMENT/THERAPY

Despite the vast amount of information accumulated regarding the basic biologic properties of HIV, the unfortunate but undeniable reality is that AIDS remains a fatal disease. Despite this fact, however, a number of management issues in children must be addressed, including breast-feeding, immunizations, treatment of acute and chronic infections, and anti-HIV therapy.

Breast Feeding/Immunizations

HIV has been isolated from breast milk, and postnatal transmission of HIV through breast feeding has been clearly documented (56,57). Because of this, it has generally been recommended in the United States that antibody-positive women should not breast feed their infants (196). This is a reasonable recommendation for industrialized nations where safe alternatives are available, but in developing nations where formulas are not readily available and the water supply is often contaminated, the WHO has recommended that breast feeding continue.

Immunization of immunocompromised patients with live, attenuated viruses may lead to serious vaccine-related infections. As a result of these concerns, the Immunization Practices Advisory Committee (ACIP) has recommended that HIV seropositive children not receive the oral polio vaccine (Sabin) or bacille Calmette-Guérin. They have reviewed the data concerning measles, mumps, and rubella (MMR) and thus far, there have been no reports of untoward events after MMR immunization of seropositive infants. Evidence suggests that MMR immunization provides some protection to children with HIV (197). Reports from Africa have shown that measles is capable of causing a devastating disease in unvaccinated HIV-seropositive children (198). The ACIP has now revised their previous recommendation not to vaccinate symptomatic HIV children by recommending that all children with HIV receive MMR at 15 months (199). HIV-seropositive children should also receive diptheria, pertussis, tetanus (DPT), inactivated polio vaccine (Salk), and *Haemophilus influenzae* type B vaccine (HIB)(Table 25.10). Pneumococcal vaccine and yearly inactivated-influenza vaccine should be

Table 25.10   Routine immunization of HIV-infected children

Vaccine	HIV Infection	
	Asymptomatic	*Symptomatic*
DTP*	yes	yes
OPV[@]	no	no
IPV⁺	yes	yes
MMR**	yes	yes
HIB⁺⁺	yes	yes
Pneumococcal	no	yes
Influenza	no	yes

*DTP   = Diphtheria and tetanus toxoids and pertussis vaccine;
@OPV   = Oral, attenuated poliovirus vaccine; contains poliovirus types 1, 2, and 3;
+IPV   = Inactivated poliovirus vaccine; contains poliovirus types 1, 2, and 3;
**MMR   = Live measles, mumps, and rubella viruses in a combined vaccine;
++HIB   = *Hemophilus influenzae* type b conjugate vaccine.

administered to symptomatic HIV children (200). Passive prophylaxis with varicella zoster immune globulin after a known exposure to varicella is required for symptomatic HIV children.

Acute/Chronic Infections

PCP is the most common opportunistic infection found in children and adults. Treatment is initiated with either oral trimethoprim and sulfamethoxazole (TMP-SMX)(20 mg/kg/d TMP and 100 mg/kg/d SMX) or intramuscular or intravenous pentamidine (4 mg/kg/d)(201). The response rate to either of these agents in adults is 60% to 80% during the first episode of infection (202). Preliminary evidence suggests that inhaled pentamidine may be equally effective (202). The use of these agents as primary prophylaxis is under investigation.

Mucocutaneous candidiasis is treated with oral ketoconazole or clotrimazole. Systemic infections require intravenous amphotericin B, and patients with CNS involvement should also receive 5-fluorocytosine.

Cytomegalovirus is the most common cause of an HIV-associated retinitis and may also cause colitis and adrenalitis. Recent reports document clinical benefit from ganciclovir (DHPG, dihydroxypropoxymethyl-guanine) although its efficacy in children is not yet established (203). Other Herpes viruses (herpes simplex and zoster) may be treated with acyclovir. Mild mucocutaneous disease can be treated orally, whereas more serious disease requires intravenous therapy.

Although children with HIV disease commonly have hypergammaglobulinemia, they have a poor specific antibody response to new antigenic challenges. In one study of patients with AIDS (10 children and 6 adults), biweekly intravenous administration of gammaglobulin decreased the number of bacterial infections (204). Although no precise recommendations exist concerning the use of gammaglobulin therapy with HIV infection, it should be considered in any patient with chronic or recurrent bacterial infections. Currently, controlled clinical trials are examining the role of gammaglobulin therapy in children with HIV.

Anti-Human Immunodeficiency Virus Therapy

At the present time, there is no definitive treatment for HIV. Of various therapeutic modalities currently available, the dideoxynucleoside analogues, which have been shown to be potent inhibitors of the essential retroviral enzyme, reverse transcriptase, appear to be the most promising. Zidovudine is now approved for treatment of adults and children with HIV. Adult studies suggest that zidovudine is effective in significantly reducing the number and severity of opportunistic infections, decreasing viral shedding, improving clinical performance, and reducing overall mortality (205,206).

Early studies with zidovudine in symptomatic HIV-infected children seem to imply similar clinical, immunologic, and neuropsychologic improvement (207–209). In one study, the continuous intravenous administration of zidovudine was related to improvement in appetite, weight gain, and decreased lymphadenopathy and hepatosplenomegaly. In addition, infected children had a decrease in total serum immunoglobulins and an increase of their population of CD4 cells (208). Of great interest was the apparent efficacy of zidovudine in reversing documented neuropsychologic deficits to premorbid levels (209). The major side effect of zidovudine is its hematologic toxicity which may limit its administration (210,211). Recently, zidovudine has also been associated with a myopathy. Another analogue, 2′,3′-dideoxycytidine (DDC), has shown significant antiviral activity, but in adults has caused a painful neuropathy after 2 to 3 months of high-dose therapy (212,213). In adult patients, alternating regimens zidovudine and DDC appear to be equally effective against HIV and reduce the toxicity of each drug (212–214).

Other strategies for antiviral therapy include monoclonal antibodies directed against an invariant portion of the CD4 binding moiety, soluble CD4, alpha interferon, ampligen (an interferon inducer), and dextran sulfate, which apparently inhibits viral binding (213,215,216). Although several different HIV vaccines are being investigated, it is still too early to know how effective they will be (217). HIV has been and remains a formidable challenge. Its ability to incorporate itself into the host-cell genome and then remain latent, regulate its own replication independent of the host cell, and alter its antigenic sites are all features contributing to the great difficulty encountered in combating HIV (169,217).

Currently, the most important and effective treatment remains prevention and education. It is essential to counsel families about the risk for future pregnancies and to review modes of transmission, reassuring them that transmission does not occur through casual contact (218).

REFERENCES

1. Gottlieb MS, Schroff R, Schanker HM, et al. *Pneumocystis carinii* pneumonia and mucosal candidiasis in previously healthy homosexual men: Evidence of a new acquired cellular immunodeficiency. N Engl J Med 1981;305:1425–1431.

2. Gottlieb MS, Schanker HM, Fan PT, et al. *Pneumocystis* pneumonia—Los Angeles. MMWR 1981;30:250–252.

3. Centers for Disease Control. Kaposi's sarcoma and *Pneumocystis* pneumonia among homosexual men—New York City and California. MMWR 1981;30:305–308.

4. Fordham Von Reyn C, Mann JM. Global epidemiology. In: AIDS—A Global Perspective [special issue]. West J Med 1987;147:694–701.

5. Curran JW, Morgan WM, Hardy AM, et al. The epidemiology of AIDS: Current status and future prospects. Science 1985;229:1352–1357.

6. Gold KD, Thomas L, Garrett TJ. Aggressive Kaposi's sarcoma in a heterosexual drug addict. N Engl J Med 1982; 307:498.

7. Moll B, Emerson EE, Small CB, et al. Inverted ratio of inducer to suppressor T-lymphocyte subsets in drug abusers with opportunistic infections. Clin Immunol Immunopathol 1982;25:417–423.

8. Vieir J1, Frank E, Spira TJ, et al. Acquired immune deficiency in Haitians: Opportunistic infections in previously healthy Haitian immigrants. N Engl J Med 1983; 308:125–129.

9. Poon M, Landay A, Prasthofer EF, et al. Acquired immunodeficiency syndrome with *pneumocystis carinii* pneumonia and *Mycobacterium avium*-intracellulare infection in a previously healthy patient with classic hemophilia. Ann Intern Med 1983;98:287–290.

10. Centers for Disease Control. Immunodeficiency among female sexual partners of males with acquired immunodeficiency syndrome (AIDS)—New York. MMWR 1983; 31:697–698.

11. Centers for Disease Control. Unexplained immunodeficiency and opportunistic infections in infants—New York, New Jersey, California. MMWR 1982;31:665–6674.

12. Oleski J, Minnefor A, Cooper R Jr, et al. Immune deficiency syndrome in children. JAMA 1983;249:2345–2349.

13. Rubinstein A, Sicklick M, Gupta A, et al. Acquired immunodeficiency with reversed T4/T8 ratios in infants born to promiscuous and drug-addicted mothers. JAMA 1983;249:2350–2356.

14. Ammann AJ, Cowan MJ, Wara DW, et al. Acquired immunodeficiency in an infant: Possible transmission by means of blood products. Lancet 1983;1:956–958.

15. Scott GB, Buck BE, Leterman JG, et al. Acquired immunodeficiency syndrome in infants. N Engl J Med 1984; 310:76–81.

16. Barre-Sinoussi F, Chermann JC, Rey F, et al. Isolation of a T-lymphotropic retrovirus from a patient at risk for acquired immunodeficiency syndrome (AIDS). Science 1983;220:868–871.

17. Montagnier L, Gruest S, Chamaret S, et al. Adaptation of lymphadenopathy associated virus (LAV) to replication in EBV-transformed B-lymphoblastoid cell lines. Science 1984;225:63–66.

18. Gallo RC, Salahuddin SZ, Popovic M, et al. Frequent detection and isolation of cytopathic retroviruses (HTLV-III) from patients with AIDS and at risk for AIDS. Science 1984;224:500–503.

19. Sarngadharan MG, Popovic M, Bruch L, et al. Antibodies reactive with human T-lymphotropic retroviruses (HTLV-III) in the serum of patients with AIDS. Science 1984; 224:506–508.

20. Popovic M, Sarngadharan MG, Read E, et al. Detection, isolation and continuous production of cytopathic retrovirus (HTLV-III) from patients with AIDS and pre-AIDS. Science 1984;224:497–500.

21. Schupbach J, Sarngadharan MG, Gallo RC. Antigens on HTLV-III infected cells recognized by leukemia and AIDS sera are related to HTLV viral glycoproteins. Science 1984;224:607–610.

22. Broder S, Gallo RC. A pathogenic retrovirus (HTLV-III) linked to AIDS. N Engl J Med 1984;311:1292–1297.

23. Petricciani JC. Licensed tests for antibody to human T-lymphotropic virus type III: Sensitivity and specificity. Ann Intern Med 1985;103:726–729.

24. Brown F. Human immunodeficiency virus. Science 1986; 232:1486.

25. World Health Organization. Special Programme on AIDS. Progress Report 2, November 1987.

26. Quinn TC. The global epidemiology of the acquired immunodeficiency syndrome. In: Report of the Surgeon General's Workshop on Children with HIV Infection and Their Families. DHHS publication, Washington DC, 1987;No.HRS-D-MC 87–1:7–10.

27. Rogers MF, Thomas PA, Starcher ET, et al. Acquired immunodeficiency syndrome in children: Report of the Centers for Disease Control National Surveillance, 1982 to 1985. Pediatrics 1987;79:1008–1014.

28. Centers for Disease Control. Acquired immunodeficiency syndrome (AIDS). Weekly Surveillance Report United States. Atlanta, September 26, 1988;1–5.

29. Hearst N, Hulley SB. Preventing the heterosexual spread of AIDS. JAMA 1988;259:2428–2432.

30. Morgan WM, Curran JW. Acquired immunodeficiency syndrome: Current and future trends. Public Health Rep 1986;101:459–465.

31. Kleinman S, The Transfusion Study Safety Study Group. The infectivity of anti-HIV positive blood components. Proceedings from the Third International Conference on AIDS, Washington, D.C., June 1–5, 1987, 101. [abstract]

32. Lange JMA, van den Berg H, Dooren LJ, et al. HTLV-III/LAV infection in 9 children infected by a single plasma donor: Clinical outcome and recognition patterns of viral proteins. J Infect Dis 1986;154:171–174.

33. Kreiss JK, Kitchen LW, Prince HE, et al. Human T cell leukemia virus type III antibody, lymphadenopathy, and acquired immunodeficiency syndrome in hemophiliac subjects. Results of a prospective study. Am J Med 1986; 80:345–350.

34. Gerberding JL, Bryant-LeBlanc CE, Nelson K, et al. Risk of transmitting the human immunodeficiency virus, cytomegalovirus, and hepatitis B virus to health care workers exposed to patients with AIDS and AIDS-related conditions. J Infect Dis 1987;156:1-8.

35. Shannon KM, Ammann AJ. Acquired immunodeficiency syndrome in childhood. J Pediatr 1984;106:332–342.

36. Rubinstein A, Bernstein L. The epidemiology of pediatric acquired immunodeficiency syndrome. Clin Immunol Immunopathol 1986;40:115–121.

37. Pahwa S, Kaplan M, Fikrig S, et al. Spectrum of human T-cell lymphotrophic virus type III infection in children: Recognition of symptomatic, asymptomatic, and seronegative patients. JAMA 1986;255:2299–2305.

38. Mok JQ, Giaquinto C, De Rossi A, et al. Infants born to mothers seropositive for human immunodeficiency virus. Lancet 1987;1:1164–1168.

39. Grosch-Worner I, Koch S, Vocks M, et al. HIV infection in children of seropositive mothers. Arch Gynecol Obst 1989;245:185–188.

40. Abrams EJ. Longitudinal study of infants born to women at risk for AIDS. Proceedings from the Fourth International Conference on AIDS, Stockholm, Sweden, June 12–16, 1988;1:442. [abstract]

41. Scott GB, Hutto C, MaKuch RW, et al. Survival in children with perinatally acquired human immunodeficiency virus type 1 infection. N Engl J Med 1989,321:1791–1796.

42. Willoughby A, Mendez H, Hittelman J, et al. Epidemiology of the perinatal transmission of human immunodeficiency virus (HIV). Proceedings from the Fourth International Conference on AIDS, Stockholm, Sweden, June 12–16, 1988;2:293. [abstract]

43. Selwyn PA, Schoenbaum EE, Davenny K, et al. Prospective study of human immunodeficiency virus infection and pregnancy outcomes in intravenous drug users. JAMA 1989; 261:1289–1294.

44. Berrebi A, Puel J, Tricoire J, et al. Influence of pregnancy on the development of HIV infection. Revue de Practicien 1990;40:113–116.

45. Sprecher S, Soumerknoff G, Puissant F, et al. Vertical transmission of HIV in 15 week fetus. Lancet 1986;2:288–289.

46. Lyman WD, Kress Y, Rashbaum WK, et al. An AIDS virus-associated antigen localized in human fetal brain. Ann N Y Acad Sci 1988;540:628–629.

47. Peutherer JF, Rebus S, Aw D, et al. Detection of HIV in the fetus: A study of six cases. Proceedings from the Fourth International Conference on AIDS, Stockholm, Sweden, June 12–16, 1988;1:436. [abstract]

48. Lapointe N, Michaud J, Pekovic D, et al. Transplacental transmission of HTLV-III virus. N Engl J Med 1985;312: 1325–1326.

49. Pyun KH, Ochs HD, Dufford MTW, et al. Prenatal infection with human immunodeficiency virus: Specific antibody responses by the neonate. N Engl J Med 1987;317: 611–614.

50. Grosch-Worner I, Helge H, Weber B. AIDS problematik in der Padiatrie. Bundesgesundhbl 1986;29:351–356.

51. Thomas PA, O'Donnell RE, Guigli P, et al. Gestational characteristics and mode of delivery of 98 children with AIDS in New York City. Proceedings from the Third International Conference on AIDS, Washington DC, June 1–5, 1987, 136. [abstract]

52. Marion RW, Wiznia AA, Hutcheon G, et al. Human T-cell lymphotropic virus type III (HTLV-III) embryopathy: A new dysmorphic syndrome associated with intrauterine HTLV-III infection. Am J Dis Child 1986;140:638–640.

53. Iosub S, Bamji M, Stone RK, et al. More on human immunodeficiency virus embryopathy. Pediatrics 1987; 80:512–516.

54. Embree J, Braddick M, Datta P, et al. Lack of correlation of maternal human immunodeficiency virus infection with neonatal malformations. Pediatr Inf Dis J 1989;8:700–704.

55. Menez-Bautista R, Fikrig SM, Pahwa S, et al. Monozygotic twins discordant for the acquired immunodeficiency syndrome. Am J Dis Child 1986;140:678–679.

56. Ziegler JB, Cooper DA, Johnson RO, et al. Postnatal transmission of AIDS-associated retrovirus from mother to infant. Lancet 1985;1:896–898.

57. Thiry L, Sprecher-Goldberger S, Jonckheer T, et al. Isolation of AIDS virus from cell-free breast milk of three healthy virus carriers. Lancet 1985;2:891–892.

58. Ward JM, Holmberg SD, Allen JR, et al. Transmission of human immunodeficiency virus (HIV) by blood transfusions screened as negative for HIV antibody. N Engl J Med 1988;318:473–478.

59. Centers for Disease Control. Prevention of acquired immune deficiency syndrome (AIDS): Report of interagency recommendations. MMWR 1983;32:101–103.

60. Centers for Disease Control. Classification system for human T-lymphotropic virus type III/lymphadenopathy-associated virus infections. JAMA 1986;256:20–25.

61. Centers for Disease Control. Classification system for human immunodeficieny virus (HIV) infection in children under 13 years of age. MMWR 1987;36:225–230.

62. Centers for Disease Control. Revision of the CDC surveillance case definition for acquired immunodeficiency syndrome. MMWR 1987;36 Suppl 1:3–15.

63. Rubinstein A. Pediatric AIDS. Curr Probl Pediatr 1986;16:365–409.

64. Weintrub PS, Scott GB. Pediatric HIV Infection. In: Leong G, Mills J, eds. Opportunistic Infections in Patients with the Acquired Immunodeficiency Syndrome. New York: Marcel Dekker, 1989,153–168.

65. Fox R, Eldred LJ, Fuchs EJ. Clinical manifestations of acute infection with human immunodeficiency virus in a cohort of gay men. AIDS Res 1987;2:35–38.

66. Hessol NA, Rutherford GW, Lifson AR, et al. The natural history of HIV. Infection in a cohort of homosexual and bisexual men: A decade of follow-up. Proceedings from the Fourth International Conference on AIDS, Stockholm, Sweden, June 12–16, 1988;1:283. [abstract]

67. Ward J, Bush TJ, Perkins HA, et al. The natural history of transfusion-associated with human immunodeficiency virus. Factors influencing the role of progression to disease. N Engl J Med 1989;321:947–952.

68. Auger I, Thomas P, DeCoruttola V, et al. Incubation periods for pediatric AIDS patients. Nature 1988;336:575–577.

69. Bernstein LJ, Krieger BZ, Novick B, et al. Bacterial infections in the acquired immunodeficiency syndrome of children. Pediatr Infect Dis 1985;4:472–475.

70. Barrett DJ. The clinician's guide to pediatric AIDS. Contemp Pediatr 1988;5:24–47.

71. Joshi VV, Oleske JM, Minnefor AB, et al. Pathologic pulmonary findings in children with the acquired immunodeficiency syndrome: A study of ten cases. Hum Pathol 1985:16:241–246.

72. Rubinstein A, Morecki R, Silverman B, et al. Pulmonary disease in children with acquired immunodeficiency syndrome and AIDS-related complex. J Pediatr 1986;108:498–503.

73. Scott GB. Natural history of HIV infection in children. In: Report of the Surgeon General's Workshop on Children with HIV infection and their Families. DHHS publication, Washington DC, 1987;No. HRS-D-MC 87–1:22–23.

74. Andiman WA, Eastman R, Martin K, et al. Opportunistic lymphoproliferations associated with Epstein-Barr viral DNA in infants and children with AIDS. Lancet 1985;2:1390–1393.

75. Shanks GD, Redfield RR, Fisher GW. Toxoplasma encephalitis in an infant with acquired immunodeficiency syndrome. Pediatr Infect Dis 1987;6:70–71.

76. Epstein LG, DiCarlo FJ Jr, Joshi VV, et al. Primary lymphoma of the central nervous system in children with acquired immunodeficiency syndrome. Pediatrics 1988;82:355–363.

77. Saulsbury FT, Bayle RJ, Wykoff RF, et al. Thrombocytopenia as the presenting manifestation of human T-lymphotropic virus type III infection in infants. J Pediatr 1986;109:30–34.

78. Rao TKS, Mallis LR, Freidman EA. Nephropathy: As the initial (only?) sign of human immunodeficiency virus (HIV) disease. Proceedings from the Fourth International Conference on AIDS, Stockholm, Sweden, June 12–16, 1988;1:402. [abstract]

79. Rao TKS, Friedman EA, Nicastri AD. The types of renal disease in the acquired immunodeficiency syndrome. N Engl J Med 1987;316:1062–1068.

80. Steinherz LJ, Brockstein JA, Robins J. Cardiac involvement in congenital acquired immunodeficiency syndrome. Am J Dis Child 1986;140:1241–1244.

81. Rodgers VD, Kagnoff MF. Gastrointestinal manifestations of the acquired immunodeficiency syndrome. West J Med 1987;146:57–67.

82. Snider WD, Simpson DM, Nielsen S, et al. Neurological complications of acquired immunodeficiency syndrome: analysis of 50 patients. Ann Neurol 1983;14:403–418.

83. Levy RM, Bredesen DE, Rosenblum ML. Neurological manifestations of the acquired immunodeficiency syndrome (AIDS): Experience at UCSF and review of the literature. J Neurosurg 1985;62:475–495.

84. Koppel BS, Wormser GP, Tuchman AJ, et al. Central nervous system involvement in patients with acquired immunodeficiency syndrome (AIDS). Acta Neurol Scand 1985;71:337–353.

85. Navia BA, Jordan BD, Price RW. The AIDS dementia complex: I. Clinical features . Ann Neurol 1986;19:517–524.

86. Petito C . Review of central nervous system pathology in human immunodeficiency virus infection. Ann Neurol 1988;23 Suppl:S54–S57.

87. Petito C, Cho ES, Lemann W, et al. Neuropathology of acquired immunodeficiency syndrome (AIDS): An autopsy review. J Neuropathol Exp Neurol 1986;45:635–646.

88. Anders KH, Guerra WF, Tomiyasu U, et al. The neuropathology of AIDS: UCLA experience and review. Am J Pathol 1988;124:537–558.

89. Nielsen SL, Davis RL. Neuropathology of acquired immunodeficiency syndrome. In: Rosenblum ML, Levy RM, Bredesen DE, eds. AIDS and the Nervous System; Vol. 8. New York: Raven Press, 1988,155–181.

90. Levy RM, Bredesen DE. Central nervous system dysfunction in acquired immunodeficiency syndrome. In: Rosenblum ML, Levy RM, Bredesen DE, eds. AIDS and the Nervous System; Vol. 3. New York: Raven Press, 1988,29–63.

91. Elder GA, Sever JL. AIDS and neurological disorders: An overview. Ann Neurol 1988;23 Suppl:S4–S6.

92. Epstein LG, Sharer LR, Joshi W, et al. Progressive encephalopathy in children with acquired immune deficiency syndrome. Ann Neurol 1985;17:488–496.

93. Belman AL, Ultmann MH, Horoupian D, et al. Neurologic complications in infants and children with acquired immune deficiency syndrome (AIDS). Ann Neurol 1985;18:560–566.

94. Epstein LG, Sharer LR, Oleske JM, et al. Neurologic manifestations of human immunodeficiency virus infection in children. Pediatrics 1986;78:678–687.

95. Epstein LG, Sharer LR, Goudsmit J. Neurological and neuropathological features of human immunodeficiency virus infection in children. Ann Neurol 1988;23 Suppl:S19–S23.

96. Epstein LG, Sharer LR. Neurology of human immunodeficiency virus infection in children. In: Rosenblum ML, Levy RM, Bredesen DE, eds. AIDS and the Nervous System; Vol. 5. New York: Raven Press, 1988,79–101.

97. Belman AL, Diamond G, Dickson D, et al. Pediatric acquired immunodeficiency syndrome: Neurologic syndromes. Am J Dis Child 1988;142:29–35.

98. Ultmann MH, Belman AL, Ruff HA, et al. Developmental abnormalities in infants and children with acquired immune deficiency syndrome (AIDS) and AIDS-related complex. Dev Med Child Neurol 1985;27:563–571.

99. Coulter DL, Chase C, McLean K. Possible neuropsychological deficits in infants with acquired immunodeficiency syndrome. Ann Neurol 1988;24:358. [abstract]

100. Davis SL, Halsted CC, Levy N, et al. Acquired immune deficiency syndrome presenting as progressive infantile encephalopathy. J Pediatr 1987;110:884–888.

101. Weiner SP, Rosenbaum F, Guerra Hanson IC, et al. A 5-year-old boy with a neurodegenerative process as the initial manifestation of human immunodeficiency virus infection. Ann Neurol 1988;24:360. [abstract]

102. Belman AL, Lantos G, Horoupian D, et al. AIDS: Calcification of the basal ganglia in infants and children. Neurology 1986;36:1192–1199.

103. Epstein LG, Berman CZ, Sharer LR, et al. Unilateral calcification and contrast enhancement of the basal ganglia in a child with AIDS encephalopathy. AJNR 1987;8:163–165.

104. Jarvik JG, Hesselink JR, Kennedy C, et al. Acquired immunodeficiency syndrome: Magnetic resonance patterns of brain involvement with pathologic correlation. Arch Neurol 1988;45:731–736.

105. Ho DD, Rota TR, Schooley RT, et al. Isolation of HTLV-III from cerebrospinal fluid and neural tissues of patients with neurologic syndromes related to the acquired immunodeficiency syndrome. N Engl J Med 1985;313:1493–1497.

106. Resnick L, Berger JR, Shapshak P, et al. Early penetration of the blood-brain-barrier by HIV. Neurology 1988;38:9–14.

107. Goudsmit J, De Wolf F, Paul DA, et al. Expression of human immunodeficiency virus anitgen (HIV-Ag) in serum and cerebrospinal fluid during acute and chronic infection. Lancet 1986;2:177–180.

108. Epstein LG, Goudsmit J, Paul DA, et al. HIV expression in cerebrospinal fluid of children with progressive encephalopathy. Ann Neurol 1987;21:391–401.

109. Smith T, Jakobsen J, Gaub J, et al. Clinical and electrophysiological studies of human immunodeficiency virus-seropositive men without AIDS. Ann Neurol 1988;23:295–297.

110. Koch T, Weintrub P, Rumsey C, et al. Early manifestations of neurologic involvement in infants with congenital HIV. Proceedings from the Fourth International Conference on AIDS, Stockholm, Sweden, June 12–16, 1988;1:437. [abstract]

111. Kairam R, Emerson R, Bamji M, et al. Median nerve sensory evoked potentials: A marker for human immunodeficiency virus-related neurologic disease. Ann Neurol 1988;24:360. [abstract]

112. Petito CK, Navia BA, Cho ES, et al. Vacuolar myelopathy pathologically resembling subacute combined degeneration in patients with the acquired immunodeficiency syndrome. N Engl J Med 1985;213:874–879.

113. Dickson DW, Belman Al, Kim, TS, et al. Spinal cord pathology in pediatric acquired immunodeficiency syndrome. Neurology 1989;39:227–235.

114. Sharer LR, Epstein LG, Michaels J, et al. HIV-l infection of the spinal cord in children with AIDS. Proceedings from the Fourth International Conference on AIDS, Stockholm, Sweden, June 12 to 16, 1988;1:436. [abstract]

115. Bredesen DE, Lipkin WI, Messing R. Prolonged, recurrent aseptic meningitis with prominent cranial nerve abnormalities: A new epidemic in gay men? Neurology 1983;33 Suppl 2:85. [abstract]

116. Levy J, Shimabukuro J, Hollander H, et al. Isolation of AIDS-associated retroviruses from cerebrospinal fluid and brain of patients with neurologic symptoms. Lancet 1985;2:586–588.

117. Hollander H, Stringari S. Human innumodeficiency virus-associated meningitis. Clinical course and correlations. Am J Med 1987;83:813–816.

118. Levy RM, Bredesen DE, Rosenblum ML. Opportunistic central nervous system pathology in patients with AIDS. Ann Neurol 1988;23 Suppl:S7–S12.

119. Miller JR, Barrett RE, Britton CB, et al. Progressive multifocal leukoencephalopathy in a male homosexual with T-cell immune deficiency. N Engl J Med 1982;307:1436–1438.

120. Post MJD, Hensley GT, Moskowitz LB, et al. Cytomegalic inclusion virus encephalitis in patients with AIDS: CT, clinical and pathologic correlation. AJNR 1986;7:275–280; AJR 1986;146:1229–1234.

121. Britton CB, Mesa-Tejeda R, Fenoglio CM, et al. A new complication of AIDS: Thoracic myelitis caused by herpes simplex virus. Neurology 1985;35:1071–1074.

122. Ryder JW, Croen K, Kleinschmidt-DeMasters BK, et al. Progressive encephalitis three months after resolution of cutaneous zoster in a patient with AIDS. Ann Neurol 1986;19:182–188.

123. Post MJD, Chan JC, Hensley GT, et al. Toxoplasma encephalitis in Haitian adults with acquired immunodeficiency syndrome: A clinical-pathologic-CT correlation. AJR 1983;140:861–868.

124. Kovacs JA, Kovacs AA, Polis M, et al. Cryptococcosis in the acquired immunodeficiency syndrome. Ann Intern Med 1985;103:533–538.

125. Henry JM, Heffner RR Jr, Dillard SH, et al. Primary malignant lymphomas of the central nervous system. Cancer 1974;34:1293–1302.

126. Rosenblum ML, Levy RM, Bredesen DE, et al. Primary central nervous system lymphomas in patients with AIDS. Ann Neurol 1988;23 Suppl:S13–S16.

127. So YT, Beckstead JH, Davis RL. Primary central nervous system lymphoma in acquired immunodeficiency syndrome: A clinical and pathological study. Ann Neurol 1986;20:566–572.

128. So YT, Choucair A, Davis RL, et al. Neoplasms of the central nervous system in acquired immunodeficiency syndrome. In: Rosenblum ML, Levy RM, Bredesen DE, eds. AIDS and the Nervous System; Vol. 13. New York: Raven Press, 1988,285–300.

129. Ziegler JL, Beckstead JH, Volberding PA, et al. Non-Hodgkin's lymphoma in 90 homosexual men: Relation to generalized lymphadenopathy and the acquired immunodeficiency syndrome. N Engl J Med 1984;311:565–570.

130. Levy RM, Bredesen D, Rosenblum ML, et al. Postmortem neuropathology in the acquired immunodeficiency syndrome (AIDS). Proceedings from the Annual Meeting of the Congress of Neurological Surgeons, New Orleans, LA, 1986. [abstract]

131. Engstrom J, Lowenstein DH, Bredesen D. Cerebral infarctions and transient neurologic deficits associated with acquired immunodeficiency syndrome. Am J Med 1989;86:528–532.

132. Bloom EJ, Abrams DI, Rodgers G. Lupus anticoagulant in the acquired immunodeficiency syndrome. JAMA 1986;256:491–493.

133. Park YD, Belman AL, Dickson D, et al. Stroke in pediatric acquired immunodeficiency syndrome. Ann Neurol 1988;24:359. [abstract]

134. Frank Y, Lim W, Kahn E, et al. Cerebral granulomatous angiitis causing multiple ischemic cerebrovascular accidents in a child with acquired immunodeficiency syndrome. Ann Neurol 1987;22:452. [abstract]

135. Miller RG, Kiprov DD, Parry G, et al. Peripheral nervous system dysfunction in acquired immunodeficiency syndrome. In: Rosenblum ML, Levy RM, Bredesen DE, eds. AIDS and the Nervous System; Vol. 4. New York: Raven Press, 1988,65–78.

136. Cornblath DR, McArthur JC, Kennedy PG, et al. Inflammatory demyelinating peripheral neuropathies associated with human T-cell lymphotrophic virus type III infection. Ann Neurol 1987;21:32–40.

137. Dalakas MC, Pezeshkpour GH. Neuromuscular diseases associated with human immunodeficiency virus infection. Ann Neurol 1988;23 Suppl:S38–S48.

138. Parry GJ. Peripheral neuropathies associated with human immunodeficiency virus infection. Ann Neurol 1988;23 Suppl:S49–S53.

139. So YT, Holtzman DM, Abrams DI, et al. Peripheral neuropathy associated with acquired immunodeficiency syndrome: Prevalence and clinical features from a population-based study. Arch Neurol 1988;45:945–948.

140. De la Monte SM, Gabuzda DH, Ho DD, et al. Peripheral neuropathy in the acquired immunodeficiency syndrome. Ann Neurol 1988;23:485–492.

141. Comi G, Medaglini S, Galardi G, et al. Subclinical neuromuscular involvement in acquired immune deficiency syndrome. Muscle Nerve 1986;9:665. [abstract]

142. Cornblath DR, McArthur JC. Peripheral neuropathies associated with HIV infection: Classification and pathogenesis. Proceedings from the Fourth International Conference on AIDS, Stockholm, Sweden, June 12–16, 1988;1:203. [abstract]

143. Lipkin WI, Parry G, Kiprov DD, et al. Inflammatory neuropathy in homosexual men with lymphadenopathy. Neurology 1985;35:1479–1483.

144. Vendrell J, Heredia C, Pujol M, et al. Guillain-Barré syndrome associated with seroconversion for anti-HTLV-III. Neurology 1987;37:544.

145. Yarchoan R, Berg G, Brouwers P, et al. Response of human immunodeficiency-virus-associated neurological disease to 3′-azido-3′-deoxythymidine. Lancet 1987;1:132–135.

146. Vishnubhakat SM, Kaplan M, Farber B, et al. Effect of azidothymidine (AZT) on peripheral neuropathy of HIV-infected patients: a prospective study. Neurology 1988;38 Suppl 1:241. [abstract]

147. Anderson V, Greco MA, Recalde AL, et al. Intestinal cytomegalovirus ganglioneuritis in children with human immunodeficiency virus infection. Pediatric Pathol 1990;10:167–174.

148. Dalakas MC, Pezeshkpour GH, Gravell M, et al. Polymyositis associated with AIDS retrovirus. JAMA 1986;256:2381–2383.

149. Simpson DM, Bender AN. Human immunodeficiency virus-associated myopathy: Analysis of 11 patients. Ann Neurol 1988;24:79–84.

150. Gonzales MF, Olney RK, So YT, et al. Subacute structural myopathy associated with human immunodeficiency virus infection. Arch Neurol 1988;45:585–587.

151. Sharer LR, Epstein LG, Cho ES, et al. Pathologic features of AIDS encephalopathy in children: Evidence for LAV/HTLV-III infection of brain. Hum Pathol 1986;17:271–284.

152. Nielsen SL, Petito CK, Urmacher CD, et al. Subacute encephalitis in acquired immune deficiency syndrome: A postmortem study. Am J Clin Pathol 1984;82:678–682.

153. Navia BA, Cho ES, Petito CK, et al. The AIDS dementia complex: II. Neuropathology. Ann Neurol 1986;19:525–535.

154. De la Monte SM, Ho DD, Schooley RT, et al. Subacute encephalitis of AIDS and its relation to HTLV-III infection. Neurology 1987;37:562–569.

155. Shaw GM, Harper ME, Hahn BH, et al. HTLV-III infection in brains of children and adults with AIDS encephalopathy. Science 1985;227:177–182.

156. Gajdusek DC, Amyx HL, Gibbs CJ, et al. Infection of chimpanzees by human T-lymphotropic retroviruses in brain and other tissues from AIDS patients. Lancet 1985;1:55–56.

157. Stoler MH, Eskin TA, Benn 5, et al. Human T-cell lymphotrophic virus type III infection of the central nervous system: A preliminary in situ analysis. JAMA 1986;256:2360–2364.

158. Wiley CA, Belman AL, Dickson D, et al. Human immunodeficiency virus within the brains of children with AIDS. Clin Neuropathol 1990;9:1–6.

159. Wiley CA, Schrier RD, Nelson JA, et al. Cellular localization of human immunodeficiency virus infection within the brains of acquired immunodeficiency syndrome patients. Proc Natl Acad Sci USA 1986;83:7089–7093.

160. Gartner S, Markovits P, Markovitz DM, et al. Virus isolation from and identification of HTLV-III/LAV-producing cells in brain tissue from a patient with AIDS. JAMA 1986;256:2365–2371.

161. Pumarola-Sune T, Navia BA, Cordon-Cardo C, et al. HIV antigen in the brains of patients with the AIDS dementia complex. Ann Neurol 1987;21:490–496.

162. Gabuzda DH, Ho DD, de la Monte SM, et al. Immunohistochemical identification of HTLV-III antigen in brains of patients with AIDS. Ann Neurol 1986;20:289–295.

163. Vazeux R, Brousse N, Jarry, et al. AIDS subacute encephalitis: Identification of HIV-infected cells. Am J Pathol 1987;126:403–410.

164. Koenig S, Gendelman HE, Orentstein JM, et al. Detection of AIDS virus in macrophages in brain tissue from AIDS patients with encephalopathy. Science 1986;233:1089–1093.

165. Najera R, Herrera MI, de Andres R. Human immunodeficiency virus and related retroviruses . West J Med 1987;147:702–708.

166. Essex M, Allan J, Kanki P, et al. Antigens of human T-lymphotropic virus type-III/lymphadenopathy-associated virus. Ann Intern Med 1985;103:700–703.

167. Gonda MA, Wong-Staal F, Gallo RC, et al. Sequence homology and morphologic similarity of HTLV-III and visna virus, a pathogenic lentivirus. Science 1985; 227:173–177.

168. Gallo RC. The AIDS virus. Sci Am 1987;256:47–56.

169. Haseltine WA, Wong-Staal F. The molecular biology of the AIDS virus. Sci Am 1988;259:52–62.

170. Rabson A, Martin M. Molecular organization of the AIDS retrovirus. Cell 1985;40:477–480.

171. Gallo R, Wong-Staal F, Montagnier L, et al. HIV/HTLV gene nomenclature. Nature 1988;333:504.

172. Levy JA. The biology of the human immunodeficiency virus and its role in neurologic disease. In: Rosenblum ML, Levy RM, Bredesen DE, eds. AIDS and the Nervous System; Vol. 16. New York: Raven Press, 1988, 327–345.

173. Cheng-Mayer C, Levy JA. Distinct biologic and serologic properties of human immunodeficiency viruses from the brain. Ann Neurol 1988;23 Suppl:S58–S61.

174. Rubsamen-Waigmann H, Becker WB, Helm EB, et al. Isolation of variants of lymphocytopathic retroviruses from the peripheral blood and cerebrospinal fluid of patients with ARC or AIDS. J Med Virol 1986;19:335–344.

175. Levy J, Kaminsky L, Morrow W, et al. Infection by the retrovirus associated with acquired immunodeficiency syndrome. Ann Intern Med 1985;103:694–699.

176. Hahn BH, Shaw GM, Wong-Staal F, et al. Genomic variation of HTLV-III/LAV, the retrovirus of AIDS. In: Fields B, Martin MA, Kamely D, eds. Genetically Altered Viruses and the Environment. New York: Cold Springs Harbor Laboratory, 1985,235–249.

177. Dalgleish A, Beverley P, Clapham P, et al. The CD4 (T4) antigen is an essential component of the receptor for the AIDS retrovirus. Nature 1984;312:763–773.

178. Klatzmann D, Champagne E, Chamaret S, et al. T-lymphocyte T4 molecule behaves as receptor for human retrovirus LAV. Nature 1984;312:767–768.

179. Levy JA, Shimabukuro J, McHugh T, et al. AIDS-associated retroviruses (ARV) can productively infect other cells besides human T-helper cells. Virology 1985;147:441–448.

180. Cheng-Mayer C, Rutka JT, Rosenblum ML, et al. The human immunodeficiency virus (HIV) can productively infect cultured human brain cells. Proc Natl Acad Sci USA 1987:84:3526–3530.

181. Sodroski J, Goh WC, Rosen C, et al. The role of HTLV-III/LAV envelope in syncytium formation and cytopathicity. Nature 1986;322:470–474.

182. Kiprov D, Busch D, Simpson D, et al. Antilymphocyte serum factors in patients with acquired immunodeficiency syndrome. In: Gottlieb M, Groopman J, eds. Acquired Immune Deficiency Syndrome. New York: AR Liss, 1984,299–308.

183. Stricker R, McHugh TM, Moody DJ, et al. An AIDS-related autoantibody reacts with a specific antigen on stimulated helper/inducer T-cells. Nature 1987;327:710–713.

184. Bredesen DE. Implications of acquired immunodeficiency syndrome for neurological pathophysiology. In: Rosenblum ML, Levy RM, Bredesen DE, eds. AIDS and the Nervous System; Vol. 18. New York: Raven Press, 1988,377–387.

185. Kalish SB, Ostrow DG, Goldsmith J, et al. The spectrum of immunologic abnormalities and clinical findings in homosexually active men. J Infect Dis 1984;149:148–156.

186. Fauci A. Immunologic abnormalities in the acquired immunodeficiency syndrome (AIDS). Clin Res 1985;32:491–499.

187. Ammann AJ. The acquired immunodeficiency syndrome in infants and children. Ann Intern Med 1985;103:734–737.

188. Ammann AJ, Schiffman G, Abrams D, et al. B-cell immunodeficiency in acquired immune deficiency syndrome. JAMA 1984;251:1447–1449.

189. Weiss SH, Goedert JJ, Sarngadharan MG, et al. Screening test for HTLV-III (AIDS agent) antibodies: Specificity, sensitivity and applications. JAMA 1985;253:221–225.

190. Borkowsky W, Krasinski K, Paul D, et al. Human immunodeficiency virus infections in infants negative for anti-HIV by enzyme-linked immunoassay. Lancet 1987;1:1168–1170.

191. Sampelayo TH, Gurbindo D, Fermosel J. Silent HIV infection periods in infants. Proceedings from the Fourth International Conference on AIDS, Stockholm, Sweden, June 12–16, 1988;1:439. [abstract]

192. Barin F, Courouce AM, Maniez M, et al. A comparison of four enzyme immunoassays (EIAs) for the detection of HIV antigen (HIVAg). Proceedings from the Fourth International Conference on AIDS, Stockholm, Sweden, June 12–16, 1988;2:80. [abstract]

193. Borkowsky W, Kransinski K, Paul D, et al. Human immunodeficiency virus type 1 antigenemia in children. J Pediatr 1989;114:940–945.

194. Pahwa 5, Kaplan M, Lim W, et al. Perinatal HIV transmission: Value of HIV antigen determination in serum. Proceedings from the Fourth International Conference on AIDS, Stockholm, Sweden, June 12–16, 1988;1:443. [abstract]

195. Epstein LG, Boucher CAB, Morrison SH, et al. Persistent human immunodeficiency virus type 1 antigenemia in children correlates with disease progression. Pediatrics 1988;82:919–924.

196. Centers for Disease Control. Recommendations for assisting in the prevention of perinatal transmission of human T-lymphotropic virus type III/lymphadenopathy associated virus and the acquired immunodeficiency syndrome. MMWR 1985;34:721–731.

197. Thomas PA, McLaughlin P, Rubinstein A, et al. Use of live vaccines in children with HTLV-III/LAV infection: Public health perspectives. Proceedings from the Second International Conference on AIDS, Paris, France, June 23–25, 1986,33. [abstract]

198. Sension MG, Quinn TC, Markowitz LE, et al. Measles in hospitalized African children with human immunodeficiency virus. Am J Dis Child 1988;142:1271–1272.

199. Centers for Disease Control. Immunization of children with human immunodeficiency virus-supplementary ACIP statement. MMWR 1988;37:181–183.

200. Centers for Disease Control. Recommendations of the Immunization Practices Advisory Committee (ACIP) immunization of children infected with human T-lymphotropic virus type III/lymphadenopathy virus. MMWR 1986;35:595–606.

201. Glatt AE, Chirgwin K, Landesman SH. Treatment of infections associated with human immunodeficiency virus. N Engl J Med 1988;318:1439–1448.

202. Wharton JM, Coleman DL, Wofsy CB, et al. Trimethoprim-sulfamethoxazole or pentamidine for *Pneumocystis carinii* pneumonia in the acquired immunodeficiency syndrome: A prospective randomized trial. Ann Intern Med 1986;105:37–44.

203. Jacobson MA, Mills J. Serious cytomegalovirus disease in the acquired immunodeficiency syndrome (AIDS): Clinical flndings, diagnosis, and treatment. Ann Intern Med 1988;108:585–594.

204. Rubinstein A, Sicklick M, Bernstein L, et al. Treatment of AIDS with intravenous gammaglobulin. Pediatr Res 1984;18:264.

205. Yarchoan R, Weinhold KJ, Lyerly HK, et al. Administration of 3′-azido-3′deoxythymidine, an inhibitor of HTLV-III/LAV replication, to patients with AIDS or AIDS-related complex. Lancet 1986;1:575–580.

206. Fischl MA, Richman DD, Grieco MH, et al. The efficacy of azidothymidine (AZT) in the treatment of patients with AIDS and AIDS-related complex: A double-blind, placebo-controlled trial. N Engl J Med 1987;317:185–191.

207. Vocks M, Cammann U, Saur S, et al. Effects of zidovudine (AZT) in children with AIDS. Proceedings from the Fourth International Conference on AIDS, Stockholm, Sweden, June 12–16, 1988;1:256. [abstract]

208. Pizzo PA, Eddy J, Falloon J, et al. Effects of continuous intravenous infusion of zidovudine (AZT) in children with symptomatic HIV infection. N Engl J Med 1988;319:884–896.

209. Moss H, Brouwers P, Wolters P, et al. Reversible neuropsychological deficits: The effect of AZT therapy in a pediatric AIDS population. Proceedings from the Fourth International Conference on AIDS, Stockholm, Sweden, June 12–16, 1988;1:440. [abstract]

210. Richman DD, Fischl MA, Grieco MH, et al. The toxicity of azidothymidine (AZT) in the treatment of patients with AIDS and AIDS-related complex. N Engl J Med 1987; 317:192–197.

211. Gelmon K, Montaner JSG, Fanning M, et al. Nature time course and dose dependence of zidovudine-related side effects: Results from the Multicenter Canadian Azidothymidine Trial. Aids 1989;3:555–561.

212. Yarchoan R, Mitsuya H, Broder 5. AIDS therapies. Sci Am 1988;259:110–119.

213. Yarchoan R, Pluda JM, Thomas RV, et al. Long-term treatment of AIDS and AIDS-related complex (ARC) with an alternating weekly regimen of AZT and 2',3'-dideoxycytidine (DDC). Proceedings from the Fourth International Conference on AIDS, Stockholm, Sweden, June 12–16, 1988;1:257. [abstract]

214. Spector SA, Ripley D, Hsia K. Human immunodeficiency virus (HIV) inhibition is prolonged by 3'-azido-3'-deoxythymidine alternating with 2',3'-dideoxycytidine compared to 3'-azido-3'-deoxythymidine alone. Antimicrob Agents Chemother 1989;33:920–923.

215. Mitsuya H, Broder 5. Strategies for antiviral therapy in AIDS. Nature 1987;325:773–778.

216. Dalgleish AG, Kennedy RC, Chanh TC, et al. Therapeutic strategies against HIV based on the CD4 molecule: Monoclonal antibody therapy, soluable CD4 and anti-idiotype vaccines. Proceedings from the Fourth International Conference on AIDS, Stockholm, Sweden, June 12–16, 1988;1: 235. [abstract]

217. Matthews TJ, Bolognesi DP. AIDS vaccines. Sci Am 1988;259:120–127.

218. Centers for Disease Control. Education and foster care of children infected with human T-lymphotropic virus type III/lymphadenopathy-associated virus. MMWR 1985;34: 517–521.

Part V

Neurologic Manifestations of Childhood Hazards

Chapter 26
Neurologic Manifestations of Substance Abuse in Children

Donna M. Ferriero

All drugs of abuse can be presumed to affect the nervous system as it develops and matures. As the use of these drugs by people of child-bearing age continues to grow, so does our understanding of their teratogenic and addictive effects on the developing nervous system and the clinical consequences of their withdrawal at the time of birth. Unfortunately, clinical studies of these problems are very difficult to pursue because maternal histories are often poor and multiple drugs may have been used and are inadequately documented. Other variables such as poor nutrition and adverse social and environmental factors may exist, and affected patients may ultimately have subtle developmental or behavioral abnormalities that are difficult to quantitate and cannot be assessed until many years have passed.

It must be remembered that direct abuse of drugs by children and adolescents is an additional problem of steadily increasing magnitude, and while this occurs at an age when danger to the developing nervous system is no longer a threat, the same spectrum of acute and long-term neurologic and systemic complications of drug abuse as exist in adults still remains.

ETHANOL

The hazards to the developing fetus of intrauterine exposure to alcohol have been recounted through time in folklore, but the first documented observation appeared in an essay by Carpenter (1849), "The use and abuse of alcoholic liquors in health and disease." He discussed the alcohol-related impairment in newborns and noted that Aristotle observed, "drunken women bring forth children like to themselves." Brown, a resident physician at the Crichton Lunatic Asylum, proclaimed, "The drunkard not only injures and enfeebles his own nervous system, but entails mental disease upon his family. His daughters are nervous and hysterical. His sons are weak, wayward, eccentric and sink insane under the pressure of excitement of some unforeseen exigency or of the ordinary calls of duty. At present I have two patients who appear to inherit a tendency to unhealthy action of the brain, from mothers addicted to drinking . . . " (1).

This report was well taken, but it was not until recent decades that additional significant clinical studies were reported. Lemoine et al. (1968) reported their study of 127 infants born to alcoholic parents and described the abnormalities associated with maternal ethanol abuse (2). Subsequent reports expanded the concept of the fetal alcohol syndrome (FAS) (3,4), and extensive animal studies have now substantiated that the teratogenic effects of ethanol seen in humans may also occur in a variety of animal species (5–7). Estimates regarding the frequency of FAS suggest that one to two live births per one thousand are affected (4). The major features of FAS are intrauterine and postnatal growth retardation, craniofacial dysmorphology (midface hypoplasia with thinned upper vermilion and hypoplastic philtrum, microphthalmia, epicanthal folds, congenital heart defects, skeletal anomalies, and central nervous system (CNS) abnormalities (Figures 26.1 and 26.2; Tables 26.1 and 26.2) (4). The CNS abnormalities include microcephaly, irritability in infancy, hyperactivity in childhood, hypotonia, delay in fine and gross motor coordination, kinetic tremor, axial ataxia, and mental retardation (3,4).

Teratogenic Effects

Although it is not clear in what manner alcohol exerts its effects to produce the fetal alcohol syndrome, it is assumed

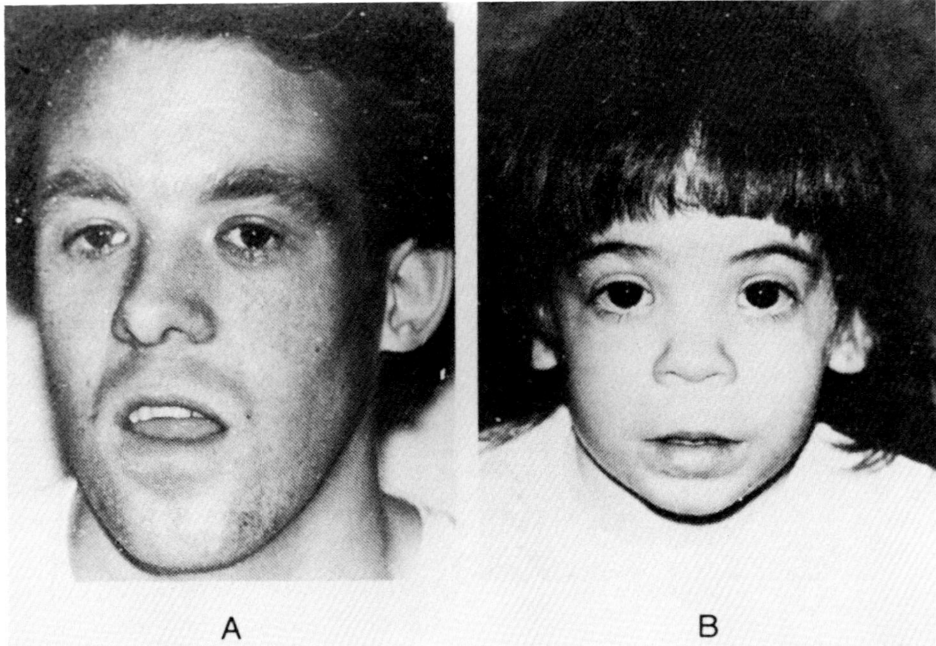

FIGURE 26.1 Patients at 17 (**A**) and 2 1/2 (**B**) years of age with facial appearance observed in fetal alcohol syndrome. Reprinted with permission from Clarren SK, et al. The fetal alcohol syndrome. N Engl J Med 1978;298:1063–1067.

that alcohol and not its metabolites cause the morphologic abnormalities. Ethanol readily crosses the placenta, and in humans fetal blood ethanol levels approximate those in maternal blood (8). The elimination of ethanol from the fetus is accomplished primarily by maternal hepatic biotransformation of ethanol, since the fetal liver has no alcohol dehydrogenase activity until 16 weeks, when its level is yet only 10% of the adult liver (9). The rate of ethanol elimination from amniotic fluid is only 1/2 that from maternal blood; thus, the amniotic fluid acts as a reservoir for ethanol. The ethanol concentrations of adult brains are similar to those of blood, but those of fetal brains have not been studied. It would be expected that concentrations would be higher, however, because of the higher water content of fetal brain (10).

At this time, it is believed that the major pathogenic affect of alcohol on the developing nervous system is on neuronal migration. The neuropathologic findings in FAS include neuroglial meningeal heterotopias, cortical neuronal disorganization, agenesis of the corpus callosum,

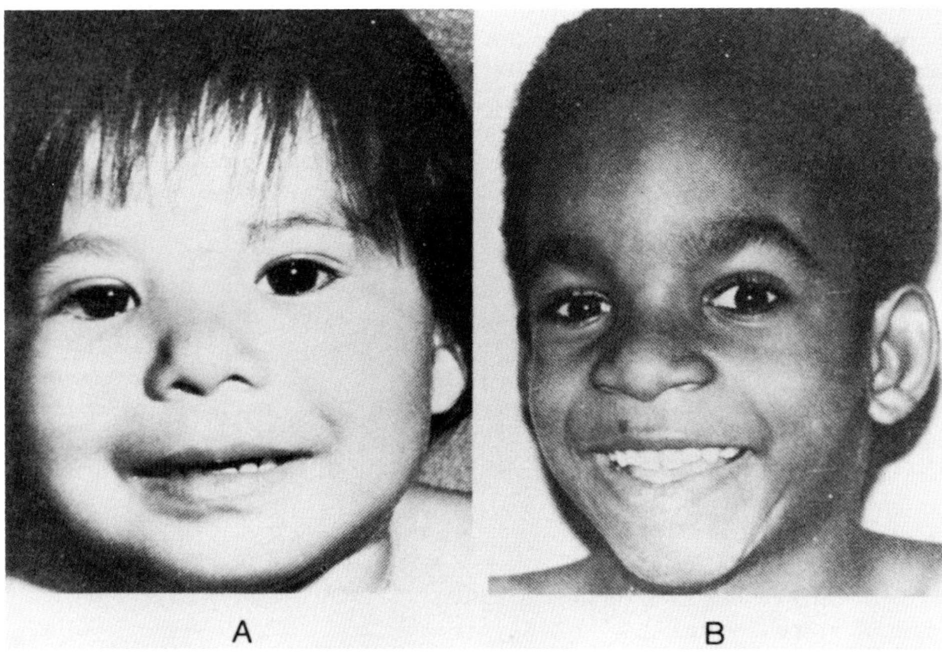

FIGURE 26.2 Patients at 1 1/2 (**A**) and 6 (**B**) years of age differing slightly from Figure 26.1 because of racial backgrounds. Reprinted with permission from Clarren SK, et al. The fetal alcohol syndrome. N Engl J Med 1978;298:1063–1067.

Table 26.1 Principal features of the fetal alcohol syndrome observed in 245 affected persons.

Feature	Manifestation
Central nervous system dysfunction	
Intellectual	Mild to moderate mental retardation*
Neurologic	Microcephaly*
	Poor coordination, hypotonia**
Behavioral	Irritability in infancy*
	Hyperactivity in childhood**
Growth deficiency	
Prenatal	< 2 SD for length and weight*
Postnatal	< 2 SD for length and weight*
	Disproportionately diminished adipose tissue**
Facial characteristics	
Eyes	Short palpebral fissures*
Nose	Short, upturned**
	Hypoplastic philtrum*
Facial characteristics	
Maxilla	Hypoplastic**
Mouth	Thinned upper vermilion*
	Retrognathia in infancy*
	Micrognathia or relative prognathia in adolescence**

*Feature seen in > 80% of patients.
**Feature seen in > 50% of patients.

Adapted with permission from Clarren SK, et al. The fetal alcohol syndrome. N Engl J Med 1978;298:1063–1067.

and cortical and cerebellar heterotopias (Figure 26.3) (11–15). On a subcellular level, reduced numbers and abnormal dendritic spines have been observed on pyramidal neurons (Figure 26.4) (16). The significance of these findings is uncertain, although the reduced number of spines may result in decreased input to the dendritic arbor and, thus, produce abnormal neuronal firing and communication (15). Other morphologic studies have shown an increased number of corticospinal neurons as well as a

delay in the time of their origin, suggesting that the normal developmental process of paring down of exuberant projections may be affected (16).

Prenatal exposure to ethanol can cause a significant decrease in glucose utilization in a variety of regions throughout the brain, especially the motor and somatosensory cortices (17). In vitro studies have shown that ethanol decreases protein synthesis and glutamate synthetase activity in glia (18). Inhibition of neurotropic factor production has also been described in chick sensory neurons at ethanol concentrations that did not affect neuronal survival or adhesion (19). These metabolic and morphologic effects provide evidence for the direct influence of ethanol on the developing central nervous system, but the elucidation of exact pathophysiologic mechanisms awaits further study.

Passive Addiction and Withdrawal

The consequences of passive addiction to alcohol in utero are manifested at birth when the infant undergoes "withdrawal" from the alcohol. The signs of withdrawal are most obvious in severely affected infants with FAS, who may display irritability, apnea, opisthotonos, tremor, and hypertonia. However, signs of passive addiction are also present in nondysmorphic children born to mothers who drank moderately or heavily during pregnancy. These infants have more tremors, hypertonia, restlessness, excessive mouthing movements, unconsolable crying, and reflex abnormalities than infants born to mothers who never drank or who stopped drinking in the second trimester (20). Most of these behaviors begin by the 3rd day of life and may continue for an undetermined period.

In cases where the mother appears intoxicated at the time of delivery, withdrawal symptoms may occur as early as 6 to 12 hours of life. The more severely affected newborn will be jittery, hypersensitive to sound, irritable, tremulous, and hypertonic. Generalized seizures are common in overtly

Table 26.2 Associated features of the fetal alcohol syndrome observed in 245 affected persons.

Area	Frequent*	Occasional**
Eyes	Ptosis, strabismus, epicanthal folds	Myopia, clinical microphthalmia, blepharophimosis
Ears	Posterior rotation	Poorly formed concha
Mouth	Prominent lateral palatine ridges	Cleft lip or cleft palate, small teeth with faulty enamel
Cardiac	Murmurs, especially in early childhood usually atrial septal defect	Ventricular septal defect, great-vessel anomalies, tetralogy of Fallot
Renogenital	Labial hypoplasia	Hypospadias, small rotated kidneys, hydronephrosis
Cutaneous	Hemangiomas	Hirsutism in infancy
Skeletal	Aberrant palmar creases, pectus excavatum	Limited joint movements, especially fingers and elbows; nail hypoplasia, especially 5th; polydactyly; radioulnar synostosis; pectus carinatum; bifid xiphoid, Klippel-Feil anomaly; scoliosis
Muscular		Hernias of diaphragm, umbilicus, or groin; diastasis recti

*Feature seen in > 80% of patients.
**Feature seen in > 50% of patients.

Adapted with permission from Clarren SK, et al. The fetal alcohol syndrome. N Engl J Med 1978;298:1063–1067.

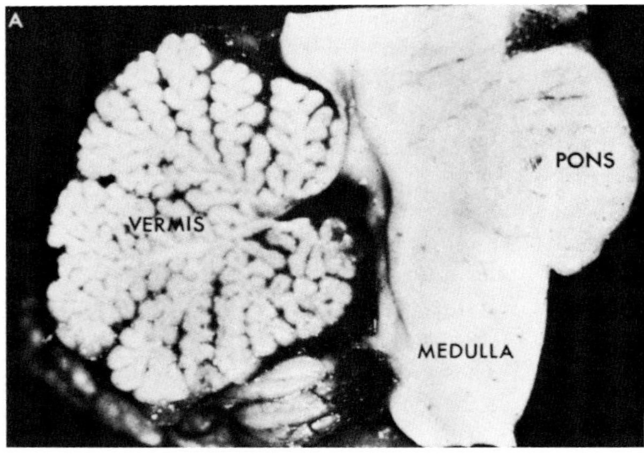

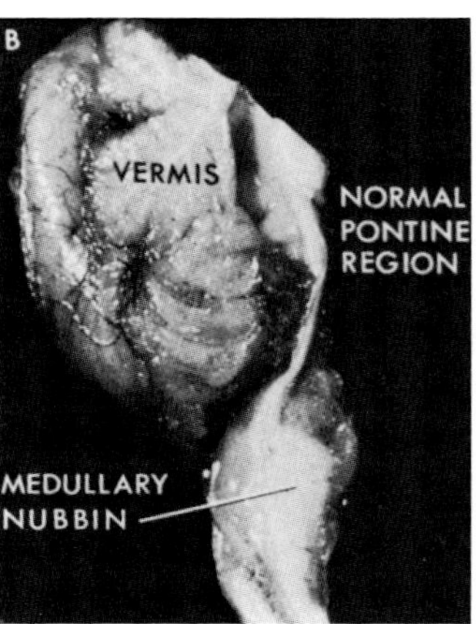

FIGURE 26.3 **A:** Normal relationship of the pons, medulla, and cerebellar vermis. **B:** The cerebellum is small and poorly formed. The pons is absent; the medulla is represented only by an aberrant nubbin of tissue. The brain stem is surrounded by glistening leptomeningeal, neuroglial heterotopia. Reproduced with permission from Clarren SK, et al. Brain malformation related to prenatal exposure to ethanol. J Pediatr 1978;92:64–67.

symptomatic infants, with tremors evolving into seizures as observed in adults (21,22). Therapy consists of short-term administration of a benzodiazepine such as lorazepam or of phenobarbital.

Late Effects

Follow-up studies of children with FAS have yielded conflicting results. A 10-year follow-up study of eleven

FIGURE 26.4 Photomicrograph of apical dendrites of layer V pyramidal neurons in consecutive segments from proximal to distal regions of cell body (1–2). **A** is control, aged 3 months; **B** is fetal alcohol syndrome at the age of 4 months. Decreased number of spines and predominance of spines with long, thin pedicles are observed in this child (Rapid Golgi method × 1,000). Reproduced with permission from Ferrer I, et al. Dendritic spine anomalies in fetal alcohol syndrome. Neuropediatrics 1987;18:161–163.

children with this syndrome revealed continued growth deficiency and dysmorphism; half of the children were of borderline intelligence while the other half were severely handicapped intellectually. The authors concluded that the degree of permanent handicap was correlated with the original extent of craniofacial abnormalities (23). In a larger prospective multidisciplinary study, however, affected children showed progressively less dysmorphism with age and a corresponding improvement in their neurologic handicap. Hyperactivity and distractibility persisted, however, despite rehabilitative treatment aimed at improving speech and sensorimotor skills (24).

Acute Ethanol Intoxication and Chronic Alcoholism

As in adults, the clinical symptoms of acute alcohol intoxication in children include sedation, ataxia, dysarthria, and disinhibition; and with increasing blood levels of alcohol, hypoglycemia, seizures, and coma may be present (25). Seizures are generalized and may occur during the intoxicated phase or during withdrawal. It should be recognized that the hypoglycemia associated with acute intoxication may also cause seizures.

The long-term sequelae of chronic alcoholism have been well described in the adult literature (26) and are not substantively different from those observed in patients who began drinking in late childhood or adolescence. All components of the nervous system are affected. Dementia can be caused by pellagra, hepatic dysfunction, cortical myelinolysis, thiamine deficiency, or the alcohol itself. Alcoholic cerebellar degeneration, central pontine myelinolysis, peripheral neuropathy, myopathy, and stroke are all associated problems in the chronic drinker.

OPIATES

Since the value of methadone for management of heroin addiction was recognized in 1965 (27), heroin addicts have been treated with methadone even throughout pregnancy, despite the fact that the use of either drug can cause neonatal addiction and withdrawal. The question of whether the effects of an opiate are less detrimental to normal fetal development than those of withdrawal from the drug in utero has been addressed by Kuwahara and Sparber (28). Fetal chicks were made opiate-dependent on day 3 of embryogenesis and subsequently exhibited profoundly depressed fetal mobility. The injection of naloxone caused a significant increase in their mobility, but also notably reduced their hatchability (28). Since similar experiments in other species corroborated these findings (29,30), it would appear that narcotic withdrawal in a developing organism may be more deleterious to its survival than continued in utero exposure to the drug.

Although experimental data have raised the possibility of impaired fetal brain growth and development resulting from the use of these drugs during pregnancy (31), clinical correlation is yet limited (32,33). As noted earlier, studies regarding intrauterine drug exposure have inherent limitations because of small patient populations, unreliable drug histories, and confounding social and environmental factors. However, despite these limitations, a number of important features have emerged since data collection began in the early 1970s.

Teratogenic Effects

The main concerns of clinicians, thus far, have been focused on the perinatal abstinence syndrome, the possibility of late effects on behavior and personality, and other associated medical problems of these high-risk infants. To date there has been little evidence that intrauterine exposure to opiates has significant postnatal sequelae for humans. In experimental animals, however, studies have repeatedly shown disturbances of brain growth, primarily by affecting macromolecular synthesis (34,35). Brain DNA, RNA, and protein synthesis are significantly decreased in the offspring of rats chronically exposed to morphine or methadone (Figure 26.5) (36). These effects seem to be independent of the nutritional deficit caused by the appetite suppressant effects of the opiates. The general pattern of growth delay observed in addicted animal pups is distinct from that caused by malnutrition. When rats exposed to opiates and their pair-fed controls were matched for ornithine decarboxylase activity, the delays were predominantly in the normal maturational decline of the brain enzyme, indicating a delay in cellular maturation in the drug-treated group (35).

Additional studies in the rat have shown disturbed synaptic development of the biogenic amines dopamine, norepinephrine, and serotonin. Available data indicate that opiates slow synaptogenesis and reduce vesicular uptake of biogenic amines, suggesting that the number of synaptic terminals is reduced, coincident with decreased brain weight and cell numbers (37).

Although animal data have shown these limitations in brain development at the cellular and biochemical level, and human data seem to support these observations, there is as yet no convincing evidence that opiates cause true malformations of the central nervous system (CNS) (38). When administered to hamsters at very high doses, opiates did cause disorders of neural tube development such as exencephaly, cranioschisis, and myelomeningocele (39), but currently there are no reports of impaired brain embryogenesis in humans caused solely by opiate exposure.

Passive Addiction and Withdrawal

The major immediate medical and neurologic problems of fetal opiate exposure arise when the narcotic-exposed neonate is born. In addition to systemic problems such as

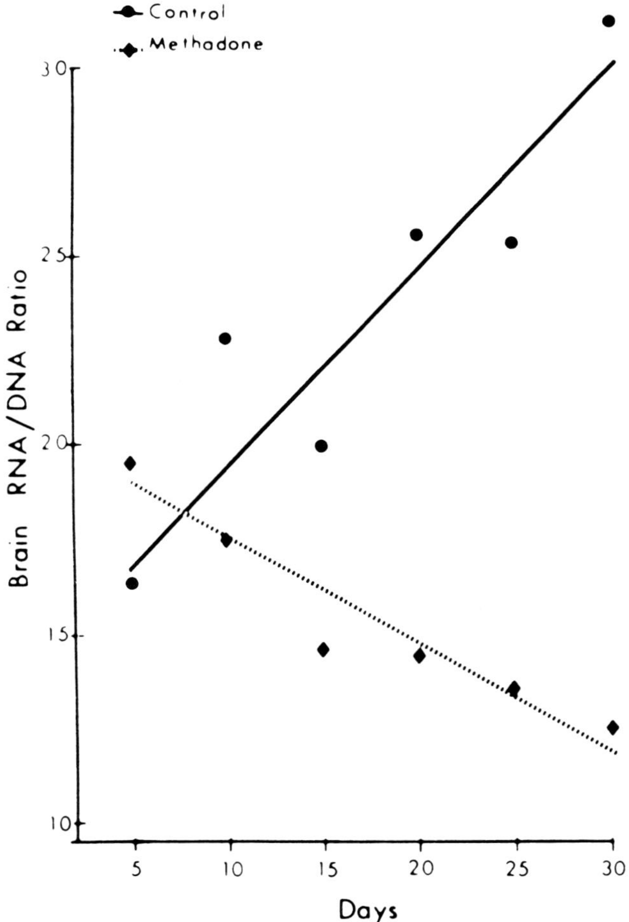

FIGURE 26.5   Ratio of brain RNA to DNA in offspring of control and treated female rats. Reproduced with permission from Peters MA. The effect of maternally administered methadone on brain development in the offspring. J Pharmacol Exp Therap 1977;203:340–346.

respiratory distress, jaundice, sepsis, and disturbed endocrine function (40), these infants may have signs of drug withdrawal (Table 26.3) (41), manifested primarily by signs of disturbed CNS function including jitteriness, hypertonia, disturbed sleep-wake cycles, irritability, and apnea (40). In one well-controlled study, opiate-addicted neonates were shown to have drug-related disorders of sleep, including decreased quiet sleep and increased active rapid eye movement (REM) sleep (42). This state of increased CNS arousal can persist from 3 to 6 months. The presence of withdrawal symptoms does not differ with respect to which opiate has been abused, although the outcome appears to be significantly better in infants born to women on supervised methadone maintenance (43). Most infants passively addicted to heroin have onset of symptoms in the first 24 hours of life, whereas methadone-exposed infants present slightly later, during the 2nd or 3rd day of life, and their symptoms last longer than those associated with heroin (44).

Seizures occur in 5% to 21% of neonates addicted to methadone and in 2% to 4% of heroin-exposed babies (45,46). In one study of 302 neonates passively addicted to narcotics, 18 had seizures that were predominantly generalized motor and myoclonic jerks. Interictal electroencephalograms (EEG) were normal, but some patients had focal or multifocal discharges preceding and accompanying clinical seizures (Table 26.4) (45). There was no apparent relationship between maternal opiate dosage and the frequency or severity of seizures (45). In one recent study, 14 neonates had seizures from opiate exposure, 12 of which were of myoclonic type. Multiple drug abuse was common, however, including cocaine, amphetamines, and barbiturates. Only five interictal EEGs were normal; the remainder showed bilateral or multifocal spike activity or unilateral sharp waves. Most abnormalities were observed when the EEG was done within 1 to 5 days of the seizure (46). Although the biochemical mechanisms of withdrawal-associated seizures are still unknown, the biochemical immaturity of neonatal brain must play a role because withdrawal seizures from opiates are rarely observed in

Table 26.3 Symptoms of drug withdrawal

W = Wakefulness
I = Irritability
T = Tremulousness, temperature variation, tachypnea
H = Hyperactivity, high-pitched persistent cry, hyperacusia, hyperreflexia, hypertonus
D = Diarrhea, diaphoresis, disorganized suck
R = Rub marks, respiratory distress, rhinorrhea
A = Apneic attacks, autonomic dysfunction
W = Weight loss or failure to gain weight
A = Alkalosis (respiratory)
L = Lacrimation

Adapted from Committee on Drugs. Neonatal drug withdrawal. Pediatrics 1983;72:895–902.

Table 26.4 Seizure types in neonatal withdrawal

Myoclonic
Generalized tonic–clonic
Multifocal clonic
Subtle (staring, blinking, lip smacking)

Seizure type in order of decreasing frequency observed in neonates withdrawing from narcotic analgesics.

Adapted with permission from Herzlinger RA, et al. Neonatal seizures associated with narcotic withdrawal. J Pediatr 1977; 91:638–641.

adults. The reduction of central catecholamine synthesis may potentiate cerebral excitability (47–49).

The types of pharmacologic agents used in the management of the withdrawal state include the sedative–hypnotic drugs (phenobarbital or diazepam), narcotic agonists (paregoric and other opium preparations), or phenothiazines (chlorpromazine). The comparative efficacy of these therapeutic approaches is yet unresolved, although one prospective randomized trial of opiates compared with CNS depressant therapy suggests that paregoric is the treatment of choice for the neonatal abstinence syndrome (50). The severity of signs of neonatal abstinence is influenced by perinatal variables such as gestational age, birth weight, Apgar score, treatment onset, and maternal factors including the length of drug use and time of last methadone dose. Comparison of the impact of either an opiate (paregoric) or a CNS depressant (phenobarbital) showed that although control of CNS, autonomic, and gastrointestinal signs did not differ between groups, 7 of the 62 neonates treated with phenobarbital had abstinence-associated seizures, while none occurred in the paregoric treated neonates. Because paregoric is also nonsedating and does not seem to alter sucking behavior, it appears to be preferred over drugs that may cause cardiorespiratory depression and feeding impairment.

Paregoric contains anhydrous morphine (0.4 mg/mL), opium alkaloids, camphor, and high concentrations of alcohol (44% to 46%), benzoic acid 4 mg/mL, and glycerine. It is administered until seizures are controlled (dose range 0.8 to 2.0 mL/kg day divided every 8 hours) and should then be tapered over the next 3 to 5 days. Tincture of opium also contains opiate alkaloids and morphine (10 mg/mL) but in a weaker alcohol preparation (17% to 21%); a 25-fold dilution contains the morphine equivalent of 0.4 mg/mL, which is the same as paregoric without the disadvantages of other additives (41). Oral preparations of morphine (2 or 4 mg/mL) containing no additives and even less alcohol (10%) are now available. Oral methadone contains chlorobutanol (0.5 mg/mL), which is a sedative, and 8% alcohol.

Parenteral diazepam contains high concentrations of propylene glycol (40%) and ethanol (10%) and is contraindicated in icteric or premature infants because of its ability to displace bilirubin from plasma protein binding sites. If used, despite these limitations, the dose is 0.04 to 0.1 mg/kg/dose every 2 to 4 hours.

Parenteral phenobarbital also contains high concentrations of propylene glycol (68%), as well as ethanol (10%) and benzyl alcohol (1.5%); phenobarbital elixirs contain 14% to 25% ethanol. Although phenobarbital is adequate for control of seizures and hyperactivity, it does not control gastrointestinal symptoms, it acts as a cardiorespiratory suppressant, and it may cause feeding impairment. If used, a maintenance dose of 8 mg/kg/day is required and should be decreased by 10% to 20%/day when the condition of the neonate has been stabilized.

Subacute opiate withdrawal, manifested as recurrent seizures, occurs in up to 80% of those who exhibit withdrawal in the perinatal period. Tremors, restlessness, and irritability with disturbed sleep states are common for 3 to 6 months after hospital discharge (51).

Other Postnatal Sequelae and Late Effects

Perhaps the most life-threatening sequelae of maternal opiate abuse are due not to narcotic withdrawal, but rather to the increased risk of the sudden infant death syndrome (SIDS) and the acquired immune deficiency syndrome (AIDS). The incidence of SIDS in these infants is five times greater than in the general population (52), and because of the generally high rate of HIV positivity in opiate-addicted mothers, transplacental passage of the virus is common. Infectivity rates are currently about 30% (53%; personal communication). The direct neurologic sequelae of passive opiate addiction and withdrawal in infants are, thus, further complicated by the potential effects of HIV invasion of the CNS (See Chapter 25).

The late effects of intrauterine opiate exposure on development are thought to be significant and are difficult to analyze, partly because of factors discussed earlier, but also because many complex variables are associated with creating a well-balanced individual. Nonetheless, this important issue has been studied in the last decade but with conflicting results.

Wilson et al. (54) matched a group of children born to heroin-addicted mothers with three comparative groups: those with postnatal exposure to a drug culture; children considered high risk on the basis of medical factors; and children of similar socioeconomic backgrounds. They found that children of the heroin-exposed group in the age range of 3 to 6 years were smaller and included a greater number of children with head circumference less than the third percentile. Although mean intelligence quotients (IQ) scores did not differ between the matched groups, the heroin-exposed children performed more poorly than the comparison groups on the general cognitive index and the McCarthy scales of children's abilities. The major deficiencies were in areas of perceptual performance, quantitative tasks, and memory. Overall, maladaptive behavior patterns, marked by impulsiveness, uncontrollable temper, and poor self-confidence, predominated in the heroin-exposed group (54).

Later studies by Wilson did not subtantiate the somatotropic growth delay observed in earlier studies of his group (55). The postnatal growth of children exposed to opiates in utero was no more impaired than that of a high-risk comparison group (56). However, even though weight and length parameters showed a "catch up" by 9 months of age, the head circumference remained significantly smaller throughout the first 2 years of life.

Some animal studies appear to have corroborated Wilson's observations of neurobehavioral alterations in these infants by showing disturbed behavioral control. One study, for example, demonstrated an impaired ability of adult rats to modulate task-oriented motor activity after prenatal exposure to methadone (57). The studies of Chasnoff, et al. appear to confirm the inability of opiate-exposed infants to perform well on interactive behaviors (58). Other prospective studies, however, have not confirmed Wilson's findings regarding neurobehavior, but the children were followed until 2 years of age, and only Bayley scales were used to interpret changes (56).

Proper prenatal and postnatal care, rather than drug exposure, may be the single most important factor in determining the outcome of patients. The full impact of drug exposure, however, cannot be ascertained until large populations of these affected children have been followed through their complete development, as in the case of ethanol-exposed children. Current figures from screening programs in Rhode Island (59) and Florida estimate that 8% to 15% of pregnant women abuse drugs. There was no difference in prevalence insofar as race or socioeconomic status was concerned, although poor black women were more likely to be reported (60).

COCAINE

There was great interest in the medical consequences of cocaine use during the 1930s, but that interest slackened and became overshadowed by other more prevalent drugs of abuse. Recently, there has been a medical reawakening to these complications because of the current epidemic of cocaine abuse. In 1986, the National Institute on Drug Abuse estimated that almost 15% of the United States population had tried cocaine and that three million people regularly abused cocaine (61). The increased use of the drug has been attributed to the greater availability of the cheaper smoked form of cocaine known as "crack," to its heightened addictive qualities, and to the fact that blood levels are achieved within seconds following its inhalation.

Because of widespread use, cocaine abuse during pregnancy is now a common problem. Prenatal morbidity is increased as more infants are exposed to the drug in utero, and reports of teratogenic effects, small for gestational age babies with microcephaly, seizures, and neonatal stroke from cocaine exposed pregnancies are increasing. Indeed, pregnancy outcomes are poor even when compared with other drug-exposed groups. An increase in spontaneous abortion, abruptio placenta, fetal wastage, prematurity, and precipitous labor have been documented (62,63). Long-term studies to determine late effects on development are in progress, but preliminary reports indicate that neurobehavioral abnormalities persist at least throughout the 1st month of life (64). The incidence of SIDS may also be increased in comparison with that of the general population (65,66), but a recent prospective study showed that when cocaine-exposed neonates were matched to a socioeconomic nondrug-exposed cohort, there was no increased risk (67). Because the cocaine story is still unfolding, most data are incomplete and are derived from series of small numbers of patients in select populations. Caution, therefore, is needed in interpreting the information.

Teratogenic Effects

Despite the limitations of studies (for example, uncontrolled variables of nutrition, and coincident ethanol consumption), certain effects of cocaine abuse have consistently been reported. It is clear that infants exposed to cocaine are smaller and that a significant number of them have decreased head circumference. Whether this reflects a decrease in neuronal size or number remains to be seen. The pathophysiology of the growth disturbance is unknown, but a recent study of pregnant ewes showed that maternal administration of cocaine produced marked dose-dependent increases in uterine vascular resistance and maternal blood pressure and decreased uterine blood flow. These abnormalities of maternal hemodynamics resulted in fetal hypoxemia, hypertension, and tachycardia (68). The impairment in fetal oxygenation suggests a plausible mechanism for decreased growth.

Reports of associated cardiac anomalies (transposition of the great vessels, hypoplastic right heart, ventricular septal defects), genitourinary tract malformations, skull defects (encephalocele, parietal bone defects), and sacral exotosis are emerging as more babies exposed to cocaine are recognized (69,70). However, a recent prospective study found no increase in teratogenicity per se, although significant intrauterine growth retardation and microcephaly were seen (71).

There are few available animal studies, but one study with mice showed teratogenic effects with low doses of cocaine (72). Exencephaly, hydronephrosis, and cryptorchidism, multiple bony abnormalities, anophthalmia,

and malformed lenses were seen. Pregnant rats given cocaine had significant reduction in fetal weight and increased fetal wastage (73). One in vitro study of the effect of cocaine on primary cultures of mouse embryonic brain cells showed that although no gross changes were evident in cell morphology, there was a slight retardation of growth as measured by total protein content. During the peak period of acetylcholinesterase activity, there was a significant decrease in activity in the cocaine group. These cumulative data suggest that cocaine can disturb neurons in the developing brain (74).

Passive Addiction and Perinatal Effects

It is now clear that cocaine causes a postnatal abstinence syndrome similar to that seen in narcotic-exposed infants. Neonates show signs of withdrawal by the 2nd day of life, characterized by irritability, jitteriness, and hypertonia. An increased frequency of abnormal sleep patterns, poor feeding, vomiting, high-pitched cry, frantic fist sucking, tachypnea, fever, loose stools, and yawning have been observed. Transient signs of CNS irritability manifested by tremors and hypertonia were seen in 87% of neonates with intravenous cocaine exposure (Table 26.5) (75). Almost half of patients had EEG abnormalities during the 1st week of life that persisted when repeated later in the neonatal period; only one child of this group had a persistently abnormal record (76).

Multiple investigators have reported neurobehavioral abnormalities as measured by the Brazelton Behavioral Scale of neonatal assessment. Depressed interactive abilities and significant impairment of organizational abilities have been noted, and visual processing, particularly, seems to be affected (75,77). Abnormal visual evoked potentials (VEP), as well as absent saccades on visual pursuit, have been observed in two small series of patients. Visual processing of faces and objects is poor, and long dull-alert periods

Table 26.5 Neurologic abnormalities during neonatal cocaine withdrawal

Abnormal sleep patterns
Tremors
Poor feeding
Hypertonia
Vomiting
Sneezing
High-pitched cry
Frantic fist sucking
Tachypnea
Yawning
Fever

Adapted with permission from Oro AS, et al. Perinatal cocaine and methamphetamine exposure: Maternal and neonatal correlates. J Pediatr 1987;111:571–578.

Table 26.6 Neurologic problems in cocaine-exposed neonates

Microcephaly
Seizures
Clinical withdrawal
Stroke
Abnormal visual processing
Germinal matrix cysts
Periventricular leukomalacia
Intraparenchymal cysts

with eyes open characterize the awake state. Auditory processing may also be affected with one study showing prolonged Wave I–V latency in infants born to cocaine-abusing mothers (78). Further studies are needed to determine whether these findings point to abnormal auditory system development or function.

Sensitive behavioral procedures in laboratory animals have demonstrated behavioral disruptions produced by withdrawal of cocaine that are independent of classic physical symptomatology (79). Therefore, even infants who are not overtly sick and symptomatic from cocaine withdrawal may exhibit subtle behavioral changes that could affect neurodevelopment.

Recent reports of stroke and CNS lesions in cocaine babies are particularly alarming (Table 26.6; Figure 26.6) (77,80). Both hemorrhagic and thrombotic cerebrovascular lesions have been reported, in addition to cystic lesions, germinal matrix cysts, and periventricular leucomalacia (Figure 26.7) (80–83).

Since the occurrence of seizures in these babies often heralds stroke, a complete neurologic evaluation is required, including adequate neuroimaging. Treatment of seizures with phenobarbital only during the symptomatic period is adequate; however, in children with CNS lesions and persistently abnormal EEGs, long-term therapy is necessary. There have been no reports of CNS vascular anomalies, but the iris vasculature has been reported as tortuous and dilated in cocaine-intoxicated babies (Figure 26.8) (84)

In adults, cocaine is detoxified by plasma and liver cholinesterases to the water-soluble metabolites benzoyl-ecgonine and ecgonine methyl-ester, which are then excreted in the urine. However, because plasma cholinesterase activity is much lower in fetuses, infants, and pregnant women (85), there is a longer half-life of the drug as it takes longer to clear from the blood. One report indicates that neonates and pregnant women metabolize cocaine via N-demethylation yielding the N-demethyl product, norcocaine, which is highly biologically active (85). These factors probably account for the increased sensitivity of small doses in these groups. Because cocaine metabolites may persist in the urine of an infant for more than 4 days, urine screening is a very effective method of detection.

Cocaine intoxication has also been reported after breast feeding and during the topical application of cocaine to indurated nipples while breast feeding. Symptoms of irritability and tremulousness occurred soon after feeding

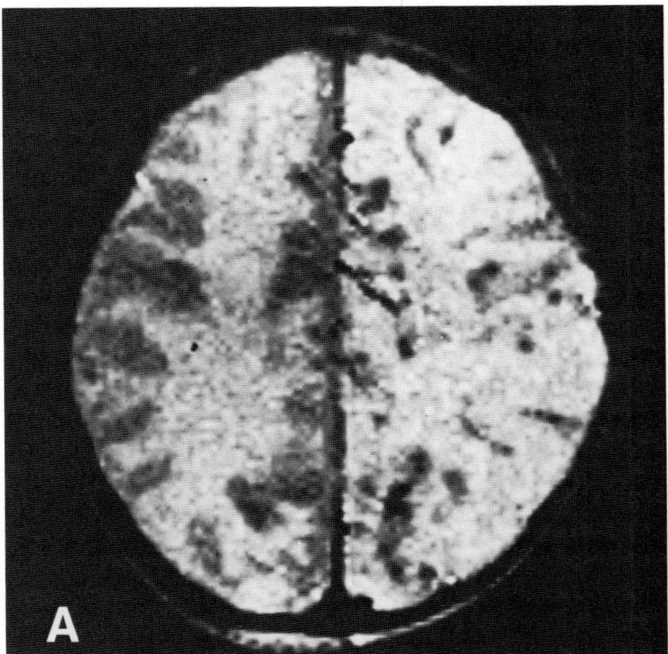
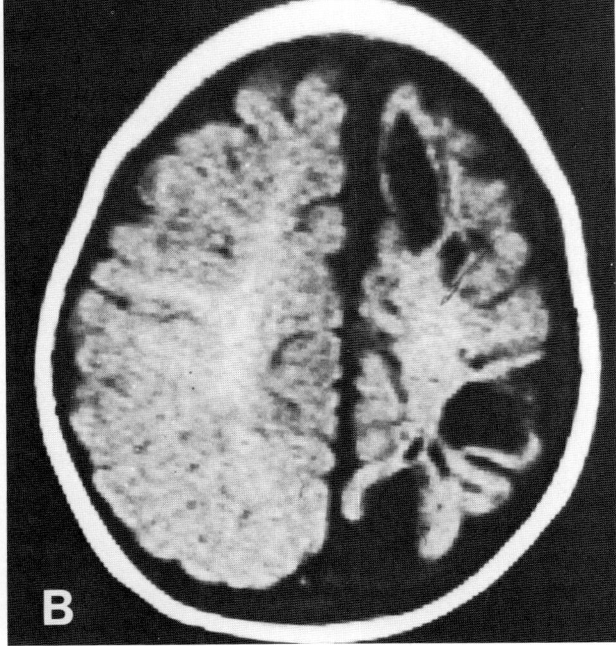

FIGURE 26.6 MRI brain scan of cocaine-exposed neonate showing edema of left cerebral hemisphere at four days (A). Follow-up MRI scan (B) at age four months shows infarction involving the anterior, middle, and posterior cerebral artery circulations. Reproduced with permission from Ferriero DM, et al. Congenital defects and stroke in cocaine-exposed neonates. Ann Neurol 1988;24:348–349 [abstract].

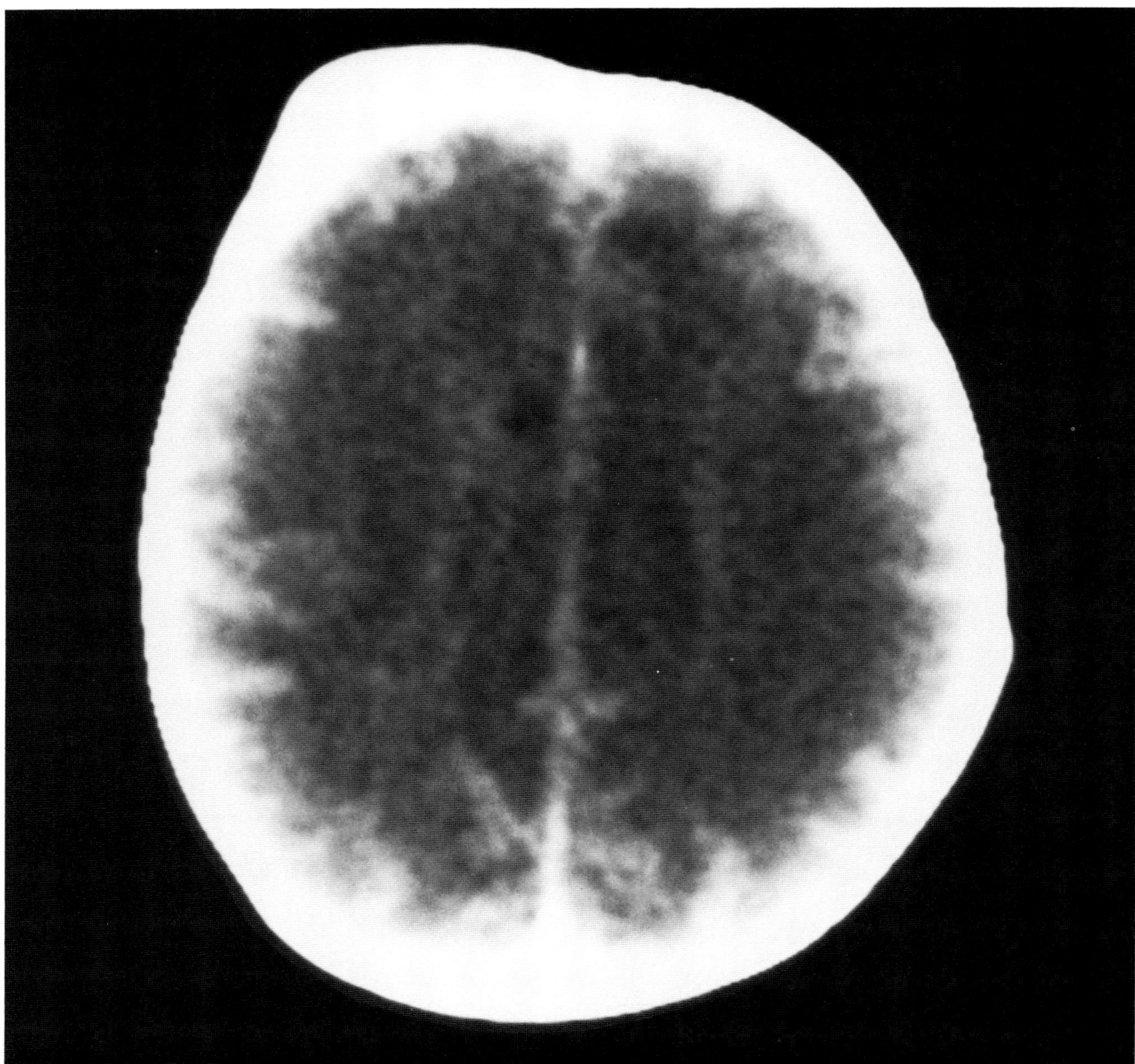

FIGURE 26.7   CT brain scan of cocaine/amphetamine-exposed neonate on the 2nd day of life, showing small intraparenchymal cyst in the right hemisphere. Reproduced with permission from Ferriero DM, et al. Congenital defects and stroke in cocaine-exposed neonates. Ann Neurol 1988;24:348–349 [abstract].

and has persisted for 48 hours after the cessation of breast feeding (86).

Late Effects

Persistent neurobehavioral abnormalities are a major concern for these drug-exposed babies. Preliminary data indicate the persistence of difficulties beyond infancy, but confirmation of this fact awaits long-term studies. The eventual outcome of infants presenting with seizures in the neonatal period is also unknown; and whether they develop epilepsy will depend, in part, on the presence and severity of an underlying CNS lesion.

The complications of cocaine abuse in adolescents are similar to those observed in the adult population. Seizures, status epilepticus, hemorrhagic (arteriovenous malformation or aneurysm rupture) or thrombotic stroke, and focal neurologic deficits have been described (87). Headache, transient loss of consciousness, and acute psychiatric dis-

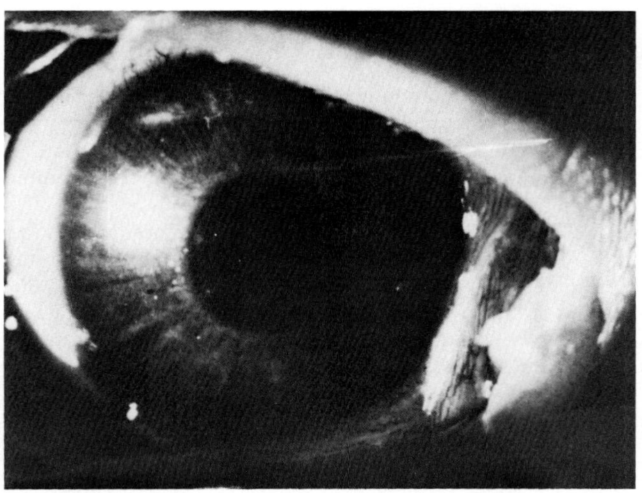

FIGURE 26.8 The superior portion of the iris showing dilated and tortuous blood vessels. Reproduced with permission from Isenberg SJ, et al. Ocular signs of cocaine intoxication in neonates. Am J Ophthalmol 1987;103:211–214.

turbances including dysphoria, agitation, assaultiveness, paranoia, psychosis, and hallucinations may occur. Although the mechanisms are unknown, the psychiatric disturbances are probably related to the effect of cocaine on the metabolism of norepinephrine, dopamine, and serotonin.

The full impact of cocaine addiction will not be realized for another decade, when the current generation of cocaine-exposed neonates will have completed their development. Careful follow-up studies of these children should then provide the necessary information regarding the late effects of cocaine on human neurodevelopment.

REFERENCES

1. Carpenter WB. Use and Abuse of Alcoholic Liquors. Boston: Crosby and Nichols, 1851. For Massachusetts Temperance Society.
2. Lemoine P, Harousseau H, Borteyru J-P, et al. Les enfants de parents alcooliques: Anomalies observées, à propos de 127 cas. Arch Fr Pediatr 1968;25:830–831.
3. Jones KL, Smith DW, Ulleland CN, et al. Patterns of malformation in offspring of chronic alcoholic mothers. Lancet 1973;1:1267–1271.
4. Clarren SK, Smith DW. The fetal alcohol syndrome. N Engl J Med 1978;298:1063–1067.
5. Chernoff GF. The fetal alcohol syndrome in mice: An animal model. Teratology 1977;15:223–230.
6. Sandor S. The influences of ethyl alcohol on developing chick embryo II. Rev Roum Embryol 1968;5:167–171.
7. Tze WJ, Lee M. Adverse effects of maternal alcohol consumption on pregnancy and fetal growth in rats. Nature 1975;257:479–480.
8. Breen JF, Loomis CW, Tranmer J, et al. Disposition of ethanol in human maternal venous blood and amniotic fluid. Am J Obstet Gynecol 1983;146:181–186.
9. Pikharainen PH, Räihä NCR. Development of alcohol dehydrogenase activity in the human liver. Pediatr Res 1967;1:165–168.
10. Erickson CK. Regular distribution of ethanol in rat brain. Life Sci 1976;19:1439–1446.
11. Dow KE, Riopelle RJ. Neurotoxicity of ethanol during prenatal development. Clin Neuropharmacol 1987;10:330–341.
12. Marcus JC. Neurologic findings in the fetal alcohol syndrome. Neuropediatrics 1987;18:158–160.
13. Wisniewski K, Dambska M, Sher JH, et al. A clinical neuropathologic study of fetal alcohol syndrome. Neuropediatrics 1983;14:197–201.
14. Clarren SK, Alvord EC, Sumi SM, et al. Brain malformation related to prenatal exposure to ethanol. J Pediatr 1978;92:64–67.
15. Ferrer I, Galofré E. Dendritic spine anomalies in fetal alcohol syndrome. Neuropediatrics 1987;18:161–163.
16. Miller MW. Effect of prenatal exposure to alcohol on the distribution and time of origin of corticospinal neurons in the rat. J Comp Neurol 1987;257:372–382.
17. Vingar RD, Dow-Edwards DL, Riley EP. Cerebral metabolic alterations in rats following prenatal alcohol exposure: A deoxyglucose study. Alcoholism Clin Exp Res 1986;10:22–26
18. Davies DL, Vermakadis A. Effects of ethanol on cultured glial cells: Proliferation and glutamine synthetase activity. Dev Brain Res 1984;16:27–35.
19. Dow KE, Riopelle RJ. Ethanol neurotoxicity: Effects on neurite formation and neurotrophic factor production in vitro. Science 1985;228:591–593.
20. Coles CD, Smith IE, Fernhoff PM, et al. Neonatal ethanol withdrawal: Characteristics in clinically normal, nondysmorphic neonates. J Pediatr 1984;105:445–451.
21. Nichols MM. Acute alcohol withdrawal syndrome in a newborn. Am J Dis Child 1967;113:714–715.
22. Robe LB, Gromisch DS, Losub S. Symptoms of neonatal ethanol withdrawal. Curr Alcohol 1981;8:484–491.
23. Streissguth AP, Clarren SK, Jones KL. Natural history of the fetal alcohol syndrome: a 10-year follow-up of eleven patients. Lancet 1985;1:85–91.
24. Spohr H-L, Steinhausen H-Chr. Follow-up studies of children with fetal alcohol syndrome. Neuropediatrics 1987;18:13–17.
25. Cummins LH. Hypoglycemia and convulsions in children following alcohol ingestion. J Pediatr 1961;58:23.
26. Messing RO, Greenberg DA. Alcohol and the nervous system. In: Aminoff MJ, ed. Neurology and general medicine. New York: Churchill Livingstone, 1989;29:533–547.

27. Dole VP, Nyswander ME. Rehabilitation of heroin addicts after blockade with methadone. NY State J Med 1966; 66:2011–2017.

28. Kuwahara MD, Sparber SB. Prenatal withdrawal from opiates interferes with hatching of otherwise viable chick fetuses. Science 1981;212:945–947.

29. Cohen MS, Rudolph AM, Melmon KL. Antagonism of morphine by naloxone in pregnant ewes and fetal lambs. Dev Pharmacol Therap 1980;1:58–69.

30. Lichtblau L, Sparber SB. Opiate withdrawal in utero increases neonatal morbidity in rat. Science 1981; 212:943–945.

31. Lichtblau L, Sparber SB. Opioids and development: A perspective on experimental models and methods. Neurobehav Toxicol Teratol 1984;6:3–8.

32. Chasnoff IJ, Burns KA, Burns WJ, et al. Prenatal drug exposure: Effects on neonatal and infant growth and development. Neurobehav Toxicol Teratol 1986;8:357–362.

33. Hutchings DE. Methadone and heroin during pregnancy: A review of behavioral effects in human and animal offspring. Neurobehav Toxicol Teratol 1982;4:429–434.

34. Seidler FJ, Whitmore WL, Slotkin TA. Delays in growth and biochemical development of rat brain caused by maternal methadone administration: Are the alterations in synaptogenesis and cellular maturation independent of baseline materal food intake? Dev Neurosci 1982;5:13–18.

35. Johannesson T, Steele WJ, Becker BA. Infusion of morphine in maternal rats at near-term—Maternal and fetal distribution and effects on analgesia, brain DNA, RNA and protein. Acta Pharmacol Toxicol 1972;31:353–368.

36. Peters MA. The effect of maternally administered methadone on brain development in the offspring. J Pharmacol Exp Therap 1977;203:340–346.

37. Slothkin TA, Whitmore WL, Salvaggio M, et al. Perinatal methadone addiction affects brain synaptic development of biogenic amino systems in the rat. Life Sci 1979; 24:1223–1230.

38. Ostrea EM, Chavez CJ. Perinatal problems (excluding neonatal withdrawal) in maternal drug addiction: a study of 830 cases. J Pediatr 1979;94:292–295.

39. Geber WF, Schramm LC. Congenital malformation of the CNS produced by narcotic analgesics in the hamster. Am J Obstet Gynecol 1975;123:705–713.

40. Bashore RA, Ketchum JS, Staisch KJ, et al. Heroin addiction and pregnancy. West J Med 1981;134:506–514.

41. Committee on Drugs. Neonatal drug withdrawal. Pediatrics 1983;72:895–902.

42. Dinges DF, Davis MM, Glass P: Fetal exposure to narcotics: neonatal sleep as a measure of nervous system disturbance. Science 1980;209:619–621.

43. Stimmel B, Goldberg J, Reisman A, et al. Fetal outcome in narcotic dependent women: The importance of the type of maternal narcotic used. Am J Drug Alcohol Abuse 1982–3; 9:383–395.

44. Rajegowda BK, Glass L, Evans HE, et al. Methadone withdrawal in newborn infants. J Pediatr 1972;81:532–534.

45. Herzlinger RA, Kandall SR, Vaughan HG. Neonatal seizures associated with narcotic withdrawal. J Pediatr 1977; 91:638–641.

46. Doberzak TM, Shanger S, Cutler R, et al. One year follow-up of infants with abstinence-associated seizures. Arch Neurol 1988;45:649–668.

47. Engel JE, Katzman R. Facilitation of amygdaloid kindling by lesions of the stria terminalis. Brain Res 1977;122:137–142.

48. Rosenman ST, Smith CB. C-catecholamine synthesis in mouse brain during morphine withdrawal. Nature 1972; 240:153–155.

49. McGinty JF, Ford DH. Effects of prenatal methadone on rat brain catecholamines. Dev Neurosci 1980;3:224–234.

50. Kandall SR, Doberzah TM, Mauer KR, et al. Opiate vs. CNS depressant therapy in neonatal drug abstinence syndrome. Am J Dis Child 1983;137:378–382.

51. Chasnoff IJ. Perinatal addiction: Consequences of intrauterine exposure to opiate and nonopiate drugs. In: Chasnoff IJ, ed. Drug Use in Pregnancy. Boston: MTP Press Ltd, 1986; 52–64.

52. Chavez CJ, Ostrea EM, Stryker JC, et al. SIDS among infants of drug dependent mothers. J Pediatr 1979;95:407–409.

53. Alroomi LG, Davidson J, Evans TJ, et al. Maternal narcotic abuse and the newborn. Arch Dis Child 1988;63:81–83.

54. Wilson GS, McGeary R, Kean J, et al. The development of preschool children of heroin-addicted mothers: A controlled study. Pediatrics 1979;63:135–141.

55. Lifschitz MH, Wilson GS, Smith EO, et al. Fetal and postnatal growth of children born to narcotic dependent women. J Pediatr 1983;102:686–691.

56. Gal P, Sharpless MK. Fetal drug-exposure-behavioral teratogenesis. Drug Intell Clin Pharm 1984:18:186–201.

57. Hutchings DE, Towey JP, Gounson HS, et al. Methadone during pregnancy: Assessment of behavioral effects in rat offspring. J Pharmacol Exp Ther 1979;208:106–111.

58. Chasnoff IJ, Hatcher R, Burns WJ. Polydrug and methadone-addicted newborns: A continuum of impairment? Pediatrics 1982;70:210–213.

59. Griffin J, Hollinshead W, Jones S. Statewide prevalence of illicit drug use by pregnant women—Rhode Island. MMWR 13 April 1990;39:225–227.

60. Chasnoff IJ, Landress HJ, Barrette ME. The prevalence of illicit drug or alcohol use during pregnancy and discrepancies in mandatory reporting in Pinellas County, Florida; N Engl J Med 1990;322:1202–1206.

61. Gawin F, Ellinwood E. Cocaine and other stimulants: Actions, abuse and treatment. N Engl J Med 1988; 318:1173–1182.

62. Chasnoff IJ, Burns WJ, Schnoll SH, et al. Cocaine use in pregnancy. N Engl J Med 1985;313:666–669.

63. MacGregor SN, Keith LG, Chasnoff IJ, et al. Cocaine use during pregnancy: Adverse perinatal outcome. Am J Obstet Gynecol 1987;157:686–690.

64. Griffith D, Chasnoff IJ, Dirkes K, et al. Neurobehavioral development of cocaine-exposed infants in the first month. Pediatr Res 1988;23:210 [abstract].

65. Riley JG, Brodsky NL, Porat R. Risk for SIDS in infants with in utero cocaine exposure: a prospective study. Pediatr Res 1988;23:454 [abstract].

66. Bauchner HC, McClain M, Frank DA, et al. Cocaine use during pregnancy and the risk of SIDS. Pediatr Res 1988; 23:319 [abstract].

67. Bauchner H, Zuckerman B, McClain M, et al. Risk of SIDS among infants with in utero exposure to cocaine. J Pediatr 1988;113:831–834.

68. Woods J, Plessinger M, Clark K. Effect of cocaine on uterine blood flow and fetal oxygenation. JAMA 1987; 257:957–961.

69. Bingol N, Fuchs M, Diaz V, et al. Teratogenicity of cocaine withdrawal in humans. J Pediatr 1987;110:93–96.

70. Madden JD, Payne TF, Muller S. Maternal cocaine abuse and effect on the newborn. Pediatrics 1986;77:209–211.

71. Hadeed A, Siegel SR. Maternal cocaine use during pregnancy: effect on the newborn infant. Pediatrics 1989;84:205–210.

72. Mahalik MP, Gautiere RF, Mann DE. Teratogenic potential of cocaine hydrochloride in CF-1 mice. J Pharm Sci 1980;69:703–706.

73. Fantel AG, MacPhail BJ. The teratogenicity of cocaine. Teratology 1982;26:17–19.

74. Matthews S, Tyrala EE, Rao GS. Effect on intra-uterine exposure of cocaine on acetylcholine esterase (ACE) in primary cultures of embryonic mouse brain cells. Pediatr Res 1988;23:418 [abstract].

75. Oro AS, Dixon SD. Perinatal cocaine and methamphetamine exposure: Maternal and neonatal correlates. J Pediatr 1987;111:571–578.

76. Doberzak TM, Shanzer S, Senie RT, et al. Neonatal neurologic and electroencephalographic effects of intrauterine cocaine exposure. J Pediatr 1988;113:758–763.

77. Ferriero DM, Wong DF, Townsend R, et al. Neurological complications in infants of cocaine abusing mothers. Neurology 1988;38:163 [abstract].

78. Shih L, Cone-Wesson B, Reddix B, et al. Effects of maternal cocaine abuse on the neonatal auditory system. Pediatr Res 1988;23:264 [abstract].

79. Carroll ME, Lac ST. Cocaine withdrawal produces behavioral disruptions in rats. Life Sci 1987;40:2183–2190.

80. Chasnoff I, Bussey M, Savich R. Perinatal cerebral infarction and maternal cocaine use. J Pediatr 1986;108:456–459.

81. Ferriero DM, Partridge JC, Wong DF. Congenital defects and stroke in cocaine-exposed neonates. Ann Neurol 1988;24:348–349 [abstract].

82. Dixon S, Bejar R. Brain lesion in cocaine and methamphetamine exposed neonates. Pediatr Res 1988;23:405 [abstract].

83. Cohen H, DeMarinis P, daSilva M, et al. Cranial sonography in infants of alkaloidal cocaine ("crack") abusing mothers. Pediatr Res 1988;23:551 [abstract].

84. Isenberg SJ, Spierer A, Inkelis SH. Ocular signs of cocaine intoxication in neonates. Am J Ophthalmol 1987;103:211–214.

85. Chasnoff IJ, Lewis DE. Cocaine metabolism during pregnancy. Pediatr Res 1988;23:257 [abstract].

86. Chasnoff IJ, Lewis DE, Squires L. Cocaine intoxication in a breast-fed infant. Pediatrics 1987;80:836–838.

87. Lowenstein DH, Massa SM, Rowbotham MC, et al. Acute neurologic and psychiatric complications associated with cocaine abuse. Am J Med 1987;83:841–846.

Chapter 27
Adverse Neurologic Effects of Chemotherapy and Radiation Therapy

Bruce H. Cohen and Roger J. Packer

Six to seven thousand children in the United States will develop cancer each year. Although cancer results in more childhood deaths than any other disease, survival rates have improved over the last few decades (1,2). Long-term disease control is now possible in the majority of patients with acute lymphocytic leukemia, Hodgkin lymphoma, primitive neuroectodermal tumors (medulloblastoma), and other childhood malignancies. Chemotherapeutic agents, advanced radiation therapy techniques, and the ability to treat complications have been, in part, responsible for improved survival. Treatment itself, however, carries with it the possibility of different types of central nervous system (CNS) damage. The standard therapeutic approach employed in treating many forms of childhood cancers is based on the principle, first outlined by Goldie and Coldman (3), that tumor drug resistance may be avoided by using as many neoplastic agents in as large a tolerated dose as possible, early in treatment. Added benefit is obtained in some treatment protocols by using chemotherapy in doses much larger than conventional amounts or by delivering the chemotherapy in other than a standard (oral or intravenous) fashion; that is, via intrathecal (IT), intraventricular, or intraarterial routes. For more efficacy, radiation therapy usually must be given in doses approximating the normal tolerance of the CNS. Newer radiation therapeutic approaches utilize significantly larger total doses, given by employing different types of radiotherapy (electron beam vs. photon), delivery systems (direct implantation), or fractionation of radiotherapy (hyperfractionation).

A variety of often poorly understood host factors also determines the degree of treatment-related neurologic sequelae. There are many well-recognized neurologic syndromes that result from specific treatments. Defining the etiology of many neurologic sequelae can be difficult especially since the deleterious effects of cancer treatment may be delayed. The clinician is often faced with a patient whose impairment may be due to tumor, multiple chemotherapeutic agents, radiation therapy acting in concert with chemotherapy, metabolic derangements due to the tumor or treatment, infection, or combinations of the above. This chapter will review the acute, subacute, and long-term neurotoxicities of radiation therapy and chemotherapy presently utilized in the treatment of childhood cancer.

RADIATION THERAPY

Therapeutic irradiation is used as a primary modality or in combination with chemotherapy in treating many childhood cancers including brain tumors, acute lymphocytic leukemia, the lymphomas, sarcomas, and others. It is also used in a palliative fashion for treating tumor pain. The dosage and techniques used in delivering radiation therapy are determined by the tumor type and extent and the age of the patient. As with any cancer treatment modality, the goal is to maximize tumor cell death and minimize the effect on the normal surrounding tissue (4,5).

The most common form of radiation therapy currently used is the photon (X-ray or gamma ray). Photons produce intracellular free radicals that interact with and damage DNA. Cell death does not occur immediately but usually occurs at the subsequent mitotic phase following irradiation, although some damaged cells may survive 1 or 2 additional cell divisions (6). Cells in the mitotic and early DNA synthetic phase are more sensitive than cells in the resting phase (7,8). Both malignant and normal cells have mechanisms for repair. In the nervous system, cells capable of division include the endothelial cell and to a lesser degree, the glial cells, especially in young children. These cell types and not the neuron itself, appear to suffer the primary damage induced by radiation. Neuronal damage follows the death of these supporting elements.

A number of factors are critical variables with respect to both the clinical response of tumors to irradiation, and to the harmful side effects. First, cell survival falls exponentially as the dose of radiation is increased. Smaller tumors respond better than larger ones. Oxygen concentration also influences cell survival, as hypoxic regions in the central necrotic portions of tumors require 2 to 3 times the radiation dose to achieve the same fraction of cell death as the better oxygenated tissue at the tumor periphery (9). The time interval between radiation dosages is also important. Most radiation therapy protocols (standard fractionation) require daily fractions of radiation 5 days a week, allowing 24 to 48 hours for cellular repair to occur. Hyperfractionation, the practice of dividing the normal total daily dose into 2 or more doses separated by 4 or more hours, takes advantage of the ability of normal cells to repair DNA damage faster than tumor cells. This theoretical advantage allows for larger total doses to be given without a corresponding increase in the damaging effects (10).

The final variable, and most important in regard both to tumor effect and neurologic damage, is the total dose and energy level of the radiation. The unit of dosage currently being used is the Gray (Gy), defined as 1 joule of energy absorbed by 1 kg of tissue (1Gy = 100 cGy = 100 rad). The energy level of the photon is determined by the source, with levels ranging from 100,000 eV to 400,000 eV (orthovoltage) to 4 to 18 x 10^6 eV (megavoltage) now being delivered with linear accelerators. Higher energy levels allow for the majority of energy transfer to occur at deeper levels, partially sparing the normal tissues in the path of the beam. Treatment dosage is based on tumor histology but is limited by tolerance of normal tissues. In the course of radiation therapy, normal tissue is exposed to a substantial degree. In treating brain tumors, the field of treatment, referred to as the target volume, depends upon the type of tumor treated. Patients with malignant tumors (medulloblastoma and germinomas, among others) that tend to

disseminate through the cerebrospinal fluid (CSF) pathways early in illness receive treatment to the entire neuroaxis. Benign tumors, or those which tend to primarily recur locally, generally receive radiation to the tumor plus a margin around the tumor (local or involved field radiation). Radiation therapy used to treat small or peripherally located brain tumors will cause less damage to normal tissue than a larger or centrally located tumor where larger beams must traverse larger volumes of normal brain. When treating nonneural tumors, radiation utilized to prevent the occurrence of late nervous system relapse (so-called presymptomatic or prophylactic radiation therapy) in malignancies such as acute lymphocytic leukemia may also include the brain and peripheral (cranial) nerves in the target volume.

The appearance of adverse neurologic effects are a function of total dosage, dose fractionation, beam energy and composition (photon, neutron, electrons, etc.), age of the patient, and use of chemotherapy (before, during, or after irradiation). Neurologic sequelae can develop during the 6 to 8 weeks course of radiation therapy (acute reactions), within a few weeks to months after the completion of radiation therapy (early delayed reactions), or several months to years after radiation therapy (late delayed reactions) (Tables 27.1, 27.2).

Acute Neurologic Toxicity of Radiation Therapy

In clinical practice, acute neurologic reactions (those seen during or immediately after the course of irradiation) are limited to patients receiving whole brain or local brain irradiation for treatment of primary or metastatic brain tumors. With current means of delivery, acute reactions are rarely seen in children receiving brain irradiation for the treatment of extracranial neoplasms, or in children receiving cranial irradiation for prophylaxis of meningeal leukemia.

Patients receiving conventional fractionation and dosage for treatment of brain tumors (160 to 200 cGy per day, 5 days per week for a total dose up to 5,500 cGy) rarely have

Table 27.1   Radiation related neurotoxicity

Acute
  Acute edema

Subacute (Early delayed)
  Somnolence syndrome
  Transient radiation myelopathy

Chronic
  Radiation necrosis
  Radiation vasculitis
  Radiation myelitis
  Mineralizing microangiopathy/dystrophic calcification
  Endocrinologic dysfunction
  Cognitive dysfunction
  Peripheral neuropathy
  Secondary tumors

Table 27.2   Overview of radiation related neurotoxicity

Type	Timing	Etiology	Symptoms/signs	Outcome	Treatment
Acute	During or immediately after RT	Peri-tumoral edema	Worsening focal signs; headache; vomiting; nausea	Spontaneous resolution	Corticosteroids
Subacute	Weeks to 3 months after RT	Transient demyelination (? oligodendroglial dysfunction)	Somnolence— 1) Somnolence lasting 3 to 10 days;	Spontaneous resolution of somnolence; ? school difficulties; seizures	None
			2) Myelitis—electric shock down spine	Spontaneous resolution	None
Chronic	Months to years post radiation	Vasculitis; oligodendroglial dysfunction; autoimmune	1) Radionecrosis—focal deficits; seizures; symptoms of increased ICP	Variable; at times stabilization; at times progression to death	Surgical resection; corticosteroids; ? heparin
			2) Large vessel occlusion—focal deficits; seizures	Variable	? Endarterectomy
			3) Mineralizing microangiopathy—focal deficits; seizures; headaches	? Cognitive damage	None
			4) Endocrinologic—growth failure; hypothyroidism; hypogonadism	Fixed endocrinology dysfunction	Replacement therapy
			5) Neurocognitive—school difficulties; memory loss; retardation	Static deficits or progressive difficulties	Special education
			6) Myelopathy—paraparesis; quadriparesis; bowel and bladder dysfunction	Stabilization or progression	None
			7) Peripheral neuropathy—cranial nerve palsies; autonomic dysfunction; weakness	Variable	None

significant acute neurotoxicity. Transient worsening of the child's signs or symptoms and elevation of intracranial pressure referrable to the tumor mass and surrounding edema infrequently occurs. It is essentially impossible to distinguish between radiation-induced neurologic deterioration and tumor progression during the acute phase of radiation therapy. Care must be taken not to incorrectly conclude that clinical or radiographic worsening during or early after completion of radiation therapy is secondary to disease, and institute needless and potentially neurotoxic therapy (Figures 27.1a, 27.1b).

Experimental evidence has not yet defined the etiology of the acute radiation reaction, although evidence suggests radiation-induced peri-tumor edema is responsible. In animal experiments, normal monkeys treated with a single exposure to 3,500 cGy of 250 kV radiation, developed white matter edema and to a lesser degree, gray matter edema comparatively late (20 to 24 weeks) after exposure.

Earlier histologic changes consisted of "astrocytic or microglial reactions, with occasional perivascular collections of mononuclear cells (11)." Although it is difficult to draw conclusions by comparing adverse reactions in normal monkey brain to human brain diseased by tumor, these results suggest the acute reaction seems not to be due to radiation damage to normal brain structures but rather to the tumor vasculature.

Acute radiation reaction seems to correlate with the dose fraction and not the total dose. This syndrome is less common and less severe with smaller dose-fractions used to treat primary brain tumors (160 to 200 cGy/day) than the larger dose fractions often used to treat brain metastases. Randomized trials have compared a number of dose-fraction regimens for treating patients with brain metastases. In 1 study patients were treated with steroids and received either 10 fractions of 300 cGy over 2 weeks, 5 fractions of 400 cGy over 1 week, or 2 fractions of 600

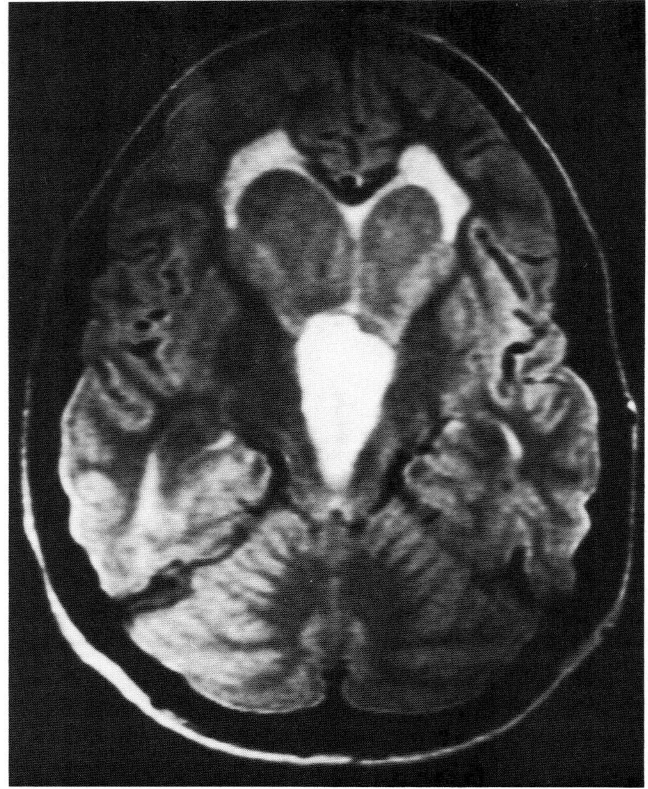

A

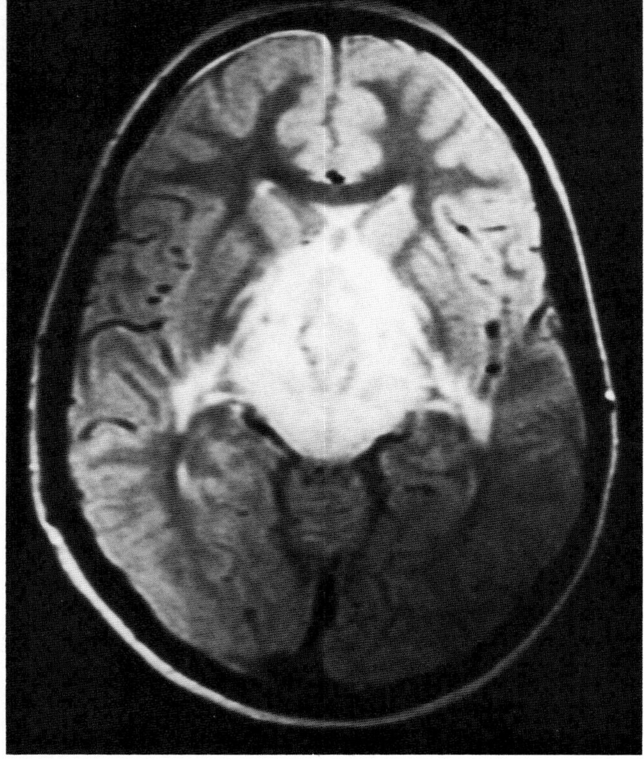

B

FIGURE 27.1A and 27.1B   Radiation induced peritumor edema. Preoperative proton density MRI of a 13-year-old girl with a hypothalamic glioma demonstrating dilated frontal horns, periventricular CSF transudation, and a hyperintense mass in the midbrain, hypothalamus, and 3rd ventricle. The bulk of the tumor was removed, and the patient began local irradiation. One week after radiation began the patient lapsed into a deep stupor. A MRI obtained showed a hyperintense region, with mass effect, extending throughout the midbrain, thalami, and basal ganglia; consistent with peritumor edema. The patient recovered with steroids, and the MRI returned to normal.

cGy over 2 days. In this study, the larger single fractions were tolerated, and although total dose was smaller in patients receiving larger dose fractions, the biologic effect of all regimens was similar (12). Young et al. (13) compared standard fractionation (3,000 cGy given in 15 treatments) to a biologically equivalent rapid course treatment consisting of 1500 rads divided into 2 treatments over 3 days. Forty nine percent of patients receiving rapid course radiation therapy developed headaches, nausea, vomiting, fevers, or herniation syndromes or both, compared to 15% in the standard treatment group. These symptoms developed within 7 days of treatment, although most occurred within 1 day. The most severe complications were in the patients with the greatest degree of neurologic impairment at initiation of therapy. Hindo et al. (14) studied patients with metastatic brain tumors receiving 1,000 cGy in a single fraction. Five of 54 patients died within 1 week of receiving a single dose of 1,000 cGy, and although these patients were moribund at the time of treatment, their deaths were hastened by radiation-induced edema.

Dexamethasone, known to be effective in treating vasogenic edema, seems to prevent or reduce symptoms, especially those symptoms caused by lower dose-fractions. It is necessary to taper dexamethasone carefully early in radiotherapy. It is unknown whether "prophylactic" steroids given prior to and early in the course of irradiation are of any benefit in reducing the incidence of acute reactions, although this type of treatment is frequently instituted. Clinical experience, however, strongly suggests that in patients dependent on steroids, especially patients with large midline or intrinsic brainstem lesions, the steroids need to be slowly tapered during radiation therapy (Table 27.3).

Early Delayed Neurotoxicity of Radiation Therapy

Early delayed reactions present a few weeks to a few months following completion of therapeutic irradiation. They are more common than acute reactions and are generally self-limiting. The 2 early delayed reactions following irradiation are the somnolence syndrome and transient radiation myelopathy.

Table 27.3   Radiation-induced acute toxicity

Reaction:
Generally limited to patients receiving treatment for brain tumors—(primary or metastatic)

Signs and symptoms:
Consistent with worsening of neurologic abnormalities or increased intracranial pressure, likely due to increased peritumoral edema

Patients most affected:
Patients with large tumors and those that have more significant neurologic impairment have more significant reactions

Toxicity:
Large dose-fractions and not the amount of total doses given seems to be responsible for the early toxicity

Therapy:
Dexamethasone may prevent or alleviate symptoms, expecially in patients receiving lower dose-fractions

The Somnolence Syndrome

This syndrome was first noted in 1929 when Druckman (15) noted 3% of 1,100 children irradiated with 150 kV X-rays (dosage in rads not calculated) for tinea capitis developed somnolence, anorexia, and headaches 6 to 8 weeks after irradiation. These effects lasted from 4 to 14 days, and after as long as 4 years of follow-up, there were no sequelae. Somnolence did not occur when the energy was reduced to 70 kV.

In 1973 Freeman et al. (16) described similar symptoms in 22 of 28 (79%) children with acute lymphocytic leukemia. Treatment consisted of either 2,400 cGy (200 cGy fractions) of craniospinal irradiation (7 children) or 2,400 cGy of cranial and 1,000 cGy of spinal radiation plus 4 doses of IT methotrexate (MTX) (21 children). Between 3 1/2 to 9 weeks after completion of irradiation, children developed anorexia and irritability, followed by 3 to 7 days of somnolence. The degree of somnolence varied from mild tiredness to greater than 20 hours of sleep per day. Lethargy was described as mild in 11 children and severe in the remaining 11 patients. Younger children had the greatest degree of somnolence. Electroencephalography (EEG) was performed in 5 children and showed generalized irregular rhythmic slowing (3 to 7 Hz). The EEG later improved, but did not normalize after symptoms resolved. In 4 of 5 children in whom CSF was examined, the protein concentration was elevated in 3 children (65, 67, and 750 mg/dL) and the white cell count was elevated at 43 mononuclear cells per mm^3 in 1 patient (3,16).

In a prospective study of 211 children with acute lymphocytic leukemia, Ch'ien et al. (17) delineated the neurologic sequelae of 49 children who remained in the study for 4 years. Children above 2 years of age were treated with 2,400 cGy of cranial irradiation and 5 doses of IT MTX. In children between 1 and 2 years of age, 2,000 cGy were given, and in those less than 1 year of age, 1,500 cGy were

delivered plus the MTX. Twenty-nine children (60%) developed somnolence associated with significant EEG slowing. Although the EEG background frequency improved, it remained persistently slow for the 4 years of the study. Only 3 of 15 (20%) children under 3 years of age developed somnolence, presumably because of reduced radiation therapy dosage. A significantly increased incidence of school difficulties and seizures developed in the children with somnolence, a finding not reported previously.

A similar syndrome occurs with patients receiving larger doses of radiation therapy for treatment of brain tumors. Hoffman and co-workers (18) reported 49 patients with malignant gliomas treated with 6,000 cGy to the tumor and 5,000 cGy to the whole brain, plus 1,3 bis (2-chloroethyl)-1-nitrosourea (BCNU). Within 18 weeks of radiation, 7 patients (14%) developed reversible exacerbation of symptoms. The exact incidence of this syndrome in children with brain tumors has not been determined, and separation of tumor-related neurologic compromise and radiation-induced somnolence is often possible only in retrospect.

It is believed that the somnolence syndrome is due to radiation-induced oligodendrocyte dysfunction with inhibition of myelin production. The latent period between the completion of radiation therapy and the onset of symptoms represents normal function of the myelin already present; the clinically symptomatic phase represents the time of myelin degeneration without regeneration and the recovery period begins as new myelin is formed (16,17). There are a few case reports of progressive neurologic dysfunction resulting in death about 3 months after irradiation, with extensive demyelination at autopsy; however, these appear to be extreme examples. This transient demyelination that results in somnolence or transient worsening of focal neurologic deficits is generally benign, and with the exception of the Ch'ien study, appears not to be predictive of future neurologic sequelae.

Transient Radiation Myelopathy

Analogous to the somnolence syndrome is transient radiation myelopathy (19,20), a frequent sequela of radiation to the neck or spinal cord. Two to 37 weeks after irradiation involving the spinal cord, patients can develop Lhermitte sign; that is, electric-shock sensations that can localize to the neck or travel down the spinal column, arms, or legs, occurring upon neck flexion. Patients rarely, if ever, develop objective neurologic signs. Autopsy of 2 patients who died of progressive cancer demonstrated astrocytosis involving the white matter, consistent with previous edema. The pathogenesis of transient radiation myelopathy is thought to be the same as with the somnolence syndrome; that is, transient radiation suppression of myelin production. This syndrome differs in initial symptoms and course from progressive radiation myelopathy.

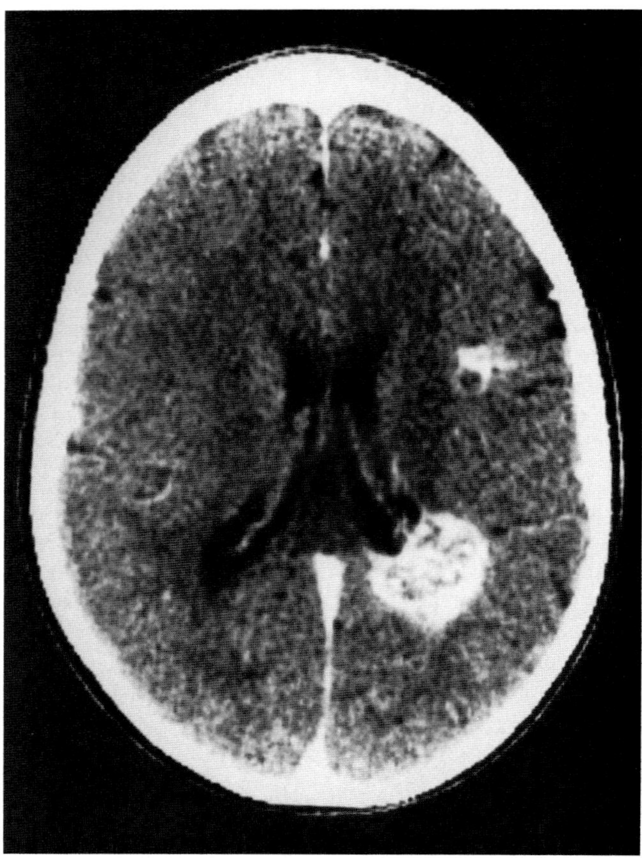

A

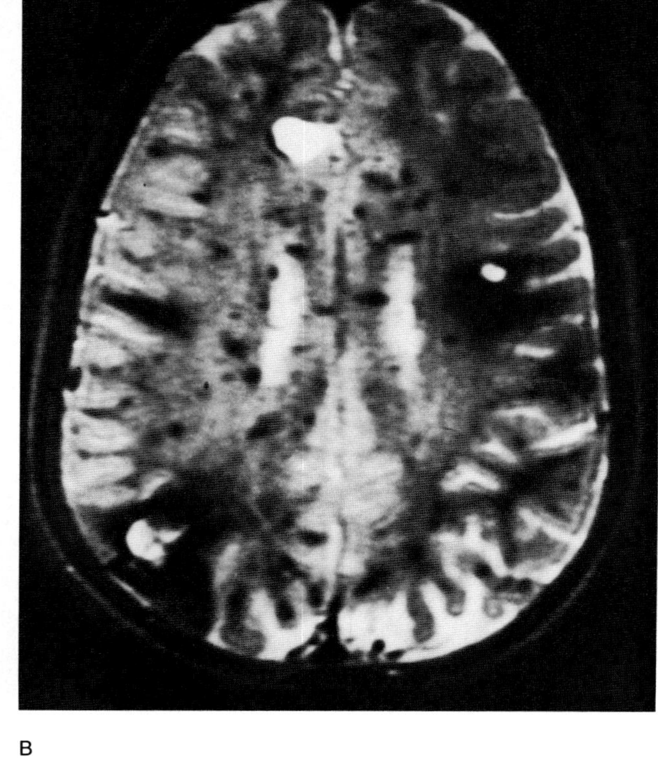

B

FIGURE 27.2   A Radiation necrosis. A 20-year-old man treated with 2,400 cGy cranial radiation and intrathecal methotrexate 10 years previously for acute lymphocytic leukemia. Contrast CT showing 2 enhancing, partially calcified masses in the subcortical white matter. **B** Radiation necrosis. Proton density MRI of the same patient 2 years later (image reversed) demonstrating numerous hypointense echoes scattered throughout the white matter consistent with multiple old hemorrhages (necrosis) and secondary calcification. Large lesions demonstrate a hyperintense core (subacute hemorrhage) surrounded by a hypointense region (old hemorrhage). The patient is employed as a telephone operator.

Delayed Neurotoxicity of Radiation Therapy

Radiation Necrosis

The most disastrous adverse neurologic sequelae of therapeutic irradiation is the development of cerebral radiation necrosis (radionecrosis). This syndrome is seen in 0.1% to 5% of patients treated with 5,000 to 6,000 cGy in 150 to 200 cGy fractions of cranial (involved field or whole brain) irradiation (5,21,22). The risk of occurrence correlates with larger total dosages; in one study 4% of patients treated with 5,000 cGy were affected (22). Although 80% of affected patients will develop symptoms within 3 years after treatment, the onset of symptoms ranges from 3 months to 19 years (5,21). Most patients reported with this syndrome have undergone radiation for an intracranial tumor, although cases have occasionally been reported in the setting of treatment for an extracranial neoplasm (23). Radionecrosis has been reported less frequently in children than adults (22). The pathologic lesion is a necrotic mass generally limited to the white matter and is in the portal of the radiation beam. Most often the lesion is focal and usually appears in the region previously occupied by the tumor (22); however, at times the lesions can be distant from the primary tumor site (Figure 27.2a, 27.2b) (24).

Signs and symptoms of radionecrosis are generally the same as those for any intracranial mass. Patients most commonly develop signs of increased intracranial pressure; namely, headaches, nausea, and vomiting. Altered sensorium, seizures, hemiparesis, papilledema, and other focal deficits have also been described. Without treatment, radiation necrosis is generally progressive and fatal.

The diagnosis of radionecrosis is often difficult to establish because both clinical and radiographic features of radiation necrosis and recurrent tumor are alike. Computerized tomography (CT) most frequently demonstrates a low density lesion in the white matter, with or without mass effect; the presence of contrast enhancement is variable and these findings are not specific for radionecrosis (22,25,26). Radionecrosis usually appears as an avascular mass on angiographic examination; however, tumors may also have a similar appearance (27,28). Only if abnormal vascular staining or neovascularization is present (suggestive of a recurrent tumor) can these entities be distinguished by cerebral angiography. Positron emission tomography (PET), allowing for determination of regional cerebral metabolism, seems to be the most promising imaging technique to distinguish between recurrent tumor and radionecrosis. Increased glucose and methionine utilization have been demonstrated in tumors compared to decreased utilization in radionecrotic lesions (29,30). Other diagnostic studies are abnormal in radionecrosis but similar abnormalities are seen with tumors. EEG frequently shows focal delta slowing overlying the radionecrotic lesion. The CSF protein concentration is usually elevated, and there is focal uptake on radionuclide scanning (28). Definite diagnosis can only be made by histologic examination.

Pathologic changes are mainly vascular in nature and generally limited to the white matter regions. The small arteries and arterioles show endothelial proliferation, hyalinization of the media, and narrowing of the lumen. A perivascular inflammatory response is variable. The white matter shows varying degrees of myelin loss, ranging from patches of myelin loss to coagulation necrosis of the entire centrum semiovale. Significant reactive astrocytosis surrounds necrotic lesions. Gray matter abnormalities, when present, are not striking (Figure 27.3) (24,28,30).

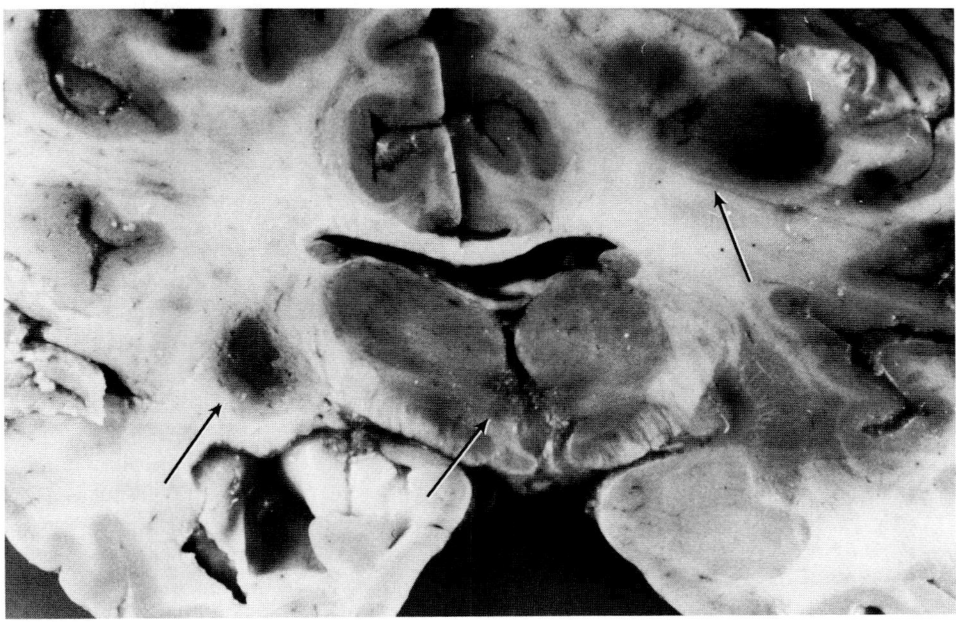

A

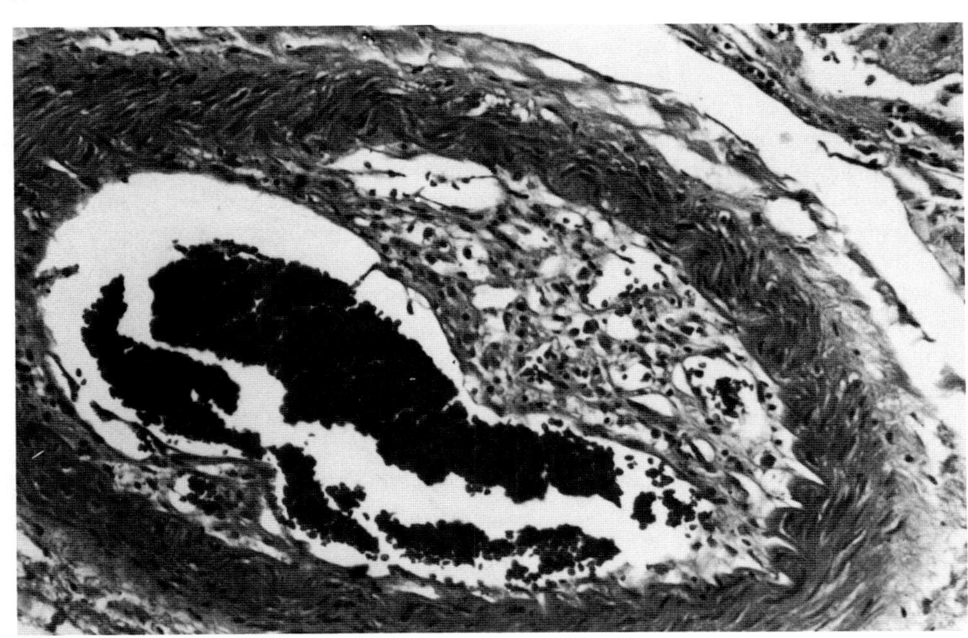

B

FIGURE 27.3 A Radiation necrosis. Coronal section through the third ventricle and thalamic nuclei demonstrating multiple areas of necrosis (arrows) secondary to vasculopathy resulting from irradiation for a posterior fossa primitive neuroectodermal tumor. **B** Radiation vasculitis. Subarachnoid artery. H&E stain. Magnification X40 before a 23% reduction. Photomicrograph of a large subarachnoid artery in a child with acute lymphocytic leukemia having received irradiation demonstrating irregular intimal thickening with slight inflammation.

The pathogenesis of radionecrosis has not been determined. Explanations include primary vascular damage with secondary tissue ischemia, primary oligodendroglial injury with subsequent demyelination, and an immunologic mechanism in which damaged glial cells release antigens that induce a hypersensitivity vasculitis. One or all of these mechanisms can occur in varying degrees in individual patients (21,24,29).

Animal experiments of normal pubescent and adult monkeys exposed to 4,000, 6,000, or 8,000 cGy in 200 cGy per day fractions of whole brain irradiation have produced pathologic lesions similar to that seen in humans. Necrotic lesions began to appear as early as 4 to 5 months after irradiation or as late as 1 to 2 years, demonstrating the element of host variability in this disorder. Pubescent monkeys treated with 4,000 cGy did not develop clinical or pathologic abnormalities. The 6,000 cGy group developed papilledema, EEG, and visual-evoked potential changes, but the scattered necrosis stabilized over time with lesions later becoming mineralized, suggestive of healing. Animals receiving 8,000 cGy had earlier development of abnormalities with a progressive course, and developed blindness, motor impairment, and abnormal behavior. The pathologic process showed confluent necrosis. Both pubescent and adult monkeys exposed to 6,000 cGy showed the same clinical and pathologic abnormalities, but this occurred earlier and with greater frequency in younger animals, suggesting that host age may be an important factor in the development of radionecrosis (11).

Treatment depends on the location of the lesion and the presence of signs suggestive of mass effect. Patients with surgically accessible masses may benefit from aggressive debulking. In some patients, excision of the radionecrotic mass can be curative, although patients may continue to develop progressive necrosis in adjacent regions. In those patients with necrosis located in deep regions, potential morbidity may preclude surgical intervention, and dexamethasone may be, at least transiently, useful in attempting to alleviate symptoms. Steroid responders usually become steroid dependent (28,31,32). A recent report demonstrated significant and long-lasting improvement in 2 adults with pathologically confirmed radionecrosis treated with heparin followed by warfarin. This finding was serendipitous as the 1st patient developed a deep vein thrombosis requiring heparin therapy and made a dramatic and long-lasting neurologic improvement. Heparin binds substances that can injure vascular endothelium and may prevent vascular injury from endogenous or exogenous substances, including radiation (33). Although interesting, more data is needed before heparin can be recommended as treatment for radionecrosis.

Children are more apt to develop necrosis in the brainstem region because of the posterior fossa location of most childhood tumors, the high dosage of irradiation utilized, and the relatively good chance of surviving many posterior fossa tumors. This region of the brain is difficult to treat

Table 27.4 Radiation-induced necrosis

Reactions:
 Occur mainly in patients being treated for brain tumors (either primary or metastatic), but may occur in children receiving radiation therapy for extracranial neoplasms

Signs and symptoms:
 Mimics an intracranial mass lesion and may be focal or diffuse

Dosage:
 Larger total radiation dose seems to correlate with the risk of occurrence and degree of pathology

Radionecrotic mass v. recurrent mass:
 Current diagnostic tests are of limited utility and only examination of pathologic material obtained at surgery is definitive. Experience with PET suggests it may be useful in such distinctions

Pathologic lesions:
 The pathologic lesion is most likely of vascular nature and dexamethasone may alleviate symptoms due to vasogenic edema, especially in patients also treated surgically

Surgery:
 Surgery may be curative if the necrotic tissue can be debulked

surgically, is intolerant of edema, and patients with brainstem involvement generally do not survive (Table 27.4) (31).

RADIATION VASCULITIS AND LARGE VESSEL OCCLUSION

A rare event following radiation therapy is the occurrence of large vessel strokes. Patients can present with typical stroke syndromes (seizures, hemiparesis, aphasia, amaurosis fugax, headache, etc.) 18 months to 30 years following radiation therapy to the head or neck. This syndrome is seen in children and adults, and the pathologic abnormality is an atherosclerotic plaque involving large arteries (27,34–37). It is likely that radiation therapy produces a spectrum of vascular injury ranging from small vessel vasculitis producing radionecrosis, to large vessel atherosclerosis causing stroke syndromes. Large vessel arterial occlusion with basal ganglia telangiectasis has been described in 2 children with neurofibromatosis irradiated for optic nerve gliomas (34). Right hemiparesis and aphasia developed in another patient 6 years after radiation therapy for a facial hemangioma. This child was found to have a stenotic left carotid artery (34). Painter, Chutorian, and Hilal (36) described 4 children with stroke syndromes previously irradiated for tumors. Three of the 4 patients had angiograms or autopsy data or both demonstrating large vessel narrowing. All 4 had evidence of mass effect suggestive of radionecrosis, but pathologic confirmation of radionecrosis was not seen in the 1 autopsied patient, and the other patients recovered in varying degrees (36).

There are no data regarding treatment for children with this condition. Eight adults in one series were treated with an endarterectomy procedure and although technically more difficult than in a typical patient, it was not associated with additional morbidity (37).

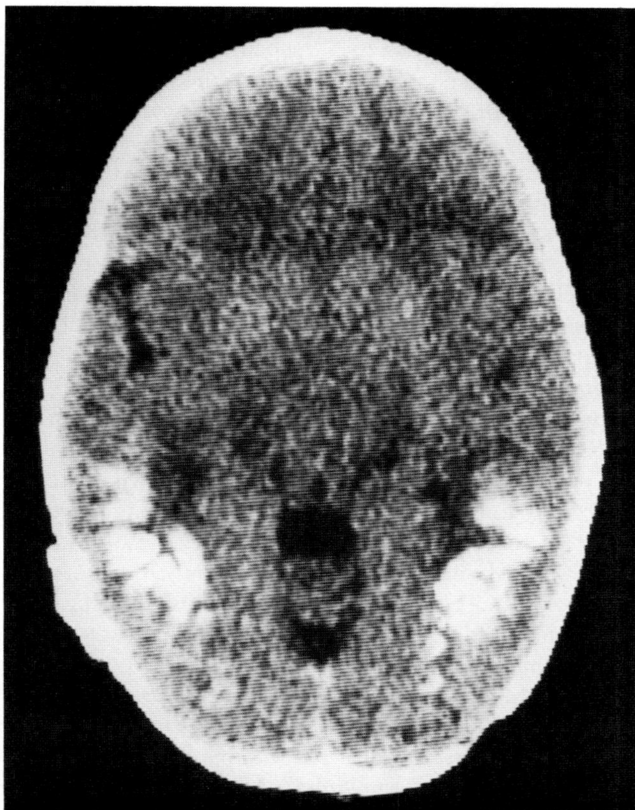

FIGURE 27.4A Dystrophic calcification. Unenhanced CT of a 5-year-old girl treated at 1 year of life with craniospinal irradiation and CCNU, CPDD, and vincristine for a malignant posterior fossa ependymoma. Calcification is present at the junction of the cortical gray and white matter in the occipital cortex corresponding to the area of brain included in the radiation boost given to the tumor bed.

Mineralizing Microangiopathy and Dystrophic Calcification

Mineralizing microangiopathy and dystrophic calcification was first described by Price and Birdwell (38) in 28 of 163 (17%) autopsied brains of children dying of acute lymphocytic leukemia at least 10 months after initial treatment. Of these 28 children, all but 4 received at least 1,500 cGy of cranial irradiation or received systemic and IT MTX. Four of 24 children in this retrospective autopsy series had histories of neurologic dysfunction that included focal seizures, transient abnormal EEGs, difficulty in walking, poor coordination, and headache. In a prior study in the same instituition (39), 21 children had not received IT MTX or radiation therapy. None of these 21 autopsied brains demonstrated this feature.

Pathologic findings include deposition of calcium in the walls of small vessels and, occasionally, occlusion of the lumina with mineralized deposits. The putamen and other basal ganglia areas were most often involved, with cortical and cerebellar gray matter occasionally involved. The pathogenesis is believed to be radiation-induced (usually greater than 2,000 cGy) small vessel injury with subsequent calcification. These calcifications are visible on CT in 26% to 80% of children after radiation therapy and IT MTX (40,41). Intrathecal MTX (39,40) or cytosine arabinoside (39) can play a role in the pathogenesis of this syndrome (41). The association between these findings and intellectual impairment or other CNS sequelae is unclear (Figure 27.4).

Radiation-Induced Endocrine Dysfunction

Endocrine dysfunction is seen in children receiving greater than 2,400 cGy of cranial irradiation for acute lymphocytic

FIGURE 27.4B Mineralizing microangiopathy/dystrophic calcification. H & E stain. Magnification X40 before a 23% reduction. Photomicrograph of a section of basal ganglia demonstrating extensive vascular and parenchymal calcification with mild gliosis following cranial irradiation for CNS leukemia.

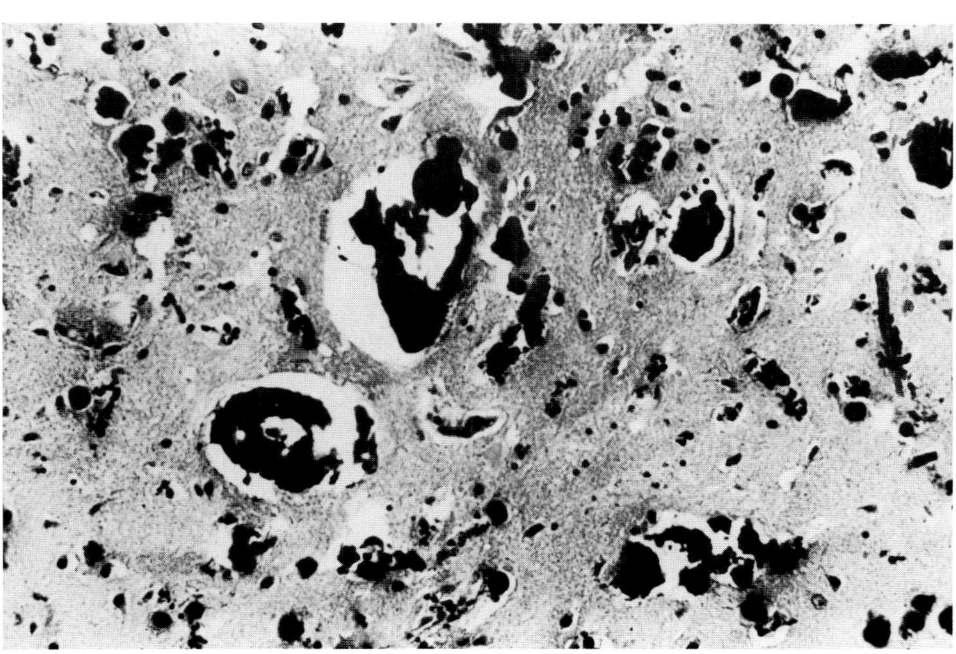

leukemia and to children receiving larger dosages of irradiation for brain tumors. Many subsets of children with brain tumors are at risk. Obviously those receiving presymptomatic whole-brain irradiation and those receiving local irradiation, where the portal includes the hypothalamus and pituitary, are at highest risk. Patients receiving isolated posterior-fossa irradiation are also at some risk because the anterior aspect of the field can extend to the posterior clinoids and include the ventromedial nucleus of the hypothalamus, the site of growth hormone releasing hormone (GHRH) production (42,43).

The largest body of data regarding endocrine dysfunction involves children with acute lymphocytic leukemia who received cranial irradiation as prophylaxis against meningeal leukemia. The available information is somewhat conflicting but suggests that 2,400 cGy affects growth hormone (GH) release but not linear growth. In one report children receiving 2,400 cGy or less demonstrated a blunted GH response to insulin-induced hypoglycemia, a response under hypothalamic control mediated by GHRH, but a normal GH response to arginine, presumed to be directly mediated by the anterior pituitary (44). Patients who received greater than 2,400 cGy had decreased GH release to both insulin-induced hypoglycemia and arginine, and control groups receiving no cranial irradiation (IT chemotherapy only) or abdominal irradiation (for Wilms tumor) had normal responses to both agents. It seems that 2,400 cGy adversely affected the hypothalamus but not the pituitary, and that higher doses were needed to destroy the pituitary cells that secrete GH. Of note, all children with abnormal responses to both insulin and arginine (those receiving greater than 2,400 cGy) were less than the 3rd percentile for height; whereas, children not irradiated and those receiving 2,400 cGy had normal mean height percentiles (43).

In another study of 25 children with acute lymphocytic leukemia, 15 children received 2,500 cGy in 10 fractions over 2 1/2 weeks, 10 children received 2,400 cGy in 20 fractions over 4 weeks, and 3 children did not receive radiation therapy. The children who received a higher dose fraction (2,500 cGy group) had significantly depressed GH response to hypoglycemia compared with the other groups. Although the most likely explanation is that the higher dose fraction contributed to this finding, this group had also received treatment prior to the other groups and the GH response may reflect increased time interval between treatment and study. Most of these children were small-statured but details were not discussed (45,46). More recent studies have not supported the findings of growth delay. Fourteen children treated with 2,000 to 2,500 rads in 10 to 15 fractions over 11 to 18 days had normal growth, and all of the 8 patients in the group tested demonstrated normal GH responses to hypoglycemia, thyroid function, cortisol response, and gonadotropin levels (47). These results have been confirmed in another study of 10 children treated with 2,400 cGy over 18 days. All children had normal linear

growth, bone age, diurnal cortisol measurements, thyroid function, and response to adrenocorticotrophic hormone (ACTH). GH response to oral glucose tolerance testing and to tolbutamide tolerance testing was normal in all but 1 child (48).

Children receiving larger dosages of cranial irradiation for treatment of brain tumors clearly develop growth impairment and other neuroendocrine abnormalities. In a recent prospective study by Duffner et al. (43), 14 children received 2,600 to 5,800 cGy of cranial, craniospinal, or posterior fossa irradiation in which the portal included the hypothalamic-pituitary axis. All had abnormal GH responses to insulin and all but one had abnormal GH responses to arginine. Ten of these patients were irradiated prior to puberty, and all had decelerated linear growth. Primary hypothyroidism developed in patients who received 3,000 cGy to the spine because the thyroid gland received direct irradiation. Children receiving at least 5,500 to cGy to the whole brain developed thyroid stimulating hormone (TSH) and ACTH abnormalities, as well as GH deficiency. In another study of children with posterior fossa medulloblastoma, these findings were not entirely confirmed, although the average dose of radiation therapy to the posterior fossa was significantly less than in Duffner and co-workers' (43) study (3,600 cGy compared to 4,400 cGy). Fourteen of 19 (73%) prepubertal patients had decreased linear growth, but only 3 of 10 children studied had abnormal GH stimulation tests. The authors concluded that this was not the result of an absolute GH deficiency, but due to impaired GH regulation or secretory pattern abnormalities not detectable by GH stimulation tests. More than 2/3 of their patients also had thyroid dysfunction, related to thyroid exposure during spinal radiation (49). The different results between these two reports may reflect the smaller radiation therapy dose or the shorter interval between radiation treatment to hormone testing in the latter study.

Gonadotropin and corticotropin levels in children treated with 2,400 cGy of cranial radiation (47,48) and those with larger doses in which the radiation portal does not involve the hypothalamus or the pituitary or both (42), are almost always normal.

Endocrine abnormalities are treatable side effects of radiation therapy and testing should be a routine part of follow-up on all brain tumor patients. Thyroid studies (T_4 and TSH) should be obtained early in treatment. If growth has been normal prior to diagnosis of the tumor, initial GH studies are not necessary. Repeat thyroid studies should be obtained every 6 months for at least 3 years, and GH stimulation studies should be obtained if linear growth falls to less than 2 standard deviations below the mean growth rate per year. Gonadotropin levels should be obtained if the child does not enter puberty at the expected age. Patients with tumors near the craniospinal axis (craniopharyngiomas, pineal region tumors, astrocytomas of the diencephalon, etc.) should receive a complete battery of studies (cortisol, prolactin, gonadotrophin, GH, T_4 and TSH) at diagnosis and should be evaluated routinely after treatment (50).

Neurocognitive Damage

Intellectual disability is a particularly distressing outcome following survival of cancer. The best studied group of patients are those children surviving acute lymphocytic leukemia, although a number of recently reported studies involve children treated for brain tumors. Intellectual impairment may take the form of dementia (loss of higher cortical functions) or the child may simply cease to acquire new cognitive skills.

Although radiation treatment seems to be the most significant factor in causing lost intellect in some groups of cancer survivors, other important factors must be considered. Children with acute lymphocytic leukemia, for example, often are treated with intrathecal methotrexate in addition to radiation therapy, and it appears that both are responsible for the pathologic change known as necrotizing leukoencephalopathy. When considering the intellect of surviving brain tumor patients, other factors must also be weighed including disruption by tumor of the normal neural pathways involved in higher cortical function, surgical intervention, CNS infections, episodes of increased intracranial pressure, and effects of chemotherapy. Cortical atrophy, as seen on CT imaging, does not correlate well with intellectual ability, and pathologic data on survivors are not available. Therefore, the studies of intellectual effects must come from statistical analyses of neuropsychologic tests (which are difficult to correlate with specific pathologic data) of surviving cohorts treated differently.

Early reports of intellectual functioning in acute lymphocytic leukemia survivors seemed encouraging. A retrospective analysis of 22 patients tested 5 years after diagnosis and treated with 2,400 cGy of cranial irradiation and 5 doses of IT MTX suggested this treatment was "destitute of prohibitive toxicity . . . ," although 1/3 of patients tested below average in some area of neuropsychologic function (51). No major neuropsychologic abnormalities were found in another group of 34 patients treated with 2,400 cGy of cranial irradiation, with or without IT MTX, although these patients were tested within 18 months of treatment (52).

More recent studies refute these data. In a retrospective report, children were treated either with 2,400 cGy of craniospinal irradiation and IT MTX or cytosine arabinoside, while others received no CNS prophylaxis. The children who received radiation therapy had full-scale intelligence quotients (IQs) 14 points lower than their siblings; whereas, those who did not receive radiation therapy had similar IQs as their siblings. Children less than 5 years old had the greatest degree of dysfunction (53). In a prospective study of patients treated with 2,400 cGy of cranial irradiation and IT MTX, progressive decline in IQ and learning deficits developed in 11 of 18 (61%) children. These deficits were more pronounced in children with initially high IQs and those diagnosed with leukemia between 2 and 5 years of age. The full decline in IQ was not apparent until 3 years or more after diagnosis (54).

Results of intelligence testing of children with brain tumors given cranial irradiation support the findings of intellectual impairment in children with acute lymphocytic leukemia after treatment with cranial radiation. Most studies investigating the cognitive effects of radiation therapy have evaluated children only with posterior fossa tumors to eliminate the effect of the tumor on cerebral function. Intelligence testing of children with medulloblastoma treated with cranial irradiation (4,000 to 5,000 cGy to the cranium and 5,000 to 5,500 cGy to the tumor bed) showed 12 of 15 (80%) had full scale IQs less than 80 and 7 children (47%) less than 70 (55). In another study of 10 children with posterior fossa tumors (6 medulloblastoma, 2 brainstem gliomas, 1 ependymoma, and 1 recurrent cerebellar astrocytoma) treated with radiation (including whole brain in 7 of 10) and chemotherapy (IT and intravenous (IV) MTX, BCNU and vincristine) showed significant IQ declines in all. The 6 children in this study with medulloblastoma were treated with 4,400 to 6,450 cGy to the posterior fossa, 3,000 to 3,719 cGy to the whole brain, and 2,000 to 3,000 cGy to the spinal cord. The range of post treatment IQs ranged from untestable (less than 20) to 107 with 3 to 6 children having IQs less than 80. The major drop in intelligence was in performance rather than verbal scores (56). Specific functional abnormalities have been studied in another group of 28 medulloblastoma patients treated with 3,500 cGy whole brain and 5,000 cGy posterior fossa irradiation (with 1/2 receiving IT MTX). Fifty-eight percent had IQs between 70 and 90 and 31% had IQs less than 70. Dysphasia, dysgraphia, and defective spatial orientation were the most frequent abnormalities noted. Twenty-six of 28 (93%) had attention deficits, negativistic behavior, and emotional regression. These patients were significantly more impaired than the nonirradiated control patients with cerebellar astrocytomas (57).

In an attempt to determine if other factors besides radiation therapy play a role in cognitive outcome of children with brain tumors, 23 consecutive surviving patients with medulloblastoma were analyzed with respect to age at diagnosis, preoperative examination, extent of disease at diagnosis, operative and postoperative course, dose of radiation therapy, and chemotherapy. All patients received craniospinal (3,600 to 4,000 cGy) and local (5,500 cGy) irradiation. Median full scale IQ was 98 (verbal IQ 102, performance IQ 90) and 14 of 23 (61%) were in a regular classroom. Factors correlating with significantly poorer cognitive outcome included age of less than 7 years at diagnosis, obtundation at presentation of illness, subtotal resection, the need for a permanent shunt, and postoperative bacterial meningitis (58). A more recent prospective study of children with posterior fossa tumors suggested that after

2,400 to 3,600 cGy of whole brain irradiation, many patients experience a significant drop in intelligence between 1 and 2 years after the completion of radiation therapy. There was a direct correlation between age at treatment and the severity of intellectual loss (58).

The mechanism of cognitive impairment is unknown. CT imaging is not useful because atrophy is frequently present in patients without any intellectual deficits. Magnetic resonance imaging (MRI) of demented children previously given radiation therapy demonstrates increased signal intensity in focal areas of white matter. In severely affected children, these focal areas appear confluent (59). Pathologic correlation of intellectual and behavioral sequelae following radiation therapy is not available and the pathophysiology is unknown (Table 27.5).

Chronic Progressive Radiation Myelopathy

Analogous to radiation necrosis, the occurrence of chronic progressive radiation myelopathy is a function of total radiation dose and dose-fractionation (60). Symptoms usually begin 5 $\frac{1}{2}$ to 30 months (mean of 14 months) following completion of radiation therapy to the spinal cord, and include numbness or pain in the legs that ascend to the trunk and arms. Bowel and bladder dysfunction are common and weakness ultimately develops. Neurologic signs usually progress to an incomplete or complete transverse myelopathy.

The syndrome is rapidly progressive during the first 6 months following onset of symptoms and then tends to progress slowly (61). The diagnosis can only be made if the following criteria are met: the area of spinal cord injury must be in the portal of tissue exposed to irradiation; and neuroimaging or surgery must exclude spinal cord or nerve root involvement with tumor or meningeal disease (62). In a review of 172 adult patients surviving for at least 18 months, who were treated with irradiation for nonneural tumors, Wara and co-workers (63) found 9 patients who developed permanent myelopathy. After analysis with respect to dose and dose-fraction, safety guidelines were proposed and have been supported by others (62,63,64). Two thousand cGy in 5 fractions, 3,000 cGy in 10 fractions,

Table 27.5   Radiation effects on cognition

Cranial radiation therapy results in cognitive impairment, and patients with brain tumors fare worse than those with leukemia.

The magnitude of cognitive impairment seems to correlate broadly with the total dose of radiation therapy and is more severe in younger children.

The use of intrathecal methotrexate may also potentiate this effect.

Intellectual deficits may not become apparent for 3 years after treatment but seem to appear earlier with higher dosages of radiation therapy.

or 5,000 cGy in 25 fractions were not associated with this syndrome, at least in the 1st 18 months following radiation therapy. Radiation myelitis appears to be quite rare in children, with only 7 cases described (65–68). The clinical descriptions are similar to those found in adults. Concominant chemotherapy appears to enhance radiation myelopathy. Actinomycin-D, a known radiation potentiating agent (69), and IT MTX (68) have been implicated in enhancing radiation myelitis.

The histologic appearance of lesions is similar to that seen in cerebral radiation necrosis. Demyelination, edema, infarction and necrosis of the cord, with necrosis of blood vessels have been seen at autopsy (65,66). In the most recent review of radiation myelitis, Goldwein (70) summarized the risk factors associated with the syndrome as: larger fraction size; shorter treatment time; higher total dose; increased length of cord treated; and other factors such as associated chemotherapy.

Radiation Injury to the Peripheral Nervous System

Clinically apparent radiation injury to the peripheral nervous system including cranial nerves, roots, plexuses, and peripheral nerves, is relatively rare (71). As with damage to the CNS, damage to the peripheral nervous system correlates with total radiation dose and dose-fraction. Patients at risk are those in which the nerve lies in the radiation portal. Radiation-induced neuropathy presents months to years after treatment, with functional impairment of the innervated muscle group or, in the case of sensory nerves, with impaired sensation. Pain may or may not be a component. The major difficulty in making this diagnosis, especially if there is a palpable or radiographic mass along the peripheral nerve, is distinguishing radiation-induced neuropathy from recurrent tumor.

Cranial Nerves

Any of the cranial nerves can be damaged by radiation therapy, although at least from the clinical viewpoint, injury is rare or at least obscured by concurrent brainstem impairment. Auditory and optic nerve damage produce the most commonly reported clinical effects. Radiation therapy involving the cochlea can produce chronic hearing loss by obliterative arteritis (72). Hearing loss is potentiated when cisplatin, a chemotherapeutic agent with associated high-frequency hearing loss at increasing cumulative dosages, is used after irradiation (73). Radiation therapy of 6,300 to 7,000 cGy in normal fractions involving orbital structures can cause visual loss from central retinal artery thrombosis (9 to 15 months latent period), maculoretinal degeneration (2 to 3$\frac{1}{2}$ year latent period), or optic nerve atrophy (4 to 5 year latent period) (74). Other cranial nerves have also been reported to be damaged by irradiation (75,76).

Peripheral Nerves

Radiation-induced peripheral neuropathy usually presents as a brachial or lumbosacral neuropathy following radiation therapy for breast or pelvic carcinomas. In general, metastatic disease causes severe pain and progressive limb dysfunction, while radiation-induced plexopathy causes mild pain with progressive paraesthesia and weakness (77–79). In the most extensive study of brachial plexopathy in cancer patients (79), those with metastatic plexopathy most likely presented with symptoms corresponding to the lower trunk (roots C8 and T1) because of the proximity of these roots to the local lymphatics. Many of these patients also had a Horner syndrome. Patients with radiation-induced plexopathy more frequently presented with signs referable to the upper trunk, primarily roots C5, C6 or C7. These roots run a longer course through radiation portals and are not protected from radiation by the clavicle, as are C8 and T1. Severe pain was the presenting complaint in 75% to 89% of patients with metastatic plexopathy and only 18% of patients with radiation-induced plexopathy. One-third of the radiation group never had pain, however, during the course of illness the majority of patients did complain of paraesthesias and hypesthesias.

Radiation injury was less likely to occur in patients treated with less than 6,000 cGy. In those treated with more than 6,000 cGy, patients presenting within 1 year of therapy tended to have radiation-induced plexopathy; no prediction could be made on patients presenting after 1 year (79). In a long-term study of 20 patients with lumbosacral plexopathy, leg weakness was the initial symptom in 12, paraesthesia in 6, and pain in 2. Symptoms progressed over months to years.

Diagnosis may be aided by myelography, CT scanning, or MR imaging. Extension of the metastatic process can also involve proximal nerve roots and involve the epidural space. Sixty-three percent of patients in one study with metastatic plexopathy had an abnormal myelogram (79). CT scanning may demonstrate a tumor mass, although a normal CT scan can be misleading. Electromyography demonstrates myokymia in patients with radiation-induced plexopathy (80,81). Surgical exploration is useful if it leads to a diagnosis of metastatic disease; however, a false-negative result is possible. There is no successful treatment for radiation-induced plexopathy (21).

The pathogenesis of the neuropathy can be due to radiation damage to the nervous tissue elements or vascular supply, or by subsequent compression of the nerve by radiation-induced fibrosis of surrounding connective tissue (21,71).

Secondary tumors of the peripheral nerve are another late complication of radiation therapy. Benign and malignant nerve sheath tumors have been reported 4 to 41 years after successful completion of radiation therapy. Malignant schwannomas have been seen in children after radiation therapy and there is a suggestion that they may be more likely to occur in patients with neurofibromatosis (82,83).

Radiation-Induced Brain Tumors

It is well known that irradiation can induce secondary malignancies. Although a rare phenomenon, as increasing numbers of children survive cancer, the rate of radiation-induced brain tumors will also probably increase. The most common forms of radiation-induced tumors are sarcomas and meningiomas. A number of studies have estimated the occurrence of secondary neoplasms of all types in cancer patients, which range from 6.5% to 12% depending upon the reporting center and length of follow-up (84–87). Secondary brain tumors arise in the field of prior irradiation. It is difficult to estimate the rate of occurrence of secondary neurologic neoplasms due to prior irradiation because of differences in concomitant chemotherapy, difficulties in defining the population at risk, and relatively small numbers of patients.

There does not appear to be a lower limit of radiation dosage that is safe with respect to secondary neoplasms. Although no longer in practice, low dose (approximately 140 cGy) irradiation was used to treat tinea capitis prior to the advent of griseofulvin. Medical records of 10,902 children irradiated for tinea capitis were reviewed and matched against two different control groups, with follow-up periods ranging from 12 to 23 years. There was a significant increased risk of both malignant and benign brain tumors. The histology of the malignant tumor types were not described; however, the benign tumors included meningioma and a craniopharyngioma (88).

Second CNS malignancies are described after radiation therapy for primary brain tumors. Brain sarcomas are reported to arise 2 1/2 to 20 years following at least 3,000 cGy. Although most cases are seen in adults treated for pituitary adenomas, it has been seen in a 14-year-old, 7 years after receiving local irradiation for a cortical astrocytoma. Brain sarcomas, when they occur, are uniformly fatal (21,27,89–92).

Meningiomas and malignant astrocytomas are also seen after therapeutic irradiation. In a recent review, 8 patients (six children) irradiated with 2,300 to 7,200 cGy for brain tumors, developed meningiomas 5 to 25 years later. In the same review, 6 children receiving 3,000 to 6,007 cGy developed astrocytomas, 5 of which were malignant astrocytomas or glioblastoma multiforme (42).

Cases of high-grade astrocytoma developing in children previously treated for acute lymphocytic leukemia are increasing in number. One example is the case of glioblastoma multiforme reported in a child with acute lymphocytic leukemia who received 2,400 cGy and IT MTX as prophylaxis against meningeal leukemia. Because intrathecal methotrexate has never been implicated to be oncogenic, radiation is a likely inducing factor (93). It has been postulated, however, that patients with acute lymphocytic leukemia can be intrinsically prone to develop a second primary tumor located in the brain, irrespective of therapy previously administered.

CHEMOTHERAPY

Major improvements have occurred over the last 20 years in treating childhood cancers. The development of chemotherapeutic agents, the use of multiple agents to treat tumors, and the awareness and ability to treat many of the side effects of chemotherapy, have resulted in prolonged survival and improved quality of life. The goal of chemotherapy is to achieve a substantial kill of tumor cells, allowing the human immune system to cope with the few remaining cancer cells. Systemic toxicity is acceptable but limits the dose of each chemotherapeutic agent. The nervous system is relatively protected from the damaging effects of chemotherapy compared to other tissues because it is protected by the blood–brain barrier, and its individual components (neurons, glia) divide slowly, if at all. However, agents that pass freely through the blood–brain barrier, those that damage cells by affecting cellular metabolism, intracellular transport (as opposed to affecting DNA replication), and those that have secondary effects on blood flow are more likely to cause nervous system damage. In addition, the nervous system is limited in its ability to repair itself compared to more commonly affected organ systems like the gastrointestinal or hemopoietic systems. The combined use of irradiation and multiple chemotherapeutic agents is now standard in many childhood tumors (medulloblastoma, rhabdomyosarcoma, acute lymphocytic leukemia, et cetera) and may cause additive toxicity; in some cases the adverse effects seem synergistic. Finally, as length of survival increases, other neurotoxic effects may become evident. A broad spectrum of chemotherapy-related neurotoxicity may be seen, ranging from encephalopathy to peripheral neuropathy (Tables 27.6 and 27.7).

Table 27.6   Chemotherapy related acute encephalopathy (189)

Methotrexate, intrathecal, high-dose (stroke-like syndrome, seizures)

Vincristine (seizures, blindness)

BCNU (high-dose, intracarotid)

5-FU (high-dose)

Ara-C (high-dose)

Cyclophosphamide (mild symptoms)

Ifosfamide (worsened symptoms with prior Cis-platinum)

Interferon (180)

Procarbazine (173)

Table 27.7   Chemotherapy related peripheral neuropathy (189)

Vincristine
Vinblastine
Etoposide (VP–16–213), (191)
Misonidazole (192, 193)
Metronidazole (192)
Procarbazine (173)
Hexamethylmelamine (173)
5-Azacytidine (194)
Cis-platinum

ANTIMETABOLITES

Methotrexate

MTX inhibits the enzyme dihydrofolate reductase by competing with folate for binding sites. Its antitumor effects include: interference with formation of tetrahydrofolate, the coenzyme necessary for methylation reactions in the synthesis of purine nucleotides and thymidylate, and impairment of DNA and RNA synthesis necessary for cellular reproduction and protein synthesis. MTX can also affect other enzyme systems related to tetrahydrofolate. It is known to inhibit glucose metabolism (phosphorylation) and glucose transport (94). Tetrahydrofolate is a necessary cofactor for the hydroxylation of the amino acids phenylalanine, tyrosine, and tryptophan into the neurotransmitters DOPA and 5-hydroxytryptophan (95,96). Impaired tetrahydrofolate synthesis can affect synthesis of these necessary neurotransmitters and result in neurotoxicity.

Methotrexate can be given orally, intravenously (in various dosages), or intraventricularly or intrathecally into the CSF space. Because MTX is water-soluble, significant penetration into the CNS is achieved only by the IV high-dose (HD-MTX) route or by direct administration into the CSF space. Leucovorin (citrovorum factor-CF) is used as an antidote to HD-MTX. Leucovorin is converted in normal cells into 5-methyltetrahydrofolate, bypassing the metabolic block (susceptible tumor cells are deficient in the enzyme needed to convert leucovorin). The level of leucovorin achieved in the CNS may not be sufficient to restore local tetrahydrofolate levels (96,97).

The clinical spectrum of MTX-induced CNS toxicity has been well defined, but the mechanism of injury is not yet fully known. Neurotoxic reactions can be classified as acute, subacute, or chronic/delayed and seem to occur primarily in patients having received HD-MTX or direct instillation of MTX into the CSF space (Table 27.8). Lower doses of IV or oral MTX can be neurotoxic, especially after prior radiation therapy. The type of toxicity seen is highly dependent on the delivery system used. The acute and subacute reactions are generally mild or reversible or both. The delayed toxicity, although rare, causes significant and generally irreversible morbidity (98,99).

Table 27.8   Methotrexate neurotoxicity

Acute	
HD-MTX:*	Vomiting, seizures, somnolence, confusion
IT MTX:+	Arachnoiditis, necrosis (with CSF flow obstruction or misplaced drug)
Subacute	
HD MTX:	Stroke-like syndrome, altered sensorium
IT MTX:	Myelopathy, seizures, cranial nerve palsies, cerebellar dysfunction, altered sensorium
Chronic/Delayed	
HD MTX:	Necrotizing leukoencephalopathy
IT MTX:	Necrotizing leukoencephalopathy

*HD-MTX = high-dose methotrexate
+IT MTX = intrathecal methotrexate

Acute/Subacute Syndromes of Intrathecal Methotrexate

Acute arachnoiditis is the earliest type of MTX toxicity and can be seen as early as 12 hours after IT administration. Headache, vomiting, fever, and meningismus are common clinical features, and can persist for up to 2 weeks. Factors such as doses, frequency and timing of doses, age, the diluent used, and presence of active CNS leukemia determine the degree of sequelae (100). CSF clearance of MTX seems to be of major importance, and factors that interfere with CSF circulation, such as the presence of CNS leukemia, appear to make sequelae more likely. Geise et al. (101) reported this syndrome in 29 of 73 courses (40%) of IT MTX given prophylactically. In Duttera's series (102), 17 of 31 patients (55%) with meningeal leukemia who received preservative-free MTX developed this syndrome. Symptoms occurred regardless of concurrent CNS irradiation. Elevation of CSF cell count, protein concentration, and increased opening CSF pressure are seen with this syndrome and resolve spontaneously (100–102). IV steroids have been used in treating severe cases (103).

Subacute encephalopathy or myelopathy can occur days to weeks after repeated courses of IT MTX (94,100, 102,104) or after HD-MTX (105). In patients receiving IT MTX, spinal cord syndromes (paresis or paralysis) and brain syndromes (seizures, altered sensorium, brain stem, or cerebellar signs) are seen days to weeks following treatment. Recovery is variable, with symptoms generally improving if the dosage is reduced or treatment eliminated. Once again, delayed clearance of MTX from the CSF or blood seems to be a major factor in causing these subacute syndromes.

Acute Dysfunction After High or Moderate Dose Methotrexate

A fully reversible syndrome is seen in 2.3% to 15% of patients receiving moderate or high-dose methotrexate with citrovorum factor rescue (HD MTX-CF) (105–108).

Allen et al. (105) reported on 4 of 158 patients who developed acute neurologic signs about 10 days following high-dose MTX (8 to 10 g/m^2) for treatment of osteogenic sarcoma. Hemiparesis, seizures, language dysfunction, and alteration in consciousness occurred and lasted approximately 3 days. Two patients had no sequelae, and the other 2 patients improved but were left with a mild hemiparesis. CT head scans were normal, and the EEG showed theta slowing in all patients, and focal sharp activity in 1. These patients received further treatment without recurrence of this syndrome (105). Martino et al. (106) described 2 patients with the same syndrome after receiving moderate-dose MTX (2.76 g/m^2). All 3 patients made a full recovery. Jaffe et al. (107) reported 9 of 60 patients (15%) undergoing treatment for osteogenic sarcoma with HD MTX-CF who experienced 14 neurologic events several hours to 20 days (average 6 days) after treatment. Neurologic deficits included varying degrees of hemiparesis (5 of 14 events), seizures (8 of 14 events), altered sensorium without seizure (3 of 14 events), aphasia (3 of 14 events), and 1 patient each with ascending paralysis and dystonia. CT head scans were normal, EEGs showed varying degrees of theta and delta slowing in 6 of 7 EEGs performed and spike and slow wave in one. CSF protein concentration was markedly elevated (88 mg/dL, 198 mg/dL) in 2 of 7 patients studied. The authors did not find elevated CSF MTX levels in these patients but reported no further neurologic events in patients once increased CF doses were given (100 mg every 3 hours) (107).

Because the CNS is comprised of mainly undividing or slowly dividing cells, impaired DNA synthesis cannot be invoked as a mechanism of acute injury although it may be a factor in chronic or delayed injury. Acute MTX sequelae are likely due to impairment of glucose metabolism or neurotransmitter synthesis (95,97,109–111). Phillips and co-workers (110,111) have demonstrated altered behavior, encephalographic slowing, and a substantial decrease in cerebral glucose metabolism in rats receiving HD-MTX. Regions of the brain that normally have the highest rate of glucose utilization had the greatest decrement after HD-MTX. Rats treated with high-dose leucovorin immediately after HD-MTX showed no decrement in regional glucose utilization.

Chronic Methotrexate Toxicity After Intraventricular Instillation

Prolonged elevated MTX concentrations in the CSF can cause severe permanent CNS injury, which is seen most frequently in the setting of intraventricular installation in patients with obstructive hydrocephalus. Shapiro et al. (112) reported 3 children with ventricular obstruction due to posterior fossa tumors who were treated with multiple doses of MTX instilled into an Ommaya reservoir. All patients developed coagulation necrosis of the brain

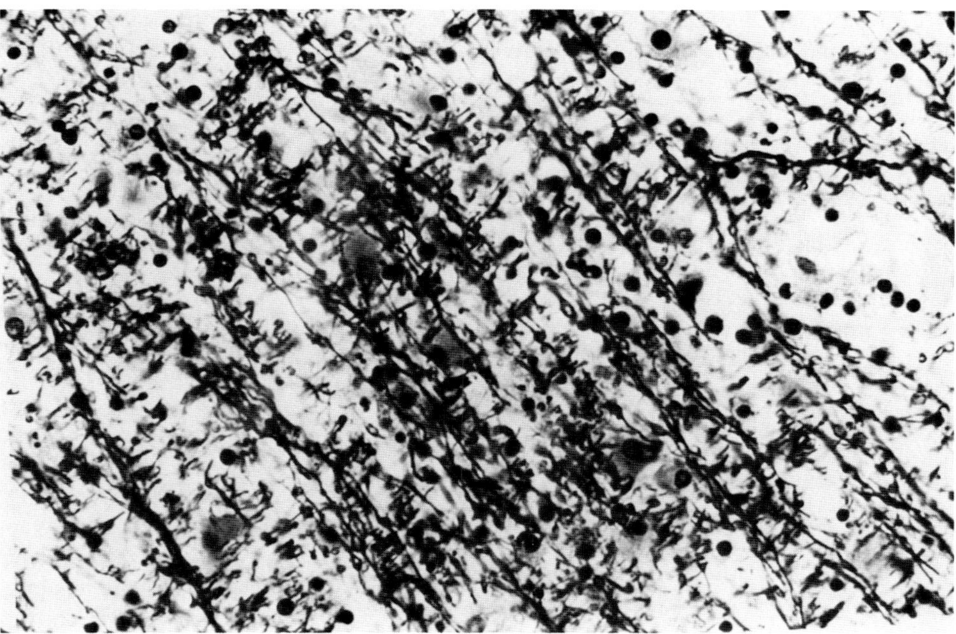

FIGURE 27.6 Methotrexate leukoencephalopathy. Luxol Blue-Cresol Violet stain. Magnification X250 before a 22% reduction. Photomicrograph demonstrating degeneration of white matter following methotrexate therapy. Note rerefaction of tissue and fragmentation of myelin sheaths.

effects. Bleyer (98) described 53 cases of necrotizing leukoencephalopathy and found 28 patients had received irradiation, IT MTX, and HD-MTX; 17 patients received irradiation and IT MTX; and 10 patients received IT MTX or HD-MTX or both. No patient with radiation alone developed this syndrome and, therefore, the development of leukoencephalopathy requires exposure to HD-MTX or IT MTX. Denominators are not given so the incidence of this syndrome in different settings cannot be determined.

Cortical Atrophy

Intrathecal methotrexate also appears to produce cerebral atrophy. Crosley et al. (118) reviewed autopsy specimens of 91 children with acute leukemia. Brain atrophy with cortical neuronal loss, the most common feature, correlated with the use of IT MTX. The presence of atrophy in patients receiving irradiation alone was similar to patients not given any irradiation. Patients receiving irradiation in addition to IT MTX did not have any greater degree of atrophy than those receiving IT MTX alone. These data suggest IT MTX is the major causative factor in producing cerebral atrophy. However, this was an autopsy series and it is difficult to correlate with MTX-induced leukoencephalopathy found in survivors (118).

Cerebellar Sclerosis

Cerebellar sclerosis is a pathologic finding consisting of atrophy and increased firmness of the cerebellum. Microscopic examination reveals neuronal loss in all layers of the cerebellum, with secondary gliosis. When the sclerosis is severe, loss of pontine and inferior olivary nuclei can also be present. There are numerous disorders associated with this pathologic finding, most often hypoxic or ischemic disease or both (118–120). This condition is also seen at autopsy in patients with cancer; however, no single or unifying etiology is known (121–123).

A recent study identified this condition in 14 of 120 children who died of cancer (124). Ten of the 12 children had acute lymphocytic leukemia, 1 had osteogenic sarcoma, and 1 neuroblastoma. Patients with this condition did not have evidence during life of isolated cerebellar dysfunction, although 2 patients had significant MTX induced-disease. Ten patients in the series received whole-brain irradiation and 11 had leptomeningeal spread of their tumor. There was no significant association between the development of cerebellar sclerosis and treatment with irradiation, IV or IT cytosine arabinoside, or IT MTX, although patients receiving IV MTX were more likely to develop this type of damage. Cerebellar sclerosis occurred more frequently in patients with acute lymphocytic leukemia than in other malignancies ($P<0.001$). The role of leptomeningeal disease is not clear, but may predispose previously treated cerebellar tissue to further ischemic injury (124).

Cytosine Arabinoside

Cytosine Arabinoside (Ara-C) is a pyrimidine analogue. The active metabolite of Ara-C arabinofuranosylcytosine triphosphate, inhibits DNA polymerase and also interferes with DNA synthesis by direct incorporation into the DNA chain. It is an effective drug against lymphomas and leukemias at varying IV dosages, and can also be injected intrathecally as treatment or prophylaxis against meningeal neoplasms. Ara-C crosses the blood–brain barrier, with CSF concentrations that are 40% that of plasma (125).

Conventional IV doses of 100 to 200 mg/m^2 had been used for many years and except for one report of 2 patients developing a sensory neuropathy with parethesias (126), Ara-C had not been associated with adverse neurologic effects. Since 1979, high-dose Ara-C (approximately 3g/m^2 every 12 hrs for 12 or more doses) has been used as primary treatment for acute nonlymphocytic leukemia and for relapsed leukemia and lymphoma. In early clinical trials high-dose Ara-C was noted to cause somnolence (127). In one of the first large studies (128,129), 49 patients (aged 16 to 79 years) were treated with high-dose Ara-C for relapsed acute leukemia. Eight of 49 patients (16.3%) developed cerebellar dysfunction consisting of dysarthria, ataxia, or dysdiadochokinesia. Three patients had severe but reversible courses, and 2 had irreversible courses. No patient became neurologically symptomatic unless a total dose of 36 g/m^2 had been reached, and the 2 most severely affected patients received 54 g/m^2. Postmortem findings of the most severely affected patient revealed a loss of the Purkinje cell layer of the cerebellum with reactive astrocytosis (128). In another study (130) 4 of 24 patients (16.7%) developed irreversible cerebellar degeneration. Ataxia, dysarthria, and oculomotor dysfunction developed 5 to 7 days into treatment, worsened over the next 3 days, and stabilized over the following 2 to 6 days. Partial improvement occurred in the subsequent 1 to 2 weeks. Three other patients developed similar but reversible cerebellar syndromes. Pathologic findings were similar to those in the previously described study with predominant Purkinje cell loss in the lateral cerebellar hemispheres.

Diffuse encephalopathies manifested by varying degrees of mental status changes and seizures may also occur (127,129,130). Expressive (Broca type) aphasia without cerebellar signs has been reported in an adult patient (129,130). A young adult developed an acute demyelinating polyneuropathy (Guillain-Barré syndrome) after receiving 36 g/m^2 of Ara-C (131).

The pathogenesis of high-dose Ara-C-induced damage in the cerebellum is not clear. Purkinje cells are postmitotic and the only known pharmacologic action of Ara-C is upon DNA synthesis. It has been postulated that Ara-C exerts its affect by interference with Purkinje cell nucleus DNA synthesis (necessary for repair, gene amplification, and turnover) (130).

There is no effective treatment for high-dose Ara-C toxicity. It has been recommended that Ara-C therapy should be stopped if neurologic symptoms occur after a cumulative dose of 24 g/m^2 has been reached (132,133).

The use of IT Ara-C is not associated with cerebellar disease (134). A spectrum of neurologic complications has been associated with the use of IT Ara-C at a dose of approximately 30 mg/m^2 including headache, meningismus, disseminated necrotizing leukoencephalopathy, central and peripheral myelinopathy, and seizures (134–137). Other factors including prior or concomitant use of irradiation, IT MTX and other medications, severe metabolic disturbances, and meningeal leukemia are usually present and

a definitive casual relationship due to Ara-C is difficult to document in most cases.

5-Fluorouracil

5-fluorouracil (5-FU) is a pyrimidine analogue that impedes DNA synthesis by inhibiting thymidylate synthetase. Neurotoxicity is characterized by a reversible cerebellar syndrome manifested by varying degrees of truncal or appendicular ataxia, dysmetria, hypotonia, coarse nystagmus, and slurred speech (99,138). The frequency is dose related and ranges from no toxicity with doses of 7.5 to 15 mg/kg a week to 7% with 20 mg/kg a week (139). Symptoms generally resolve in 1 to 6 weeks after the drug is stopped (99). High-dose 5-FU (0.8 to 1.9 g/m^2 given every 2 weeks) is associated with similar cerebellar symptoms but also causes cortical symptoms including confusion, memory impairment, and dementia. This occurred in more than 50% of patients in one series. Cortical symptoms slowly resolved over 2 months after cessation of therapy (140). The mechanism of toxicity is not known, but is possibly related to the degradation products fluorocitrate and fluoroacetate (141). The spectrum of toxicity is similar to that of cytosine arabinoside, and it is speculated that a similar mechanism of toxicity exists.

ALKYLATING AGENTS

Cyclophosphamide

Cyclophosphamide is an alkylating agent used in the treatment of acute leukemias, lymphomas, sarcomas, neuroblastomas, and in some brain tumors. At conventional dosages, there is no significant neurologic toxicity. Rapid IV infusion has been associated with the sensation of being drunk, but this effect lasted only minutes (142). Visual blurring was reported in 5 of 29 children (17%) receiving 750 mg/m^2 every other day for 5 doses. In 2 children, symptoms occurred within minutes, the other 3 developed symptoms 24 hours later. Symptoms lasted less than an hour in 3, but took 3 days to resolve; and the remaining 2 patients took 2 weeks to resolve (143).

Ifosfamide/MESNA

Ifosfamide is a relatively new chemotherapeutic agent, although initial clinical trials took place in the early 1970s (144). It is an analogue of cyclophosphamide with activity against tumors resistant to cyclophosphamide (145) and has been used in a number of phase II trials in children with malignant solid tumors (including brain tumors). Currently, MESNA (sodium 2-mercaptothane sulfate) is used in conjunction with ifosfamide and serves to protect the bladder from toxic catabolites of ifosfamide, which may produce hemorrhagic cystitis. The dose of ifosfamide used in the largest childhood clinical studies was 1,600 mg/m^2/day administered intravenously over 15 minutes for a 5 day period and given every 3 to 5 weeks (145,146).

Neurotoxicity associated with the use of ifosfamide MESNA is frequent and severe, although is most often reversible. Symptoms occur during treatment and include mental status changes that range from irritability and confusion to coma, cerebellar dysfunction, weakness, cranial nerve dysfunction, and seizures. Thirteen of 61 patients (21%) developed neurotoxicity during 20 of 143 (14%) treatment courses. EEGs showed progressive slowing of background frequencies to the delta range, followed by high-voltage rhythmic delta activity; however, this did not correlate with severity of clinical neurotoxicity. Spike activity was present in 1 patient who later had a seizure. Symptoms invariably resolve within 72 hours of completion of the 5 day course. Recurrence of neurotoxicity was not invariable when children received further treatment (145,146).

The etiology of this neurotoxicity is not clear, but MESNA does not seem to be the primary cause. No neurologic toxicity was seen in normal adult volunteers given 250 mg/kg of MESNA divided over 4 days, a larger dose than used clinically (147). Degradation products of ifosphamide have been implicated. Ifosfamide is oxidized to chloracetaldehyde, a compound similar to acetaldehyde and the neurotoxic metabolite of ethyl alcohol, which requires liver aldehyde dehydrogenase for its degradation. Impairment of hepatic function limits removal of this toxic metabolite and enhances toxicity. Adult clinical studies have demonstrated increased risk of neurotoxicity in patients with low serum albumin (indicative of hepatic dysfunction) or elevated serum creatinine (148,149). In children, significant neurotoxicity correlated closely with more than 300 mg/m^2 cumulative dosage of prior cis-platinum (CPDD) (150). It is yet unclear if this is due to CPDD-related neurotoxicity alone or possibly a synergistic effect of CPDD. It is not known if prior cranial irradiation significantly increases the risk of neurotoxicity.

Toxicity is enhanced in the presence of abnormal hepatic or renal function. Termination of treatment is warranted if toxicity is severe (146), and although prior ifosfamide MESNA-induced encephalopathy does not preclude further treatment (145,146) close monitoring is advised. In addition, alternate day dosing of ifosfamide may decrease toxicity (150).

The Nitrosoureas

BCNU [1,3-bis-(2-chloroethyl)-1-nitrosurea], CCNU [1-(2-chlorethyl)-3-cyclohexyl-1-nitrosourea], and PCNU [1-(2-chlorethyl)-3-(2,6-dioxo-3-pipridyl)-1-nitrosourea] are alkylating agents that also inhibit protein synthesis and DNA repair. The nitrosoureas are used to treat brain tumors, Hodgkin and other lymphomas, and a number of carcinomas. They are highly lipid-soluble and penetrate the blood–brain barrier. Systemic administration of the nitro-

soureas at conventional doses is not associated with neurologic side effects, with the exception of potentiating the side effects of radiation therapy (138). High-dose BCNU has been used in patients with progressive malignancies and for preparation prior to bone-marrow transplantation. In a report where 4 patients received up to 3450 mg/m^2 (none received prior radiation therapy), 3 died of a progessive, subacute encephalopathy 25 to 47 days after receiving high-dose BCNU. Autopsy revealed foci of swollen axis cylinders without an inflammatory response and coagulation necrosis. The authors comment on the similar appearance between this pathology and that seen in radiation necrosis and MTX leukoencephalopathy (151). This process is less frequently encountered in dosages less than 1500 mg/m^2 (152,153).

Recently, BCNU and PCNU have been administered by intracarotid infusion for treatment of primary or metastatic brain tumors (154,155). Infusion of either agent into the ophthalamic artery is well known to cause permanent blindness. In a study of 37 adults with brain tumors, 111 intra-arterial infusions of BCNU (100 mg/m^2/dose) caused transient confusion in 14 patients, transient cortical blindness in 1 patient and hemiparesis in another (156). Immediate and delayed seizures have also been reported with intracarotid BCNU (157). Intraarterial PCNU (60 to 110 mg/m^2) has been associated with transient focal neurologic deficits (focal numbness, hemiparesis, focal seizures, impaired speech) in 10 of 17 patients (59%), permanent worsening of the neurologic condition in 1 patient, and a seizure in 1 patient (154).

HEAVY METALS

Cisplatin (Cis-Platinum)

Cisplatin (CPDD), a heavy metal compound, inhibits DNA synthesis by cross linking DNA, mainly at the guanine base. It is used for treating many types of brain tumors and other solid tumors. Peripheral neuropathy and ototoxicity are the major neurologic sequelae from IV CPDD, although papilledema and retrobulbar neuritis have also been reported.

The development of peripheral neuropathy appears to be dose related. Usual dosages of CPDD are on the order of 60 to 100 mg/m^2, given at monthly intervals for 8 to 12 months. In an extensive adult study, 22 of 24 patients (92%) treated with CPDD and adriamycin developed a polyneuropathy. Distal extremity numbness developed in 58% of patients by the 6th dose. Vibratory sensation was most affected, with joint position, touch, and pin sensation less affected. Deep-tendon reflexes were often decreased, most severely at the ankles. Strength was not affected. Patients first became symptomatic after receiving a cumulative dose of 300 mg/m^2, and all affected patients had developed symptoms by the time they had received 500 to 600 mg/m^2. The effect of concomitant administration of adriamycin in this study is not known and may have synergistic effects; however, adriamycin alone does not produce a sensory neuropathy. Patients were not followed long enough to comment on recovery (158). Similar findings are reported in another adult study with the symptom of Lhermitte sign developing in 40% of patients. In this study, where 15 patients were available for long-term follow-up, 13 of 15 made incomplete improvement and 2 did not improve (159). Pathologic examination in biopsied sural nerves showed a decrease in large diameter myelinated fibers, axonal degeneration, and segmental demyelination (158). The specific mechanism of CPDD-induced neuropathy is not known; however, all of the heavy metals can induce a peripheral neuropathy. The significance of this adverse effect in children is not clear, probably because many treatment protocols using CPDD also use vincristine; which causes an earlier, more severe, sensorimotor neuropathy.

Ototoxicity due to CPDD is well described. Tinnitus occurs in about 9%, symptomatic hearing loss in 6%, and high-frequency hearing loss on audiometric examination in 24% of patients (160). In a childhood study, 23 patients received 90 mg/m² every 3 weeks. At a cumulative dose of 270 mg/m², half had a significant hearing loss at 8,000 Hz. Significant loss at 2,000 Hz (speech frequency) occurred in 30% of children at 540 mg/m² and in 50% at 810 mg/m². Recovery did not occur in a 15 month follow-up period (161). The ototoxic effect of CPDD is enhanced by prior irradiation when the cochlea was within the irradiation field (73,162). This effect can be anticipated, and audiograms should be obtained in young children and all patients previously treated with radiation therapy involving the auditory nerve prior to each dose of CPDD.

A few case reports exist associating CPDD with reversible increased intracranial pressure and papilledema (163), permanent or transient retrobulbar neuritis (163,164), and seizures (165). Intracarotid CPDD has been used to treat brain tumors and is associated with severe encephalopathy (166,167). In addition to direct neurologic toxicity, CPDD interferes with renal function causing wasting of sodium and magnesium that can result in tetany and seizures.

OTHERS

Vincristine

Vincristine and vinblastine are vinca alkaloids that serve as effective chemotherapeutic agents by inhibiting the formation of microtubules and arresting mitosis (168). Vincristine is more commonly used in childhood cancers and its dose-limiting toxicity is limited to the peripheral nervous system (PNS); however, there are reported CNS effects. Most series describing vincristine neurotoxicity include primarily adult patients; childhood studies on vincristine neurotoxicity are not as comprehensive. In general, children tend to tolerate vincristine better than adults; this is especially true for patients treated prior to adolescence. All peripheral nerves can be affected including cranial and autonomic nerves. Peripheral neuropathy can appear after only 1 or 2 treatments and initially manifests as loss of the Achilles reflex. This effect is virtually universal in patients treated with repeated doses of vincristine (169,170). With further treatment, children will lose the patellar reflex, and reflexes in the arms will be variably diminished or lost. Maximum reflex loss occurs approximately 17 days after a single dose, with resolution in 1 to 3 months (170).

Early symptoms include paresthesias and pain. Approximately 1/2 of treated patients will experience paresthesias, usually in the hands and feet, which will tend to resolve after discontinuation of the drug. Pain, especially jaw pain, occurs in 6% to 8% of patients (169,170). Despite these bothersome symptoms, overt sensory signs are infrequent and minor, and usually resolve after therapy is stopped (169–171).

Cranial neuropathy is less common. In one series, ptosis occurred in 5 of 50 (10%), sixth nerve palsy in 3 of 50 (6%), and seventh nerve palsy in 2 of 50 (4%) patients treated with vincristine (170). In another report 5 of 392 patients (1.2%) treated with this drug developed vocal cord paralysis (169).

Weakness can follow loss of reflexes, especially in those patients treated with multiple doses. The foot and toe dorsiflexors and foot evertors are most commonly affected first, with more proximal muscles and wrist and finger extensors becoming involved if therapy is continued (169,170,172). Weakness has occurred in 1/4 to 1/3 of adults treated (169–172). Although weakness is partially or completely reversible, recovery can take months. Significant weakness is an indication to reduce or withhold the dosage until signs resolve. Muscle cramps can occur in the recovery phase of illness and be quite bothersome; they tend to respond to dantrolene or other muscle relaxants.

Autonomic dysfunction, especially abdominal pain and constipation, is common early in treatment and occurs in about 1/2 of patients. (170). Anticipatory or prophylactic treatment with laxatives can reduce symtoms. Urinary symptoms and orthostatic hypotension are also reported. Clinical trials of thiamine (173), vitamin B_{12} (173), folinic acid (174) and vitamin B_6 (175) have failed to reduce vincristine peripheral neuropathy.

The syndrome of inappropriate antidiuretic hormone secretion (SIADH) has been described in children treated with vincristine (176–179) and results in seizures due to hyponatremia. Seizures have occurred in patients after vincristine administration in which hyponatremia was not present. The pathogenesis of such seizures is unclear and treatment is supportive.

L-Asparaginase

L-Asparaginase (L-Asp) is an enzyme found throughout nature that hydrolyzes L-asparagine into aspartate and

Table 27.9 Overview of chemotherapy related neurotoxicity (98,99,138,173,189) excluding methotrexate

Drug	Acute/Subacute	Chronic
Cytosine arabinoside intrathecal	Meningitis; seizures; radiculitis; myelitis; brain necrosis (if intraparenchymal infusion)	Leukoencephalopathy; myelitis; peripheral neuropathy
Intravenous high-dose	Cerebellar ataxia; encephalopathy	Cerebellar ataxia; ? demyelinating polyneuropathy
5-Fluorouracil		
Intravenous low-dose	Cerebellar syndrome	
Intravenous high-dose	Cerebellar syndrome; encephalopathy	reversible encephalopathy
Cyclophosphamide	Visual blurring; sensation of alcohol intoxication	———
Ifosfamide	Encephalopathy; cerebellar ataxia; weakness; cranial nerve dysfunction; seizures	? encephalopathy
BCNU		
Intraarterial	Focal brain necrosis; blindness; seizures; encephalopathy	Blindness; seizures; encephalopathy; brain necrosis
Intravenous high-dose	———	Progressive brain necrosis
Cis-platinum		
Intraarterial	Encephalopathy; blindness	Blindness; progressive brain necrosis
Intravenous	Increased intracranial pressure; seizures; retrobulbar neuritis	Peripheral neuropathy; ototoxicity[b]
Vincristine	Muscle cramps; paresthesias; jaw pain; cranial neuropathy, peripheral neuropathy (sensory and motor); autonomic neuropathy; constipation: reversible	Peripheral neuropathy
L-Asparaginase	Metabolic encephalopathy; cerebral vascular accidents due to thrombosis or hemorrhage	Sequelae of cerebral vascular accidents
Actinomycin D	Myelitis[a]; focal necrosis[a]	Myelitis[a]; focal deficits[a]
Interferon (190)	Encephalopathy	———
Procarbazine (195)	Encephalopathy; peripheral neuropathy; ataxia, autonomic neuropathy; psychosis with high dosages	———
VP–16–213 (191)	Peripheral neuropathy	———
Misonidazole (9,192,193)	Peripheral neuropathy	———
Metronidazole (192)	Peripheral neuropahty	———
Thiotepa		
Intrathecal	Radiculitis; weakness	Radiculitis; myelitis; weakness
5-Azacytidine (192)	Encephalopathy; weakness; myopathy	———
Mechlorethamine (196) (nitrogen mustard)		
Intravenous	Encephalopathy (rare)	———
Intracarotid	Seizures; coma; hearing loss	hearing loss; vestibular dysfunction

[a]occurs when used with concomitant radiotherapy, or after radiotherapy
[b]enhanced by radiotherapy

ammonia and has some ability to hydrolyze glutamine into glutamate and ammonia. Protein synthesis is, therefore, inhibited in tumor cells unable to synthesize L-asparagine. The main use of L-Asp is in the induction phase of childhood acute lymphocytic leukemia. Because it is a large protein, L-Asp does not cross the blood–brain barrier. The neurotoxicity is not a direct effect of the drug but rather the metabolic derangements or clotting abnormalities, inducing cerebrovascular accidents.

One early study reported 25% to 50% of patients receiving L-Asp developed an acute encephalopathy at variable IV doses of the drug (99). This high incidence has not been seen in more recent studies utilizing intramuscular administration of the drug. The encephalopathy can consist of mild lethargy and confusion; however, it may progress to seizures, stupor, or coma (179). This syndrome occurs in the first few days after initiation of L-Asp therapy. The encephalopathy is reversible in almost all patients and treatment can continue if symptoms are mild (99,173,180). The etiology is believed to be metabolic, as elevated systemic levels of aspartate, glutamate, and ammonia occur soon after treatment is begun. These compounds readily cross the blood–brain barrier in toxic concentrations and can interfere with entry into the CNS of other essential amino acids. The CNS levels of asparagine have been shown to be depleted (181), and this may serve as an additional explanation for the encephalopathy. Electroencephalography demonstrates diffuse slowing that normalizes as symptoms clear (173,180,182).

The other adverse neurologic effect of L-Asp is a coagulopathy-induced cerebral hemorrhage or thrombosis (Figure 27.7) (183,184). This is not common but potentially serious. L-Asp has been shown to induce low levels of fibrinogen, factors IX and XI, antithrombin, and plasminogen, with subsequent clotting abnormalities producing hemorrhagic and thrombotic strokes. Thrombosis usually occurs in the sagittal sinus or surface cortical veins and can result in focal seizures, hemiparesis, and severe mental status changes. In one study, 4 of 194 (2%) children receiving L-Asp developed cerebrovascular accidents. Patients acutely developed seizures, focal deficits, or mental status changes after the ninth dose of L-Asp during induction therapy. One of the 2 patients with sagittal sinus thrombosis died, and the other with a partial thrombosis recovered fully. The other 2 patients had subcortical infarcts and

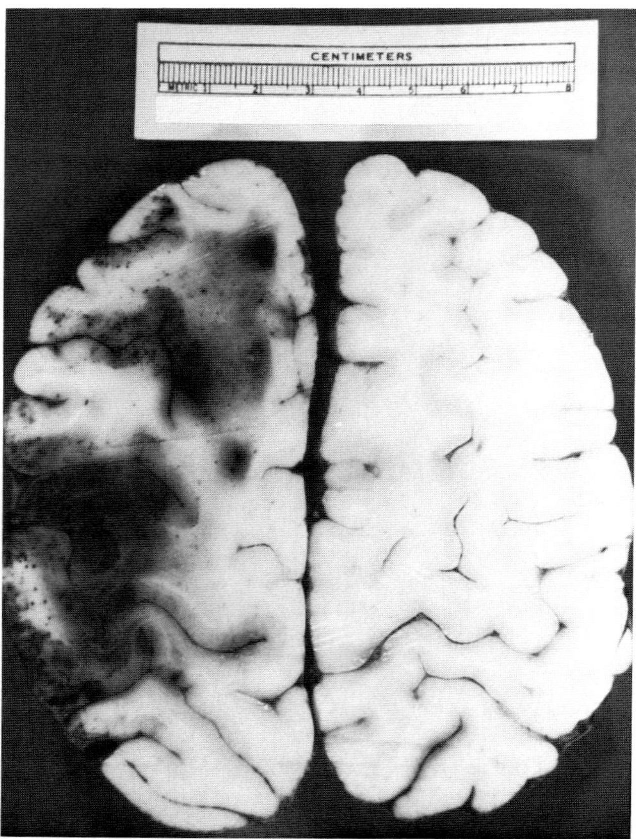

FIGURE 27.7 L-asparaginase venous thrombosis. Transverse section of cerebral hemispheres approximately 2 centimeters below the vertex. Note multiple areas of cortical and subcortical hemorrhagic necrosis secondary to extensive venous thrombosis following L-asparaginase therapy.

recovered without neurologic deficits. Treatment is supportive and repletion of clotting factors with fresh frozen plasma can be helpful. Recurrence of symptoms after recovery did not occur in patients receiving additional L-Asp (185).

Antiemetics

Although not anticancer agents, antiemetics are often necessary adjuncts to chemotherapeutic protocols. Phenothiazines (promethazine, prochlorperazine, chlorpromazine) and other compounds exert antiemetic effects through dopamine antagonism within the medullary chemoreceptor trigger zone. Sedation is a common side effect of all these drugs. Acute extrapyramidal reactions can occur soon after their IV administration and include involuntary movements, torticollis, oculogyric crisis, forced protrusion of the tongue, facial grimacing, and akathisias (involuntary restlessness).

Of all the drugs used as antiemetic agents, metoclopramide has been reported as the most neurotoxic. Metoclopramide, at dosages equal to or above 2 mg/kg has been reported in children to induce akathisias in 9 to 27 (33%) and extrapyramidal reactions in 4 of 27 (15%) (186). These adverse reactions of antiemetic agents are usually easily treated with IV diphenhydramine (1 mg/kg) and can be reduced in frequency and severity if concomitant diphenhydramine is given.

BONE-MARROW TRANSPLANTATION

Bone-marrow transplantation is a relatively new technique that is being increasingly applied to the treatment of cancer. It is also used for children with other medical conditions including aplastic anemia and various metabolic diseases. Bone-marrow transplantation requires the use of immunosuppressant and antineoplastic agents that predispose patients to infection, thrombocytopenia, and potential neurotoxicity. Recent information has suggested that a variety of childhood malignancies, especially various forms of leukemia, respond well to transplantation techniques. Although not a truly isolated form of therapy, because of the multiple neurotoxic agents used in transplantation regimens, complications following transplantation warrant a separate discussion.

Bone-marrow transplantation allows the use of potentially lethal doses of chemotherapeutic agents or radiation or both to eradicate systemic malignancy. Most transplant regimens require the use of total body irradiation; doses of radiation ranged from between 300 and 1,000 cGy. Such irradiation on top of previous neurotoxic treatment can result in a host of neurologic deficits. Newer transplant regimens have eliminated the use of total body irradiation and have instead substituted multiple chemotherapeutic agents such as melphalan, VM-26, doxorubicin, cis-platinum, associated with cortical or brain stem dysfunction. Patients without ventricular obstruction did not develop encephalopathy and the authors concluded that this syndrome was due to prolonged brain exposure to toxic doses of MTX. Packer et al. (113) reported encephalopathy (altered sensorium, hemiparesis, aphasia) in 2 patients after receiving MTX instilled into the brain parenchyma via a misplaced catheter tip. One patient improved after shunt revision and treatment with systemic steroids, but the other did not. Clearly, adequate CSF flow dynamics, either with a normal ventricular system or adequate shunting, must be ensured prior to administration of intraventricular MTX.

Leukoencephalopathy

The chronic form of MTX toxicity typically presents as a delayed leukoencephalopathy of variable severity that may be static or progressive (97–114). These chronic sequelae develop months to years after treatment and are seen usually in a variety of settings: patients with acute lymphocytic leukemia who had received prophylactic IT MTX with or without cranial irradiation; patients with brain tumors treated with irradiation and IT MTX or HD-MTX; patients with meningeal dissemination treated with IT MTX with or without radiation; and patients with osteogenic sarcoma treated with HD-MTX (114). The most distressing aspect of this syndrome is that many patients are apparently cured of their tumor by the time symptoms become apparent. Symptoms include dementia, memory dysfunction, pseudobulbar signs, ataxia, spasticity, seizures, coma, and death. CT demonstrates cerebral atrophy and diffuse white matter hypodensity (Figure 27.5) (114).

Pathologic changes are seen in patients receiving MTX alone, regardless of having also received irradiation, and the extent of injury seems to correlate with the total dosage of MTX. Changes are limited to the white matter and consist of multiple scattered, noninflammatory foci, or necrotic degeneration with varying amounts of mineralization, reactive astrocytosis, and necrotizing microangiopathy. When severe, axonal swelling and extensive demyelination occur, the focal areas of necrosis become confluent (Figure 27.6) (114–117).

Although the mechanism of injury is not yet defined in humans, the generally accepted theory, as proposed by Price and Jamison (115), is that methotrexate interferes with the metabolism of myelin-supporting structures in the CNS. Prior irradiation damages the endothelial cells, comprising the blood–brain barrier, and can allow for additional MTX to diffuse into the CNS, causing further damage (115).

The difficulty in determining whether MTX is the sole cause of this syndrome or just one of many factors is that few patients receive MTX alone. Radiation therapy, the presence of meningeal leukemia, and either method of giving MTX (HD-MTX and IT MTX) likely have synergistic

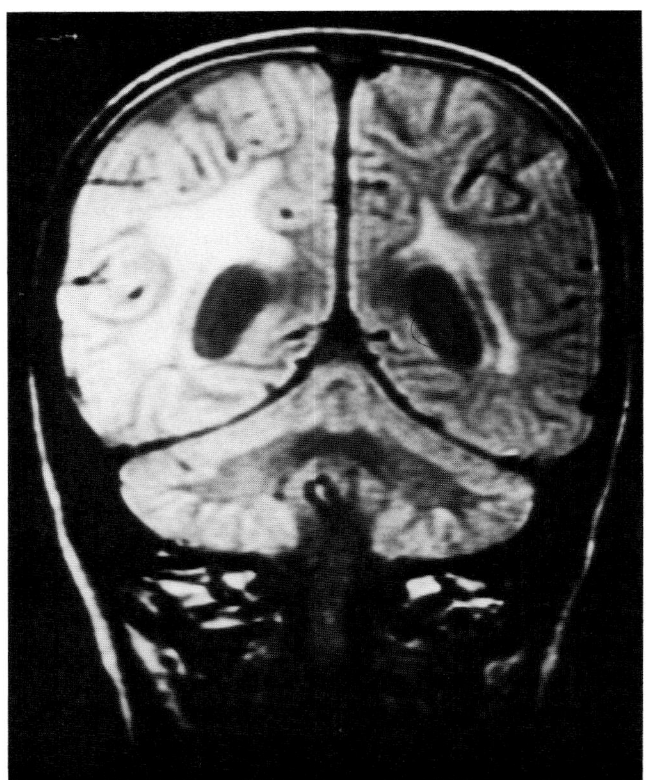

A

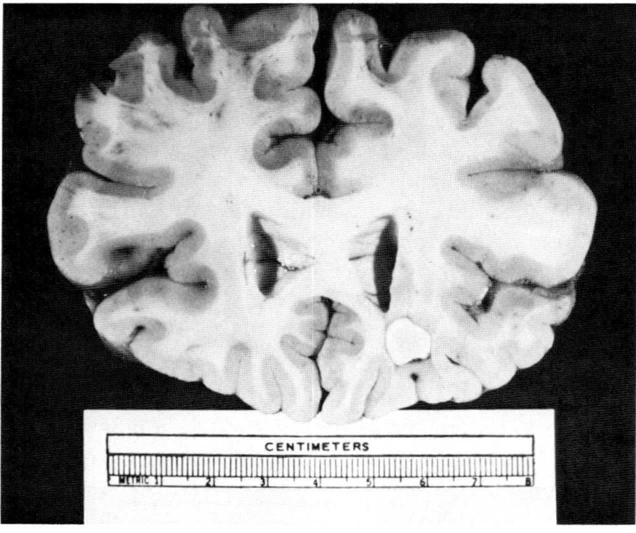

B

FIGURE 27.5 A Methotrexate leukoencephalopathy. Proton density MRI of a 14-year-old boy treated with intrathecal methotrexate for acute lymphocytic leukemia. Abnormal hyperintense signal from subcortical white matter is present more in the right hemisphere but also seen in the left. **B** Methotrexate leukoencephalopathy. Coronal section through the frontal lobe of a 6-year-old boy showing sharply demarcated areas of necrosis in the right subcortical white matter. This lesion in chronic and characterized by partial calcification of the necrotic focus. Note the mild cortical atrophy evidenced by widened sulci.

nitrogen mustard, vincristine or cyclophosphamide, or both. Some of these drugs have intrinsic neurotoxicity that can be additive or synergistic with previously given neurotoxic agents.

Early reports, primarily dealing with adults following bone-marrow transplantation reported few, if any, neurologic complications. In 1982 Patchell et al. (187) described a 60% incidence of neurologic complications following bone-marrow transplantation in a mixed adult–pediatric population. The majority of complications were metabolically induced. Wiznitzer et al. (188) in 1984, reported the incidence of neurologic difficulties in 60 consecutive children undergoing bone-marrow transplantation, including patients with malignancies, aplastic anemia, and metabolic disease. Twenty-six patients (43%) had CNS dysfunction including infections in 8, cerebrovascular accidents in 5, the later development of CNS leukemia in 7, and metabolic encephalopathies in 5. Neuropsychologic dysfunction was present in 4 of 5 long-term survivors evaluated. Seventy-four percent of patients who underwent postmortem examination had structural CNS damage. CNS dysfunction was more common in patients with lymphoreticular malignancies. The toxicities seemed to be due to the additive toxicity of bone-marrow transplantation regimens and immunosuppression on top of previous neurotoxic treatment. Children who had previously received whole-brain radiotherapy or large doses of methotrexate seem to be the most likely to develop neurologic toxicity. Peripheral nervous system involvement was also found, but less frequently. This included cranial nerve dysfunction primarily secondary to CNS infection and neurologic deficits following herpetic infection. The development of graft-versus-host disease in patients following transplantation was not found to predispose to increased neurologic toxicity (188).

ACKNOWLEDGMENTS

Supported in part by the Preuss Foundation and the Chatlow Foundation. We would like to thank Dr. Jonathan L. Finlay for his editorial assistance and Dr. L. Rorke for supplying the neuropathologic photomicrographs. We would also like to thank Linda Cella for her secretarial assistance.

REFERENCES

1. Young JL, Jr., Heise HE, Silverberg E, et al. Cancer incidence, survival and mortality for children under 15 years of age. New York, American Cancer Society Professional Education Publication, September 1978.

2. Miller RW, Mickey FW. Decline in U.S. childhood cancer mortality, 1950 thru 1980. JAMA 1984;215:1567–1570.

3. Goldie JH, Coldman AJ. A mathematical model for relating the drug sensitivity of tumors to their spontaneous mutation rate. Cancer Treat Rep 1979;63:172.

4. Kun LE. Principles of radiation therapy. In: Cohen ME, Duffner PK, eds. Brain Tumors in Children. Principles of Diagnosis and Treatment. New York: Raven Press, 1984;47–70.

5. Sheline GE. Irradiation injury of the human brain: a review of clinical experience. In: Gilbert HA, Kagan AR, eds. Radiation Damage to the Nervous System. A Delayed Therapeutic Hazard. New York: Raven Press, 1980;39–58.

6. Doida Y, Otada S. Radiation induced mitotic delay in cultured mammalian cells L5178Y. Radiat Res 1969;38:513.

7. Denakamp J. Fowler JF. Cell proliferation kinetics and radiation therapy. In: Becker FE, ed. Cancer—A Comprehensive Treatise. New York: Plenum Publishing 1977;101–137.

8. Whitmore GF, Gulyas S, Botond J. Radiation sensitivity throughout the cell cycle and its relationship to recovery. In: Cellular Radiation Biology. Baltimore: Williams & Wilkins, 1965;423–431.

9. Hall EJ. Cell survival curves. Radiosensitivity and cell age in the mitotic cycle. In: Hall EJ, ed. Radiobiology for the Radiologist, 2nd ed. Hagerstown: Harper & Row, 1978;36–82.

10. Shukovsky LJ, Fletcher GH, Montague ED, et al. Experience with twice-a-day fractionation in clinical radiotherapy. Am J Roentgenol 1976;126:155–162.

11. Caveness WF. Experimental observations: Delayed necrosis in normal monkey brain. In: Gilbert HA, Kagan AR, eds. Radiation Damage to the Nervous System. A Delayed Therapeutic Hazard. New York: Raven Press, 1980;1–38.

12. Kramer S, Hendrickson F, Zelen M, et al. Therapeutic trials in the management of metastatic brain tumors by different time/dose fraction schemes of radiation therapy. Monogr Natl Cancer Inst 1977;46:213–221.

13. Young DF, Posner JB, Chu F, et al. Rapid course radiation therapy of cerebral metastases: Results and complications. Cancer 1974;34:1069–1076.

14. Hindo WA, DeTrana FA III, Lee MS, et al. Large dose increment irradiation in treatment of cerebral metastases. Cancer 1970;26:138–141.

15. Druckmann A. Schlafsucht als Folge der Röntgenbestrahlung: Beitrag zur strahlenempfindlichkeit des gehirns. Strahlentherapie, 1929;33:382–384.

16. Freeman JE, Johnston PDG, Voke JM. Somnolence after prophylactic cranial irradiation in children with acute lymphoblastic leukaemia. Br Med J 1973;4:523–525.

17. Ch'ien CT, Aur RJA, Stagner S, et al. Long-term neurological implications of somnolence syndrome in children with acute lymphatic leukemia. Ann Neurol 1980;8:273–277.

18. Hoffman WF, Levin VA, Wilson CB. Evaluation of malignant glioma patients during the post irradiation period. J Neurosurg 1979;50:624–628.

19. Boden G. Radiation myelitis to the cervical cord. Br Med J 1948;2:79–94.

20. Jones A. Transient radiation myelopathy (with reference to Lhermitte's sign of electrical paresthesia). Br J Radiol 1964;37:727–744.

21. Glass JP, Foley KM. Harmful effects of radiation. In: Asbury AK, McKhann GM, McDonald WI, eds. Diseases of the Nervous System. Clinical Neurobiology. Philadelphia: W.B. Saunders, 1986;1188–1202.

22. Mikhael MA. Dosimetric calculations in the diagnosis of radiation necrosis of the brain. In: Gilbert HA, Kagan AR, eds. Radiation Damage to the Nervous System. A Delayed Therapeutic Hazard. New York: Raven Press, 1980;54–91.

23. Glass JP, Hwang TL, Leavens ME, et al. Cerebral radiation necrosis following treatment of extracranial malignancies. Cancer 1984;54:1966–1972.

24. Shewmon DA, Masdeu JC. Delayed radiation necrosis of the brain contralateral to original tumor. Arch Neurol 1980; 37:592–594.

25. Mikhael MA. Radiation necrosis of the brain: Correlation between computed tomography, pathology and dose distribution. J Comput Assist Tomogr 1978;2:71–80.

26. Mikhael MA. Radiation necrosis of the Brain: Correlation between patterns on computed tomography and dose of radiation. J Comput Assist Tomogr 1979;3:241–249.

27. Deck MDF. Imaging techniques in the diagnosis of radiation damage to the central nervous system. In: Gilbert HA, Kagan AR, eds. Radiation Damage to the Nervous System: A Delayed Therapeutic Hazard. New York: Raven Press, 1980;107–127.

28. Martins AN, Johnston JS, Henry JM, et al. Delayed radiation necrosis of the brain. J Neurosurg 1977;47:336–345.

29. Patronas NJ, DiChiro G, Brooks RA, et al. Work in progress: (^{18}F) fluordeoxyglucose and positron emission tomography in the evaluation of radiation necrosis of the brain. Radiology 1982;144:885–889.

30. O'Tuama LA, Williams JA, LaFrance ND, et al. Role of "C-L-methionine" positron emission tomography (PET) in the care of children with brain tumors. Ann Neurol 1986; 20:422.

31. Groothuis DR, Vick NA. Radionecrosis of the central nervous system: The perspective of the clinical neurologist and neuropathologist. In: Gilbert HA, Kagan AR, eds. Radiation Damage to the Nervous System: A Delayed Therapeutic Hazard. New York: Raven Press, 1980: 93–106.

32. Edwards MS, Wilson CB. Treatment of radiation necrosis. In: Gilbert HA, Kagan AR, eds. Radiation Damage to the Nervous System: A Delayed Therapeutic Hazard. New York: Raven Press, 1980;129–143.

33. Rizzoli HA, Pagnanelli DM. Treatment of delayed radiation necrosis of the brain. A clinical observation. J Neurosurg 1984;60:589–594.

34. Hilal SK, Solomon GE, Gold AP, et al. Primary cerebral arterial occlusive disease in children. II. Neurocutaneous syndromes. Radiology 1971;99:87–94.

35. Wright TL, Bresnan MJ. Radiation-induced cerebrovascular disease in children. Neurology 1976;26:540–543.

36. Painter MJ, Chutorian AM, Hilal SK. Cerebral vasculopathy following irradiation in childhood. Neurology 1975;25: 189–194.

37. Silverberg GD, Britt RH, Goffinet OR. Radiation-induced carotid artery disease. Cancer 1978;40:130–137.

38. Price RA, Birdwell DA. The central nervous system in childhood leukemia. III. Mineralizing microangiopathy and dystrophic calcification. Cancer 1978;42:717–728.

39. Price RA, Jamieson PA. The central nervous system in childhood leukemia. II. Subacute leukoencephalopathy. Cancer 1975; 35:306–318.

40. McIntosh S, Fischer DB, Rothman S, et al. Intracranial calcifications in childhood leukemia. J Pediatr 1977;91:909–913.

41. Davis PC, Hoffman JC, Pearl CS, et al. CT evaluation of effects of cranial irradiation therapy in children. AJNR 1986;7:639–644.

42. Cohen ME, Duffner PK. Long-term clinical effects of radiation and chemotherapy. In: Brain Tumors in Children. Principles of Diagnosis and Treatment. New York;Raven Press, 1984;308–327.

43. Duffner PK, Cohen ME, Anderson SW, et al. Long-term effects of treatment on endocrine function in children with brain tumors. Ann Neurol 1983;14:528–532.

44. Dickinson MS, Berry DH, Dickenson BA, et al. Differential effects of cranial irradiation on growth hormone response to arginine and insulin infusion. J Pediatr 1978;92:754–756.

45. Shalet SM, Beardwell CG, Morris-Jones PH, et al. Growth hormone deficiency after treatment of acute leukemia in children. Arch Dis Child 1976;51:489–492.

46. Shalet SM, Beardwell CG, Twomey JA, et al. Endocrine function following the treatment of acute leukemia in childhood. J Pediatr 1977;90:920–923.

47. Swift PGF, Kearney PJ, Dalton RG, et al. Growth and hormonal status of children treated for acute lymphoblastic leukemia. Arch Dis Child 1978;53:890–894.

48. Fisher JN, Aur RJA. Endocrine assessment in childhood acute lymphocytic leukemia. Cancer 1982;49:145–151.

49. Oberfield SE, Allen JC, Pollak J, et al. Long-term endocrine sequelae after treatment of medulloblastoma: Prospective study of growth and thyroid function. J Pediatr 1986; 108:219–223.

50. Duffner PK, Cohen ME, Thomas PRM, et al. The long-term effects of cranial irradiation on the central nervous system. Cancer 1985;56:1841–1846.

51. Verzosa MS, Aur RJA, Simone JV, et al. Five years after central nervous system irradiation of children with leukemia. Int J Radiat Oncol Biol Phys 1976;1:209–215.

52. Soni SS, Marten GW, Pitner SE, et al. Effects of central nervous system irradiation on neuropsychologic functioning of children with acute lymphocytic leukemia. N Engl J Med 1975;293:113–118.

53. Moss Ha, Nonnis ED, Poplack DG. The effects of prophylactic treatment of the central nervous system on the intellectual functioning of children with acute lymphocytic leukemia. Am J Med 1981;71:47–52.

54. Meadows AT, Massari DJ, Fergusson J, et al. Declines in IQ scores and cognitive dysfunctions in children with acute lymphocytic leukaemia treated with cranial irradiation. Lancet 1981;1:1015–1018.

55. Raimondi AJ, Tomita T. Advantages of "total" resection of medulloblastoma and disadvantages of full head post-operative radiation therapy. Child's Brain 1979;5:550–551.

56. Duffner PK, Cohen ME, Thomas P. Late effects of treatment on the intelligence of children with posterior fossa tumors. Cancer 1983;51:233–237.

57. Hirsch JF, Reiner D, Czernichow P, et al. Medulloblastoma in childhood. Survival and functional results. Acta Neurochir 1979;48:1–15.

58. Packer RJ, Bruce DA, Atkins TA, et al. Factors impacting on neurocognitive outcome in long-term survivors of primitive neuroectodermal tumors/medulloblastoma (PNET-MB). Ann Neurol 1986;20:396–397.

59. Packer RJ, Zimmerman RA, Bilaniuk LT. Magnetic resonance imaging in the evaluation of treatment related central nervous system damage. Cancer 1986;58:635–640.

60. Kagan AR, Wollin M, Gilbert HA, et al. Comparison of the tolerance of the brain and spinal cord to injury by radiations. In: Gilbert HA, Kagan AR, eds. Radiation Damage to the Nervous System: A Delayed Therapeutic Hazard. New York: Raven Press, 1980;183–190.

61. Reagan TJ, Thomas JE, Colby MY. Chronic progressive radiation myelopathy. Its clinical aspects and differential diagnosis. JAMA 1968;203:128–132.

62. Pallis CA, Lewis S, Morgan RL. Radiation myelopathy. Brain 1961;84:460–479.

63. Wara WM, Phillips TL, Sheline GE, et al. Radiation tolerance of the spinal cord. Cancer 1975;35:1558–1562.

64. Eyster EF, Wilson CB. Radiation myelopathy. J Neurosurg 1970;32:414–420.

65. Ballweg GP, Donnenfeld H, Chusid JG. Subacute radiation myelopathy in a 12 year old boy. Child's Brain 1976; 2:195–201.

66. Sundaresan N, Gutierrez FA, Larsen MB. Radiation myelopathy in children. Ann Neurol 1978;4:47–50.

67. Littman P, Rosenstock JG, Bailey C. Radiation myelitis following craniospinal irradiation with concurrent actinomycin-D therapy. Med Pediatr Oncol 1978;5:145–151.

68. Cohen ME, Duffner PK, Terplan K. Myelopathy with severe structural derangement associated with combined modality therapy. Cancer 1983;52:1590–1596.

69. D'Angio GS, Farber S, Maddock CL. Potentiation of x-ray effects by actinomycin-D. Radiology 1959;73:175–177.

70. Goldwein JW. Radiation myelopathy: A review. Med Pediatr Oncol 1987;15:89–95.

71. Kinsella TI, Weichselbaum RR, Sheline GE. Radiation injury of cranial and peripheral nerves. In: Gilbert HA, Kagan AR eds. Radiation Damage to the Nervous System: A Delayed Therapeutic Hazard. New York: Raven Press, 1980; 145–153.

72. Borsanyi S, Blanchard CL. Ionizing radiation and the ear. JAMA 1962;181:958–961.

73. Granowetter L, Rosenstock JG, Packer RJ. Enhanced cisplatinum neurotoxicity in pediatric patients with brain tumors. J Neurooncol 1983;1:293–297.

74. Shukousky LJ, Fletcher GH. Retinal and optic nerve complications in high dose irradiation technique of ethmoid sinus and nasal cavity. Radiology 1972;104:629–634.

75. Cheng VST, Shultz MD. Unilateral hypoglossal nerve atrophy as a late complication of radiation therapy of head and neck carcinoma. Cancer 1975;35:1537–1544.

76. Berger PS, Bataini JP. Radiation-induced cranial nerve palsy. Cancer 1977;40:152–155.

77. Bagley FH, Walsh JW, Cody B, et al. Carcinomatosis versus radiation-induced brachial plexus neuropathy in breast cancer. Cancer 1978;41:2154–2157.

78. Thomas JE, Colby MY. Radiation-induced or metastatic brachial plexopathy? A diagnostic dilemma. JAMA 1972; 222:1392–1395.

79. Kori SH, Foley KM, Posner JB. Brachial plexus lesions in patients with cancer: 100 cases. Neurology 1981; 31:45–50.

80. Thomas JE, Cascino TE, Earle JD. Differential diagnosis between radiation and tumor plexopathy of the pelvis. Neurology 1985;35:1–7.

81. Albers JW, Allen AA, Bastrow JA, et al. Limb myokymia. Muscle Nerve 1981;4:494–504.

82. Foley KM, Woodruff JM, Posner JB. Radiation-induced malignant schwannomas. Neurology 1975; 25:354.

83. Foley KM, Woodruff JM, Ellis FT, et al. Radiation-induced malignant and atypical peripheral nerve sheath tumors. Ann Neurol 1980;7:311–318.

84. Li FP, Cassady JR, Jaffe N. Risk of second tumors in survivors of childhood cancer. Cancer 1975; 35:1230–1235.

85. Li FP. Second malignant tumors after cancer in childhood. Cancer 1977;40:1899–1902.

86. Meadows AT, D'Angio GS, Evans AE, et al. Oncogenesis and other late effects of cancer treatment in children. Radiology 1975;114:175–180.

87. Haselow RE, Nesbit M, Dehner LP, et al. Second neoplasms following megavoltage radiation in a pediatric population. Cancer 1978;42:1185–1191.

88. Modan B, Mart N, Baidatz D, et al. Radiation-induced head and neck tumors. Lancet 1974;23:277–279.

89. Kramer S. The hazards of therapeutic irradiation of the central nervous system. Clin Neurosurg 1968;15:301–318.

90. Noetzli M, Malamud N. Post irradiation fibrosarcoma of the brain. Cancer 1962;15:617–662.

91. Schrantz JL, Araoz CA. Radiation-induced meningeal fibrosarcoma. Arch Pathol 1972;92:26–31.

92. Waltz TA, Brownell B. Sarcoma: A possible late result of effective radiation therapy for pituitary adenoma: A report of two cases. J Neurosurg 1966;24:901–907.

93. Chug CK, Stryker JA, Cruse R, et al. Glioblastoma multiforme following prophylactic cranial irradiation and intrathecal methotrexate in a child with acute lymphocytic leukemia. Cancer 1981;47:2563–2566.

94. Gagliano R, Costani J. Paraplegia following intrathecal methotrexate: Report of a case and review of the literature. Cancer 1976;37:1663–1668.

95. Levine RA, Miller LP, Lovenberg W. Tetrahydrobioptein in striatum: Localization in dopamine terminals and role in catecholamine synthesis. Science 1981;214:919–921.

96. Metita BM, Shapiro WR, Rosen G, et al. Distribution of folate following methotrexae - leukovorin rescue regimen in cancer patients. In:Kisliuk RL, Brown GM, eds. Chemistry and Biology Pteridines. New York: Elsevier North-Holland, 1979;677–682.

97. Abelson HT. Methotrexate and central nervous system toxicity. Cancer Treat Rep 1978;62:1999–2001.

98. Bleyer WA. Neurologic sequelae of methotrexate and ionizing radiation. A new classification. Cancer Treat Rep 1981;65:89–98.

99. Weiss HD, Walker MD, Wiernik PH. Neurotoxicity of commonly used neoplastic agents. N Engl J Med 1974;291: 75–81,127–133.

100. Pizzo PA, Poplack DG, Bleyer WA. Neurotoxicities of current leukemia therapy. Am J Pediatr Hematol Oncol 1979;1: 127–140.

101. Geise CF, Bishop Y, Frei E. Toxic effects of intrathecal methotrexate (IT MTX) in central nervous system (CNS) prophylaxis of leukemic children: Clinical and morphologic studies. Proc Am Cancer Res 1974;15:77.

102. Duttera MJ, Bleyer WA, Pomeroy TC, et al. Irradiation, methotrexate toxicity and the treatment of meningeal leukemia. Lancet 1973;2:703–707.

103. Price RA. Histopathology of CNS leukemia and complications of therapy. Am J Pediatr Hematol Oncol 1979;1: 21–30.

104. Saiki JH, Thompson S, Smith F, et al. Paraplegia following intrathecal chemotherapy. Cancer 1972;29:370–374.

105. Allen JC, Rosen G, Mehta BM, et al. Leukoencephalopathy following high-dose IV methotrexate chemotherapy with leukovorin rescue. Cancer Treat Rep 1980;64:1261–1271.

106. Martino RL, Benson AB, Merritt JA, et al. Transient neurologic dysfunction following moderate-dose methotrexate for undifferentiated lymphoma. Cancer 1984;54:2003–2005.

107. Jaffe N, Takaue Y, Anzai Y, et al. Transient neurologic disturbances induced by high-dose methotrexate treatment. Cancer 1985;56:1356–1360.

108. Packer RJ, Grossman RI, Belasco J. High-dose systemic methotrexate: Associated neurologic dysfunction. Med Pediatr Oncol 1983;11:159–161.

109. Kaminskas E, Nussey AC. Effect of methotrexate and of environmental factors on glycolysis and metabolic energy state in cultured Ehrlich ascites carcinoma cells. Cancer Res 1978;38:2989–2996.

110. Phillips PC, Berger CA, Arnold JC, et al. High-dose leukovorin reverses high-dose methotrexate-induced depression of regional cerebral metabolic rate for glucose in the rat. Ann Neurol 1985;18:404.

111. Phillips PC, Thaler HT, Berger CA, et al. Acute high-dose methotrexate neurotoxicity in the rat. Ann Neurol 1986;20:583–589.

112. Shapiro WR, Chernik NL, Posner JB. Necrotizing encephalopathy following intraventricular instillation of methotrexate. Arch Neurol 1973;28:96–102.

113. Packer RJ, Zimmerman RA, Rosenstock J, et al. Focal encephalopathy following methotrexate therapy. Arch Neurol 1981;38:450–452.

114. Shapiro WR, Allen JC, Horter BC. Chronic methotrexate toxicity to the central nervous system. Clin Bull 1980;10:49–52.

115. Price RA, Jamieson PA. The central nervous system in childhood leukemia. II. Subacute leukoencephalopathy. Cancer 1975;35:306–318.

116. Rubinstein LJ, Herman MM, Long TF, et al. Disseminated necrotizing leukoencephalopathy: A complication of treated central nervous system leukemia and lymphoma. Cancer 1975;35:291–305.

117. Hendlin B, DeVivo DC, Torack R, et al. Parenchymatous degeneration of the central nervous system in childhood leukemia. Cancer 1974;33:468–482.

118. Crosley CJ, Rorke LB, evans A, et al. Central nervous system lesions in childhood leukemia. Neurology 1978;28:678–685.

119. McHenry LC, Ewald RA, Talbert WM, et al. Bilateral cortical cerebellar sclerosis. Arch Pathol 1964;78:665–672.

120. Roseman NP, Shapiro MB, Wolf PA. Sclerotic atrophy of the cerebellum: A clinicopathological survey. J Neuropathol Exp Neurol 1978;37:174–191.

121. Winkelman MD, Hines JD. Cerebellar degeneration caused by high-dose cytosine arabinoside: A clinicopathological study. Ann Neurol 1983;14:520–527.

122. Olsen ME, Chernik NL, Posner JB. Infiltration of the leptomeninges by systemic cancer. Arch Neurol 1974;30:122–137.

123. Price RA, Johnson WM. The central nervous system in childhood cancer. I. The arachnoid. Cancer 1973;31:520–533.

124. Wiznitzer M, Packer RJ, Rorke LB, et al. Cerebellar sclerosis in pediatric cancer patients. J Neurooncol 1987;4:353–360.

125. Ho DHW, Frei E. Clinical pharmacology of 1-B-D-arabino-furanosyl arabinoside. Clin Pharmacol Ther 1974;12:944–954.

126. Russell JA, Powles RL. Neuropathy due to cytosine arabinoside. Br Med J 1974;4:652.

127. Rudnick SA, Gadman EC, Capizzi RL, et al. High-dose cytosine arabinoside in refractory acute leukemia. Cancer 1979;44:1189–1193.

128. Lazarus HM, Herzig RH, Herzig GP, et al. Central nervous system toxicity of high-dose systemic cytosine arabinoside. Cancer 1981;48:2577–2582.

129. Watson PR, Brubaker LH, Yaghmai F. Severe central nervous system toxicity from high-dose cytarabine: Expressive aphasia occurring after the second day of treatment. Cancer Treat Rep 1985;69:313–314.

130. Winkelman MD, Hines JD. Cerebellar degeneration caused by high-dose systemic cytosine arabinoside. Ann Neurol 1982;12:77.

131. Johnson NT, Crawford SW, Sargur M. Acute acquired demyelinating polyneuropathy with respiratory failure following high-dose systemic cytosine arabinoside and marrow transplantation. Bone Marrow Transplant 1987;2:203–207.

132. Herzig RH, Wolff SN, Lazarus HM, et al. High-dose cytosine arabinoside therapy for refractory leukemia. Blood 1983;62:361–369.

133. Yung WKA, Hwang T, Martinez-Prieto J, et al. Neurotoxicity of high-dose Ara-C and intracarotid chemotherapy. Prog Exp Tumor Res 1985;29:183–189.

134. Benger A, Browman GP, Walker IR, et al. Clinical evidence of a cumulative effect of high-dose cytarabine on the cerebellum in patients with acute leukemia: A leukemia Intergroup report. Cancer Treat Rep 1985;69:240–241.

135. Rubinstein LJ, Herman MM, Long TF, et al. Disseminated necrotizing leukoencephalopathy: A complication of treated central nervous system leukemia and lymphoma. Cancer 1975;35:291–305.

136. Mena H, Garcia JH, Velandia F. Central and peripheral myelinopathy associated with systemic neoplasia and chemotherapy. Cancer 1981;48:1724–1737.

137. Eden OB, Goldie W, Wood T, et al. Seizures following intrathecal cytosine arabinoside in young children with acute lymphoblastic leukemia. Cancer 1978;42:53–58.

138. Young DF, Posner JB. Nervous system toxicity of chemotherapeutic agents. In: Vinken PJ, Bruyn GW, eds. Handbook of Clinical Neurology. II. Neurologic Manifestations of Systemic Diseases. New York, North-Holland Publishing, 1980;91–131.

139. Moertel CG, Reitemeier RJ, Bolton CF, et al. Cerebellar ataxia associated with fluorinated pyrimidine therapy. Cancer Treat Rep 1964;41:15–18.

140. Howell SB, Pfeifle CE, Wung WE. Effect of allopurinol on the toxicity of high-dose 5-fluorouracil administered by intermittent bolus injection. Cancer 1983;51:220–225.

141. Koenig H, Patel A. The acute cerebellar syndrome in 5-fluorouracil chemotherapy: A manifestation of fluoroacetate intoxication. Neurology 1970;20:416.

142. Tashima CK. Immediate cerebral symptoms during rapid intravenous administration of cyclophosphamide. Cancer Chemother Rep 1975;59:441–432.

143. Kende G, Sirkin SR, Thomas PRM, et al. Blurring of vision. A previously undescribed complication of cyclophosphamide therapy. Cancer 1979;44:69–71.

144. Cohen MH, Creaven RJ, Tejada F, et al. Phase I clinical trial of ifosfamide (NSC-109724). Cancer Chemother Rep 1975;59:751–755.

145. Pratt CB, Horowitz ME, Meyer WH, et al. Phase II trial of ifosfamide in children with malignant solid tumors. Cancer Treat Rep 1987;71:131–135.

146. Pratt CB, Green AA, Horowitz ME, et al. Central nervous system toxicity following the treatment of pediatric patients with ifosfamide/MESNA. J Clin Oncol 1986;4:1253–1261.

147. Luce JK. MESNA Background and Clinical Summary. Columbus, Ohio, Adria Laboratories, October 4, 1983.

148. Meanwell CA, Kelly KA, Blackledge G. Avoiding ifosfamide/MESNA encephalopathy. Lancet 1986;2:406.

149. Perren TJ, Turner RC, Smithe IE. Encephalopathy with rapid infusion ifosfamide/MESNA. Lancet 1987;1: 390–391.

150. Pratt CB. Personal communication. December 15, 1987.

151. Burger PC, Kamenar E, Schold SC, et al. Encephalomyelopathy following high-dose BCNU therapy. Cancer 1981; 48:1318–1327.

152. Schold SC, Fay JW. Central nervous system toxicity from high-dose BCNU treatment of systemic cancer. Neurology 1980; 30:429.

153. Johnson DB, Thompson JM, Corwin JA, et al. Prolongation of survival for high-grade malignant gliomas with adjuvant high-dose BCNU and autologous bone marrow transplantation. J Clin Oncol 1987;5:783–789.

154. Cascino TL, Byrne TN, Deck MDF, et al. Intra-arterial BCNU in the treatment of metastatic brain tumors. J Neurooncol 1983;1:211–218.

155. Steward DJ, Grahovac Z, Russel NA, et al. Phase I study of intracarotid PCNU. J Neurooncol 1987;5:245–250.

156. Bremer AM, Kleriga E, Nguyen TQ, et al. Complications associated with intra-arterial BCNU administered in combination with vincristine and procarbazine for the treatment of malignant brain tumors. J Neurooncol 1984;2:219–132.

157. West CR, Avellanosa AM, Barua NR, et al. Phase II study on malignant gliomas of the brain treated with intra-arterial BCNU in combination with vincristine and procarbazine. Proc Am Assoc Cancer Res 1980;21:482.

158. Roelofs RI, Hrushesky W, Rogin J, et al. Peripheral sensory neuropathy and cisplatin chemotherapy. Neurology 1984; 34:934–938.

159. Ongerboer de Visser BW, Tiessens G. Polyneuropathy induced by cisplatin. Prog Exp Tumor Res 1985; 29:190–196.

160. Van Hoff DD, Schilsky R, Reichert CM, et al. Toxic effects of cisdichlorodiammineplatinum (II) in man. Cancer Treat Rep 1979;63:1527–1531.

161. McHaney VA, Thibadean G, Hoyes FA, et al. Auditory function of children receiving cis-platinum chemotherapy. Proc Am Assoc Cancer Res and ASCO 1981;22:401.

162. Baranak CC, Wetmore RF, Packer RJ. Cis-platinum ototoxicity after radiation treatment: An animal model. J Neurooncol 1988;6:261–267.

163. Ostrow S, Hahn D, Wiernk PH, et al. Ophthalmologic toxicity after cis-dichlorodiammineplatinum (II) therapy. Cancer Treat Rep 1978;62:1591–1594.

164. Beche R, Schutt P, Osieka R, et al. Peripheral neuropathy and ophthalmologic toxicity after treatment with cis-dichlorodiammine platinum II. J Cancer Res Clin Oncol 1980;96:219–221.

165. Berman IJ, Mann MP. Seizures and transient cortical blindness associated with cis-platinum (II) diamminedichloride (PDD) therapy in a thirty year old man. Cancer 1980; 45:764–766.

166. Steward D, Wallace S, Leavens M, et al. Phase I study of intracarotid cis-diamminodichloroplatinum in patients with intracerebral tumors. Proc Am Assoc Cancer Res 1981; 22:189.

167. Neuwelt EA, Glasberg M, Frenkel E, et al. Neurotoxicity of chemotherapeutic agents after blood–brain barrier modification: Neuropathological studies. Ann Neurol 1983; 14:316–324.

168. Owellen RJ, Hartke CA, Dickerson RM, et al. Inhibition of tubulin-microtubule polymerization by drugs and the vinca alkaloid class. Cancer Res 1976;36:1499–1502.

169. Holland JF, Schorland C, Gailani S, et al. Vincristine treatment of advanced cancer: A cooperative study of 392 cases. Cancer Res 1973;33:1258–1264.

170. Sandler SG, Tobin W, Henderson ES. Vincristine-induced neuropathy: A clinical study of fifty leukemic patients. Neurology 1969;19:367–374.

171. Rosenthal S, Kaufman S. Vincristine neurotoxicity. Ann Intern Med 1974; 80:733–734.

172. Radley WG, Lassman L, Pearce GW, et al. The neuromyopathy of vincristine in man: Clinical, electrophysiological and pathological studies. J Neurol Sci 1970;10:107–131.

173. Kaplan RS, Wiernik PH. Neurotoxicity of antineoplastic drugs. Semin Oncol 1982;9:103–1390.

174. Thomas LL, Braat PC, Somers R, et al. Massive vincristine overdose: Failure of leukovoran to reduce toxicity. Cancer Treat Rep 1982;66:1967–1969.

175. Jackson DV, Pope EK, McMahan RA, et al. Clinical trial of pyridoxine to reduce vincristine neurotoxicity. J Neurooncol 1986;4:37–41.

176. Fine RN, Clarke RR, Shore NA. Hyponatremia and vincristine therapy—syndrome possibly resulting from inappropriate antidiuretic hormone secretion. Am J Dis Child 1966; 112:256–259.

177. Slater LM, Wainer RA, Serpick NA. Vincristine neurotoxicity with hyponatremia. Cancer 1969;23:122–125.

178. Cutting WO. Inappropriate secretion of antidiuretic hormone secondary to vincristine therapy. Am J Med 1971; 51:269–271.

179. Robertson GL, Bhoopalan N, Zelbowitz LJ. Vincristine neurotoxicity and abnormal secretion of antidiuretic hormone. Arch Intern Med 1973;132:717–720.

180. Land VJ, Sutow WW, Fernback DJ, et al. Toxicity of L-asparginase in children with advanced leukemia. Cancer 1972;30:339–347.

181. Riccardi R, Holcenberg J, Glaubiger D, et al. L-asparaginase pharmacokinetics and L-asparagine in the cerebral spinal fluid. Proc Am Assoc Cancer Res 1980;21:366.

182. Moure JMB, Whitecar JP, Bodey GP. Electroencephalogram changes secondary to asparaginase. Arch Neurol 1970; 23:365–368.

183. Priest JR, Ramsey NK, Latchaw RE, et al. Thrombotic and hemorrhagic strokes complicating early therapy for childhood acute lymphoblastic leukemia. Cancer 1980;46: 1548–1554.

184. Cairo MS, Lazarus K, Gilmore RL, et al. Intracranial hemorrhage and focal seizures secondary to use of L-asparaginase during induction therapy of acute lymphocytic leukemia. J Pediatr 1980;97:829–833.

185. Packer RJ, Rorke LB, Lange BJ, et al. Cerebrovascular accidents in children with cancer. Pediatrics 1985; 76:194–201.

186. Allen JC, Gralla R, Reilly L, et al. Metoclopramide: Dose-related toxicity and preliminary antiemetic studies in children receiving cancer chemotherapy. J Clin Oncol 1985; 8:1136–1141.

187. Patchell RA, White CL, Clark HW, et al. Central nervous system complications of bone marrow transplantation: A clinical and pathological study (abstract). Ann Neurol 1982;12:80.

188. Wiznitzer M, Packer RJ, August CS, et al. Neurologic complications of bone marrow transplantation in childhood. Ann Neurol 1984;15:569–576.

189. Packer RJ, Meadows AT, Rorke LB, et al. Long-term sequelae of cancer treatment on the central nervous system in childhood. Med Pediatr Oncol 1987;15:241–253.

190. Rohatiner AZS, Prior P, Burton A, et al. Central nervous system toxicity of interferon. Prog Exp Tumor Res 1985; 29:197–202.

191. O'Dwyer RJ, Leyland-Jones B, Alonso MT, et al. Etoposide (VP–16–213) current status of an active anticancer drug. N Engl J Med 1985;312:692–700.

192. Bradley WG, Karlsseon IJ, Rassol GG. Metronidazole neuropathy. Br Med J 1977; 2:610–611.

193. Melgaard B, Sand Hasen H, Kamieniecka Z, et al. Misonidazole neuropathy: A clinical, electrophysiological and histological study. Ann Neurol 1982;12:10–17.

194. Weisman SJ, Berkow RL, Weetman RM, et al. 5-azacytidine: Acute central nervous system toxicity. Am J Pediatr Hematol Oncol 1985;86–88.

195. Van Eys J, Pack CR, Baram T. Phase I trial of procarbazine as a 5-day continuous infusion in children with central nervous system tumors. Cancer Treat Rep 1987;71:973–974.

196. Segal GM, Duckert LG. Reversible mechlorethamine-associated hearing loss in a patient with Hodgkin's disease. Cancer 1986;57:1089–1091.

Chapter 28
Craniospinal Trauma in Children

Michael S. B. Edwards and Philip H. Cogen

This chapter focuses on the pathophysiology, neuropathology, clinical presentation, treatment, and outcome after craniospinal trauma in children (aged 3 to 11 years) and adolescents (aged 11 to 18 years).

HEAD TRAUMA

Head trauma is the most common cause of death in children (1). This is an especially grim statistic because, unlike other major causes of childhood morbidity and mortality, head injury is potentially preventable. With intracranial injuries ranging from minor to fatal accounting for some 100,000 hospital admissions and 6,000 to 12,000 reported deaths each year (1–3), their impact on the health care system is major. While morbidity rates in the range of 0.3% to 1.0% are reported for minor head injuries in children (4), mortality rates for severe head injuries vary from 9.0% to 33% (2,5–7). This variation in mortality rates among individual series is in part a consequence of differences in the age of patients, the patient's condition on admission, the nature of the injury, and the length of time after injury until arrival at the reporting hospital. The variations also result from studies that pool data obtained from children of all age groups. Additional evidence of the importance of pediatric head injury in the spectrum of childhood trauma is that 80% of significant trauma in children involves an intracranial injury and that, in 60% of those children, their head trauma represents the most serious injury (8).

Pathophysiology

The fragility of the skull, softness of the brain parenchyma, and trauma associated with birth contribute to head injuries in newborns and neonates. Skull fractures, both linear and depressed, may be the result of a difficult birth caused by cephalopelvic disproportion or the use of instrumentation, such as forceps or suction extractors (9,10) or both. Intracranial or extracranial hematomas occur in 25% of cases of significant skull fracture in neonates. The most common type of hematoma is a cephalohematoma, a collection of blood between the skull and the pericranium bounded by normal suture lines. It is usually asymptomatic unless it is large enough to produce anemia because of the volume of blood lost, or if it calcifies, producing a disfiguring mass. Focal neurologic deficit may occur if depressed bone fragments penetrate the dura and injure the underlying brain tissue. Subarachnoid and/or intraventricular blood may be the result of a difficult delivery, but major intraventricular hemorrhage is usually associated with prematurity, maternal eclampsia, disproportion in the fetal head size, or significant coagulopathy (9).

In infants, the soft consistency of the unmyelinated brain and fragility of the cerebral bridging veins make the child vulnerable to a subdural hematoma. The incidence of subdural hematoma is highest in infants and elderly adults and has the same poor prognosis in both age groups (3). Infants and toddlers are often brought to a physician for evaluation of head injury after falling from their crib, changing table, or parent's bed, or less frequently after a motor vehicle accident (8). Unfortunately, many infants and toddlers who receive a head injury are the victims of so-called nonaccidental trauma or child abuse (11). Abused children may present with irritability or lethargy, a bulging fontanel, retinal hemorrhages, bruises on the head or body, or fractures of long bones or ribs. They usually do not have a clinical history consistent with the severity of the injury shown by the physical and neurologic examination. Evidence for repeated episodes of injury, such as healing fractures or acute and chronic subdural blood, is also suggestive of child abuse. Seizures may result from cortical irritation produced by subarachnoid or subdural blood. It is important to consider child abuse as the cause of head injury in all infants and young children because future episodes are potentially preventable. Doubts about the veracity of the history of head injury in a young child, or the appearance of signs of child abuse on either physical or radiologic examination should be investigated before planning the child's discharge from the hospital (9,11,12).

Older children and adolescents are most often injured from falls; in motor vehicle, pedestrian, or bicycle accidents; or, less often, during sports activities (2,13). Because of the thickness and immobility of the skull in these children, most of the insult from trauma is borne by the brain parenchyma and vasculature. This may be manifested clinically by a concussive state associated with loss of consciousness at the time of the accident, and by retrograde amnesia for events about the time of the injury (14). Even minor head injuries, without causing focal neurologic deficit, may produce a brief loss of consciousness and possibly retrograde amnesia for the period surrounding the injury (4). Seizures may occur at the time of initial impact and are most common during the first 24 hours after a head injury (15).

Significant intracranial hematomas are less common in older children and adolescents than in adults, except for those injured in high-speed motor vehicle or bicycle accidents (16). Epidural hematomas, which occur very seldom in infants, increase slowly in incidence throughout childhood and reach their peak during adulthood. Subdural hematomas, most commonly seen in infants and the elderly, are rarely seen in adolescents. Subarachnoid bleeding may result from even minor injuries (17). Skull fractures are often linear and should raise the suspicion of underlying epidural blood if the fracture line crosses a major dural artery, such as the middle meningeal artery, or a dural venous sinus. A child with a basilar skull fracture may present with cranial nerve deficits if the temporal bone is involved, and there may be cerebrospinal fluid (CSF) leakage through the nose and/or ear if the dura and arachnoid have been lacerated. Severe basilar skull fractures, especially those producing traumatic blindness, can lacerate the carotid artery or its branches or produce a dissection of the carotid or vertebral arteries, resulting in cerebral ischemia with transient or permanent motor weakness or death from massive intracranial or extracranial hemorrhage (16).

Neuropathology

Significant injury to the brain in infants younger than 6 months old characteristically produces tears in the white matter because of the lack of myelination and the soft consistency of the brain parenchyma (18). Traumatic injury in older children can damage crossing axons in the corpus callosum, which will be seen as distinct areas of hemorrhage on neuroimaging studies (16).

The most common response of the child's brain to significant injury is the development of diffuse cerebral swelling, the mechanism of which is not completely clear. It has been shown that diffuse swelling develops in a significantly greater number of children than adults with similar types of head injuries (18). Studies measuring cerebral blood flow in children immediately and several days after head injury have shown a relative hyperperfusion and intravascular congestion, suggesting that the cerebral swelling is caused by an increase in intravascular blood volume and not only by a change in vascular permeability (vasogenic edema) leading to an increase in free water (19–21). A better term for this event is therefore *cerebral hyperemia*. The hyperperfusion and cerebral swelling may occur in as short a time as several minutes after injury or as long as 24 hours later. Control of the associated increased intracranial pressure (ICP) is of paramount importance in the management of these children. The ability to regulate and reduce raised ICP is one of the most important predictors of the outcome after head injury (2,7,19). Diffuse cerebral swelling may also produce cellular hypoxia and hypoglycemia, producing cytotoxic edema which aggravates the initial brain insult (19).

Diffuse axonal injury (DAI) resulting from damage to the axon (Figure 28.1) may accompany diffuse cerebral swelling and hyperperfusion or may occur as an isolated event (20). The outcome from this type of direct neuronal injury is variable; severe DAI often results in permanent neurologic deficit. Similar but less dramatic pathologic events have been shown to occur following minor head injury in experimental animals, using horseradish peroxidase as a marker of cell mobility and disruption (22). These experimental findings may explain the clinical observation of significant neurologic dysfunction occurring in association with lesser degrees of head trauma in children (4). Direct injury to the brain stem has also been proposed as an important pathologic concomitant of significant pediatric head trauma; however, magnetic resonance imaging (MRI) techniques have shown that this type of pathologic finding rarely occurs as an isolated event. When present, damage to brain stem long tracts and cranial nerve nuclei is usually associated with prolonged coma and permanent neurologic deficit.

The cerebral vasculature of the developing brain is vulnerable to trauma. In the infant, tearing of the fragile veins bridging to the sagittal sinus results in an acute subdural hematoma. The underlying cerebral cortex undergoes an acute inflammatory response, which may lead to cerebral edema that eventually involves the entire hemisphere. It is not clear, however, whether this marked cerebral swelling is a direct response to the presence of the hematoma or if the hematoma is only a marker of a more severe direct parenchymal injury.

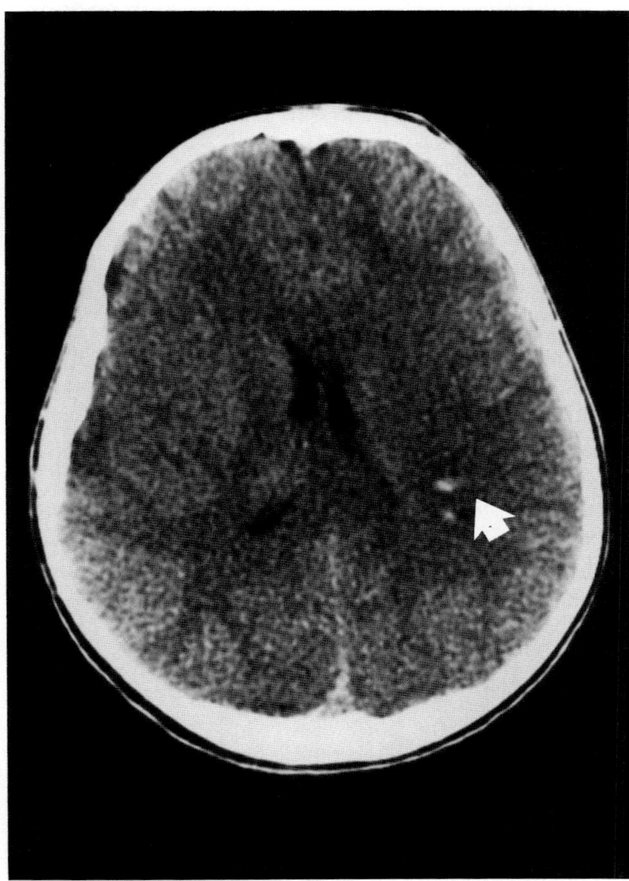

FIGURE 28.1   Axial CT brain scan without contrast agent following severe closed head injury. The dense lesions in the white matter (arrow) represent hemorrhage associated with diffuse axonal injury (DAI). The patient was a 6-year-old boy who was comatose with contralateral hemiparesis.

A rare but potentially devastating vascular complication of head injury is venous thrombosis, with propagation of clotted blood into the sagittal sinus producing venous infarction, diffuse cerebral edema, and permanent neurologic sequelae (17). Hypotension from associated systemic injuries significantly worsens the prognosis of the child following a head injury. Hypotension is associated with blood loss from intracranial hemorrhage only when there has been massive intraventricular hemorrhage in an infant, or a tear in a major venous sinus (10).

Arterial pathology may result from head trauma. Traumatic interruptions of the blood supply to the brain range from focal lesions, such as the shearing of small arterial branches, to dissection of the larger intracranial or extracranial arteries resulting in ischemia (17). Intracranial infarction may be produced or aggravated by systemic hypotension. Increased ICP may cause arterial vascular occlusion or impaired venous drainage with concomitant cerebral vascular congestion. Fractures of the temporal bone may tear the middle meningeal artery, producing an epidural hematoma. Epidural and subdural hematomas

also occur in the posterior fossa, where sudden changes in vital signs and respiratory arrest may be the result of brain stem compression (23).

Fractures of the skull base may produce direct injury to the cranial nerves. Fractures of the temporal bone in the middle fossa most often injure the seventh and/or eighth cranial nerves. However, in general, the first and sixth cranial nerves are the most commonly injured, the former by shearing forces along its delicate attachment to the floor of anterior fossa and the latter as a result of its long intracranial course. A CSF fistula may result from a skull fracture that lacerates the dura and entraps the arachnoid between the edges of the fractured bone. In some children, the interposition of arachnoid through a fracture may prevent healing of the bone edges, producing a leptomeningeal cyst or growing fracture of childhood.

Blood in the intraventricular or subarachnoid space may lead to obstruction of CSF pathways, producing hydrocephalus. It is clinically important to distinguish this etiology from the *ex vacuo* ventricular dilatation resulting from loss of tissue secondary to brain atrophy with a compensatory increase in the CSF space (13).

Neurologic Presentation

The presenting signs and symptoms of head trauma depend on the age of the child as well as on the mechanism of injury. Neonates who have had significant head injury during delivery show, at or shortly after birth, evidence of cardiorespiratory instability, bulging of the fontanel, irritability, and seizures. Physical examination may reveal an obvious depressed skull fracture (24). Poor suck and/or feeding responses, persistent bradycardia, or apnea are common signs of increased ICP (9). Older infants with increased ICP, whether from hemorrhage or post-traumatic hydrocephalus, have an increasing head circumference, bulging of the anterior fontanel, and separation of the calvarial sutures.

For infants and toddlers, child abuse may be inferred from repeated episodes of injury such as soft tissue bruises, new and healing fractures of the ribs and long bones, seizures, lethargy, or hyperirritability associated with bulging of the fontanel (11,25). Ophthalmologic examination may reveal retinal hemorrhages. Subarachnoid, subdural, or intracranial hemorrhage may be seen on computed tomographic (CT) brain scans or MRI. Seizures, ranging from a single convulsion to status epilepticus, may be a prominent presenting sign of child abuse. While the history elicited may be that of a "shaken baby," experimental studies suggest that a contact injury is necessary to produce the forces that result in the clinical presentation of most of these infants (12).

Head trauma in older children and adolescents presents with signs and symptoms that differ from those in infants and toddlers because of the thickness of the calvarium and the advanced maturity of the central nervous system (13). Patients who have repeated episodes of nausea and/or projectile vomiting or confusion and lethargy following injury require admission to the hospital. Minor head trauma presenting as a concussion is the most common type of childhood injury seen in most emergency rooms (2).

Although more than 90% of seizures following head injury occur during the first 24 hours after impact, they may occur several days after the initial injury (15). A single seizure in a child who is otherwise neurologically intact infrequently requires long-term anticonvulsant treatment, particularly if the seizure is within the first few minutes following the initial impact. The incidence of long-term seizures is higher in children who have intracranial mass lesions, prolonged coma, and/or depressed skull fractures that produce dural and brain lacerations. If there is a change in neurologic function associated with subsequent convulsions, additional neurologic evaluation is warranted.

The percentage of head-injured children who harbor mass lesions varies in the reported series from 10% to 40% and depends on the age range of the children reported and the acuteness of evaluation following injury (1–3,5–7). Epidural hematomas, which increase in incidence with advancing age of the patients (3), may present with signs of increased ICP immediately after injury, but these signs may be delayed during a lucid interval until several hours after the initial trauma. Factors increasing the risk of developing an epidural hematoma include a linear skull fracture that crosses the course of the middle meningeal artery or a major dural venous sinus, a change in mental status after several hours following injury, and a history of having incurred a high velocity impact. A large subgaleal hematoma, particularly in the temporal area, should alert the physician to the possibility of an epidural hematoma. The definitive diagnosis is based on a CT brain scan made without contrast agent (26).

Depressed skull fractures may be visible through an open laceration or may be palpable by gentle pressure in the area of injury (27). The presence of a subperiosteal hematoma may mimic that of a depressed fracture. Compound depressed skull fractures consist of an open laceration with displaced fragments of bone and require surgical debridement. Skull fractures from a head injury may not be apparent on physical examination if they are linear and are not depressed. Signs of a basilar skull fracture include bruising over the mastoid (Battle sign) or around the eyes (raccoon sign) (16). Fractures crossing the middle cranial fossa (temporal bone) may produce dysfunction of the seventh and/or eighth cranial nerves. Fractures through the cribriform plate and anterior fossa may be associated with CSF rhinorrhea, while those involving the temporal bone may produce CSF otorrhea.

Leakage of CSF is apparent from the persistent drainage of clear fluid from the nose or ear. The fluid tests positive for glucose, although it must be differentiated from tears and mucous which also are glucose-positive. The definitive diagnosis of a CSF leak is a persistent, copious leakage of watery fluid that is position-dependent. The fluid may be sent for analysis, including cell count, protein content, or serum protein electrophoresis, if the diagnosis is in doubt, but if there is sufficient fluid for such laboratory studies it is probably more worthwhile to pursue a neuroradiologic evaluation immediately.

Acute subdural hematomas resulting from head injury usually present with obvious signs of increased ICP at the initial examination. These findings include a depressed response to stimuli, increased blood pressure, and decreased pulse rate (Cushing sign), respiratory irregularity, pupillary asymmetry, and contralateral hemiparesis — all evidence of impending cerebral herniation. The pupillary dilatation is always on the side of the intracranial mass lesion in cases of cerebral herniation, although an ipsilateral hemiparesis may be seen from pressure across the tentorium with compression of the contralateral cerebral peduncle (Kernohan notch phenomenon) (16). Children with acute subdural hematoma should undergo immediate evacuation of the hematoma and be treated for the increased ICP.

Diffuse increased ICP following head injury may present with a picture similar to that of an intracerebral mass lesion, with either focal neurologic findings or evidence of generalized cerebral dysfunction. A CT brain scan is the most reliable way to determine whether there is a surgical mass lesion present (20).

Delayed effects from head injury in children may be subtle in onset. In infants, communicating hydrocephalus caused by arachnoidal scarring from a previous intracranial hemorrhage presents as progressive enlargement of the head circumference and bulging of the anterior fontanel (9). These same findings may be seen in association with a chronic subdural hematoma (28). Additional clinical signs in both of these conditions include poor feeding response, lethargy or irritability, nausea and vomiting, and seizures. Older children with delayed onset of hydrocephalus or chronic subdural hematomas may, after their injury, have a slow recovery of or late decline in mental status, persistent vomiting, or onset of new neurologic deficit (13) (Figure 28.2). In children with large chronic subdural hematomas, focal deficits such as hemiparesis may occur. As the acute subdural blood liquefies, well-developed and highly vascular membranes develop around the hematoma cavity. The amount of fluid in the cavity may increase because of a new hemorrhage from the surrounding membranes, often following a minor episode of head injury. These events lead to an increase in the mass effect of the hematoma and the appearance of new neurologic findings (28). CSF leak may appear days or weeks after the initial injury and may go unnoticed by the child, parents, or physician until an episode of meningitis initiates an evaluation of its etiology.

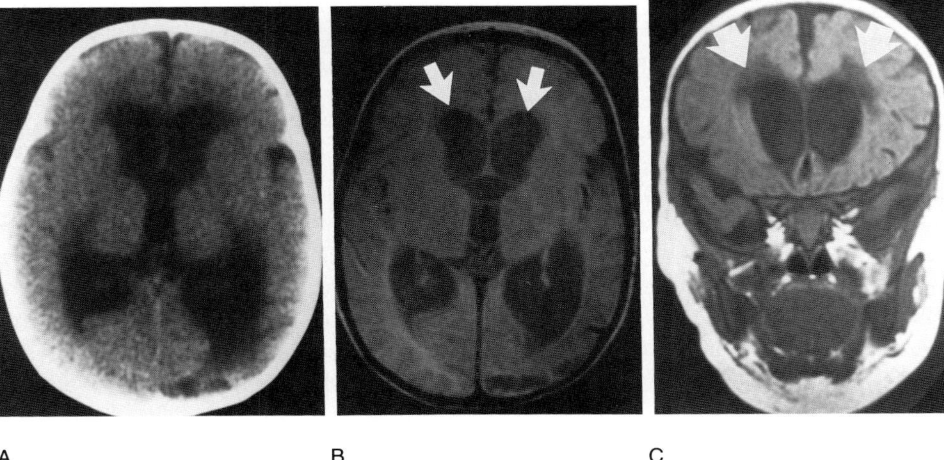

FIGURE 28.2   A: Axial CT brain scan without contrast agent in a 2-month-old male infant with posttraumatic hydrocephalus. The entire ventricular system is dilated. **B, C:** T1-weighted axial and coronal MR images better demonstrate the transependymal flow of cerebrospinal fluid (arrows). The child's irritability and vomiting resolved following the placement of a shunt.

A   B   C

General Diagnostic Considerations

The degree and complexity of the diagnostic evaluation of a child with head injury should be predicated on the index of suspicion for significant pathology, as based on the mechanism of injury, if it is known, and the clinical presentation of the child. Recent studies have shown that plain radiographs of the skull give little information and are not indicated for most head injuries (29). Even for cases in which a depressed skull fracture is suspected, a noncontrast CT scan is superior to radiographs in delineating the nature of the bone injury and in assessing the intracranial compartment and need for surgical intervention. At present, the CT brain scan is the best diagnostic test in the initial evaluation of a head-injured child (26). Computed tomography permits the evaluation of the bony calvarium, the soft tissues of the scalp, and the brain parenchyma. The brain parenchyma may demonstrate only edema, manifested by a diffuse decrease in signal, or edema associated with focal or diffuse intracranial hemorrhage. The presence of subarachnoid, subdural, epidural, and/or intracerebral blood is easily detected by increased signal intensity, allowing rapid and appropriate treatment (26). Intracranial hemorrhage observed on the CT brain scan in association with retinal hemorrhages may confirm a diagnosis of child abuse (30). In infants, ultrasonography is useful for demonstrating intracranial hemorrhage and/or hydrocephalus and is a reliable noninvasive method of routine follow-up review.

There is little or no indication for lumbar puncture in the acutely head-injured patient because this may cause cerebral herniation if the child has significant mass effect from edema or hemorrhage. Lumbar puncture may be necessary at a later time to evaluate a child with a fever to exclude a diagnosis of infection. The use of angiography is warranted in patients with more complex deficits, such as traumatic blindness, to exclude secondary vascular injury such as carotid or vertebral dissection, embolization, or transection (16). MRI has proved useful in the detection of more subtle lesions and in the correlation of overall outcome from head injury (31). However, the necessity of keeping the child motionless during imaging makes it a procedure best suited for follow-up evaluations. With improvements in the technology, however, MRI may eventually replace CT as the initial neuroradiologic test.

The decision to perform CT and/or to admit the child to the hospital is best addressed on an individual case basis, but general guidelines can be outlined (32). For infants, when it is difficult to obtain a history or when the family's report of the injury is not reliable, it is best to admit the child to the hospital. If the head injury has been severe enough to produce either a loss of consciousness or a seizure, or if there is a question about the nature of the injury, hospital admission is advisable. When it is necessary to sedate the child to perform a CT scan, it is advisable to arrange an overnight admission to the hospital. General indications for a CT brain scan in older head-injured children include significant alterations in mental status, focal neurologic deficit, suspicion of a depressed skull fracture, CSF leak, persistent projectile vomiting, and deterioration of neurologic function. Indications for admission to the hospital involve the presence of any of the findings just outlined or an abnormal CT scan. For a child with a lesser degree of injury, the presence of a responsible family member with the ability to observe the child's status also influences the decision to admit to the hospital (2).

Immediate Diagnosis and Treatment

The appropriate treatment modalities for a head-injured child depend on proper initial triage and assessment of the extent of injury. For newborns and infants, ultrasound imaging is helpful to determine the presence of hydrocephalus and of an intracranial hematoma, whether extra-axial or intraventricular. Significant intracranial hemorrhage in children of this age may produce a drop in the hematocrit and secondary hypovolemia, requiring transfusion. The presence of large volumes of blood in the ventricles and subarachnoid spaces also may signify the acute or delayed appearance of hydrocephalus.

If there is progressive dilatation of the ventricles consistent with hydrocephalus, serial lumbar punctures and the oral administration of Diamox (25 mg/kg every 24 hr divided into 3 doses) are frequently useful in the initial treatment of hydrocephalus. If lumbar punctures yield only small amounts of CSF, are technically difficult, or are required for more than 10 to 14 days because of persistence of hydrocephalus, then a ventricular access device may be inserted to aid in the drainage of CSF. This device may be subsequently converted into a shunt if necessary. Acute epidural or subdural hematomas associated with significant mass effect require immediate surgical evacuation.

Older children sustaining minor head injuries without neurologic deficit or loss of consciousness may be carefully observed and treated with mild analgesics that have no sedative effects, such as acetaminophen, and with antiemetics such as trimethobenzamide. Phenothiazine compounds and their derivatives, which can lower the seizure threshold, should not be used to treat the nausea and vomiting that occurs after head injury. If there is no improvement in the child's condition after several hours, or if there is a deterioration in neurologic status at any time, a CT scan should be performed.

Serious head injuries require a more aggressive approach. The use of the Glasgow coma scale (GCS), as modified for children (Table 28.1), is helpful in delineating the severity of head injury and the results of treatment (9). This scale gives a total of 1 to 4 points for ocular movement, 1 to 3 points for vocalization, and 1 to 4 points for motor response. It does not require an ability to follow verbal commands and therefore can be used to evaluate infants and young children (9). The GCS should be recorded for every apparently seriously head-injured child at the initial examination and serially at frequent intervals thereafter,

Table 28.1   Modified Glasgow coma score (gcs) for children*

Ocular response
    4 pursuit
    3 pupils reactive, extraocular motion intact
    2 pupils nonreactive or extraocular motion impaired
    1 pupils nonreactive and extraocular motion absent

Verbal response
    3 crying
    2 spontaneous breathing
    1 apnea

Motor response
    4 flexion and extension
    3 withdrawal from painful stimulation
    2 hypertonia
    1 flaccid

*Maximum score assignable is 11, minimum score assignable is 3. Reprinted with permission from Childs Brain 1984;11:12–35.

along with the vital signs. A child with a GCS of less than 6 on admission to the hospital is considered to have had a severe head injury.

The initial treatment of seriously head-injured children consists of measures to ensure adequate cardiorespiratory function and to lower ICP. Upon the child's arrival in the emergency room, the first assessment is of the vital signs, with particular attention to blood pressure, pulse, and respiratory effort and pattern. Symptoms of hypovolemia and shock should alert the physician to loss of blood elsewhere in the body as a result of associated injury. Determination of the source of bleeding and appropriate treatment is mandatory for optimal survival. Because the outcome is poorest for children with severe head injury who are hypotensive when they arrive at the emergency room (2,7), it is mandatory to establish good venous access to provide adequate fluid replacement and maintain blood pressure. Adequate airway control is essential and an endotracheal tube may be introduced even if medications to paralyze and sedate the patient are necessary.

The initial neurologic examination should include simple mental status testing (alertness, response to voice, vocalization); evaluation of pupillary size, shape, and reactivity; and motor movement, both spontaneous and with stimulation, including an assessment of muscle tone. The presence of corneal reflexes is easily tested and may be evaluated at the same time as the pupils are being checked.

Increased ICP, which occurs in all significantly head-injured patients, should be treated initially by measures that include elevating the head of the bed to 45° to improve venous return, and hyperventilation to a low pCO_2 level in the range of 24 to 28 mm Hg. An intravenous bolus injection of 20% mannitol (0.5 to 1.0 mg/kg) should be given. The child should then have a CT brain scan or be taken directly to the operating room if there is loss of consciousness associated with a lateralizing finding, such as a dilated and unreactive pupil. The lower incidence of surgical mass lesions in head-injured children suggests that a CT scan should precede surgical exploration in most cases (2,3,7,16).

The most common finding on CT scans of children with head injury is diffuse cerebral hyperemia, without a focal hematoma. ICP usually is elevated, appearing on CT scans as diffuse regions of low density in the brain parenchyma, together with compression of the ventricular system and a decrease in size of the perimesencephalic cistern, suggesting brain stem compression (26). Treatment of diffuse cerebral hyperemia without a focal hematoma should include elevation of the child's head, hyperventilation, fluid restriction to 1/2 to 2/3 of maintenance requirements, and placement of an ICP monitor to guide management strategies. Monitoring of the ICP is of prognostic benefit because a sustained ICP greater than 40 mm Hg associated with a GCS of less than 5 has been shown to be invariably fatal (7,21). ICP monitors may be placed in the epidural or subdural space or within the ventricle (33). The epidural monitor has the advantage of not transgressing the dura, thereby lowering the risk of infection and hemorrhagic complications. However, the pressure tracing from an epidural pressure monitor may not reflect the ICP accurately. Intraventricular monitors have the advantage of allowing drainage of CSF to treat increased ICP and are preferred when there is significant intraventricular hemorrhage and associated hydrocephalus. However, cannulation of the ventricular system may be difficult to perform if the ventricles are collapsed from diffuse increased ICP or if they are shifted as a result of focal cerebral swelling.

A subdural ICP monitor, such as a subarachnoid bolt or fiberoptic device, inserted through a twist-drill hole in the skull, is the most frequently used monitor for head-injured children (7). Insertion can be performed at the child's bedside using local and intravenous anesthetics. A fiberoptic device is preferable because a screw or bolt is easily occluded by blood and intracranial debris.

In addition to the treatment measures already outlined, it is important that the patient be kept comfortable to control increased ICP. Often, in an attempt to allow for serial neurologic examinations, head-injured children are not sedated. This is frightening to the child, particularly if he or she has an endotracheal tube in place. It is reasonable to use short-acting sedative/tranquilizing agents such as morphine (0.05 to 0.1 mg/kg) or vecuronium (0.1 mg/kg) for sedation and paralysis because they are easily reversed if a question of neurologic deterioration arises. If, despite these measures, the ICP is sustained at a level over 20 mm Hg for several minutes, or remains elevated and is associated with a change in neurologic status, then efforts to increase hyperventilation to maintain pCO_2 in the range of 19 to 24 mm Hg should be undertaken. If this effort is ineffective in controlling the ICP, then 20% mannitol (0.5 to 1.0 g/kg) may be administered as an intravenous bolus injection at intervals as frequent as every hour, if necessary, until serum osmolality reaches 300 to 320 mOsm. Other diuretics, such as furosemide (1 mg/kg), may be used as well, with careful attention directed to electrolyte balance (Na 130 to 150 mEq/L; K 3 to 5 mEq/L) (16).

If these measures fail to maintain the ICP at 20 mm Hg or less, barbiturate coma may be instituted (3,16). A loading dose of 10 to 20 mg/kg of pentobarbital should be given as a slow intravenous drip, followed by an intravenous infusion of 3 to 5 mg/kg until burst-suppression is noted on electroencephalographic monitoring. The drug infusion should be maintained at that level until the ICP is controlled for 24 to 48 hours, and then gradually withdrawn. Side effects of pentobarbital, such as hypotension and cardiac dysfunction, may require the use of Swan-Ganz monitoring and the administration of vasopressor drugs, such as dopamine (5 to 10 μg/kg/min), especially in younger children.

In addition to careful clinical monitoring in an intensive care unit, follow-up studies should include serial CT brain scans to assess the severity and course of the cerebral hyper-

emia and to monitor the child for the possibility of delayed intracranial complications, such as hemorrhage into an ischemic area of brain, hydrocephalus, pneumocephalus, or infection. A precipitous change in neurologic function or inability to control the ICP may be the warning sign of a delayed intracranial hemorrhage and calls for an emergency CT brain scan (26) (Figure 28.3).

All children who have had a severe head injury (GCS less than 6) should receive prophylactic anticonvulsants because the incidence of posttraumatic seizures is as great as 25% (15). Phenytoin is usually the drug of choice, and a loading dose (15 to 20 mg/kg) may be administered intravenously with minimal side effects; the loading dose of phenytoin

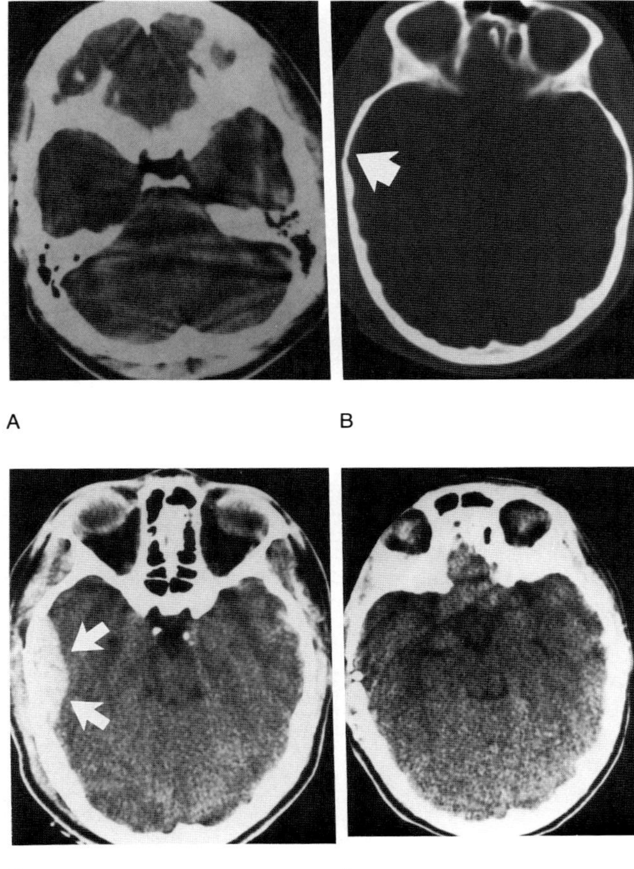

FIGURE 28.3   **A:** Axial CT brain scan, without contrast agent, obtained immediately following a severe closed head injury in a 15-year-old girl. There is no evidence of hematoma. A device to monitor intracranial pressure (ICP) was placed and the pressure initially well-controlled by hyperventilation and sedation. **B:** Bone windows from the same CT scan show a right temporal fracture across the distribution of the middle meningeal artery (arrow). **C:** Axial CT scan, without contrast agent, of the same patient obtained 10 hours later when the ICP was no longer controllable. A large, acute epidural hematoma is seen underlying the temporal fracture line (arrows). **D:** Postoperative axial CT scan without contrast agent following emergency evacuation of the hematoma. The underlying brain has expanded again. The child made an excellent recovery.

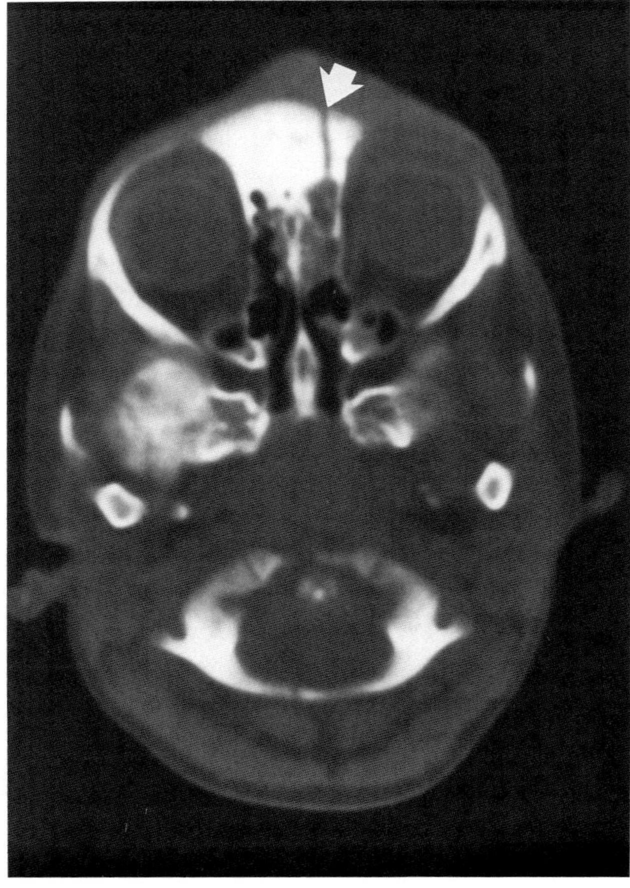

A

FIGURE 28.4 A: Axial CT brain scan without contrast agent, obtained following head trauma in a 4-year-old boy with cerebrospinal fluid rhinorrhea. A fracture through the anterior frontal bone is clearly shown (arrow).

should be followed by a maintenance dose (5 to 10 mg/kg divided into two or three doses daily), with monitoring of serum levels thereafter. Phenobarbital (15 to 30 mg/kg loading dose, 5 mg/kg maintenance dose thereafter) is also useful, but may produce drowsiness or hyperactivity. During the recovery stage, the anticonvulsant may be changed to carbamazepine (10 to 20 mg/kg divided into three or four doses daily) or phenobarbital; carbamazepine is the drug of choice considering its low incidence of long-term side effects. The medication should be continued for 3 to 6 months if no areas of cortical damage are demonstrated by imaging studies and up to 1 year if the child has had major parenchymal injury. A history of convulsions following head injury may prompt continuation of anticonvulsants until a 2- to 3-year seizure-free period has occurred.

Pneumocephalus may occur after a significant basilar skull fracture, with or without the development of clinical CSF rhinorrhea or otorrhea. The onset of pneumocephalus several days following an injury may account for a deterioration in the patient's condition. Intracranial air should be gradually absorbed; the persistence of significant pneumocephalus suggests that there is a fistula into the subarachnoid space requiring further evaluation. The initial management of a traumatic CSF leak is observation, as most fistulas resolve spontaneously. If there is copious CSF drainage or if the leak persists for more than 2 to 3 days, then placement of a lumbar spinal drain permits diversion of the CSF and a decrease in the ICP, which often allows the fistula to seal. If there is persistent CSF leakage after the drain is clamped, of if leakage recurs after a delay, a diagnostic imaging study should be performed. An MRI brain study is particularly useful in delineating the site of the leak by showing the presence of fluid levels in the paranasal sinuses or middle ear (Figure 28.4). The detail of bone may

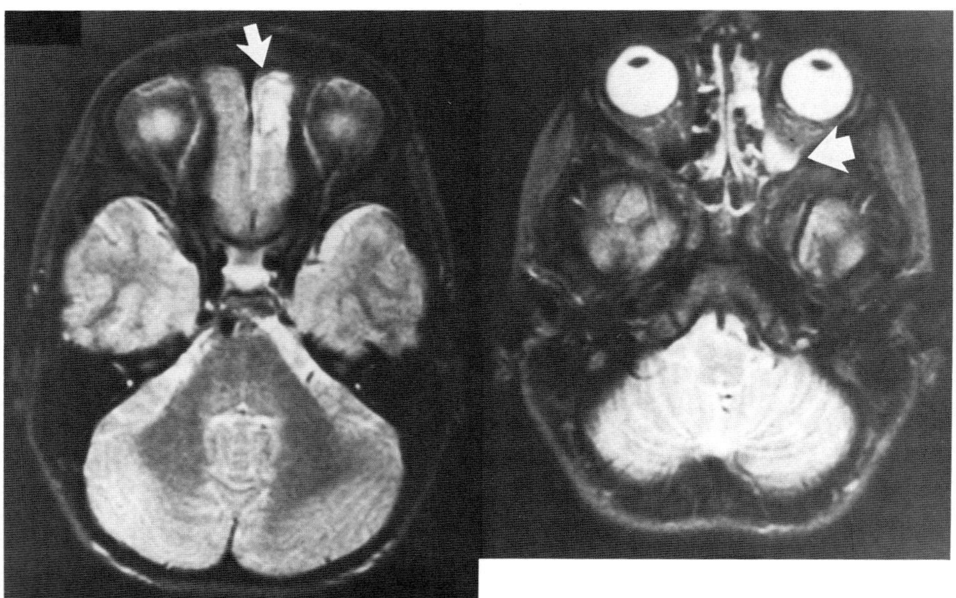

B   C

FIGURE 28.4 B: Axial MR image of the same child. An area of encephalomalacia (arrow) in the frontal cortex overlying the fracture is apparent. **C:** MR image through the frontal sinuses of the same child. The sinus underneath the fracture has an air-fluid level (arrow), indicating the presence of a CSF leak. The child was operated on through a bifrontal craniotomy and the site of the fistula was identified and patched.

be better visualized with a CT scan and, if there is an active leak, metrizamide may be instilled in the subarachnoid space and the site of the leak demonstrated on a scan. If the site of the fistula is visualized and accessible, it should be repaired through a craniotomy with microsurgical patching of the defects in dura and bone. Left unrepaired, the fistula will allow persistent CSF leakage with the risk of meningitis. If the fracture is too extensive or inaccessible for a direct repair, a ventriculoperitoneal or lumboperitoneal shunt may be inserted to divert the CSF.

Treatment of chronic subdural hematoma does not in general require craniotomy, as the relatively liquid blood may be easily drained through trephinations (28). In infants, these fluid collections may be tapped by needle through the anterior fontanel and the fluid sent for culture after each aspiration. The fluid collection should be tapped if there is evidence of a large fluid accumulation observed at ultrasonography or at CT, if the child's head circumference is enlarging, or if there is clinical evidence of increased ICP. Drainage may be required on a daily basis or only every 2 to 3 days. If after 10 days to 2 weeks the fluid collections have not resolved, then the best treatment appears to be shunting of the fluid to the peritoneum or atrium. Bilateral collections may be treated initially with a unilateral shunt and a second system added if there is persistence of the contralateral fluid collection.

A ventriculoperitoneal or ventriculoatrial shunt may be necessary to treat post-traumatic hydrocephalus. Progressive ventricular enlargement may be seen on serial ultrasonograms and/or CT or MRI of the head. CT or MRI studies are helpful in differentiating high-pressure hydrocephalus from ventricular enlargement caused by primary brain damage (*ex vacuo* hydrocephalus). Transependymal flow of CSF into the brain parenchyma shown on CT scan or MRI studies suggests that the ventricular enlargement is associated with increased intraventricular pressure and that a shunt may benefit the patient (See Figure 28.2). Defects in the skull are treated by a cranioplasty, performed either with methyl methacrylate or autologous split cranial bone. If there has been an infection at the site of the bone defect, the reconstruction is delayed for 1 year after the completion of antibiotic treatment. Children who develop a leptomeningeal cyst in the fracture site require repair of the dura as well as the overlying bone (Figure 28.5).

Outcome

The outcome of treatment for infants and children who suffer head injury is better in all series than the outcome for head-injured adults, with the exception of those children who develop acute subdural hematomas (3). A 50% to 60% mortality rate from this condition has been reported for all age groups. The mortality from severe head trauma in children has been reported to be as low as 9% in one series (21), but this study may be in a biased sample, as the patients were drawn from a large, tertiary care setting and they generally presented more than 24 hours after their initial injury. The overall mortality rates of severe pediatric head injury at our acute care trauma center is 30% to 40%, which correlates favorably with rates in most other series of patients with a similar severity of injury (7). The highest mortality rates are in children who, on their admission to the hospital, are flaccid with fixed and dilated pupils (21) and in those with a syndrome of diffuse hyperemia and focal hemorrhage (31) (Figure 28.6). These figures are still significantly better than those for similarly injured adults, however, in whom mortality rates are as high as 50% to 60% following severe head trauma (3).

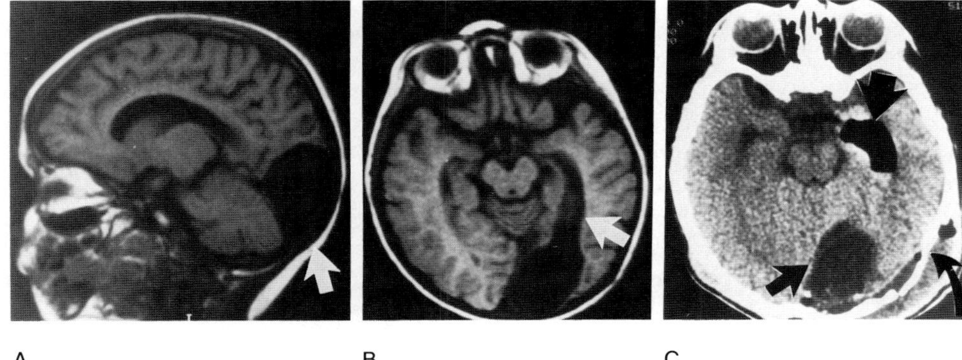

A   B   C

FIGURE 28.5 A: Sagittal MRI head study in an 18-month-old boy 8 months after head trauma associated with an occipital fracture. The child presented with an enlarging, soft mass in the region of the previous fracture. A well-demarcated fluid collection represents a leptomeningeal cyst (arrow). **B:** Axial MR image of the same child shows a connection between the cyst and the occipital horn of the ventricle (arrow). This indicates that there is an area of porencephaly as well as the entrapped arachnoid. A defect in the occipital bone was seen at the site of the lesion at operation. **C:** Postoperative axial CT scan made without contrast agent. The entrapped arachnoid has been resected and the dura repaired. The porencephalic cavity is well-visualized (small arrow). Intraventricular air is present (large arrow). The defect in the bone has been repaired with autologous bone harvested from the child's calvarium (curved arrow).

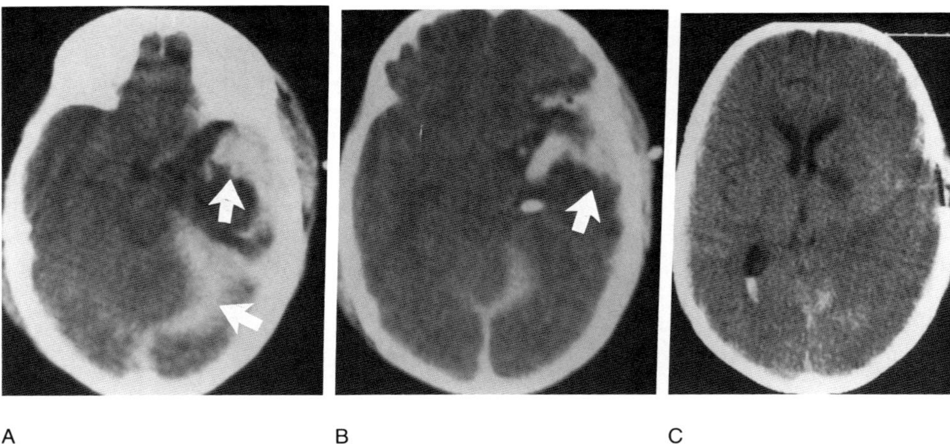

A   B   C

FIGURE 28.6   A: Axial CT brain scan without contrast agent, obtained in a 9-year-old boy following head injury, shows a large subdural and intracranial hematoma (arrows). The child underwent emergency evacuation of the hemorrhage and an intracranial monitor was placed. The intracranial pressure (ICP) initially was well-controlled. **B:** Axial CT scan without contrast agent obtained 48 hours later when the ICP began to rise. There has been a recurrent hemorrhage into the contused temporal lobe (arrow). Emergency reoperation was undertaken. **C:** Axial CT scan without contrast agent, obtained approximately 1 week later, shows resolution of most of the hemorrhage but persistence of brain swelling. Despite aggressive treatment, including barbiturate coma, the child died from the uncontrollable increased ICP.

The long-term effects of head injury are often most obvious in infants and children because their longer lifetime and the effects of the injury on their schooling make deficits more easily recognized. The overall morbidity in children is less than that in comparable adult series, provided that any coma was less than 3 months in duration (13,16). However, when assessed by neuropsychologic study, the majority of significantly head-injured children have deficits in cognitive functions or learning skills. Because of these deficits, the child may require special schooling (2,4,9,14, 34,35).

The developing neuroendocrine system of the infant and child requires evaluation following significant head-injury, particularly if hypothalamic damage is suspected or if there has been prolonged coma. Visual and auditory assessments, including evoked-potential evaluations, are mandatory to detect deficits that may be subtle but contribute significantly to the recovery of the child. Physical and occupational therapy may be needed to improve strength, range of motion, and coordination. The integration of all of these factors is best performed in a chronic, comprehensive pediatric rehabilitation unit.

Conclusions

Head trauma is a regrettably common cause of morbidity and mortality in children. While many injuries are the result of a fall or motor vehicle accident, the incidence of nonaccidental trauma has increased. Minor head injury, as defined by a brief postconcussive state, may cause permanent cognitive impairment. Severe head injuries are associated with permanent neurologic deficits, seizures, hydrocephalus, and disorders of memory, learning, and endocrine function. Although the outcome from head trauma is better in the pediatric than in the adult population, intensive, aggressive treatment is necessary immediately following the injury and in the subsequent comprehensive rehabilitation during recovery.

SPINAL CORD TRAUMA*

Approximately 7,000 to 8,000 spinal cord injuries occur each year in the United States. Although over 50% of these injuries occur in individuals less than 25 years of age, the incidence of severe spinal cord injury is low in infancy, childhood, and early adolescence. It has been estimated that only 2% to 10% of spinal cord injuries occur in children younger than 15 years old. Spinal cord injury is twice as common in male as in female children. There is a peak incidence in the summer months. The majority of these injuries are the result of motor vehicle accidents; however, in infants and young children, falls account for a significant number. The mortality rate varies from 10% to 59% depending on the series reviewed and emphasizes the severity of this problem. The immature spine is subject to different types of injury than is the adult spine (36–40).

*Portions of this section were adapted with permission from Edwards MS, Cogen PH. Spinal Trauma. In: Dieckmann RA, Grossman M, eds. Pediatric Emergency Medicine. A Clinician's Reference. Philadelphia: JB Lippincott, 1991:267.

Anatomy and Biomechanics of the Immature Spine

Significant differences exist in the anatomy and biomechanics of the adult and pediatric spine that account for the characteristic patterns of spinal injury seen in children. The laxity of the major ligamentous structures of the child's spine allows for an unusually high degree of spinal mobility. For most children the ligamentous characteristics of the adult spine are not obtained until 8 years of age. In addition, the cervical musculature, which plays an important role in the stability and alignment of the adult spine, is poorly developed in the child. Forces at the time of injury capable of distracting the spine are not well checked because of the above factors. Last, the articular facets of the pediatric spine are more horizontally positioned than in the adult spine. In infancy, they may be as low as 30°, increasing to 70° by 10 years of age. All of these factors contribute to an increased physiologic mobility of the pediatric spine and may allow subluxation to occur with surprisingly little force.

The spine of an infant is primarily cartilaginous and ossifies progressively throughout childhood. Therefore, injuries in infants and young children tend to be avulsions or epiphyseal separations rather than true fractures. Odontoid injuries in children usually produce a separation through the basilar synchondrosis and into the body of C2. Injuries in this age group are essentially splits in the cartilaginous endplates and routinely heal well with spontaneous fusion, as opposed to odontoid-waist fractures in adults which often require surgical fusion.

The fulcrum for flexion–extension is different in children than in adults. In adults, flexion and extension produces the greatest motion at the C5-C6 level. In children, the greatest amount of motion is at the C2-C3 level, and the fulcrum gradually moves caudally with increasing age. The motion characteristics of the adult spine are usually reached by 8 to 10 years of age. The anatomic and biomechanical features of the immature spine make the upper cervical spinal segments from C1 to C3 particularly vulnerable to injury.

Modes of Injury and Clinical Presentations

Neonates

Intrapartum spinal cord injury is a rare phenomenon (Figure 28.7) (41,42). It is most often associated with a difficult delivery and/or breech presentation. The injury results from longitudinal stretching and hyperextension of the vertebral column. The clinical presentation depends on the level of spinal cord injury. The common level of involvement is the mid to lower cervical and upper thoracic spine. Pathologic examination in most instances reveals spinal cord transection with subsequent atrophy. Plain radiographs of the spine are usually normal, although on rare occasions they may demonstrate a vertebral dislocation. Myelography especially in conjunction with CT may reveal spinal cord swelling. The use of MRI will help in determining whether cord swelling is due to edema or hemorrhage. High cervical spinal cord lesions with quadriparesis may initially appear to represent a congenital neuromuscular disorder. Other differential diagnoses include congenital spinal cord tumor and hypoxic ischemic encephalopathy. The prognosis is dependent on the severity and level of spinal cord injury. High cervical cord injuries carry a worse prognosis because of the effects on ventilation. Despite high complete lesions, several children have been reported to have survived and are productive adults. A few infants with what initially appeared to be complete transections of the spinal cord have made near complete recoveries. Therefore, all infants, despite the initial severity of their spinal cord lesion, should

FIGURE 28.7   A: Sagittal MRI (T1-weighted) demonstrates the site of cervical cord injury (curved arrow). B: Axial MRI (arrow) demonstrates cord narrowing at the site of maximum stretch injury.

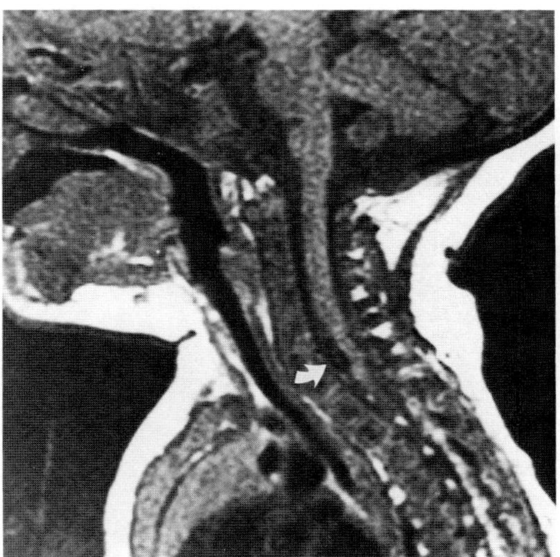

A

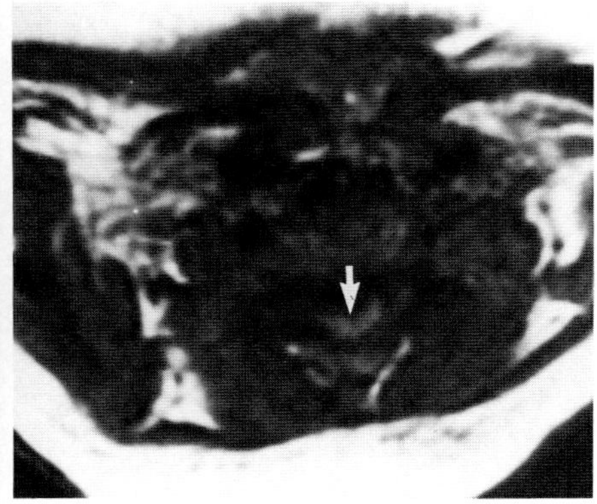

B

receive aggressive supportive care and be observed closely for recovery. Surgical exploration is rarely if ever indicated for these lesions. Possibly, with the increased use of MRI, infants with extradural cord compression may be found and considered as candidates for surgical intervention.

Infants and Children

Although infants and children show similar anatomic patterns of spinal cord injury to those in adults, the frequency and clinical presentation often are markedly different. In adults, 85% of fractures and dislocations in the cervical region occur below the C3 vertebral level, whereas in children, only 30% occur below this level. There is a tendency for young children to suffer a disproportionately large percentage of high cervical injuries (36,37). In addition, locked facets, which are frequent in adults, do not occur in children.

Injuries that occur rarely in adults are seen more frequently in children. For example, rotatory subluxation, an injury that is rare in adults, is a relatively common problem in the infant and young child. It is usually the result of minor trauma associated with the sudden rotation and twisting of the neck beyond its normal range. The child presents with painful torticollis and local tenderness to palpation in the posterior neck region over the C1-C2 spinous processes. The diagnosis is confirmed by open mouth radiographs, that demonstrate the odontoid processes asymmetrically placed between the lateral articular masses of the atlas. Reduction is usually achieved by light cervical traction using 3 to 5 pounds of weight. If reduction cannot be achieved using traction or if subluxation recurs after traction has been discontinued, an atlantoaxial fusion may be required.

Atlantooccipital dislocation is rarely recognized clinically because it usually produces cervicomedullary compression leading to respiratory arrest and death. Nine of 13 reported cases have been in children younger than 18 years of age. The shallow articular surfaces of the atlas and the small size of the occipital condyles in children make the stability of this region almost entirely dependent on ligamentous integrity. In addition, the relatively large head of infants and the weakness of the cervical musculature make infants especially vulnerable to this type of injury. The mechanism that produces this injury is extreme hyperextension in association with lateral flexion. The diagnosis is made on plain radiographs when there is malalignment of the odontoid with respect to the anterior aspect of the foramen magnum and of the posterior arch of the atlas with respect to the posterior edge of the foramen magnum. MRI demonstrates the severity of cord injury (Figure 28.8). The initial treatment is supportive care and ventilatory support. Initial spinal stability and realignment are achieved with a halo apparatus followed by an occipital cervical fusion.

The frequency of odontoid fracture in childhood is unknown. Controversy exists as to whether os odontoidium is an anatomic abnormality or a result of trauma. In the infant and young child the transverse ligament is stronger than the incompletely ossified dens so that with traumatic subluxation the atlantodental interval (ADI) is usually maintained. Most odontoid fractures in children are similar to epiphyseal separations that occur in the long bones. Similarly, they will readily heal if their position is reestablished and immobilization maintained (43).

It is postulated that an unrecognized fracture in the young child with subsequent fibrous replacement of the bone is the primary mechanism by which os odontoidium develops (44,45) (Figure 28.9). There are two varieties of os odontoidium. In the orthotopic variety the ossicle lies in place of the normal dens and moves with the axis and atlas. In the dystopic variety the os lies near the base of the clivus and moves with the clivus or fuses with it; the anterior arch of C1 is hypertrophied and the posterior arch is hypoplastic. Neurologic signs are insidious in almost 50% of patients, while the other 50% present with the acute onset of neurologic dysfunction. Neck pain is a major feature in

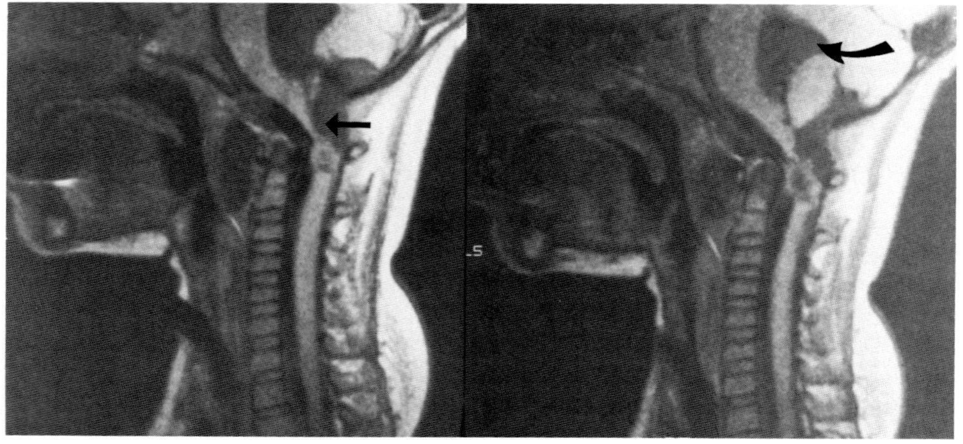

FIGURE 28.8 **A:** Sagittal MRI (T1-weighted) cervicomedullary junction postatlantooccipital dislocation in a 5-year-old boy who survived his injury. There is near complete transection of the cervicomedullary junction (arrow). **B:** MRI at a slightly different sagittal location. Dilatation of the fourth ventricle (hydrocephalus) has developed from posttraumatic basilar arachnoiditis (curved arrow). Cystic changes in the cervicomedullary cord are observed.

A

B

FIGURE 28.9 A: Lateral cervical extension radiograph of a 14-year-old male following a fall from a bicycle. There appears to be good alignment of the cervical spine. **B:** Lateral cervical flexion radiograph of the same patient. There is 14 mm of anterior subluxation of C1 on C2 (arrow). The status of the odontoid process is undetermined. **C:** Sagittal MRI (T1-weighted) of the cervical spine in flexion. There is no evidence of cord compression. There is evidence of an abnormality of the odontoid process (os odontoideum) (arrow). **D:** Sagittal MRI of the cervical spine in extension. There is no evidence of cord compression. However, there is posterior displacement of the odontoid process and increased soft tissue indenting the spinal subarachnoid space (arrow).

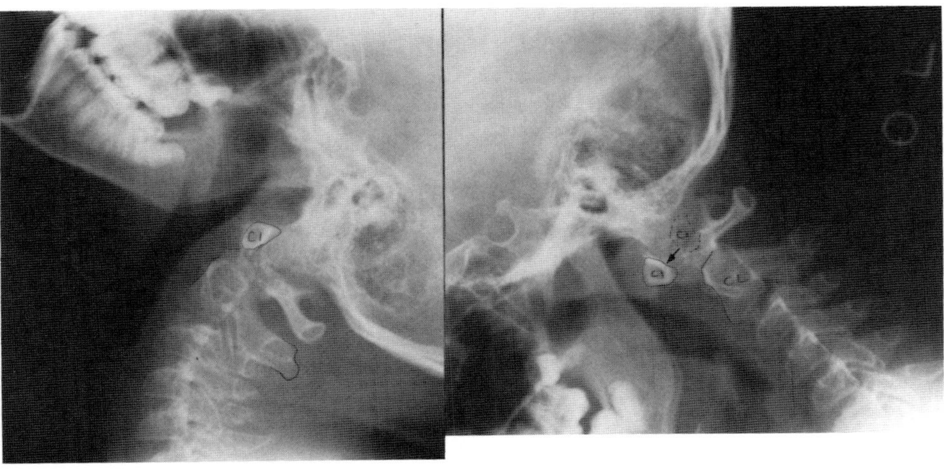

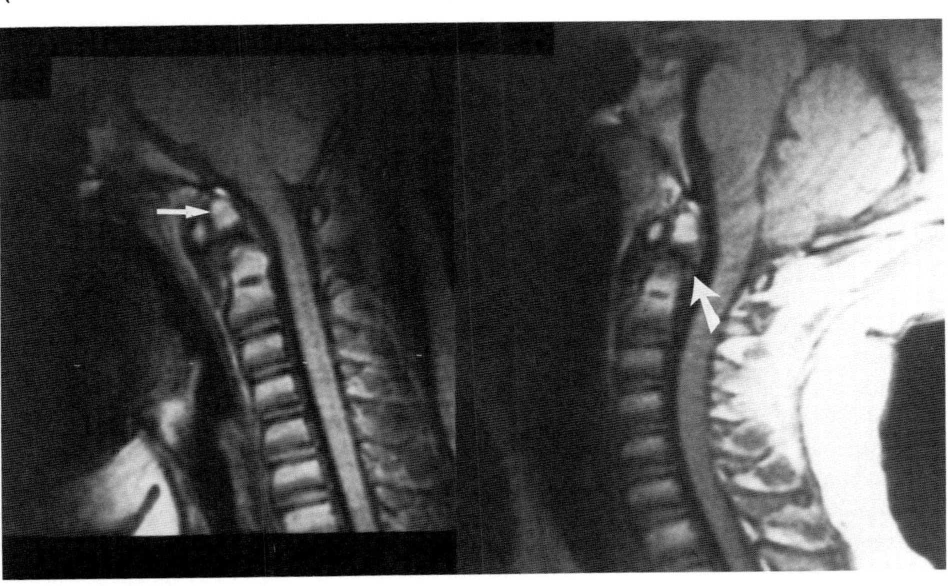

2/3 of patients. Treatment depends on whether cord compromise occurs on flexion or extension. If the lesion is reducible with positioning or traction, then stabilization is important. If it is nonreducible, then an anterior or posterior decompression followed by a stabilization procedure is necessary. The orthotopic os requires a C1-C2 posterior fusion, whereas the dystopic variety usually requires a occipitocervical fusion. In the infant and child, fractures of the pedicles of C2 (hangman's fracture), lower cervical spine fractures, and thoracolumbar fractures are rare.

Older Children and Adolescents

The spinal motion characteristics of the adult are usually obtained by 8 years of age but on occasion not until the age of 12 years. At this age the spine is ossified, the ligaments and joint capsules have lost their laxity, the facets have assumed a vertical orientation, and the cervical paraspinal musculature is much stronger. Spinal injuries assume an adult pattern and the majority occur in the lower cervical segments. The injuries that occur are predominantly wedge compression fractures and anterior subluxation and dislocation caused by axial loading and hyperextension. Also, thoracolumbar fractures become relatively more common due to flexion–rotation injuries caused by motor vehicle accidents. These injuries in children are managed in a fashion similar to those in adults.

Special Situations

Certain children with congenital abnormalities have an increased incidence of spinal injury. Children with Down syndrome have an abnormally increased laxity of the transverse ligament that tends to cause anterior subluxation of C1 on C2 (46). In addition, approximately 6% of children with Down syndrome have an odontoid abnormality, such as aplasia, hypoplasia, or divided dens, which serves to further increase the risk of C1-C2 subluxation. Up to 15% of children with Down syndrome will have radiologic evidence of C1-C2 subluxation greater than or equal to 5 mm; however, the majority are asymptomatic (47). If the incidence of subluxation is truly this high, many children with Down syndrome would be expected to suffer a spinal cord injury. However, despite the involvement of diving and gymnastics in the Special Olympics over the past 15 years, there has not been a reported case of spinal cord injury (48).

In the majority of patients suffering spinal injury, neurologic dysfunction was present prior to the injury. Therefore, children with neurologic dysfunction and subluxation of C1 on C2 of greater than 5 mm should undergo a posterior fusion of C1-C2. Children with asymptomatic subluxation of greater than 5 mm should be restrained from participating in activities that favor maximal neck flexion such as contact sports, somersaults, and trampoline exercises. Because Burke et al. (46) reported that 7 of 32 patients who initially were free of subluxation developed significant subluxation and instability over a 13-year period, all children with Down syndrome should be observed for neurologic dysfunction and/or neck pain in a longitudinal fashion. Other children with a predisposition to spinal cord injury are those with dwarfism (e.g., Morquio syndrome, achondroplasia, or spondyloepiphyseal dysplasia) that are associated with ligamentous laxity, spinal stenosis, spinal kyphosis, and/or stenosis of the foramen magnum (49).

The phenomenon of spinal cord injury without associated radiographic abnormality (SCIWORA) has been estimated to occur in 16% to 66% of children younger than 8 years of age with severe spinal injuries (49–54). The most common cause is vehicular accidents. The pathophysiology remains uncertain but may be related to severe flexion or hyperextension injuries with subsequent ischemic damage to the spinal cord. The extreme degree of ligamentous laxity may predispose the pediatric spine to severe subluxation at the time of injury that subsequently spontaneously reduces itself. This subluxation may produce mechanical damage to the cord and thus produce neurologic deficits. The diagnosis of this entity requires a complete radiographic series including flexion–extension views. CT, often with the addition of intrathecal contrast, and/or MRI is usually necessary to rule out spinal cord compression as the etiology. In most cases these diagnostic tests are normal or demonstrate a partial block at the time of the initial injury (54). MRI performed from 1 to 3 months after injury may demonstrate atrophy of the spinal cord if there is neurologic residual (Figure 28.10). Approximately 50% of children with SCIWORA will have a late onset of neurologic deterioration from 30 minutes to 4 days (mean 1.2 days)

after the injury. The paralysis usually develops rapidly once it begins and most frequently culminates in a complete cord lesion. The pathophysiology of delayed cord injury is undetermined at present.

Traumatic infarction accounted for 8% of spinal cord injuries in children at the Hospital for Sick Children, Toronto (55). In this group of 8 children an injury involving the chest or abdomen was the initiating event. The children were typically neurologically intact at presentation but developed a profound and usually complete paraplegia within hours or days, and only 2 of the 8 patients demonstrated any neurologic recovery. Plain spine radiographs and myelograms were normal; however, spinal angiography performed in one patient demonstrated occlusion of the anterior spinal artery. Surgical intervention is not warranted in these patients.

Interestingly, delayed spinal deformity despite a long follow-up period was not observed in the series by Pang and Wilberger (53). Recently, Pang and colleagues reported recurrent spinal cord injury in 8 of a series of 42 SCIWORA patients during their 2-month postinjury immobilization period (56). The children most susceptible to reinjury were those who initially sustained a mild or transient cord injury and who rapidly recovered and resumed normal activities. Based on this observation Pang and associates recommend patients' strict compliance with neck immobilization in a rigid cervical brace for 3 months and restriction of both contact and noncontact sports.

The long-term prognosis for patients with SCIWORA is poor (53–56). Children with complete lesions and those with severe incomplete lesions do not recover (54). The initial neurologic status is the major predictor of the extent of recovery.

The "burning hands" syndrome described by Maroon in 1977 is primarily seen in children (55,57). This was initially described in high school football players suffering a neck injury. It is characterized by burning dysesthetic pain in the hands and fingertips and occasionally in the feet. The pathophysiology is thought to be a central cord contusion (central spinothalamic tract) secondary to hyperextension of the cervical spine. Any athlete with spinal trauma and complaints of paresthesias or dysesthesias in the extremities, even without neck pain, should be treated and managed as if a fracture or dislocation were present. A careful radiologic evaluation is necessary because more than 50% of children with these symptoms have a cervical fracture or dislocation.

Radiologic Evaluation

The radiologic evaluation of the infant or child suspected of having a spinal cord injury is the same as for an adult. Plain anterior–posterior (AP) and lateral radiographs of the cervical and/or the thoracolumbar spine should be obtained first. Flexion and extension views of the spine should be

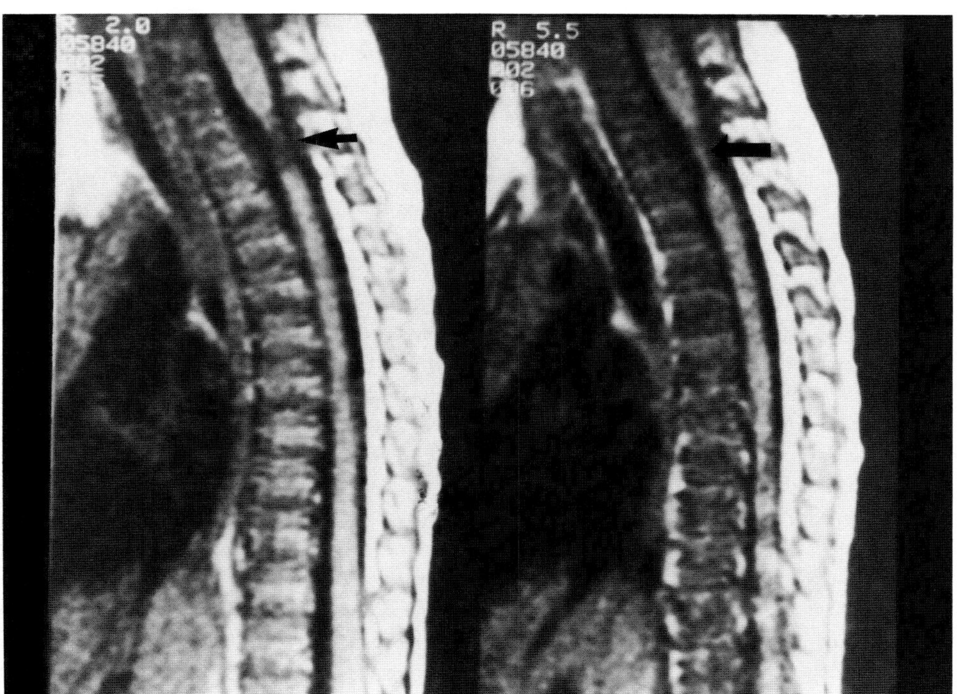

FIGURE 28.10 **A:** Sagittal MRI of a 12-month-old child rendered paraplegic in an automobile accident. The initial neurodiagnostic studies including CT myelography were normal. This MRI obtained 3 months postinjury demonstrates severe spinal cord atrophy at the T4–T6 level (arrow). **B:** Sagittal MRI at a different level showing near complete transection of the cord (arrow). The changes must be due to atrophy of spinal cord tissue because the initial studies demonstrated a normal diameter thoracic spinal cord.

A

B

obtained if the initial static radiographs do not reveal subluxation or dislocation. These films must be obtained with caution, especially in the infant and young child in whom passive motion of the spine must be utilized. If muscle spasm restricts neck motion the dynamic studies should be repeated when spasm has resolved and full flexion and extension is possible. CT with bone window settings is helpful in determining the location and extent of bone injury, especially in the upper cervical spine where neural arch fractures may not be detected by plain radiographs. CT may be particularly helpful in defining synchondrosis from fracture. Myelography is essential if there is evidence of neurologic dysfunction. The sensitivity is increased by using intrathecal water-soluble contrast in conjunction with CT (CT myelography). If a block to the flow of intrathecal contrast is identified, the upper and lower extent of the block must be determined by placing contrast in the subarachnoid space through a C1-C2 puncture. In many instances, CT without and with intrathecal contrast is being replaced by MRI. However, for the present the child requiring physiologic monitoring or ventilatory support is more safely evaluated using CT techniques.

The radiographic appearance of the pediatric spine is complicated by the normal occurrence of multiple epiphyseal plates, incomplete ossification, and hypermobility due to ligamentous laxity (58,59). Epiphyseal plates are ubiquitous in infants and children, and a complete knowledge of their appearance and time of resolution is not essential to the evaluation of the pediatric spine. However, important anatomic points need to be remembered. At birth the atlas (C1) has three ossification centers, one for the body of the

vertebrae and one for each of the neural arches. Therefore, in 80% of neonates the anterior arch of C1 will appear to be discontinuous. The neural arches usually close by the 3rd year of life to form a complete ring and subsequently fuse to the body of C1 by the age of 7 years. The axis (C2) has four centers of ossification: one for the odontoid process, one for the vertebral body, and one for each neural arch. In all children less than 3 years of age and in 50% of children less than 5 years of age, the dens is separated on plain radiographs from the body of C2 by a broad cartilaginous band that corresponds to an intervertebral disk. This radiolucent line may be visualized until 11 years of age and should not be misinterpreted as a fracture. The previously described ligamentous laxity and the horizontal position of the facet joints allows for excess mobility in the pediatric spine. In adults, the normal distance on plain radiographs from the anterior arch of C1 to the odontoid process (the ADI) is 3 mm or less. In the infant and child, the ADI may increase to 5 mm due to the laxity of the supporting transverse ligamentous structures. In addition, 40% of plain lateral radiographs in normal children under the age of 8 years show C2 shifted forward and tilted downward in relation to C3. More than 50% of these children have a 3 mm or greater degree of forward displacement. This "pseudosubluxation" can be differentiated from true subluxation by forced hyperextension. In true subluxation the anterior displacement cannot be reduced, whereas with pseudosubluxation the displacement is always easily reduced. Last, immature vertebral bodies are wedged anteriorly, and this should not be mistaken for a compression fracture. By the age of 10 years, the pediatric spine has taken on the attributes of the adult spine anatomically and radiographically and should be assessed and treated as an adult spine.

Treatment

Pathophysiology

There is little other than prevention that can significantly reduce the effects of the primary injury to the spinal cord. The primary event produces immediate disruption of the spinal gray and white matter. The subsequent progression of neurologic dysfunction is the result of a series of mechanisms (secondary injury) set in motion by the primary injury and develops over a period of hours or days.

The secondary injury likely involves a series of pathologic processes occurring either concurrently or in series, some of which may be the initiating factors for other injurious events. Reduction of spinal cord blood flow following trauma may produce extracellular ion flux, decreased oxygen and glucose utilization, production of toxic free radicals, lipid peroxidation, and possibly release of neuropeptides. The exact sequence and interrelationship of these events is unknown. Pharmacologic treatments targeted at reversing or substantially reducing the secondary injury. Despite encouraging experimental results, there is no unequivocal proof of their clinical efficacy (60,61).

Initial Management

Management at the site of injury should include immobilization. If an athletic helmet is in place it should be left alone. The level of consciousness should be assessed, as should perfusion and ventilation. If ventilation is judged to be inadequate, cardiopulmonary resuscitation (CPR) should be started. The child should be placed on a spinal board and the head sandbagged during transport to a pediatric neurosurgical facility.

On arrival in the emergency room the child should be maintained in the supine position and the head supported. Patients with suspected cervical injuries should be placed in a semirigid plastic collar (soft collar or sandbags for infants) and a long spine board used if a thoracic or lumbar fracture is suspected. The ventilatory status must be assessed. The neck should not be flexed in order to establish an airway. Rather, the use of a jaw thrust or simple suction of secretions should be considered. If inadequate oxygenation is suspected, the use of supplemental oxygen and monitoring of arterial blood gases or the use of a pulse oximeter should be instituted. If oxygenation is inadequate despite those techniques, an endotracheal tube should be established using a *nasotracheal* route. Perfusion status needs to be assessed concurrently. Hemorrhagic shock should be treated with volume replacement. Hypotension

and a slow pulse secondary to loss of sympathetic tone (i.e., venous pooling in the lower extremities) may indicate a high cervical spinal cord injury. Volume replacement or vasopressor drugs will usually resolve the hypotension.

Neurologic assessment of the spinal cord injury is frequently complicated by head trauma and a reduced level of consciousness. Management of the head injury should take precedence over the spinal cord injury. The child's head injury should be ranked on the GCS (Table 28.1) or a pediatric modification of the GCS. Identification of the neurologic deficit is particularly difficult in the infant, young child, and uncooperative patient. The examiner should try to define a motor and/or sensory level. In the uncooperative patient a level to pin sensation may be the only modality detectable. Also helpful is a change in skin temperature with warmth below the level of injury secondary to vasodilatation or finding a sweat level with absence of sweating (warm, dry skin) below the level of injury. In the cooperative patient a complete sensory and motor examination including evaluation of the superficial and deep tendon reflexes should be performed and documented. It is imperative that rectal sphincter tone and perianal sensation be assessed. The evaluation of the bulbocavernosus reflex will give insight into the presence or absence of spinal shock. The findings of complete motor and sensory paralysis with persistence of the bulbocavernosus reflex is a bad prognostic finding indicating that spinal shock cannot account for the paralysis.

In all children with neurologic dysfunction an indwelling bladder catheter should be inserted to prevent severe bladder distention and to evaluate fluid balance and renal function. Children with cervical or upper thoracic spinal cord injuries usually develop an ileus; therefore, a nasogastric tube should be placed to prevent abdominal distention, regurgitation, and possible aspiration. Cervical and upper thoracic injuries producing paralysis and sensory loss may mask an intra-abdominal process such as a perforated viscus; therefore, all patients suspected of having abdominal trauma should be evaluated with abdominal CT and/or peritoneal lavage.

The initial radiologic evaluation depends on the site of suspected spinal injury. Cervical vertebral injuries should be evaluated first by a cross-table lateral radiograph. All seven cervical vertebrae must be visualized. In order to do this it may be necessary to pull the patient's shoulders down or to obtain a lateral swimmer's view. If the lateral radiograph is normal, then an AP radiograph should be obtained along with an open mouth view to evaluate the odontoid. If all of these tests show normal results and a cervical spine injury is still suspected, flexion–extension views should be obtained with a physician in attendance.

Evaluation of the thoracic spine requires that AP and lateral radiographs be obtained and all 12 thoracic vertebrae be visualized. Similarly, AP and lateral radiographs of all five lumbar vertebrae and the sacrum should be obtained to evaluate the lumbosacral spine adequately. Standard chest, abdominal, and long-bone radiographs should be obtained as indicated from the medical history and physical examination. Plain CT with bone windows is frequently helpful in defining an abnormality suspected on the basis of plain radiographs.

Stiff or molded cervical collars can provide additional support but, in general, are of little value for the infant or young child. Pediatric soft cervical collars designed for infants and young children should be available. If an acutely unstable spinal fracture is identified, skeletal traction should be applied early in the child's management. In older children, Gardner-Wells tongs or a halo device may be applied in minutes. However, in infants, especially those younger than 18 months, the cranium is too thin and soft to safely place an external fixation device as described. Traction may be applied safely by placing two 1-cm trephinations in both parietal bones through which wires can be passed and connected to skeletal traction. In adolescents and older children, reduction of the cervical spine is accomplished by placing approximately 5 pounds of weight on the traction apparatus for each spinal level involved (i.e., C4-C5 subluxation = 20 pounds, C5-C6 subluxation = 25 pounds, and so on). However, this amount of weight is inappropriate for the young child and infant for whom from 1 to 3 pounds per segment added slowly is a more rational plan considering the known ligamentous laxity in this age group. Because locked facets rarely if ever occur in children, reduction is usually easily accomplished in the acute phase of the injury. It must be emphasized that life-threatening injuries, respiratory depression, hypotension, and severe hemorrhage must be rapidly treated and take priority over the spinal cord injury.

Surgical Management

The same controversies that exist concerning the management of the adult with a spinal cord injury — such as operative versus nonoperative treatment, the efficacy of acute surgery, and the most appropriate surgical approach and technique — exist for children as well. Early surgical intervention is only infrequently necessary (36,37,54). Children with residual distal neurologic function who fail to improve or develop progressive neurologic deterioration are surgical candidates. Acute surgical intervention should be considered for those children with an incomplete myelopathy with persistent spinal deformity and for children with complete neurologic loss below the level of injury when the possibility exists to preserve or recover the function of an important nerve root. Last, children with an anterior cord syndrome on neurologic examination in whom CT and/or myelography or MRI demonstrate anterior cord compression should undergo decompression. Except for the above situations the decision to operate is usually based on orthopedic rather than neurosurgical considerations. For example, unstable fracture dislocations are operated on for internal fixation when the patient's condition permits, the

goal being early ambulation and rehabilitation. Those children with total and complete cord injury will not benefit from surgical intervention.

Surgical intervention, particularly in the child with a residual neurologic deficit, may produce acute and/or chronic spinal instability. Of considerable importance in planning the management of the child with an injury to the spinal column is the injury or subsequent treatment on spinal growth. Spinal injuries that damage the epiphyseal plates may cause an incomplete cessation of longitudinal growth or an asymmetric stimulation of epiphyseal growth resulting in scoliosis or kyphosis (62). Girls younger than 12 years and boys younger than 14 years of age with cervical or thoracic injuries are at greatest risk with up to a 90% incidence of spinal deformity developing after injury. Close follow-up should be maintained throughout the child's period of maximum growth; proper bracing should be applied and surgical intervention undertaken when necessary to prevent a severe progressive spinal deformity.

When surgical intervention for spinal fusion is undertaken it is imperative that the fusion be limited to allow for axial growth and maximum physiologic mobility. This goal is best accomplished when the surgical exposure is limited to only the segments to be fused. Children fuse very rapidly; if unnecessary vertebral segments are exposed and the soft tissues surrounding them are stripped from the bone, they may become incorporated in a more extensive multilevel (creeping) fusion than had been originally planned.

Rehabilitation

Although spinal cord injury with severe residual neurologic dysfunction is uncommon in children, the consequences are particularly devastating because of the long life expectancy. It must also be recognized that children with spinal cord injury have special needs because of their potential for continued physical, intellectual, psychologic, and social growth. The goals of rehabilitation are to optimize the child's neurologic recovery, to provide skills that compensate for lost or impaired functions, and to permit the fullest functional development possible. This is best accomplished in a pediatric rehabilitation center where a multidisciplinary approach is available.

Bladder management is one of the most critical factors in determining a child's social acceptance and in determining long-term survival. Clean intermittent catheterization is the preferred method of management, and when used in conjunction with anticholinergic medications the majority of patients can be made continent. Children as young as 5 years of age can be taught clean intermittent catheterization. Continued urologic management is important in reducing the long-term morbidity and mortality from spinal cord injury.

Worsening of neurologic function is not part of the natural history of spinal cord injury. Any loss of neurologic function, especially ascending paralysis, should instigate a careful search for a surgically correctable cause, particularly a posttraumatic syrinx. MRI is the diagnostic test of choice but may not be feasible if metallic rods were placed for spinal stabilization.

Spinal cord injury usually produces spasticity that becomes clinically more apparent within a few weeks of the event. Although flexor spasms may occur early, extensor spasms may eventually predominate and interfere with residual voluntary motor function, sitting in a wheelchair, and transferring positions. If associated with pain they may prevent rehabilitation. Oral pharmacologic agents such as baclofen, diazepam, and dantrolene sodium have shown minimal effectiveness in ameliorating these symptoms. Intrathecal baclofen has recently shown effectiveness in adults (63), and intrathecal morphine is under investigation. Selective dorsal rhizotomy has shown effectiveness in treating spasticity secondary to static encephalopathy and is also being used in selected patients.

Last, the importance of sexual development and function in the adolescent is critical and should not be underestimated. Adolescents may need professional help to develop confidence in their sexuality. They should be assured that persons with spinal cord injury can and do engage in sexual activity and that there are satisfying options for them.

Conclusions

Spinal cord injury in children fortunately is not common. It is important to maintain a high index of suspicion to prevent a delay in diagnosis and treatment. The pathophysiology, clinical presentation, initial and definitive management, and sequelae are different in children than in adults. Many spinal cord injuries in children are preventable with proper use of safety equipment, such as infant car seats, and educational programs that encourage recreational safety.

REFERENCES

1. Amacher AL. Pediatric head injury: A national tragedy. Concepts Pediatr Neurosurg 1985;6:76–83.
2. Kraus JF, Fife D, Conroy C. Pediatric brain injuries: The nature, clinical course, and early outcomes in a defined United States population. Pediatrics 1987;79:501–508.
3. Luerssen TG, Klauber MR, Marshall LF. Outcome from head injury related to the patient's age. J Neurosurg 1988; 68:409–416.
4. Casey R, Ludwig S, McCormick MC. Morbidity following minor head injury in children. Pediatrics 1986;78:497–503.
5. Alberico AM, Ward JD, Choi SC, et al. Outcome after severe head injury. J Neurosurg 1987;67:648–656.
6. Bruce DA. Outcome following head trauma in children. In: Shapiro K, ed. Pediatric Head Trauma. Mount Kisco, NY: Futura 1983;213–223.
7. Berger MS, Pitts LH, Lovely M, et al. Outcome from severe head injury in children and adolescents. J Neurosurg 1985; 62:194–199.
8. Mayer T, Walker ML, Johnson DG, et al. Causes of morbidity and mortality in severe pediatric trauma. JAMA 1981; 245:719–721.
9. Raimondi AJ, Hirschauer J. Head injury in the infant and toddler. Childs Brain 1984;11:12–35.
10. Garza-Mercado R. Intrauterine depressed skull fractures of the newborn. Neurosurgery 1982;10:694–698.
11. Billmire ME, Myers PA. Serious head injury in infants: Accident or abuse? Pediatrics 1985;75:340–342.
12. Duhaime A-C, Gennarelli TA, Thibault LE, et al. The shaken baby syndrome. J Neurosurg 1978;48:679–688.
13. Brink JD, Imbus C, Woo-Sam J. Physical recovery after severe closed head trauma in children and adolescents. J Pediatr 1980;97:721–727.
14. Levin HS, Eisenberg HM, Wigg NR, et al. Memory and intellectual ability after head injury in children and adolescents. Neurosurgery 1982;11:668–674.
15. Hahn YS, Fuchs S, Flannery AM, et al. Factors influencing post-traumatic seizures in children. Neurosurgery 1988; 22:864–868.
16. Raphaely RC, Swedlow DB, Downes JJ, et al. Management of severe pediatric head trauma. Pediatr Clin North Am 1980; 27:715–728.
17. Samson D. Traumatic lesions of the cerebral vasculature. In: Edwards MSB, Hoffman HJ, eds. Cerebral Vascular Disease in Children and Adolescents. Baltimore: Williams and Wilkins 1988;195–203.
18. Ordia IJ, Strand R, Gilles F, et al. Computerized tomography of contusional clefts in the white matter in infants. J Neurosurg 1981;54:696–698.
19. Bruce DA. Clinical care of the severely head injured child. In: Shapiro K, ed. Pediatric Head Trauma. Mount Kisco, NY: Futura, 1983;27–44.
20. Bruce DA, Alavi A, Bilaniuk L, et al. Diffuse cerebral swelling following head injuries in children: The syndrome of "malignant brain edema." J Neurosurg 1981;54:170–178.
21. Bruce DA, Schut L, Bruno LA, et al. Outcome following severe head injuries in children. J Neurosurg 1978;48: 679–688.
22. Povlishock JT, Becker DP, Cheng CLY, et al. Axonal change in minor head injury. J Neuropathol Exp Neurol 1983;42: 225–242.
23. Ammirati M, Tomita T. Posterior fossa epidural hematoma during childhood. Neurosurgery 1984;14:541–544.
24. Eisenberg D, Kirschner SG, Perrin EC. Neonatal skull depression unassociated with birth trauma. AJNR 1984;143: 1063–1064.
25. Kirschner RH, Stein RJ. The mistaken diagnosis of child abuse. Am J Dis Child 1985;139:873–876.
26. Bruce DA, Schut L. The value of CAT scanning following pediatric head injury. Clin Pediatr 1980;19:719–726.
27. Steinbok P, Flodmark O, Martens D, et al. Management of simple depressed skull fractures in children. J Neurosurg 1987;6:506–510.
28. McLaurin RL. Chronic subdural hematoma in infants. Contemp Neurosurg 1980;2:1–7.
29. Masters SJ, McClean PM, Arcarese JS, et al. Skull x-ray examinations after head trauma. N Engl J Med 1987;316:84–91.

30. Cohen RA, Kaufman RA, Myers PA, et al. Cranial computed tomography in the abused child with head injury. AJNR 1985;6:883–888.

31. Levin HS, Amparo E, Eisenberg HM, et al. Magnetic resonance imaging and computerized tomography in relation to the neurobehavioral sequelae of mild and moderate head injuries. J Neurosurg 1987;66:706–713.

32. Feuerman T, Wackym PA, Gade GF, et al. Value of skull radiography, head computed tomographic scanning, and admission for observation in cases of minor head injury. Neurosurgery 1988;22:449–454.

33. Venes J. Intracranial pressure monitoring in perspective. Childs Brain 1980;7:236–251.

34. Filley CM, Cranberg LD, Alexander MP, et al. Neurobehavioral outcome after closed head injury in childhood and adolescence. Arch Neurol 1987;44:194–198.

35. Farmer MY, Singer AS, Mellits ED, et al. Neurobehavioral sequelae of minor head injury in children. Pediatr Neurosci 1988;13:304–309.

36. Wilberger JE. Spinal Cord Injuries in Children. Mount Kisco: Futura, 1986.

37. Hill SA, Miller CA, Kosnik EJ, et al. Pediatric neck injuries. A clinical study. J Neurosurg 1984;60:700–706.

38. Kewalramani LS, Kraus JF, Sterling HM. Acute spinal-cord lesions in a pediatric population: Epidemiological and clinical features. Paraplegia 1980;18:206–219.

39. Kewalramani LS, Tori JA. Spinal cord trauma in children. Neurologic patterns, radiologic features, and pathomechanics of injury. Spine 1980;5:11–18.

40. Ruge JR, Sinson GP, McLone DG, et al. Pediatric spinal injury: The very young. J Neurosurg 1988;68:25–30.

41. Byers RK. Spinal-cord injuries during birth. Develop Med Child Neurol 1975;17:103–110.

42. Adams C, Babyn PS, Logan WJ. Spinal cord birth injury: Value of computed tomographic myelography. Pediatr Neurol 1988;4:105–109.

43. Hadley MN, Browner C, Sonntag VKH. Axis fractures: A comprehensive review of management and treatment in 107 cases. Neurosurgery 1985;17:281–290.

44. Fielding JW, Hensinger RN, Hawkins, RJ. Os odontoideum. J Bone J Surg 1980;62A:376–383.

45. Menezes AH. Os odontoideum — pathogenesis, dynamics and management. Concepts Pediatr Neurosurg 1988;8:133–145.

46. Burke SW, Roberts JM, Johnston CE, et al. Chronic atlantoaxial instability in Down syndrome. J Bone Joint Surg Am 1985;67A:1356–1360.

47. Pueschel SM, Scola FH. Atlantoaxial instability in individuals with Down syndrome: Epidemiologic, radiographic, and clinical studies. Pediatrics 1987;80:555–560.

48. Davidson RG. Atlantoaxial instability in individuals with Down syndrome: A fresh look at the evidence. Pediatrics 1988;81:857–880.

49. Bethem D, Winter RB, Lutter L, et al. Spinal disorders of dwarfism. Review of the literature and report of eighty cases. J Bone J Surg 1981;63A:1412–1425.

50. Burke DC. Traumatic spinal paralysis in children. Paraplegia 1974;11:268–276.

51. Burke DC. Spinal cord trauma in children. Paraplegia 1971;9:1–14.

52. Walsh JW, Stevens DB, Young AB. Traumatic paraplegia in children without contiguous spinal fracture or dislocation. Neurosurgery 1983;12:439–445.

53. Pang D, Wilberger JE. Spinal cord injury without radiographic abnormalities in children. J Neurosurg 1982;57:114–129.

54. Hadley MN, Zabramski JM, Browner CM, et al. Pediatric spinal trauma. Review of 122 cases of spinal cord and vertebral column injuries. J Neurosurg 1988;68:18–24.

55. Choi JU, Hoffman HJ, Hendrick EB, et al. Traumatic infarction of the spinal cord in children. J Neurosurg 1986;65:608–610.

56. Pollack IF, Pang D, Sclabassi R. Recurrent spinal cord injury without radiographic abnormalities in children. J Neurosurg 1988;69:177–182.

57. Maroon JC. "Burning hands" in football spinal cord injuries. JAMA 1977; 238:2049–2051.

58. Bailey DK. The normal cervical spine in infants and children. Radiology 1952;59:487–500.

59. Cattell HS, Filtzer DL. Pseudosubluxation and other normal variations in the cervical spine in children. A study of one hundred and sixty children. J Bone Joint Surg (Am) 1965;47:1295–1309.

60. Faden AI, Jacobs TP. High dose corticosteroid therapy in experimental spinal injury: Increased mortality and failure to improve neurologic recovery. Neurology 1983;33 Suppl 2:192.

61. Faden AI. Pharmacologic therapy in acute spinal cord injury: Experimental strategies and future directions. In: Becker DP, Povlishok JT, eds. Central Nervous System Trauma Status Report 1985. Bethesda, MD: NINCDS 1985;481–485.

62. Mayfield JK, Erkkila JC, Winter RB. Spine deformity subsequent to acquired spinal cord injury. J Bone Joint Surg 1981;63A:1401–1411.

63. Penn RD, Kroin JS. Long-term intrathecal baclofen for treatment of spasticity. J Neurosurg 1987;66:181–185.

Part VI

Disorders of
Conscious States

Chapter 29
Sleep Disorders of Children

Christian Guilleminault

The incidence and prevalence of sleep disorders in children are still unclear. Many surveys do not report results separately by age, presenting instead overall frequencies for a wide age range, and prevalence found at a certain age does not necessarily correspond with findings at earlier or subsequent testing periods. Furthermore, the frequency used to define a problem; that is, the number of times per week or months the problem occurs, is often not described, making comparisons across studies difficult. What may be considered as within the wide range of the "normal" by one, may be considered as "pathologic" by another. However, children themselves are aware of having a "sleep problem" or a "sleep disorder" much more often than anticipated. Among the unexpected results of a telephone survey in the San Francisco area were that although 58% of the 6- to 14-year-old children and 56% of the 15- to 19-year old teenagers reported a sleep problem at that time (1), few sought medical attention for the problem, and most were not concerned about it. These findings were corroborated by those of White et al. in 1983 (2). To better survey sleep disorders, one must have a good understanding of the normal development of the sleep-wake cycle in infancy, valid definitions of syndromes, and a classification of sleep-wake disorders whose validity has been tested on large numbers of subjects. In 1979, the "diagnostic classification of sleep and arousal disorders in adults" (3) was published by the Association of Sleep Disorders Centers and tested by multi-center studies. An effort was made to try to apply, with some adaptation, this classification. Disorders of excessive daytime sleepiness (EDS), disorders of initiating and maintaining sleep, disorders of the sleep-wake schedule, and the parasomnias can be recognized in school-aged children, at least in Western society where children must comply with school and social time schedules. This classification is less useful, however, when discussing younger children. A neonate has no consolidated sleep and is not adapted to a 24-hour rhythm. The speed at which a newborn infant adapts his sleep-wake schedule to a day-night cycle depends on many factors, some directly related to maturation of the central nervous system (CNS) and other control systems, and some related to environmental elements.

DEVELOPMENT OF SLEEP AND WAKEFULNESS

During the first 6 months of life the two sleep states, rapid eye movement (REM) and non-rapid eye movement (NREM) sleep, evolve. Sleep consolidates, that is becomes condensed into fewer periods of longer duration, with a higher probability of wakefulness during the day and sleep at night. During the newborn period, infants spend two-thirds of the 24-hour period asleep (4); by 6 months, they spend half of their time asleep and half awake. The proportion of the 24-hour period spent in REM sleep is gradually reduced from one-third to one-fourth of sleep time (5,6). NREM sleep (usually called "Quiet" sleep at this age) shows much refinement during that period of time (5,6). Electroencephalographic (EEG) figures, which allow further subdivision of NREM sleep state in stages classified from 1 to 4 (7), are progressively more easily recognizable; and the classification as "Quiet," "Indeterminate," and "Active" (REM) sleep, necessary to use in scoring premature and newborn infant sleep states, is changed by 3 months of age. NREM sleep stages 1–2 and stages 3–4 (delta sleep) can be scored, based on EEG patterns (7). Even if theta waves are a prominent feature of young infant sleep onset, the 4 sleep stages defined in adult NREM sleep can be scored without difficulty by 6 months of age (6). Though NREM sleep shows much refinement and subdivision, its proportion of time during the 24-hour cycle stays strikingly constant over this developmental period. The gradual reduction of REM sleep is balanced by an increase in the proportion of time spent in wakefulness during the 24-hour period. During the first 6-month period of life, the organization of the sleep cycle also changes (5,8). At birth, infants fall asleep after being fed and immediately enter REM sleep. With aging, the number of sleep onsets decreases over time as sleep consolidates. Simultaneously, the proportion of sleep onset REM sleep periods (SOREMPs) also decreases (5). For example, of ten sleep onsets during one 24-hour period at 3 weeks of age, an infant is likely to have 6.4 SOREMPs. By 6 months of age, the ratio is 0.6 SOREMP in three sleep onset periods. There is the progressive development of a long sleep period during the night and a consolidated long wake period, usually in the afternoon, peaking in the late afternoon or early evening just before the onset of the "long sleep period" (5). By 6 months of age, the basic nocturnal sleep structure that will persist throughout life is present. There is a shorter NREM-REM sleep cycle (60–70 minutes) than will be noted later on, but there is already a slight prominence of delta sleep in the earlier nocturnal sleep cycles, a trend that will accentuate within the following year. There is a great variability, depending on children, cultures, socioeconomic environment, for example, as far as age of termination of daytime napping. For example, some Western countries such as France and Switzerland have afternoon "rest periods" for children up to 4 or 5 years of age in state-controlled kindergartens. It is, however, normal that during the 5th year of age, kindergarten children do not take afternoon naps. Also, afternoon naps are not planned in most western countries' school systems in the equivalent of first grade, where children are between 6 and 7 years of age. Carskadon's investigations (9) have demonstrated that in Tanner stage 1 (prepubertal) children 7 to 11 years of age, alertness during the daytime is maximal, with multiple sleep latency test (MSLT) scores of between 17 to 20; i.e., maximum alertness (10). Coble et al. (11) and Carskadon (9) have found closely related values; viz., between 6 to 10 years of age, children in the United States spend between 8 1/2 and 9 1/2 hours asleep at night and do not take naps. This is in sharp contrast to what is noted during adolescence. Society often expects a reduction in total sleep time with adolescence. Carskadon et al. (12,13) demonstrated that older adolescents do not present a reduced "need" for sleep at night. All groups, when given the opportunity, averaged around 9 hours of nocturnal sleep (12,14). Older adolescents, sleeping 7 hours or less, most probably develop a "sleep debt," which may explain the low MSLT scores, that is, "sleepiness" scores noted by Carskadon in her experiments (12–14). However, it is safe to state that adolescents in their late teens are most commonly excessively sleepy (15). This sleepiness must not be considered as related to a pathologic syndrome, but rather is essentially related to the adolescent way of life. It also emphasizes the need to assure standardized nocturnal sleep monitoring

conditions when a disorder of excessive sleep is suspected at this age.

DISORDERS OF EXCESSIVE SLEEPINESS

As already mentioned, age and developmental status are important factors when considering "pathologic sleepiness." Disorders of excessive sleepiness (DOES) develop for a wide variety of reasons. Daytime sleepiness may be only one of many problems certain children have including the following: children with neurologic problems; organic brain syndrome (with or without mental retardation); or epilepsy often seen early in life in specialized sleep clinics. Most commonly, daytime sleepiness is ignored until teachers complain about the problem.

Objective Determination of Excessive Daytime Sleepiness

A good interview examining the child's sleep-wake habits and schedules is mandatory in sleep disorders medicine. This interview must be completed by establishing a "sleep log." The sleep log can be obtained through standardized sleep diaries or simple, regular parental notes. The information must be collected for a minimum of 1 week, and parents and/or child must note at least time of "sleep onset" and "sleep offset" for naps and nocturnal sleep, periods of somnolence or marked desire for sleep, periods of food intake, and exercise. The sleep log may already provide clues concerning abnormal sleep-wake schedule problems or may lead to simple counseling. It will help to organize the day-night schedule of the child before administering the most commonly used objective test, the MSLT (15–18). Before giving the MSLT, nocturnal sleep time must be stabilized for a few days at home, and a minimum of 8 1/2 hours of nocturnal sleep time (more in younger children) must be assured. The child must come to the sleep laboratory the night before the MSLT for monitoring during sleep to assess causes of nocturnal sleep disturbances in order to objectively determine the nocturnal sleep structure. The MSLT consists of 5 tests administered at 2-hour intervals from 0930 to 1730 hours. Each test, if negative (i.e., no sleep occurs), lasts for 20 minutes. If the child falls asleep during the 20-minute testing period, he is left to sleep for a maximum of 15 minutes, to record the possible early appearance of REM sleep that is, within 15 minutes of sleep onset. If this is noted, a SOREMP is recorded. This is an abnormal sleep pattern that is registered simultaneously with the presence of absence of abnormally short sleep latencies. Between each test, great efforts must be made to keep the child awake. In adults and postpubertal teen-agers normal tests indicate a mean sleep latency of at least 10 minutes. At 7 years and older (prepubertal children) a longer sleep latency is expected, most commonly equal to or above 15 minutes. Children are more sleepy during pubertal years. However, a mean sleep latency of at least 10 minutes is expected.

Another Objective Measurement Approach: Ambulatory Monitoring During the 24-Hour Period

Before standardization of the MSLT, 24-hour continuous monitorings in a laboratory situation were performed to evaluate EDS. Development of cassette-type recorders has allowed children to be monitored in real-life situations. Because this test and the MSLT are not administered under the same experimental conditions, they are considered complementary to each other. The MSLT has the advantage of being performed under standardized, even if artifically imposed, conditions. The continuous monitoring indicates what happens in a real-life situation. Analysis of EEG (C_3/A_2-C_4/A_1), electrooculogram (EOG), and chin electromyogram (EMG) will allow determination of drowsiness and light sleep (stage 1 NREM), for example.

Causes of Excessive Daytime Sleepiness

Children presenting with neurologic problems with or without mental retardation and with or without epilepsy may present with EDS, but these periods of daytime somnolence are often interrupted by periods of insomnia, and these children present a sleep-wake schedule disorder rather than EDS proper (Table 29.1).

Obstructive Sleep Apnea Syndrome

The obstructive sleep apnea syndrome (OSAS) (19–21), with its associated symptoms of EDS, abnormal daytime behavior (hyperactivity to pathologic shyness and withdrawal), learning problems, morning headaches, frequent upper airway infections, and failure to thrive or obesity, has in common with partial but continuous sleep-related upper airway obstructions, the element of heavy snoring at night.

Enlarged tonsils and adenoids are very often found in both cases. However, the enlarged lymphoid tissues play only a partial role in the development of the syndrome (19,22–24), for retrognathia , micrognathia, or the not so obvious moderate retroposition of the vertical branch of

Table 29.1 Most common causes of excessive daytime sleepiness (EDS)

Complete or partial upper airway obstruction during sleep
Narcolepsy
EDS associated with neuromuscular disorder
Central nervous system hypersomnia
Periodic hypersomnia (rare)
EDS related to medical treatment

the mandible, cleft palate or its repair, enlarged tongue and/or fatty infiltration of the neck will be frequently seen with enlarged tonsils and adenoids. These anatomic abnormalities may render specialists cautious about the possible reappearance of snoring and partial airway obstruction, particularly in postpubertal male adolescents after testosterone surge. The nocturnal polygraphic recording, at times performed with esophageal balloon if continuous but only partial upper airway obstruction without oxygen saturation drop is present, will confirm the diagnosis. Images of the upper airway that will give a picture of the anatomic configuration of the region are needed, such as cephalometric radiographs, computed tomographic scans, and fluoroscopy (24–26), coupled with endoscopic evaluation. Diverse respiratory function tests will confirm that no associated lung problem such as broncho-pneumo dysplasia, and cystic fibrosis is noted.

Narcolepsy

If narcolepsy (27–29) is the second most common cause of EDS in the pubertal and postpubertal years, it is uncommon in the prepubertal period. When seen in the latter, cataplexy, the abrupt and reversible decrease or loss of muscle tone, is frequently associated very early on with the daytime sleepiness. It may even precede the onset of EDS. Cataplexy, most frequently elicited by emotions such as laughter, anger, surprise, or abrupt strain, and seen during social activities as in games or school can involve the entire voluntary musculature, with the exception of the ocular muscles and the diaphragm, or be limited to the muscles of the head and neck or to the jaw. In a typical attack, the jaw sags, the head falls forward, the arms drop to the side, and the knees release. The patient may collapse to the floor, injuring himself in the process. But the attacks may be more subtle, lasting 1 to 2 seconds, and may involve a weakness or—a step further—a buckling of the knees or an isolated sagging of jaw or shoulders that may be hard to recognize. In the initial stage of the attack, consciousness remains intact. If the cataplectic attack is prolonged, hallucinations may occur and the patient may even enter REM sleep.

Hypnagogic hallucinations at sleep onset, whether during daytime nap or nocturnal sleep, may be unpleasant and sometimes very frightening. They may, however, be lacking in the very early phases of the disease, or may be absent or very limited throughout the life of the narcoleptic patient.

Sleep paralyses are very closely related to cataplexy. Their appearance at sleep onset or upon awakening is the peculiarity of these temporary and completely reversible episodes of abrupt muscle weakness.

The daytime sleepiness can present itself with different patterns and patients may report uncontrollable episodes of sleep occurring several times daily, more often in association with monotonous tasks. The sleepiness may develop gradually, and subjects may be perfectly aware of it. A possible mode of entry is the impossibility of waking up in the morning, and if awakened, presenting typical symptoms of "sleep drunkenness," with confusion, disorientation, and even aggressiveness. Sleep drunkenness is not, per se, a symptom of narcolepsy; it is a symptom of EDS. The daytime sleepiness presented by narcoleptics is related to repetitive micro-sleeps that may occur in subjects with their eyes open. The presence of SOREMPs at MSLT on at least two of the five tests, and frequently at onset of nocturnal sleep, will support the diagnosis of narcolepsy in association with a positive history of cataplexy if the test is appropriately performed; the subject is off medications influencing REM sleep for at least 15 days, and a systematic urine drug screen is given on the test day. In rare prepubertal cases, SOREMPs may be lacking, or only one may be seen at the five sleep latency tests. One must not hesitate to repeat the MSLT within 4 to 6 months in case of doubt (29,30).

There is a genetic factor in most, but not all, human cases. Testing for the human leucocyte antigen (HLA) DR and DQ may help in confirming the genetic origin of the narcolepsy, and testing of parents and siblings may indicate the side of the family from which the HLA-DR-DQ linked gene comes. Most genetic narcoleptics are HLA-DR2 (DR$_w$15) DQ$_w$6 D$_w$2, independent of their racial background. The presence of HLA-DR2 DQ$_w$6 alone does not, by any means, imply narcolepsy. There is currently more and more evidence, but no complete proof, that the HLA gene is not the narcoleptic gene (or, at least, not the only gene involved). The genetic transmission of narcolepsy, which was highly suspected for years, was strongly supported by the Japanese discovery of a link between the presence of the HLA DR$_2$ DQWI gene, located on the small arm of the sixth chromosome, and the presence of narcolepsy in humans (31–35). Several genetic models have been proposed, including a multifactorial mode of inheritance. Currently, even if a recessive transmission has been demonstrated in narcoleptic Labradors and Dobermans, two of the breeds presenting canine narcolepsy (28,36–38), the mode of genetic transmission is still unresolved, even if indirect investigations favor, once again, a multifactorial mode of inheritance with associated intervention of environmental factors (39,40). Investigation of canine narcolepsy has demonstrated a significant involvement of alpha-1-adrenoceptor in the development of cataplexy, coupled with a muscarinic cholinergic brainstem receptor impairment (28).

Excessive Daytime Sleepiness Associated with Neuro-Muscular Disorder

In prepubertal years, EDS may be more commonly associated with an unrecognized or undiagnosed neuromuscular disorder than with narcolepsy. The most common yet undiagnosed disorder seen in a sleep clinic with symptoms of daytime sleepiness is myotonic dystrophy (MD). The cause of EDS in MD is not always readily apparent. Undoubtedly, some MD patients may already present with alveolar hypoventilation and even central apnea due to their muscle disease involving respiratory accessory muscles and perhaps the diaphragm. Some patients even present with typical obstructive apneas, and the nocturnal sleep fragmentation related to their breathing disorder could be responsible for the daytime sleepiness. Certain MD patients, however, have minimal or no breathing problems and still present abnormal SOREMP at MSLT. The existence of an independent sleep disorder linked to MD is thus considered; MD could induce a disorder of sleep and its central controls by an as yet unknown mechanism.

Central Nervous System Hypersomnia

CNS hypersomnia is not a disorder commonly seen in the perpubertal years. It is probably a syndrome of diverse etiologies of which two are clearly identified: hypersomnia associated with hydrocephalus, particularly communicating hydrocephalus, and the progressive development of daytime sleepiness immediately following infectious mononucleosis, Guillain-Barré syndrome, or certain types of infectious hepatitis, or atypical pneumonia. The reasons why certain individuals may develop EDS following a viral infection involving Epstein-Barr and perhaps some ECHO or other viruses are unclear (41). Montplaisir et al. have tried to perform systematic HLA typing similar to that done in narcolepsy. The Canadian data has indicated a CNS hypersomniac subgroup with a predominance of HLA-DR typing; however, these results are very preliminary (28). Even if CNS hypersomnia is clearly seen in the teen-age years and may lead to significant disability, the pathophysiologic mechanisms are poorly understood.

Periodic Hypersomnia

The Kleine-Levin syndrome is a rare entity and one should always question this diagnosis, as intermittent sleepiness could be the first indication of the future establishment of a daily syndrome as described above. The Kleine-Levin syndrome is seen in teen-aged boys, often at the end of puberty. Symptoms are recurring episodes of daytime sleepiness, hyperphagia, and abnormal behavior of 1 to 2 weeks' duration. Its evolution is variable, and it may, though not always, improve spontaneously after 20 years of age (42).

Menstruation-linked periodic hypersomnia (43) is also rare but more common than the Kleine-Levin syndrome. It occurs most commonly within months or during the first 2 years after the appearance of menstruation. The recurrent episodes last 6 to 10 days and usually end when the menses occur. Generally, birth control pills control the symptoms, which often reappear if medication is interrupted. Symptoms frequently spontaneously disappear when the patient reaches her twenties or after pregnancy (43).

DISORDERS OF THE SLEEP/WAKE SCHEDULE

These disorders are common and are the cause of many complaints of lack of nocturnal sleep and/or excessive daytime sleepiness. They may appear very early in life and be responsible for the so-called "sleepless child."

Sleepless Child and Schedule Disturbances

The ultradian rhythm of alternating sleep cycles has a period of only 50 minutes during infancy. It increases slowly throughout childhood and adolescence, reaching 90 minutes during adulthood (44–46). Circadian controls of the sleep-wake cycle and temperature rhythm begin between 5 and 8 weeks of age in the full-term newborn. Initially, entrainment of sleep-wake cycles appears to be influenced more by feeding schedules than by light-dark cues. Initially, infants appear to "free-run," independent of their day-night cycle, following their genetic rhythm, which for the majority is approximately 25 hours (range 23 to 27 hours) (8). The development of stable sleep-wake and eating schedules emerges progressively, and these schedules are related to the relationship of the infant and parents in infants without brain insults (8,47).

Although some infants sleep through the night from birth, most do not; most neonates wake up every 20 minutes to 6 hours throughout the day and night. Some will cry, others will not. In normal infants, the longest sleep and longest wake periods emerge near 3 months of age and are very well established by 6 months (between 1900 and 0007 hours) (5). However, normal children wake up at night. Klackenberg's longitudinal study showed that 34% of 4- to 5-year-old children were still waking up at night, although only 3% were considered "poor sleepers" (48–50). These normal patterns must be taken into account before considering a pattern as "pathologic."

The relation of sleep problems to habits and parental responsiveness is difficult to quantify. As stated by Richman, "one must be concerned less with factors which might have caused the sleep difficulty, such as neonatal irritability and parental responsiveness following a difficult birth, than with those currently maintaining the problem" (51). Ferber noted (46), the causes of sleeplessness in infants and toddlers must be categorized pragmatically in terms of the patterns present at time of clinical visit. In young children, the two most important factors are those of particular habits associated with sleep transitions and excessive nighttime feedings. In older children, no longer sleeping in a crib, sleep problems are more often related to parents' poor and inconsistent limit-setting. "Biological factors may make it more likely for parents to reinforce wakings, but if wakings are not reinforced, they diminish and are replaced by more sleep" (46). A child waking under a set of conditions different from those present at bedtime may have difficulty returning to sleep until these conditions are reestablished.

The infant may never have an opportunity to learn to settle by himself at sleep onset, or may have forgotten it. The proposed therapeutic approaches emphasize the need to create consistent bedtime rituals and patterns of nighttime interventions which lead to less and less parental intervention at sleep onset and gradual decrease of parental contact. These programs often require support and counseling for the parents during the training period. Similarly, the nighttime feeding habits may be very much responsible for the so-called "sleepless" infant. It must be remembered that by 6 months of age, an infant has the ability to obtain satisfactory nutrition during the daylight hours and to sleep through the night without sensation of hunger. Repeat feedings during the night condition the infant to become hungry at those times and to develop night sleep difficulties. Eliminating night feedings and letting the child learn to fall asleep on his own usually resolve many of the "sleepless" infant's problems (52). Between 4 and 8 years of age, the problems are more of bedtime difficulties than nocturnal sleep disruption. Often it appears that limits are set in an inconsistent manner, with one parent at times undermining the tentative limit-setting of the other. The causes of the difficulties in limit-setting by both parents have to be appreciated and well evaluated to effect changes in the child's behavior. Some of the night setting problems are related to the child's social stresses. They are most often linked to the family stresses, but personal, particularly school-related adaptation problems must also be evaluated.

Special Problems

"Colicky" Infant

Colic in infants has been defined by Illingworth (53) as "violent rhythmical, screaming attacks which did not stop when the infants were picked up and for which no cause . . . could be found."

As indicated by Weissbluth (54), colic is "an extreme form of normal crying along with agitated wakefulness." The periodic crying disappears between 3 and 4 months of age, but the colic many have induced a pattern of response in the parents that may be responsible for persistence of a sleep disturbance, and a switch from a "colic" behavior to an "abnormal settling" behavior, as described above, may be seen.

Infant With a "Brain Insult" or Other Neurologic Problems

Irregular sleep-wake rhythm is often observed in extensively brain-impaired children (55). The most severe is seen in bedridden infants with very limited response to external stimuli. Most acerebrate children develop dispersed sleep with no clearly delineated NREM or REM sleep (56). No circadian or a poor circadian rhythmicity can be seen. If a rhythm can be noted, it is of a decreased amplitude (57). There is always a temptation to use drugs in these cases, but hypnotics are not the solution.

Children with severe or moderate mental retardation tend to lack normal social relationships with their families and their immediate environment. They may present significant sleep-wake disorders with a leading complaint of "abnormal wakefulness" during the middle of the night. If monitoring of rectal temperature for several days can be obtained and/or simultaneous monitoring of body movements, it will be confirmed that these children often have a poorly defined circadian rhythm with a low acrophase, or a free-running rhythm (58,59). In the worst cases, an irregular sleep-wake rhythm is noted. These rhythm abnormalities are worse when blindness is associated with mental retardation (60). Okawa and Sasaki have also reported prolonged (that is longer than 24 hours) rhythm from 2 to 6 days (57).

These circadian rhythm disturbances in brain-injured and/or mentally retarded children are brought to medical attention more because of the parental nocturnal disturbances that they induce than because of the possible daytime sleepiness. However, the sleep-wake disturbances may have a detrimental impact on the training of these already handicapped children. Once again, hypnotic medications are often prescribed in large quantities with, at times, very little impact on the nocturnal behavior. Following Czeisler et al.'s (61,62) report on the effect of light on the sleep-wake cycle, we tried a non-drug treatment approach on five children between the ages of 3 and 6 years with a history of mental retardation with and without brain insult (unpublished observation). In one case, a temperature cycle obtained with parental cooperation demonstrated the presence of a 24-hour rhythm of very low amplitude. Each child was subsequently placed under very strict feeding schedules, a fixed lights-out time, late for the children's age of 2200 hours, a fixed wake-up schedule of 0630 hours with, however, the possibility of extending sleep up to 0700 hours, but no later, and the exclusion of daytime naps, which caregivers denied. Parents were asked to build light panels using "Vitalite"™ full-spectrum light tubes and that a minimum of 8,000 Lux be provided in one room where each child was kept for 2 hours from the time of immediate waking. If the day was sunny and it was possible for the parents, the child was placed outside under full sun. This light therapy, currently also tried as an adjuvant in the treatment of adult depression, was much more successful in controlling the sleep-wake disorder than was any previously tried drug. This treatment has been followed for a minimum of 8 months and a maximum of 24 months. There was no trial to perform a single or double blind study using low intensity light. Parents have been so satisfied with the results that they have refused to interrupt the light treatment to see if the child would present a reappearance of symptoms. One of the 5 children presented an abnormal night an average of one night every ten nights despite the light treatment.

Delayed Sleep Phase Syndrome

The delayed sleep phase syndrome (DSPS), described by Weitzman et al. (63), is often seen in adolescents. The most important factor responsible for the syndrome seems to be that the underlying circadian clock has a free-running rate closer to 25 than to 24 hours. An individual always finds it easier to stay up later at night and sleep later in the morning than the reverse. Moore-Ede et al. (64) hypothesized that a reduced phase advance capability could be caused by a low amplitude advance portion of the phase response curve. In the DSPS, the child or adolescent complains of having difficulty falling asleep in the evening, or just goes to bed late, but cannot get up in the morning. If forced to go to bed earlier than usual, for example, near 2200 hours, the child or adolescent cannot fall asleep before 0200 or 0300 hours and cannot get up before 1000 to 1200 hours. Chronotherapy (65) has been proposed for this disorder. It involves a difficult week of rescheduling sleep, delaying sleep by 3 hours every 24 hours, with a sleep period of 7 1/2 hours and rotation of the sleep period until bedtime is "in phase" again with the nighttime period. This difficult sleep-wake rescheduling has been a valid therapeutic approach. However, since 1987 we have been using the phototherapy as described above, with lights kept between 8,000 and 12,000 lux as recommended by Czeisler et al. (62). Results have been as good as with chronotherapy. Light therapy was often pursued on a daily basis for 2 to 3 months. It may be possible to interrupt the treatment earlier, but data are lacking.

The primary circadian pacemaker is located in the nucleus suprachiasmaticus (66,67), and a direct connection between the pineal and melatonin-containing neurons and the suprachiasmatic neurons has been well shown through lesion experiments in rodents and other mammals. It is supposed that similar cells and pathways are involved in the circadian controls in humans, but this is still mostly unproven and is based on very indirect evidence (64).

PARASOMNIAS

The term nonrapid eye movement (NREM) parasomnia, or dyssomnia, refers to a group of acute, episodic, physical phenomena generally seen during, or exacerbated by, nocturnal sleep. The most common problems are sleepwalking, nightmares, night terrors, and head banging. Enuresis was previously classified under this term, but more recent work has demonstrated that classic "idiopathic" nocturnal enuresis occurs throughout the night, being evenly distributed throughout sleep (68–70).

The parasomnias occur after sleep onset, disrupting NREM sleep, usually stage 4 (delta) sleep. As Klackenberg (50,71) and Richman (72) clearly demonstrated with the normative data from longitudinal studies, many children experience a few of these episodes, usually linked to a specific age or state of maturity during the prepubertal years, but occurring infrequently in a normal population. Pathology is suspected when the frequency persists over time. Exceptionally, the parasomnias can be related to a very specific cause, such as temporal lobe epilepsy, migraine headaches, or OSAS. As there is a continuum between what is seen in a normal population and what is considered pathologic, the incidence and prevalence of pathologic parasomnias is unknown. All published studies have emphasized the frequent positive family histories for such behavior (73–76). Broughton questioned the pathophysiologic mechanisms behind these disorders and arrived at the concept of "disorders of arousal" (77). Paroxysmal in nature and occurring when coming out of NREM sleep, most commonly stage 4 (delta) sleep, they are characterized by a lack of responsiveness to the environment, automatic actions, and retrograde amnesia (78). Confusion and disorientation are customary, and the subject typically has only a vague, partial memory of the event, although children often remember some terrifying element if they are completely awake after the event. Young children may be able to provide only an indication of fear, but older children may convey a vivid and elaborate description of the nightmarish, hallucinatory content. The degree of retrograde amnesia varies, therefore, with the child's age, the intensity of the child's confusion during the event, and the elapsed time between event and report.

Night Terror, Nightmare, and Sleepwalking

During an episode of night terror or sleepwalking, the child's behavior is stereotypical (78). He may evince bodily movements, sit up with glassy eyes, and present manifestations of extreme autonomic nervous system (ANS) discharge, with tachycardia, tachypnea, perspiration, and vocalizations indicating distress. He may walk or rush about with a fearful expression. Even if stationary, the child may exhibit confusion and disorientation. If someone tries to restrain him, the combination of intense fear, confusion, disorientation, and reflex escape behavior may lead the child to struggle violently against the interference. It is during this escape behavior that accidents may occur, such as walking through a glass window or falling down the stairs. At other times, children just scream for a few seconds up to 20 minutes, unresponsive to parental solicitations.

There is a tendency to link this abnormal behavior to known syndromes, but one must insist on the fact that epilepsy is exceptionally associated with and the cause of the parasomnia (79,80). Epileptic events can be suspected when there is a combination of features, particularly violent acts and stereotypical behavior not limited to the first third of the night. Abnormal critical EEG discharges will affirm the diagnosis (80). A problem is the not infrequent anteromesio-temporal focus, more commonly right than left, that may be difficult to demonstrate, but none of the clinical patterns are characteristic of epilepsy. Even if the classic nonepileptic parasomnia is most commonly seen during the first third of the night, before 0100 hours, and out of delta sleep, it is possible to see typical parasomnia out of stage 3 and even stage 2 NREM sleep. It is possible to note them later in the night, particularly if two or more episodes occur during the same night; and violence, as already mentioned, may be seen during typical parasomnia. The diagnosis of an epileptic disorder must always be questioned, and as already shown, known epileptic children have a tendency to present nonepileptic parasomnia. It would be preferable to consider that a brain insult may favor the appearance of parasomnias in a certain number of cases. It is with this in mind that one must consider the association between migraine and somnambulism (81,82). It is known that sleep is much more disturbed during migraine headaches, particularly nocturnal migraines, and the sleep disturbance would favor the parasomnia. A similar hypothesis is considered to explain the association between obstructive sleep apnea and somnambulism (83).

When one considers nightmares (or "dream anxiety attacks" which arise out of REM sleep and where the child is aware of his actual surroundings immediately upon awakening), night terrors, and sleepwalking, one must remember that current external stresses or new developmental spurts often precipitate the event by reactivating old traumas; that is, those partly dormant but still unassimilated.

If doubt exists, it is important to perform not only a sleep-deprived, awake-sleep, EEG with nasopharyngeal leads, but also all-night polygraphic monitoring using the 10–20 electrode placement and video camera to simultaneously monitor the child's behavior. Most commonly the "pathologic" parasomnias will be controlled with a nondrug approach. We have used psychotherapy (83) and behavior modification programs with good results, but hypnosis has also given positive results (84). In certain cases, considering the clinical severity of the problem and the risks of physical injury, medications may be needed as a first treatment step. The most commonly used and probably most effective drug has been diazepam (2 to 10 mg/bedtime). Medications such as other benzodiazepines and carbamazepine have also been tried with beneficial results. It is important, however, to know how to progressively decrease the drug intake once a good relationship has developed between patient and psychotherapist.

Headbanging

A very difficult and often poorly controlled problem is chronic headbanging, jactatio capitis nocturnus. There is a general agreement that drugs often have a poor, if any, impact on the symptom, and the response to psychotherapy and behavior modification programs, for example, is much more limited than with the other parasomnias. Two types of headbanging are considered: one occurring after an arousal from sleep; that is, appearing in a wake state even though a confused state of wakefulness; and the other starting or persisting for long periods during stages 1 and 2 NREM sleep. To distinguish between the two requires a systematic nocturnal sleep monitoring. Although data are still scarce, it would seem that medications preventing and/or decreasing arousals during sleep might have some positive effects on the wake-related headbanging. This type of repetitive movement may also be related to other rhythmic movements seen at sleep onset in many infants between 2 and 5 years of age. A combination of restructuring sleep onset rituals, psychotherapy, and initial administration of drugs may be able to control this parasomnia.

CONCLUSIONS

Sleep disorders are undoubtedly frequent in children and adolescents and may be related to multiple organ dysfunction. The controls of our vital functions are different during wake, NREM, and REM sleep. Our autonomic nervous system exercises a very different balance on all of our organs, depending on our state of alertness. Medications given during wake states will also impact on CNS control settings during NREM and REM sleep. The only response to these iatrogenic or pathologic disturbances of the controls of our biologic functions during NREM and REM sleep will be a sleep disorder. All physicians who care for children must be able to ask the appropriate questions concerning sleep and sleep behavior during systematic evolution of children. It must be remembered that parents may not pay attention to a sleep-related symptom or may not give it a physiologic meaning. Sleep disorders must be considered as an alarm, for a more general health problem may be hidden and its first manifestation may occur during NREM and REM sleep. Sleep medicine may prevent further progression of an illness, recognizing an early phase of the disease and preventing the appearance of unexplained respiratory, cardiac, gastro-esophageal, and other problems during the daytime. Sleep-related investigations allow the scrutiny of biologic functioning during the two other states of alertness, NREM and REM sleep, which together represent between 33 and 60% of the life of a young human being.

REFERENCES

1. Welstein C, Dement WC, Redington D, et al. Insomnia in the San Francisco Bay area: A telephone survey. In: Guilleminault C, Lugaresi E, eds. Sleep/wake Disorders: Natural History, Epidemiology, and Long-Term Evolution. New York: Raven Press, 1983:73–86.
2. White L, Hahn P, Mitler MM. Sleep questionnaire. In: Chase MH, Walter DF, eds. Adolescents in Sleep Research. Los Angeles: UCLA Brain Research Institute/Brain Information Service, 1983:9.
3. Association of Sleep Disorders Centers. Diagnostic classification of sleep and arousal disorders. Sleep 1979;2:1–137.
4. Anders T, Emde R, Parmelee AH, eds. A Manual of Standardized Terminology, Techniques and Criteria for Scoring States of Sleep and Wakefulness in Newborn Infants. Los Angeles: UCLA Brain Information Service/Brain Research Institute, 1971.
5. Coons S, Guilleminault C. The development of sleep-wake patterns and nonrapid eye movement sleep stages during the first six months of life in normal infants. Pediatrics 1982; 69:793–798.
6. Coons S, Guilleminault C. Development of consolidated sleep and wakeful periods in relation to the day/night cycle in infancy. Dev Med Child Neurol 1984;26:169–176.
7. Guilleminault C, Souquet M. Sleep states and related pathology. In: Korobkin R, Guilleminault C, eds. Advances in Perinatal Neurology. New York: Spectrum, 1979:225–247.
8. Kleitman N. Sleep and Wakefulness, 2nd ed. Chicago: University of Chicago Press, 1983.
9. Carskadon MA, Keenan S, Dement WC. Nighttime sleep and daytime sleep tendency in preadolescents. In: Guilleminault C, ed. Sleep and Its Disorders in Children. New York: Raven Press, 1987:43–52.
10. Carskadon MA, Harvey K, Duke P, et al. Pubertal changes in daytime sleepiness. Sleep 1980;2:453–460.
11. Coble PA, Kupfer DJ, Reynolds, CF III, et al. EEG sleep of healthy children 6 to 12 years of age. In: Guilleminault C, ed. Sleep and Its Disorders in Children. New York: Raven Press, 1987:29–41.
12. Carskadon MA, Dement WC. Sleepiness in the normal adolescent. In: Guilleminault C, ed. Sleep and Its Disorders in Children. New York: Raven Press, 1987:53–66.
13. Carskadon MA, Orav EJ, Dement WC. Evolution of sleep and daytime sleepiness in adolescents. In: Guilleminault C, Lugaresi E, eds. Sleep/Wake Disorders: Natural History, Epidemiology, and Long-Term Evolution. New York: Raven Press, 1983:201–216.
14. Carskadon MA, Dement WC. Effects of a daytime nap on sleepiness during sleep restriction. Sleep Res 1986;15:69.
15. Carskadon MA, Harvey K, Dement WC. Sleep loss in young adolescents. Sleep 1981;4:299–312.
16. Carskadon MA, Dement WC. The multiple sleep latency test: What does it measure? Sleep 1982;5:S67–S72.
17. Richardson GS, Carskadon MA, Flagg W, et al. Excessive daytime sleepiness in man: Multiple sleep latency measurement in narcoleptic and control subjects. Electroencephalogr Clin Neurophysiol 1978;45:621–627.
18. Van den Hoed J, Kraemer H, Guilleminault C, et al. Disorders of excessive daytime somnolence: Polygraphic and clinical data for 100 patients. Sleep 1981;4:23–38.
19. Guilleminault C. Obstructive sleep apnea syndrome in children. In: Guilleminault C, ed. Sleep and Its Disorders in Children. New York: Raven Press, 1987:213–224.
20. Guilleminault C, Eldreidge FL, Simmons FB, et al. Sleep apnea in eight children. Pediatrics 1976;58:28–31.

21. Guilleminault C, Winkle R. A review of 50 children with OSAS. Lung 1981;159:275–287.

22. Piecuch JF. Costo-chondral grafts to temporo-mandibular joints. In: Abstracts and Proceedings of the Annual Meeting of the American Association of Oral and Maxillofacial Surgeons, Chicago, 1978 [abstract 38].

23. Kuo PC, West RR, Bloomquist DS, et al. The effect of mandibular osteotomy in three patients with hypersomnia sleep apnea. Oral Surg 1979; 48:385–392.

24. Riley R, Guilleminault C, Herran J, et al. Cephalometric analyses and flow volume loops in obstructive sleep apneic patients. Sleep 1983;6:303–311.

25. Walsh JK, Katsantonis P, Schweitzer RP, et al. Somnofluoroscopy: Cineradiography observation of obstructive sleep apnea. Sleep 1985;8:294–297.

26. Suratt PM, Dee P, Atkinson RL, et al. Fluoroscopy and computed tomography features of the pharyngeal airway in obstructive sleep apnea. Am Rev Respir Dis 1983; 127:487–492.

27. Guilleminault C. Narcolepsy and its differential diagnosis. In: Guilleminault C, ed. Sleep and Its Disorders in Children. New York: Raven Press 1987:181–194.

28. Guilleminault C. Narcolepsy. Sleep 1986;2:291.

29. Guilleminault C. Disorders of excessive daytime sleepiness. In: Guilleminault C, ed. Sleep and Its Disorders in Children. New York: Raven Press, 1987:177–179.

30. Navelet Y, Anders TF, Guilleminault C. Narcolepsy in children. In: Guilleminault C, Dement WC, Passouant P, eds. Narcolepsy. New York: Spectrum, 1976:171–177.

31. Honda Y, Asaka A, Tanaka Y, et al. Discrimination of narcoleptic patients by using genetic markers and HLA. Sleep Res 1983;12:254 [abstract].

32. Honda Y, Doi Y, Juji T, et al. Narcolepsy and HLA: Positive DR2 as a prerequisite for the development of narcolepsy. Folia Psychiatr Neurol Jpn 1984;38:360–367.

33. Honda Y, Doi Y, Juji T, et al. Positive HLA-DR2 finding as a prerequisite for the development of narcolepsy. Folia Psychiatr Neurol Jpn 1985;39:203–204.

34. Langdon N, Welsh KI, Van Dam M, et al. Genetic markers in narcolepsy. Lancet 1984;2:1178–1180.

35. Billiard M, Seignalet J. Extraordinary association between HLA-DR2 and narcolepsy. Lancet 1985;1:226–227.

36. Mefford IN, Baker TL, Boehme RE, et al. Narcolepsy: Biogenic amine deficits in an animal model. Science 1983; 220:629–632.

37. Boehme RE, Baker TL, Mefford IN, et al. Narcolepsy: Cholinergic receptor changes in animal model. Life Sci 1984; 34:1825–1828.

38. Baker T, Mitler M, Foutz A, et al. Diagnosis and treatment of narcolepsy in animals. In: Kirk RW, ed. Current Veterinary Therapy, Vol. VIII: Small Animal Practice. Philadelphia: Saunders, 1983:755–759.

39. Thomson G. The mode of inheritance of the HLA-linked gene predisposing to narcolepsy. Tissue Antigens 1985;26: 201–203.

40. Guilleminault C, Mignot E, Grumet FC. Familial patterns of narcolepsy. Lancet 1989;2:1376–1379.

41. Guilleminault C. Disorders of excessive sleepiness. Ann Clin Res 1986;17:209–219.

42. Critchley M. Periodic hypersomnia and megaphagia in adolescent males. Brain 1962;85:627–656.

43. Billiard M, Guilleminault C, Dement WC. A menstruation-linked periodic hypersomnia, Kleine-Levin syndrome or a new clinical entity? Neurology 1975;25:436–443.

44. Parmelee AH. Ontogeny of sleep patterns and associated periodicities in infants. In: Faulkner E, Kretchmer N, Ross E, eds. Pre- and Postnatal Development of the Human Brain. Basel: Karger, 1974:298–311.

45. Anders TF. State and rhythmic processes. J Am Acad Child Psychiatry 1978;17:401–420.

46. Ferber R. The sleepless child. In: Guilleminault C, ed. Sleep and Its Disorders in Children. New York: Raven Press, 1987: 141–163.

47. Anders TF. Biological rhythms in development. Psychosom Med 1982;44:61–72.

48. Klackenberg G. Sleep behaviour studied longitudinally. Acta Paediatr Scand 1982;71:501–506.

49. Karlberg P, Klackenberg G, Klackenberg-Larsson I, et al. The development of children in a Swedish urban community: A prospective, longitudinal study; introduction, design and aims of the study. Acta Paediatr Scand 1968, Suppl 187.

50. Klackenberg G. Incidence of parasomnias in children in a general population. In: Guilleminault C, ed. Sleep and Its Disorders in Children. New York: Raven press, 1987:99–113.

51. Richman N. A community survey of characteristics of one- to two-year-olds with sleep disruptions. J Am Acad Child Psychiatry 1981;20:281–291.

52. Ferber R, Boyle MP. Nocturnal fluid intake: A cause of, not treatment for, sleep disruption in infants and toddlers. Sleep Res 1983;12:243.

53. Illingworth RS. "Three months" colic. Arch Dis Child 1954; 29:167–174.

54. Weissbluth M. Sleep and the colicky infant. In: Guilleminault C, ed. Sleep and Its Disorders in Children. New York: Raven Press, 1987:129–140.

55. Okawa M, Takahashi K, Sasaki H. Disturbance of circadian rhythms in severely brain-damaged patients correlated with CT findings. J Neurol 1986;233:274–282.

56. Sasaki H, Tamagawa K, Okawa M. Sleep of "acerebrate" patients. Clin Electroencephalogr 1978;20:672–676.

57. Okawa M, Sasaki H. Sleep Disorders in Children. New York: Raven Press, 1987:269–290.

58. Meier-Koll A, Hall U, Hellwing U, et al. A biological oscillator system and the development of sleep-waking behavior during early infancy. Chronobiologie 1978;5: 425–440.

59. Wever RA. The Circadian System of Man: Results of Experiments Under Temporal Isolation. New York: Springer-Verlag, 1979.

60. Miles LE, Wilson MA. High incidence of cyclic sleep wake disorders in the blind. Sleep Res 1977;6:192.

61. Czeisler CA, Richardson GS, Zimmerman JC, et al. Entrainment of human circadian rhythms by light dark cycles: A reassessment. Photochem Photobiol 1981;34:239–247.

62. Czeisler CA, Allan JS, Strogatz SH, et al. Bright light resets the human circadian pacemaker independent of the timing of the sleep-wake cycle. Science 1986;233:667–671.

63. Weitzman ED, Czeisler Ca, Coleman RM, et al. Delayed sleep phase syndrome: A chronobiologic disorder with sleep onset insomnia. Arch Gen Psychiatry 1981;38:737–746.

64. Moore-Ede MC, Sulzman FM, Fuller CA. The Clocks That Time Us. Cambridge: Harvard University Press, 1982.

65. Czeisler CA, Richardson GS, Coleman RM, et al. Chronotherapy: Resetting the circadian clocks of patients with delayed sleep phase insomnia. Sleep 1981;4:1–21.

66. Moore RY, Eichler VB. Loss of a circadian adrenal corticosterone rhythm following suprachiasmatic lesions in the rat. Brain Res 1972;42:201–206.

67. Stephan FK, Zucker I. Circadian rhythms in drinking behavior and locomotor activity of rats are eliminated by hypothalamic lesions. Proc Natl Acad Sci USA 1972;69:1583–1586.

68. Nino-Murcia G, Keenan SA. Enuresis and sleep. In: Guilleminault C, ed. Sleep and Its Disorders in Children. New York: Raven Press, 1987:253–267.

69. Mikkelsen EJ, Rapoport JL, Nee L, et al. Childhood enuresis. I. Sleep patterns and psychopathology. Arch Gen Psychiatry 1980;37:1139–1144.

70. Rapoport JL, Mikkelsen EJ, Zavadil A, et al. Childhood enuresis. II. Psychopathology, plasma tricyclic concentration and enuretic effect. Arch Gen Psychiatry 1980;37:1146–1152.

71. Klackenberg G. Somnambulism in childhood: Prevalence, course and behavioral correlation. Acta Paediatr Scand 1982;71:495–499.

72. Richman N. Surveys of sleep disorders in children in a general population. In: Guilleminault C, ed. Sleep and Its Disorders in Children. New York: Raven Press, 1987:115–127.

73. Abe K, Shimakawa M. Predisposition to sleep walking. Psychiatr Neurol 1966;152:306–312.

74. Bakwain H. Sleep walking in twins. Lancet 1970;2:446–447.

75. Kales A, Soldatos CR, Bixler EO, et al. Herediatary factors in sleep walking and night terrors. Brt J Psychiatry 1980;137:111–118.

76. Hallstrom R. Night terror in adults through three generations. Acta Psychiatr Scand 1972;48:350–352.

77. Broughton RJ. Sleep disorders: Disorders of arousal? Science 1978;159:1070–1078.

78. Gastaut H, Broughton RJ. A clinical and polygraphic study of episodic phenomena during sleep. Biol Psychiatry 1965;7:197–221.

79. Tassinari CA, Mancia D. Della Bernadina B, et al. Pavor nocturnus of nonepileptic nature in epileptic children. Electroencephalogr Clin Neurophysiol 1972;33:603–607.

80. Pedley TA, Guilleminault C. Episodic nocturnal wanderings responsive to anticonvulsant drug therapy. Ann Neurol 1977;2:30–35.

81. Barabas G, Ferrari M, Schemp P, et al. Childhood migraine and somnambulism. Neurology 1983;33:948–949.

82. Dexter JD. The relationship between stage II-IV and REM sleep and arousals with migraine. Headache 1975;29:101–106.

83. Guilleminault C. Disorders of arousal in children: Somnambulism and night terrors. In: Guilleminault C, ed. Sleep and Its Disorders in Children. New York: Raven Press, 1987:243–252.

84. Reid WH. Treatment of somnambulism in military trainees. Am J Psychiatry 1975;29:101–105.

Chapter 30
Coma in Childhood

Roger P. Simon

Coma is a symptom and not a disease entity. The underlying causes of coma may vary from a benign and completely reversible syndrome, as in the case of a sedative drug overdose, to a reflection of catastrophic central nervous system (CNS) injury, as in subarachnoid hemorrhage. Further, potentially reversible disease states that manifest as coma, like hypoglycemia, require prompt, accurate diagnosis if an optimal outcome is to be assured. Accurate analysis of the clinical signs of coma will reliably reflect the anatomic and physiologic process that is producing the CNS dysfunction and will, therefore, also dictate the investigative and therapeutic interventions appropriate in a given clinical situation. Knowledge of the anatomic substrate of consciousness, the analysis of the relevant signs accessible during examination, and the differential diagnosis of unconsciousness based on the neurologic examination are reviewed.

ANATOMY OF CONSCIOUSNESS

Consciousness requires both arousal and awareness. Arousal is mediated by the reticular activating system of the brain stem; awareness requires the functioning of the cerebral cortex. Arousal may occur without awareness in the setting of diffuse bihemispheric injury that may occur, for example, from anoxic encephalopathy or following bihemispheric cerebral infarction. This injury results in a persistent vegetative state (1) in which the patient is awake (reticular function of the brain stem) but not aware (hemispheric function). Alternatively, a brain stem infarction may eliminate the possibility of arousal while leaving the potential of cerebral hemispheric function intact. Such lesions of the reticular formation eliminate arousal and produce the state of coma; a sleep-like state in which eye closure is the hallmark.

The reticular activating system is located diffusely within the brain stem. Its caudal end is in the midpons at the level of the trigeminal nerve. Brain stem lesions below this level do not produce coma. Such low brain stem lesions, however, result in transection of descending motor pathways for limb and cranial nerve function and thereby render the patient quadriparetic and mute while awake and aware, the so-called locked-in state (2). Such patients are recognized by volitional vertical eye movement, a motor function subserved by the midbrain. The rostral extent of the reticular formation responsible for consciousness extends to the hypothalamus and thalamus. Bilateral hypothalamic lesions, however, usually produce a state of hypersomnolence rather than coma, but bilateral thalamic lesions, such as those produced by occlusion of perforating thalamic arteries, result in coma.

Cortical function responsible for awareness is multifocally located within the cerebral hemispheres. In the main, the level of consciousness is proportional to the amount of functioning cortical tissue present, and consciousness fades in proportion to the volume of cerebral cortex removed (3). Accordingly, extensive bilateral lesions of the cerebral hemispheres are required in order to produce unconsciousness. Some data exist, mainly from intracarotid barbiturate injections for localization of the lateralization of language function in the brain, which support a special role for consciousness in the dominant cerebral hemisphere (4). This is not commonly clinically recognized, although it has been reported (5). Bihemispheric dysfunction produces unconsciousness rather than coma. Although these patients are unaware of their surroundings, eye opening and spontaneous eye movements occur.

PATHOPHYSIOLOGY OF COMA

Unconsciousness is the result of dysfunction of both cerebral hemispheres. Coma, however, occurs only with compromise of the brainstem reticular formation. Such reticular formation compromise is the result of only three disease processes: when the brain stem is compromised by an expanding mass (like a tumor) or destructive process (such as a stroke or a demyelinating process); during the metabolic dysfunctional state of organ-system failure, electrolyte/osmolar dysfunction, or as the result of extrinsically administered drugs; electrical dysfunction of the brain resulting (usually transiently) from a generalized seizure disorder.

Hemispheric Mass Lesions

Hemispheric masses (e.g., tumor, infarction, abscess, hematoma) begin in or over one cerebral hemisphere. Unconsciousness and finally coma are produced by the sequential compromise of the contralateral hemisphere, the rostral brain stem, and finally the caudal brain stem. The mechanism of this progressive CNS dysfunction is described as transtentorial herniation. This term refers to the physical movement of cerebral parenchyma from one intracranial compartment to another, that is, from the supratentorial compartment to the infratentorial compartment. A pressure differential between the two compartments—and not the overall intracranial pressure per se—produces the herniation. The pressure differential is essential, because diffusely increased intracranial pressure (in the range of 900 to 1000 mm H_2O) will produce headache but not clouding of the sensorium or altered consciousness (6).

In transtentorial herniation from a hemispheric mass, clinical CNS dysfunction progresses in a rostral-caudal manner in that somnolence first occurs with involvement of diencephalic (thalamic) structures, pupillary function becomes compromised with midbrain involvement, inducible eye movements are next paralyzed with involvement at the pontine level, and finally respiratory and cardiac function are altered as the medulla is affected (Figure 30.1)(7). Two forms of transtentorial herniation have been described: central and uncal (8). With central herniation, a bilateral symmetric rostral-caudal compromise occurs; with uncal herniation, the asymmetric mass forces the uncus (the most medial portion of the temporal lobe) against the brain stem (at the midbrain level) as the initial stage of the herniation events. A clear distinction between these two types of herniation probably does not occur (9,10). Clinically, a combination of the two herniation types is most commonly observed, with an initial asymmetry of motor system dysfunction referable to the initial localization of the mass in one of the two hemispheres. Midbrain compromise occurs subsequently, beginning ipsilateral to the mass. Later, the herniation process progresses in a symmetric manner.

Brain Stem Lesions

Expanding lesions within the posterior fossa produce coma by mass effect and upward transtentorial herniation.

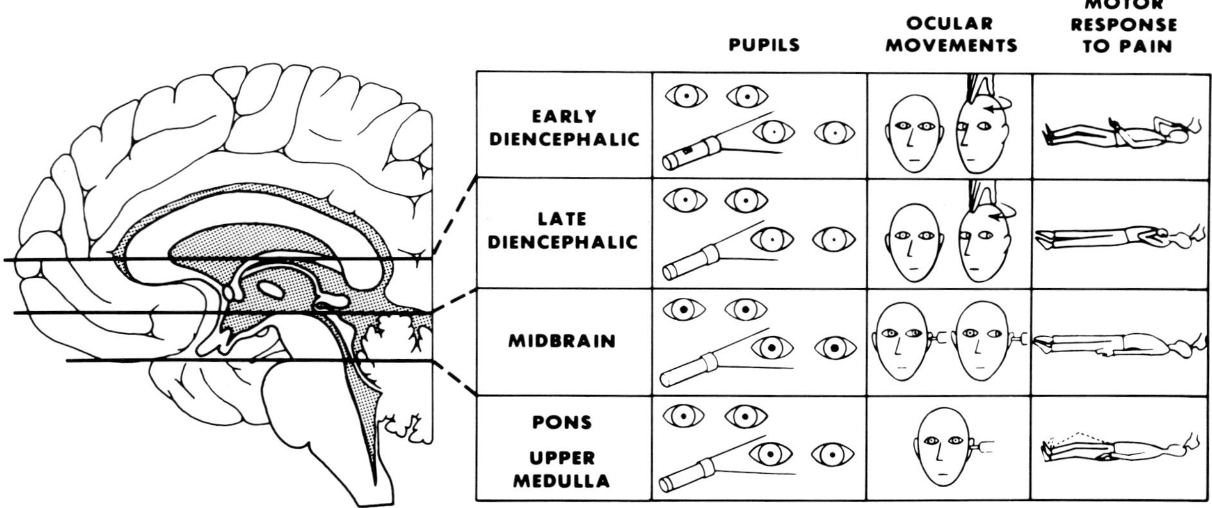

FIGURE 30.1   This schema relates each of the physical signs to be evaluated—pupillary response, doll's eyes maneuver, and pain response—to the area of the brain that is affected. Reprinted by permission from Mills J, Ho MT, Salber PR, et al.: Current Emergency Diagnosis and Treatment. East Norwalk, CT: Appleton & Lange, 1983.

Although this syndrome often goes unrecognized, coma with decerebrate posturing and abnormal eye movements can precede midbrain compromise in accordance with the caudal-rostral progression of abnormalities. Common examples are hemorrhages, tumors, or infarction of the cerebellum.

Compromise of the brain stem reticular formation can occur and produce coma in the absence of upward herniation. Basilar artery embolus and the rupture of a brain stem arteriovenous malformation are vascular causes. Cerebellar and pontine gliomas constitute common mass lesions in children; rare causes in the first years of life include Leigh disease. Basilar artery migraine can also result in confusion and even deep coma. The clinical examination can demonstrate major compromise of brain stem structures to include an absence of the pupillary light reflex (11). In our experience, patients in coma with basilar migraine have recovered completely within hours to a day.

METABOLIC LESIONS

Anoxia and Ischemia

Anoxia

Anoxia (inadequate oxygenation) is distinct from ischemia (impairment of blood flow). Pure hypoxia ($PaO_2 > 20$ to 40 mm Hg) without ischemia for up to 40 minutes is compatible with a good outcome (12–14). Diffuse nervous system injury from anoxia usually is the result of superimposed ischemia. Hypoxia ($PaO_2 < 20$ to 40 mm Hg) results in a centrally mediated fall of blood pressure and cardiac output with resultant superimposed ischemia. Accordingly, the terms *anoxia* and *ischemia* are not synonymous, but have marked distinctions as regards prognosis.

Ischemia

A failure of cerebral perfusion can result from systemic illness producing hypotension, from cardiac arrhythmias with a resultant fall in cardiac output, or from an increase in intracranial pressure that exceeds the arterial perfusion pressure (e.g., Reye syndrome or subarachnoid hemorrhage). The neuropathologic changes induced by ischemia occur in one of two patterns. Impairment of cerebral blood flow first affects regions of the cerebral cortex with an end-arterial distribution (Figure 30.2). This results in so-called watershed infarctions, which have their major expression between the anterior and middle cerebral arteries and the middle and posterior cerebral arteries. In the parietal area, such watershed infarction produces neurologic deficits of the arms with preferential sparing of the legs and face. Posterior watershed infarctions result in occipital lobe ischemia with cortical blindness. Posterior cerebral/middle cerebral ischemia may affect the medial temporal lobe and

result in the phenomenon of Korsakoff syndrome of short-term memory loss. Watershed infarction also occasionally affects the spinal cord with resultant paraparesis.

Global ischemia followed by reperfusion of the brain, as in cardiac arrest, results in a different pattern of neuronal injury; viz., that of involvement of the selectively vulnerable cell groups of hippocampus, cortex, thalamus, striatum, and cerebellum. Prominent neuronal loss in the cortical mantle (so-called laminar necrosis) may result in prolonged coma with depression or absence of electroencephalographic (EEG) activity but with preserved brain stem function; viz., the syndrome of neocortical death. The region of selective vulnerability appears to be related to excitatory amino-acid receptors pathologically stimulated by an increase in extracellular glutamate, which results from global ischemia. The pattern of the excitatory receptor populations is probably responsible for the unique susceptibility of the neonatal striatum to perinatal asphyxia with the resultant static encephalopathy ("cerebral palsy")(15). The excessive stimulation by excitatory amino-acid neurotransmitters produces intracellular calcium accumulation, which may itself be toxic to neurons. This pathophysiology has suggested a treatment for ischemic syndromes, either with calcium-channel blockade or pharmacologic blockade of postsynaptic glutamate receptors (16). Barbiturates have not proved to be protective during ischemia in primate models (17) or in humans (18).

Clinical Features

Cardiac arrest and drowning are the most common causes of anoxic-ischemic injury in children. With cardiac arrest, asystole of 4 to 8 seconds in the upright position and 12 to 15 seconds in the supine position is necessary to produce coma. Prodromal symptoms include weakness, light-headedness, tinnitus, nausea, and dimming of vision. With asystole of 15 to 20 seconds, tonic posturing occurs, the minimal expression of which is jaw clenching. After a minute or more, both urinary and fecal incontinence are seen. The pupils become fixed and unreactive 2 to 4 minutes after asystole (19).

Following cardiac resuscitation, the prognosis as regards the CNS depends on the duration of cerebral hypoperfusion, the resulting signs on examination, and the rapidity of their normalization. As regards the brain stem, pupillary unresponsiveness and lack of inducible lateral eye movements are poor prognostic signs; in the motor system,

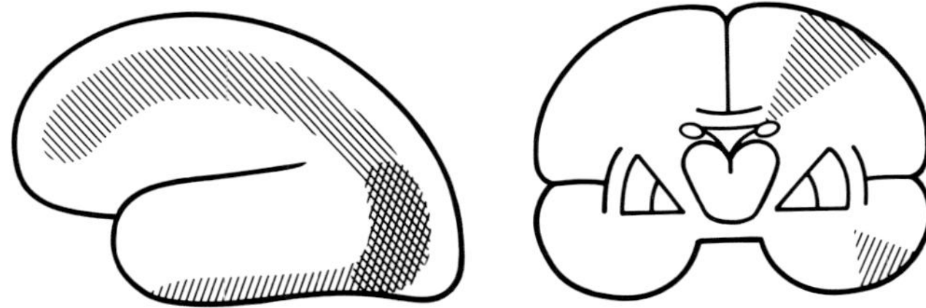

FIGURE 30.2   Distribution of "watershed" infarctions.

flaccidity is worse than decorticate or decerebrate posturing, and appropriate localization of pain is the best feature.

In 210 adults studied prospectively, the absence of pupillary light reflexes at the initial examination was incompatible with a good recovery, that is, independent function. At 24 hours after resuscitation, the persistent lack of flexor or extensor motor responses and the lack of orienting, or at least conjugate roving eye movements, was associated with eventual independent function in a single patient only (20).

In 636 children resuscitated from cardiac arrest, cortical function was assessed clinically by responsiveness and by the EEG. An estimated duration of cerebral hypoperfusion of 10 to 30 seconds was uniformly associated with rapid cortical recovery; with 3 to 4 minutes, preserved EEG activity was seen, and rapid recovery usually followed. With 5 to 8 minutes, persistent slowing was seen on EEG, and no patients made a full recovery. At 8 to 10 minutes, burst suppression was seen on the EEG, and all patients died. With greater than 10 minutes of circulatory impairment, a flat (isoelectric) EEG was seen, and death followed in all cases (21).

In cases of near drowning, increasing immersion time is associated with a decreasing prognosis for recovery. A favorable outcome has been reported with immersion times as long as 20 minutes in some reports (22); whereas, other reports have concluded that immersion times of greater than 6 minutes are always associated with severe damage (23). Additional poor prognostic signs are an arterial pH of less than 7, low rectal temperature on admission, need for cardiopulmonary resuscitation in the emergency room, seizures, fixed pupils, flaccid motor tone, and lack of response to pain. A favorable prognosis suggested by Pearn (24) is spontaneous breathing (the first gasp) occurring within 20 minutes. The theoretic differences between freshwater and salt-water immersion and warm-water versus cold-water drowning appear to have minimal correlates with neurologic recovery (25,26).

Hypoglycemia

The most common causes of hypoglycemia include in infants, inadequate glycogen stores; in children younger than 5 years, ketotic hypoglycemia; in patients older than 5 or 6 years, islet cell adenoma. The symptoms of hypoglycemia are diffuse and correlate poorly with serum glucose concentrations. The time course of neurologic changes following insulin-induced coma has been described (Table 30.1)(27). Physiologically, these clinical features suggest a rostral-caudal pattern of dysfunction. In adults, confusion was seen with glucose concentrations of 9 to 60 mg/dL, stupor with concentrations of 8 to 59 mg/dL, and coma with concentrations of 2 to 28 mg/dL (28). Accordingly, absolute serum glucose levels may not be reliable indicators of the cause of coma in a given patient. Hypoglycemia prior to coma may also produce an agitated state, seizures, and lat-

Table 30.1 Signs and symptoms of hypoglycemia after insulin administration

Time after Insulin Administrations	Symptoms
30 min	Perspiration; salivation; somnolence; excitement and restlessness; tachycardia if stimulated (bradycardia if somnolent)
2–3 hr	Loss of contact with environment; myoclonus; primitive reflexes (gasping, sucking); reactive, dilated pupils
4–5 hr	Comatose; depressed responses to pain; roving eye movements; tonic and torsional muscular spasms; extensor plantar responses
5–6 hr	Decerebrate rigidity
6–7 hr	Small pupils; bradycardia; flaccid tone; depressed reflexes

The time course of neurologic changes seen after insulin administration for the purposes of inducing "insulin shock." Modified from Himwich HE. Hypoglycemia and brain metabolism. Assoc Res Nerv Ment Dis 1953;32:345–371.

eralized deficits. Hypothermia is an extremely common accompaniment of hypoglycemia and may be an important clinical clue in a given patient. In coma, decerebrate posturing may be seen, which is usually symmetric and accompanied by intact pupillary light reflexes, a constellation of findings that strongly suggest a metabolic cause.

Hypoglycemic coma can persist for up to 90 minutes without irreversible changes occurring in the brain (27). Symptoms from hypoglycemia commonly resolve within minutes of administration of glucose, but more prolonged syndromes followed by good recovery have been described (29). Residual neurologic damage in severe hypoglycemia is highly similar, both clinically and neuropathologically, to that seen in anoxia (30). Specifically, dementia, Korsakoff syndrome, ataxia, and spasticity may occur.

Liver Dysfunction

Hepatic encephalopathy and coma commonly occur in the setting of obvious acute or chronic hepatic dysfunction. Hepatic encephalopathy, however, also occurs without intrinsic liver failure in the setting of urea cycle deficits early in life, resulting in developmental delay and seizures. Hyperammonemia, either congenital or due to intestinal absorption in patients with ureterosigmoidostomy, may produce intermittent encephalopathy lasting days to weeks (Table 30.2)(31,32). In addition, congenital intra- and extra-hepatic shunts can produce hepatic encephalopathy in the presence of normal liver-function tests (33). Hepatic encephalopathy usually occurs insidiously, but may be relatively acutely precipitated by a protein load (like gastrointestinal hemorrhage) in the setting of marginal hepatic function and can be seen intermittently in some of the organic acidemias (Table 30.2)(31).

Table 30.2 Inborn errors of metabolism associated with episodic coma

Organic Acidemias and Amino Acidurias* (Acidosis and Anion Gap with Ketosis)	Age of Onset
Intermittent maple syrup urine disease	Infancy to adolescence
Intermittent late-onset leucinosis	Childhood and later
Methylmalonic aciduria	Childhood and later
Isovaleric aciduria, beta-methylcrotonyl-glycinuria, propionic acidemia, and ketotic hyperglycinemia	Childhood and later

Hyperammonemias	Age of Onset
Argininosuccinic aciduria	2 to 6 years
Ornithine transcarbamylase deficiency	Early infancy to juvenile
Citrullinemia	1st year of age
Hyperlysinemia	Infancy

From Adams RD, Lyon G. Neurology of Hereditary Metabolic Diseases of Children. New York: McGraw-Hill, 1982.
*See chapters 1 and 3.

Acute hepatic failure with fatty degeneration and associated encephalopathy is termed Reye syndrome (34) (see chapter 14). Patients commonly have had a preceding varicella or influenza B viral infection, especially when associated with salicylate use. A seasonal incidence (November through April), with the peak number of cases occurring in February has been noted. The syndrome may begin with protracted vomiting and delirium, progressing to deep coma within 2 days. Seizures are common, but are self-limited. During coma, decerebrate posturing may occur but focal neurologic signs are rare. On examination, sustained hyperventilation can be seen, and hepatomegaly is usually noted. The laboratory examination is notable for elevated serum transaminases and arterial ammonia concentrations. The prothrombin time is prolonged, but the serum bilirubin is normal. The presence of icterus makes the diagnosis of Reye syndrome doubtful. Plasma glucose concentration is often decreased because of hepatic failure, and the hypoglycemia will be reflected in the cerebrospinal fluid (CSF). The CSF protein and cell count are usually normal. The degree of hepatic dysfunction is not well correlated with CSF findings. The CNS abnormalities are best correlated with cerebral edema and intracranial pressure. Treatment is directed toward the control of intracranial pressure, with the goal of maintaining cerebral perfusion pressure (systemic arterial pressure minus intracranial pressure) at greater than 50 mm Hg. An intracranial pressure monitor should be inserted and the patient intubated to permit hyperventilation (pCO_2 below 22 mm Hg). In addition, the body temperature should be maintained at a normal level. Serum osmolality should be below 320 mOsm/L, and serum glucose concentration should be maintained between 150 and 200 mg/dL.

The major toxic cause of acute hepatic failure with coma is acetaminophen overdose (35). Children younger than 5 years of age appear to be relatively resistant, however. Hep-

atic dysfunction and resultant hepatic encephalopathy occur 3 to 5 days following ingestion. The history is usually that of nausea, vomiting, anorexia, and diaphoresis occurring for 12 to 24 hours following the ingestion. This is followed by a quiescent phase of 1 to 4 days, during which time hepatic enzymes, serum bilirubin, and prothrombin time become progressively abnormal. Hepatic encephalopathy is introduced by the return of anorexia, nausea, and malaise with the addition of jaundice, hypoglycemia, stupor, and coma. Renal failure and cardiomyopathy may be associated.

The examination in patients with hepatic coma shows that pupillary responses are well-preserved as are inducible eye movements by the doll's eyes maneuver. Symmetric decorticate or decerebrate posturing is common. The symmetry of the motor posturing in the presence of intact pupillary response suggests a metabolic cause in these patients. Occasional abnormal eye movements such as ocular bobbing, dysconjugate lateral gaze, and tonic eye deviation have occasionally been reported (36). Seizures occur but are rare (37) except when caused by the underlying hepatic disorder, such as amino acidurias or hyperammonemias (31).

In hepatic encephalopathy, respiratory alkalosis is present except in the presence of an overriding metabolic acidosis, as occurs in some inborn errors of metabolisms (e.g., amino acidosis, hyperammonemias). When present, this is an extremely helpful laboratory sign. The role of alkalosis in the development of the encephalopathy is uncertain, because correction of the ventilatory dysfunction by mechanical means does not alter the encephalopathy (38). The prognosis of patients with hepatic coma depends on the underlying liver disease. With return of hepatic function, most patients awaken without neurologic abnormalities.

The toxic factor in hepatic coma remains uncertain. Ammonia is increased and clearly toxic to the metabolic function of the brain, but arterial ammonia levels correlate only in a general way with the severity of the encephalopathy. This observation has led to the speculation that there are other causes of hepatic encephalopathy such as an alteration of blood-brain barrier, increased concentration of blood serotonin, the presence of false neurotransmitters, and an alteration in blood amino-acid content. The hyperammonemia in the CNS results in increased glutamate by combining with alpha-ketoglutarate. Glutamate is converted to glutamine in brain astrocytes, which are induced in chronic hyperammonemia. Although the role of these substances in the generation of hepatic encephalopathy remains uncertain, virtually all patients with hepatic encephalopathy have elevated CSF concentrations of glutamine and alpha-ketoglutarate; the former is a commonly used confirmatory laboratory test (Figure 30.3)(39). Cerebral edema is not a factor in the genesis of hepatic encephalopathy unless liver failure is sudden, as in the case of fulminate hepatic necrosis or Reye syndrome (40–42).

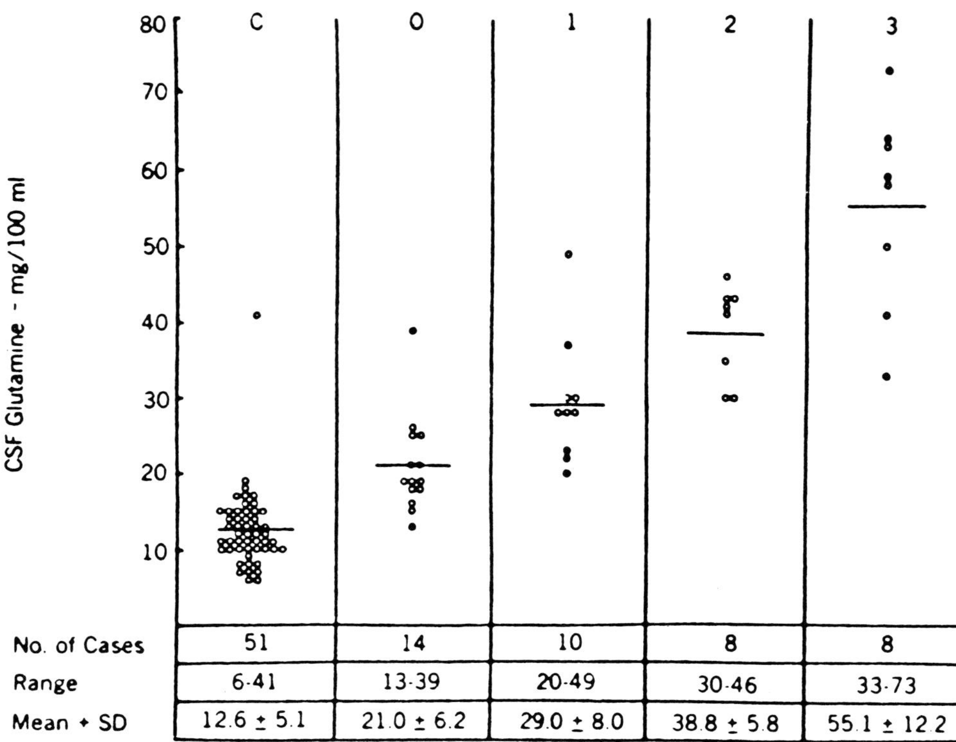

FIGURE 30.3 Cerebrospinal fluid glutamine levels in controls (C), patients with liver disease, and those with various grades of clinical encephalopathy (0 to 3). Reprinted with permission from Hourani BT, Hamlin EM, Reynolds TB. Cerebrospinal fluid glutamine as a measure of hepatic encephalopathy. Arch Intern Med 1971;127: 1033–1035. Copyright 1971, American Medical Association.

Renal Failure

Uremic encephalopathy is subacute in onset; myoclonus, seizures, and tetany precede unconsciousness. Penicillin in high doses may precipitate myoclonus, seizures, and coma in renal failure (43,44). With acute renal failure in children, the elevation of systemic blood pressure to levels of 160/100 mm Hg or higher may result in altered consciousness due to the induction of hypertensive encephalopathy.

The identity of the toxin in uremia is uncertain. The plasma blood urea nitrogen (BUN) levels correlate poorly with mental state. A child with delirium secondary to renal failure has been reported with a BUN of 48 mg/dL (45). Alternatively, BUN values greater than 200 mg/dL may occur without alteration of consciousness, and dialysis may produce improvement of uremic encephalopathy without an alteration in the BUN level (46). Brain edema may occur in uremic encephalopathy, and an alteration in blood-brain barrier permeability has been one suggested means of entrance of systemic toxins into the brain (47). Acidosis does not appear to explain uremic encephalopathy because the CSF pH is usually normal (48).

Pulmonary Failure

Pulmonary encephalopathy is caused by CO_2 narcosis and occurs in acute and chronic forms. Chronically elevated CO_2 levels are better tolerated, with no alteration in mental function observed with $PaCO_2$ concentrations of 50 to 60 mm Hg. Acidosis is a frequent correlate of acute or chronic pulmonary failure, but correction of the acidosis does not reverse the encephalopathy. Clinical features include headache, tremor, myoclonus, and asterixis; seizures are quite rare. Vascular engorgement in the retina and papilledema occur in approximately 10% of patients (45). As with other metabolic encephalopathies, brainstem reflexes, including pupillary function and eye movements, are normal.

The pathogenesis of pulmonary encephalopathy appears related to CSF (but not systemic blood) acidosis (49). Increased intracranial pressure in patients with papilledema may also be a factor in the encephalopathy of pulmonary failure.

Myoclonus, seizures, and coma have been induced by rapid correction of $PaCO_2$ in patients with chronic pulmonary failure. The pathophysiology of these events is probably explained by the resultant cerebral alkalosis producing vasoconstriction and a leftward shift of the oxyhemoglobin dissociation curve (50).

Hypothermia

Common causes of hypothermia, especially in infants, include sepsis, exposure, hypoglycemia, and, in older children, drug overdose, hepatic encephalopathy, hyperthyroidism, and renal failure. Rare causes include diencephalic epilepsy and Shapiro syndrome associated with agenesis of the corpus callosum. Acute alcohol intoxication and Wernicke encephalopathy are common causes in adults, but rare in childhood. Although the associated illnesses inducing hypothermia may alter consciousness, a fall in body temperature may produce coma and even result in a mistaken diagnosis of death. The degree of neurologic abnormality attributable to hypothermia alone in a given patient is not entirely predictable, but may be inferred from reported studies of accidental hypothermia and refrigeration of normal subjects (51,52). With hypothermia alone, mentation is usually preserved until a temperature of 93°F (34°C) occurs; subsequently, a progressive cognitive decline occurs. Pupillary light reaction becomes sluggish at approximately 90°F (30°C), and pupils become unreactive below 80°F (26.5°C). Reflex (decorticate or decerebrate) posturing is exceedingly uncommon in coma due to hypothermia when uncomplicated by other metabolic disorders. Similarly, abnormalities of ocular movements and extensor plantar responses are unlikely to be directly related to hypothermia. Recovery from coma secondary to hypothermia is determined by the underlying disease state as neurologic abnormalities are completely reversible. Transient choreoathetosis may be seen days or several weeks after profound hypothermia induced during cardiopulmonary bypass surgery in children.

Hyperthermia

Hyperthermia results from fever, overexertion in high environmental temperatures (heat stroke), and as a result of untoward reaction to dopamine antagonists; viz., neuroleptic malignant syndrome (53), or malignant hyperthermia seen especially in children with congenital myopathies.

Encephalopathy of hyperthermia may be insidious or relatively sudden in onset and occurs with temperatures of 42°C to 43°C or higher (107.6°F to 109.5°F)(54). Reflex eye movements and pupillary reactivity are unaltered; convulsions may occur. Permanent residual abnormalities following hyperthermia are common and include particularly cerebellar ataxia as well as dementia and hemiparesis. Hyperthermic injury to the brain appears to occur because cerebral oxygen consumption declines at temperatures above 42°C (55).

Disorders of Osmolality

Altered consciousness is found in patients with serum osmolality less than approximately 260 mOsm/kg or greater than 330 to 350 mOsm/kg. Serum osmolality (mOsm of solute/kg) can be readily calculated (56): 2 [Na] + glucose/18 + BUN/2.8. Because cell membranes do not partition urea, BUN level does not contribute to the effect of osmolality in the brain (57).

Hypo-osmolality

Clinically, disorders of hypo-osmolality are those of decreased serum sodium or increased free water. Hyponatremia from diarrhea and dehydration is the most common cause of hypo-osmolality in children; additional causes include dialysis dysequilibrium, correction of diabetic ketoacidosis, congestive heart failure, renal failure, and inappropriate antidiuretic hormone secretion. Serum sodium values must be below 120 mEq/L to alter consciousness, and most symptomatic patients have levels below 110 mEg/L. The rate of fall of serum sodium, however, is the most important factor (58).

Clinical features in hypo-osmolar states include altered mentation, increased intracranial pressure, and seizures (59). Brain stem function (the pupillary light reflex and eye movements) is normal. Experimentally, intracellular edema is produced by hyponatremia, but the precise mechanism of altered consciousness remains uncertain. Brain swelling occurs clinically, but does not correlate with the severity of the encephalopathy. Experimentally, the rate of fall of serum sodium correlates with the degree of increased brain water (58).

Although there is a lack of clarity surrounding this issue, experimental and clinical data strongly support the risk of precipitation of central pontine myelinolysis following rapid correction of hyponatremia (60). Although it is uncertain exactly the rate at which serum sodium can be safely elevated, and the ability to accurately control the rise in serum sodium is imprecise, the goal should be an elevation in serum sodium no more than 12 mmol/L over the first 24 hours with an even more gradual elevation subsequently. If the patient is convulsing continually, the risks of rapid saline administration versus prolonged seizures must be weighed. If hypertonic saline is used, small volumes (100 mL bottles) will prevent accidental infusion of large quantities of sodium.

Hyperosmolality

Elevation in plasma osmolality is the result of hypernatremia or hyperglycemia. Hypernatremia is caused by hypertonic dehydration, homemade formulas especially in the setting of diarrhea, excessive diuresis, severe burns, or hypothalamic dysfunction with resultant diabetes insipidus. Hyperosmolality resulting from hyperglycemia occurs in the setting of diabetic nonketotic hyperosmolality and diabetic ketoacidosis.

Clinically, hyperosmolality produces the features of dehydration (e.g., loss of skin turgor, hypotension). Neurologic findings include altered mentation, tremor, myoclonus, and rarely focal deficits occur. Brain stem function (pupillary reactivity and eye movements) is normal. Seizures may occur in patients with hypernatremia during the rehydration phase (61). In patients with hyperglycemic hyperosmolality, focal seizures, with or without alteration of consciousness, who do not respond to anticonvulsant drugs are extremely common (62).

The pathophysiology of cerebral dysfunction from hyperosmolar states remains uncertain. Dehydration produces cellular shrinkage, which results in mechanical abnormalities by tearing small blood vessels. Intradural, subarachnoid, and intracellular hemorrhages may occur. Dehydration may also result in venous sinus thrombosis, especially in infants. Coma in patients with diabetic ketoacidosis may occur during the correction phase. Experimentally, the rapid decrease in blood glucose concentration produces increased intracranial pressure, which is seen in rapid correction of ketoacidosis.

Drug-Induced Coma

Sedative drug intoxication is a common cause of coma in childhood; tricyclics and benzodiazepines are next in frequency. The syndrome of evolution of these drug-induced comas is distinct. Initially, intoxication and a delirious state occur; this is followed by obtundation and coma. By the time obtundation is present, inducible lateral eye movements (doll's eyes) become paralyzed in the setting of maintained pupillary reaction. This combination of preserved pupillary light reflexes associated with paralyzed eye movements is characteristic of drug-induced coma. Occasionally, early transient decorticate decerebrate posturing may occur, but the pupillary and eye movement signs noted strongly support drug intoxication as the cause (63). Hypothermia is a common feature of sedative drug-induced coma. A similar clinical picture is seen with phenothiazine-induced coma as well as with coma from narcotics, the latter characteristically producing very miotic pupils and providing an easy diagnosis. These small pupils, however, may be mimicked by organophosphate poisoning, which also may result in coma.

Lithium intoxication is characterized by myoclonus, tremor, and seizures. Cocaine, phencyclidine hydrochloride, and methamphetamine usually produce aggressive paranoid states with hallucinations rather than coma.

Overdosage of iron supplements may produce coma in children because of resultant hypotension or a postulated direct effect of iron on the brain. The CNS effects appear 12 to 48 hours following ingestion (64). A late effect of lead ingestion, occurring most often in children younger than 5 years of age, is increased intracranial pressure, which may induce obtundation and coma (65). Gasoline sniffing (tetraethyl lead poisoning) induces tremor and cerebellar signs rather than coma.

Salicyclate poisoning may result in disorientation, convulsions, and coma. Associated findings include hyperventilation, sweating, dehydration, and fever. Metabolic acidosis is present (66).

Meningeal Inflammation

Bacterial and viral meningitis and meningeal irritation from subarachnoid hemorrhage most often produce a syndrome of metabolic encephalopathy; that is, impaired consciousness with preserved pupillary reactivity and eye movements. Such metabolic (or more clearly stated, diffuse) dysfunction in the setting of signs of meningeal irritation (neck stiffness, Brudzinski sign of reflex knee flexion with neck flexion) documents that the "metabolic" encephalopathy is the result of a meningeal process. Meningeal signs may not be present before the 2nd year of life.

NEUROLOGIC EXAMINATION AND DIFFERENTIAL DIAGNOSIS

The neurologic examination of the comatose patient is confined to the brain stem; viz., the thalamus, midbrain, pons, and medulla (See Figure 30.1)(7). Thus, attention is directed to the evaluation of the pupils (a midbrain function), eye movements (mainly pontine function), the motor response to a painful stimulus (diffusely represented within the brain stem), and some attention to ventilatory and cardiac function (medullary function).

Pupils

Unreactive pupils result from midbrain compromise. Lesions affecting both sympathetic and parasympathetic systems characteristically produce midposition (5 mm) unreactive pupils. In children, however, pupils are larger than those of adults. Accordingly, unreactive pupils in children may be larger than the midposition pupils in adults. Oval pupils and pupils displaced from the center of the iris may be seen with structural midbrain abnormalities (67). Seizures may transiently produce anisocoria with the pupil ipsilateral or contralateral to the hemispheric seizure focus dilating and reacting sluggishly to light. This abnormality is seen during the fit and persists for some minutes or even hours following the epileptic event (68,69).

Metabolic versus structural dysfunction as the cause for coma requires special attention to pupillary reactivity. Pupillary sparing is the hallmark of a metabolic encephalopathy. With rare exceptions such as glutethimide intoxication or severe anoxia/ischemia, metabolic causes of coma spare pupillary reactivity while impairing low brainstem functions of reflex motor movements and ventilation. Experimentally, pure anoxia as opposed to ischemia does not produce pupillary dilation; the pupils remain either unchanged in size or constricted (70). With pure experimental ischemia, pupillary constriction is initially seen, evolving to dilatation with cardiac outputs of less than 70% of normal. Following death, the pupils return to midposition (71).

Tiny pupils (1 mm) occur with intrapontine structural abnormalities (pontine infarction or hemorrhage) and are often associated with ocular bobbing. These entities are rare in children. Tiny reactive pupils are also seen with narcotic overdose and poisoning with cholinesterase inhibitors, which are usually found in insecticides. Small, unreactive pupils (2 to 3 mm) can also occur with hypothermia (51). With the exceptions noted, bilateral symmetric reactive pupils are seen in patients with metabolic coma until the very late stage.

Eye Movements

Evaluation of eye movements in coma is especially useful as the neuroanatomy responsible for oculomotor function in the brain stem traverses the reticular formation responsible for consciousness (from midpons, the pontine gaze center, and sixth nerve nucleus responsible for lateral gaze, up the medial longitudinal fasciculus to the midbrain and third nerve responsible for medial rectus function).

In patients with coma, conjugate roving eye movements (consisting of slow, random, usually horizontal movements), seen with or without eyelid closure occur with diffuse CNS dysfunction; for example, anoxic encephalopathy or persistent vegetative state of any cause. These slow eye movements of constant velocity cannot be mimicked voluntarily, and their presence, therefore, excludes volitional unresponsiveness. Occasionally, the eye movements stop, and a patient with persistent vegetative state will seem to be "looking at" an examiner or a person in the room. Cessation of roving gaze is therefore open to misinterpretation.

Horizontal gaze deviation occurs with large hemispheric lesions, in which the eyes are directed to the side of the lesion. In brain stem lesions, the eyes are directed away from the lesion and toward the hemiparesis. During seizures of focal cortical onset, the eyes are driven away from the side of the lesion.

The integrity of the brain stem, and by extrapolation the reticular formation, can be evaluated by inducing lateral eye movements on examination. The doll's eyes maneuver (rocking the head slowly back and forth) induces movements within the semicircular canals that drive the eyes from side to side. A stronger stimulus is that of infusing a quantity of ice water (25 to 50 mL) against the tympanic membrane of one ear. This induces an inhibitory input from the vestibular system and will cause the eyes to move toward the direction of the ice water in a patient whose brain stem is intact.

Induction of full conjugate lateral gaze attests to the integrity of the brain stem reticular formation and therefore excludes a structural reticular abnormality as the cause of coma. Inducible ocular abduction without adduction suggests lesions within the brain stem involving the medial longitudinal fasciculus. With ice water oculovestibular testing, this response can also be seen in barbiturate-induced coma (72).

Vertical gaze deviation can be seen with lesions of the posterior diencephalon or midbrain like pinealomas or craniopharyngiomas. In patients with coma, impairment of inducible upward gaze during flexion-extension movements of the head (vertical doll's eyes) are also seen with lesions in the same area.

In patients with reactive pupils and a symmetric examination, a differentiation can be made between exogenous and endogenous metabolic causes of coma by evaluation of eye movements. Exogenous causes of coma (drugs) paralyze eye movements early while preserving pupillary reflexes. Coma caused by endogenous toxins (organ-system failure) preserve both pupillary light reflex and inducible eye movements until late in their course.

Motor Signs

It is essential to assess motor function in comatose patients, and induction of a painful stimulus is required to produce a motor-system response. Failure to induce a painful stimulus markedly reduces the data available from the neurologic evaluation. Although the precise anatomic level correlating with the various motor responses is imprecise, three degrees of motor dysfunction will be seen sequentially as abnormalities proceed in a rostral to caudal manner (Figure 30.1)(7). The highest level of response is the localization of the painful stimulus (the patient reaches in the direction of the area of induced pain). In the presence of lesions that have progressed to approximately the level of the thalamus, decorticate posture (reflex flexion in the upper extremities and extension in the lower extremities) is found. With lesions approximately at the midbrain level or below, decerebrate posturing is seen (reflex extension of both arms or legs). At the pontine level and below, flaccidity is the rule.

The presence of the induced motor response to pain is noted, as well as the symmetry or asymmetry of the motor movements. Posturing is routinely seen in coma produced by expanding hemispheric mass lesions. Because these lesions begin in one hemisphere and progress in a rostral-caudal fashion, the induced posturing from a hemispheric mass will be asymmetric; for example, purposive on one side of the body and decorticate on the other, or decorticate on one side and decerebrate on the other. The motor abnormality will be maximal in the limbs contralateral to the hemisphere of origin for the mass lesion.

In patients with metabolic disorders, posturing is less common, but can be seen especially in those with hepatic failure. In this case, however, the posturing is symmetric. Symmetric posturing may also occur in patients with hypoglycemia, uremia, and, occasionally, transiently in the early stages of sedative hypnotic drug overdose (63,73,74). Anoxia/ischemia is the most common metabolic cause of posturing, and the persistence of such posturing into the 2nd day makes a functional outcome highly unlikely in adults (20). In young children, no large studies regarding this point exist, but experience suggests a more favorable outcome.

Myoclonus, either spontaneous multifocal myoclonus or massive myoclonic jerks that are induced by stimulation, is seen in patients with coma, usually of metabolic cause. Multifocal myoclonus is seen particularly in patients with renal failure, especially if also receiving penicillin, barbiturate withdrawal, and CO_2 narcosis. Massive generalized myoclonus may be spontaneous or stimulus induced and is most common following anoxia/ischemia.

Ventilation

Abnormal ventilatory patterns commonly occur in coma of both structural and metabolic cause. Of the typical ventilatory patterns in patients with coma (Cheyne-Stokes, neurogenic hyperventilation, apneustic ventilation, and ataxic ventilation), only the last is correlated with the location of structural CNS dysfunction. This ventilatory pattern is found most often with medullary abnormalities (75).

In patients with metabolic encephalopathies, certain characteristic patterns are seen. Hepatic encephalopathy is most often associated with respiratory alkalosis. This acid-base pattern can also be seen early in sepsis and occurs in psychogenic hyperventilation as well. Respiratory acidosis occurs most often in sedative drug overdoses. Metabolic acidosis is found in salicylate intoxication, hyperosmolar coma, diabetic ketoacidosis, uremic encephalopathy, lactic acidosis, and late in sepsis. Metabolic alkalosis is rare in coma.

BRAIN DEATH*

The criteria for brain death in adults (76) and children (77) both require documentation of irreversibility and cessation of brain function. The most important requirement in this regard is that the diagnosis is known and is adequate to explain brain death. Reversible metabolic disorders, sedative hypnotic drugs, paralytic agents, hypothermia (less than 32.3°C), and hypotension must be excluded. The examination of the brain must document a lack of function at each anatomic level:

1. Cerebral hemispheres: unresponsiveness
2. Midbrain: pupillary unreactivity to a bright light
3. Pons: lack of inducible eye movements by ice water caloric stimulation. Absent corneal reflex.
4. Medulla: absence of bulbar muscle function or reflexes

*See Chapter 31

most easily tested by an absence of reflex swallowing on tugging on the endotracheal tube. Apnea (vide infra).
5. No motor response to pain (purely spinal reflex responses may be permitted).

Apnea is confirmed by the lack of a spontaneous ventilatory effort in the face of a maximum CO_2 drive to ventilation (CO_2 greater than 60 mm Hg). This testing is safely accomplished by disconnecting the patient from the ventilatory equipment and delivering high flow oxygen (6 L/min) through a catheter passed down the endotracheal tube. This apneic oxygenation will assure an adequate pO_2 while the pCO_2 is permitted to rise. In apnea, pCO_2 rises approximately 3 mm Hg per minute; the required duration of the apnea test can therefore be estimated from the beginning pCO_2 (Table 30.3).

An EEG is recommended for patients younger than 1 year of age (78), but for older children and adults, this is not required (76,79). To confirm brain death, the EEG must document an absence of cerebral electrical activity above background artifact. The study is optimally performed with widely spaced (10 cm) electrodes (not always possible in the very young); it must be performed with maximum amplifier gain and must include a recorded response (or lack of same) to stimulation (pain).

Ancillary tests are useful and may decrease the required duration of observation or confirm brain death when the history and diagnosis are uncertain. Most useful are cerebral angiography or cerebral radionuclide angiography. Documentation of the absence of cerebral circulation during these studies confirms brain death. The value of the latter study in patients younger than 2 months of age remains uncertain as does digital subtraction angiography, xenon computed tomography, and ultrasound or Doppler techniques to estimate cerebral blood flow or velocity. The usefulness of evoked responses in this setting is controversial as well.

Table 30.3 Brain death*

Age	Number of Examinations	Interval	EEG
7 d–2 mths	2	48 hr	+, +
2 mths–1 yr	2	48 hr	+, or radionuclide angiography
> 1 yr	1	12–24 hr	−

*Recommendations according to age groups for number of examinations required, the interval between these examinations, and the neccessity of an EEG at each examination, or an alternate confirmatory study.

REFERENCES

1. Feinberg, WM, Ferry PC. A fate worse than death: The persistent vegetative state in childhood. Am J Dis Child 1984; 138:128–130.

2. Kotagal S, Rolfe U, Schwarz KB, et al. "Locked-in" state following Reye's syndrome. Ann Neurol 1984; 15: 599–601.

3. Chapman LF, Wolff HJ. The cerebral hemispheres and the highest integrative functions of man. Arch Neurol 1959; 1:357–424.

4. Serafetinides EA, Hoare RD, Driver MV. Intracarotid sodium amylobarbitone and cerebral dominance for speech and consciousness. Brain 1965; 88:107–130.

5. Albert ML, Silverberg R, Reches A, et al. Cerebral dominance for consciousness. Arch Neurol 1976; 33:453–454.

6. Ethelberg S, Jensen VA. Obscurations and further time related paroxysmal disorders in intracranial tumors: Syndrome of initial herniation of parts of brain through tentorial incisure. Arch Neurol Psych 1952; 68:130–149.

7. Simon RP. Stupor and coma. In: Mills J, Ho MT, Salber PR, et al., eds. Current Emergency Diagnosis and Treatment. Los Altos: Lange Medical Publications, 1983, 73–88.

8. McNealy DE, Plum F. Brainstem dysfunction with supratentorial mass lesions. Arch Neurol 1962; 7:10–32.

9. Ropper AH. Lateral displacement of the brain and level of consciousness in patients with an acute hemispheric mass. N Engl J Med 1986; 314:953–958.

10. Feldman E, Gandy SE, Becker R, et al. Magnetic resonance imaging demonstrates descending transtentorial herniation. Neurology 1988; 38:697–701.

11. Bickerstaff ER. Improvement of consciousness in migraine. Lancet 1961; 2:1057–1059.

12. Brierley JB, Graham DI. Hypoxia and vascular disorders of the central nervous system. In: Adams JH, Corsellis JAN, Duchen LW, eds. Greenfield's Neuropathology; 4th ed. New York: John Wiley, 1984, 125–207.

13. Levy DE, Bates D, Caronna JJ, et al. Prognosis in nontraumatic coma. Ann Intern Med 1981;94:293–301.

14. Weinberger LM, Gibbon MH, Gibbon JH Jr. Temporary arrest of the circulation to the central nervous system, II. Pathologic effects. Arch Neurol Psychiatry 1940; 43:961–986.

15. Greenamyre T, Penney JB, Young AB, et al. Evidence for transient perinatal glutamatergic innervation of globus pallidus. J Neurosci 1987;7:1022–1103.

16. Meldrum BS, Evans MC, Swan JH, et al. Protection against hypoxic/ ischaemic brain damage with excitatory amino acid antagonists. Med Biol 1987; 65:153–157.

17. Gisvold SE, Safar P, Hendrick HHL, et al. Thiopental treatment after global ischaemia in pigtailed monkeys. Anesthesiology 1984; 60:88–96.

18. Brain resuscitation clinical trial I study group. Randomized clinical study of thiopental loading in comatose survivors of cardiac arrest. N Engl J Med 1986; 314:397–403.

19. Engel GL. Fainting, 2nd ed. Springfield, Illinois: Charles C Thomas, 1962.

20. Levy DE, Caronna JJ, Singer BH, et al. Predicting outcome from hypoxic-ischemic coma. JAMA 1985;253:1420–1426.

21. Pampiglione G, Chaloner J, Harden A, et al. Transitory ischemia/anoxia in young children and the prediction of quality of survival. Ann NY Acad Sci 1978; 315:281–292.

22. Kruus S, Bergstrom L, Suutarinen T, et al. The prognosis of near-drowned children. Acta Pediatr Scand 1979; 68:315–322.

23. Peterson B. Morbidity of childhood near-drowning. Pediatrics 1977; 59:364–370.

24. Pearn J. The management of near drowning. Br Med J 1985; 291:1447–1452.

25. Pearn J. Neurological and psychometric studies in children surviving freshwater immersion accidents. Lancet 1977; 1:7–9.

26. Fandel I, Bancalari E. Near-drowning in children: Clinical aspects. Pediatrics 1976; 58:573–579.

27. Himwich HE. Hypoglycemia and brain metabolism. Assoc Res Nerv Ment Dis 1953; 32:345–371.

28. Malouf R, Brust JCM. Hypoglycemia: Causes, neurological manifestations, and outcome. Ann Neurol 1985; 17:421–430.

29. MacCuish AC, Munro JF, Duncan LJP. Treatment of hypoglycemic coma with glucagon, intravenous dextrose and mannitol infusion in 100 diabetics. Lancet 1970; 2:946–949.

30. Richardson JC, Chambers RA, Heywood PM. Encephalopathies of anoxia and hypoglycmia. Arch Neurol 1959; 1:178–190.

31. Adams RD, Lyon G. Neurology of hereditary metabolic diseases of children. New York: McGraw-Hill, 1982.

32. Edwards RH. Hyperammonemic encephalopathy related to uretero sigmoidostomy. Arch Neurol 1984; 41:1211–1212.

33. Raskin NH, Price JB, Fishman RA. Portal-systemic encephalopathy due to congenital intrahepatic shunts. N Engl J Med 1964; 270:225–229.

34. Rogers MF, Schonberger LB, Hurwitz ES, et al. National Reye syndrome surveillance, 1982. Pediatrics 1985; 75:260–264.

35. Rumack BH. Acetaminophen overdose in young children. Am J Dis Child 1984; 138:428–433.

36. Rai G, Buxton-Thomas M, Scanlon M. Ocular bobbing in hepatic encephalopathy. Br J Clin Pract 1976; 30:202–205.

37. Adams RD, Foley JM. The neurological disorder associated with liver disease. Res Publ Assoc Res Nerv Ment Dis 1953; 32:198–237.

38. Posner JB, Plum F. Toxic effects of carbon dioxide and acetazolamide in hepatic encephalopathy. J Clin Invest 1980; 39:1246–1258.

39. Hourani BT, Hamlin EM, Reynolds TB. Cerebrospinal fluid glutamine as a measure of hepatic encephalopathy. Arch Intern Med 1971;127:1033–1035.

40. Anastacio M, Hoyumpa DDV Jr, Avant G, et al. Hepatic encephalopathy. Gastroenterology 1978; 76:184–195.

41. Canalese J, Gimson A, Davis C, et al. Controlled clinical trial of dexamethasone and mannitol for cerebral oedema of fulminant hepatic failure. Gut 1982; 23:625–629.

42. Groflin UB, Tholen H: Cerebral edema in the rat with galactosamine-induced severe hepatitis. Experientia 1978; 34:1501–1503.

43. Fossieck B, Parker RH. Neurotoxicity during intravenous infusion of penicillin: A review. J Clin Pharmacol 1974; 14:504–512.

44. Sackellares JC, Smith DB. Myoclonus with electrocerebral silence in a patient receiving penicillin. Arch Neurol 1979; 36:857–858.

45. Plum F, Posner JB. The Diagnosis of Stupor and Coma; 3rd ed. Philadelphia: FA Davis, 1980.

46. Merrill JP, Legrain M, Hoigne R. Observations on the role of urea in uremia. Am J Med 1953; 14:519–520.

47. Hicks JM, Young DS, Wooton DP. The effect of uremic blood constituents on certain cerebral enzymes. Clin Chim Acta 1964; 9:228–235.

48. Arieff AI, Guisado R, Massry SG, et al. Central nervous system pH in uremia and the effects of hemodialysis. J Clin Invest 1976; 58:306–311.

49. Posner JB, Plum F. Spinal-fluid pH and neurologic symptoms in systemic acidosis. N Engl J Med 1967; 277: 605–613.

50. Rotherman EB, Safar P, Robin ED. CNS disorder during mechanical ventilation in chronic pulmonary disease. JAMA 1964; 189:993–996.

51. Fishbeck K, Simon RP. Neurologic manifestations of accidental hypothermia. Ann Neurol 1981; 10:384–387.

52. Fay T, Smith GW. Observations on reflex responses during prolonged periods of human refrigeration. Arch Neurol Psychiatry 1941; 45:215–222.

53. Mueller PS, Vester JW, Fermaglich J. Neuroleptic malignant syndrome. Successful treatment with bromocriptine. JAMA 1983; 249:386–388.

54. Ebaugh FG, Barnacle CH, Ewalt JR. Delirious episodes associated with artificial fever: A study of 200 cases. Am J Psych 1936; 43:191–215.

55. Nemoto EM, Frankel HM. Cerebral oxygenation and metabolism during progressive hyperthermia. Am J Physiol 1970; 219:1784–1788.

56. Gennari FJ: Serum osmolality, uses and limitations. N Engl J Med 1984; 310:102–105.

57. Feig PU, McCurdy DK. The hypertonic state. N Engl J Med 1977; 297:1444–1454.

58. Arieff AI, Llach F, Massry SG: Neurological manifestations and morbidity of hyponatremia: Correlation with brain water and electrolytes. Medicine 1976; 55:121–129.

59. Fishman RA. Neurological manifestations of hyponatremia. In: Vinken PJ, Bruyn GW, Klawans HL, eds. Handbook of Clinical Neurology; Vol. 28. Amsterdam: North-Holland, 1976, 495–505.

60. Laureno R, Karp BI. Pontine and extrapontine myelinolysis following rapid corrections of hyponatraemia. Lancet 1988; 1:1439–1441.

61. Morris-Jones PH, Houston IB, Evans RC. Prognosis of the neurological complications of acute hypernatremia. Lancet 1967; 2:1385–1389.

62. Singh BM, Strobos RJ. Epilepsia partialis continua associated with nonketotic hyperglycemia: Clinical and biochemical profile of 21 patients. Ann Neurol 1980; 8:155–160.

63. Greenberg DA, Simon RP. Flexor and extensor postures in sedative drug-induced coma. Neurology 1982; 32:448–451.

64. Lacouture PG, Wason S, Temple AR, et al. Emergency assessment of severity in iron overdose by clinical and laboratory methods. J Pediatr 1981: 99:89–91.

65. Chisholm J, Barltrop D. Recognition and management of children with increased lead absorption. Arch Dis Child 1979; 54:249–262.

66. Hill JB. Salicylate intoxication. N Engl J Med 1973; 288: 1110–1113.

67. Fisher CM. Ocular bobbing. Arch Neurol 1964;11:543–546.

68. Pant SS, Benton JW, Dodge PR. Unilateral pupillary dilation during and immediately following seizures. Neurology 1966; 16:837–840.

69. Zee DS, Griffin J, Price DL. Unilateral pupillary dilation during advesive seizures. Arch Neurol 1974; 30:403–405.

70. Jordanov J, Ruben H: Reliability of pupillary changes as a clinical sign of hypoxia. Lancet 1967; 2:915–917.

71. Binnion PF, McFarland RJ. The relationship between cardiac massage and pupil size in cardiac arrest in dogs. Cardiovasc Res 1967; 3:915–917.

72. Simon RP. Forced downward ocular deviation: Occurrence during oculovestibular testing in sedative drug-induced coma. Arch Neurol 1978; 35:450–458.

73. Conomy JP, Swash M. Reversible decorticate and decerebrate postures in hepatic coma. N Engl J Med 1968; 278: 876–879.

74. Himwich HE. Brain Metabolism and Cerebral Disorders. Baltimore: Williams and Wilkins, 1951.

75. North JB, Jennett S. Abnormal breathing patterns associated with acute brain damage. Arch Neurol 1974; 31:338–344.

76. Barber J, Becker D, Behrman R, et al. Guidelines for the determination of death: Report of the medical consultants on the diagnosis of death to the President's Commission for the Study of Ethical Problems in Medicine and Biomedical and Behavioral Research. JAMA 1981; 246:2184–2186.

77. Guidelines for the determination of brain death in children: Task force for the determination of brain death in children. Neurology 1987; 37:1077–1078.

78. Alvarez LA, Moshé SL, Belman AL, et al. EEG and brain death determination in children. Neurology 1988; 38: 227–230 .

79. Pallis C. The arguments about the EEG. Br Med J 1983; 286:284–287.

Chapter 31
Brain Death in Infants and Children

Stephen Ashwal and Sanford Schneider

The determination and management of brain death in children has evolved independently in many medical centers without universal acceptance of the validity of specific criteria. All physicians agree that maintaining life support systems after the unequivocal documentation of brain death is futile and inhuman; yet justified controversy and dialogue persists. The problem of brain death in children is examined from multiple perspectives including: historic, epidemiologic, findings on neurologic examination, application and validity of neurodiagnostic testing, assessment of the newborn, current recommendations for brain death determination, parental concerns, and organ donation.

In 1959 Mollaret and Goulon (1) introduced the term "coma depasse" (a state beyond coma) to describe an absolute loss of sensory, motor, conscious, and vegetative functions of the brain. Subsequently in 1986 an Ad Hoc Committee of the Harvard Medical School Faculty proposed various criteria defining brain death to include coma, apnea, lack of spontaneous movements or movement to stimuli over one hour, and absence of elicitable reflexes. Reflex activity includes pupillary, ocular movement following caloric irrigation, blinking response, corneal reflex, pharyngeal reflex, swallowing, yawning, and vocalization (2). A prerequisite of brain death under these conditions was the exclusion of hypothermia and the presence of central nervous system (CNS) depressants. These criteria had to persist for 24 hours. Two isoelectric electroencephalograms (EEGs) performed 24 hours apart were proposed as being of confirmative value, but they were not thought to be essential in the declaration of brain death (3). In 1971, brain death criteria proposals emphasized the importance of both etiology of brain injury and the documentation of persistent apnea in the diagnosis of brain death (4). Nine years later, the National Institute of Neurologic and Communicative Disorders and Stroke (NINCDS) Collaborative Study of Brain Death reported on the evaluation of 503 patients with profound coma and apnea (5). The major findings of this study included a review of neurologic, neuropathologic, and electroencephalographic findings. It was found that the loss of pupillary light reflex, vestibular reflex to caloric tympanic stimulation, and oculocephalic and corneal reflexes were highly predictive of death.

The combined findings of coma, apnea, absence of cephalic reflexes, and electrocerebral silence were usually associated with the pathologic features characteristic of the respirator brain. There were postmortem specimens in the study, however, that lacked typical features of the pathology of a respirator brain despite electrocerebral silence. Other neuropathologic examinations of brains, however, were typical of a respirator brain although continuous biologic activity had been recorded by the EEG.

The EEG was considered important in determining brain death and its use was recommended. Although an isoelectric EEG did not always anticipate total brain destruction, it did always predict a fatal outcome except for 2 patients with drug intoxication (5,6). The study also emphasized that if cerebral activity was recorded by EEG an individual could not be considered brain dead. Moreover, it was found that 28% of all patients had detectable barbiturate or nonbarbiturate sedatives that could suppress EEG activity and that 30% of these patients were not initially suspected of drug intoxication. An additional 30% of patients received other CNS depressant drugs for therapeutic reasons. The report concluded that a drug screen and EEG were mandatory prior to the pronouncement of brain death.

Cerebral radioisotopic blood flow techniques were shown to have similar reliability to 4 vessel angiography in determining the absence of cerebral blood flow (CBF) and correlated well with clinical and EEG findings of brain death (7).

The Conference of Medical Royal Colleges and their faculties in the United Kingdom (1976) emphasized that "permanent functional death of the brain stem contitutes brain death" and that this should be diagnosed only in a defined context of irreversible structural brain damage and

Table 31.1 President's Commission guidelines for the determination of brain death

An individual presenting the findings in either section A (cardiopulmonary) or section B (neurological) is dead. In either section, a diagnosis of death requires that both *cessation of functions*, as set forth in subsection 1, and *irreversibility* as set forth in subsection 2 be demonstrated.

(A) An individual with irreversible cessation of circulatory and respiratory functions is dead.
   (1) Cessation is recognized by an appropriate examination.
   (2) Irreversibility is recognized by persistent cessation of functions during an appropriate period of observation or trial of therapy or both.

(B) An individual with irreversible cessation of all functions of the entire brain, including the brain stem, is dead.
   (1) Cessation is recognized when evaluation discloses findings of (a) and (b).
      (a) Cerebral functions are absent.
      (b) Brain stem functions are absent.
   (2) Irreversibility is recognized when evaluation discloses findings of (a), (b), and (c).
      (a) The cause of coma is established and is sufficient to account for the loss of brain functions.
      (b) The possibility of recovery of any brain function is excluded.
      (c) The cessation of all brain functions persists for an appropriate period of observation or trial of therapy or both.

Other Factors:
- Complicating conditions, such as drug and metabolic intoxication and hypothermia (core temperature below 32.2°C) should be excluded.
- The presence of shock should alert the physician to be particularly cautious in applying neurologic criteria to determine death.
- Children: The brains of infants and young children have increased resistance to damage and may recover substantial functions even after exhibiting unresponsiveness on neurologic examination for longer periods compared with adults.
- Physicians should be particularly cautious in applying neurologic criteria to determine brain death in children younger than 5 years (10).

Table 31.2 Guidelines for the determination of brain death in children*

A. History   determine the cause of coma to eliminate remediable or reversible conditions

B. Physical examination criteria
   1. Coma and apnea
   2. Absence of brain stem function
      (a) Midposition or fully dilated pupils
      (b) Absence of spontaneous oculocephalic (doll's eye) and caloric-induced eye movements
      (c) Absence of movement of bulbar musculature, corneal, gag, cough, sucking and rooting reflexes
      (d) Absence of respiratory effort with standardized testing for apnea
   3. Patient must not be hypothermic or hypotensive
   4. Flaccid tone and absence of spontaneous or induced movements excluding activity mediated at spinal cord level
   5. Examination should remain consistent for brain death throughout the predetermined period of observation

C. Observation period according to age

(1) 7 days to 2 months	Two examination and EEGs 48 hours apart
(2) 2 months to 1 year	Two examination and EGGs 24 hours apart or one examination and an initial EEG showing ECS combined with a radionuclide angiogram showing no CBF, or both
(3) more than 1 year	Two examinations 12 to 24 hours apart; EEG and isotope angiography are optional

*Reprinted with permission from Journal of Pediatrics 1987; 110:15−19.[13]

after certain specified conditions were excluded (8). They emphasized that loss of brain stem function could be assessed clinically, and that the EEG was not necessary for the diagnosis of brain death. In 1979, a second memorandum identified brain stem death as the sine qua non of death (9).

In 1982 guidelines for the determination of death were published in the United States (Table 31.1). This Commission's report recognized that adult criteria might not be applicable to children because of developmental factors, a possible greater tolerance to asphyxia as noted in animal models, and the clinical recognition that infants and children occasionally demonstrated surprisingly significant recovery despite prolonged coma (10,11). The age of 5 years and above was selected as suitable for applying adult criteria, although this age selection reflected no known specific phenomena reported in younger children.

In 1987 guidelines for the determination of brain death in children were published by an ad hoc task force committee, comprised of representatives from the American Academy of Neurology, American Academy of Pediatrics, American Bar Association, American Neurological Association, Child Neurolgy Society, and the NINCDS (Table 31.2). These guidelines emphasized the importance of the history and clinical examination, specifically investigating the etiology of coma to ensure that any remedial or reversible conditions were eliminated (12). Age-related observation periods, including specific neurodiagnostic testing, were recommended for children under 1 year of age. In children over the age of 1 year, laboratory testing was not always considered to be a requisite of diagnosis, although repeated clinical examinations over 12 or more hours were recommended. Excluded from these guidelines were criteria for preterm infants and term infants less than 7 days of age. These 2 groups were excluded because of lack of sufficient data to develop accurate guidelines. Alternative criteria have also been prepared by an ad hoc committee from the Boston Children's Hospital and in our earlier reports (13,14), all of which have received specific commentary (15–17).

EPIDEMIOLOGY OF BRAIN DEATH IN CHILDREN

Incidence of Brain Death

The incidence of brain death in children is unknown. Of 503 patients in the NINCDS Collaborative Study on Brain Death, 8.6% of patients were less than 10 years and 11.6% were between 10 and 19 years of age (18). In a recent study of 26,640 pediatric patients hospitalized over a 5-year period, the diagnosis of brain death was established in 58 patients out of a total of 761 deaths, suggesting an incidence of 7.6% (19). From previous studies of pediatric brain death, an estimation of age incidence can be ascertained (Table 31.3). Of these patients, eight (5%) were premature. Brain death was most commonly diagnosed in infants under 1 year of age. After 5 years of age, the incidence of brain death decreased. The relatively low incidence in the 10 to 18 year age group was surprising, considering the frequency of suicide, trauma, and vehicular accidents in this population.

The primary admission diagnoses in children with brain death were retrospectively calculated from available data in 253 patients (Table 31.4). The results were quite different from that observed in the NINCDS collaborative study (18). Closed head trauma, typically associated with motor

Table 31.3   Age distribution in children with brain death

	#	(%) of Patients
Premature	8	(5%)
Term Infants	10	(4%)
0 to 4 mo	22	(10%)
4 to 12 mo	30	(14%)
1 to 2 yr	37	(17%)
2 to 5 yr	71	(32%)
5 to 10 yr	17	(8%)
10 to 18 yr	22	(10%)
	219	(100%)

Data from references 20 to 39.

Table 31.4   Admission diagnosis in children with suspected brain death

	#	(%) of Patients
Closed head trauma	64	(25%)
Near-drowning	30	(12%)
Infection—meningitis(11), encephalitis(5), abscess(2), unknown(11)	29	(11%)
Asphyxia	20	(8%)
Near miss SIDS	15	(6%)
Nonaccidental trauma	13	(5%)
Metabolic diseases—Reye syndrome(8), acute encephalopathy(2), hepatic failure(2), adrenogenital syndrome(1), urea cycle defect(1)	14	(5%)
Cerebrovascular disease	10	(4%)
Aspiration	5	(2%)
Strangulation/suffocation	5	(2%)
Hydrocephalus	5	(2%)
Smoke inhalation	5	(2%)
Cardiac arrest—epiglottitis, status epilepticus, cardiac disease, unknown	4	(2%)
Intra/Post operative	2	(1%)
Miscellaneous—asthma, dehydration, (1 each) malignant hyperthermia, neuroblastoma, myelodysplasia, hemolytic uremic syndrome, prosthetic valve emboli, air embolus, exsanguination, status epilepticus, tumor	11	(5%)
Newborn—asphyxia(11), meningitis(2), aspiration(1)	14	(5%)
Premature—intraventricular hemorrhage(3), asphyxia(2), meningitis(2)	7 7	(3%) (3%)
Total	253	(100%)

*Data from references 20 to 39.

vehicle accidents, was the most common clinical problem leading to brain death (25%), followed by near drowning (12%), and asphyxia (8%). The majority of children with the diagnosis of asphyxia, however, usually were suffering from septic shock, post cardiorespiratory arrest of undetermined etiology, sudden infant death syndrome (SIDS), or acute encephalopathy with herniation. Nonaccidental trauma due to child abuse, occurred in 5% of deaths. In these patients, even after confirmation of brain death, discontinuation of ventilator support or organ donation is frequently prolonged because of potential medicolegal or procedural problems. Brain death occurring in patients with CNS infection, such as meningitis, was usually associated with an acute severe fulminating disease with brain death occurring within the first 2 to 3 days of hospitalization. Similarly, infants with near miss (SIDS) (6%) suffered an acute anoxic encephalopathy and developed malignant cerebral edema with herniation within 2 to 3 days of admission. Neonatal asphyxia was also related to both intrauterine and perinatal factors and was more common in the term than preterm infant. Congenital malformations, aside from hydrocephalus, were not typically associated with brain death.

Prognosis of Pediatric Brain Death

Temporal events of 223 brain dead children have been reviewed (Table 31.5). Forty-five percent of patients were declared dead following an estimated interval of 1.7 days from the time of brain death diagnosis, and in the majority of these patients, life support systems were discontinued. The interval between the diagnosis of brain death and removal of life support systems ranged from 14 to 144 hours with an average of 45 hours (14). In contrast, those children who were brain dead on ventilator support had prolonged survival until cardiac arrest occurred (average 17.3 days). Some children were maintained with ventilator support for periods as prolonged as 6 months with serial computed tomography (CT) scans demonstrating liquefaction necrosis of the cerebrum (32). One of the 223 patients with suspected, but not confirmed, brain death recovered, and 2 other patients survived with severe neurologic residua. These figures contrast with those of the NINCDS collaborative study, in which 69% of 503 patients died from cardiac reasons, 23% were brain dead, and 5% recovered completely, primarily because 23 of these 26 patients were found to have drug intoxication. In contrast to children, adults with brain death usually died within 2 days after the diagnosis was established and no patients survived beyond 4 weeks.

There have been no reports of children surviving who met adult brain death criteria on neurologic examination (11). These criteria include an absence of spontaneous activity, specific cranial nerve dysfunction, cardiac response to ocular compression, decerebrate or decorticate posturing and apnea. Fifteen comatose children, from 3 months to 6 years of age, who fulfilled these criteria for 3 days ultimately died (31). A 3-day time period was selected in this study because a previous report of a 35-week preterm infant with brain stem failure for 3 days survived with mild developmental delay (31). This infant, however,did not satisfy all criteria for brain death and had only mild EEG abnormalities (34).

Table 31.5 Outcome of pediatric patients with brain death

Outcome	# of Patients	Estimated Interval from Brain Death Diagnosis (Days)
Cardiac death	110	17.3
Brain death	101	1.7
Death but mechanism uncertain	9	——
Incomplete recovery	2	——
Complete recovery	1	——

This does not include 2 patients who survived for 70 and 201 days before spontaneous cardiac arrest (Drake et al. 1986, Rowland et al. 1983). Data compiled from references 20 to 39.

NEUROLOGIC EXAMINATION IN PEDIATRIC BRAIN DEATH

Initial Presentation

Limited information is available concerning the neurologic examination of children with suspected brain death. In one recent series of 61 children with suspected brain death, 85% of patients arrived at the emergency room in cardiopulmonary arrest and required prolonged resuscitation (20). Of these 61 patients 91% were apneic; the remaining patients rapidly deteriorated and required assisted ventilation. Seventy-five percent of patients had absent pupillary reflexes; minimal responses to deep pain were observed initially in 48%, and the remaining patients had no response to deep pain. Deep tendon reflexes were initially absent in 71% of these children. Hypothermia was observed in 51% with a rectal temperature less than 35.5°C. A modified Glasgow coma scale, (normal: 15, minimal: 3), of these children 24 hours after arrival was 3.5 (Table 31.6). All patients ultimately developed fixed dilated pupils and, at the time of apnea testing and confirmation of brain death, had no elicitable brain stem reflexes.

Brain Stem Examination

Early neurodevelopmental factors should be considered in assessing the validity of cranial nerve testing in infants with suspected brain death (40). The pupillary light reflex is uniformly absent before 29 to 30 weeks of gestation, developing by 32 weeks gestational age. In addition, the pupils are quite miotic. Similarly, the oculocephalic response may not

Table 31.6 Modified Glasgow Coma Scale*

Observation	Score
Eye Opening	
Spontaneous	4
To noise	3
To pain	2
None	1
Motor response	
Obeys commands	6
Localizes pain	5
Withdraws	4
Abnormal flexion	3
Extension response	2
None	1
Verbal response	
Oriented	5
Confused conversation	4
Inappropriate words	3
Incomprehensible sounds	2
None	1

*Lowest score, 3; best score, 15; (from Lockman LA. Impairment of Consciousness. In: Swaiman KF, ed. Pediatric Neurology: Principles and Practice. St. Louis: C. V. Mosby, 1989;157–167.)

be elicitable prior to 32 weeks gestation and is frequently difficult to elicit since many infants delivered at 28 to 32 weeks gestation are intubated. Caloric stimulation, used to evaluate auriculo-ocular function, is also difficult to perform in infants because of the small external auditory canal, immaturity of vestibular function and, in some infants, possible ototoxicity secondary to hyperbilirubinemia, sepsis, meningitis, or prolonged administration of ototoxic antibiotics. Assessment of cranial nerves IX to XII is frequently limited by intubation or maintenance neuromuscular blockers.

Moreover, it is also not clear whether failure of all brain stem reflexes is necessary to diagnose brainstem death. The President's Commission did not recommend testing of cranial nerve responses, stressing the documentation of apnea. In the NINCDS collaborative study, 141 of 459 unresponsive patients who died had one or more preserved brain stem reflexes and no single brain stem reflex was discriminative enough to identify all persons with some preserved reflexes (18). The combination of pupillary light, oculocephalic, and vestibular reflexes had the greatest discriminative power, but still failed to identify 4% of comatose and apneic patients who had other active brain stem reflexes. Although this phenomena has not been studied in infants and children, it is our impression that nearly all children who are apneic have lost all cranial nerve function.

Cerebral Unresponsivity

The clinical definition of unresponsivity is a poorly characterized component of the neurologic examination of children. Standardization by using a modified Glasgow coma scale (See Table 31.6) may be helpful (20,41). In one series of 61 children with suspected brain death, a modified Glasgow coma scale score at 24 hours was 3.5 and did not improve over the subsequent 48 to 72 hours (20). The predictive value of unresponsivity in infants and young children may be less than in adults. It is well-recognized by physicians caring for young children that recovery occasionally occurs under circumstances where unresponsiveness has been present for prolonged periods, and even when serious structural nervous system dysfunction is present. Thus, if the neurologic assessment is uncertain or inconsistent in young infants and children under 1 year of age, supportive laboratory documentation, including EEG and CBF determinations should be considered.

Determination of Apnea

Sustained absence of spontaneous respiration is the single most important criterion for determining brain death. Testing for apnea by temporary disconnection of respiratory support must: allow adequate time for pCO_2 to increase to respiratory stimulation levels, provide adequate

ozygenation, and generate no adverse cardiovascular responses (25).

Several protocols have been recommended for apnea testing in adults (28). The Harvard Medical School Ad Hoc Committee (1968) suggested a 3-minute test period of withholding ventilatory support with the patient on room air. The Conference of Royal Colleges and Faculties of the United Kingdom (1976) recommended administering a mixture of 5% carbon dioxide and oxygen for 5 minutes, followed by disconnecting the ventilator while delivering cannula oxygen into the trachea. A pCO_2 exceeding 50 mm Hg was considered an adequate stimulatory drive for respiration. The President's Commission for the Study of Ethical Problems in Medicine (1982), suggested ventilation with oxygen for 10 minutes followed by ventilator withdrawal and passive oxygen flow for an additional 10 minutes achieving a pCO_2 of at least 60 mm Hg.

The apneic threshold (minimum pCO_2 at which respiration begins) depends on many factors. Although the threshold in healthy adults is less than 40 mm Hg, anesthetic agents, narcotics, sedatives, and certain disease states, as well as changes in altitude above sea level, may alter the carbon dioxide tension at which respiratory effort begins. Schafer and Caronna (42) described 3 patients suspected of brain death who resumed spontaneous breathing at pCO_2 levels of 45 to 56 mm Hg and suggested that apnea could only be diagnosed when a pCO_2 above 60 mm Hg failed to stimulate breathing. In contrast, Ropper et al. (43) found a pCO_2 of 39 mm Hg capable of respiratory stimulation in patients thought to be brain dead and concluded from their study of 7 adult patients that 44 mm Hg is a satisfactory end point for apnea testing.

In infants and children, the apneic threshold has yet to be determined (25). Two recent studies on apnea testing in brain dead children have been reported. Outwater and Rockoff (28) administered 100% oxygen for 5 minutes to 10 patients, ages 10 months to 15 years, before discontinuing ventilation but continued oxygen flow via the endotracheal tube for 5 minutes. Mean pCO_2 (39.4 mm Hg) increased to 59.5 mm Hg due to a pCO_2 increase of 8.3 mm Hg during the 1st minute and 4.0 mm Hg per minute over the entire test period; pO_2 remained over 200 mm Hg in all patients and heart rate remained stable. Rowland et al. (25) performed 16 apnea tests on 9 patients, ages 4 months to 13 years, 4 of whom had detectable phenobarbital levels between 10 and 25 mg/dL. These patients received 100% oxygen for 10 minutes; after discontinuing the ventilator, oxygen was delivered at 6 L/min through a catheter into the length of the endotracheal tube during the 15-minute study period. These patients were moderately hyperventilated before the apnea test with a mean pCO_2 of 28 mm Hg; pCO_2 increased 4.4, 3.4, and 2.6 mm Hg per minute at 5, 10, and 15 minutes. Arterial pCO_2 at the end of 15 minutes ranged from 40 to 116 mm Hg, and by 15 minutes, 14 of 16 patients had pCO_2 levels greater than 60 mm Hg. Two patients had pCO_2 levels of 110 and 116 mm Hg with pH determinations of 6.92 and 6.98. Arterial pO_2 remained above 100 mm Hg and in 12 of 16 patients it was above 200 mm Hg. Mild alterations of pulse or blood pressure or both were also observed in 6 patients but were not serious and were reversible. Both studies recommended using a pCO_2 threshold of 60 mm Hg with preoxygenation periods of 5 to 10 minutes, as well as apnea test periods of either 5 or 10 minutes. Because there appears to be significant variability among patients in reference to utilization of oxygen and other factors controlling carbon dioxide production and diffusion, individual increases in CO_2 tension (mm Hg/min) are quite variable. Thus, duration of apnea testing initially should be 10 minutes before reinstituting artificial ventilation and if the pCO_2 level is less than 60 mm Hg, a repeat study should be performed over 15 minutes. The results of apnea testing of patients who are hypothermic or receiving medications that suppress respiration, are not valid for documenting apnea. They can, however, still be performed under such circumstances because the presence of respiratory effort, (that is, a negative test) would eliminate brain death as a diagnosis.

NEURODIAGNOSTIC STUDIES IN PEDIATRIC BRAIN DEATH

Electroencephalography

Electrocerebral silence (ECS), defined as "no electrocerebral activity over 2 microvolts (µv)", has been utilized in the United States for confirmation of brain death (18). Guidelines formulated by the American EEG Society include: a minimum of 8 scalp and ear reference electrodes; electrode resistances under 10,000 but over 100 ohms; test for integrity of the recording system by deliberately creating electrode artifact; interelectrode distances of at least 10 cm; gain increased during most of the recording from 7 µv to 2 µv/mm; use of 0.3 or 0.4 sec time constants during part of the recording; recording of electrocardiogram (ECG) and extracerebral potentials by electrodes on the dorsum of the right hand; tests for reactivity to pain, loud noise, and light; a 30 minute total recording time; recording by a qualified technician; repeating the recording if ECS result is doubtful; and telephone transmitted EEGs are not appropriate for determination of ECS (44).

Technical Problems in Pediatric EEGs

Technical problems encountered in performing EEGs, as well as the nature and types of artifacts found, have been reviewed and summarized extensively (18,45,46). In infants and children, other unique aspects of EEG recording must also be considered including: shorter interelectrode distances; external artifacts in newborn and pediatric intensive care units; rapid cardiac and respiratory rates of infants and children compared to adults; shorter distances between heart and brain making ECG contribution disproportionately larger in children; reduced amplitude of cortical potentials in premature and newborn infants; uncertain effects of hypothermia or CNS depressant drugs on EEG activity; longer duration of effect of CNS depressant drugs in infants and children; greater tendency for suppression burst patterns in infants with neurologic disorders; lack of availability of personnel to perform and neurologists capable of interpreting pediatric EEGs; and congenital CNS malformations, such as hydranencephaly, that can be associated with ECS.

Reversible Electrocerebral Silence

Reversible ECS has been documented in a variety of circumstances including CNS depressant drugs, hypothermia, cardiovascular shock, and metabolic encephalopathy.

In children, drugs capable of producing ECS include barbiturates, diazepam, clonazepam, and phenytoin. Various intravenous (IV) anesthetic agents (thiopental, ketamine, midazolam) and IV narcotics (morphine sulphate, meperidine, fentanyl), as well as several inhalation anesthetics (halothane and isoflurane) may also suppress cortical activity. The most common drug responsible for reversible ECS is phenobarbital, as it is widely used for seizure control and in cerebral resuscitation protocols. Although the therapeutic range for phenobarbital is 20 to 40 µg/mL, the minimum level that would not induce ECS has not been established in infants and children. Based on our clinical experience, phenobarbital levels above 25 to 35 µg/mL may suppresss the EEG (47).

Previous studies in adults have suggested that ECS will not occur until the temperature falls below 20°C, and a core temperature greater than 32.2°C (90°F) has been regarded as prerequisite for reliably determining brain death with the aid of the EEG (48). In children, suppression of EEG activity does not appear until 24°C (64.4°F), and complete loss of EEG activity does not occur until the temperature is below 18°C (64.4°F) (49). In the NINCDS collaborative study, only 12 of 503 patients were hypothermic and most of the patients could be warmed to temperatures acceptable for EEG recording. From our experience, the average temperature at the time of EEG recording for brain death confirmation has been 97.3 ± 1.4°F, suggesting that hypothermia is unlikely to be a significant problem for pediatric EEG recordings in most hospital settings.

Postcardiorespiratory arrest ECS may be reversed when cerebral perfusion improves. In longitudinal studies (50) of post resuscitation neurologic function in 37 adult patients who regained consciousness and 88 patients who remained unconscious, it was observed that ECS activity reappeared at first intermittently and then continuously within 10 minutes to 8 hours after restoration of circulation. We have observed in at least 3 young infants, a similar interval of 8 to 10 hours post cardiac arrest in which initial ECS changed to a diffuse low voltage background with survival of the infants in a persistent vegetative state.

Disturbances in serum electrolytes, acid-base balance, blood gases, and severe hepatic and renal dysfunction, as well as certain inborn errors of metabolism, have all been thought to contribute to the development of ECS. The exact role of these metabolic and endocrine disorders has not been well established in children. Thus, in the young infant in whom the etiology of brain death is uncertain, evaluation for metabolic diseases, including urea cycle enzyme defects, disorders of lactic, amino and organic acid metabolism should be considered.

Value of the EEG in Determination of Brain Death

In the absence of hypothermia, depressant drugs, and toxic–metabolic factors, an EEG obtained shortly after the clinical determination of brain death is predictive of brain death. In the NINCDS collaborative study, only 2 of 87 individuals with ECS survived; both had exogenous drug intoxication. Additional illuminative data from the collaborative study showed that 41% of patients had ECS on their initial EEG; in 22% ECS occurred within the next several days, and if ECS first occurred within 4 days after the initial neurologic insult, the patient rarely survived over 24 hours (18).

Retrospective data compiled from several pediatric studies and totaling 165 patients showed that the initial EEG was isoelectric in 60% to 100% of children, averaging 82% of the total (Table 31.7). Except for 3 previous case reports, children whose initial EEG demonstrated ECS also had ECS upon repeat study (36,50). In 1 patient, return of EEG activity was believed to be inconclusive by the authors and probably represented muscle artifact. In 2 other infants, a 6-week-old with seizures and apnea and a term infant with asphyxia, repeat EEGs 24 hours after the initial finding of ECS showed definite return of activity. At the time of the repeat EEG studies, however, neither infant was clinically brain dead. Both had some respiratory effort, pupillary activity, and spontaneous movement. We believe

there are no other authenticated reports of infants or children who had return of EEG activity or who achieved clinical recovery after the initial EEG was isoelectric. The unlikelihood of ECS reversibility has also been observed in adults and according to Chatrian (45), close scrutiny of those cases with reversible ECS has never actually shown a fully acceptable example of recovery. Thus, the available data in children indicates that one EEG with electrocerebral silence should be sufficient laboratory confirmation of brain death providing the above caveats are observed (39).

In infants and children with suspected brain death whose initial EEGs demonstrated activity, it is probable that a subsequent EEG will become isoelectric. In one recent study, 14 of 47 children with clinically suspected brain death initially maintained electrocortical activity; repeated EEGs were performed in 9 of these patients with 6 showing ECS at 48 and 72 hours (20). The remaining 3 patients had cardiorespiratory deaths. Similar findings have been noted by other investigators (30). Therefore, if the neurologic examination remains unchanged, an infant or child who is clinically brain dead but has some initial EEG activity will probably progress to ECS or the patient will deteriorate and die from cardiorespiratory failure. If the child survives, the neurologic prognosis is usually that of a persistent vegetative state.

Various established brain death criteria recommendations have not included mandatory demonstration of ECS. In the NINCDS collaborative study, 8% to 40% of patients meeting different criteria for brain death showed EEG activity (18). In 1969, 1 year after the Harvard criteria were established, the Harvard committee was "unanimous in its belief that an electroencephalogram was not essential to a diagnosis of irreversible coma, but that it would provide valuable supporting data" (3). Pallis (51), in his review of brain death, suggested that "the main argument about the EEG is conceptual, not technical." Thus, advocates for ECS documentation seek to diagnose the biologic death of the whole brain. In contrast, those who claim that EEG is unnecessary seek to diagnose brain death as a functional unit that is death of the brain as a whole associated principally with brain stem death. This was emphasized by Pallis

Table 31.7 Initial and follow-up EEG in children with brain death

Author	# of Pts*	EEG #1 % of Pts with ECS	EEG #2 in Pts with ECS on EEG #1	EEG #2 in Pts with Activity on EEG #1
Alvarez et al. (1988)	52	100%	100% ECS	———
Thompson et al. (1987)	6	100%	100% ECS	———
Drake et al. (1986)	47	70%	70% ECS	77% ECS 23% Activity
Coker et al. (1986)	11	100%	100% ECS	———
Furgiuele et al. (1984)	10	91%	———	1 pt's EEG in 6 mo.: low voltage
Holzman et al. (1983)	18	61%	100% ECS	1/7:ECS
McMenamin & Volpe (1983)	3	100%	———	———
Ashwal & Schneider (1979)	5	0%	———	100% activity
Ashwal et al. (1977)	11	82%	100% ECS	1 pt:ECS
Green & Lauber (1972)	2	100%	0% ECS	———
Total	165			

*Pts = patients

in examination of the prognostic value of EEG in patients with or without brain stem function. In over 1,000 patients with apnea, coma, absent brain stem reflexes, and ECS, asystole developed within several days in all patients. In 147 similar patients who had EEG activity, the prognosis was identical. However, 26 patients who demonstrated brain stem function and ECS survived. Such findings again suggest limitations of the EEG. In 1979, we reported 5 patients, ages 28 weeks to 30 months, with apnea, coma, and absent CBF by angiography or radionuclide imaging who had persistent low voltage EEG activity (32). Neurologic examination remained unchanged, EEG activity persisted and all patients died 2 to 32 days after the initial clinical diagnosis of brain death. In more recent studies, we have found ECS in only 8 out of 17 preterm and term infants who were clinically brain dead (47). Thus, in children as well as adults, EEG may not correlate with the neurologic examination or CBF determinations, and in contrast to adults, survival in infants with absent brain stem function and some EEG activity may be prolonged. Chatrian, in his recent extensive review of the electrophysiologic evaluation of brain death, noted that the diagnosis of brain death can be determined "by good history and competent clinical examination and the EEG is of value in helping to expedite the clinical diagnosis, decreasing chances of error, and providing confirmatory objective proof in those cases in which such objective proof is thought to be desirable (45)." He also suggested that reliance on the clinical examination is better suited for those hospitals in which EEG, other laboratory facilities, or related professional and technical skills are either inadequate or lacking. As aptly stated by Pampiglione and coworkers (52), "no EEG investigation at all is better than unreliable and misleading services" in the assessment of brain death.

Brain Stem Auditory-Evoked Responses

The role of brain stem auditory-evoked responses (BAER) in the laboratory evaluation of comatose or suspected brain dead children is still controversial. Lutschg et al. (53) examined BAERs in 43 comatose children and found that absence of evoked responses indicated a poor outcome while prolonged latencies occurred in 1/3 of patients who recovered completely. In those children who were clinically brain dead, BAER revealed bilateral loss of all components or occasional persistence of wave I. In another study, 10 clinically brain dead children, ages 2 months to 17 years, demonstrated no waves or only wave I, which was in contrast to 13 comatose children who had a recordable BAER (23). However, the absence of BAER in a comatose, apneic infant is not predictive of brain death as recently reported in 2 infants, ages 12 and 37 weeks (24). Taylor et al. (54) also reported a 33-month-old child who lost all brain stem evoked potentials, did not fulfill clinical criteria of brain death, and recovered. In another recent study, 3 of 17

comatose children survived with either absent BAER or only the presence of waves I/III; 2 of the children had minimal neurologic abnormalities and 1 was in a vegetative state (55). These 3 patients, a 3-year-old near-drowning victim, a 10-day-old with propionic acidemia, and a 3-year-old involved in a motor vehicle accident probably were not brain dead clinically at the time of evaluation. These studies, however, suggest that BAER can indicate severe but potentially reversible brain stem dysfunction in children. BAER should not be used at present as confirmatory laboratory criteria of brain death. Currently, the somatosensory-evoked response has not been studied in children suspected of brain death, although evidence from adult studies suggests that this technique may be potentially of greater clinical use than BAER (56). Combining repetitive somatosensory responses with the EEG may increase the sensitivity of either test and allow clinical conclusions as the location or mechanisms of cerebral dysfunction (57).

Radionuclide Imaging

Demonstration of the complete absence of CBF in both children and adults is undeniable evidence of brain death (7,14,37,58). Cerebral angiography, radionuclide angiography, Doppler ultrasonography, CT with contrast injection, and xenon computed tomography (XeCTCBF) have all been useful in determining the state of CBF. Currently, radionuclide angiography is the preferred technique, as it has been shown to be sensitive and correlates well with angiography; it is practical in its technical application at the bedside in both children and adults (7,20,26,30,58,59).

At least 129 infants and children with brain death have been evaluated by radionuclide angiography, demonstrating absence of CBF; only 1 patient survived for several months (Table 31.8). In contrast, 6 of 27 patients with clinically suspected brain death but positive cerebral flow survived for short periods. Three of these patients died from cardiac arrest, 1 became brain dead, and the other 2 lived for several months with severe neurologic disablilities. Isotopic scanning is thus useful, particularly in patients in whom hypothermia and high serum barbiturate levels exist. In studies by Holzman et al. (30), 4 of 7 patients so treated who had isoelectric or suppressed EEGs but intact CBF recovered some neurologic function.

The absence of CBF in brain death is due primarily to low cerebral perfusion pressure and secondarily to release of vasoconstrictors from vascular smooth muscle and the brain parenchyma. In the majority of children we have studied, cerebral perfusion pressure has been below 20 to 30 mm Hg at the time of brain death and documentation of absent CBF. Four of 24 brain dead children with intracranial pressure monitoring, however, had persistently high cerebral perfusion pressures greater than 45 to 50 mm Hg at the time that no CBF was observed (14). Holzman et al. observed the same phenomena in 4 patients, ages 8 months

Table 31.8   Cerebral blood flow and velocity studies in children with brain death*

Author	CBF Method	# Patients No Flow	# Patients Recovered	# Patients + Flow	# Patients Recovered
Alvarez et al. (1988)	Scintigraphy	0	0	0	0
Thompson et al. (1987)	Scintigraphy	5	0	1	1
Drake et al. (1986)	Scintigraphy	27	0	15	0
Coker et al. (1986)	Scintigraphy	53	0	2	1
Schwartz et al. (1984)	Scintigraphy & angiography	9	0	—	—
Holzman et al. (1983)	Scintigraphy	10	0	8	4
Ashwal & Schneider (1979)	Scintigraphy & angiography	5	0	—	—
Ashwal et al. (1977)	Scintigraphy	10	0	1	1
Parvey & Gerald (1976)	Angiography	4	0	—	—
Ahman et al. (1987)	Doppler	28	0	4	—
McMenamin & Volpe (1983)	Doppler	6	0	—	—
Furgiuele et al. (1984)	Cranial Ultrasound	11	0	—	—
TOTAL		168	0	31	7

*Data from references 20–39

to 3 years (30). Such findings indicate that several mechanisms are involved in the loss of CBF during brain death, as only a moderate percentage are related to marked elevation of intracranial pressure.

Concern about validation of radionuclide imaging techniques in the newborn has been raised, especially in view of several recent reports of preterm and term infants with reduced CBF values who survived with relatively intact neurologic function. In one series of premature infants, Xenon[133] cerebral flow values averaged 12 mL/min/100 g in 24 of 42 infants; in another small study of preterm infants using positron emission tomography (PET), flow values ranged from 7 to 11 mL/min/100 g (60,61). None of these patients were clinically brain dead. In a study of eight brain dead adults, stable XeCTCBF measured 1.6 ± 2.0 mL/min/100 g (62). In another study of 9 clinically brain dead children, 1 month to 11 years of age, CBF determined by XeCTCBF was compared to radionuclide imaging techniques. All patients showed no flow by radionuclide imaging and had XeCTCBF values of 1.29 ± 1.6 mL/min/100 g (37). Although none of these patients were preterm infants, 3 were 1 month, 7 weeks, and 3 months of age. Both the adult and pediatric XeCTCBF investigations showed that CBF at the time of brain death was less than 2 mL/min/100 g and that this value correlated with the absence of flow by radionuclide imaging. Therefore, it is likely that radionuclide imaging, available in most hospitals, is valid in infants for estimating absent CBF.

Pediatric patients have also been reported who are clinically brain dead, yet have CBF (64). In the studies reported by Drake et al. (20), 15 of 47 children suspected of brain death had CBF as determined by radionuclide imaging. Of the 9 patients with both EEG activity and cerebral flow, 3 were unchanged at 48 and 72 hours; whereas, isoelectric EEG tracings and absent cerebral flow developed in the remaining 6 patients within 72 hours. In contrast, 4 of the 6 restudied patients who originally had CBF with ECS showed no CBF on a second study. The remaining 2 patients died of cardiorespiratory arrest; 1 on day 1 and the

other 43 days later. In more recent studies, 5 of 16 preterm and term infants who were clinically brain dead had CBF as measured by radionuclide imaging (47). Altman et al. (61) also reported 2 suspected brain dead newborn infants who had preserved CBF documented by PET scanning with ECS (63). In these infants, phenobarbital and diazepam had been administered with a phenobarbital level of 42 μg/mL in one patient. These patients were taken off respiratory support and neuropathologic examination was consistent with diffuse neuronal necrosis and the clinical diagnosis of brain death. Overall, these studies suggest that CBF may be detectable in infants and children and, to a much lesser extent, in adults who are clinically brain dead. In those patients who have ECS and CBF, a repeat CBF study is likely to document the loss of CBF within 24 hours.

Pulsed Doppler Ultrasound Cranial Ultrasonography

In the newborn and young infant, both Doppler and real time cranial ultrasonography have been used to determine the absence of CBF. McMenamin and Volpe (29) reported 6 brain dead infants, 28 to 40 weeks gestation, who had characteristic deterioration of Doppler wave forms in the anterior cerebral arteries including: loss of diastolic flow, appearance of retrograde flow during diastole, diminution of systolic flow in the anterior cerebral artery, and no detectable flow in the anterior cerebral artery, despite flow in the common carotid artery.

Intracranial pressures measured in 4 of 6 infants with the Ladd pressure monitor were elevated (17 to 21 mm Hg) and EEGs obtained in 3 infants showed ECS. All patients died spontaneously or had respiratory support discontinued. Although cerebral and isotopic angiography were not performed to verify Doppler results, postmortem examinations in all patients revealed severe cerebral damage consistent with but not necessarily typical of those reported in brain death.

In other studies with pulsed Doppler ultrasound, 19 of 23 brain dead children older than 4 months showed a characteristic velocity pattern with a single sharp systolic peak followed by a rapid negative deflection below baseline, sharply rebounding to forward flow in early to mid-diastole with gradual tapering at the end of diastole to the zero baseline or below (38). Eight of the 19 patients with this wave form also demonstrated absent CBF by radionuclide angiography. Infants under 4 months of age who were studied had atypical wave forms suggesting that use of the pulsed Doppler technique in the newborn period is not yet a reliable method.

Real time cranial ultrasonography, which demonstrated the absence of pulsatile movements of the anterior and middle cerebral arteries, was found to correlate with the absence of brain function and ECS in 11 infants, 38 weeks to 20 months of age (27). Cranial ultrasonography was believed to be most useful in the neonatal period because of alterations of the neurologic examination by hypothermia, medications, or neuromuscular paralytic agents used to facilitate mechanical ventilation. In this study, alternative techniques of flow determination were not performed to validate these findings. Thus, although of unique potential, both doppler and cranial ultrasonography need further validation to determine their usefulness and reliability in brain death determination.

Stable Xenon Computed Tomographic Cerebral Blood Flow

XeCTCBF is a noninvasive method capable of measuring local CBF (mL/min/100 g) in selected brain regions that has recently been utilized in evaluating brain death. In 8 adult patients with clinical brain death, XeCTCBF averaged 1.6 ± 2.0 mL/min/100 g (62). This technique has been applied to children with suspected brain death with our studies in 10 clinically brain dead patients showing an average XeCTCBF of 1.63 ± 1.6 mL/min/100 g (22,37). Recent animal studies have also suggested that CBF greater than 15 mL/min/100 g was adequate to preserve tissue viability; whereas, average flow values above 19 mL/min/100 g were adequate to maintain normal cerebral function (65). Thus, CBF values in infants and children older than 2 months below 10 mL/min/100 g are probably indicative of cerebral death. Because previous studies of preterm infants have shown low CBF (7 to 12 mL/min/100 g) with good recovery, however, the minimal CBF needed to confirm the clinical diagnosis of brain death in infants has yet to be determined (60,61). The minimal survival CBF may well vary with gestational age.

XeCTCBF has also been helpful in demonstrating that residual dural sinus activity is not due to extracranial collateral flow but very low flow through the intracranial circulation (22). Whereas residual dural sinus activity was believed initially to be inconsistent with a diagnosis of brain death, our recent studies have shown that CBF in patients with sinus flow is still below 2 mL/min/100 g (37).

BRAIN DEATH IN THE NEWBORN

Brain death is a rare phenomenon in the newborn period. Recent data indicate that there are approximately 40,000 infant deaths, compared to 3.76 million live births, per year in the United States (66). Our statistics at Loma Linda University Medical Center reflect that only 1% of all infant deaths required a diagnosis of brain death. Therefore, we roughly estimate a relatively rare total annual incidence in the US of 400 infants requiring a neurologic diagnosis of brain death.

Determination of brain death in preterm and term infants has been complicated by lack of data in this population, as well as the unique physiology of the cerebral circulation in the perinatal period (15). Determination of both the cessation and irreversibility of cerebral function are also more difficult to assess in the newborn because of the problems defining the extent and causes of coma. In infants, the primary event causing cerebral injury usually occurs in utero and data concerning the nature and severity of this insult is difficult to obtain and may not be reliable. Other factors, such as hypotension, medication effects, and other organ involvement, especially in the hypoxic/ischemic infant, can complicate the neurologic examination. In addition, various brain imaging techniques do not truly assess the potential reversibility of hypoxic ischemic insults in the newborn; and other diagnostic studies, including EEG or radionuclide imaging, may be difficult to interpret or lack sufficient accumulation of data to be valid. Other factors relating to the clinical examination should be considered. These include the immaturity of certain developmental reflexes used to assess cerebral and brain stem function, such as pupillary reactivity, vestibular function, ventilatory control, state of alertness or consciousness, and other brain stem reflexes. As stressed by Volpe, there have also been several atypical cases of survival in preterm and term infants thought initially to meet clinical criteria for brain death (15). Additional problems relate to EEG criteria and the observation that normal EEG patterns in the preterm and term infant are of such relatively low voltage and may be readily suppressed after asphyxia or when anticonvulsant medication is used. There is also the observation noted previously that premature and term infants may have relatively low CBF, yet survive reasonably neurologically intact.

Our recent studies of 17 newborn infants, 16 of whom had both EEG and CBF studies, are of interest in view of these problems (Table 31.9). In this series, 4 infants were preterm with gestational ages 29 to 36 weeks, 8 infants were term less than 7 days of age, and 5 infants were 1 to 4 weeks of age (47). In this series, ECS (9 of 17 patients) or absent CBF (12 of 17) provided laboratory confirmation

Table 31.9 EEG and CBF studies in 16 brain dead neonates

		EEG Activity	
		(+)	*(−)*
Cerebral			
Blood	(+)	1	4
Flow	(−)	7	5

(+), Present; (−) absent. (−) EEG = electrocerebral silence.

and in only 4 of 16 patients did both studies support the clinical diagnosis of brain death. It was also observed that ECS in the absence of barbiturates, hypothermia, or cerebral malformations was indicative of brain death if the examination remained unchanged over 24 hours. In addition, absence of CBF in conjunction with either initial ECS or persistence of clinical brain death for 24 hours was predictive of brain death. We also noted that in these infants, phenobarbital levels above 25 to 35 μg/mL appeared to suppress EEG activity.

Based on the clinical review of these 17 infants, we observed that term infants, remaining clinically brain dead for 2 days and preterm infants brain dead for 3 days, never recovered spontaneous respirations and could only survive on ventilator support. Thus, confirmation of brain death can nearly always be established in the newborn, solely on a clinical basis, and EEG and CBF studies are usually not necessary. Such studies, however, do have confirmatory value and can potentially shorten the time interval necessary to establish the diagnosis of brain death in the newborn. It is likely that the current Task Force Guidelines (12) can include the preterm and term infant, and that the diagnosis of brain death in the newborn can usually be determined by clinical assessment.

Current Guidelines for Brain Death Determination in Children

Guidelines for the determination of brain death in infants over 7 days of age and children were proposed in the 1987 report of the Ad Hoc Task Force Committee (Table 31.2). As emphasized in these criteria, the most important factor in assessing brain death is determination of the cause of coma to insure the absence of any remedial or reversible condition.

Clinical Evaluation

At the time of clinical evaluation, children must not be significantly hypothermic. In children, the core body or rectal temperature generally is 1° greater than the oral temperature. Normal core body temperatures range from 36.1°C (97°F) to 37.2°C (99°F). In addition, the patient should not be hypotensive or cardiovascularly unstable.

The critical portions of the clinical examination include the determination of apnea and absence of brain stem reflexes. Prior to apnea testing, the patient should receive 100% oxygen for at least 5 minutes and have a pCO₂ in the normal range (30 to 45 mm Hg). During apnea testing, the patient should receive 100% oxygen into the endotracheal tube and be disconnected from ventilator support for 10 minutes. A pCO₂ greater than 60 mm Hg without respiratory effort is sufficient proof of apnea. If the pCO₂ is not greater than 60 mm Hg after 10 minutes, the patient should then be disconnected from the ventilator for 15 minutes or until the pCO₂ is greater than 60 mm Hg.

Testing for the absence of brain stem reflexes should include the following: pupillary, no direct or consensual response to bright light; oculocephalic, no lateral or vertical eye movements in response to head turning; corneal response, no blink reflex to light touch; auriculo-ocular, no movement or blink response to loud noise; vestibulo-ocular, no eye movement response to cold water caloric-tympanic membrane stimulation; and gag reflex, no gag response to palatal, pharyngeal, or tracheal stimulation by endotracheal tube movement. Various spinal reflexes, such as deep tendon reflexes, withdrawal, and plantar responses that may indicate integrity of spinal cord function should not be misconstrued as brain stem activity.

Coma must also be assessed. The patient with brain death exhibits complete loss of consciousness, vocalization, volitional activity, and any purposeful response to externally applied stimuli including pain, light, and noise. Frequently, a modified Glasgow coma scale is useful in assessing the depth of coma in patients with suspected brain death (Table 31.6).

Blood and Urine Studies

These studies exclude toxic or metabolic disorders and should include arterial blood gases, serum electrolytes, calcium, blood glucose, blood urea nitrogen (BUN), creatinine, aspartyl serum transferase (AST), lactate dehydrogenase (LDH), serum ammonia, and lactate. In specific clinical situations, a urine metabolic or organic acid screen may be indicated. A urine toxicology screen also is recommended at any age.

Observation Periods According to Age

The Task Force Committee guidelines have suggested different observation periods and neurodiagnostic studies, depending on the age of the child. Based on our personal clinical experience, our guidelines are somewhat different in terms of time intervals and need for neurodiagnostic studies. Our current recommendations for the period of observation to confirm brain death include: preterm infants: 3 days; term infants to 2 months: 2 days; two months to 1 year: 24 hours; and over 1 year: 12 to 24 hours.

EEG and CBF Studies in Conjunction with Clinical Brain Death

An EEG is obtained using the recording procedures established by the American Association of Electroencephalographers (44). If the patient has received phenobarbital, the level must be less than 25 µg/mL for accurate interpretation of ECS (44). If the EEG is isoelectric in a child over 2 months of age, this finding is believed to be sufficient confirmatory criteria and a repeat study is not necessary (12). If the initial EEG in a younger child is isoelectric and a CBF study reveals no flow, then sufficient laboratory criteria are present to confirm irreversible brain death (12). If either the initial EEG shows ECS or if the CBF study shows no flow and the infant remains clinically brain dead for 24 hours, repeat studies are not necessary and the patient can be declared brain dead.

If the initial EEG demonstrated activity, CBF studies still should be obtained because infants may maintain minimal electrocortical activity without significant CBF and can be considered brain dead. If the CBF study shows no flow in an infant over 2 months of age, this is sufficient to confirm brain death. If the infant is less than 2 months old and the clinical exam is unchanged after 24 hours then brain death is established.

PARENTAL CONFLICTS, CONCERNS AND INTERACTIONS

Parents cannot acutely perceive that their child is near death. The vast majority of clinical situations are acute; namely, trauma, near drowning, and asphyxia. Parents are not preconditioned to deal with accepting the need to discontinue respirator support under these emotional circumstances, much less discuss potential organ donation. These emotional forces must be recognized and accepted by the treating physician. If the initial impression is grim, one should realistically discuss this without delay. The physician should use his or her accumulated knowledge and prior experience in rapidly educating parents to understand the clinical diagnosis, the pitfalls and dilemmas of treatment, and the anticipated outcome. The diagnosis must be established quickly. Understand that knowledge of the etiology and pathophysiology of the child's coma is far more useful than any specific laboratory test in discussions of prognosis with the parents. The physician must address every question raised by parents, relatives, and friends that seemingly conflict with prior discussions. Explain that return of deep tendon reflexes and withdrawal in the brain dead patient is mediated at the spinal cord level and is not due to improvement of cortical function. Include families to be part of the decision-making process, but never allow parents to feel totally responsible for the ultimate decision to discontinue respiratory support. Most parents do not want their child existing as a profoundly brain damaged,

comatose, respirator dependent child ultimately succumbing to infection or cardiac arrest. Parents should depend on physician guidance in this decision-making process. The physician should not coerce or be indecisive toward these grieving families, but should remain sympathetic and supportive. The physician's personal feelings, ethics, and religious beliefs should not be promulgated in discussions with parents grieving over the impending death of their, until recently, normal child. Since the act of discontinuing respirator support is so emotionally traumatic, the attending physician must be available and responsive to the needs and inevitable feelings of guilt experienced by the parents. During these discussions regarding the futility of continued support, the possibility of potential organ donation may be raised. If the child is not a potential donor (infection, prolonged ischemia), it is imperative to discuss why donation was not possible so parents do not later feel that organ donation was overlooked.

BRAIN DEATH AND TRANSPLANTATION

Transplantation of organs is not new, as renal transplantation has been successful for over 30 years. However, transplantation of hearts, lungs, and livers, particularly in infants, is recent and experience in donor collection is only now starting to accumulate. Consequently, unique situations arise for which there are no present solutions. Anencephalics, theoretically ideal donors, are controversial donors because of the difficulty in declaring the brain stem dead before irreversible hypoxia has occurred in body organs. Another example are infants with spinal muscular atrophy (Werdnig-Hoffmann syndrome) who cannot be declared brain dead while maintained on respirators, despite their inevitable death. It appears that donor organs will continue to be largely supplied by acute trauma victims under the circumstances previously described. Thus, the supply of neonatal donors will never be adequate for the number of potential recipients.

A recently completed study at Loma Linda University reviewed 50 brain dead children for suitability as cardiac donors (67). Prior to death, these patients were screened by echocardiograms and fractionated creatine kinase determinations. Thirty-three hearts were examined postmortem and 19 would have been suitable for transplantation. Interestingly, prolonged cardiac arrest did not generally preclude donor selection. Near drowning patients tended to have severe cardiac ischemia, while child abuse victims usually were excellent potential donors.

Brain death from child abuse is a unique circumstance since consent for organ donation may well come from the abuser(s). Also, release of donor tissue by the local coroner or medical examiner (and possibly their presence at donor surgery) must be obtained after declaring the child brain dead, while continuing to maintain cardiac function by mechanical ventilation. To salvage these organs, transplant surgeons, child neurologists, and pediatricians need to establish an advanced working relationship with their respective coroners to ensure donation. This arrangement is particularly important since child abuse, unfortunately, remains one of the common causes of brain death in young children.

Our experience is that parents are more willing to consider donation if discussion initiated early in the process of declaring a child brain dead. This dialogue should be initiated and continued by the responsible physician. An overly zealous approach should be avoided as this may solidify parental guilt and a common belief that their child's suffering will somehow continue if organs are removed after death. The National Organ Transplant Act of 1987 requires hospitals in the US to have an in-house mechanism for requesting donation of organs.

After a child considered suitable for organ donation is declared brain dead, the parents, previously briefed on the value of organ donation, should be asked to allow donation, providing a suitable need has been identified. An adamant refusal should be accepted without further coercing of grieving parents who have previously been adequately informed and educated in the need for pediatric donor organs. With the parents concurrence, arrangements should be made with a transplant team to remove the organ(s) or transfer the respirator dependent body to a transplant center. Donor parents should not be expected to be liable for any of the expenses of organ removal, transportation, or increased funeral costs.

Education needs to replace isolated individual media pleas for organs. Parents need to understand that, however remote the possibility, their children may need to be an organ donor, as well as a recipient.

Maintenance of the Brain Dead Child for Organ Donation

The loss of neuroendocrine and neurovascular function in the brain dead patient must be treated if successful organ donation is feasible. Diabetes insipidus secondary to insufficient antidiuretic hormone production and release has been observed recently in 14 of 16 brain dead children (68). Treatment with vasopressin has been recommended. Because vasopressin is a potent vasoconstrictor, low-dosage therapy is recommended (3 to 5 units intramuscularly and 0.05 to 0.1 units/kg IV) to avoid ischemic injury to potential organs (69). Physiologic dosages of corticosteroids should also be considered because of the deterioration of the pituitary–adrenal axis with impaired synthesis and release of adrenocorticotropic hormone (ACTH). Adequate ventilatory support to maintain organ function is also important. Hyperoxia (pO_2 greater than 150 mm Hg) can induce pulmonary edema in lung allografts; whereas, hypoxia (pO_2 less than 60 mm Hg) may cause tissue ischemia. Little is known about maintenance of ideal donor temperature prior to transplantation. In addition, treatment and prevention of infection probably will further minimize cardiovascular instability. There are also numerous social, ethical, religious, and legal concerns to consider after the diagnosis of brain death has been established. Thus, the time period in which a decision is made to discontinue ventilatory support or to donate an organ will vary. Respect for the physical being of the brain dead child, and providing appropriate grief counselling and support for the parents and their families are all of critical importance. Often overlooked is the emotional needs of the nursing, support, and physician staff who care and grieve for these children. Discuss your thoughts and the reasons for your actions so your fellow workers do not feel as if they are toiling in the dark without direction.

A final word on brain death. Brain death diagnosis in children is a new concept. Further evolution is to be anticipated, discussed, amended, and ultimately accepted. We hope the prudent reader will not accept this chapter as the final word but will selectively, but continuously, expand their knowledge of brain death in children.

REFERENCES

1. Mollaret P, Goulon M. Le coma depasse. Rev Neurol 1959; 101:3–15.
2. Beecher HK. A definition of irreversible coma. Report of the Ad Hoc Committee of Harvard Medical School to examine the definition of brain death. JAMA 1968;205:337–340.
3. Beecher HK. Definition of irreversible coma. N Engl J Med 1969;281:1070–1071.
4. Mohandas A, Chou SN. Brain Death: A clinical pathological study. J Neurosurg 1971;35:211–218.
5. The NINCDS Collaborative Study of Brain Death, Monograph No. 24, NIH Publ. No. 81–2286,1980.
6. Goldensohn ES. The relationship of the EEG to the clinical examination in determining brain death. Ann NY Acad Sci 1978;315:137–142.
7. Korein J, Braunstein P, George A, et al. Brain death. I. Angiographic correlation with a radioisotope bolus technique for evaluation of cerebral blood flow. Ann Neurol 1877;2: 195–205.
8. Conference of Medical Royal Colleges and their faculties in the UK: Diagnosis of death. Br Med J 1976;2:1187–1188.
9. Conference of Medical Royal Colleges and their Faculties in the UK: Diagnosis of death. Br Med J 1979;1:332.
10. Guidelines for the determination of death: Report of the medical consultants on the diagnosis of death to the President's Commission for the study of ethical problems in medicine and biomedical and behavioral research. Neurology 1982; 32:393–399.
11. Moshe SK, Alvarez LA. Diagnosis of brain death in children. J Clin Neurophysiol 1986;3:239–249.
12. Guidelines for the determination of death in children. Pediatrics 1987;80:298–300.
13. Ad Hoc Committee on Brain Death, The Children's Hospital, Boston: Determination of brain death. J Pediatr 1987; 110:15–19.
14. Ashwal S, Schneider S. Brain death in children: Part I and Part II. Pediatr Neurol 1988;2:5–10, 69–77.

15. Volpe JJ. Commentary—Brain death determination in the newborn. Pediatrics 1987;80:293–297.

16. Freeman JM, Perry PC. New brain death guidelines in children: Further confusion. Pediatrics 1988;81:301–303.

17. Shewmon DA. The probability of inevitability: The inherent impossibility of validating criteria for brain death or 'irreversibility' through clinical studies. Stat Med 1987;6: 535–553.

18. Walker AE. Cerebral Death, 3rd ed. Baltimore: Urban and Schwarzenberg, 1985:206.

19. Doroshow RW, Saukel GW, Ashwal S. Availability and selection of pediatric cardiac donors. American Heart Association 59th Scientific Session, 1986.

20. Drake B, Ashwal S, Schneider S. Determination of cerebral death in the pediatric intensive care unit. Pediatrics 1986;78: 107–112.

21. Coker SB, Dillehay GL. Radionuclide cerebral imaging for confirmation of brain death in children: The significance of dural sinus activity. Pediatr Neurol 1986;2:43–46.

22. Thompson JR, Ashwal S, Schneider S, et al. Comparison of cerebral blood flow measurements by Xenon computed tomography and dynamic brain scintigraphy in clinically brain dead children. 13th Symposium Neuroradiologicum. Acta Radiol Suppl (Stockh) 1987;369: 675–679.

23. Steinhart CM, Weiss IP. Use of brainstem auditory evoked potentials in pediatric brain death. Crit Care Med 1985;13: 560–562.

24. Dear PRF, Godfrey DJ. Neonatal auditory brainstem response cannot reliably diagnose brainstem death. Arch Dis Child 1985;60:17–19.

25. Rowland TW, Donnelly JH, Jackson AH. Apnea documentation for determination of brain death in children. Pediatrics 1984;74:505–508.

26. Schwartz JA, Baxter J, Brill DR. Diagnosis of brain death in children by radionuclide cerebral imaging. Pediatrics 1984; 73:14–18.

27. Furgiuele TL, Frank LM, Riegle C, et al. Prediction of cerebral death by cranial sector scan. Crit Care Med 1984;12:1–3.

28. Outwater KM, Rockoff MA. Apnea testing to confirm brain death in children. Crit Care Med 1984;12:357–358.

29. McMenamin JB, Volpe JJ. Doppler ultrasonography in the determination of neonatal brain death. Ann Neurol 1983; 14:302–307.

30. Holzman BH, Curless RG, Sfakianakis GN, et al. Radionuclide cerebral perfusion scintigraphy in determination of brain death in children. Neurology 1983;33:1027–1031.

31. Rowland RW, Donnelly JH, Jackson AH, et al. Brain death in the pediatric intensive care unit. Am J Dis Child 1983; 137:547–550.

32. Ashwal S, Schneider S. Failure of electroencephalography to diagnose brain death in comatose patients. Ann Neurol 1979; 6:512–517.

33. Ashwal S, Smith AJK, Torres F, et al. Radionuclide bolus angiography: A technique for verification of brain death in infants and children. J Pediatr 1977;91:722–728.

34. Pasternak JF, Volpe JJ. Full recovery from prolonged brainstem failure following intraventricular hemorrhage. J Pediatr 1979;95:1046–1049.

35. Parvey LS, Gerald B. Arteriographic diagnosis of brain death in children. Pediatr Radiol 1976;4:78–82.

36. Green JR, Lauber A. Recovery of activity in young children after ECS. J Neurol Neurosurg Psychiatry 1972;35: 103–107.

37. Ashwal S, Schneider S, Thompson J. Xenon computed tomography measuring cerebral blood flow in the determination of brain death in children. Ann Neurol 1989;25:539–546.

38. Ahman PA, Carrigan TA, Carlton D, et al. Brain death in children: Characteristic common carotid arterial velocity patterns measured with pulsed doppler ultrasound. J Pediatr 1987; 110:723–728.

39. Alvarez LA, Moshe SL, Belman AL, et al. EEG and brain death determination in children. Neurology 1988;38: 227–230.

40. Sher PK. Neurological examination of the premature infant. In: Swaiman KF, Wright FS, eds. The Practice of Pediatric Neurology. St. Louis: C.V. Mosby, 1982:22–23.

41. Lockman LA. Impairment of Consciousness. In: Swaiman KF, ed. Pediatric Neurology Principles and Practice. St. Louis: C.V. Mosby, 1989:157–167.

42. Schafer JA, Caronna JJ. Duration of apnea needed to confirm brain death. Neurology 1978;28:661–666.

43. Ropper AH, Kennedy SK, Russell L. Apnea testing in the diagnosis of brain death. J Neurosurg 1981;55:942–946.

44. American Electroencephalographic Society, Guidelines in EEG 1–7 (revised 1985). J Clin Neurophysiol 1986;3: 131–168.

45. Chatrian GE. Electrophysiologic evaluation of brain death: A critical appraisal. In: Aminoff MJ, ed. Electrodiagnosis in Clinical Neurology. New York: Churchill-Livingstone, 1986: 669–736.

46. Bennett DR, Hughes JR, Korein J, et al. Atlas of electroencephalography in coma and cerebral death. New York: Raven Press, 1976:244.

47. Ashwal S, Schneider S. Brain death in the newborn: Clinical, EEG and blood flow determinations. Pediatrics 1989;84 429–437.

48. Hicks RC, Poole JL. Electroencephalographic changes with hypothermia and cardiopulmonary bypass in children. J Thorac Cardiovasc Surg 1981;81:781–786.

49. Jorgensen EO, Malchow-Moller A. Cerebral prognostic signs during cardiopulmonary resuscitation. Resuscitation 1978; 6:217.

50. DeOliveira WM, DeOliveira MLJ, Pereira IE, et al. Reavaliacao dos criterios clinicos e electroencefalograficos de determinacao da morte cerebral na crianca. Arq Neuropsiquiatr 1984;42:25–31.

51. Pallis C. ABC of brainstem death: The arguments about the EEG. Br Med J 1983;286:284–287.

52. Pampiglione G, Chaloner J, Harden A, et al. Transitory ischemia/anoxia in young children and the prediction of quality of survival. Ann NY Acad Sci 1978;315:281.

53. Lutschg J, Pfenninger J, Lundin HP, et al. Brainstem auditory evoked potentials and early somatosensory evoked potentials in neuro-intensively treated comatose children. Am J Dis Child 1983;137:421–426.

54. Taylor MJ, Houston BD, Lowry NJ. Recovery of auditory brainstem responses after a severe hypoxic ischemic insult. N Engl J Med 1983;309:1169–1170.

55. De Merlier JL, Taylor MJ. Evoked potentials in comatose children: Auditory brainstem responses. Pediatr Neurol 1986; 2:31–34.

56. Goldie WD, Chaippa KH, Young RR, et al. Brainstem auditory and short-latency somatosensory evoked responses in brain death. Neurology 1981;31:248–256.

57. Ganes T, Lundar T. EEG and evoked responses in comatose patients with severe brain damage. Electroencephalogr Clin Neurophysiol 1988;69:6–13.

58. Goodman JM, Heck LL, Moore BD. Confirmation of brain death with portable isotope angiography: A review of 204 consecutive cases. Neurosurgery 1985;16:492–497.

59. Vernon DD, Holzman BH. Brain death: Considerations for pediatrics. J Clin Neurophysiol 1986;3:251–265.

60. Greissen G. Cerebral blood flow in preterm infants during the first week of life. Acta Paediatr Scand 1986;75:43–51.

61. Altman DI, Powers WJ, Perlman JM, et al. Cerebral blood flow requirements for brain viability in newborn infants is lower than in adults. Ann Neurol 1988;24:218–226.

62. Darby JM, Yonas H, Gur D, et al. Xenon-enhanced computed tomography in brain death. Arch Neurol 1987;44:551–554.

63. Altman DI, Perlman JM, Powers WJ, et al. Preservation of brainstem and cerebral blood flow (CBF) in two asphyxiated newborn infants with clinical brain death. Pediatr Res 1987; 21:487A.

64. Toffol GJ, Lansky LL, Huges JR, et al. Pitfalls in diagnosing brain death in infancy. J Child Neurol 1987;2:134–138.

65. Powers WJ, Grub RL, Darriet D, et al. Cerebral blood flow and cerebral metabolic rate of oxygen requirements for cerebral function and viability in humans. J Cereb Blood Flow Metab 1985;5:600–608.

66. Wegman MD. Annual summary of vital statistics—1986. Pediatrics 1987;80:817–827.

67. Doroshow RW, Saukel GW, Ashwal S. Availability and selection of donors for pediatric heart transplantation. N Engl J Med 1988, In press.

68. Outwater KM, Rockoff MA. Diabetes insipidus accompanying brain death in children. Neurology 1984;34:1243–1246.

69. Blaine EM, Tallman RD, Frolicher D, et al. Vasopressin supplementation in a porcine model of brain-dead potential organ donors. Transplantation 1984;38:459–464.

INDEX

The letter *f* following a page number indicates a figure; the letter *t* following a page number indicates a table; page numbers in boldface indicate major discussions.